DVD CONTENTS

PROCEDURE 9
Total Shoulder Arthroplasty
Robert U. Hartzler, John W. Sperling, and Robert H. Cofield

Complete surgical total shoulder arthroplasty procedure
Surgical approach to the shoulder
Placement of humeral component
Trial reduction of humeral component and soft tissue balancing
Placement of glenoid component
Wound closure

PROCEDURE 13
Open Treatment of Anterior-Inferior Multidirectional Instability of the Shoulder
Katie B. Vadasdi, Chad J. Marion, and Louis U. Bigliani

Elevation and separation of subscapularis from anterior joint capsule
Arthrotomy and elevation of anterior capsule
Capsular shift and reconstruction

PROCEDURE 17
Arthroscopic Treatment of Posterior-Inferior Multidirectional Instability of the Shoulder
Chad J. Marion, Katie B. Vadasdi, and Christopher S. Ahmad

Arthroscopic dissection of posterior inferior labrum with an arthroscopic elevator
Preparation of posterior inferior glenoid rim with an arthroscopic rasp
Preparation of posterior inferior glenoid rim with an arthroscopic shaver
Drilling for inferior suture anchor
Placement of inferior suture anchor
Transferring suture limb to a separate portal
Passing suture passing through labrum
Passing suture through labrum
Tying suture over labrum

PROCEDURE 32
Hemiarthroplasty for Proximal Humerus Fracture
Steven M. Klein, Mark A. Mighell, and Mark A. Frankle

Operative technique for hemiarthroplasty for four part proximal humerus fracture

PROCEDURE 33
Surgical Treatment of Scapular Fractures
Donald H. Lee

Anterior shoulder incision: Marking of incision of anterior deltopectoral incision
Clavipectoral fascia: Dissection of clavipectoral fascia
Subscapularis release 1: Anterior shoulder exposure, release of subscapularis medial to its insertion on the lesser tuberosity
Subscapularis release 2: Anterior shoulder exposure, completion of the release of the subscapularis
Glenoid fracture exposure: Exposure of glenoid fracture from anterior approach
Posterior glenoid fracture exposure with probe: Posteriorly exposed scapular fracture with probe place from an anterior approach into fracture site
Posterior scapular incision 1: Skin marking for posterior scapular incision
Posterior scapular incision 2: Surgical incision for posterior approach to the scapula
Acromial fracture dissection 1: Surgical dissection of the acromion
Acromial fracture dissection 2: Surgical exposure of the acromial fracture
Acromial fracture dissection 3: Further exposure of the acromial fracture
Posterior fascial incision 1: Posterior approach to scapula, fascial dissection
Posterior fascial incision 2: Posterior approach to scapular, fascial dissection
Scapular spine dissection 1: Posterior scapular exposure, dissection of scapular spine
Scapular spine dissection 2: Posterior scapular exposure, completion of dissection of scapular spine
Scapular medial border dissection 1: Posterior scapular exposure, dissection of medial border of scapula
Scapular medial border dissection 2: Posterior scapular exposure, completion of dissection of medial border of scapula
Infraspinatus-teres minor dissection: Judet posterior exposure of the scapula with elevation of infraspinatus and teres minor
Scapular fracture exposure 1: Posterior exposure of scapular body fracture with removal of fracture callous
Scapular fracture exposure 2: Posterior exposure of scapular body fracture with removal of fracture callous
Posterior scapular plate: Placement of U-shaped contoured pelvic reconstruction plate along inferior scapular spine, posterior scapular neck, and lateral border of scapula body
Superior glenoid screw 1: Percutaneous placement of Kirschner wires prior to placement of cannulated screws for fixation of glenoid fracture
Superior glenoid screw 2: Drilling over Kirschner wires for cannulated screws

Superior glenoid screw 3: Placement of cannulated screws for fixation of glenoid fracture
Acromial fracture fixation 1: Placement of Kirschner wires in acromion for placement of cannulated screws
Acromial fracture fixation 2: Drilling and placement of cannulated screws
Acromial fracture fixation 3: Placement of second cannulated screw
Acromial fracture fixation 4: Placement of cerclage wire for tension band wire fixation for acromial fracture
Subscapularis repair: Anterior wound closure, repair of subscapularis
Infraspinatus repair 1: Posterior wound closure—repair of infraspinatus and teres minor
Infraspinatus repair 2: Posterior wound closure—repair of infraspinatus and teres minor
Infraspinatus repair 3: Posterior wound closure—repair of infraspinatus and teres minor
Deltoid trapezius repair 1
Deltoid trapezius repair 2
Final wound closure 1: Fascial wound closure of posterior wound
Final wound closure 2: Posterior wound closure

PROCEDURE 43

Radial Head Fractures: Radial Head Replacement

Donald H. Lee and John M. Erickson

Incision: Surgical incision for radial head replacement
Arthrotomy 1: Arthrotomy of radiocapitellar joint
Arthrotomy 2: Arthrotomy of radiocapitellar joint with exposure of radial head fracture, removal of radial head fragments
Head sizing: Using excised radial head to determine radial head implant size
Radial neck resection: Dissection and resection of radial neck using oscillating saw
Broach: Broaching the proximal radial neck
Trial stem insertion: Insertion of trial radial head stem
Trial head insertion: Insertion of trial radial head
Set screw insertion: Placement of set screw for trial radial head implant
Intraoperative fluoroscopy: Fluoroscopic examination following placement of trial radial head implant
Final stem insertion: Insertion of final radial head implant stem
Final head insertion: Insertion of final radial head component onto radial stem
Final fluoroscopy: Final fluoroscopic examination following placement of radial head implant
Annular ligament repair: Wound closure, repair of annular ligament
Fascial repair: Wound closure, fascial repair

PROCEDURE 56

Distal Humerus Fractures, Including Isolated Distal Lateral Column and Capitellar Fractures

Jeffry T. Watson

Patient positioning, surgical approach for a distal humeral fracture, including olecranon osteotomy and exposure of fracture
Provisional and final fixation of distal humeral fracture
Repair of olecranon osteotomy and wound closure

PROCEDURE 57

Radial Head Fractures: Open Reduction and Internal Fixation

Donald H. Lee and John M. Erickson

Radial head fracture drawing incision: Skin marking for lateral exposure of radiocapitellar joint
Radial head fracture incision: Skin incision for exposure of radiocapitellar joint
Radial head fracture fascial incision: Fascial incision and arthrotomy of radiocapitellar joint
Radial head fracture arthrotomy: Arthrotomy of the radiocapitellar joint with exposure of the radial head fracture
Radial head fracture fragment identification: Identification and mobilization of radial head fracture fragments
Radial head fracture reduction: Reduction of radial head fracture fragments
Radial head fracture tripod screw: Screw fixation of radial head fracture
Radial head fracture fluoroscopic view 1: Lateral fluoroscopic examination of radial head following fixation of the radial head
Radial head fracture fluoroscopic view 2: Anteroposterior fluoroscopic examination of the radial head following fixation of the radial head
Radial head fracture final fixation: Appearance of radial head following fixation of fracture and video showing location of safe zone based on Lister's tubercle and radial styloid
Radial head fracture safe zone: Location of safe zone for hardware placement based on Lister's tubercle and radial styloid and appearance of radial head fracture following fixation of the radial head
Radial head fracture annular ligament repair: Wound closure, repair of the annular ligament
Radial head fracture fascial repair: Wound closure, fascial repair

PROCEDURE 62

Soft Tissue Coverage I: Radial Forearm Flap

Wesley P. Thayer and R. Bruce Shack

Soft Tissue Coverage II: Latissimus Dorsi Flap

Wesley P. Thayer and R. Bruce Shack

Soft Tissue Coverage III: Posterior Interosseous Flap

Wesley P. Thayer and R. Bruce Shack

Soft Tissue Coverage IV: Brachioradialis Muscle Flap

Wesley P. Thayer and R. Bruce Shack

Soft Tissue Coverage V: Reverse Lateral Arm Flap

Wesley P. Thayer and R. Bruce Shack

Surgical dissection of the radial forearm flap
Surgical dissection of latissimus dorsi flap
Surgical dissection of the posterior interosseous flap
Surgical dissection of the brachioradialis flap
Surgical dissection of the reverse lateral arm flap
Surgical dissection of flexor carpi ulnaris flap

OPERATIVE TECHNIQUES

shoulder and elbow

surgery

OPERATIVE TECHNIQUES

shoulder and elbow surgery

Donald H. Lee, MD
Professor of Orthopaedic Surgery
Vanderbilt Orthopaedic Institute
Vanderbilt University School of Medicine
Nashville, Tennessee

Robert J. Neviaser, MD
Professor and Chairman
Department of Orthopaedic Surgery
George Washington University
Medical Center
Washington, DC

ELSEVIER
SAUNDERS

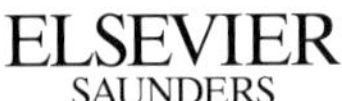

1600 John F. Kennedy Blvd.
Ste 1800
Philadelphia, PA 19103-2899

OPERATIVE TECHNIQUES: SHOULDER AND ELBOW SURGERY ISBN: 978-1-4160-3278-6

Notices

Knowledge and best practice in this field are constantly changing. As new research and experience broaden our understanding, changes in research methods, professional practices, or medical treatment may become necessary.

Practitioners and researchers must always rely on their own experience and knowledge in evaluating and using any information, methods, compounds, or experiments described herein. In using such information or methods they should be mindful of their own safety and the safety of others, including parties for whom they have a professional responsibility.

With respect to any drug or pharmaceutical products identified, readers are advised to check the most current information provided (i) on procedures featured or (ii) by the manufacturer of each product to be administered, to verify the recommended dose or formula, the method and duration of administration, and contraindications. It is the responsibility of practitioners, relying on their own experience and knowledge of their patients, to make diagnoses, to determine dosages and the best treatment for each individual patient, and to take all appropriate safety precautions.

To the fullest extent of the law, neither the Publisher nor the authors, contributors, or editors, assume any liability for any injury and/or damage to persons or property as a matter of products liability, negligence or otherwise, or from any use or operation of any methods, products, instructions, or ideas contained in the material herein.

International Standard Book Number 978-1-4160-3278-6

Acquisitions Editor: Daniel Pepper
Publishing Services Manager: Pat Joiner-Myers
Design Direction: Steven Stave

Printed in the United States of America

Last digit is the print number: 9 8 7 6 5 4 3 2 1

I would like to dedicate this book to my wife, Dawn, and our children David, Dana, Diane, Daniel, and Dustin for all their support and joy that they provide. I also dedicate this book to my parents, Kwan and Kay, for their guidance.

I would like to thank my co-editor Robert Neviaser for all the advice and encouragement that he has provided over the years. Finally, thank you to all our co-authors who have shared their time and knowledge with us.

Donald H. Lee, MD

To my wife, Anne, *"the wind beneath my wings,"* and my children (Niki, Rob, Ian, and Andy) and grandchildren (Isabel, Mac, Bozie, Kenzie, J.B., Maddie, Geordie, A.J., and Katie), the rest of my *"raisons d'être."* Finally, to my father, Julius S. Neviaser, MD, a pioneer and giant of shoulder surgery.

Robert J. Neviaser, MD

CONTRIBUTORS

Julie E. Adams, MD, MS
Assistant Professor of Orthopaedic Surgery, University of Minnesota, Minneapolis, Minnesota
Arthroscopy of the Elbow: Setup and Portals; Elbow Arthritis and Stiffness: Open Treatment; Elbow Arthritis and Stiffness: Arthroscopic Treatment; Surgical Reconstruction of Longitudinal Radioulnar Dissociation (Essex-Lopresti Injury)

Christopher S. Ahmad, MD
Associate Professor, Orthopaedic Surgery, Columbia University College of Physicians and Surgeons; Assistant Attending, Orthopaedic Surgery, New York Presbyterian Hospital, New York, New York
Arthroscopic Treatment of Posterior-Inferior Multidirectional Instability of the Shoulder

James R. Andrews, MD
Program Director, Orthopedic Sports Medicine Fellowship, American Sports Medicine Institute, Birmingham, Alabama
Ulnar Collateral Ligament Reconstruction Using the Modified Jobe Technique; Lateral Ulnar Collateral Ligament Reconstruction

Robert M. Baltera, MD
Assistant Clinical Professor, Orthopaedic Surgery Department, Indiana University Medical Center, Indianapolis, Indiana
Repair and Reconstruction of the Ruptured Triceps

Eric D. Bava, MD
Shoulder Service, The Carrell Clinic, Dallas, Texas
Humeral Hemiarthroplasty with Biologic Glenoid Resurfacing

Louis U. Bigliani, MD
Frank E. Stinchfield Professor and Chairman, Columbia University Medical Center; Director of Orthopaedics, New York-Presbyterian Hospital/ Columbia University, New York, New York
Open Treatment of Anterior-Inferior Multidirectional Instability of the Shoulder

Julie Y. Bishop, MD
Assistant Professor, Department of Orthopaedic Surgery, Chief, Division of Shoulder Surgery, The Ohio State University, Columbus, Ohio
Open Reduction and Internal Fixation of Three- and Four-Part Proximal Humerus Fractures

Pascal Boileau, MD
Professor and Chairman, Department of Orthopaedic Surgery, Medical University of Nice, Nice, France
Arthroscopic Biceps Tenodesis

Wayne Z. Burkhead, MD
Clinical Professor, Department of Orthopaedic Surgery, University of Texas Southwestern Medical School; Shoulder Service, The Carrell Clinic, Dallas, Texas
Humeral Hemiarthroplasty with Biologic Glenoid Resurfacing

Jonathan E. Buzzell, MD
Nebraska Orthopaedic Hospital; OrthoWest, Omaha, Nebraska
Open and Arthroscopic Suprascapular Nerve Decompression

Kyle A. Caswell, DO
Chief Resident, Tulane University School of Medicine; PGY 5 Resident, Tulane University Medical Center, New Orleans, Louisiana
Arthroscopic Treatment of Calcific Tendinitis in the Shoulder

Neal C. Chen, MD
Lecturer, University of Michigan, Ann Arbor, Michigan
Operative Fixation of Symptomatic Os Acromiale

Tyson Cobb, MD
Director of Hand Center of Excellence, Orthopaedic Specialists, Davenport, Iowa
Endoscopic Cubital Tunnel Release

Robert H. Cofield, MD
Professor Emeritus, Mayo Clinic College of Medicine, and Mayo Clinic, Rochester, Minnesota
Total Shoulder Arthroplasty

Mark S. Cohen, MD
Professor, Director, Orthopedic Education, and Head, Section of Hand and Elbow Surgery, Department of Orthopedic Surgery, Rush University Medical Center, Chicago, Illinois
Lateral Epicondylitis: Arthroscopic and Open Treatment

Edward V. Craig, MD, MPH
Professor of Clinical Orthopaedic Surgery, Weill Cornell Medical School; Attending Surgeon, Hospital for Special Surgery, New York, New York
Open Distal Clavicle Excision

Lynn A. Crosby, MD
Professor and Director of Shoulder Surgery, Department of Orthopaedic Surgery, Medical College of Georgia, Augusta, Georgia
Humeral Head Resurfacing Arthroplasty

Leah T. Cyran, MD
Shoulder Service, The Carrell Clinic, Dallas, Texas
Humeral Hemiarthroplasty with Biologic Glenoid Resurfacing

Matthew Denkers, MD, FRCSC
Assistant Professor, Division of Orthopaedic Surgery, McMaster University; Associate Staff, Service of Orthopaedic Surgery, Department of Surgery, Hamilton Health Sciences, Hamilton, Ontario, Canada
Arthroscopic Treatment of Traumatic Anterior Instability of the Shoulder

Allen Deutsch, MD
Clinical Assistant Professor, Baylor College of Medicine; Faculty Staff, St. Luke's Episcopal Hospital, Houston, Texas
Rotator Cuff Repair: Arthroscopic Technique for Partial-Thickness or Small or Medium Full-Thickness Tears

Christopher C. Dodson, MD
Assistant Professor of Orthopaedic Surgery, Thomas Jefferson University; Attending Orthopaedic Surgeon, Division of Sports Medicine, Rothman Institute, Philadelphia, Pennsylvania
Anterior Glenohumeral Instability Associated with Glenoid or Humeral Bone Deficiency: The Latarjet Procedure

Jason D. Doppelt, MD
Resident, Department of Orthopaedic Surgery, George Washington University, Washington, DC
Intramedullary Fixation of Clavicle Fractures

Mark C. Drakos, MD
Attending Orthopaedic Surgeon, Sports Medicine and Foot and Ankle Surgery, North Shore-Long Island Jewish Health System, New Hyde Park, New York
SLAP Lesion: Arthroscopic Reconstruction of the Labrum and Biceps Anchor

George S. M. Dyer, MD
Clinical Instructor in Orthopaedic Surgery, Harvard Medical School; Hand and Upper Extremity Service, Department of Orthopaedic Surgery, Brigham and Women's Hospital, Boston, Massachusetts
Open Treatment of Complex Traumatic Elbow Instability

Benton A. Emblom, MD
Sports Medicine Fellow, American Sports Medicine Institute, Birmingham, Alabama
Ulnar Collateral Ligament Reconstruction Using the Modified Jobe Technique

John M. Erickson, MD
Upper Extremity Surgeon, Raleigh Hand Center, Raleigh, North Carolina
Radial Head Fractures: Radial Head Replacement; Radial Head Fractures: Open Reduction and Internal Fixation; Operative Treatment of Olecranon Bursitis

Evan L. Flatow, MD
Lasker Professor and Chairman of Orthopaedic Surgery, The Leni and Peter May Department of Orthopaedic Surgery, Mount Sinai Medical Center, New York, New York
Open Unconstrained Revision Shoulder Arthroplasty

Mark A. Frankle, MD
Chief of Shoulder and Elbow Surgery, Florida Orthopaedic Institute, Tampa, Florida
Hemiarthroplasty for Proximal Humerus Fracture

Leesa M. Galatz, MD
Associate Professor, Department of Orthopaedic Surgery, Washington University School of Medicine; Associate Professor, and Shoulder and Elbow Fellowship Director, Washington University Orthopedics; Barnes-Jewish Hospital, St. Louis, Missouri
Arthroscopic Repair of Massive Rotator Cuff Tears

Andrew Green, MD
Associate Professor, and Chief of Division of Shoulder and Elbow Surgery, Warren Alpert Medical School, Brown University, Providence, Rhode Island
Open Treatment of Acute and Chronic Acromioclavicular Dislocations

Jeffrey A. Greenberg, MD, MS
Clinical Assistant Professor, Department of Orthopedics, Indiana University; Partner and Fellowship Director, Indiana Hand to Shoulder Center, Indianapolis, Indiana
Repair of Distal Biceps Tendon Ruptures

Robert U. Hartzler, MD
Resident, Department of Orthopedic Surgery, Mayo Clinic, Rochester, Minnesota
Total Shoulder Arthroplasty

Hill Hastings II, MD
Clinical Professor, Orthopaedic Surgery, Indiana University Medical Center, and Indiana Hand to Shoulder Center, Indianapolis, Indiana
Total Elbow Arthroplasty: Discovery Minimally Constrained Linked System; Total Elbow Arthroplasty for the Treatment of Complex Distal Humerus Fractures

Robert Hollinshead, MD, FRCSC
Clinical Professor, Division of Orthopaedic Surgery, and Adjunct Professor, Faculty of Kinesiology, University of Calgary; Associate Staff, Service of Orthopaedic Surgery, Department of Surgery, Peter Lougheed Centre, Alberta Health Services, Calgary, Alberta, Canada
Arthroscopic Treatment of Traumatic Anterior Instability of the Shoulder

Joseph P. Iannotti, MD, PhD
Department Chair and Professor of Orthopaedic Surgery, Cleveland Clinic, Cleveland, Ohio
Arthrodesis of the Shoulder

Frank W. Jobe, MD
Co-Founder, Kerlan-Jobe Orthopaedic Clinic, Los Angeles, California
Medial Epicondylitis: Open Treatment

Kristofer J. Jones, MD
Resident, Department of Orthopaedic Surgery, Hospital for Special Surgery, New York, New York
Anterior Glenohumeral Instability Associated with Glenoid or Humeral Bone Deficiency: The Latarjet Procedure

Jesse B. Jupiter, MD
Hansjorg Wyss AO Professor of Orthopedic Surgery, Harvard Medical School; Division of Hand and Upper Extremity Service, Massachusetts General Hospital, Boston, Massachusetts
Open Reduction and Internal Fixation of Acute Midshaft Clavicular Fractures

Anne M. Kelly, MD
Assistant Professor of Clinical Orthopaedics, Department of Orthopaedics, Weill Cornell Medical Center; Assistant Attending Orthopaedic Surgeon, Hospital for Special Surgery, New York, New York
Open Distal Clavicle Excision

W. Ben Kibler, MD
Medical Director, Shoulder Center of Kentucky, Lexington Clinic, Lexington, Kentucky
Scapular Surgery I: Eden-Lange Transfer for Trapezius Muscle Palsy; Scapular Surgery II: Pectoralis Major Transfer for Serratus Anterior Palsy; Scapular Surgery III: Rhomboid/Latissimus Dorsi Transfer for Serratus Anterior Palsy

Steven M. Klein, MD
Hospital Staff Physician, Gundersen Lutheran Hospital, La Crosse, Wisconsin
Hemiarthroplasty for Proximal Humerus Fracture

Zinon T. Kokkalis, MD
Fellow, Hand and Upper Extremity Surgery, Allegheny General Hospital, Pittsburgh, Pennsylvania
Surgical Decompression for Radial Tunnel Syndrome

Marc S. Kowalsky, MD
Assistant Attending Orthopaedic Surgeon, Department of Orthopaedic Surgery, Lenox Hill Hospital, New York, New York
Arthroscopic Repair of Massive Rotator Cuff Tears

Sumant G. Krishnan, MD
Clinical Assistant Professor, University of Texas Southwestern Medical Center, Dallas, Texas; Clinical Assistant Professor, and Director, Shoulder Fellowship, Baylor University Medical Center; Visiting Professor, Shoulder Surgery, International Orthopaedic and Traumatological Institute, Arezzo, Italy; Shoulder Service, The Carrell Clinic, Dallas, Texas; North Central Surgical Center, Baylor University Medical Center, Dallas, Texas
Humeral Hemiarthroplasty with Biologic Glenoid Resurfacing; Open and Arthroscopic Suprascapular Nerve Decompression

John E. Kuhn, MD, MS
Associate Professor, Vanderbilt University Medical School; Chief of Shoulder Surgery, Vanderbilt University Medical Center, Nashville, Tennessee
Sternoclavicular Joint Reconstruction Using Semitendinosus Graft

Donald H. Lee, MD
Professor of Orthopaedic Surgery, Vanderbilt Orthopaedic Institute, Vanderbilt University School of Medicine, Nashville, Tennessee
Surgical Treatment of Scapular Fractures; Radial Head Fractures: Radial Head Replacement; Total Elbow Arthroplasty for the Treatment of Complex Distal Humerus Fractures; Revision Total Elbow Arthroplasty; Radial Head Fractures: Open Reduction and Internal Fixation; Operative Treatment of Olecranon Bursitis

William N. Levine, MD
Professor of Clinical Orthopaedic Surgery, Columbia University; Vice Chairman, Columbia University Medical Center, New York, New York
Acromioplasty

David M. Lutton, MD
Clinical Instructor of Orthopaedic Surgery, The George Washington University School of Medicine; Attending Orthopaedic Surgeon, The George Washington University Hospital, Washington, DC
Open Unconstrained Revision Shoulder Arthroplasty

Leonard C. Macrina, MSPT, SCS, CSCS
Champion Sports Medicine, Birmingham, Alabama
Ulnar Collateral Ligament Reconstruction Using the Modified Jobe Technique

Kevin J. Malone, MD
Assistant Professor, Department of Orthopaedic Surgery, Case Western Reserve University, MetroHealth Medical Center, Cleveland, Ohio
Submuscular Ulnar Nerve Transposition

Alfred A. Mansour III, MD
Pediatric Orthopaedic Fellow, The Children's Hospital; Sports Medicine Fellow, Steadman Hawkins Clinic, Denver, Colorado
Sternoclavicular Joint Reconstruction Using Semitendinosus Graft

Milford H. Marchant, Jr., MD
Sports Medicine—Orthopaedic Surgery, Bay Area Orthopaedics & Sports Medicine, Annapolis, Maryland
Medial Epicondylitis: Open Treatment

Chad J. Marion, MD
Orthopaedic Surgeon, Pacific Medical Centers, Seattle, Washington
Open Treatment of Anterior-Inferior Multidirectional Instability of the Shoulder; Arthroscopic Treatment of Posterior-Inferior Multidirectional Instability of the Shoulder

George M. McCluskey III, MD
Clinical Professor, Department of Orthopaedic Surgery, Medical College of Georgia, Augusta, Georgia; Clinical Assistant Professor, Department of Orthopaedic Surgery, Tulane University School of Medicine, New Orleans, Louisiana; Director, St. Francis Shoulder Center, and Director, St. Francis Shoulder Fellowship Program, Columbus, Georgia
Open Treatment of Posterior-Inferior Multidirectional Shoulder Instability

Patrick J. McMahon, MD
Adjunct Associate Professor, Department of Bioengineering, University of Pittsburgh; McMahon Orthopedics & Rehabilitation, Pittsburgh, Pennsylvania
Adhesive Capsulitis

Steven W. Meisterling, MD
Sports Medicine Fellow, American Sports Medicine Institute, Birmingham, Alabama
Lateral Ulnar Collateral Ligament Reconstruction

Mark A. Mighell, MD
Shoulder and Elbow Surgery, Florida Orthopaedic Institute, Tampa, Florida
Hemiarthroplasty for Proximal Humerus Fracture

Joseph Mileti, MD
Assistant Clinical Professor of Orthopaedics, The Ohio State University; Shoulder Service, Riverside Methodist Hospital, Ohio Orthopaedic Center, Columbus, Ohio
Open Reduction and Internal Fixation of Three- and Four-Part Proximal Humerus Fractures

Anthony Miniaci, MD, FRCSC
Professor of Surgery, Cleveland Clinic Lerner College of Medicine at Case Western Reserve University, and Cleveland Clinic, Cleveland, Ohio
Treatment of the Unstable Shoulder with Humeral Head Bone Loss

Anand M. Murthi, MD
Attending Orthopaedic Surgeon, and Chief, Shoulder and Elbow Surgery, Department of Orthopaedics and Sports Medicine, Union Memorial Hospital, Baltimore, Maryland
Arthroscopic Distal Clavicle Resection

Robert G. Najarian, MD
Assistant Professor in Clinical Orthopaedics, The Ohio State University, Columbus, Ohio
Treatment of the Unstable Shoulder with Humeral Head Bone Loss

Andrew S. Neviaser, MD
Assistant Professor, Department of Orthopaedic Surgery, George Washington University Medical Center, Washington, DC
Open Repair of Rotator Cuff Tears; Mini-Open Biceps Tenodesis

Robert J. Neviaser, MD
Professor and Chairman, Department of Orthopaedic Surgery, George Washington University Medical Center, Washington, DC
Open Repair of Rotator Cuff Tears; Mini-Open Biceps Tenodesis; Intramedullary Fixation of Clavicle Fractures

Michael J. O'Brien, MD
Assistant Professor of Orthopedic Surgery, Tulane University School of Medicine; Tulane University Medical Center, New Orleans, Louisiana
Arthroscopic Treatment of Calcific Tendinitis in the Shoulder; Elbow Arthroscopic Débridement for Osteochondritis Dissecans

Stephen J. O'Brien, MD, MBA
Associate Professor of Clinical Orthopaedic Surgery, Weill Cornell Medical College; Vice Chairman, Department of Sports Medicine, Associate Attending of Orthopaedic Surgery, and Assistant Scientist, Hospital for Special Surgery, New York, New York
SLAP Lesion: Arthroscopic Reconstruction of the Labrum and Biceps Anchor

Jason Old, MD, FRCSC
Assistant Professor, University of Manitoba; Pan Am Clinic, Winnipeg, Manitoba, Canada
Arthroscopic Biceps Tenodesis

A. Lee Osterman, MD
Professor and Chairman, Division of Hand Surgery, Department of Orthopaedic Surgery, Thomas Jefferson University; President, The Philadelphia Hand Center, Philadelphia, Pennsylvania
Surgical Reconstruction of Longitudinal Radioulnar Dissociation (Essex-Lopresti Injury)

Rick F. Papandrea, MD
Assistant Clinical Professor in Orthopaedics, Medical College of Wisconsin, Milwaukee; Partner, Orthopaedic Associates of Wisconsin, Waukesha, Wisconsin
Hemiarthroplasty of the Distal Humerus; Radiocapitellar Replacement

Maxwell C. Park, MD
Clinical Faculty, Orthopaedic Biomechanics Laboratory, VA Long Beach Healthcare System, Long Beach, California Department of Orthopaedic Surgery, Southern California Permanente Medical Group, Woodland Hills, California
Arthroscopic Treatment of Anterior-Inferior Multidirectional Instability of the Shoulder

Nata Parnes, MD
Director of Orthopedics, Carthage Area Hospital, Carthage, New York
Open Reduction and Internal Fixation of Acute Midshaft Clavicular Fractures

William Thomas Payne, MD
Department of Orthopaedic Surgery, University of Colorado, Denver, Colorado
Repair of Distal Biceps Tendon Ruptures

Matthew L. Ramsey, MD
Associate Professor of Orthopedic Surgery, Thomas Jefferson University, Philadelphia, Pennsylvania
Elbow Arthroscopic Débridement for Osteochondritis Dissecans

Bradley S. Raphael, MD
Resident, Hospital for Special Surgery, New York, New York
Open Distal Clavicle Excision

Herbert Resch, MD
Professor, and Head of Department of Trauma Surgery and Sports Injuries, Paracelsus Medical University, Salzburg, Austria
Percutaneous Fixation of Proximal Humerus Fractures

David Ring, MD, PhD
Associate Professor of Orthopaedic Surgery, Harvard Medical School; Orthopaedic Hand and Upper Extremity Service, Massachusetts General Hospital, Boston, Massachusetts
Open Treatment of Complex Traumatic Elbow Instability

Felix H. Savoie III, MD
Lee Schlesinger Professor of Orthopaedic Shoulder, Elbow and Sports Surgery, Tulane University School of Medicine; Tulane University Medical Center, New Orleans, Louisiana
Arthroscopic Treatment of Calcific Tendinitis in the Shoulder

Jason J. Scalise, MD
Clinical Faculty, The CORE Institute, Phoenix, Arizona
Arthrodesis of the Shoulder

Robert J. Schoderbek, Jr., MD
Orthopaedic Specialists of Charleston, Roper St. Francis Sports Medicine, Charleston, South Carolina
Lateral Ulnar Collateral Ligament Reconstruction

Jon K. Sekiya, MD
Associate Professor, University of Michigan, Ann Arbor, Michigan
Operative Fixation of Symptomatic Os Acromiale

R. Bruce Shack, MD
Professor and Chair of Plastic Surgery, Vanderbilt University Medical Center, Nashville, Tennessee
Soft Tissue Coverage I: Radial Forearm Flap; Soft Tissue Coverage II: Latissimus Dorsi Flap; Soft Tissue Coverage III: Posterior Interosseous Flap; Soft Tissue Coverage IV: Brachioradialis Muscle Flap; Soft Tissue Coverage V: Reverse Lateral Arm Flap

Anup A. Shah, MD
Clinical Fellow, Harvard Shoulder Service, Massachusetts General Hospital, Boston, Massachusetts
Rotator Cuff Repair: Arthroscopic Technique for Partial-Thickness or Small or Medium Full-Thickness Tears

Seth Sherman, MD
Resident, Hospital for Special Surgery, New York, New York
Open Distal Clavicle Excision

Jack T. Shonkwiler, BA
Medical Illustrator, Jersey City, New Jersey
SLAP Lesion: Arthroscopic Reconstruction of the Labrum and Biceps Anchor

Ross A. Shumar, MD, Maj USAF
Staff Orthopaedic Surgeon, United States Air Force Academy, Colorado Springs, Colorado
Humeral Head Resurfacing Arthroplasty

David H. Sonnabend, MBBS, MD, BSc (Med), FRACS, FA Orth A
Professor in Orthopaedic Surgery, Department of Orthopaedic Surgery, University of Sydney, Royal North Shore Hospital; Shoulder Surgeon, Sydney Shoulder Specialists, Sydney, Australia
Rotator Cuff Repair: Open Technique for Partial-Thickness or Small or Medium Full-Thickness Tears

Dean G. Sotereanos, MD
Professor, Drexel University School of Medicine; Vice Chairman, Department of Orthopaedic Surgery, Allegheny General Hospital, Pittsburgh, Pennsylvania
Surgical Decompression for Radial Tunnel Syndrome

John W. Sperling, MD, MBA
Professor of Orthopedics, Mayo Clinic College of Medicine, and Mayo Clinic, Rochester, Minnesota
Total Shoulder Arthroplasty

Scott P. Steinmann, MD
Professor of Orthopedic Surgery, Mayo Clinic, Rochester, Minnesota
Arthroscopy of the Elbow: Setup and Portals; Elbow Arthritis and Stiffness: Open Treatment; Elbow Arthritis and Stiffness: Arthroscopic Treatment

Robert J. Strauch, MD
Professor of Clinical Orthopaedic Surgery, Columbia University; Attending, New York Presbyterian Hospital, New York, New York
Surgical Approaches for Open Treatment of the Elbow I: Posterior Approach; Surgical Approaches for Open Treatment of the Elbow II: Posterolateral (Kocher) and Kaplan Approaches to the Radial Head; Surgical Approaches for Open Treatment of the Elbow III: Anterior Approaches; Surgical Approaches for Open Treatment of the Elbow IV: Anteromedial (Hotchkiss) Approach

Eric S. Stuffmann, MD
Fellow, Hand and Upper Extremity Surgery, Allegheny General Hospital, Pittsburgh, Pennsylvania
Surgical Decompression for Radial Tunnel Syndrome

Christopher M. Stutz, MD
Fellow, Hand and Microvascular Surgery, Department of Orthopaedics, Washington University in St. Louis, St. Louis, Missouri
Total Elbow Arthroplasty for the Treatment of Complex Distal Humerus Fractures

Mark Tauber, MD
Assistant Professor, and Consultant, Department of Trauma Surgery and Sports Injuries, Paracelsus Medical University, Salzburg, Austria
Percutaneous Fixation of Proximal Humerus Fractures

Samuel A. Taylor, MD
Clinical Associate in Orthopaedic Surgery, Weill Cornell Medical College; Resident in Orthopaedic Surgery, Hospital for Special Surgery, New York, New York
SLAP Lesion: Arthroscopic Reconstruction of the Labrum and Biceps Anchor

Wesley P. Thayer, MD, PhD
Assistant Professor of Plastic Surgery, Vanderbilt University Medical Center, Nashville, Tennessee
Soft Tissue Coverage I: Radial Forearm Flap; Soft Tissue Coverage II: Latissimus Dorsi Flap; Soft Tissue Coverage III: Posterior Interosseous Flap; Soft Tissue Coverage IV: Brachioradialis Muscle Flap; Soft Tissue Coverage V: Reverse Lateral Arm Flap

Scott Thompson, MD
Resident, PG-3, Columbia University Medical Center, New York, New York
Acromioplasty

James E. Tibone, MD
Professor, University of Southern California Keck School of Medicine; Associate, Kerlan-Jobe Orthopaedic Clinic, Los Angeles, California
Arthroscopic Treatment of Anterior-Inferior Multidirectional Instability of the Shoulder

Thomas E. Trumble, MD
Professor, Department of Orthopaedics and Sports Medicine, University of Washington, Seattle, Washington
Submuscular Ulnar Nerve Transposition

Katie B. Vadasdi, MD
Orthopaedic Surgeon, Orthopaedic and Neurosurgery Specialists, Greenwich, Connecticut
Open Treatment of Anterior-Inferior Multidirectional Instability of the Shoulder; Arthroscopic Treatment of Posterior-Inferior Multidirectional Instability of the Shoulder

Peter S. Vezeridis, MD
Clinical Fellow in Orthopaedic Surgery, Harvard Medical School; Orthopaedic Surgery Resident, Harvard Combined Orthopaedic Residency Program, Massachusetts General Hospital, Boston, Massachusetts
Open Bankart Procedure for Recurrent Anterior Shoulder Dislocation

Thanapong Waitayawinyu, MD
Department of Orthopaedics, Thammasat University, Pathumthani Klong Luang, Thailand
Submuscular Ulnar Nerve Transposition

Gilles Walch, MD
Centre Orthopedique Santy, Lyon, France
Rotator Cuff Tear Arthroplasty: Open Surgical Treatment

Bryan Wall, MD
The CORE Institute, Phoenix, Arizona
Rotator Cuff Tear Arthroplasty: Open Surgical Treatment

Russell F. Warren, MD
Professor, Orthopaedic Surgery, Weill Cornell Medical College; Attending Orthopaedic Surgeon, Hospital for Special Surgery, New York, New York
Anterior Glenohumeral Instability Associated with Glenoid or Humeral Bone Deficiency: The Latarjet Procedure

Jeffrey D. Watson, MD
Chief Resident, Department of Orthopaedic Surgery, University of Maryland School of Medicine, Baltimore, Maryland
Arthroscopic Distal Clavicle Resection

Jeffry T. Watson, MD
Assistant Professor of Orthopaedics, Vanderbilt University Medical Center, and Vanderbilt Orthopaedic Institute, Nashville, Tennessee
Distal Humerus Fractures, Including Isolated Distal Lateral Column and Capitellar Fractures

Douglas R. Weikert, MD
Associate Professor, Orthopaedic Surgery, Division of Hand and Upper Extremity Surgery, Vanderbilt University, Nashville, Tennessee
Total Elbow Arthroplasty for the Treatment of Complex Distal Humerus Fractures

Neil J. White, MD, FRCS(C)
Hand and Microvascular Fellow, Department of Orthopaedic Surgery, Columbia University Medical Center, New York, New York
Surgical Approaches for Open Treatment of the Elbow I: Posterior Approach; Surgical Approaches for Open Treatment of the Elbow II: Posterolateral (Kocher) and Kaplan Approaches to the Radial Head; Surgical Approaches for Open Treatment of the Elbow III: Anterior Approaches; Surgical Approaches for Open Treatment of the Elbow IV: Anteromedial (Hotchkiss) Approach

Gerald R. Williams, Jr., MD
Professor, Orthopaedic Surgery, Jefferson Medical College; Chief, Shoulder and Elbow Service, Rothman Institute, Philadelphia, Pennsylvania
Operative Treatment of Two-Part Proximal Humerus Fractures

Allan A. Young, MBBS, MSpMed, PhD, FRACS (Orth)
Senior Lecturer in Orthopaedic Surgery, Department of Orthopaedic Surgery, University of Sydney, Royal North Shore Hospital; Shoulder Surgeon, Sydney Shoulder Specialists, Sydney, Australia
Rotator Cuff Repair: Open Technique for Partial-Thickness or Small or Medium Full-Thickness Tears

Bertram Zarins, MD
Augustus Thorndike Clinical Professor of Orthopaedic Surgery, Harvard Medical School; Emeritus Chief of Sports Medicine Service, Massachusetts General Hospital, Boston, Massachusetts
Open Bankart Procedure for Recurrent Anterior Shoulder Dislocation

PREFACE

Operative Techniques: Shoulder and Elbow Surgery is intended to provide a clear and well illustrated step-by-step review of state-of-the art of shoulder and elbow surgical procedures as described by some of the most respected surgeons in this field. As opposed to traditional book chapters, this book concentrates on surgical techniques that provide the orthopedic surgeon with the finer surgical points, tips, and pitfalls. It will also help give ancillary medical care providers the insight into how these procedures are performed. This book, a continuation of the series of Operative Techniques books provided by Elsevier, concentrates on shoulder and elbow surgical procedures.

Each chapter is constructed in a similar fashion. The surgical indications, physical examination, appropriate imaging studies, surgical anatomy, and treatment options are reviewed. The surgical technique portion of each chapter includes recommendations on surgical positioning, surgical portals and exposure, and step-by-step descriptions of the surgical procedure. Illustrations, surgical photographs, and in some cases, videos of the surgical procedure accompany the detailed surgical descriptions. The postoperative rehabilitation, the expected outcomes, and an annotated reference list are also provided. Throughout each chapter, surgical pearls, pitfalls, and controversies are discussed. We hope that these detailed surgical descriptions and discussion provide surgeons with an easily accessible, comprehensive reference that will provide surgical insight, increase surgical efficiency, and minimize complications when performing these operative procedures.

We are fortunate to have a distinguished group of contributing authors and want to express our deep appreciation to them for sharing their time and expertise in providing their contributions to this book. We would also like to acknowledge Daniel Pepper, Berta Steiner, and Julie Daniels for their invaluable assistance in making this book possible.

We hope you enjoy this book and that it is helpful to you.

Donald H. Lee, MD
Robert J. Neviaser, MD

FOREWORD

Education in the field of medicine includes many things, developing professionalism, acquiring a sense of human needs, incorporating knowledge from many sources, applying the basic sciences, studying in depth focused problems and solutions, integrating patient-based indications, understanding structural deficiencies, knowing what medicine and surgery have to offer, assimilating all these things and making a judgment about what should be done to help a patient. All this is so complex. Why aren't there books that just tell you how to do it! Early in one's career this is so useful. Later in one's career it's always helpful to see how other skilled people approach a procedure, and recognize ways one can improve techniques to address a problem. The learned editors of this volume have stepped up and formulated a book focusing on when and how to do it.

The experienced editors have selected the most commonly performed procedures and offered information that will be helpful to almost anyone in any stage of his or her career. The shoulder segment focuses on rotator cuff and other tendon-related problems, fractures, arthritis, and instability. Similarly the elbow has the material on musculotendinous attachment problems, fractures, arthritis, and instability. These are supplemented by information on how to handle nerve lesions and stiffness. An extra in the elbow area are chapters on approaches and on soft tissue coverage. Surgeons performing procedures contained in this book may be generalists or may have a focused background in trauma, sports, or adult reconstruction. But, no matter from what direction one approaches shoulder and elbow surgery, one can learn from others in the discipline who may have a different subspecialization—plus the bonus of having added input from experts with one's own background and direction.

Applied anatomy is a foundation for surgery. It is strange but true that the usual anatomy texts often don't contain the useful anatomy that one would apply for surgical procedures. In this text, that applied anatomy is carefully displayed. It is wonderful to have a step-wise approach to surgery, but also to have subtleties explained. A number of problems can be approached by open surgery or by arthroscopic surgery. Many are primary cases, but some are revision procedures.

This is a kind of textbook that one would want to pick up, read and set down, pick up and read again, and on and on as one approaches cases in practice. It seems to me that this is the kind of book one would want to have on the shelf rather than in a library. This book will have repeated use by a surgeon operating in these anatomic regions. Another bonus is the limited and focused literature on each procedure, allowing a surgeon to expand knowledge even more when addressing a specific situation.

Kudos yet again to these insightful, selfless editors and the talented authors who have devoted their energy and time to putting this user-friendly book together.

Robert H. Cofield, MD
Professor of Orthopedics
Mayo Clinic College of Medicine
Emeritus Chairman, Department of Orthopedic Surgery, Mayo Clinic
Past-President
American Shoulder and Elbow Surgeons
Past-Chairman, International Board of Shoulder and Elbow Surgery
Emeritus Editor-in-Chief, *Journal of Shoulder and Elbow Surgery*

CONTENTS

SECTION I

SHOULDER
Rotator Cuff

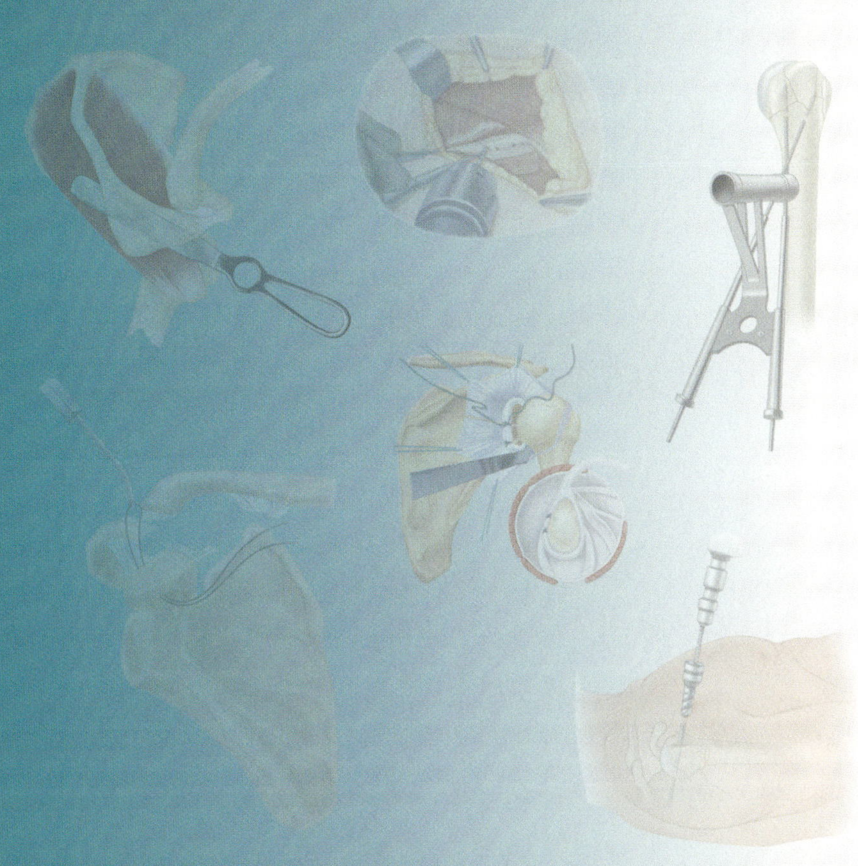

PROCEDURE 1

Acromioplasty

William N. Levine and Scott Thompson

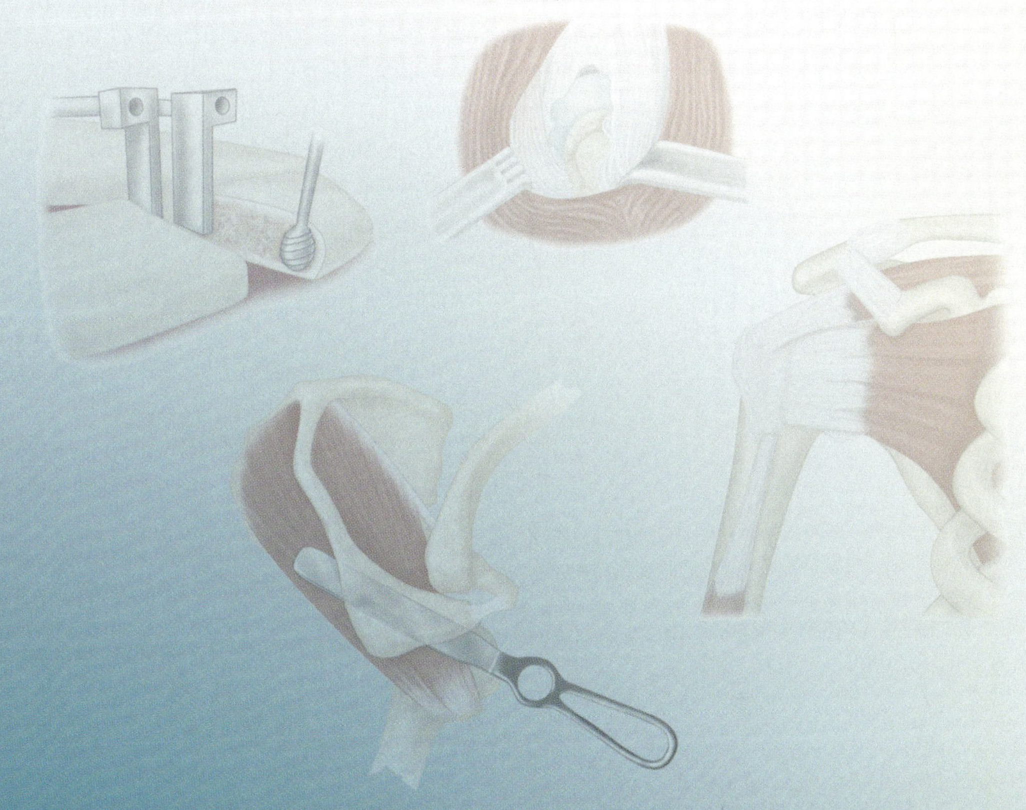

Pitfalls

- *Massive rotator cuff tears with early proximal humeral migration*

Controversies

- Some authors have advocated *no acromioplasty* in any condition. This is highly controversial and not well supported by the literature over the last 30 years, however.

Treatment Options

- Open acromioplasty
- Arthroscopic acromioplasty

Indications

- Symptomatic anterosuperior shoulder pain consistent with "impingement syndrome"
- In association with symptomatic rotator cuff tears that are not massive
- In association with partial-thickness rotator cuff tears, especially on the bursal side

Examination/Imaging

- A complete shoulder examination should be performed, but the following tests are critical:
  - The Neer sign (Fig. 1): pain on passive forward elevation of the shoulder while the examiner uses one hand to prevent scapular rotation. Pain is usually elicited in the arc between 70° and 120°.
  - The Neer impingement test: injection of local anesthetic beneath the anterior acromion with the elimination of pain with forward elevation.
  - The Hawkins sign (Fig. 2): pain with forward flexion of the humerus to 90° and then passive internal rotation.
  - Acromioclavicular (AC) joint examination
    - This joint is important to rule out as another possible contributor to pain.
    - Two tests are most sensitive: direct tenderness to palpation over the AC joint; and a positive cross-arm adduction maneuver in which the patient experiences pain over the AC joint with cross-arm adduction.

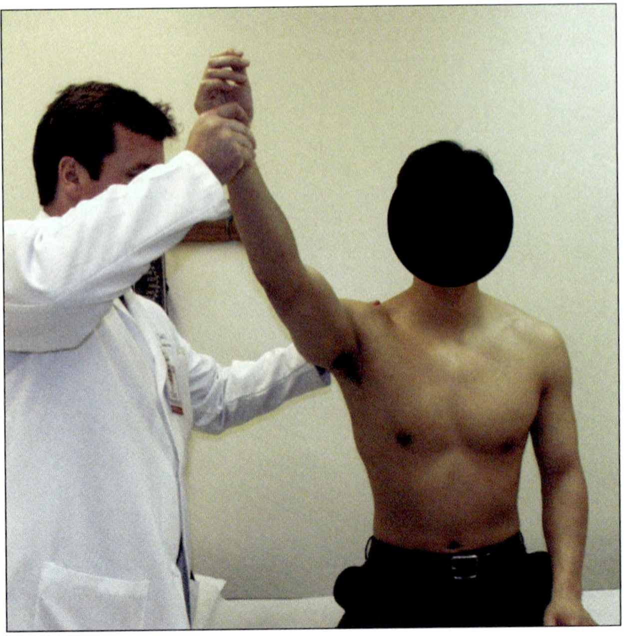

FIGURE 1

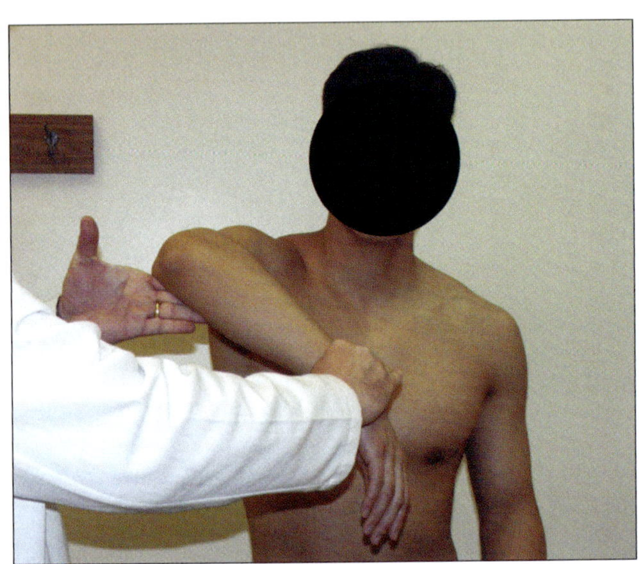

FIGURE 2

- Imaging
  - Plain films
    - True anteroposterior (Fig. 3A), scapular outlet (Fig. 3B), and axillary lateral (Fig. 3C) views should be obtained in all patients.
    - The outlet view will demonstrate the acromial morphology and any acromial pathology (spurs).
  - Magnetic resonance imaging (MRI)
    - MRI evaluates the integrity of the rotator cuff and biceps tendon.
    - MRI also identifies bony anomalies such as os acromiale (*arrow*), significant spurs, tuberosity cysts, or degenerative changes in the AC or glenohumeral joints (Fig. 4).

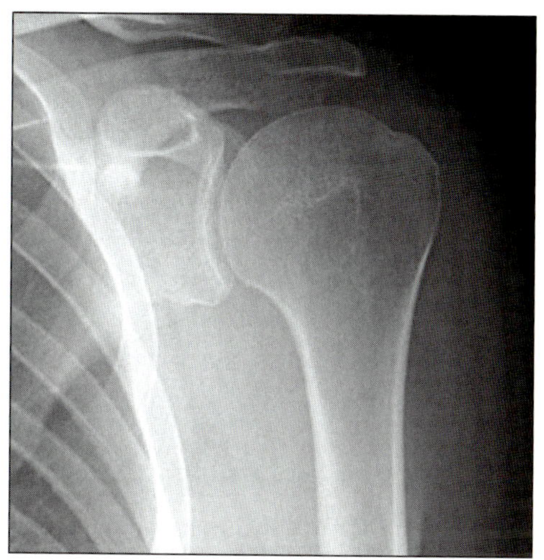

A

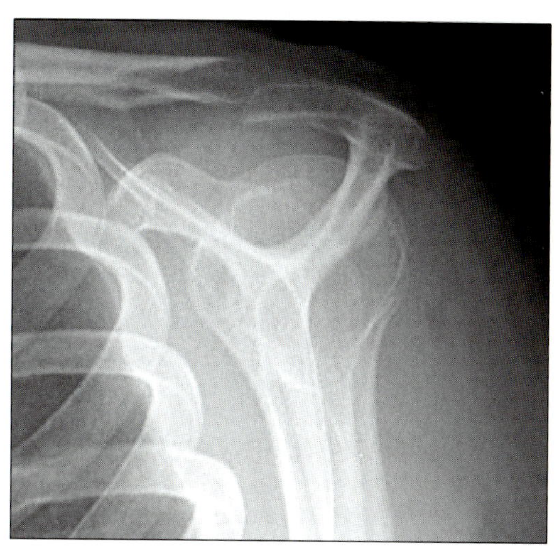

B

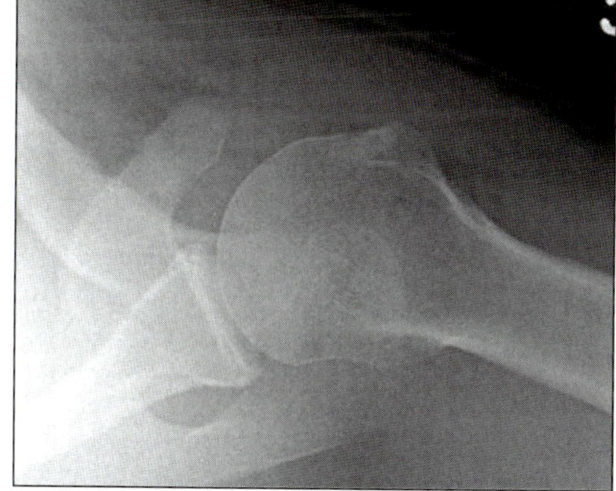

C

FIGURE 3

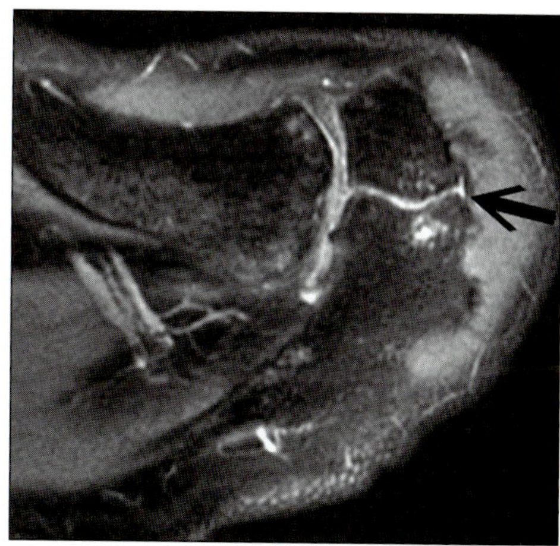

FIGURE 4

PEARLS

- *Use of a hydraulic arm positioner is invaluable to allow the arm to be placed in any position desired by the surgeon and obviates the need for an assistant (see Fig. 6).*
- *The beach chair position is preferred if rotator cuff repair or conversion to an open procedure is necessary.*

PITFALLS

- *Avoid overdistraction in the lateral decubitus or beach chair position as this can lead to brachial plexus stretch injury.*
- *In the beach chair position, ensure that the patient is brought far lateral to avoid mechanical block of access to the shoulder by the operating table.*

Equipment

- Hydraulic-controlled armholder
- Specific beach chair with table with back that slides from one side to the other to allow unencumbered access to the operative shoulder

Controversies

- Lateral decubitus versus beach chair position. For this procedure there is no clear superiority. However, we prefer beach chair since this procedure is usually performed in conjunction with a rotator cuff repair. We prefer lateral decubitus position for labral and capsulorrhaphy procedures.

Surgical Anatomy

- With the arm in anatomic position, the supraspinatus tendon, the anterior portion of the infraspinatus tendon, and the long head of the biceps lie anterior to the acromion (Fig. 5).
- Elevation of the arm in internal rotation or in the anatomic position causes these structures to pass under the anterior portion of the acromion and the coracoacromial ligament (CAL).
- Bone spurs on the anterior surface of the acromion may lead to impingement on the cuff, resulting in cyclic microtrauma with repetitive overhead use of the arm.

Positioning

- Arthroscopy can be performed with the patient placed in either the beach chair or in the lateral decubitus position. We prefer the beach chair position for this procedure.
- A hydraulic arm positioner is helpful to maintain the arm in the desired position throughout the procedure (Fig. 6).
- The coracoid process, AC joint, acromion, and distal clavicle are palpated and outlined with a marking pen (Fig. 7).

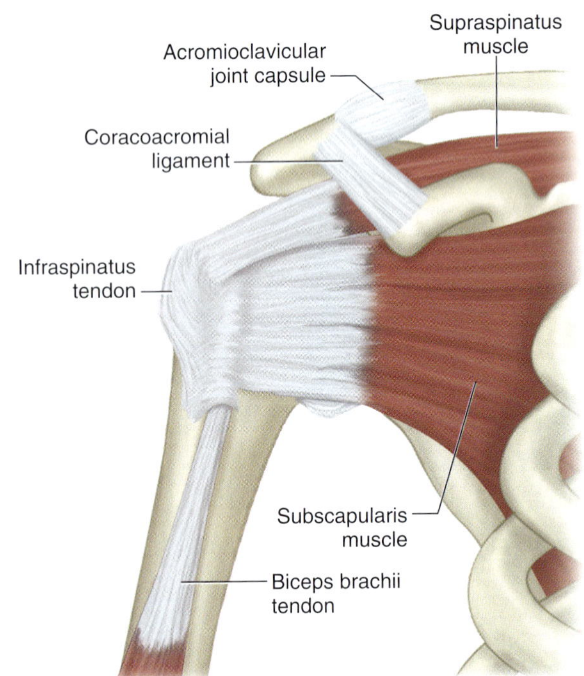

FIGURE 5

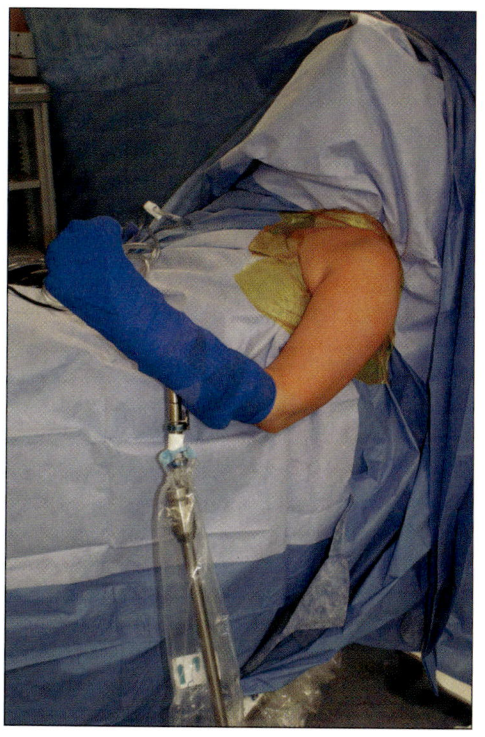

FIGURE 6

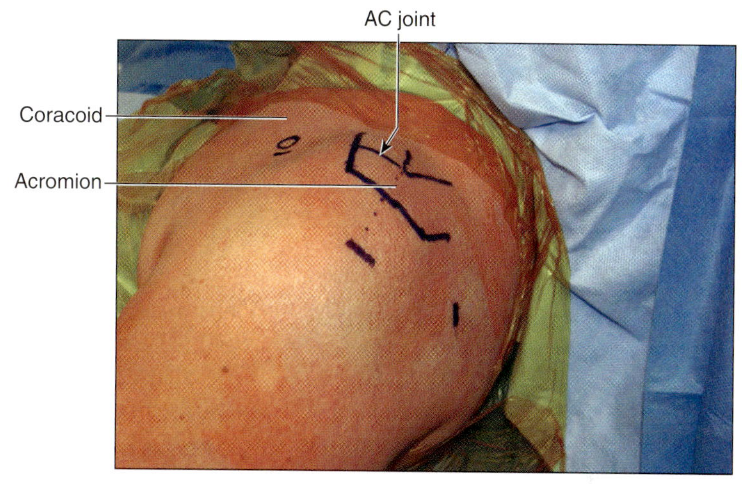

FIGURE 7

Portals/Exposures

- The posterior portal is placed at the "soft spot" located approximately 1 cm medial and 1–2 cm inferior to the posterolateral corner of the acromion (Fig. 8).
- While viewing from the posterior portal, the anterior portal is placed lateral to the coracoid process, in the rotator interval between the supraspinatus and subscapularis (see Fig. 8).
- A third midlateral portal is placed using a spinal needle under visualization of the arthroscope, 3 cm lateral to the acromial edge and parallel to the undersurface of the acromion (see Fig. 8).

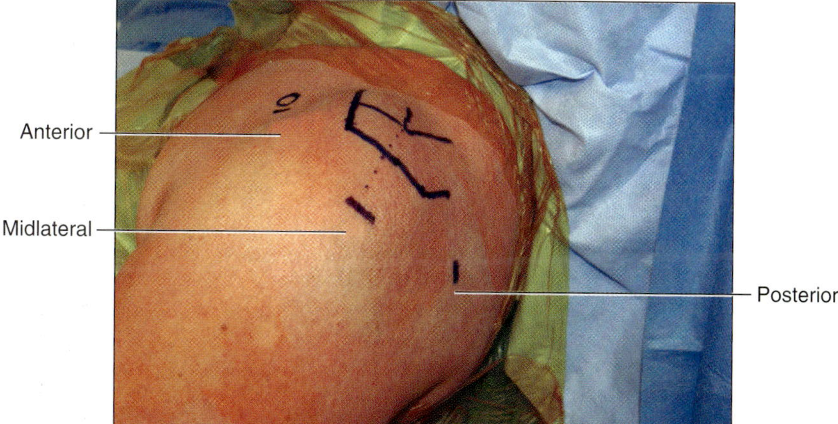

FIGURE 8

PEARLS

- *Make the posterior portal slightly more lateral in impingement/rotator cuff cases.*
- *Make the anterior portal slightly more superior in AC resection cases.*

PITFALLS

- *Do not make portals before traction is applied, especially in lateral decubitus cases.*

PEARLS

- *Become facile with the diagnostic component to allow more time for advanced procedures.*

PITFALLS

- *Do not place the arm in a beach chair hydraulic holder until the arthroscope is introduced into the joint to avoid possible inadvertent "transhumeral" scope placement.*

Procedure

STEP 1

- Diagnostic glenohumeral arthroscopy is performed from the posterior portal, evaluating for loose bodies, synovitis, and fraying or tearing of the biceps tendon, labrum, glenohumeral ligaments, or rotator cuff.
- The entire articular surface of the humeral head and glenoid is also examined by rotating the arthroscope superiorly and the humeral head into internal and external rotation.
- The right shoulder is seen through the posterior portal in Figure 9.

STEP 2

- The arthroscope is introduced into the subacromial space from the posterior portal.
- A shaver is inserted from the midlateral portal and used to perform a bursectomy.
- The soft tissues from the undersurface of the acromion are débrided, extending from 2.5 cm posterior to the anterior edge of the acromion to the CAL.
- The bursal "veil" is identified and resected to increase visualization. The *arrows* in Figure 10 point to the superior and inferior aspects of the bursal veil.

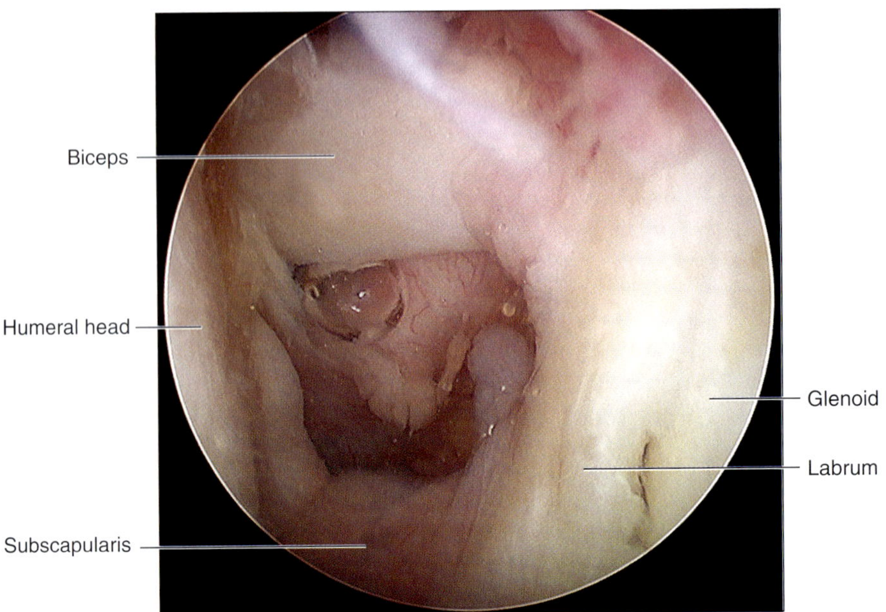

FIGURE 9

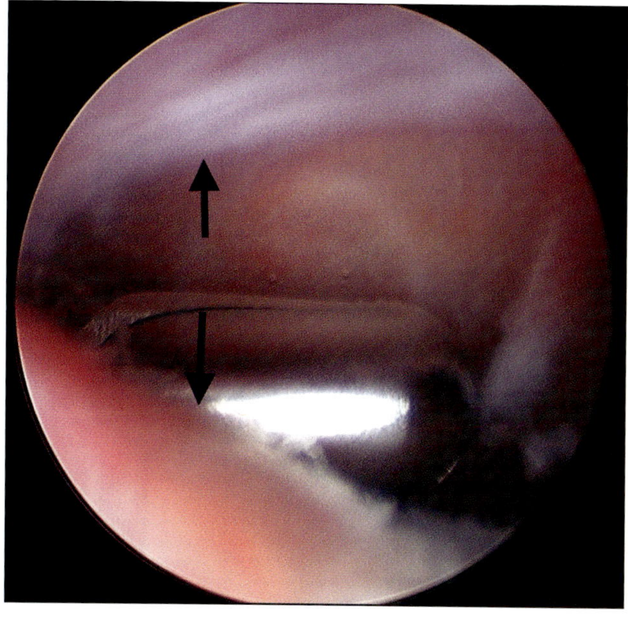

FIGURE 10

Step 3

- The CAL is completely detached from its acromial end, exposing the acromial spur. The *double-ended arrow* in Figure 11 indicates the size of the spur.
- An anterior acromioplasty is performed viewing from the posterior portal while using an arthroscopic shaver or burr via the lateral portal.
  - The shaver or burr is used to begin the acromioplasty from the anterolateral aspect of the acromion, working toward the anteromedial aspect.

Instrumentation/ Implantation

- Standard 4.0-mm arthroscope

Pearls

- *Sweep the subacromial bursa with the blunt scope obturator/ sheath to "create a space" within the bursa to aid in visualization.*
- *The bursal veil demarcates the anterior one third and posterior two thirds of the acromion. By removing the bursal veil early in the procedure, the subacromial "space" is easily visualized and exposed (see Video 1).*

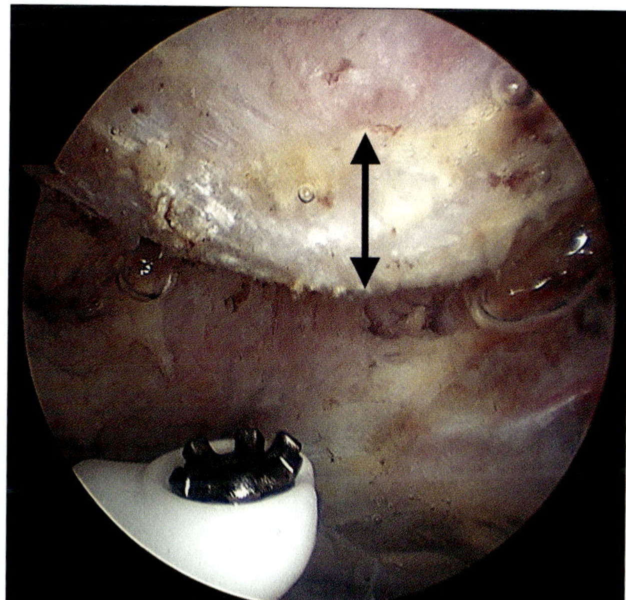

FIGURE 11

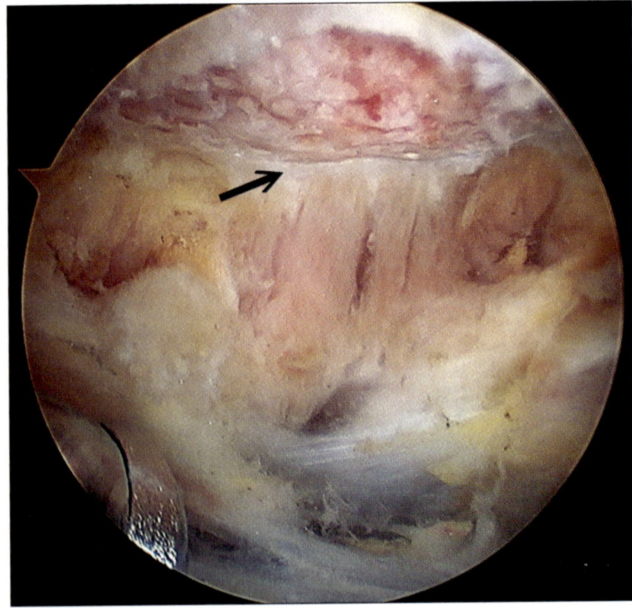

FIGURE 12

- The anterior third of the undersurface of the acromion is resected using the anterior deltoid periosteal fibers (Fig. 12; *small arrow* points to the white deltoid periosteum) as a guide to indicate an adequate resection of the spur while preserving the deltoid insertion and avoiding compromise of the deltoid origin.
- The entire anterior edge of the acromion is débrided to remove any protruberances.

Step 4

- The AC joint should be resected only if the examiner elicited tenderness to palpation or AC joint pain with cross-body adduction preoperatively.
- Radiographic assistance in decision making on the AC joint should not be relied upon in general due to the high incidence of "abnormal findings" on preoperative radiographs and MRIs. However, edema in the lateral clavicle and/or medial acromion in a T_2-weighted MRI is highly suspicious of a symptomatic AC joint.

Postoperative Care and Expected Outcomes

- Postoperatively, the arm can be supported using a sling usually for no more than 2 days.
- Pendulum exercises may be started on postoperative day 1.

Pitfalls

- *Never begin shaving "blindly" if you cannot see. Take a moment to triangulate and, if you cannot visualize the shaver, then repeat Step 1 above.*

Instrumentation/Implantation

- Be prepared for biceps tenodesis, labral repair, and of course rotator cuff repair.

Controversies

- Some surgeons have suggested a limited bursectomy due to its potential adjunct in soft tissue healing. However, we disagree with this and favor a thorough bursectomy for visualization and therapeutic purposes.

PEARLS

- *Always ensure that the arthroscope is positioned correctly (not obliquely oriented) to avoid oblique acromioplasties.*

PITFALLS

- *Avoid deltoid detachment at all costs.*
- *Ensure smooth, even resection by viewing from the posterior and midlateral portals.*

Instrumentation/ Implantation

- Aggressive shaver or burr

Controversies

- Some believe that violation of the AC joint may lead to postoperative symptoms in the joint, although this remains very controversial.

- Active and passive elevation may be started between postoperative days 1 and 4.
- Isometric exercises of the deltoid and rotator cuff may begin by the fourth day.
- Starting in the second postoperative week, light exercises against resistance may be started.
- Patients are encouraged to use the arm as normally as possible with the exception of athletics or overhead work.
- Patients are expected to return to activities of daily living within the first few days after surgery, and those who have desk jobs can return to work in 2–3 days.
- Most patients have full return of active range of motion by 3 weeks. Patients whose jobs require heavy lifting or repetitive overhead activity take 6 weeks or longer.
- Return to overhead sports is allowed after 6 weeks.

Evidence

Altchek DW, Warren RF, Wickiewicz TL, Skyhar MJ, Ortiz G, Schwarz E. Arthroscopic acromioplasty: technique and results. J Bone Joint Surg [Am]. 1990;72:1198-207.

This study described the technique and results of arthroscopic acromioplasty on 40 patients over a 2-year period. After a minimum follow-up of 12 months, all but one patient had improvement in pain. Seventy-three percent of patients had good or excellent results; 10% of patients had a failed result.

Andrews JR, Carson WG, Ortega K. Arthroscopy of the shoulder: technique and normal anatomy. Am J Sports Med. 1984;12:1-7.

This paper reviewed the technique for shoulder arthroscopy.

Bigliani LU, Levine WN. Subacromial impingement syndrome. J Bone Joint Surg [Am]. 1997;79:1854-68.

The authors reviewed the current concepts in the etiology, diagnosis, and treatment of impingement syndrome.

Ellman H, Kay SP. Arthroscopic subacromial decompression for chronic impingement: two to five year results. J Bone Joint Surg [Br]. 1991;73:395-8.

This study analyzed the long-term results of 65 cases of arthroscopic subacromial decompression for impingement syndrome without full-thickness rotator cuff tears.

Gartsman GM. Arthroscopic acromioplasty for lesions of the rotator cuff. J Bone Joint Surg [Am]. 1990;72:169-80.

This study compared the results of arthroscopic acromioplasty for subacromial impingment in 165 patients without rotator cuff tears (100 patients), with partial tears (40 patients), and with complete tears (25 patients). Acromioplasty was found to be effective in patients with no tear or with a parital tear. Patients with massive rotator cuff tears had unsatisfactory results.

Hawkins RJ, Kennedy JC. Impingement syndrome in athletes. Am J Sports Med. 1980;8:151-8.

This paper provided an overview of shoulder impingement in athletes, including functional anatomy, differential diagnosis, physical examination, and treatments based on stage of the disease.

Neer CS. Anterior acromioplasty for the chronic impingement syndrome in the shoulder. J Bone Joint Surg 1972;54:41-50.

The author reported on 50 shoulders of 47 patients treated with anterior acromioplasty over the course of 5 years. There was an average follow-up of 2.5 years. He also described the anatomy and pathophysiology of symptomatic impingement syndrome.

Potter HG, Birchansky SB. Magnetic resonance imaging of the shoulder: a tailored approach. Tech Shoulder Elbow Surg. 2006;6:43-56.
Seeger LL, Gold RH, Bassett LW, Ellman H. Shoulder impingment: MR findings in 53 shoulders. AJR Am J Roentgenol 1988;150:343-7.

In these papers, the authors reviewed MRI scans of 107 shoulders in 96 patients; those who had undergone invasive procedures prior to imaging were not included. A total of 53 shoulders with impingement syndrome were identified.

Tennent TD, Beach WR, Meyers JF. A review of the special tests associated with shoulder examination. Am J Sports Med. 2003;31:154-60.

This article reviews the specific tests described to identify rotator cuff problems.

PROCEDURE 2

Rotator Cuff Repair

Allan A. Young and David H. Sonnabend

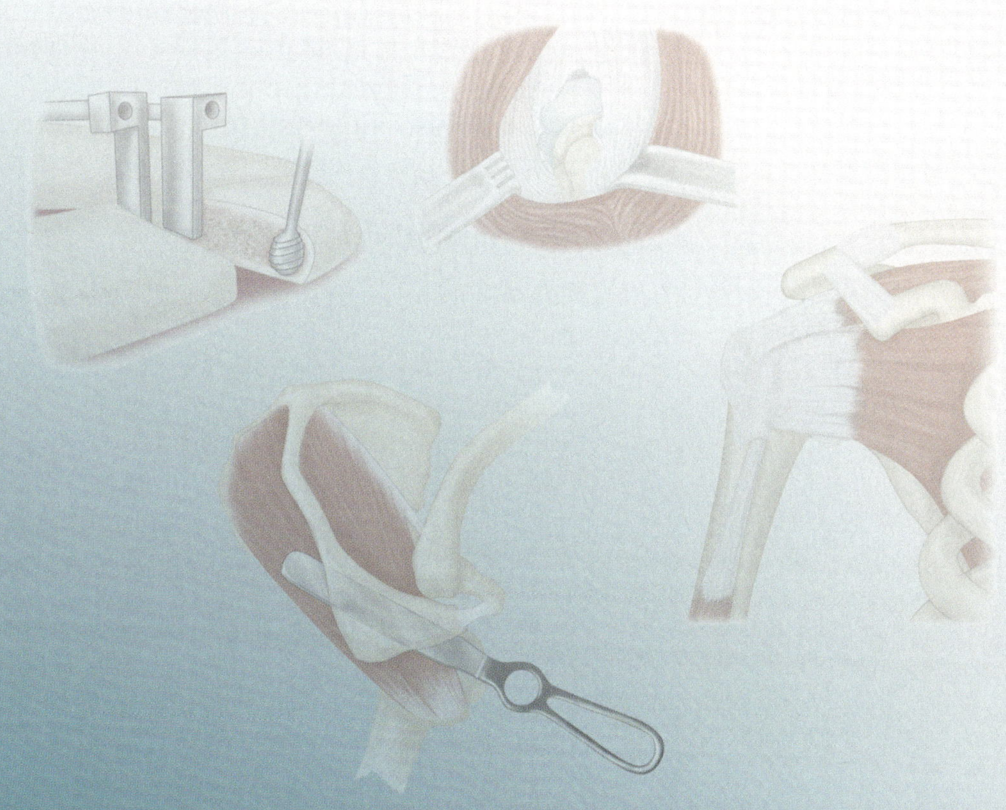

Open Technique for Partial-Thickness or Small or Medium Full-Thickness Tears

Indications

- Rotator cuff repair is indicated in patients with a documented tear ± subacromial impingement syndrome who remain symptomatic despite 3–6 months of nonoperative management.
- Acute repair is indicated in younger symptomatic patients (<50 years) following trauma.
- Repair is also indicated for revision of failed previous (arthroscopic or open) rotator cuff repair.

Examination/Imaging

- Examination of the rotator cuff should specifically include
  - Identifying muscle wasting via observation and palpation.
  - Documenting passive and active shoulder range of motion.
  - Looking for signs of impingement syndrome.
  - Acromioclavicular (AC) joint and biceps examination.
  - Assessment of cuff strength. Note that reduced power may be secondary to cuff tear, neurologic abnormality, or pain. A subacromial injection of local anesthetic often eliminates pain and allows a true assessment of strength.
- Plain radiographs
  - A true anteroposterior view is used to assess for subacromial spurring, calcification of the coracoacromial (CA) ligament, cystic changes of the greater tuberosity, and associated AC joint pathology. The acromiohumeral interval may be reduced in larger tears (normal value 7–14 mm; <5 mm suggests significant cuff tear).
  - The supraspinatus outlet view reveals acromial morphology.
  - The axillary view is useful in diagnosing an os acromiale.
- Magnetic resonance imaging (MRI)
  - MRI provides the best assessment of rotator cuff pathology and has been demonstrated to have a

Pitfalls

- *Irreparable rotator cuff tears.*
  - *The Goutallier classification, based on the extent of muscle atrophy and fatty infiltration on computed tomography or magnetic resonance imaging, is a useful guide (Goutallier et al., 2003).*
  - *Also, retraction to the level of the glenoid is generally considered irreparable.*
- *Elderly patients with poor cuff tissue/healing potential.*
- *Nonsteroidal anti-inflammatory drugs (Cohen et al., 2006) and smoking (including nicotine patches [Galatz et al., 2006]) have been shown to inhibit healing and should be considered relative contraindications.*
- *It should be emphasized to patients that results of surgical repair are more predictable for pain relief than for restoration of strength or function.*
- *Patients should be made aware of the expected duration of convalescence following cuff repair.*

Controversies

- Aggressive surgical treatment in younger or high-demand patients is increasingly recommended, based on the likelihood of tear progression and knowledge that smaller tears have increased intrinsic healing potential.
- Treatment of partial-thickness rotator cuff tears is generally reserved for symptomatic tears of greater than 50% or 6 mm of tendon thickness; however, treatment should be considered with greater than 25% or 3 mm in younger or high-demand patient.

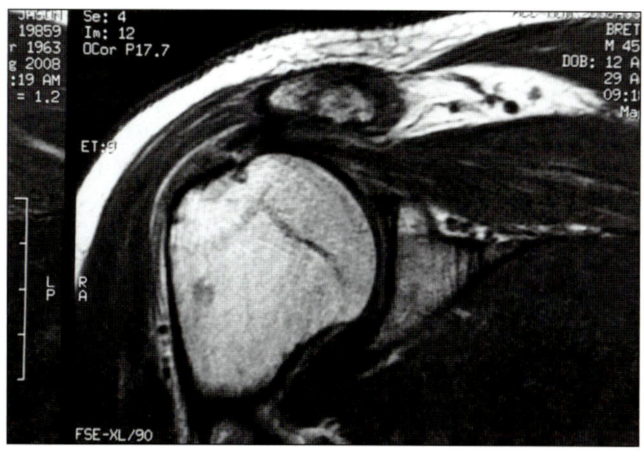

FIGURE 1

high degree of sensitivity and specificity, as seen for the full-thickness tear of the supraspinatus in Figure 1. MRI also provides information regarding the size of the tear and degree of retraction, the presence of muscle atrophy/fatty degeneration and coexistent shoulder pathology, thereby enhancing both preoperative planning and prognostication. It is better than ultrasound for identifying partial-thickness tears, particularly articular-sided tears.

- We typically utilize MRI without contrast; however, arthrography may be helpful in differentiating partial- from full-thickness tears and also in predicting the degree of tearing in partial-thickness tears.

■ Ultrasound
- Ultrasound is quicker and cheaper than MRI; however, the accuracy is extremely operator dependent. In experienced hands, ultrasound can be an effective diagnostic tool for assessing rotator cuff tears.
- An occasional indication is the patient with suspected cuff pathology who is not willing to undergo the prolonged convalescence following cuff repair. In this setting a decompression alone may be appropriate, and ultrasound is useful to confirm significant impingement.

Treatment Options

- Nonoperative management remains the mainstay of treatment for rotator cuff tears. We routinely prescribe physical therapy concentrating on posterior capsular stretching, scapular stabilization, and progressive rotator cuff strengthening.
- Another option is judicious use of subacromial cortisone injections—typically no more than two injections over a 6-month period.
- Arthroscopic and mini-open arthroscopic-assisted techniques have evolved and gained popularity for managing rotator cuff pathology.

Surgical Anatomy

- The rotator cuff is composed of blended tendons from four muscles: the supraspinatus, infraspinatus, teres minor, and subscapularis (Fig. 2A).
  - The subscapularis originates from the anterior surface of the body of the scapula and inserts onto the lesser tuberosity.
  - The supraspinatus originates from the fossa superior to the scapula spine, while the infraspinatus originates from the fossa below the spine. The teres minor originates from the dorsal surface of the lateral scapula border. Each of these three muscles inserts onto the greater tuberosity.
- The insertional footprint of the supraspinatus has recently been re-evaluated and found to be smaller than previously recognised (Mochizuki et al., 2008). It is triangular in shape, with an average medial-to-lateral length of 6.9 mm and an average anterior-to-posterior width of 12.6 mm (Fig. 2B). The footprint of the infraspinatus is trapezoidal in shape, with an average medial-to-lateral length of 10.2 mm and an average maximum anterior-to-posterior width of 32.7 mm.

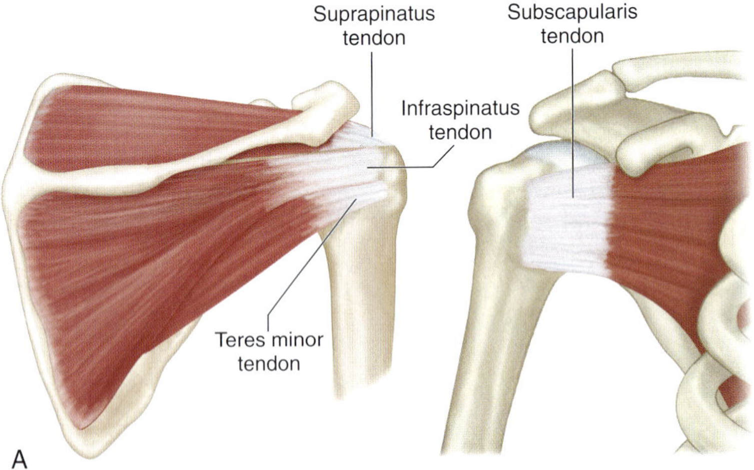

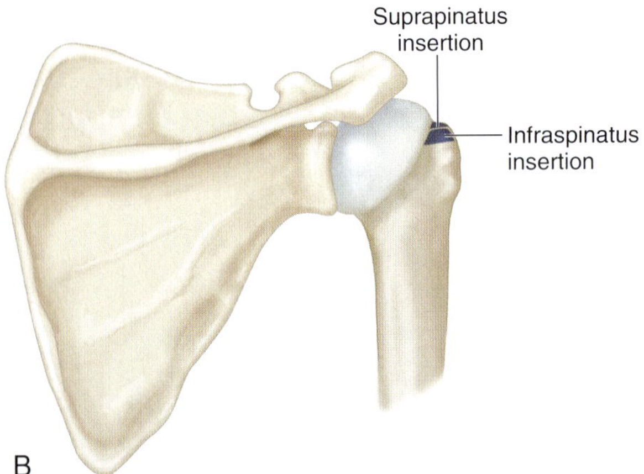

FIGURE 2 B

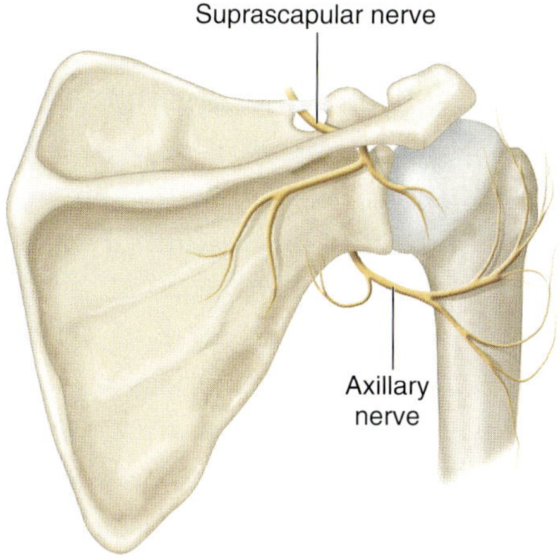

FIGURE 3

- The coracohumeral ligament originates from the lateral border of the base of the coracoid process and blends with the tendon of the supraspinatus before inserting into the greater tuberosity.
- The axillary nerve is typically located 5 cm (range, 3–7 cm) distal to the acromion (Fig. 3); therefore, splitting of the deltoid muscle should be limited to 4 cm.
- The suprascapular nerve traverses the suprascapular notch and passes around the spine of the scapula (see Fig. 3).
  - The distance between the superior glenoid margin and the suprascapular notch is typically 3 cm, and that between the posterior glenoid margin and the scapular spine is 2 cm.
  - The suprascapular nerve is at risk during surgical release of the rotator cuff, and therefore instruments should not extend further than 1.5 cm medial to the glenoid.

PEARLS

- *The use of a limb positioner (e.g., Spider arm positioner [Tenet, Calgary, Canada]) can be a useful adjunct to surgery.*
- *It is essential that the operated shoulder is hanging free over the side of the table so that the arm can be put through a complete range of motion.*

PITFALLS

- *Care must be taken to ensure that the patient is securely positioned on the operating table and the head is supported. Intermittent traction on the arm is occasionally required during the procedure to assist with exposure and can result in the position of the patient inadvertently changing during the case. We use a seatbelt to secure the patient to the table, tilt the entire operating table away from the operated side by a few degrees, and make sure the head is secure.*

Positioning

- The patient is place in the beach chair position with the operative arm draped free (Fig. 4).
- The patient should be placed at the near edge of the operating table with the shoulder freely mobile in all directions. The mattress should overlap the edge of the table to prevent neurovascular compression.
- A neurologic headrest allows easier assistant access, especially with large patients. The head should be rotated away from the operated side to also enhance access to the shoulder.
- A pillow is placed under the knees and silicone jelly pads under each heel.
- Intraoperative intermittent pneumatic calf compressive devices are utilized.

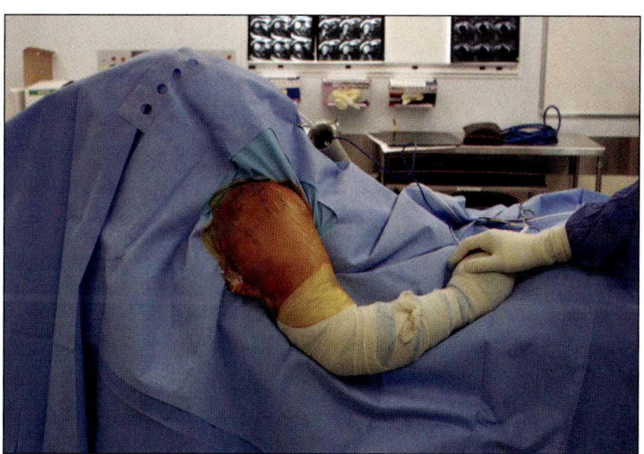

FIGURE 4

Pearls

- *Prior to making the skin incision, local infiltration of subcutaneous tissues with a vasoconstricting agent (e.g., bupivacaine 2.5 or 5 mg/ml plus adrenaline 5 μg/ml) is useful to assist with control of intraoperative bleeding.*
- *If doubt exists regarding the ability to repair a tear, although usually not a concern in small and medium tears, then care should be taken to preserve the CA ligament. In this setting, a limited deltoid split may be performed initially to allow assessment of reparability of the tear prior to extending the approach and detaching the deltoid and CA ligament.*

Pitfalls

- *Care must be taken when developing the anterior skin flap because there is a tendency to inadvertently dissect into a tissue plane deep to the anterior deltoid muscle fibers.*
- *In order to ensure a reliable repair of the deltoid and thereby avoid potential dehiscence, care must be taken to detach the deltoid aponeurosis and not the fleshy portion of the muscle. The cuff of tissue available for repair is always smaller than anticipated, which is why we recommend an incision at least 1 cm posterior to the anterior acromial border. The presence of a large acromial spur can give the wrong impression of the anterolateral corner of the acromion, leading to an incision that is too anterior. Ensure that the distinct "white" appearance of the aponeurosis is clearly exposed by removing any overlying soft tissue, which usually includes some adherent fat.*

Portals/Exposures

- A number of different skin incisions and approaches have been suggested for open repair. We favor a skin incision in line with the midpoint of the distal clavicle and extending parallel to the anterior border of the acromion (Fig. 5). The incision commences just distal to the AC joint and extends approximately 3–4 cm distal to the acromion.
- Electrocautery is used to control bleeding, and the dissection is continued to the deltotrapezial fascia.
- Full-thickness subcutaneous skin flaps of approximately 3–5 cm are created on both sides of the incision and similarly extended proximally and distally (Fig. 6).
- The AC joint and anterior border of the acromion are palpated. An incision is made in the deltotrapezial fascia 1 cm posterior to the anterior border of the AC joint and acromion (Fig. 7; forceps point toward

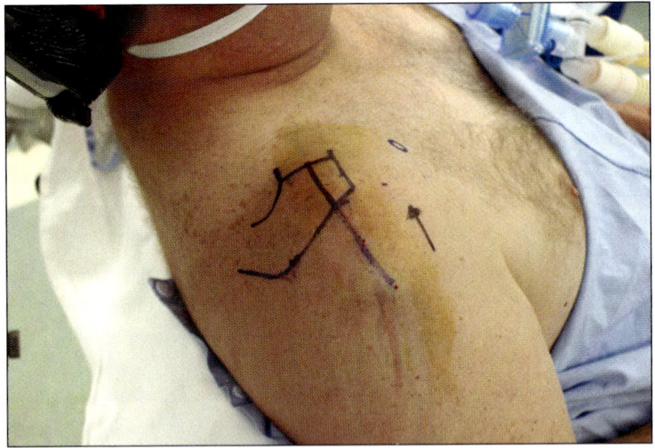

FIGURE 5

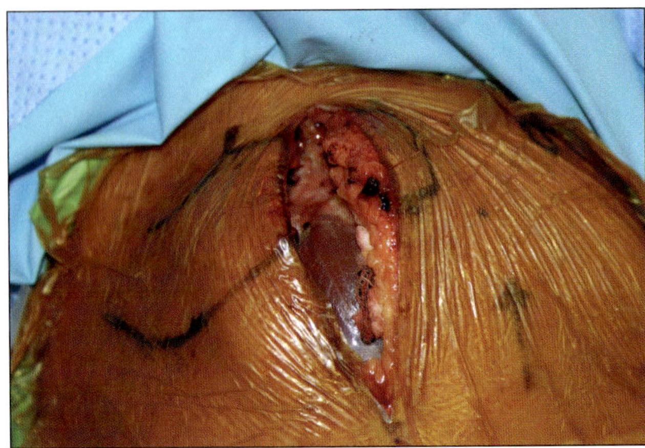

FIGURE 6

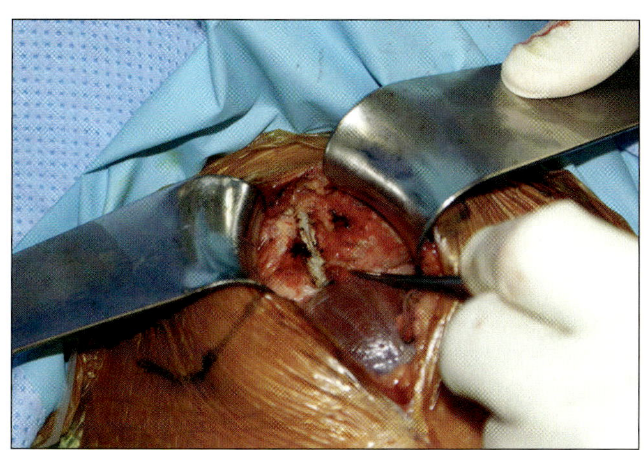

FIGURE 7

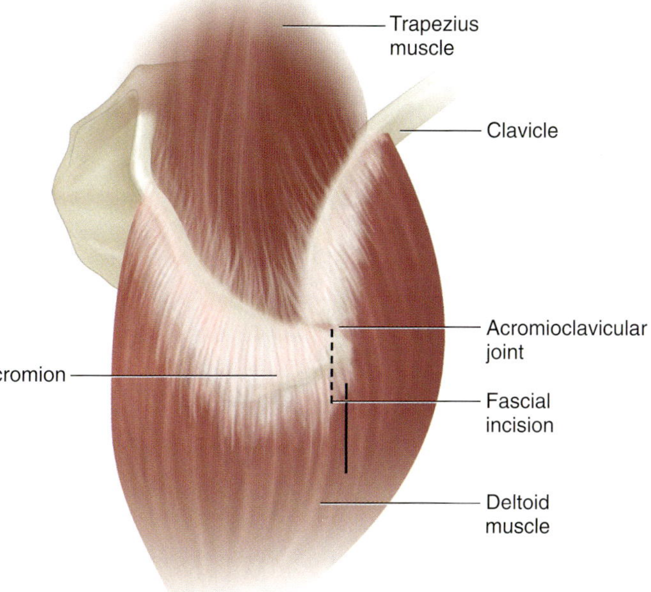

the anterolateral corner of the acromion). This incision commences just proximal to the AC joint and continues for up to 4 cm into the deltoid muscle, parallel to its fibers.

- The deltoid insertion is carefully elevated subperiosteally from the anterior acromion to the level of the AC joint (Fig. 8).
  - Elevation of the deltoid attachment is assisted by placing a pair of curved scissors through the split in the deltoid and directing them under the acromion. Opening the blades of the scissors provides retraction on the deltoid insertion and allows visualization of the undersurface of the deltoid insertion (Fig. 9).

Pitfalls—cont'd

- *The deltoid split should not be extended more than 4 cm to avoid axillary nerve injury. A suture can be tied at the distal end of the deltoid split to prevent inadvertent propagation during surgery.*

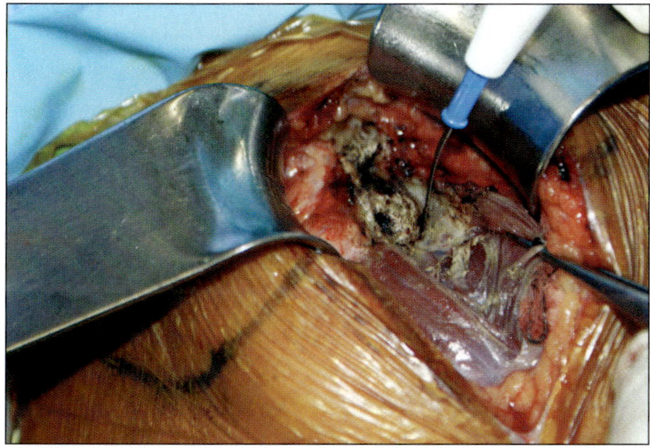

FIGURE 8

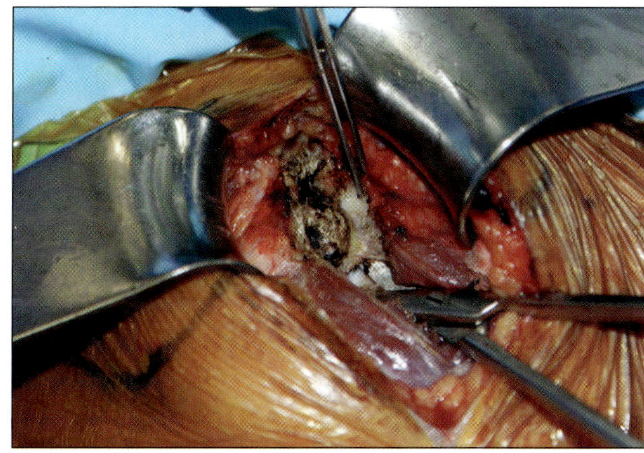

FIGURE 9

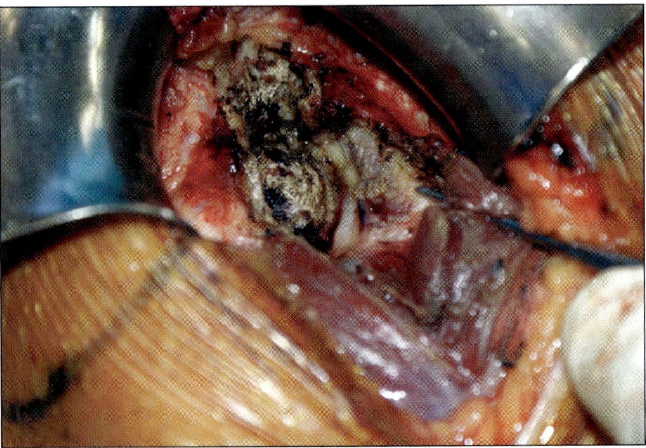

FIGURE 10

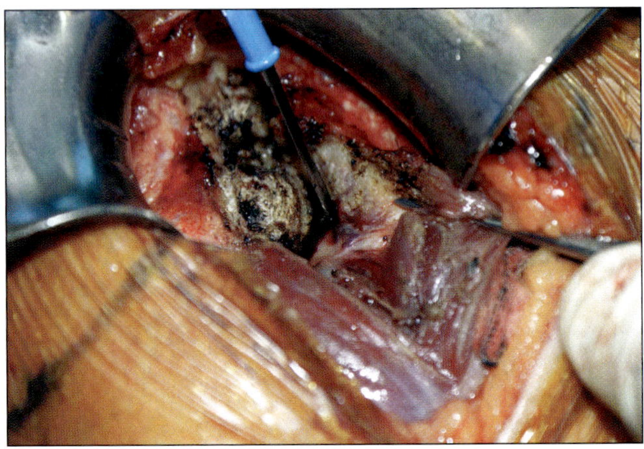

FIGURE 11

- A vessel (acromial branch of the thoracoacromial artery) is consistently found at this location (*asterisk* in Fig. 10) and can be a source of troublesome bleeding if not cauterized.

- The CA ligament is identified and its acromial insertion is detached, maximizing its length (Fig. 11).
- Subdeltoid and subacromial adhesions can be significant and interfere with exposure of the rotator cuff. Blunt dissection with the index finger is usually sufficient to break down adhesions; the finger should be allowed to sweep freely from anterior to posterior beneath both the acromion and the deltoid.

Controversies

- Some authors recommend complete resection of the CA ligament as part of rotator cuff repair. While we do not subscribe to the "no decompression for cuff repair" philosophy, we recognize that the CA ligament does have an important role, particularly in the setting of a failed cuff repair that may progress to a massive tear. In these cases, the CA ligament resists anterosuperior escape of the humeral head. By detaching but not excising the ligament, it can be reapproximated to the anterior acromion and AC joint capsule at the completion of open repair.

Procedure

Step 1

- Acromioplasty is performed.
  - At this stage, any acromial spur or ossification of the CA ligament is removed. A palpable ridge marks the anterior-most edge of the "true" acromion.
  - A large Darrach retractor is inserted under the acromion and toward its posterior margin. Using the instrument as a lever, the humeral head is displaced inferiorly, thereby providing an excellent view of the subacromial space.
  - A bone rongeur is used to resect the anterior edge of the acromion. This exposes cancellous bone, which helps with seating of the chisel or saw.
  - A thin sharp chisel is used to perform the acromioplasty (Fig. 12); alternatively, a small oscillating saw may be used. The chisel is aimed to resect the undersurface of the anterior third of the acromion until it is flat and flush with the remaining acromion.

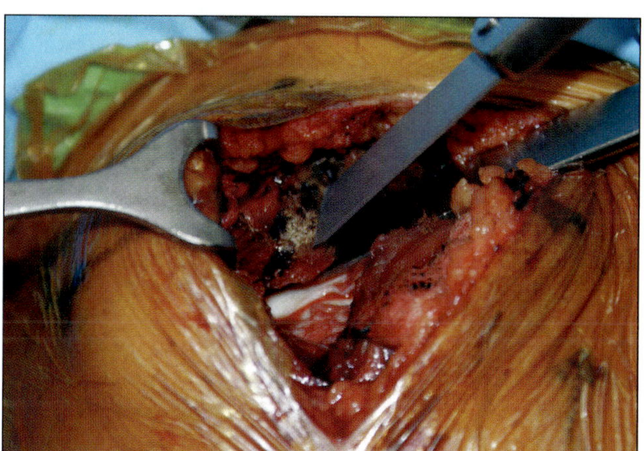

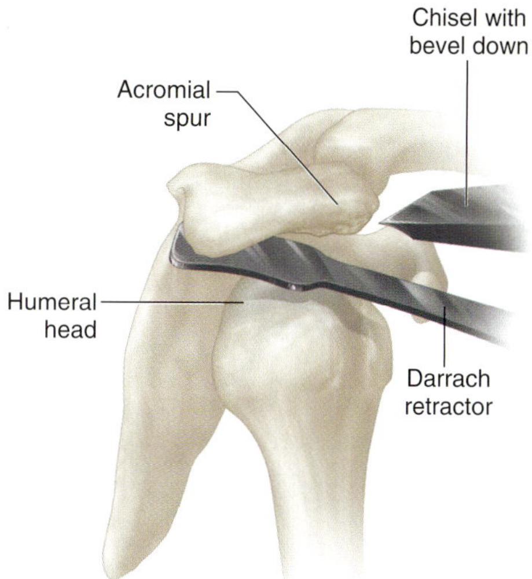

FIGURE 12

Pearls

- *Careful use of electrocautery to detach a few fibers of the deltoid from the lateral margin of the anterior acromion facilitates the exposure for the acromioplasty and minimizes the risk of leaving a lateral bony ridge (Fig. 15).*

Pitfalls

- *Care must be taken while using the chisel with the bevel facing down to avoid inadvertent superior propagation of the cut into the acromion, resulting in excessive resection. Using the chisel with the bevel uppermost is safer; however, we have found that the bevel-down technique gives a more precise cut and smoother acromial undersurface.*
- *Be aware of the risk of acromial fracture during retraction with the Darrach, particularly in women and elderly patients with relatively osteoporotic bone. Positioning the Darrach retractor beyond the posterior margin of the acromion is safer and results in a more effective lever.*

Instrumentation/ Implantation

- Darrach retractor
- Czerny retractor
- Bone rongeurs
- Chisel

- A rasp or bone file can be used to smooth out the acromial resection.
- Attention is paid to the undersurface of the AC joint.
  - A blunt, double-pronged (Czerny) retractor is extremely useful at this stage. One of the tines is placed deep to the deltoid and the other superficial to the deltoid at its insertion on the acromion (Fig. 13). The instrument is then used as a lever to expose the undersurface of the acromion (Fig. 14).
  - Any significant inferior osteophytes or spurs are excised with the chisel or bone rongeur.

- Very rarely is a formal distal clavicle excision required as part of a rotator cuff decompression and repair (<2% of cases in the senior author's experience).

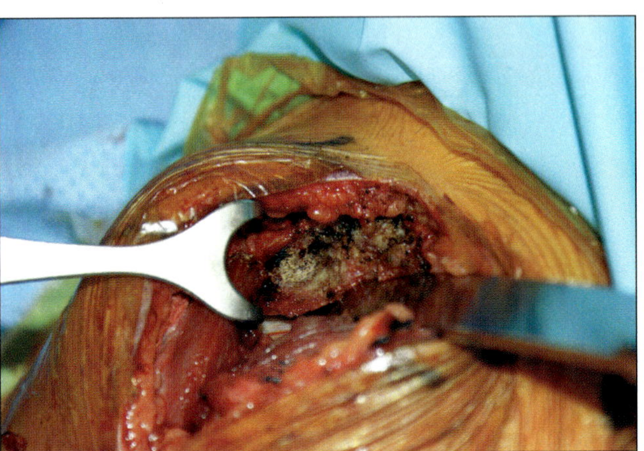

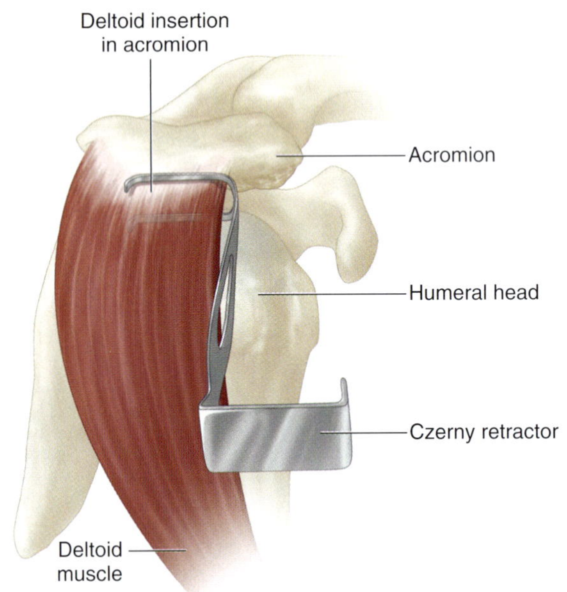

FIGURE 13

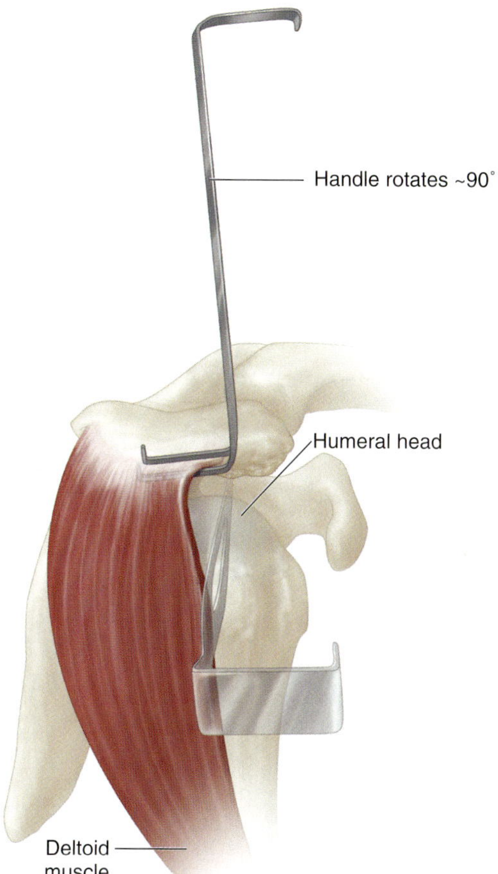

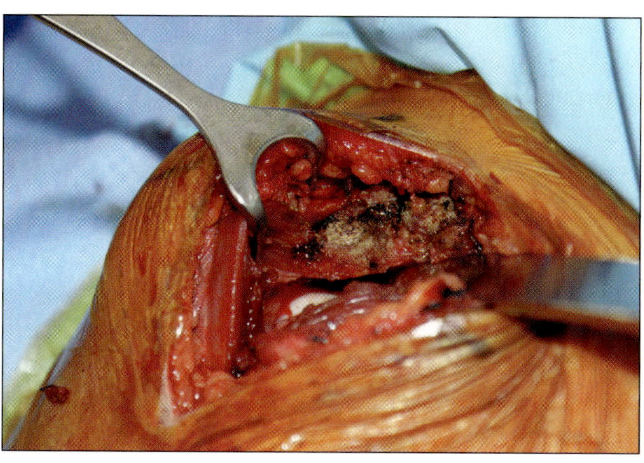

FIGURE 14

- If the patient has a symptomatic AC joint preoperatively, a fibrocartilaginous disc and adjacent cortical margins can be achieved with large rongeurs.
- If bone-to-bone contact persists, particularly posteriorly, formal resection of 5–10 mm of clavicle may be considered.

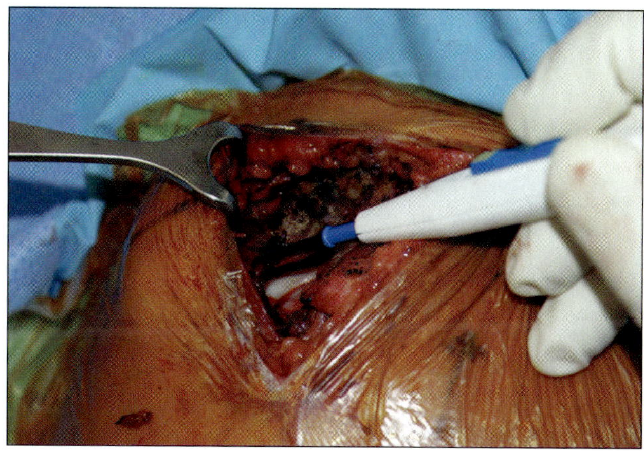

FIGURE 15

Controversies

- The role of acromioplasty in rotator cuff repair has been the subject of debate and is beyond the scope of this chapter. In almost all cases, other than the rare young patient undergoing acute repair, we recommend acromioplasty. While we recognize most acromial spurs are the result of rather than the cause of cuff failure, we note the symptomatic benefits of decompression.
- The subacromial bursa has been shown to take part in the healing process following rotator cuff repair. It is a source of cellular proliferation during cuff repair and has also been shown to express important extracellular matrix molecules, suggesting advantages to retaining the bursa during cuff repair. Alternatively, the bursa has also been shown to express high levels of proinflammatory cytokines and metalloproteinases, prompting others to recommend excision of the bursa during cuff repair. We limit bursal resection to the minimum required for adequate exposure (Fig. 16; forceps identify the bursa).

Step 2

- Tear assessment
  - The rotator cuff tear is assessed for location, shape, size, thickness, quality, and mobility of the remaining tendon, and presence of any associated tendon delamination. Figure 17 shows a full-thickness tear of the supraspinatus measuring 1–3 cm (i.e., medium tear).
  - The long head of the biceps tendon is assessed, in particular looking for any evidence of tendinopathy or instability.
  - The subscapularis tendon insertion is also assessed by observing through the supraspinatus tear and retracting on the biceps/rotator interval tissue.
- Biceps tenodesis (or tenotomy)
  - If the decision has been made to treat the biceps tendon, it is released near its glenoid attachment using a pair of curved scissors.
  - A biceps tenodesis is typically preferred to a simple tenotomy.
    - The transverse ligament is divided and the biceps sheath identified and opened. The biceps tendon is removed and tagged with a suture.
    - The elbow is placed in full extension and a point is marked on the tendon with electrocautery at the superior limit of the groove. The bicipital groove is decorticated using a chisel and rongeur, or with a motorized burr.
    - The biceps tendon is sutured into the groove using three transosseous #2 Ethibond sutures. The excess biceps tendon remaining proximally is excised.
- Releases
  - Releases are not typically required in partial and small tears of the supraspinatus; however, they may be required in medium tears depending on the mobility of the cuff. One of the important principles of cuff surgery is to obtain a repair that is not under undue tension, so the tendon being repaired should be able to be easily advanced to its site of bony repair.
  - A smooth Darrach elevator is passed medially and used in a sweeping motion to release any adhesions superficial to the supraspinatus and infraspinatus (Fig. 18).

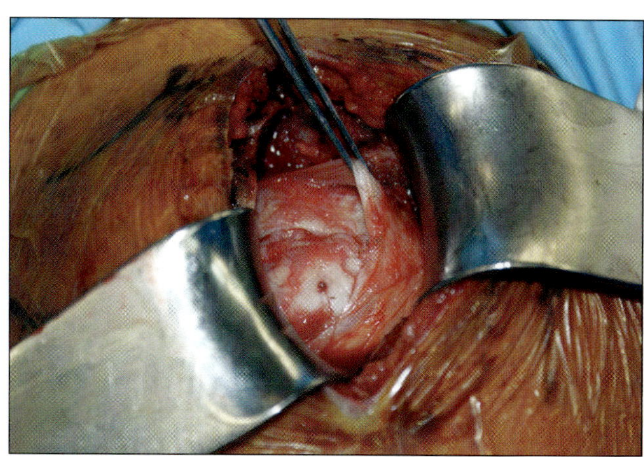

FIGURE 16

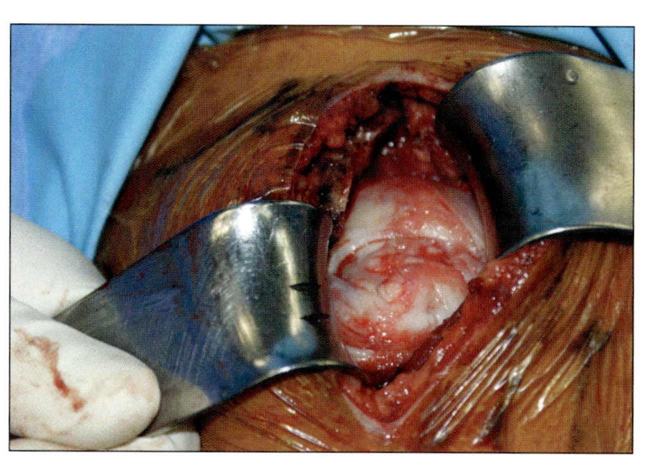

FIGURE 17

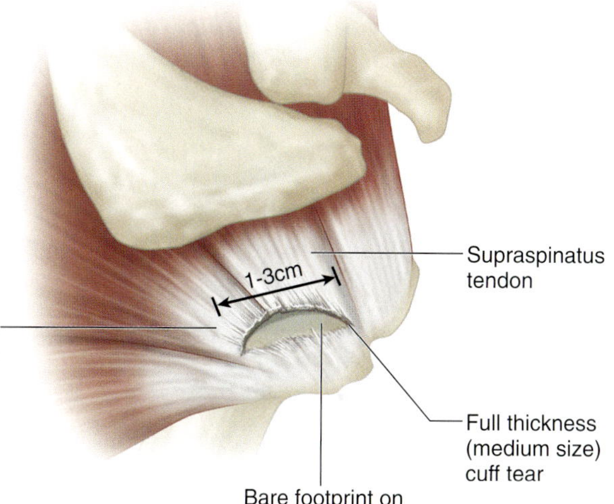

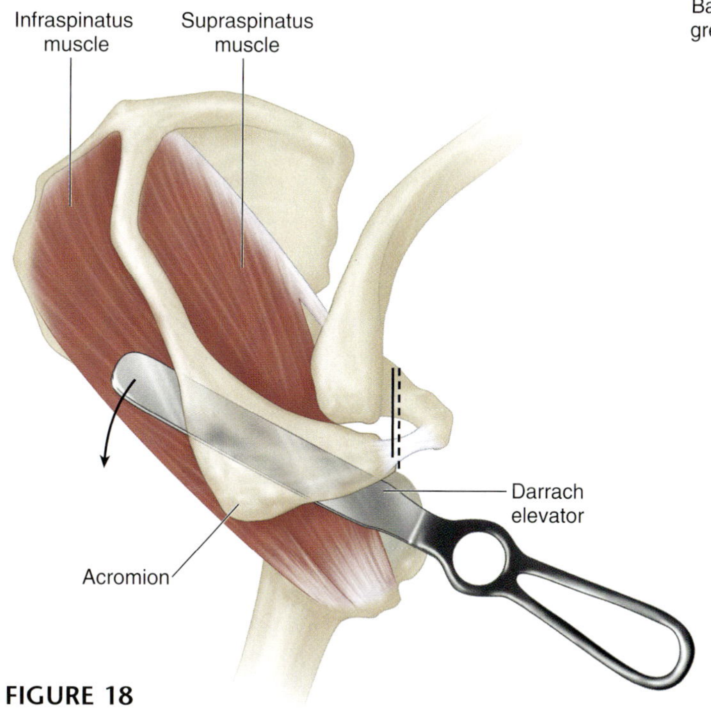

FIGURE 18

Pearls

- *Assessment is enhanced by pulling the cuff laterally and seeing where it sits best in varying degrees of humeral rotation.*
- *Allow approximately 1 cm or so of "overlengthening" while performing a biceps tenodesis. This lessens the tension on the repair and reduces the risk of failure.*

Pitfalls

- *The suprascapular nerve is in close proximity during the intra-articular release, and therefore it is recommended that all instruments remain less than 1.5 cm medial to the glenoid.*

Controversies

- Biceps pathology can be addressed by either tenotomy or tenodesis. While we often perform simple tenotomy to address biceps pathology in other settings, we prefer a tenodesis when performing a concomitant open cuff repair. The convalescent period in a sling following cuff repair is 6 weeks, which accommodates the biceps tenodesis (i.e., no added morbidity). The additional surgical time required to perform a tenodesis is worthwhile to avoid the occasional cosmetic deformity associated with tenotomy.

- If necessary, an intra-articular release is performed.
    - Gentle longitudinal traction is placed on the arm to inferiorize the humeral head and superior retraction on stay sutures placed in the edges of the cuff tear serve to enhance visualization (Fig. 19). Alternatively, a small Fukuda retractor can be positioned through the cuff defect and against the inferior glenoid margin to lever the humeral head downward and forward.
    - Using a pair of long scissors, the capsule is punctured just peripheral to the posterosuperior labrum and the resultant hole enlarged by opening the blades (Fig. 20A). This creates a defect in the capsule large enough to allow insertion of a small Darrach retractor.
    - This retractor is then used in a sweeping motion to perform the intra-articular release (Fig. 20B).
- The coracohumeral ligament is palpated with the arm in adduction and external rotation. If it tightens excessively with this maneuver or with lateral traction on the stay suture(s), it should be released from the coracoid using electrocautery.

Step 3

- Humeral preparation
    - The rotator cuff can be repaired "onto" or "into" bone.
    - For repair of small tears, the supraspinatus footprint on the greater tuberosity is débrided to bleeding bone using either a bone rongeur or motorized burr. The tendon is then repaired "onto" bone.
    - For more significant tears, including medium tears, a bony trough is prepared in the footprint of the greater tuberosity just lateral to the articular margin (Fig. 21).
        - It is important that the trough extends from a point immediately adjacent to intact tendon insertion posteriorly and extends the full length of the tear.
        - The trough is typically prepared with bone rongeurs or a motorized burr to a depth of approximately 5 mm. The width of the trough should match the tendon thickness, typically 5–10 mm. The medial edge of the trough should be trimmed so that the reattached tendon passes over a smooth edge.
- Tendon preparation
    - Débridement of the edge of the tendon is kept to a minimum, if performed at all. Every millimeter of length is useful, particularly in a tight repair, and

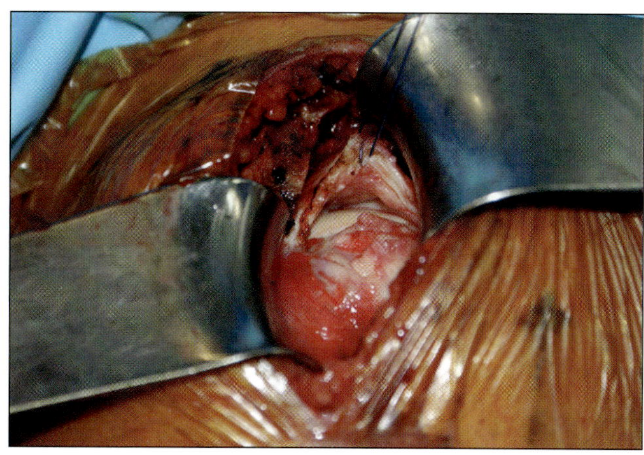

FIGURE 19

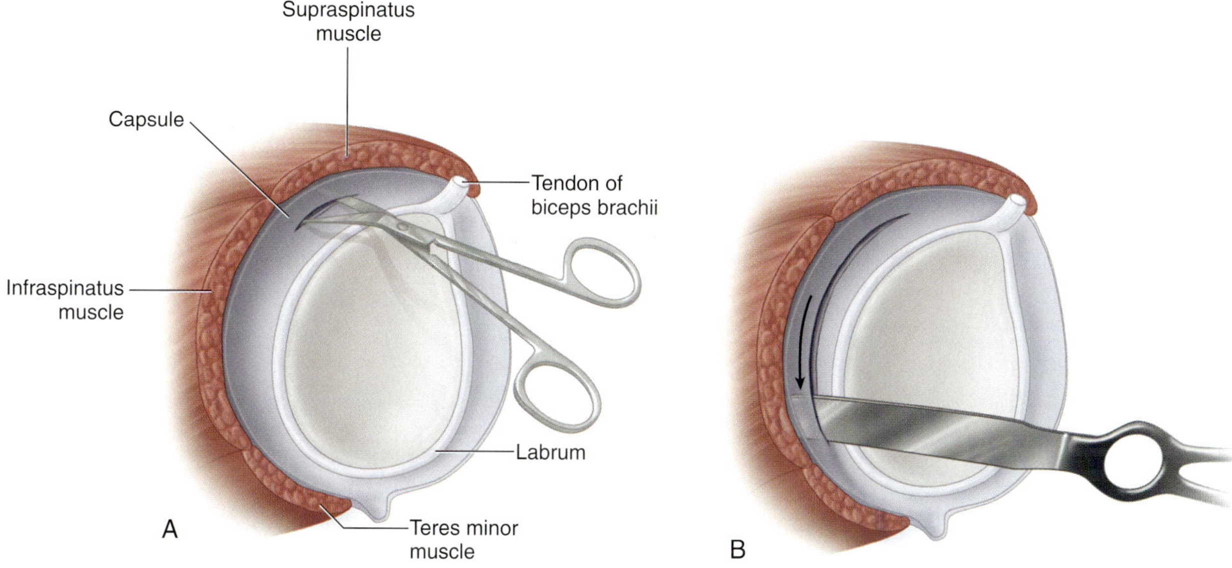

FIGURE 20

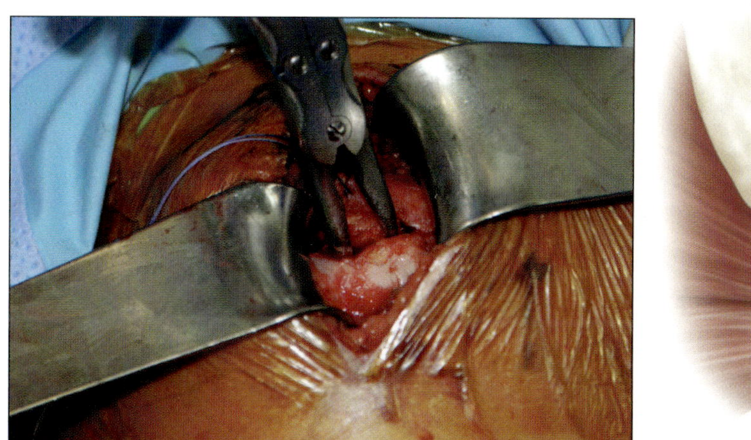

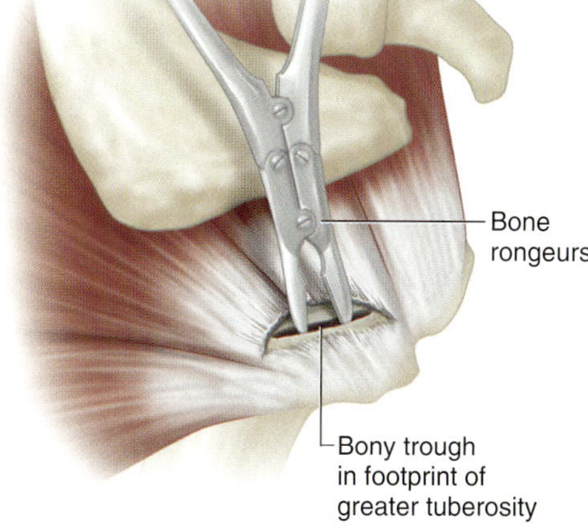

FIGURE 21

Pearls

- *In the case of a partial-thickness tear, an initial diagnostic arthroscopy may assist in deciding if the tear warrants completion and repair.*
- *Several stay sutures or traction sutures can be used to "manipulate" the tear to determine the optimal positioning and configuration. This is more relevant in larger tears, but can be a useful technique in medium tears.*

Pitfalls

- *It is important to have a repair that is not under excessive tension, or it will likely fail. If the lateral excursion of the tendon is limited despite performing the described releases, then the humeral trough can be medialized up to 1 cm onto the articular surface.*

no benefit has been shown by resecting the tendon edge.
- Deep surface laminations often retract farther than the superficial layer, and intra-articular release, as described earlier, may be necessary. Curettage of the delamination removes the thin layer of synovial cells found on either side of the tear, which enhances healing potential. An absorbable suture such as #1 Vicryl is used in an interrupted fashion to close the layers of the delamination.
- Occasionally, a very thin atrophic deep layer is present, and this can be resected rather than repaired.

- Repair of partial tears
  - Open repair of partial tears typically involves completion of the tear to a full-thickness defect. Using a scalpel blade or electrocautery, the remaining cuff is detached from its insertion into the greater tuberosity. In bursal-sided tears, this is straight forward. In articular-sided tears, however, identifying the tear can sometimes be difficult. By careful palpation of the cuff footprint, a defect in the tendon can usually be felt. The usual location is immediately posterior to the long head of the biceps tendon.
  - Once a partial tear has been completed, repair progresses similarly as for a full-thickness tear.
  - Some small superficial partial-thickness tears may be repaired onto the intact deep surface without tear completion. Suture anchors may be useful in this very occasional setting.

Controversies

- Repair of the rotator cuff tendon is performed either into a bony trough or onto the greater tuberosity. It is commonly stated that cuff tendon heals to bone similarly with either technique, a belief largely based on a single study in healthy goats (St. Pierre et al., 1995). We recommend creation of a bony trough for the following reasons:
  - It increases the surface area for tendon-to-bone repair.
  - It maintains some tendon-to-bone apposition in the event of suture creeping, which is inevitable.
  - It makes for a smoother repair construct, enabling better gliding under the CA arch.
  - We believe that the bone marrow released by creating a cancellous trough is a prominent source of stem cells capable of participating in the repair.

> **PEARLS**
>
> - *To avoid dog ears and achieve a smoother repair, the most anterior and posterior sutures should be positioned a little closer to the edge of the tendon.*
> - *In most situations, sutures can be passed directly through the greater tuberosity without the requirement for predrilling holes. A large needle is used and held very close to its tip with the needle holder when attempting to penetrate the cortex. This ensures that the applied force is in a straight line and perpendicular to the bone surface. A small mallet can be used to strike the needle holder to aid penetration.*

STEP 4

- Placement of sutures
  - Sutures are passed directly through the lateral aspect of the greater tuberosity using a needle. Alternatively, holes can be drilled. A staggered pattern is used, allowing preferably 1 cm, but at least 5 mm, between needle holes.
  - Typically four to six holes will be required for repair of a small or medium tear, thereby allowing two or three sutures.
  - For repair onto a decorticated footprint, a simple over-and-over suture pattern with a #2 braided suture is utilized. To reinforce the hold of the suture in poor-quality tendon, a Mason-Allen suture configuration is recommended.
  - For repair into a bony trough, a horizontal mattress suture using #2 braided suture is used.
    - A curved needle is passed through the greater tuberosity into the bony trough (Fig. 22).
    - The needle is then passed from superficial to deep through the tendon approximately 5–10 mm from its edge (Fig. 23).

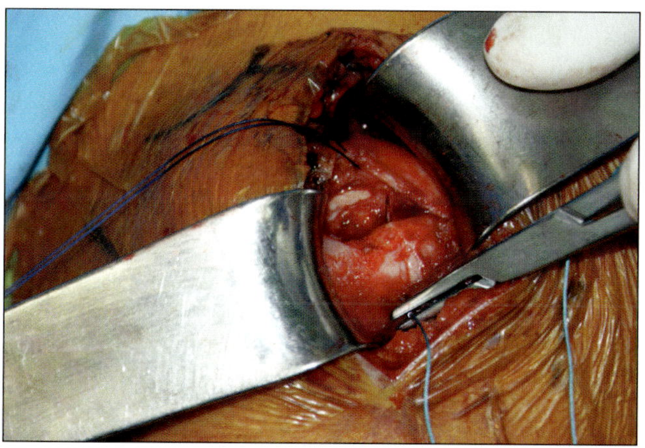

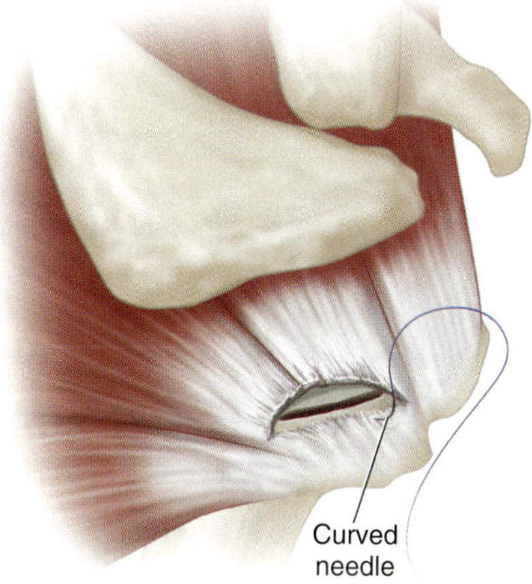

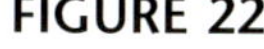
FIGURE 22

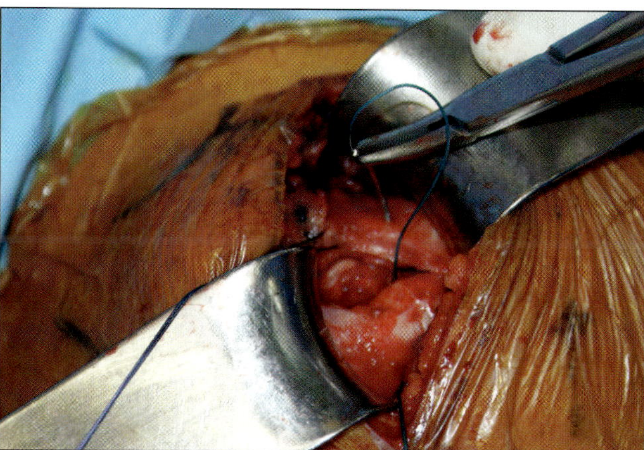

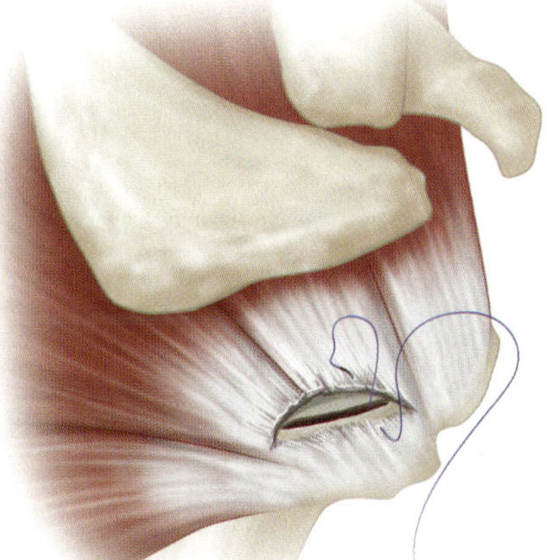

FIGURE 23

PEARLS—cont'd

- *To prevent sutures cutting through soft or weak bone, a small (usually three-hole) plate can be utilized to enhance suture fixation. Sutures exiting from the lateral aspect of the proximal humerus are threaded through the holes in the plate and then tied over the plate.*

- The needle is then passed back through the tendon from deep to superficial, at the same distance from the edge but 5 mm posterior (or anterior) to the initial passage (Fig. 24).
- The needle is then passed through the bony trough to exit through the lateral cortex (Fig. 25).
- When traction is applied on both suture limbs, the mattress suture pulls the edge of the cuff into the trough and results in a smooth transition from cuff to greater tuberosity (Figs. 26 and 27).
- The above steps are repeated for subsequent sutures depending on the size of the tear and the quality of the repair (Figs. 28 to 30).

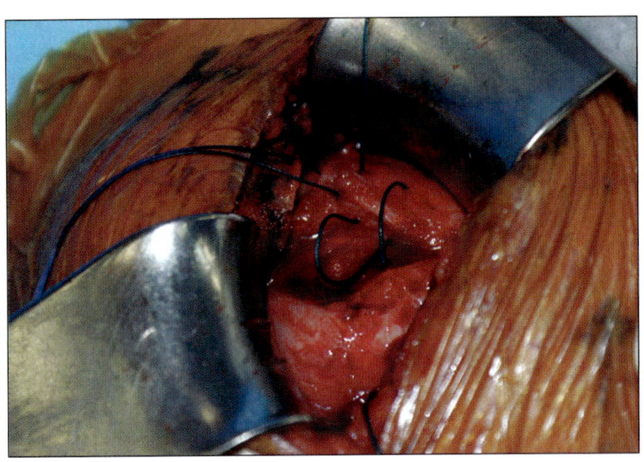

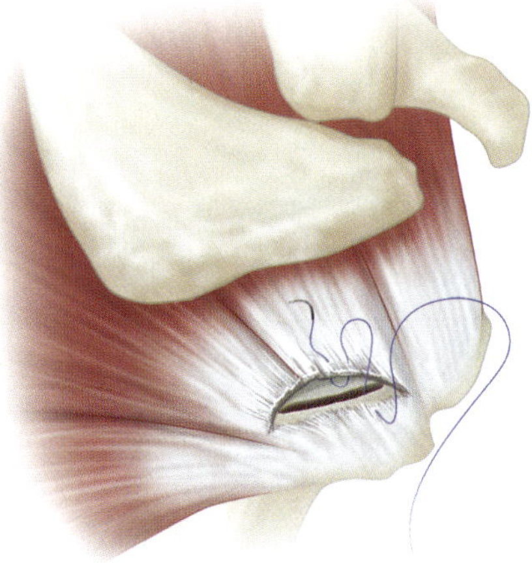

FIGURE 24

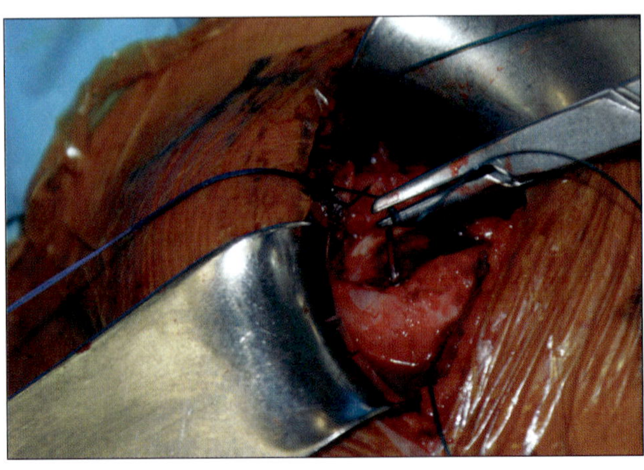

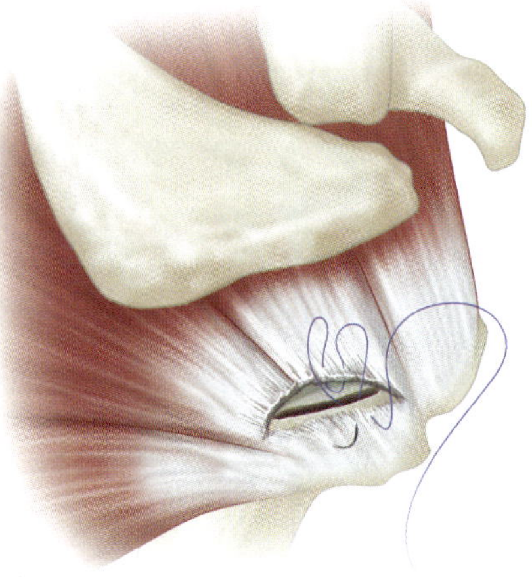

FIGURE 25

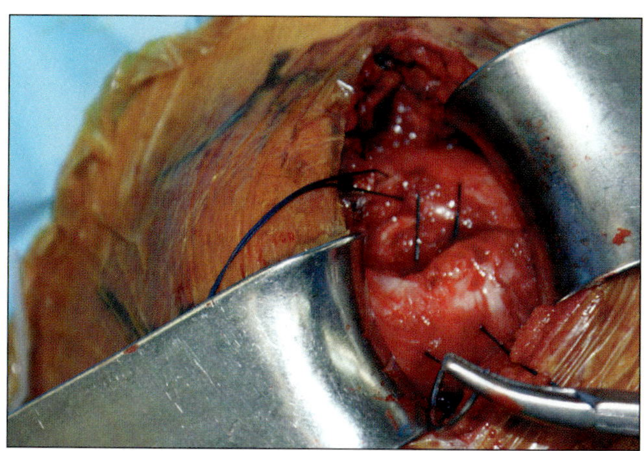

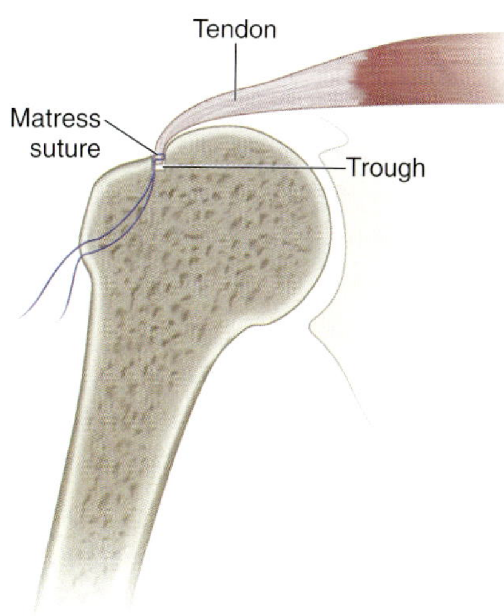

FIGURE 26

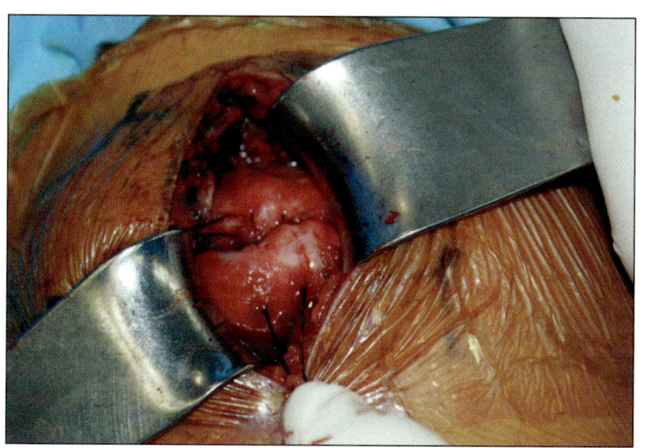

FIGURE 27

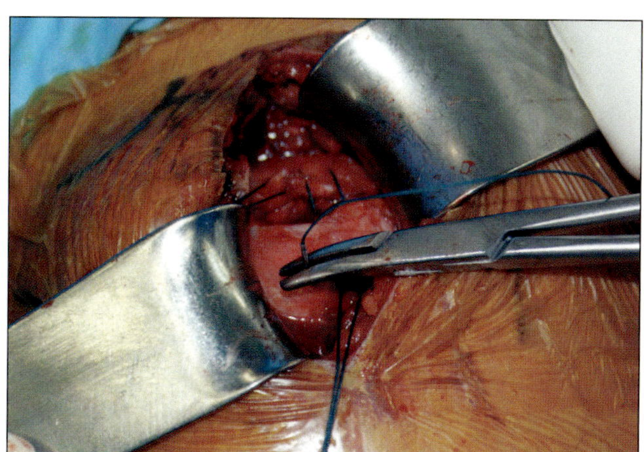

FIGURE 28

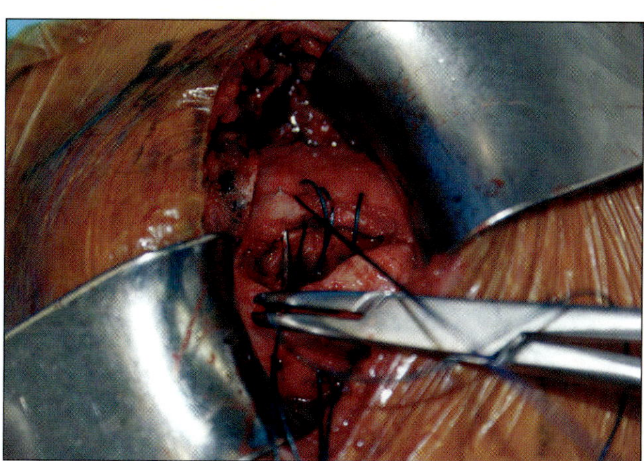

FIGURE 29

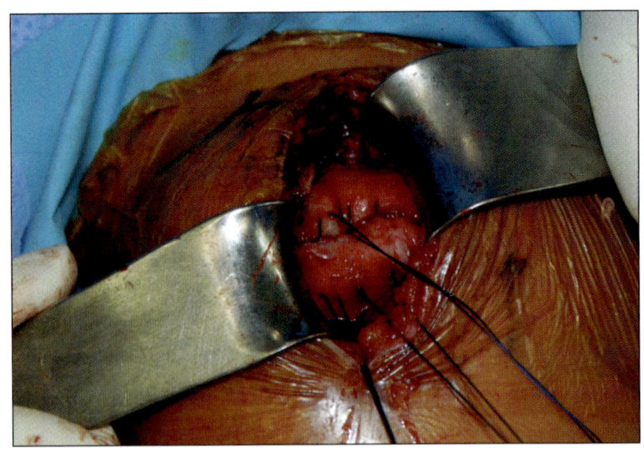
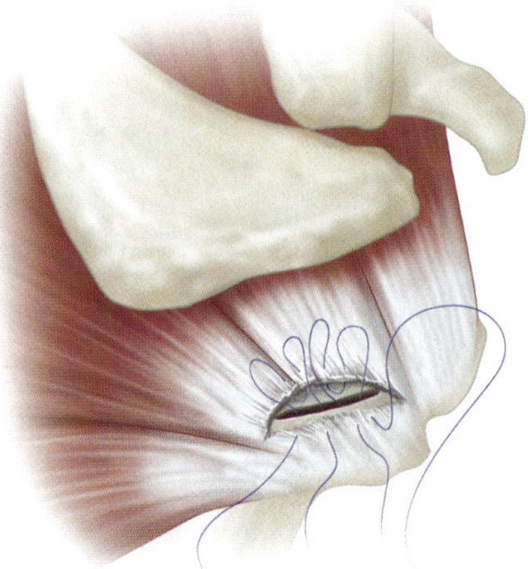

FIGURE 30

- Tying of sutures
  - Tying of sutures is performed after all sutures have been passed (Fig. 31).
  - Simultaneous traction is placed on all suture limbs to provisionally assess the quality and appearance of the repair construct.
  - Traction is maintained on available suture limbs during tying of each suture to ensure optimal tendon-to-bone apposition. Additionally, the arm is positioned in abduction during tying of sutures to assist with obtaining a firm repair construct. Sutures are cross-tied to enhance fixation (Fig. 32).
- The final repair construct is assessed (Fig. 33). Additional side-to-side sutures can be used to reinforce the repair or deal with any "dog ears."

Step 5

- Deltoid repair
  - A drain is placed into the subacromial space (Fig. 34).

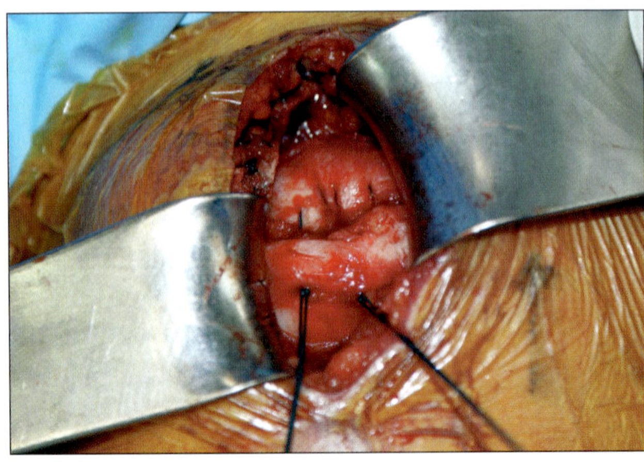
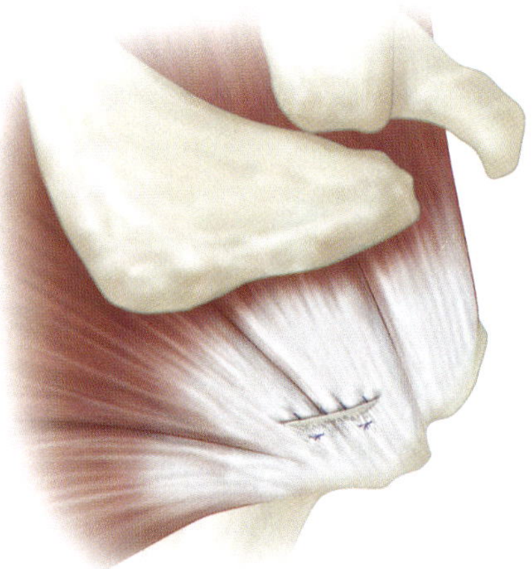

FIGURE 31

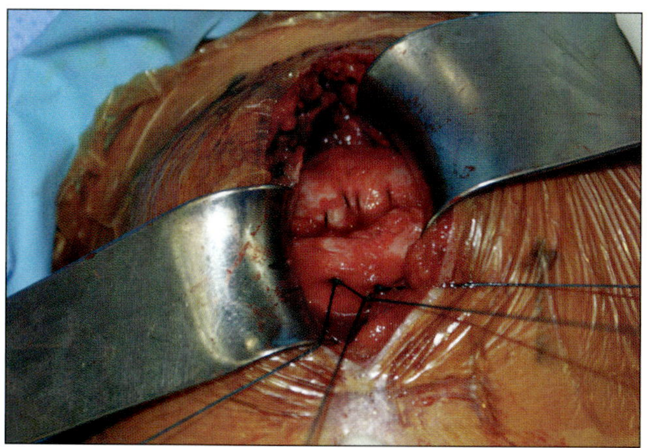

FIGURE 32

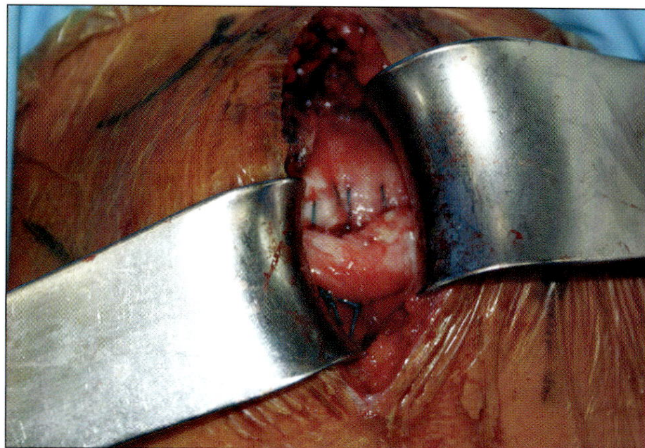

FIGURE 33

- No. 2 Ethibond sutures are used to repair the deltotrapezial fascia.
  - To strengthen the repair, the most medial suture is additionally placed through the AC joint capsule/ligaments (Fig. 35).

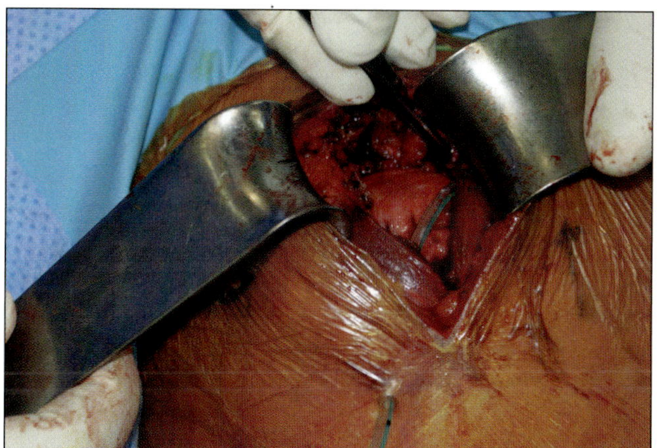

FIGURE 34

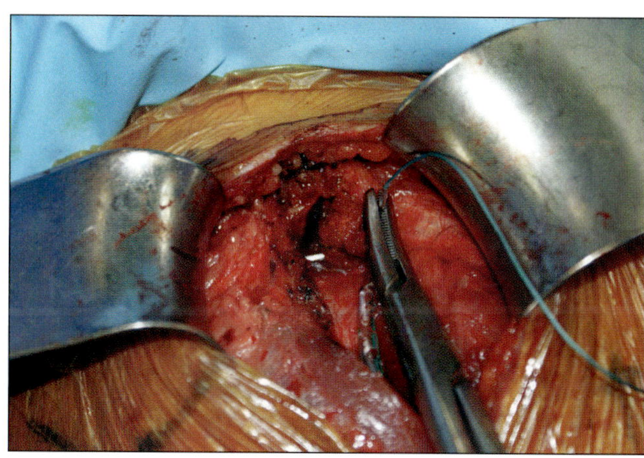

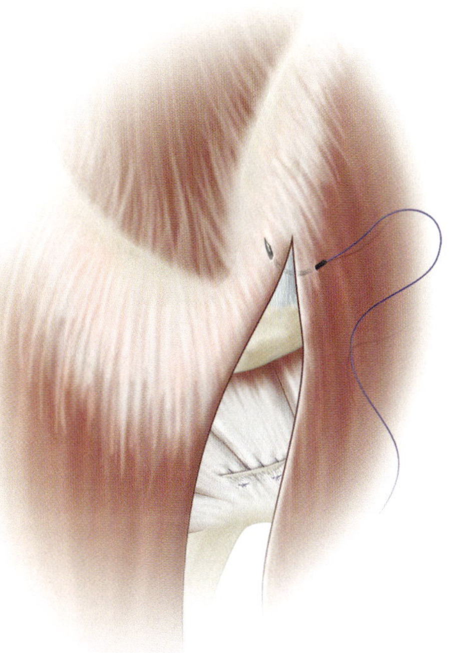

FIGURE 35

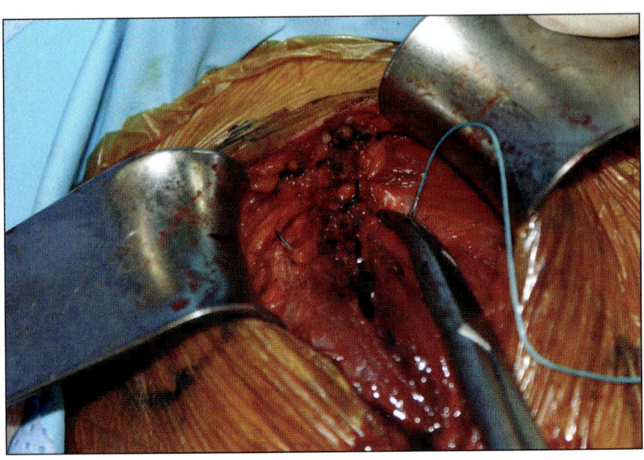

FIGURE 36

- The remaining two to three more laterally placed sutures are additionally passed through the acromion, at least 1 cm from its anterior edge (Figs. 36 and 37).
- The deltoid split is repaired side to side using interrupted #1 Vicryl sutures.

■ The subcutaneous tissue is closed with 2-0 Vicryl and the skin closed with a 3-0 subcuticular suture (Fig. 38).

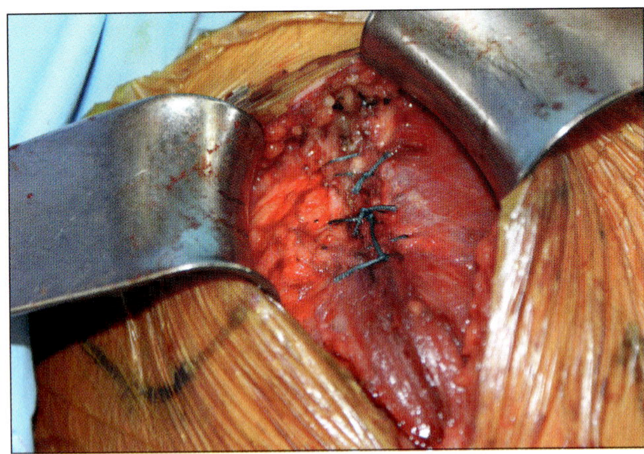

FIGURE 37

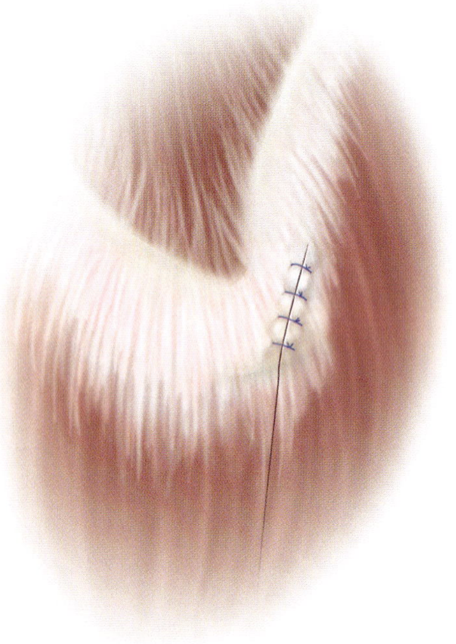

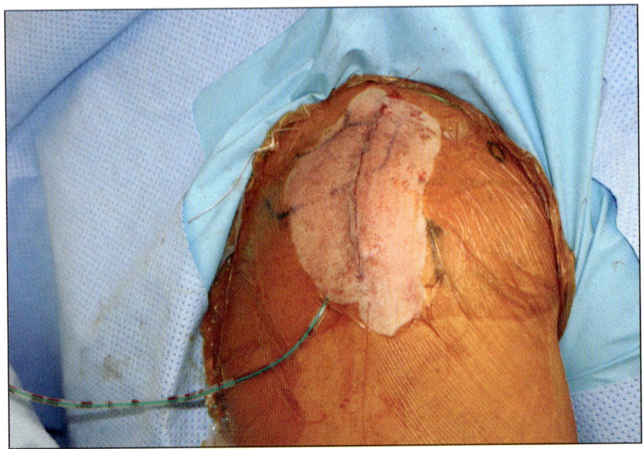

FIGURE 38

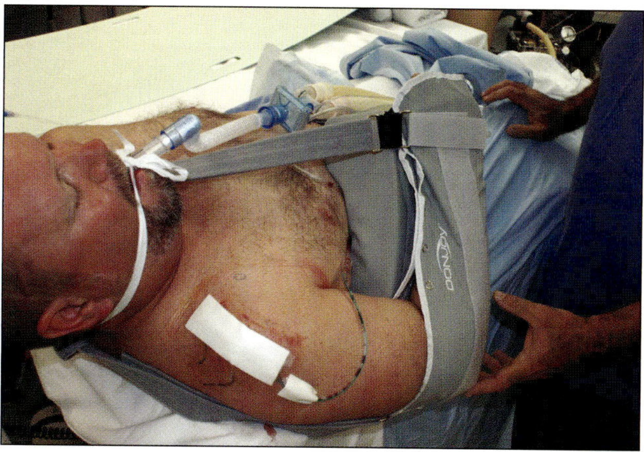

FIGURE 39

Postoperative Care and Expected Outcomes

- A sling with a 10° abduction pillow is typically applied postoperatively (Ultra Sling; Donjoy) (Fig. 39). In the occasional case with increased tension noted across the repair site, a sling with a larger abduction pillow is used (Ultra Sling II AB; Donjoy).
- A Cryo Cuff (Aircast) is applied postoperatively to assist with hemostasis and analgesia.
- The sling is worn for 6 weeks postoperatively.
- Active wrist and elbow motion is encouraged immediately, unless a biceps tenodesis has been performed, in which case elbow flexion is limited to passive only.
- Shoulder range of motion is passive only during the initial 6 weeks, with forward elevation in the plane of the scapula to 90–100°. At 90° of forward elevation (i.e., at the horizontal), additional external rotation of approximately 20° may be performed if comfortable.
- Active-assisted and active shoulder range of motion is commenced at 6 weeks, and resistance exercises are avoided until at least 12 weeks following surgery.

Evidence

Cohen DB, Kawamura S, Ehteshami JR, Rodeo SA. Indomethacin and celecoxib impair rotator cuff tendon-to-bone healing. Am J Sports Med. 2006;34:362-9.

In this laboratory study, the authors performed acute cuff repairs on 180 rats and divided them into three treatment groups: Control, traditional NSAID (Indomethacin) and COX-2 specific NSAID (celecoxib). Five cuff repairs in total failed, all in NSAID treated rats. Biomechanical testing demonstrated lower failure loads in both NSAID groups and histological examination demonstrated decreased collagen organization in both NSAID groups. The authors concluded that both traditional and COX-2 specific NSAIDS significantly inhibited tendon to bone healing.

Galatz LM, Silva MJ, Rothermich SY, Zaegel MA, Havlioglu N, Thomopoulos S. Nicotine delays tendon-to-bone healing in a rat shoulder model. J Bone Joint Surg [Am]. 2006;88:2027-34.

In this laboratory study, the authors performed acute cuff repair on 72 rats and then delivered either saline or nicotine by osmotic subcutaneous pumps. The authors found that nicotine caused a delay in tendon to bone healing and was associated with inferior mechanical properties.

Goutallier D, Postel JM, Gleyze P, Leguilloux P, Van Driessche S. Influence of cuff muscle fatty degeneration on anatomic and functional outcomes after simple suture of full-thickness tears. J Shoulder Elbow Surg. 2003;12:550-4.

The authors performed pre-operative assessment of fatty infiltration according to the Goutallier grading system (1-5) in 220 shoulders undergoing rotator cuff repair. Cuff integrity was then assessed with MRI or CT arthrogram at a mean of 37 months. The likelyhood of a recurrent tear was greater for tendons with fatty infiltration greater than grade 1. The authors concluded that fatty degeneration is an important prognostic factor in rotator cuff surgery. (Level IV evidence [case series])

Longo UG, Franceschi F, Ruzzini L, Rabitti C, Morini S, Maffulli N, Denaro V. Histopathology of the supraspinatus tendon in rotator cuff tears. Am J Sports Med. 2008;36:533-8.

In this laboratory study, the authors collected supraspinatus tendon biopsies from 88 patients undergoing arthroscopic cuff repair and also from 5 patients at autopsy following cardiovascular related deaths. The authors found that the macroscopically intact supraspinatus tendon is degenerated as well, suggesting that a failed healing response is not limited to the ends of the torn tendon. Therefore, during cuff repair, the authors concluded that it is not necessary to excessively freshen the torn tendon to bleeding tissue.

Mochizuki T, Sugaya H, Uomizu M, Maeda K, Matsuki K, Sekiya I, Muneta T, Akita K. Humeral insertion of the supraspinatus and infraspinatus: new anatomical findings regarding the footprint of the rotator cuff. J Bone Joint Surg [Am]. 2008;90:962-9.

In this laboratory study, the authors dissected 113 shoulders from 64 cadavers. The authors reported significant advances in our understanding regarding anatomical insertions of the supraspinatus and infraspinatus on the greater tuberosity. The supraspinatus footprint is much smaller than previously believed, and this area of the greater tuberosity is actually occupied by a substantial amount of the infraspinatus.

St. Pierre P, Olson EJ, Elliott JJ, O'Hair KC, McKinney LA, Ryan J. Tendon-healing to cortical bone compared with healing to a cancellous trough: a biomechanical and histological evaluation in goats. J Bone Joint Surg [Am]. 1995;77:1858-66.

In this laboratory study, 28 goats underwent bilateral tenotomy and subsequent reattachment of the infraspinatus tendon. Shoulders were randomized to undergo either tendon to cortical bone repair or repair of the tendon to a cancellous trough. Biomechanical and histological results at 6 and 12 weeks were similar. The authors concluded that tendon to bone healing was similar for repair to cortical or cancellous bone.

PROCEDURE 3

Rotator Cuff Repair

Allen Deutsch and Anup A. Shah

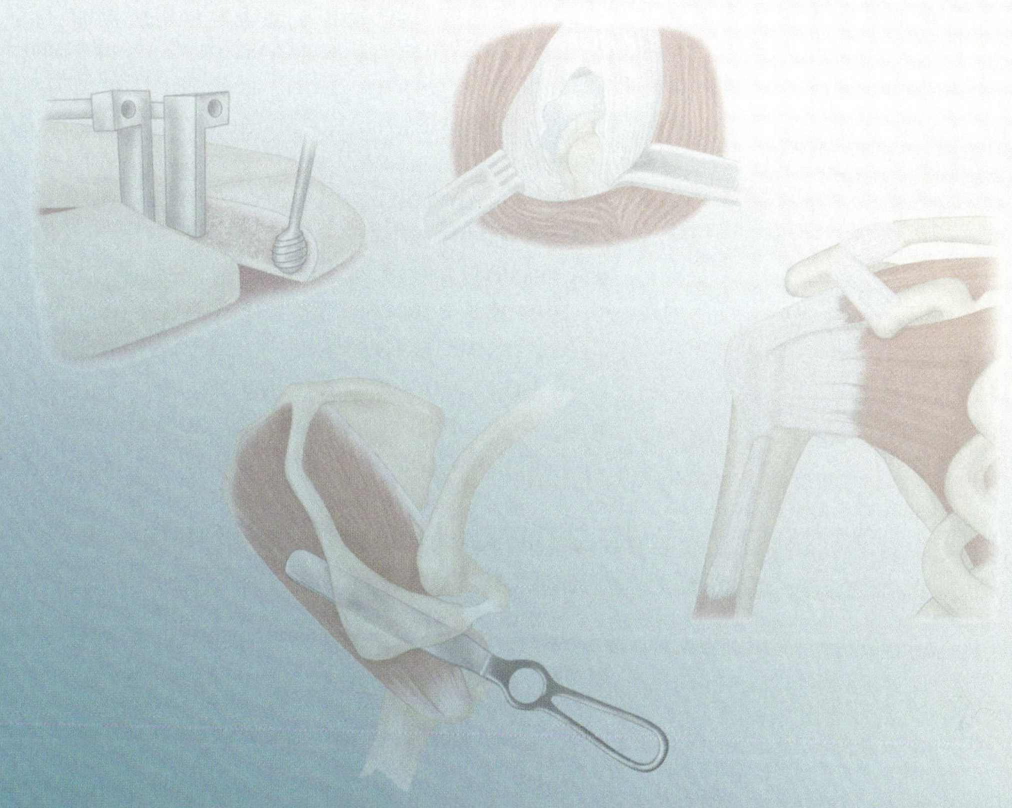

Arthroscopic Technique for Partial-Thickness or Small or Medium Full-Thickness Tears

Indications

- The primary indication is a symptomatic rotator cuff tear confirmed on imaging (magnetic resonance imaging [MRI], ultrasound, or arthrogram) with activity-related pain, night pain, and loss of function unresponsive to nonoperative treatment.
- Lack of strength alone is less of an indication; however, strength can be improved after surgical repair.
- Often concomitant subacromial impingement syndrome exists.
- Consider distal clavicle excision if there is tenderness over the acromioclavicular (AC) joint and/or inferior osteophytes (from radiographs) possibly contributing to impingement syndrome.
- If 50% or more of the tendon thickness is involved upon arthroscopic examination, repair is indicated.

Pitfalls

- *False expectation of increasing strength*
- *Active infection*
- *Frozen shoulder*
- *Unwilling or unable to follow rehabilitation program*
- *Cervical radiculopathy*
- *Suprascapular nerve palsy*
- *Unrecognized need for acromioplasty*
- *Missed AC joint pathology*

Controversies

- Failure of 3–6 months of conservative treatment
- Duration of nonoperative treatment for asymptomatic full-thickness tears is controversial due to the risk for tear progression. Serial imaging is advocated to assess tear progression.

Examination/Imaging

- Inspection: Note any atrophy of the cuff musculature or scapular dyskinesia.
- Palpation: Assess subacromial, scapuloclavicular joint, AC joint, and generalized shoulder.
  - Note pain at anterior acromion and deep to lateral deltoid.
- Evaluation: range of motion, strength, provocative tests
  - Assess for painful arc of motion, or pain with resisted forward elevation or abduction.
  - Check for positive impingement signs (Neer and Hawkins).
  - Assess forward elevation, external rotation, and internal rotation.
  - Assess subscapularis function with abdominal compression test or lift-off maneuver.
  - Check external rotation lag signs to rule out massive tear.
  - Subacromial injection may relieve pain with impingement syndrome, but weakness will persist with a cuff tear.

Treatment Options

- Nonoperative treatment of partial-thickness tears may allow return to work activities, but progression to a full-thickness tear may occur.
- Disadvantages of the open and mini-open repair techniques include deltoid morbidity, stiffness, pain, and poor cosmesis.

  - Neck examination must be performed to assess radicular symptoms.
- Plain films
  - Obtain anteroposterior, scapular Y, and axillary lateral views.
  - Identify greater tuberosity cystic changes, sclerosis, or bony changes.
  - Assess for calcific tendinitis.
  - Identify acromial morphology to plan the resection during acromioplasty. The plain film of a right shoulder scapular Y view in Figure 1 shows an inferior spur projecting from the undersurface of a type III acromion (*arrow*).
  - Assess for os acromiale.
  - Assess AC joint pathology.
  - Assess the glenohumeral space and any bony changes.

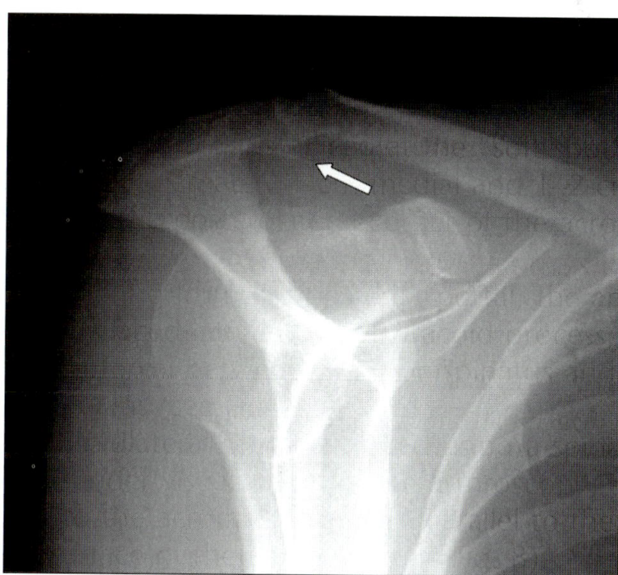

FIGURE 1

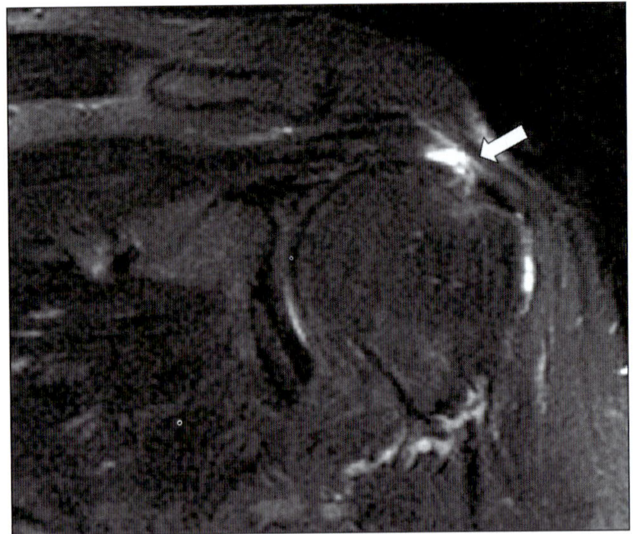
A

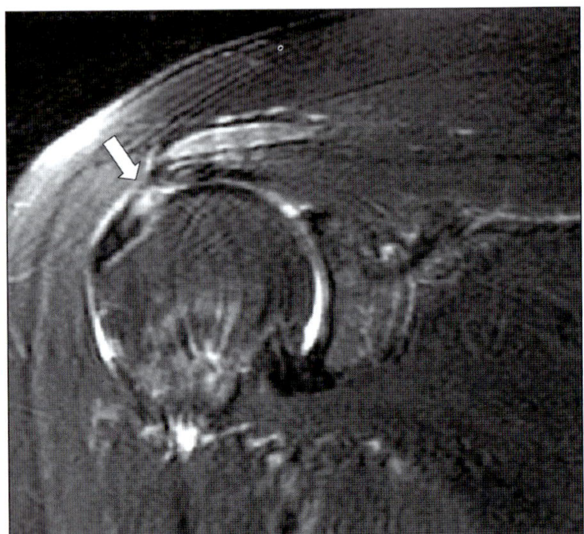
B

FIGURE 2

- MRI
  - Noncontrast studies have a high degree of accuracy in detecting full-thickness lesions. The coronal oblique MRI view of a left shoulder in Figure 2A shows a full-thickness tear of the supraspinatus tendon (*arrow*).
  - Contrast may be used to increase sensitivity in identifying partial-thickness tears. The coronal oblique MRI view of a right shoulder in Figure 2B demonstrates a partial-thickness undersurface tear of the supraspinatus tendon (*arrow*).
  - Coronal oblique and sagittal plane images are used to assess the supraspinatus and infraspinatus tendons for tear size, tendon involvement, amount of retraction, and fatty infiltration of the muscle belly.
  - Axial plane images are used to assess the subscapularis tendon.
- Ultrasound
  - Ultrasound is well tolerated and cost-effective.
  - It has a high degree of accuracy in detecting both partial- and full-thickness lesions. The coronal plane ultrasound image of a left shoulder in Figure 3 shows the absence of cuff tissue at the greater tuberosity footprint indicative of a full-thickness rotator cuff tear (*yellow arrow*).
  - It is user dependent and has a long learning curve, and there is reduced sensitivity in obese patients or patients with severely restricted shoulder movement.

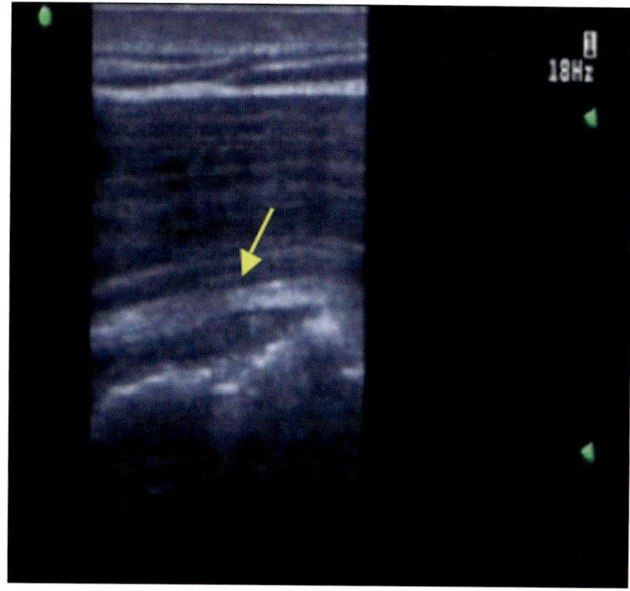

FIGURE 3

Surgical Anatomy

- Muscles/Tendons (Fig. 4)
  - The supraspinatus (supraspinatus fossa), infraspinatus (infraspinatus fossa), and teres minor (lateral border of scapula) all insert into the greater tuberosity.
  - The subscapularis (subscapularis fossa) inserts into the lesser tuberosity.
  - Cuff footprint: the medial-to-lateral width of the cuff insertion onto the tuberosities spans approximately 12–20 mm.

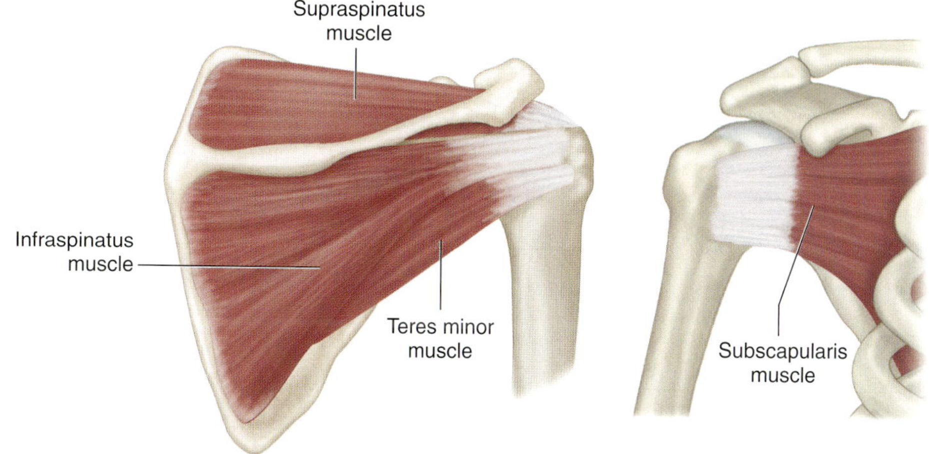

FIGURE 4

Pearls

- *Don't "drape yourself out."*
- *Protect the patient's head, neck, ears, eyes, popliteal fossa, heels, and thighs.*
- *Flex the patient's hips and knees to prevent nerve damage.*
- *A specialized arthroscopy table provides access to the posterior shoulder.*

Pitfalls

- *Failure to flex the torso upright to 70° will cause the surgeon to work "uphill."*
- *Improper draping.*
- *Positioning the torso in the full upright position while keeping the patient hypotensive to reduce bleeding should be used with caution in hypertensive patients to avoid cerebral ischemia.*

Equipment

- Operating table: Skytron 6500 with beach chair shoulder positioner (Grand Rapids, MI)
  - Right and left sides of table back are removable for full access to posterior shoulder.
- McConnell Arm Positioner (McConnell Manufacturing Company, Greenville, TX)

Controversies

- The lateral decubitus position may be used for arthroscopic repair, but conversion to mini-open or open techniques can be more difficult, and it is difficult to manipulate the extremity during the repair.

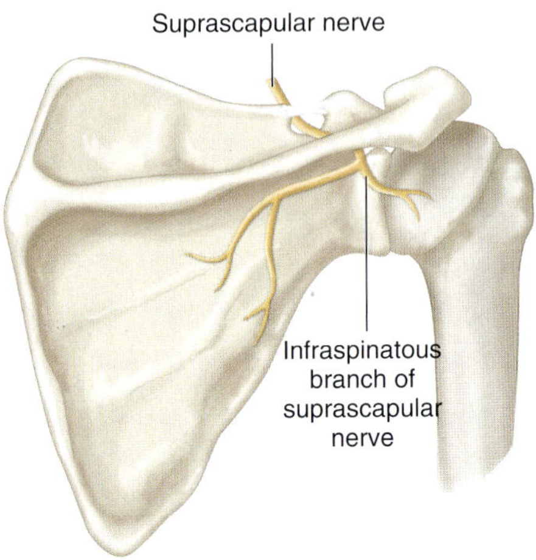

FIGURE 5

- Nerves (Fig. 5)
  - The suprascapular nerve is approximately 1.5 cm from the origin of the long head of the biceps; this is significant if cuff mobilization is performed.
  - The infraspinatus branches are approximately 2 cm from the posterior glenoid rim; this is significant if cuff mobilization is performed.
- Vessels
  - The acromial branch of the thoracoacromial artery should be cauterized during acromioplasty and the coracoacromial (CA) ligament release to achieve hemostasis.

Positioning

- The patient is placed in the standard beach chair position with the torso 70° upright and the hips and knees flexed to relieve pressure on the sciatic nerve, with popliteal fossa free of pressure. The head and neck are protected in neutral position (Fig. 6).
- The entire extremity must be draped free. Anteriorly, the drapes should extend from the ipsilateral nipple to the sternoclavicular joint and superiorly along the base of neck. Posteriorly, the drapes should extend along the medial border of the scapula. Inferiorly, they should extend along the chest wall below the axilla and along the inferior third of the pectoralis muscle.
- We use an operating table (Skytron 6500 with beach chair shoulder positioner) that allows the head and neck to be held by a padded holder; the right and left sides may be removed independently to provide full access to the posterior shoulder.

Pearls

- *Draw anatomic landmarks.*
- *Use a spinal needle to establish portals to ensure proper placement.*
- *The lateral portal should be parallel to undersurface of acromion.*
- *Lateral portal viewing essential to confirm repair of delaminated tears.*

Pitfalls

- *Portal placement is critical for visualization of the tear during suture passage.*
- *Portals placed close to the acromial edge prevent access for instrumentation.*
- *The anterior portal must be lateral to the coracoid to avoid neurovascular injury.*

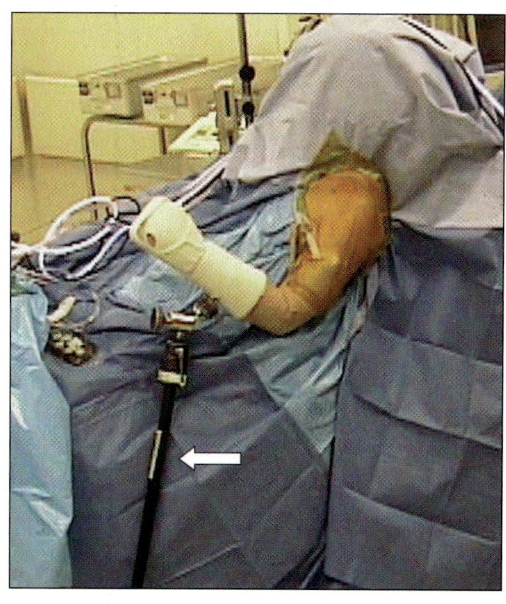

FIGURE 6

- We use a McConnell mechanical armholder to manipulate the upper extremity and apply traction to the arm to improve visualization. In Figure 6, the forearm is held by the McConnell armholder with the shoulder in neutral rotation.

Portals/Exposures

- Three standard portals are used (Fig. 7; AL, anterolateral portal).
  - Posterior portal ("P" in Fig. 7)
    - Approximately 2 cm inferior and medial to the posterolateral tip of the acromion ("a" in Fig. 7)

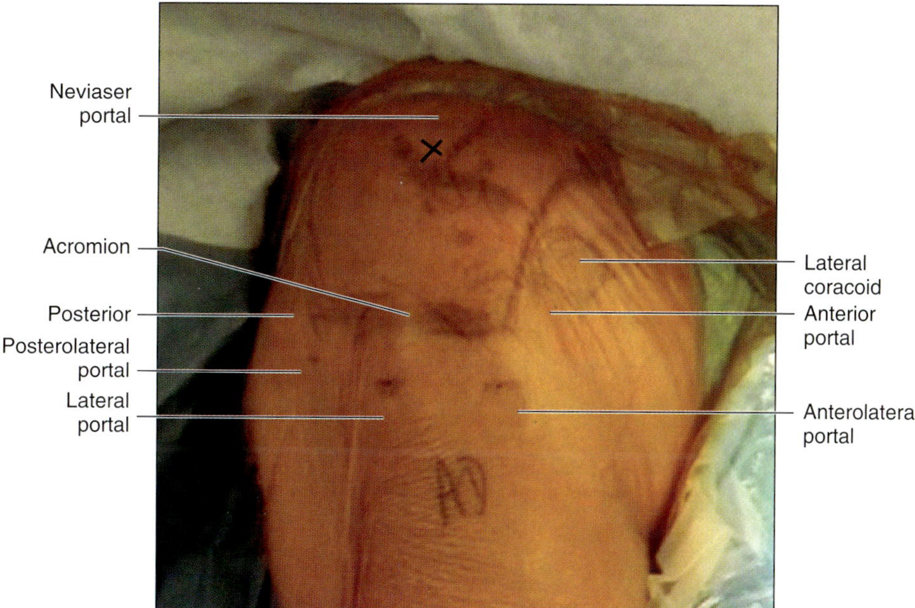

FIGURE 7

Instrumentation

- Metal cannula (scope) and two plastic cannulas
- Stryker pump (Stryker, Kalamazoo, MI) and pressure transducer for precise fluid management
- Clear twist-in cannula with a dam used during suture passage and knot tying
- Smooth cannula placed in rotator interval

Controversies

- We do not use a cannula during suture passage.
- Identical ingress and egress tracts are important. This is best accomplished by direct visualization of the ingress/egress tract during suture retrieval and device insertion (see Step 5 of Procedure). Figure 8 shows a view of the left shoulder from the posterior portal with a Scorpion suture punch (*straight arrow*) entering the subacromial space from the lateral portal via the identical tract used to retrieve the suture (*curved arrow*).

    - Viewing portal for glenohumeral joint and subacromial space during acromioplasty
    - Working portal for retrograde suture passage and acromioplasty
  - Lateral portal ("L" in Fig. 7)
    - Approximately 2 cm posterior to the anterior acromion and 2–4 cm inferior to the acromion
    - Viewing portal during antegrade suture passage and to assess undersurface of acromion during acromioplasty
    - Working portal for acromioplasty and knot tying
  - Anterior portal ("A" in Fig. 7)
    - In rotator interval, lateral to the coracoid ("c" in Fig. 7)
    - Established under spinal needle guidance
    - Viewing portal during knot tying
    - Working portal during retrograde suture passage
- Accessory portals
  - Posterolateral portal ("PL" in Fig. 7)
    - At the posterolateral acromion, approximately 2 cm inferior to the acromion
    - Viewing portal during antegrade suture passing and knot tying
  - Modified Neviaser portal ("N" in Fig. 7)
    - At the junction of the scapular spine and posterior aspect of the AC joint
    - Established under spinal needle guidance
    - Working portal during retrograde suture passage
  - Anchor portals along edge of acromion
    - For anchor placement at "deadman's angle" (45° to tuberosity surface)

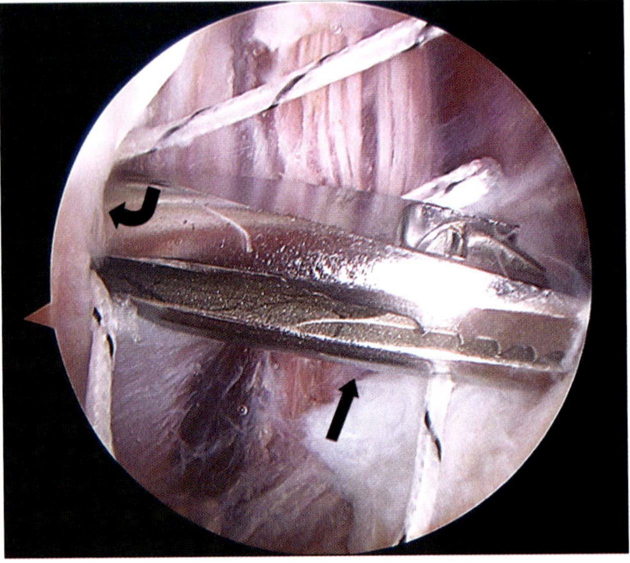

FIGURE 8

Pearls

- *Perform a complete bursectomy to expose the lateral cuff insertion and possible bursal-sided tear.*
- *View the cuff insertion through the lateral portal, rotating shoulder as needed.*

Pitfalls

- *Keep pump pressure and flow low to prevent extravasation into the soft tissues.*

Instrumentation/ Implantation

- 30° arthroscope
- Motorized pump for fluid management
- Motorized shaver
- Arthroscopic probe
- Arthroscopic punches
- Arthroscopic guillotine suture cutters (most valuable for use with high-strength sutures)
- Switching sticks

Controversies

- Some surgeons use gravity flow instead of a motorized pump.

Pearls

- *Raise pump pressure and flow to reduce bleeding during bony resection and return to a lower setting once complete to avoid extravasation.*
- *Place inferior traction on the arm through the mechanical armholder.*

Procedure

Step 1: Diagnostic Arthroscopy

- Diagnostic arthroscopy of the glenohumeral joint and subacromial space
  - An initial examination is made under anesthesia to assess range of motion.
  - Any intra-articular abnormalities, such as biceps or labral pathology, chondromalacia, loose bodies, and synovitis, are noted and addressed.
- Diagnostic arthroscopy of the subacromial space
  - A blunt-tipped trocar is penetrated through the posterior portal to the depth of the CA ligament upon initial insertion into the subacromial space to avoid problems with visualization due to the bursal tissue.
  - The lateral portal is established under spinal needle guidance.
  - A shaver is swept medially and laterally to separate bursal tissue and detach any adhesions between cuff and acromion.
  - All bursal tissue is removed to provide complete visualization of the entire cuff.
  - The subacromial space is inspected, noting the presence of bursal-sided cuff tearing, impingement lesion of the CA ligament, and hypertrophic and/ or hyperemic changes of the bursal tissue.

Step 2: Subacromial Decompression and Acromioplasty

- The CA ligament is released using a radiofrequency ablation device.
- The anterior two thirds of the acromion is skeletonized.
- An acromioplasty is performed with a motorized burr.
  - The goal of the acromioplasty is to achieve a flat type I acromion morphology to reduce abrasion of the repaired tendon.
  - The acromion is viewed from the posterior portal (Fig. 9A) with the burr in the lateral portal (Fig. 9B).
  - A template for bone resection is created at the lateral aspect of the acromion and followed medially until bone is resected.
  - The acromion is viewed from the lateral portal with the burr in the posterior portal, and the undersurface of the posterior acromion is used as a template to confirm that a flat type I acromion has been achieved (Fig. 9C).

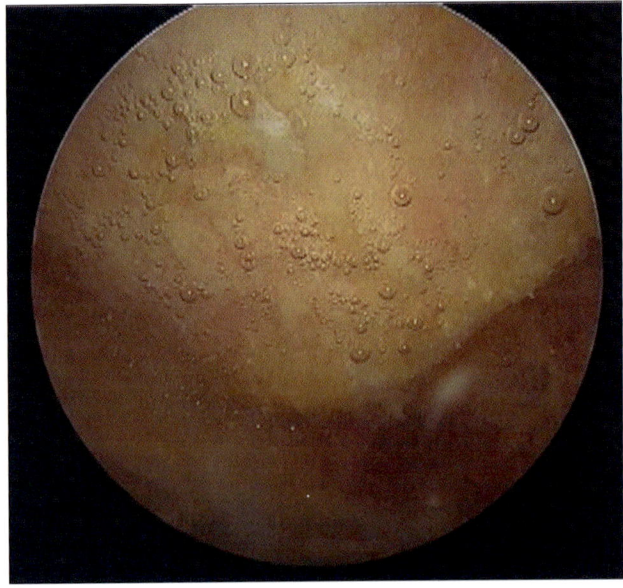

A

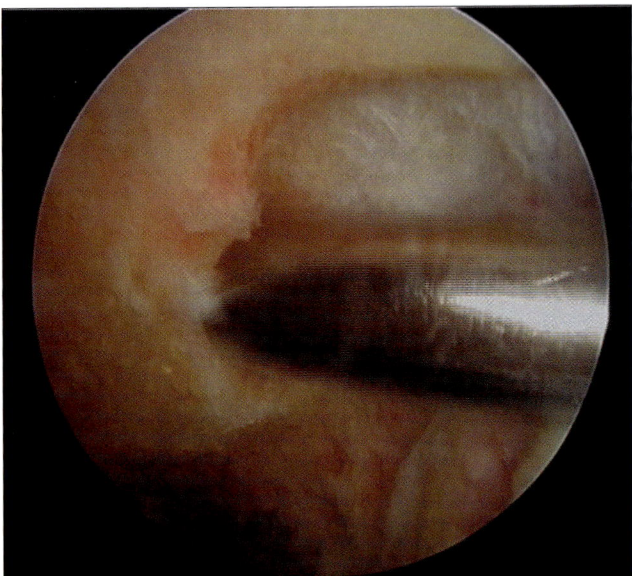

B

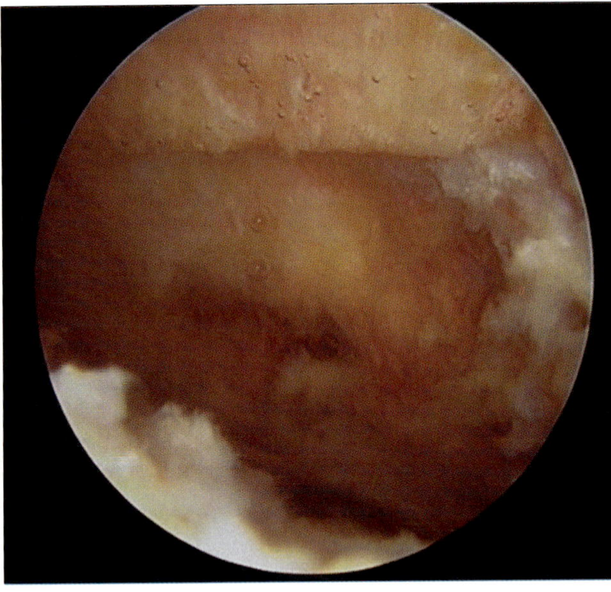

C

FIGURE 9

Pitfalls

- *Perform the acromioplasty in a timely fashion to prevent over-extravasation of fluid into tissues.*
- *Prior to the acromioplasty, confirm tear reparability.*
- *Avoid acromioplasty in patients with an irreparable tear to prevent anterior superior humeral head escape.*

Step 3: Identification of Tear Characteristics and Tear Mobilization

- The arthroscope is placed in the subacromial space through the lateral portal for a "50-yard-line" view of the cuff tear.
  - Partial tears usually involve the articular surface.
- After débridement of degenerative cuff tissue, tear size and thickness are determined by measuring the amount of exposed tuberosity.
- Tear size is measured with the tip of a cannula, shaver, or calibrated probe.
  - Partial tears that are greater than 6 cm in thickness or 50% thickness should be repaired.
  - Small full-thickness tears usually involve the supraspinatus tendon and are less than 1 cm in size.

Instrumentation/ Implantation

- Radiofrequency tissue ablation device; we prefer the ArthroCare 90° probe tip (ArthroCare Corporation, Austin, TX).
- Motorized burr; we prefer a barrel burr for uniform removal of the acromial spur.

Controversies

- There are studies that show no difference in clinical outcome whether or not an acromioplasty is performed (Gartsman and O'Connor, 2004), prompting some surgeons to avoid performing an acromioplasty.

  - Medium full-thickness tears are 1–3 cm in size and may involve the full width of the supraspinatus tendon as well as a portion of the anterior aspect of the infraspinatus tendon.
- Tear characteristics are identified (Burkhart et al., 2001), including medial retraction, tissue thickness and quality, and tear geometry and asymmetry.
  - Crescent-shaped, U-shaped, L-shaped, and reverse L-shaped tears may be identified.
  - The geometry of the tear will guide the mobilization techniques used.
- A suture retriever is used to grasp the end of the tendon and assess mobility of the cuff.
- The intra-articular capsular reflection above the biceps anchor is released in both acute and chronic tears to improve cuff mobility (Fig. 10). This may be accomplished with an electrocautery tip or an elevator, with care not to penetrate medially more than 1.5 cm to protect the adjacent suprascapular nerve.
- From the subacromial space, all bursal adhesions between the acromion and cuff are released.
- In more chronic and retracted tears, more aggressive mobilization techniques may be necessary. When there is asymmetric retraction with more retraction in the anterior aspect of the tear, the coracohumeral ligament and rotator interval are released. If there is more retraction in the posterior aspect of the tear, a posterior interval release is performed. (See Procedure 6 for detailed explanation of these techniques.)

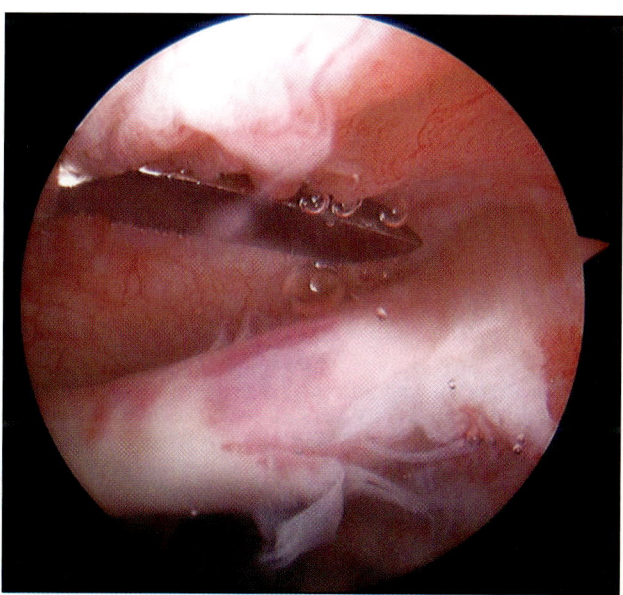

FIGURE 10

Pearls

- *When assessing cuff mobility, use a suture retriever without teeth or pass a traction suture through the lateral cuff margin.*

Pitfalls

- *If a soft tissue elevator is used to mobilize the intra-articular capsular attachments to the cuff, do not penetrate more than 1.5 cm medial to the biceps anchor to avoid injury to the suprascapular nerve and artery.*

Instrumentation/Implantation

- Suture retriever without teeth to avoid injury to the cuff tissue
- Soft tissue elevator
- Arthroscopic punches
- Arthroscopic probe

Pitfalls

- *Be wary of overzealous decortication: it weakens anchor fixation and may result in anchor pullout.*
- *Anchor pullout strength is greatest with metal twist-in corkscrew anchors.*
- *Cortical bone adjacent to the articular margin is most dense.*

Instrumentation/Implantation

- Metal corkscrew-type anchors are loaded with either two or three high-strength sutures for single-row repairs and dual-row repairs.
- Bioabsorbable metal-tipped 4.5-mm PushLock anchors (Arthrex Corp, Naples, FL) are used for dual-row repairs.

Step 4: Tuberosity Preparation and Anchor Placement

- All soft tissue is removed from the tuberosity surface using a shaver and burr.
- The burr is used in reverse to remove the most superficial layer of cortical bone to provide a healing bed for the repair.
- The site and angle of insertion are localized using a spinal needle. Figure 11 shows a view of the right shoulder with a spinal needle (*white arrow*) placed at the anterolateral aspect and along the edge of the acromion. The inset shows a spinal needle (*white arrow*) at a 45° angle to the tuberosity.
- A 3-mm incision is placed in the skin to allow passage of anchors and any punches, tamps, or drills.
- An anchor is passed into tuberosity bone under direct visualization.
  - In hard bone, a mallet is used to tap the anchor until bone purchase is achieved.
  - In osteoporotic bone, there may not be a need for the use of a mallet.
- The anchor is placed at a "deadman's angle" (45° to the tuberosity surface) to maximize pullout strength.
- The anchor is placed at the lateral-most aspect of the tuberosity to maximize surface area coverage at the repair site.
- The eyelet of the anchor is aligned for optimum sliding of sutures during knot tying.
  - For mattress sutures, the eyelet should be parallel to the tuberosity.
  - For simple sutures, the eyelet should be perpendicular to the tuberosity.
- The number of anchors used depends on the type of tear.

Step 5: Suture Passage

- Suture punches have articulating jaws that grasp and penetrate the cuff tissue.
  - After loading the suture into the device, it is passed in an antegrade fashion by deploying a needle through the cuff. Figure 12 shows a view of the right shoulder from the lateral portal with a Scorpion suture punch passed through the anterolateral portal (see inset view). The needle (*white arrow*) is passed through the cuff with the Scorpion seen in the foreground (*black arrow*).
  - The dimensions of the jaws of each device define the maximum depth through which suture can be passed.

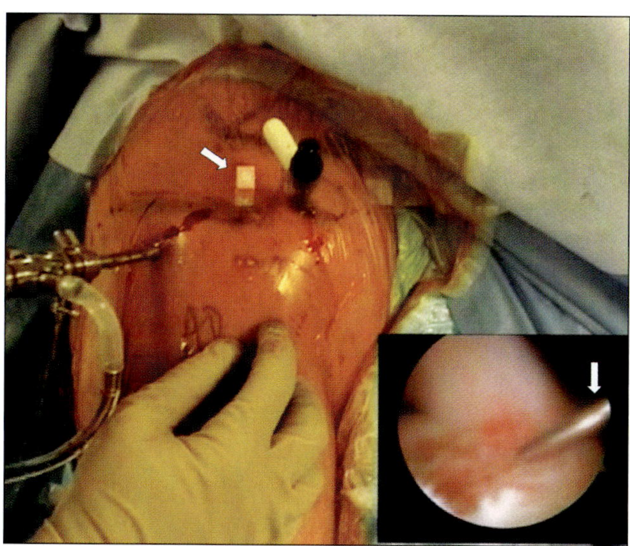

FIGURE 11

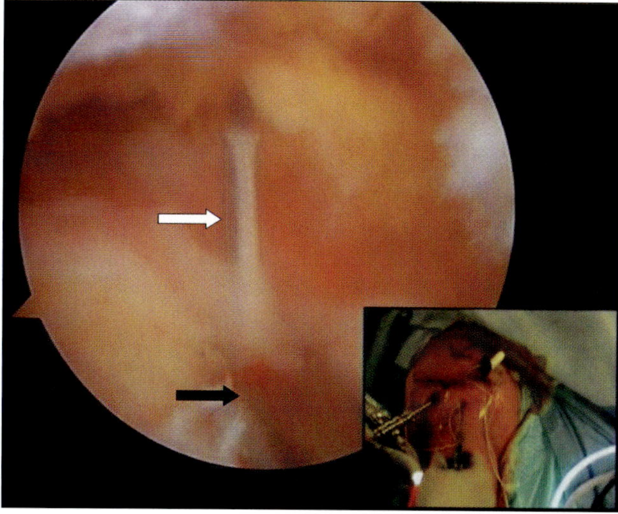

FIGURE 12

Controversies

- Some surgeons prefer to use absorbable anchors in the tuberosity. Newer biocomposite anchors offer the advantage of being resorbed and promote bone formation within the implant profile.

- Penetrating suture graspers retrieve sutures in a retrograde fashion and have the ability to enter the cuff at any point.
  - In the view of a left shoulder from the lateral portal in Figure 13A, a BirdBeak suture grasper passed through the posterior portal is grasping a FiberWire suture for a retrograde suture passage.
  - In the view of a right shoulder from the posterior portal in Figure 13B, a monofilament passing stitch (*arrowhead*) is passed through an 18-gauge spinal needle (*green arrow*). A toothed suture grasper (*black arrow*) is passed through a grey cannula (*white arrow*) in the rotator interval.

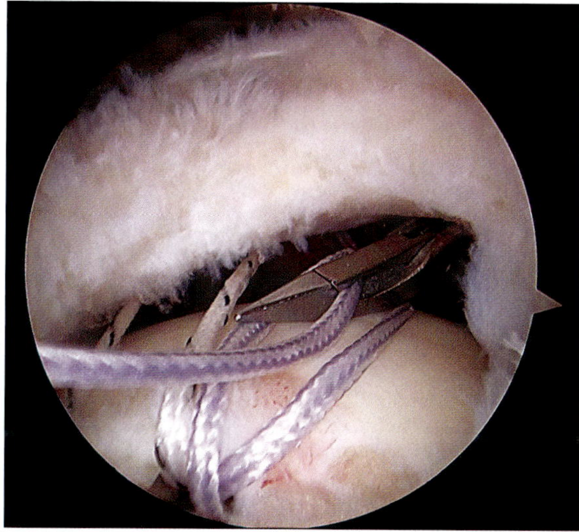

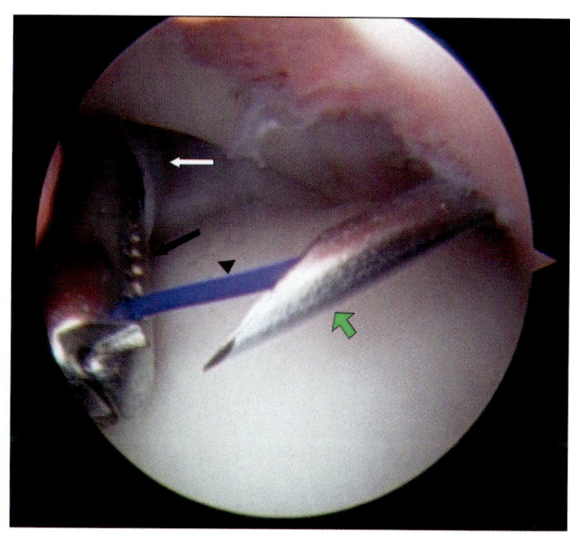

A B

FIGURE 13

Pearls

- *Use an 18-gauge spinal needle to pass a monofilament passing stitch through the cuff to minimize iatrogenic injury from larger bore suture-passing devices.*
- *A gentle curve may be placed at the distal end of the needle to help with suture passage.*
- *High-strength sutures such as FiberWire (Arthrex) and Orthocord (DePuy-Mitek, Raynham, MA) are less susceptible to injury than Ethibond (Ethicon) during suture handling, around radiofrequency energy, and with sharp instrumentation. They help prevent suture breakage during knot tying (Deutsch and Taylor, 2006).*

Pitfalls

- *It is critical to use the lateral or anterolateral portal as a viewing portal during suture passage in order to ensure incorporation of both layers of delaminated tears within the repair.*

- Spinal needle suture passage involves an additional step of using a shuttle stitch but is the least traumatic to the cuff tissue.
- The ideal "bite" of tissue to incorporate in the repair is approximately 12–15 mm to allow coverage of the footprint and prevent suture cutout (Deutsch, 2006).

Step 6A: Repair Techniques for Partial-Thickness Tears

- Most partial-thickness rotator cuff tears are on the articular side. Figure 14 shows a partial undersurface tear identified with a needle.
- The undersurface tear is débrided until all degenerative tissue is removed.
- Once all degenerative tissue has been débrided, the depth of the tear thickness should be assessed using a calibrated probe (Fig. 15).
- The amount of the exposed tuberosity should be measured.
- Options for articular-surface partial-thickness rotator cuff tear treatment include
  - Débridement alone
    - Less than 50% of tendon depth
    - Sedentary patients
    - No structural abnormalities
  - Débridement with subacromial decompression
    - Less than 50% of tendon depth
    - Positive structural abnormality
  - Arthroscopic repair with subacromial decompression
    - Greater than 50% of tendon depth
    - Active patients

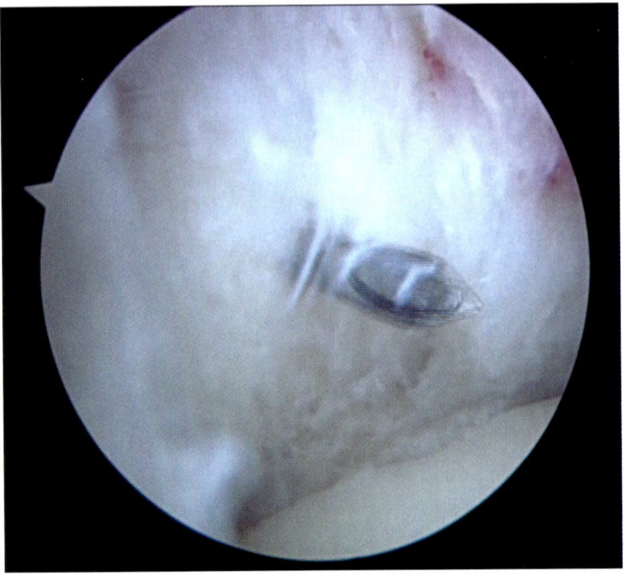

FIGURE 14

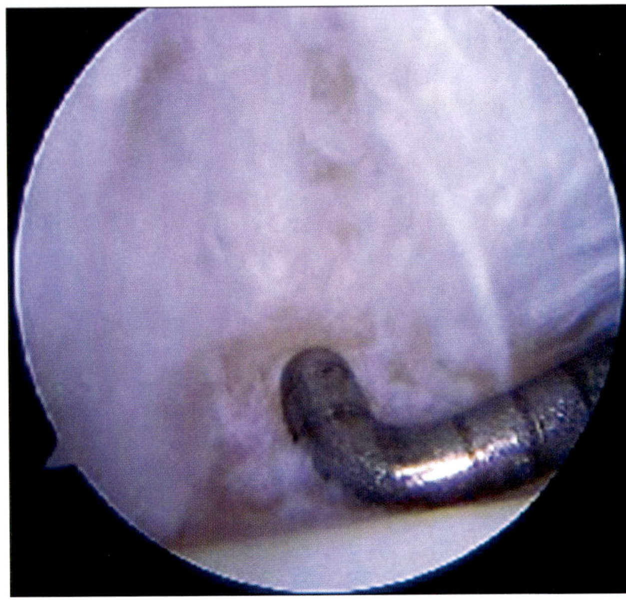

FIGURE 15

Instrumentation/ Implantation

- Suture punches: Scorpion (Arthrex) or Espressew (DePuy-Mitek) (see Fig. 12)
- Penetrating-type of suture graspers: nondisposable BirdBeak (Arthrex) or disposable SutureLasso (Arthrex) (see Fig. 13A)
- Spinal needle (see Fig. 13B)
- Suture grasper with teeth to grasp end of suture passed with spinal needle or suture punches

Controversies

- Type of suture-passage device is important. Smaller and smoother tips create more symmetric holes in the tendon, leading to decreased suture cutout (Chokshi et al., 2006).
- In cases of poor tissue quality, consider passing the stitch from a spinal needle.

Pearls

- *The shaver blade should be placed tangential to the tendon surface during débridement to remove unhealthy tissue and preserve intact cuff.*
- *The use of a spinal needle is the least traumatic to the cuff tissue during suture passage.*
- *Confirm with lateral viewing that the biceps has not been inadvertently incorporated.*
- *A triple-loaded anchor may be used to pass the limbs of the third suture in a mattress configuration to close the longitudinal split created in the cuff.*

- A cannulated needle is used to pass monofilament suture at the tear site to help identify the location of the tear when viewed from the subacromial space.
- The arthroscope is placed in the subacromial space.
  - The subacromial bursa is removed to provide full visualization of the entire cuff and to help prevent problems during suture retrieval and knot tying.
  - The cuff is assessed as to whether there is bursal-sided involvement to the articular-surface tear.
    - If there is bursal-sided involvement associated with articular surface tearing, the intact tissue is taken down and the tear converted to full thickness with generous débridement of degenerative tissue.
    - If no bursal-sided involvement is confirmed, the arthroscope is placed back into the intra-articular space.
- Three options are available for repairing articular-surface partial-thickness tears: conversion to full-thickness tear, small full-thickness window technique using spinal needle for suture passage, and trans-tendon partial articular-surface supraspinatus tendon avulsion (PASTA) technique.
- Conversion to Full-Thickness Tear
  - May be used
    - For large lesions that involve the entire supraspinatus tendon
    - For poor or very thin tissue quality
    - When creation of a small window will not provide enough access for tuberosity preparation or insertion of multiple anchors
  - A spinal needle is used to perforate the intact bursal surface.
  - Placement of the spinal needle is confirmed to be parallel to the surface of the exposed tuberosity and at the most lateral aspect of the cuff insertion.
  - Using the end of the spinal needle as a blade, the cuff tissue is cut in an anteroposterior direction until the tear is full thickness.
  - The blunt-tipped metal trocar of the arthroscopic cannula is used to perforate through the full-thickness lesion that was created.
  - The shaver is passed through the full-thickness lesion and all soft tissue from the tuberosity and all degenerative tissue at the undersurface of the cuff is débrided.
  - If necessary, a punch is used to take down any lateral cuff attachment to provide access for anchor placement and soft tissue and tuberosity débridement.

- The remainder of the repair is performed in the same manner described for a full-thickness tear (see Steps 6B and 6C).

■ Small Full-Thickness Window Technique
- The arthroscope is placed in the intra-articular space.
- A spinal needle is used to perforate the intact bursal surface. Figure 16A shows a view from the posterior portal of the left shoulder with a spinal needle passed through the subacromial space through the partial-thickness cuff lesion.
- Placement of the spinal needle is confirmed to be at a 45° angle to the surface of the exposed tuberosity and at the most lateral aspect of the cuff insertion.
- Using the end of the spinal needle as a blade, the cuff tissue is cut in a medial-to-lateral direction until there is a full-thickness longitudinal split in the cuff of at least 5 mm in size.
- The blunt-tipped metal trocar of the arthroscopic cannula is used to perforate through the full-thickness lesion that was created.
- The shaver and burr are passed through the window created in the lateral cuff to débride the degenerative tissue at the undersurface of the cuff and to prepare the tuberosity (Fig. 16B).
- A double-loaded anchor is passed through the window at a 45° angle at the lateral-most aspect of the tuberosity, and anchor stability in the bone is confirmed.
- A single limb of each suture is passed through the cuff for a simple suture configuration. Figure 16C shows a view from the posterior portal of the left shoulder with sutures from an anchor passed through the window.
  - ◆ Sutures may be passed with a suture punch with the scope in the subacromial space or may be passed using an 18-gauge spinal needle.
  - ◆ If using the 18-gauge spinal needle, it is passed along the edge of the acromion to penetrate the cuff (Fig. 16D). A monofilament suture is passed and retrieved with a toothed grasper through a cannula placed in the anterior portal.
- Cutting the stitch with the needle can be avoided by pulling the needle out of the cuff once the stitch is grasped.
- The suture is retrieved from the anchor with a nontoothed grasper (Fig. 16E) and the suture is shuttled through the cuff using a passing stitch.

Pitfalls

- *Do not jeopardize articular cartilage and healthy cuff when using a burr or shaver when preparing the tuberosity adjacent to a partial-thickness tear. If necessary, proceed to the window technique to prepare the tuberosity and pass anchors.*

Controversies

- Choice of repair technique depends on patient age and activity level, tissue quality, and surgeon experience.
- Elderly patients with poor tissue quality usually are not amenable to trans-tendon repair.
- If the trans-tendon technique is used, minimize multiple insults to intact cuff with passage of the drill, punch, anchor, and suture-passing devices.

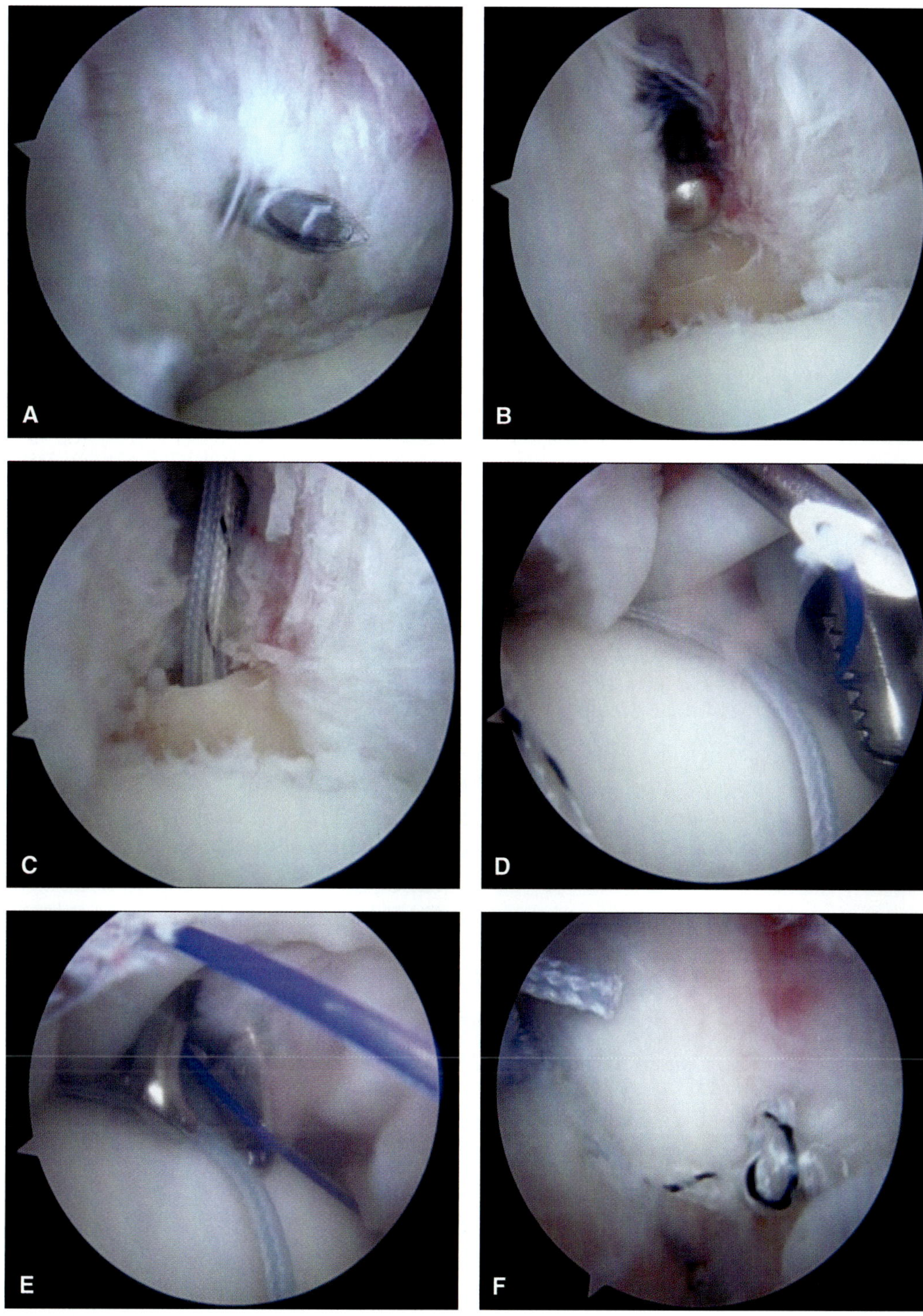

FIGURE 16

- After each suture is passed, the scope is placed in the subacromial space and knots are tied to repair the cuff. Figure 16F shows a subacromial view from the lateral portal showing the final repair of the cuff.

Pearls

- *Triple-loaded anchors provide an additional point of fixation for added security and strength to the repair.*
- *Place the anchors in the lateral-most aspect of the footprint to maximize repair site surface area (Deutsch, 2006).*
- *If using high-strength suture in thin, poor-quality tissue, consider using a combination of mattress sutures with simple sutures medial to the mattress sutures to simulate a Mason-Allen technique to prevent suture cutout from the cuff.*

Pitfalls

- *Prior to knot tying, assess tendon mobility to avoid overtensioning the repair. If necessary, adjust the amount of tissue included in the repair. Overtensioning may lead to stiffness, pain, and dysfunction (Murray et al., 2002).*

- Trans-tendon Partial Articular-Surface Supraspinatus Tendon Avulsion (PASTA) Technique
  - The arthroscope is placed in the intra-articular space.
  - The exposed surface of the tuberosity is prepared adjacent to the tear.
  - A spinal needle is used to perforate the intact bursal surface to confirm the placement at a 45° angle to the articular margin of the humeral head.
  - The anchor is passed through the cuff and into the medial footprint adjacent to the articular surface (Fig. 17A).
  - Both limbs of each suture are passed in a mattress configuration using a spinal needle and monofilament passing stitch to shuttle the sutures from the anchor through the cuff, as described above.
  - The sutures are tied with the arthroscope in the subacromial space. Figure 17B shows a subacromial view from the anterior portal of a repaired tendon using the trans-tendon PASTA repair.

Step 6B: Single-Row Anchor Repair for Small Full-Thickness Tears

- A full-thickness tear that is less than 1.5 cm can be repaired using a single-row anchor technique with a double- or triple-loaded anchor placed at the lateral aspect of the tuberosity with a simple suture configuration.

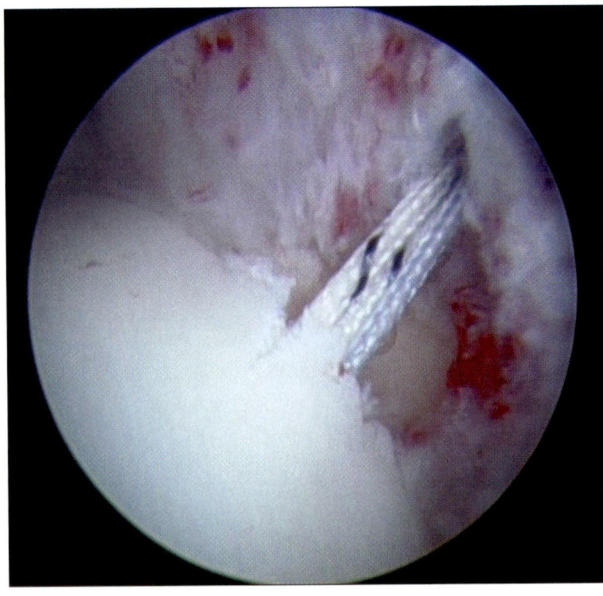

A

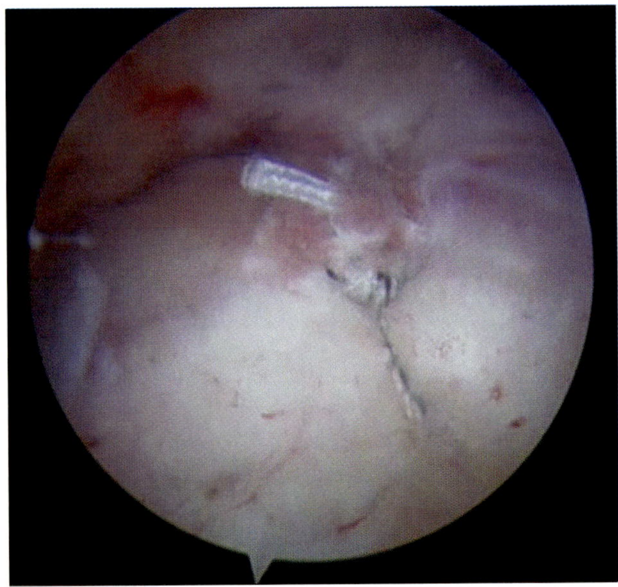

B

FIGURE 17

Controversies

- For single-row repair techniques, the site of anchor placement has been variously advocated to be adjacent to the articular margin of the humeral head to reduce overtensioning the repair; at the lateral-most aspect of the footprint in order to maximize repair site surface area coverage; or in the lateral tuberosity, which places the arthroscopic knots further away from the subacromial space.
- Suture configurations include simple, mattress, or modified Mason-Allen sutures (MAC stitch). The arthroscopic Mason-Allen configuration was not biomechanically stronger than other configurations. The MAC stitch combines a mattress stitch with a simple suture placed behind it to prevent suture cutout to simulate the Mason-Allen suture configuration.

- The arthroscope is placed in the intra-articular space.
- All degenerative tissue is débrided with a shaver placed through the full-thickness defect.
- The tuberosity is prepared.
- The arthroscope is placed in the subacromial space through the lateral portal.
- An accessory anterolateral portal is created using spinal needle guidance.
- The arthroscope is placed through the accessory anterolateral portal to view the cuff.
- Any degenerative tissue in the posterior aspect of the cuff that was not visualized with the scope in the intra-articular space is débrided.
- The number of anchors needed is determined based on assessment of tear size, the presence of delamination, tissue quality, and tendon mobility.
- Single-row anchor repair
  - The arthroscope is placed through the lateral portal in the subacromial space.
  - Using spinal needle guidance, an accessory portal is created along the edge of the acromion for suture passage.
  - A triple-loaded anchor is passed into the lateral-most aspect of the tuberosity and checked for stability.
  - The anchor eyelet is aligned so that the sutures can slide for a simple suture configuration with three limbs medial and three limbs lateral.
  - The most anterior of the three medial sutures is retrieved with a smooth-tipped suture retriever through the anterolateral portal. A cannula may be used during suture passage but is not required.
  - The suture is loaded onto the suture punch, passed back into the subacromial space, and passed through the cuff along the anterior margin of the tear.
  - The remaining two medial sutures are passed in a similar fashion, with each suture limb approximately 5–8 mm posterior to the previous suture.
  - The arthroscope is passed through the anterior portal and a clear cannula is passed through the lateral or anterolateral portal.
  - Each pair of suture limbs is retrieved from posterior to anterior and each set is tied to repair the cuff to the tuberosity.

Step 6C: Dual-Row Anchor Repair for Medium Full-Thickness Tears

- All dual-row repair techniques utilize a medial row and a lateral row of anchors to re-create the native cuff footprint.
- The dual-row technique offers the advantage of increasing tendon-bone contact area (Kim et al., 2005).
- A retracted 1.5- to 3-cm tear that is easily mobilized to the lateral aspect of the tuberosity can be repaired using a dual-row anchor technique. Use one or two anchors at the medial footprint using a mattress suture configuration and either one or two anchors laterally using a simple suture configuration. Alternatively, one or two PushLock or Versalok (DePuy-Mitek) anchors may be used laterally to execute the "transosseous equivalent" technique.
  - For 1.5-cm tears, one triple-loaded anchor is used medially and one anchor laterally.
  - For 2-cm tears, two double-loaded anchors are used medially and one or two anchors laterally. Figure 18A shows a subacromial view from the lateral portal demonstrating the "50-yard-line" view of a 2-cm supraspinatus tear. In the inset, an arthroscope is passed through the lateral portal.
  - For 3-cm tears, two triple-loaded anchors are used medially and two anchors laterally.
- The arthroscope is placed through the lateral portal in the subacromial space (see Fig. 18A inset).
- Using spinal needle guidance, an accessory portal is created along the edge of the acromion for suture passage. In Figure 18B, a spinal needle (*black arrow*) is passed along the anterolateral edge of the acromion into the subacromial space. In the inset, a subacromial view shows the spinal needle (*black arrow*) at the articular margin of the footprint.
- The anchor is passed at the medial aspect of the tuberosity along the articular margin. If two anchors are placed, they should be spaced approximately 1–1.5 cm apart and checked for stability.
- The anchor eyelet is aligned so that the sutures can slide for a mattress suture configuration with a set of limbs medial and lateral.
- The most anterior of the medial sutures is retrieved with a smooth-tipped suture retriever through the anterolateral portal. A cannula may be used during suture passage but is not required.
- The suture is loaded onto the suture punch, passed back into the subacromial space, and passed through the cuff along the anterior margin of the tear. Figure

Pearls

- *Determine the number of anchors to use based on tear size and tendon mobility. In general, use one anchor for every 1 cm of tear size.*
- *The advent of triple-loaded anchors allows for an additional point of fixation per anchor compared with double-loaded anchors. This minimizes the number of anchors placed in the tuberosity and provides additional strength to the repair.*
- *Lateral traction on the second set of mattress sutures helps reduce the cuff to the footprint during knot tying.*

Pitfalls

- *Always check cuff mobility after releases are performed. If the cuff will not reduce to the lateral aspect of the tuberosity or reduction requires high tension on the tissue, consider using single-row repair to avoid overtensioning the cuff, which may result in postoperative contracture or suture cutout through articular cartilage, bone, or the cuff.*

Controversies

- The transosseous equivalent technique creates greater contact pressure against the footprint, but overtensioning may result in strangulation of blood supply to healing cuff tissue.

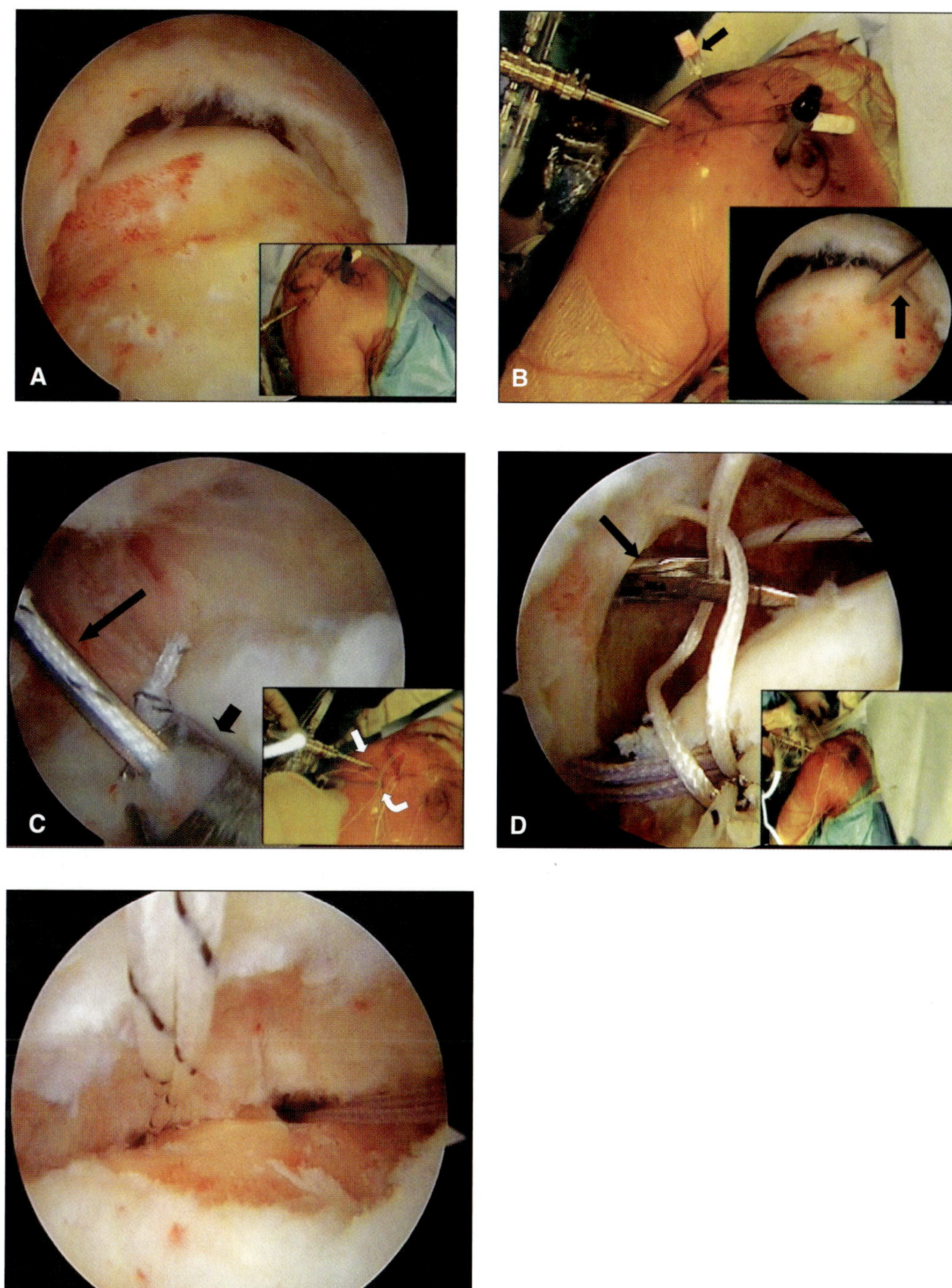

FIGURE 18

18C shows a subacromial view from the lateral portal with a Scorpion suture punch (*short black arrow*) used to pass the suture through the cuff with its needle (*long black arrow*). The inset shows an outside view of the arthroscope in the lateral portal (*straight white arrow*) and the Scorpion passed through the anterolateral portal (*curved white arrow*).

- The remaining sutures are passed in a similar fashion with each suture limb approximately 5–8 mm posterior to the previous suture.

- Alternatively, sutures may be passed in a retrograde fashion through the posterior cuff using a BirdBeak or similar penetrating suture retriever (Fig. 18D, *black arrow*).

- After the medial anchor(s) and sutures have been passed, the arthroscope is placed into the anterior portal and a twist-in clear cannula is placed through the anterolateral or lateral portal.
- Each pair of suture limbs is retrieved and knots are tied to approximate the cuff to the medial footprint. Figure 18E shows a subacromial view from the lateral portal of the footprint after medial mattress sutures have been tied. In this patient, two triple-loaded anchors were passed at the medial row but only two sets of sutures from each anchor were used. The third set of sutures from each anchor can be seen exiting from the anchors.
- If a lateral row of simple sutures is utilized for the repair, the suture limbs are cut once knots are tied.
  - The arthroscope is passed into the lateral portal (Fig. 19A, inset) and spinal needle guidance is used for passage of one or two triple-loaded anchor(s) at the lateral-most aspect of the tuberosity (Fig. 19A).
  - One limb of each pair of sutures is sequentially passed through the lateral edge of the cuff margin using a suture punch device until all sutures are passed.
  - The arthroscope is passed into the anterior portal and a clear cannula is passed through the lateral portal. Each set of sutures is retrieved and tied until all are tied, and then the excess suture is cut with a guillotine suture cutter. Figure 19B shows a subacromial view from the anterior portal of a completed repair with a medial row of mattress sutures (M) and a lateral row of simple sutures (L).
- If the transosseous equivalent technique is utilized for repair, the suture limbs should not be cut after tying the knots for the medial row.
  - The arthroscope is placed in the anterolateral portal.
  - One limb from each pair of mattress sutures is retrieved through the lateral portal so that they pass over the top of the cuff. These suture limbs should be passed through the eyelet of the metal-tipped PushLock anchor.
  - The PushLock anchor loaded with the suture limbs is passed through the lateral portal so that it rests perpendicular against the lateral cortex of the greater tuberosity. Figure 20A shows a subacromial

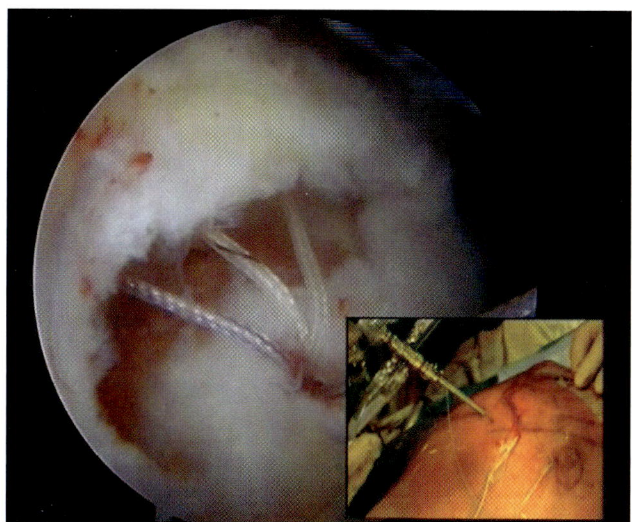

A

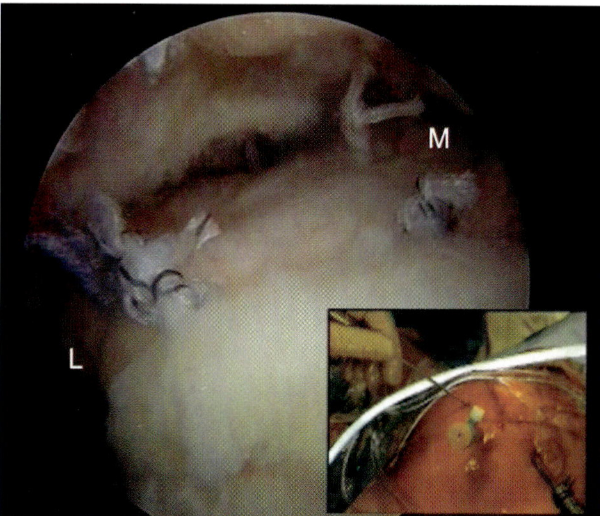

B

FIGURE 19

view from the anterolateral portal of suture limbs from the medial mattress sutures (*white arrow*) passed through the eyelet of a metal-tipped PushLock anchor (*black arrow*) aligned against the lateral cortex of the tuberosity.

- Tension of the suture limbs is adjusted over the cuff and then the anchor is malleted into the cortex until seated, which locks the sutures with interference fit against the cortex. Figure 20B shows a subacromial view from the lateral portal of the completed transosseous equivalent repair.
- A guillotine suture cutter is used to cut excess sutures.

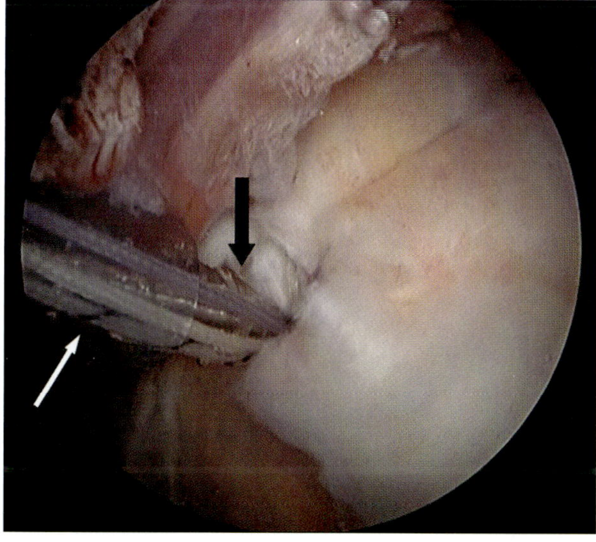

A

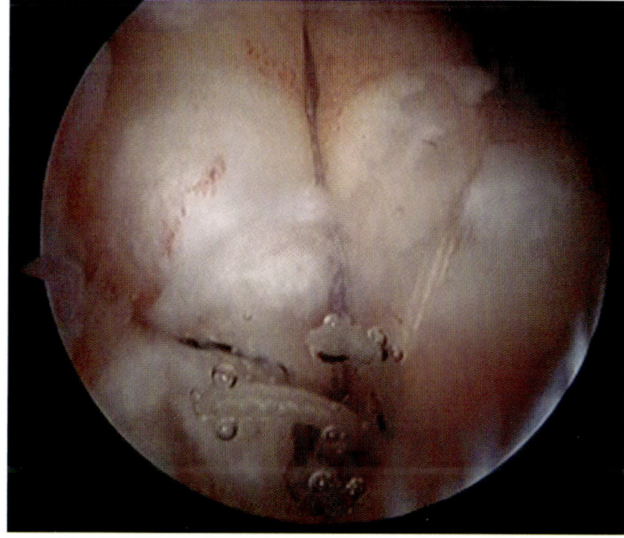

B

FIGURE 20

PEARLS

- *Tie through the lateral portal while viewing through the anterior portal. This allows easier retrieval of posterior sutures.*

Instrumentation/ Implantation

- Knot pusher
- Guillotine suture cutter

PEARLS

- *Adjust the rehabilitation protocol to prevent arthrofibrosis.*
- *Add table slides and more aggressive stretching within the first 4 weeks if the patient has*
  - *Diabetes*
  - *Less than 90° forward flexion*
  - *Dual-row or PASTA repair*
- *Educate the patient about the goals of surgery to decrease false expectations and provide understanding of the time line.*

PITFALLS

- *Not protecting repair with sling*
- *Failure to communicate with therapist*
- *Starting resistive exercises too early*

STEP 7: KNOT TYING

- We prefer a sliding square knot as the first throw that is reinforced by two alternating half-hitches on the post. The post is switched and two more alternating half-hitches are thrown.

Postoperative Care and Expected Outcomes

- For partial-thickness and small full-thickness tears, elements of the rehabilitation protocol begin at the following times (Deutsch et al., 2006):
  - Pendulum exercises: postoperative day 1
  - Supine passive internal and external rotation exercises: postoperative day 8
  - Table slides (closed chain forward elevation): postoperative day 28
  - Active-assisted forward elevation and deltoid isometrics: postoperative week 7
  - Strengthening of periscapular muscles: postoperative week 8
  - Waist-level Theraband isotonic strengthening: postoperative week 12
  - Abduction and forward elevation Theraband strengthening: postoperative week 16
  - Recreational sports and unrestricted work activities: 6 months
- For medium full-thickness tears, elements of the rehabilitation protocol begin at the following times (Deutsch et al., 2006):
  - Pendulum exercises: postoperative day 1
  - Supine passive internal and external rotation exercises: postoperative day 8
  - Table slides (closed chain forward elevation): postoperative day 28
  - Active-assisted forward elevation exercises and deltoid isometrics: postoperative week 8 for 2-cm tears and week 12 for 3-cm tears
  - Strengthening of periscapular muscles: postoperative week 8
  - Waist-level Theraband isotonic strengthening: postoperative week 14 for 2-cm tears and week 18 for 3-cm tears
  - Abduction and forward elevation Theraband strengthening: postoperative week 22 for 2-cm tears and week 26 for 3-cm tears
  - Recreational sports and unrestricted work activities: 8 months for 2-cm tears and 12 months for 3-cm tears

Controversies

- For partial-thickness and small full-thickness tears, we allow active internal and external rotation at waist level by the patient.

- Clinical outcome following repair of partial-thickness tears has been reported as excellent (Deutsch, 2007). Structural integrity and clinical outcome have been reported to be excellent using both single-row and dual-row repair techniques for small and medium full-thickness tears by several authors, with significant improvements in visual analog pain and satisfaction scores and in American Shoulder and Elbow Surgeons (ASES) functional scores with return to work and recreational activities (Deutsch, 2007; Gartsman et al., 1998; LaFosse et al., 2008).

Complications

- Persistent pain
  - Nonhealing of poor-quality cuff tissue
  - Structural failure
  - Inadequate decompression, missed AC joint arthritis, and/or biceps pathology
- Re-tear
  - Usually associated with poor tissue quality, elderly patients, multitendon tears, or tears with significant retraction.
  - If tear recurs with symptoms, revision may be warranted.
- Stiffness
  - May be caused by overtensioning the repair or prolonged immobilization (Burkhart et al., 1997).
  - Avoid repair in patients with adhesive capsulitis. In these patients, delay cuff repair until motion is regained.

Evidence

Burkhart SS, Danaceau SM, Pearce CE. Arthroscopic rotator cuff repair: analysis of results by tear size and by repair technique—margin convergence versus direct tendon-to-bone repair. Arthroscopy. 2001;17:905-12.

This study indicated that arthroscopic rotator cuff repair can achieve good and excellent results in the majority of patients. U-shaped tears repaired by margin convergence had results similar to those of crescent-shaped tears repaired directly by a tendon-to-bone technique. (Level III evidence [case series])

Burkhart SS, Johnson TA, Wirth MA, Athanasiou KA. Cyclic loading of transosseous rotator cuff repairs: "tension overload" as a possible cause of failure. Arthroscopy. 1997;13:172-6.

The authors found that rotator cuff tears repaired with a "tension overload" of the muscle-tendon units will eventually fail until the normal resting lengths of the muscle-tendon units are restored. Therefore, cuffs should be repaired without tension in possible. Additionally, transosseous tunnels should extend distal to weak, metaphyseal bone for better fixation. (laboratory study)

Chokshi BV, Kubiak EN, Jazrawi LM, Ticker JB, Zheng N, Kummer FJ, Rokito AS. The effect of arthroscopic suture passing instruments on rotator cuff damage and repair strength. Bull Hosp Joint Dis. 2006;63:123-5.

After repairing cuff reattachments with four devices (SutureLasso, straight BirdBeak, Viper, and Mayo needle), the authors found that the SutureLasso and Mayo needle repairs failed at higher loads. It was thought that the larger holes caused by the BirdBeak and Viper compromised the strength of the cuff, leading to failure at lower loads. (laboratory study)

Deutsch A. Arthroscopic repair of partial-thickness tears of the rotator cuff. J Shoulder Elbow Surg. 2007;16:193-201.

This prospective study documented successful clinical outcomes of arthroscopic repair of significant partial-thickness rotator cuff tears. (Level II evidence [prospective trial])

Deutsch A. Arthroscopic rotator cuff repair: the effect of depth of suture passage on three-dimensional repair site surface area and load to failure using single-row anchor fixation. Paper presented at the Seventy-third Annual Meeting of the American Academy of Orthopaedic Surgeons, Chicago, IL, March, 2006.

The author found a linear relationship between the amount of cuff included in the repair and repair site surface area coverage and repair strength.

Deutsch A, Guelich D, Mundanthanam G, Govea C, Labiss J. The effect of rehabilitation on cuff integrity and range of motion following arthroscopic rotator cuff repair: a prospective, randomized study of a standard and decelerated rehabilitation protocol. Paper presented at the Twenty-third Closed Meeting of the American Shoulder and Elbow Surgeons, Chicago, IL, September 2006.

The authors advocated the use of a decelerated rehabilitation protocol with no forward elevation until after 4 weeks postoperatively to prevent repair failure. This protocol was not associated with an increased risk of postoperative stiffness. (Level I evidence [prospective randomized trial])

Deutsch A, Taylor M. A prospective comparison of Ethibond vs. FiberWire Suture for Arthroscopic Rotator Cuff Repair. Study presented at the Seventy-third Annual Meeting of the American Academy of Orthopaedic Surgeons, Chicago, IL, March, 2006.

Gartsman GM, Khan M, Hammerman SM. Arthroscopic repair of full-thickness tears of the rotator cuff. J Bone Joint Surg [Am]. 1998;80:832-40.

In this study, arthroscopic repair of full-thickness tears of the rotator cuff produced satisfactory results. While a technically demanding procedure, the method offers smaller incisions, access to the glenohumeral joint, and less soft tissue dissection.

Gartsman GM, O'Connor DP. Arthroscopic rotator cuff repair with and without arthroscopic subacromial decompression: a prospective, randomized study of one year outcomes. J Shoulder Elbow Surg. 2004;13:424-6.

In this study of patients with a type II acromion undergoing an arthroscopic rotator cuff repair, functional outcome as measured by ASES scores was not affected by performing an arthroscopic acromioplasty. (Level I evidence [prospective randomized trial])

Kim DH, Elattrache NS, Tibone JE, Jun BJ, Delamora SN, Kvitne RS, Lee TQ. Biomechanical comparison of a single-row versus double-row suture anchor technique for rotator cuff repair. Am J Sports Med. 2006;34:407-14.

The authors found that double-row repair improved the strength and stiffness and decreased gap formation and strain when compared to a single-row repair. (laboratory study)

LaFosse L, Brzoska R, Toussaint B, Gobezie R. The outcome and structural integrity of arthroscopic rotator cuff repair with use of the double row suture anchor technique: surgical technique. J Bone Joint Surg [Am]. 2008;90:275-86.

In this prospective series of 105 shoulders with supraspinatus with or without infraspinatus rotator cuff tears repaired with a double-row suture anchor technique, the authors concluded that the double-row technique resulted in a lower failure rate than was previously reported. (Level II evidence [prospective review])

Murray TF, Lajtai G, Mileski RM, Snyder SJ. Arthroscopic repair of medium to large full-thickness rotator cuff tears: outcome at 2- to 6-year follow-up. J Shoulder Elbow Surg. 2002;11:19-24.

The authors reported that, at 39 months' follow-up, 44 of 45 patients were satisfied with their arthroscopic rotator cuff repair. (Level II evidence [retrospective review])

PROCEDURE 4

Open Repair of Rotator Cuff Tears

Andrew S. Neviaser and Robert J. Neviaser

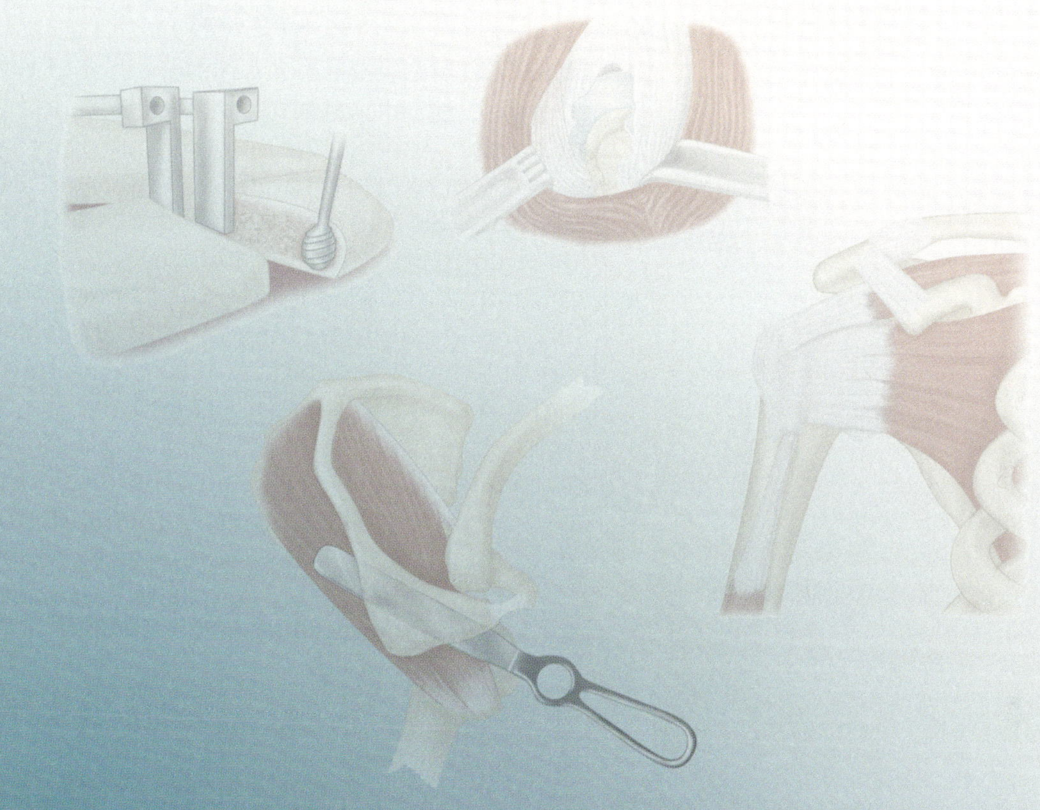

Figures 8A, 13A, 17A, and 24A reprinted with permission from Neviaser RJ, Neviaser AS. Open repair of massive rotator cuff tears: tissue mobilization techniques. In Zuckerman JD (ed). Advanced Shoulder Reconstruction. Chicago: American Academy of Orthopaedic Surgeons, 2007:175-183.
Figure 18 reprinted with permission from Neviaser RJ. Tears of the rotator cuff. Orthop Clin North Am. 1980;11:295-306.
Figure 19 reprinted with permission from Neviaser JS. Ruptures of the rotator cuff of the shoulder: new concepts in the diagnosis and operative treatment for chronic ruptures. Arch Surg. 1971;102:483-5.
Figures 20 and 21 reprinted with permission from Neviaser JS, Neviaser RJ, Neviaser TJ. The repair of chronic massive ruptures of the rotator cuff by use of a freeze dried rotator cuff graft. J Bone Joint Surg [Am]. 1978;60:681-4.
Figures 25 and 27A reprinted with permission from Neviaser RJ, Neviaser TJ. Transfer of the subscapularis and teres minor for massive defects of the rotator cuff. In Bayley I, Kessel L (eds). Shoulder Surgery. Heidelberg: Springer-Verlag, 1982:60-69.

Pitfalls

- *Cuff tear arthropathy is a contraindication to rotator cuff repair.*
- *Advanced fatty infiltration of cuff muscles (Goutallier stage 3 or 4) seen on MRI or arthro-CT portends poor outcomes and is a relative contraindication to repair.*
- *Active infection is a contraindication.*

Controversies

- Elderly, low-demand patients with large or massive tears and severe fatty infiltration may benefit from cuff débridement, limited subacromial decompression, and biceps tenotomy.
- In younger patients with irreparable tears, consideration should be given to grafts or tendon transfers (discussed later).

Treatment Options

- Pain relief is the primary objective of all treatment, and restoration of function a secondary goal. Therefore, nonoperative treatment should be directed at relieving pain.
- Subacromial steroid injection is often more effective and immediate in its relief than are nonsteroidal anti-inflammatory drugs.
- Physical therapy should be instituted when pain permits and involves two aspects: stretching and strengthening of the rotators and elevators.
- Surgery is undertaken if nonoperative treatment does not sufficiently reduce pain.

Indications

- Open repair is indicated for any painful rotator cuff tear, especially massive ones that are refractory to nonoperative treatment.
- Impaired shoulder function is also an indication, although postoperative functional outcomes are less predictable than reduction of pain.
- Acute, traumatic tears are an indication for early operative intervention.

Examination/Imaging

- A standard shoulder examination should be performed on all patients, including range of active and passive motion, elevation for atrophy (Fig. 1), weakness in external rotation, lift-off and abdominal press tests (Fig. 2A and 2B), and positive provocative rotator cuff tests (Fig. 3A and 3B).
- Radiographs should include anteroposterior views in internal and external rotation, and an axillary view.
  - An outlet view should be taken to determine the type of acromion (i.e., I–III) and the need for acromioplasty.
  - Acromioclavicular (AC) joint changes and narrowing of the acromial humeral interval can be determined from plain radiographs.
- Additional preoperative studies include magnetic resonance imaging (MRI) or ultrasound.

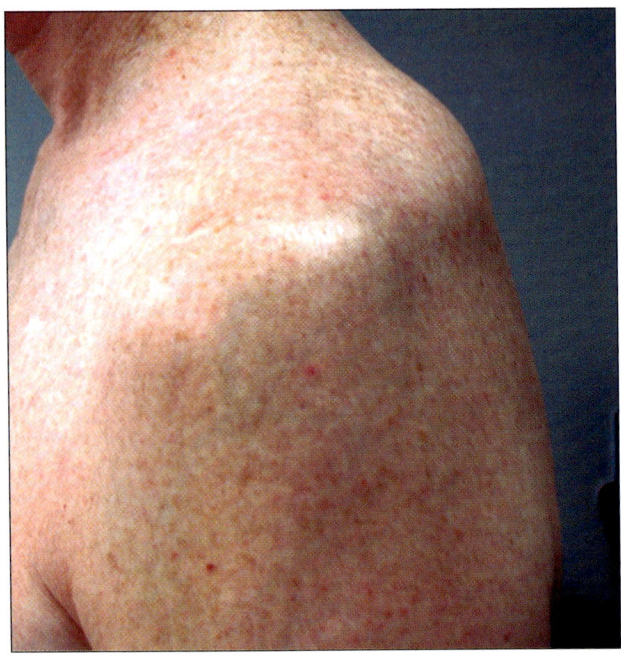

FIGURE 1

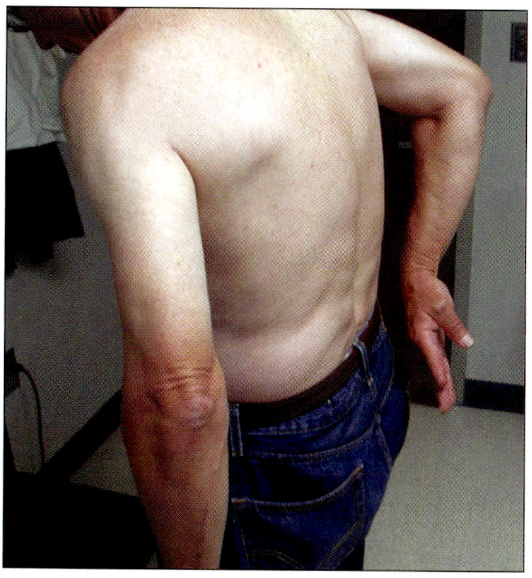
A

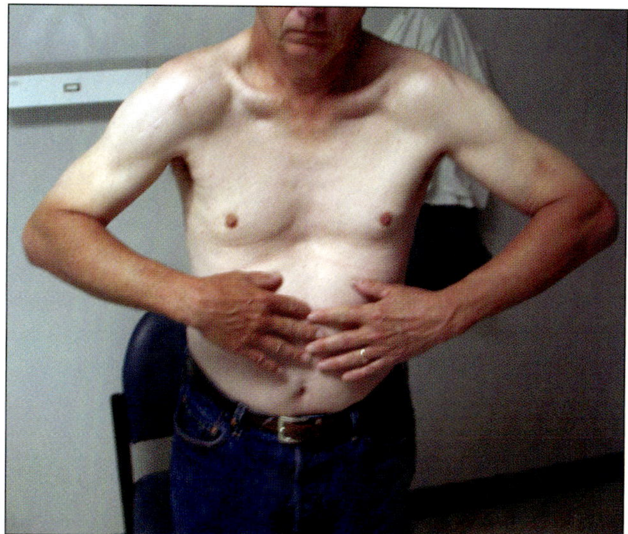
B

FIGURE 2

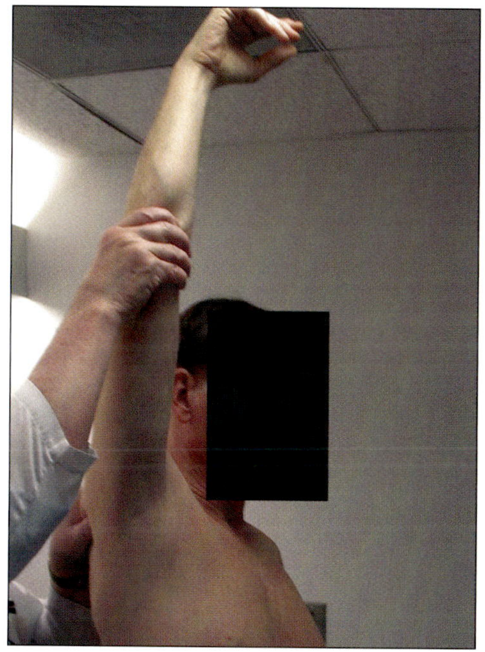
A

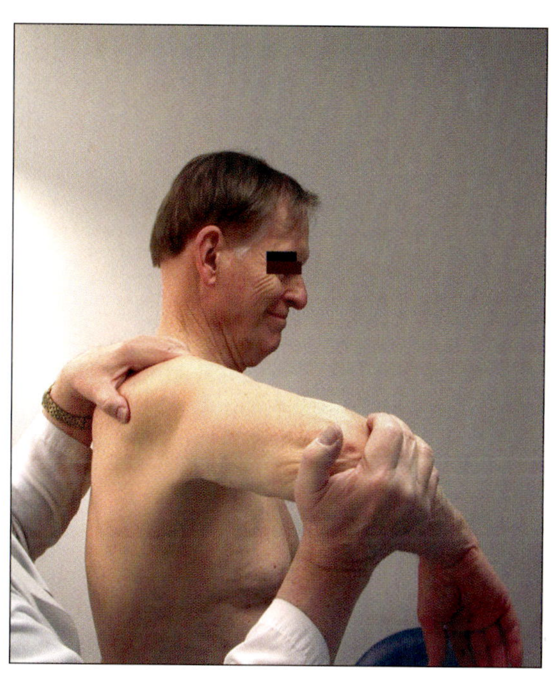
B

FIGURE 3

- MRI is the current gold standard for imaging the rotator cuff. Number of and which tendons are involved (Fig. 4A–C), atrophy and fatty degeneration of cuff muscles, and quality of the articular cartilage can be determined from MRI for preoperative planning.
- Ultrasound is an inexpensive alternative to MRI but is highly institution and operator dependent.

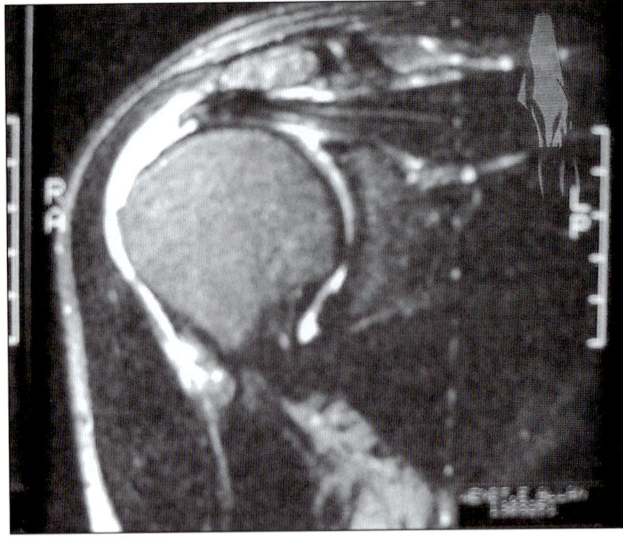
A

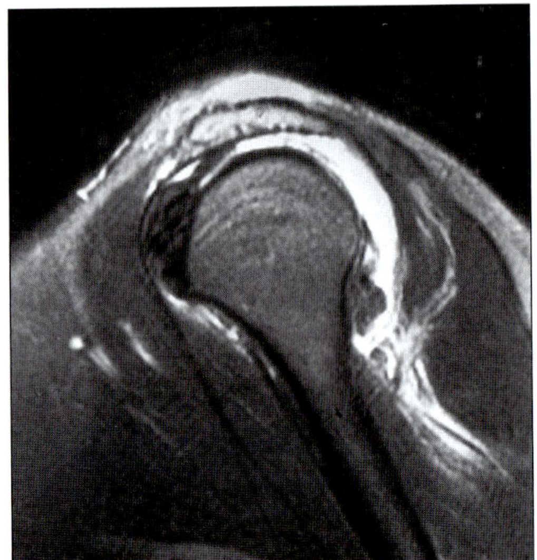
B

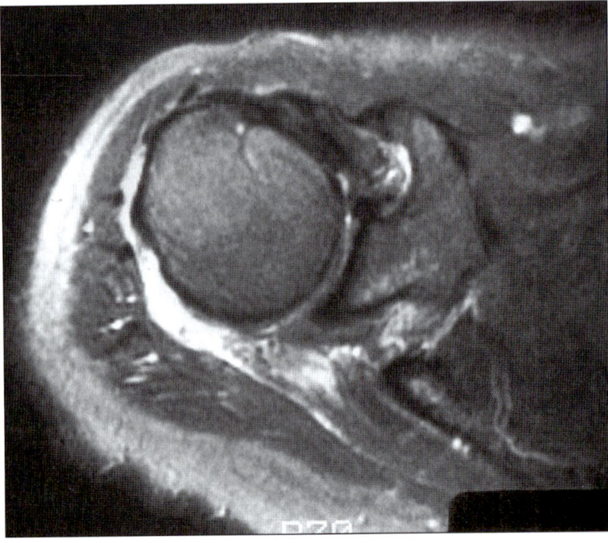
C

FIGURE 4

Surgical Anatomy

- The glenohumeral joint is supported by four soft tissues layers alternating between muscle and fascia (Cooper et al., 1993).
  - The first, most superficial layer encountered after dissection through the skin and subcutaneous tissues includes the muscles of the pectoralis major and the deltoid.
    - The deltoid originates broadly from the acromion and the lateral clavicle. Its three heads coalesce to insert on the deltoid tubercle of the lateral humerus.
    - The pectoralis major has origins on both the sternum and the clavicle and inserts on the proximal humeral shaft immediately lateral to the tendon of the long head of the biceps.

- Beneath this muscular layer is layer two, consisting of the clavipectoral fascia anteriorly and the thick posterior scapular facia posteriorly. Included within this second layer is the coracoacromial ligament, which traverses between the inferior surface of the anterior acromion and the coracoid, completing the otherwise bony acromial arch. The subdeltoid bursa is the deepest portion of layer two and allows the unhindered gliding of the rotator cuff beneath the acromial arch.
- The rotator cuff is the third layer encountered and consists of the muscles, and confluence of tendons, of the subscapularis, the supraspinatus and infraspinatus, and the teres minor.
  - The posterior rotator cuff muscles, the teres minor and infraspinatus, take origin from the inferolateral border of the scapula and the infraspinatus fossa, respectively. They insert onto the greater tuberosity; the infraspinatus inserts into the middle facet and posterolateral portion of the superior facet, while the teres minor inserts onto the inferior facet.
  - The superior rotator cuff muscle is the supraspinatus, which originates from the supraspinatus fossa and also inserts on the greater tuberosity superior facet, anterior and slightly medial to the infraspinatus.
  - The largest of the rotator cuff muscles, the subscapularis, originates from the subscapular fossa and is the only muscle to insert on the lesser tuberosity.
  - The transverse humeral ligament also attaches to the lesser tuberosity, bridges the intertubercular groove, and inserts onto the greater tuberosity. Deep to this ligament, within the groove, lies the tendon of the long head of the biceps. This tendon can be traced retrograde superiorly entering the glenohumeral joint capsule at the superolateral margin of the rotator interval (described below) to its origin on the supraglenoid tubercle. Its synovium is confluent with that of the glenohumeral joint, and intra-articular processes such as osteoarthritis or adhesive capsulitis will affect this tendon as well.
  - The triangular space between the anterior border of the supraspinatus and superior border of the subscapularus lateral to the coracoid constitutes the rotator interval.

- Layer four is the glenohumeral joint capsule, which is usually adherent to the tendinous portions of the rotator cuff except in the area of the rotator interval and the inferior axillary fold.

- Innervation of the most superficial muscles, the deltoid and the pectoralis major, is supplied by the axillary nerve and the medial and lateral pectoral nerves, respectively.
  - The axillary nerve arises from the posterior cord of the brachial plexus and traverses the anterior surface of the subscapularis, turning posteriorly at its inferior margin. It passes beneath the glenohumeral joint before exiting the quadrangular space and entering the deep surface of the deltoid.
  - Mobilization of the subscapularis muscle during anterior rotator cuff repair requires identification and protection of the axillary nerve.
  - This nerve also provides innervation to the teres minor.
- The suprascapular nerve innervates the supraspinatus and infraspinatus. It branches from the upper trunk of the brachial plexus, traverses obliquely across the superior border of the scapula and passes deep to the transverse scapular ligament in the suprascapular notch. After supplying the supraspinatus (typically via two motor branches), the nerve travels through the spinoglenoid notch to innervate the infraspinatus.
- The subscapularis receives innervation from the upper and lower subscapular nerves.

Positioning

- The patient is placed in a sitting position (Fig. 5A) with the arm draped free (Fig. 5B), allowing for complete mobility and access.
- This position is more upright than the beach chair position, allowing the surgeon to look down on the cuff from above.
  - This facilitates seeing posterosuperiorly, as well as superiorly and anteriorly.
  - It also permits better access to the posterior part of the infraspinatus and the teres minor.

Pearls

- *A table with a removable section on the side of the surgery facilitates access to the entire shoulder, anteriorly and posteriorly.*

Portals/Exposures

Arthroscopic Subacromial Decompression and Mini-Open Cuff Repair

- A standard posterior viewing portal is established. The glenohumeral joint is examined with particular

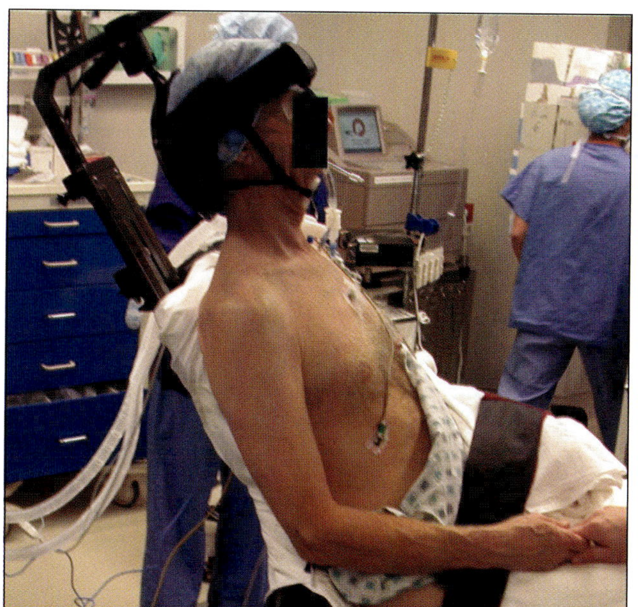

A

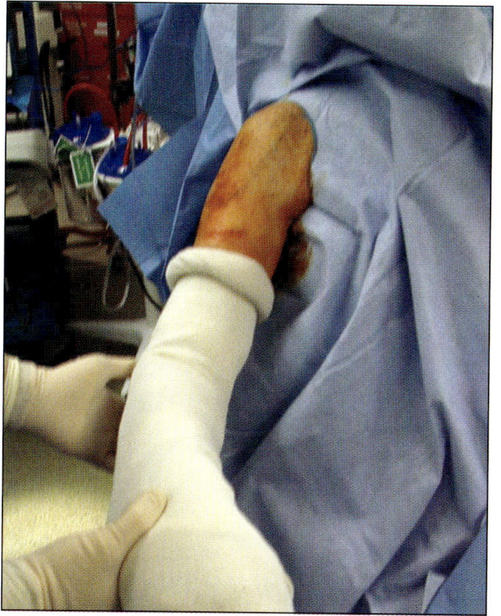

B

FIGURE 5

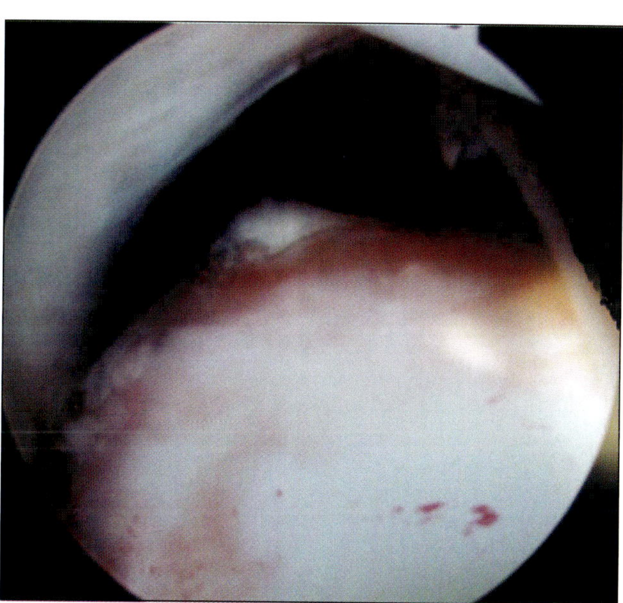

FIGURE 6

attention given to the biceps tendon. Any intra-articular procedures considered necessary can be completed at this time. The cuff defect is examined from the articular side (Fig. 6). The arthroscope is then moved to the subacromial space, still from a posterior portal, and the defect is examined from above.

- The bursa is resected sufficiently to expose the tear margins. An acromioplasty can be performed at this time, and traction stitches are placed in the torn tendon (described below).

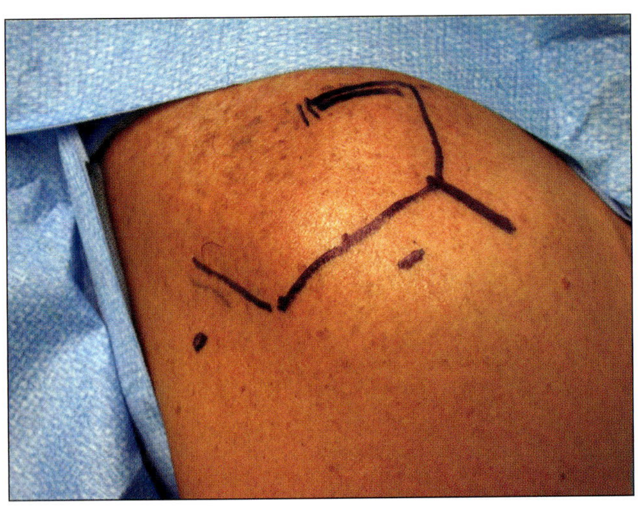

FIGURE 7

- An incision 1.5-2 cm in length is made at the anterolateral corner of the acromion (Fig. 7). The deltoid is split in line with its fibers. Narrow retractors are placed under the acromion and anteriorly, giving full exposure of the tear.

Open Repair

- An incision is made beginning superiorly at the posterior aspect of the AC joint, continuing over the top of the joint, and ending at a point just lateral to the tip of the coracoid (Fig. 8A and 8B).
- The deltoid muscle is split in line with its fibers only as far as the tip of the coracoid (Fig. 9A and 9B).

Pitfalls

- *For arthroscopic subacromial decompression and mini-open cuff repair, the deltoid is not detached from the acromion, and care should be taken not to cross the tendinous origin transversely with the dissection (i.e., detaching the deltoid origin).*
- *For open repair, the origin of the deltoid is not incised as repair of it back to the acromion often results in postoperative detachment and a defect that can led to loss of shoulder function.*

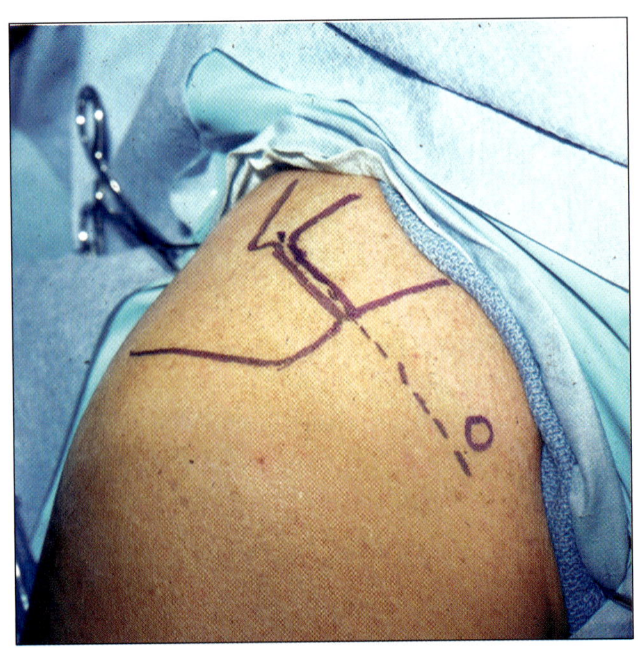

A

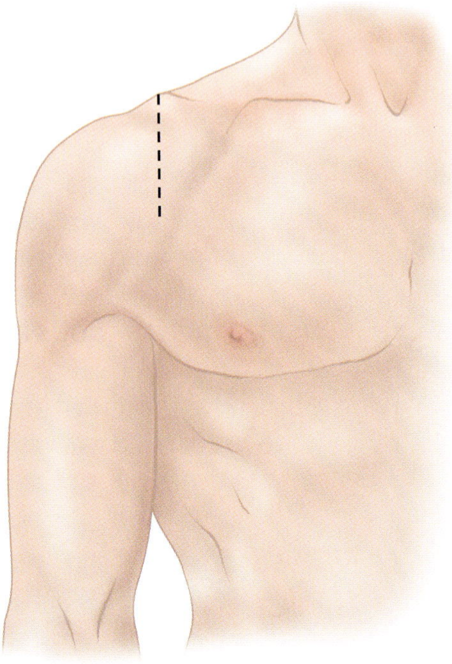

B

FIGURE 8

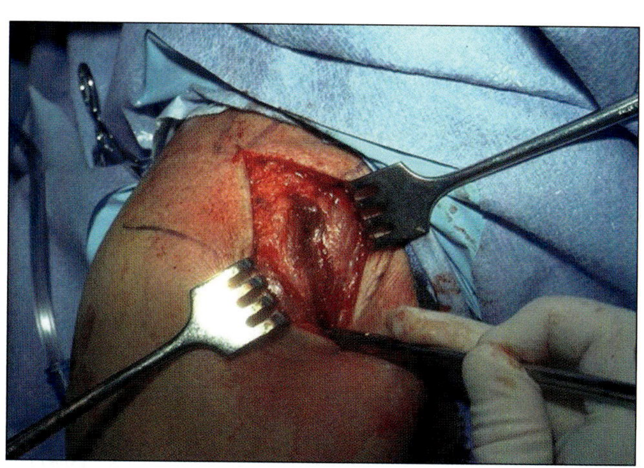
A

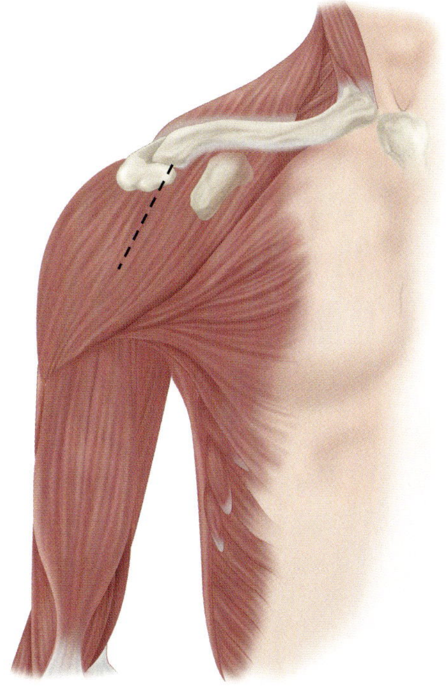
B

FIGURE 9

- The deltotrapezial aponeurosis and the superior AC ligament are sharply incised, exposing the AC joint.
- Using a sharp knife blade, 1 cm of the deltoid origin is dissected subperiosteally off the lateral clavicle. It is also dissected from the anterior, superior, and undersurface of the acromion out to the anterolateral corner of the acromion (Fig. 10A and 10B).

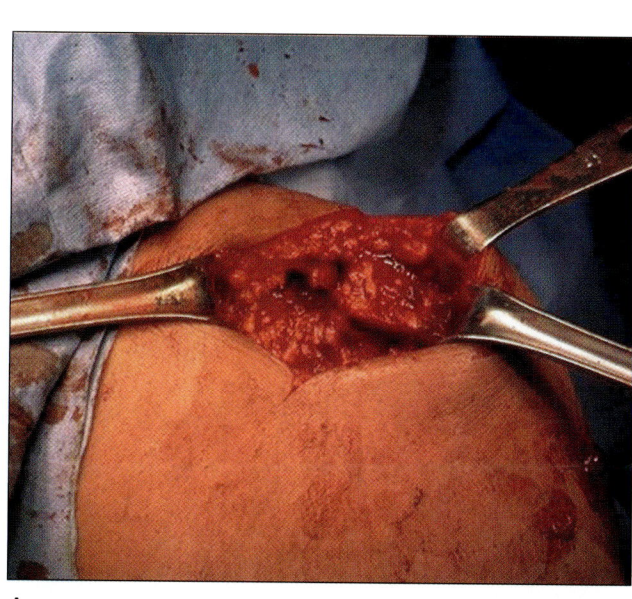
A

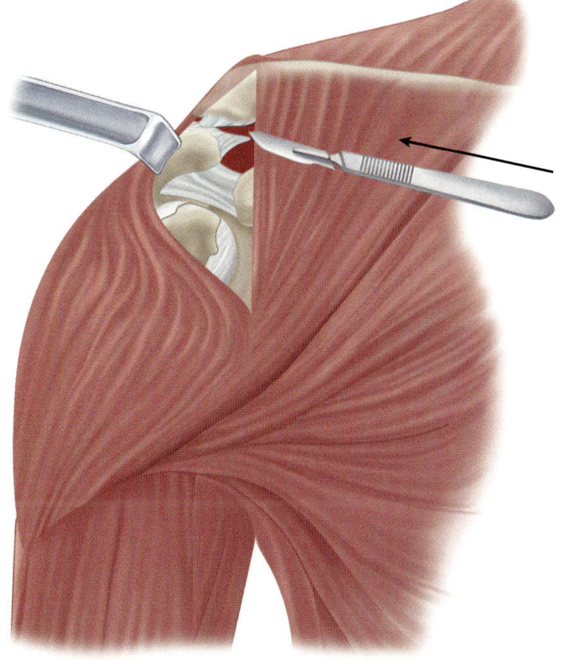
B

FIGURE 10

- The bursa is incised, undermined, and reflected. The tear in the cuff can now be seen.

PITFALLS

- *Releasing the CA ligament when the tear cannot be repaired or the repair is tenuous risks creating anterior-superior instability.*

Procedure: Mini-Open Repair

STEP 1

- After the posterior viewing portal is established, the joint inspected, and the bursa cleared from the tear, the anterior-inferior surface of the acromion, and the coracoacromial (CA) ligament are addressed.
- A standard lateral portal is established in line with the posterior margin of the clavicle. Through this portal, an electrocautery wand is inserted.
  - If the cuff tear is repairable, the CA ligament is released. If there is concern that the cuff tear may not be amenable to repair, the CA ligament should be left intact to prevent later anterior-superior escape.
  - The anterior and anterolateral margins of the acromion are clearly defined with the electrocautery.
- A burr is used to perform an acromioplasty to the same degree that is done in the open technique (i.e., create a type I acromion) (Fig. 11).

STEP 2

- Through the lateral portal, a suture punch is used to place traction sutures through the edge of the torn tendons.
- Using these sutures to apply traction, a small elevator is introduced through the lateral portal and used to

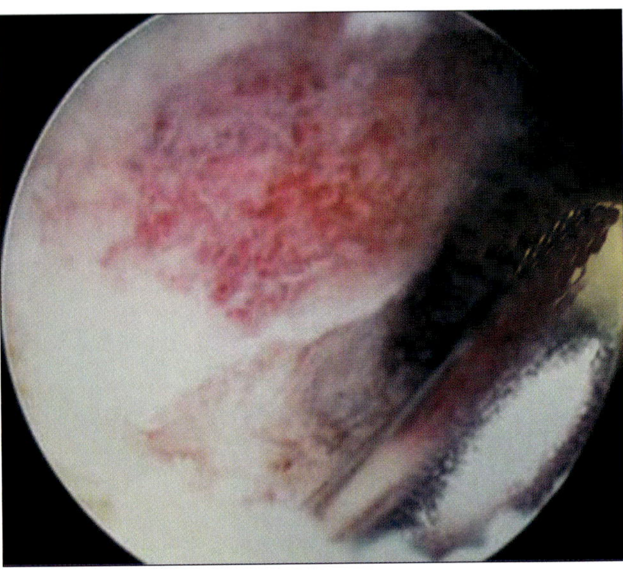

FIGURE 11

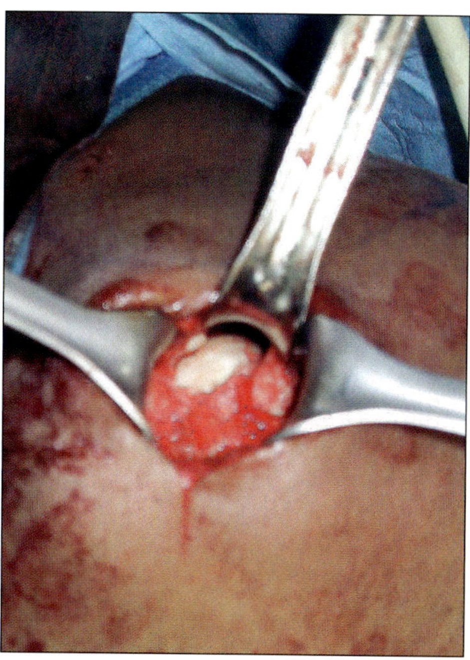

FIGURE 12

free the surrounding adhesions on both surfaces of the cuff. The degree of mobility achieved can then be easily assessed.

STEP 3

- The anterolateral incision is then made, the deltoid is split, and retractors are placed under the acromion and anteriorly to expose the tear (Fig. 12).
- Fixation of the cuff to the tuberosity is the same as described for open repairs (see below).

PITFALLS

- *Excising more than 1 cm of the outer clavicle is not necessary and can result in clavicular instability.*

Procedure: Open Repair

STEP 1

- After exposure of the AC joint, the lateral 7-8 mm of the clavicle can be resected using a reciprocating saw (Fig. 13A and 13B). A trapezoidal portion of the bone is removed, taking care not to disrupt the posterior capsule.
  - The base of the trapezoid is posterior to prevent acromioclavicular contact in this region.
- Treatment of the CA ligament is done on the same basis as in mini-open repair. With the exposure in an open repair, the surgeon has the additional option of dissecting the ligament from the undersurface of the acromion to achieve maximal length (Fig. 14) and repairing it back to the acromion through drill holes at the end of the procedure if the cuff repair is tenuous.

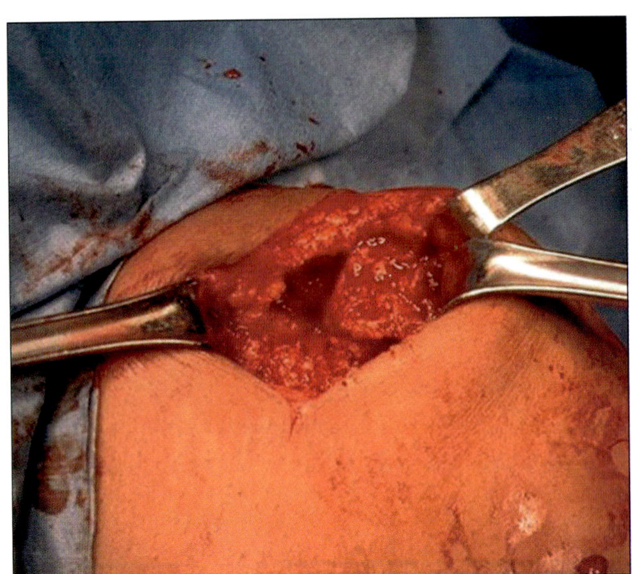

A

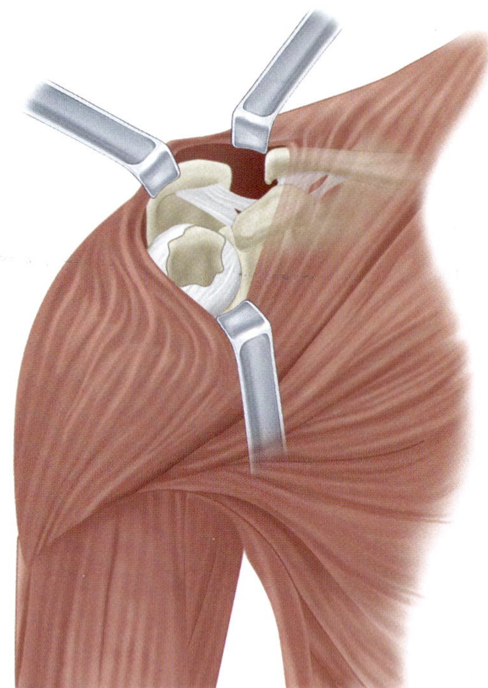

B

FIGURE 13

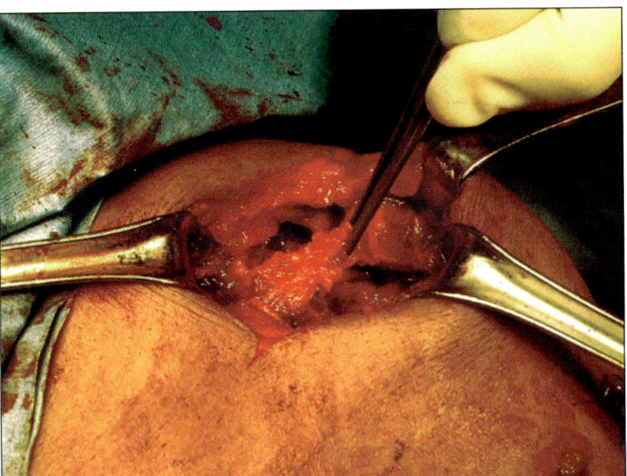

FIGURE 14

Step 2

- Using the recipricating saw, an acromioplasty is performed by removing the anterior-inferior surface from the medial articular margin to the anterolateral corner. Approximately 1 cm of bone should be removed (depth). The goal again is to create a type I or flat acromion.

Step 3

- The edges of the torn tendons are identified and débrided sharply to remove diseased tendon. This should not be done to a bleeding tendon edge as

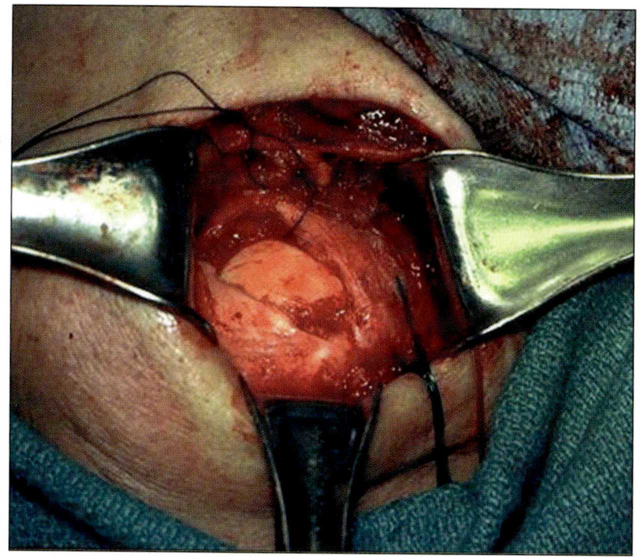

FIGURE 15

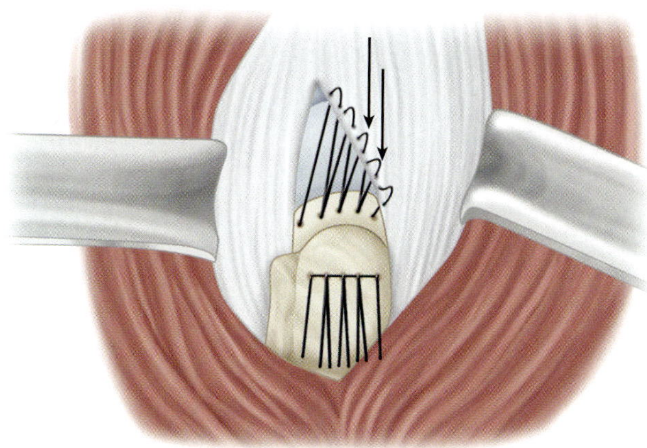

FIGURE 16

healthy tendons do not readily bleed. Simply removing the grossly diseased portion until tendon fibers appear (Fig. 15) is sufficient and usually requires excising only a few millimeters.

- Traction sutures are placed in the edges of the cuff (Fig. 16). Blunt mobilization is done using an elevator, dissecting scissors, and/or the surgeon's finger by applying traction through these sutures and releasing the subacromial adhesions.
  - Mobilization is a critical step, and as the musculotendinous unit is gradually released, additional sutures are placed successively more medially until the apex of the tear is clearly identified.
- If sufficient mobilization is not achieved with this method, interval releases are necessary. These are completed by incising between the supraspinatus and the subscapularis and between the infraspinatus and the teres minor. This releases the subacromial adhesions and restores the differential gliding between adjacent tendons.

Step 4

- When the cuff is mobile enough to be reduced to the greater tuberosity, a shallow trough (essentially a decortication more than a true trough) is made at the anatomic neck adjacent to the greater tuberosity.
- Bone tunnels are made entering the trough and exiting the lateral cortex of the greater tuberosity.
- Modified Mason-Allen sutures are placed in the cuff and passed through the bone tunnels.

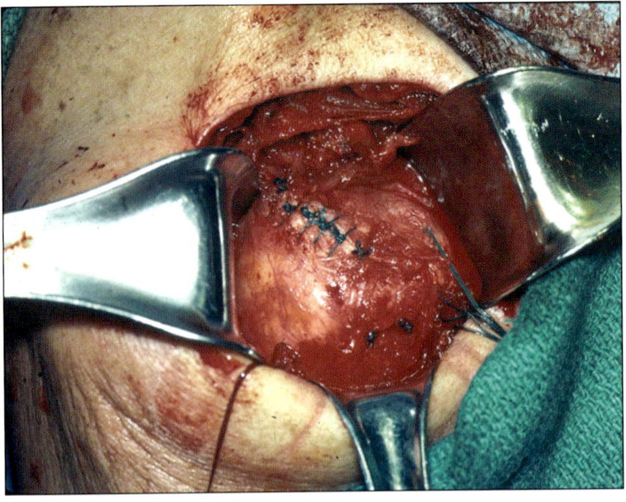

A

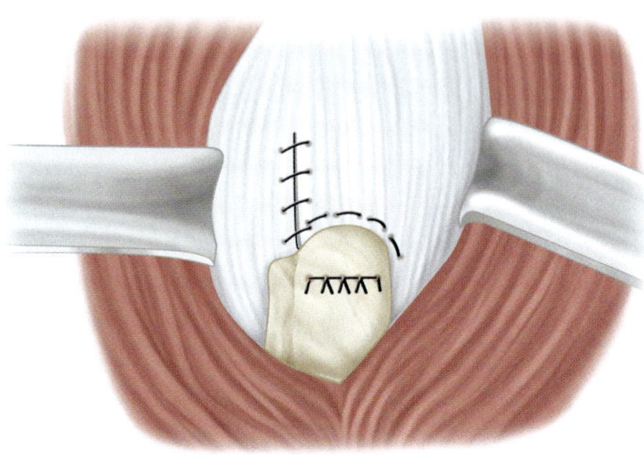

B

FIGURE 17

- Suture anchors can also be used in a double-row fashion instead of the bone tunnels.
- The arm is placed in slight internal rotation and abduction and the sutures are tied in this position.
- The longitudinal split is repaired in a side-to-side fashion (Fig. 17A and 17B).

Procedure: Open Reconstruction—Grafting

- If, after interval releases, the cuff cannot be restored to the greater tuberosity, leaving a residual defect of modest size, an interpositional graft using the biceps tendon can be used to close the defect. Use of this or any graft, however, requires that the musculotendinous motor be functional, not fixed and immobile. If there is no springy give with applied traction to the tendon or the muscle has significant fatty atrophy on the preoperative MRI, then grafting will not be effective.

Step 1

- The biceps tendon is tenodesed to the transverse humeral ligament in the bicipital groove using three figure-of-8, nonabsorbable #1 sutures (see Procedure 20).
- It is then transected above the most proximal suture and released from its origin at the supraglenoid tubercle.

Step 2

- The tendon graft is filleted (Fig. 18) and trimmed to fit the defect. The cuff itself can also be contoured

Pearls

- *The same requirement of a functioning musculotendinous unit applies to these grafts.*

Pitfalls

- *If the native residual cuff muscles are not functional, as determined by the presence of extensive fatty infiltration on preoperative imaging or the lack of mobility at surgery after adequately attempted mobilization, grafting should not be undertaken as it is doomed to fail. To succeed, grafting needs a functioning, mobile motor unit.*

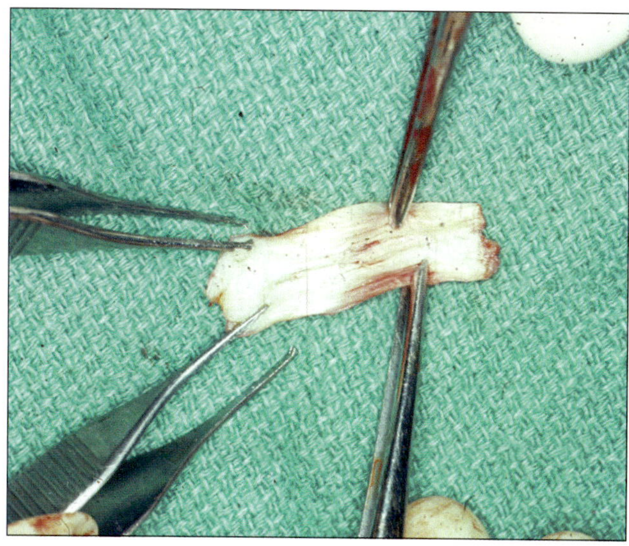

FIGURE 18

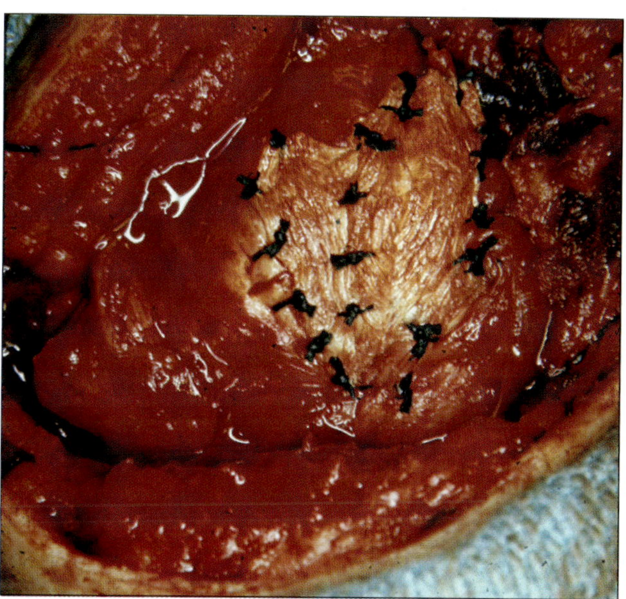

FIGURE 19

to accommodate the graft. It is fixed to the cuff with sutures and to the trough as described above (Fig. 19).

- Defects that are too large to be covered with the biceps can be filled with freeze-dried cadeveric rotator cuff grafts.

- To make the graft soft and pliable, it is soaked in sterile saline for approximately 30 minutes (Fig. 20).
- The graft is then contoured to the defect and secured with #1 nonabsorbable sutures to the tendon edge. It is secured to the humerus in the same manner described for biceps grafting (Fig. 21).

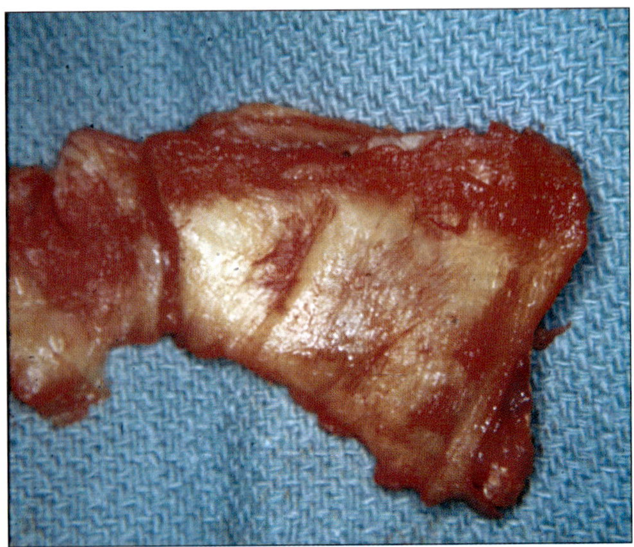

FIGURE 20

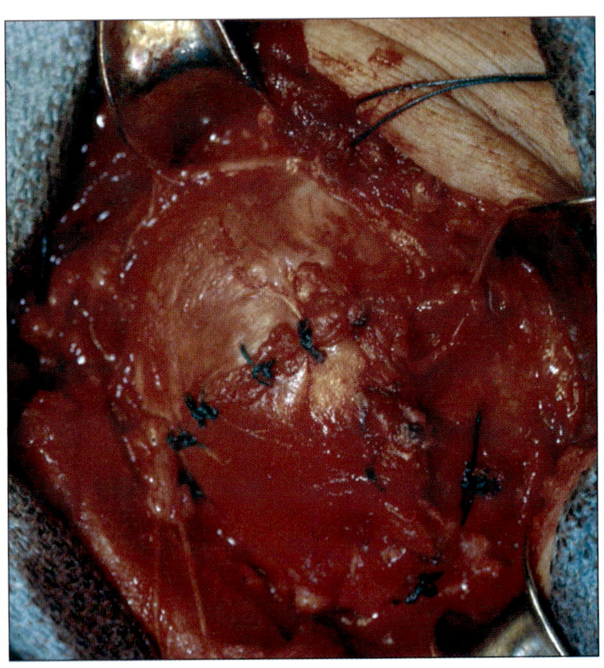

FIGURE 21

Procedure: Open Reconstruction—Local Tendon Transfers

- If the cuff cannot be closed by direct repair and the muscle-tendon unit is not sufficiently fuctional for grafting, local tendon transfers can be used.
- The subscapularis and teres minor can be used for local tendon transfers. The latissimus and teres major are also available.
- These techniques require a complete open exposure.

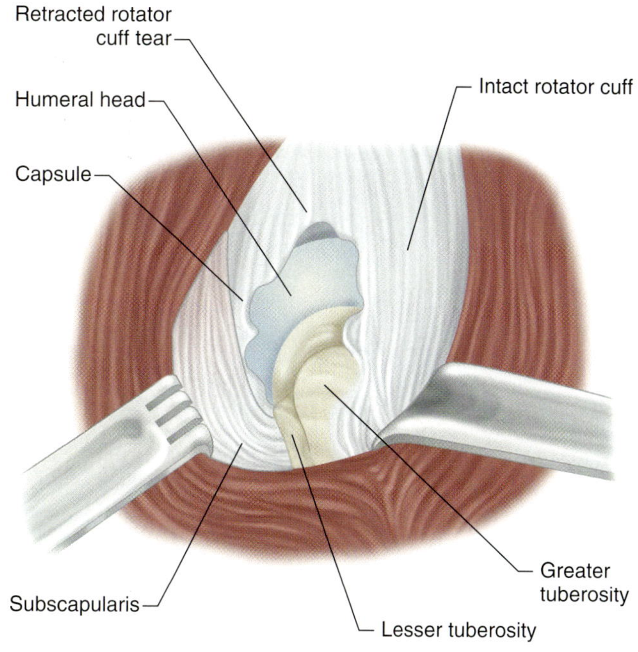

FIGURE 22

Subscapularis Transfer

- The subscapularis is separated from the anterior capsule by identifying the interval between these structures at the musculotendinous junction and dissecting laterally toward the insertion on the lesser tuberosity (Fig. 22).
- When separation is complete, the tendon is then released from its insertion. A traction suture is placed, and the subscapularis is mobilized (Fig. 23).

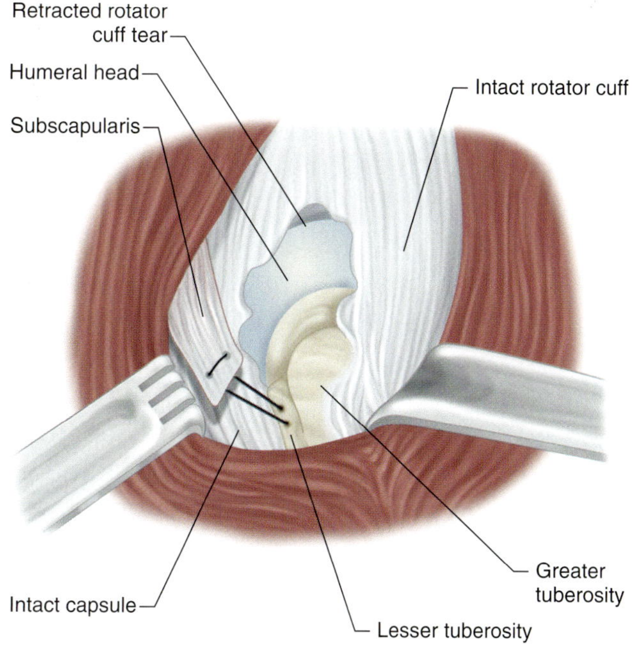

FIGURE 23

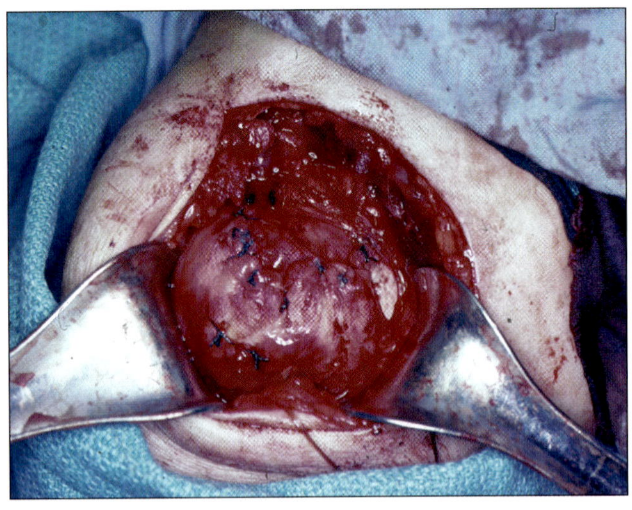

A

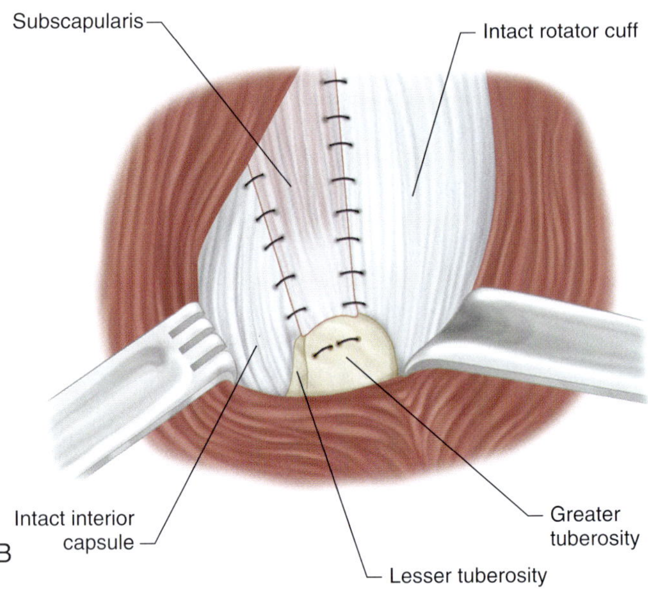

B

FIGURE 24

- The subscapularis is transferred superiorly, closing the residual defect. The superior border is sutured to the residual cuff, its lateral end to the greater tuberosity, and its inferior border to the superior edge of the anterior capsule (Fig. 24A and 24B).

Transfer of the Teres Minor and Subscapularis

- If the subscapularis transfer alone does not provide adequate coverage, the teres minor can be transferred superiorly from its more posterior position in combination with the subscapularis transfer as just described.
- After the subscapularis has been separated, detached, and mobilized, the teres minor tendon is freed from the posterior capsule in a fashion similar to that described for the subscapularis, beginning at the musculotendinous junction and moving toward the insertion (Fig. 25).
- The tendon is detached from the tuberosity, and the muscle-tendon unit is bluntly mobilized and rotated anterosuperiorly to meet the subscapularis, which has also been rotated superiorly (Fig. 26).
- The tendons are sutured together fixed to the greater tuberosity via a trough and bone tunnels. The inferior border of the tendon is fixed to the superior portion of the capsule (Fig. 27A and 27B).

Latissimus Dorsi Transfer

- The patient is placed in the lateral decubitus position with the affected shoulder and arm up. The shoulder and arm are draped free with the prepped surgical

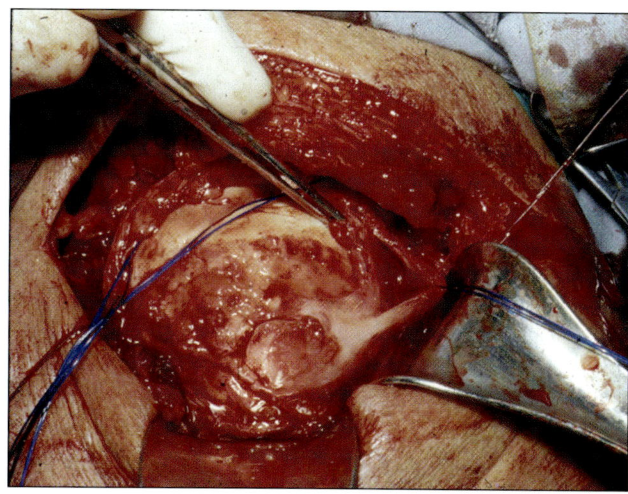

FIGURE 25

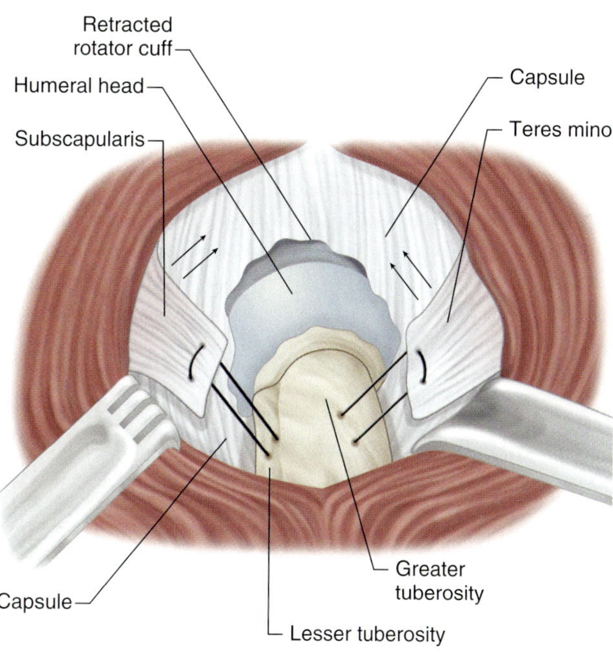

FIGURE 26

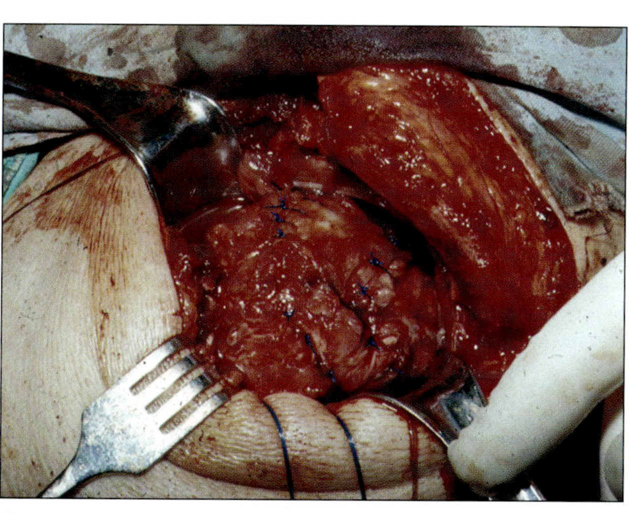

A

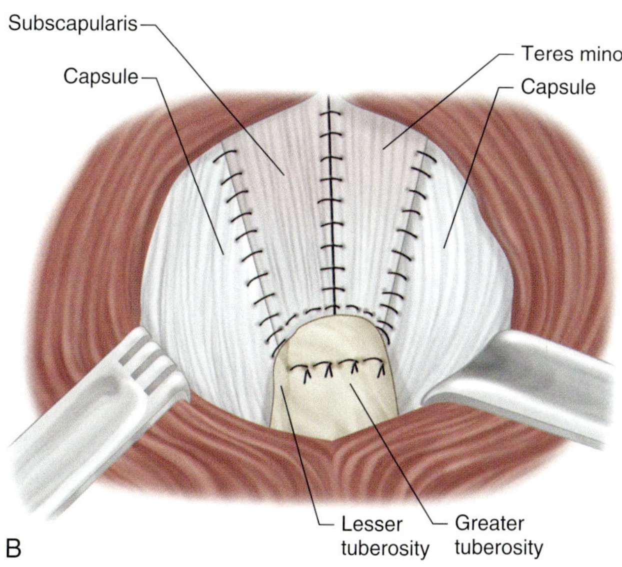

B

FIGURE 27

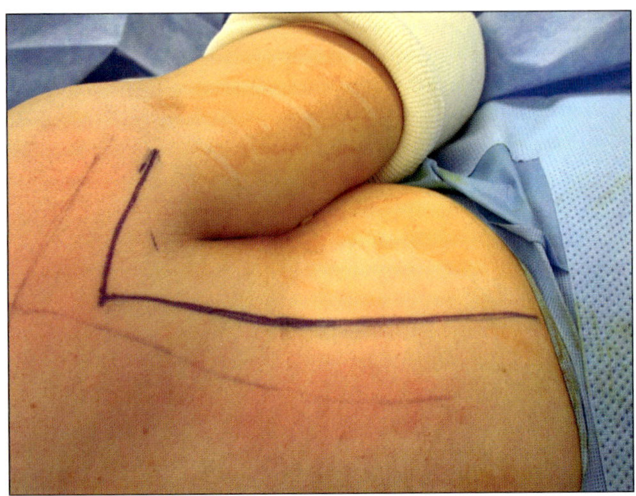

FIGURE 28

area wide enough to permit access to the latissimus dorsi muscle, as well as the anterior part of the shoulder.

- An incision is made on the back over the latissimus muscle (Fig. 28). After undermining the flaps, the latissimus dorsi muscle is identified and traced proximally to its insertion on the lesser tuberosity. Maximal length of the tendon all the way to its humeral attachment can be enhanced by internally rotating the shoulder in some abduction.
- The tendon is then detached at its insertion on the humerus (Fig. 29A and 29B), with care being taken to avoid injuring the radial nerve, which passes just beneath the tendons of the latissimus and teres major. The muscle is then mobilized bluntly and

Pitfalls

- *If the anterior and/or posterior capsules are taken with the teres minor and subscapularis tendons transferred, and not left undisturbed, shoulder instability will ensue.*
- *If the subscapularis is not intact, the latissimus transfer cannot be done. Therefore, the status of the subscapularis must be assessed by both physical examination (lift-off test and abdominal press test) and MRI.*

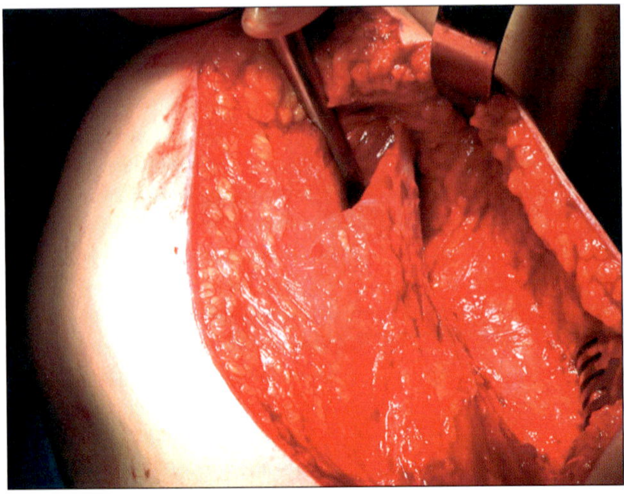

A

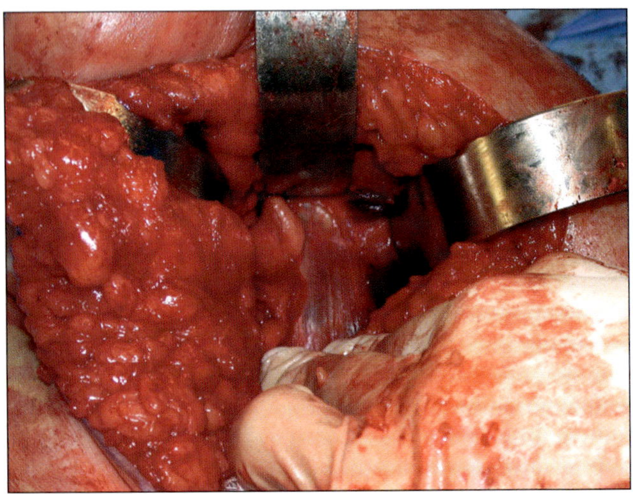

B

FIGURE 29

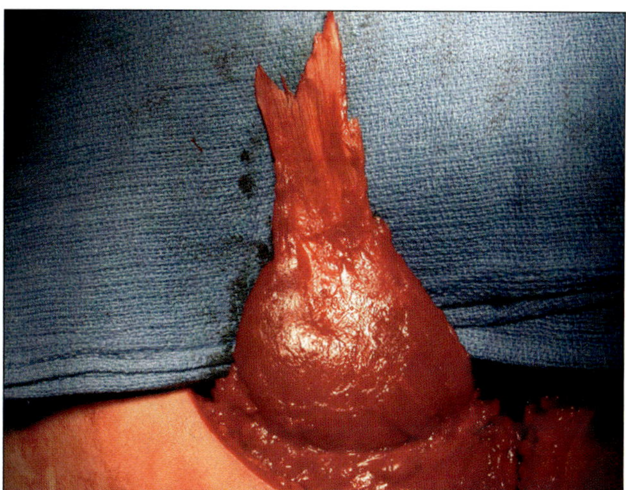

FIGURE 30

carefully well back toward its origin, constantly protecting the neurovascular bundle. This must be preserved, although gentle, careful mobilization of the bundle can provide some additional length to the musculotendinous unit (Fig. 30).

- An anterolateral mini-open approach is made to the anterior and superior cuff, allowing access to the cuff tear and the subscapularis. With an elevator or other blunt technique, a tunnel is developed under the deltoid from posterior to anterior. It must be wide enough to allow easy passage of the latissimus under the deltoid without constricting it. A traction suture is placed into the tendon of the latissimus and is used to pull the latissimus via its tendon under the deltoid to appear in the anterior exposure (Fig. 31). It is then advanced farther so that it reaches the upper border of the intact subscapularis.

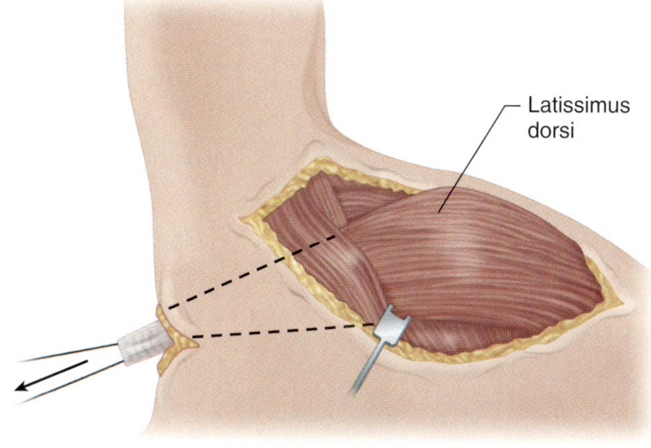

FIGURE 31

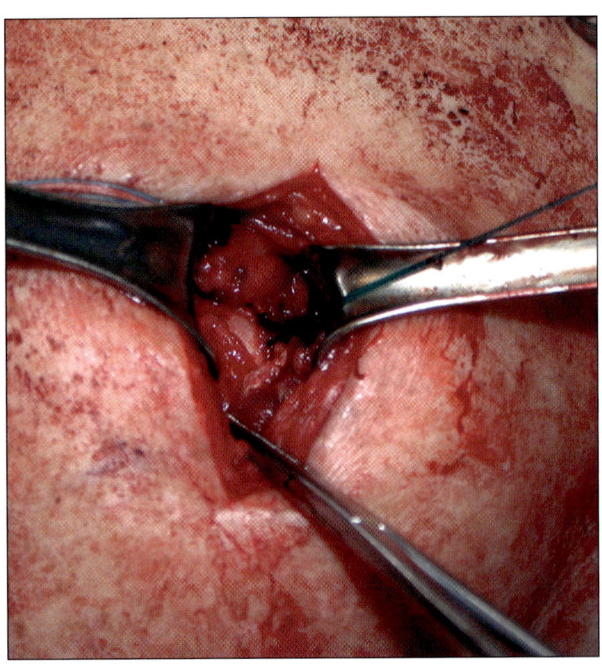

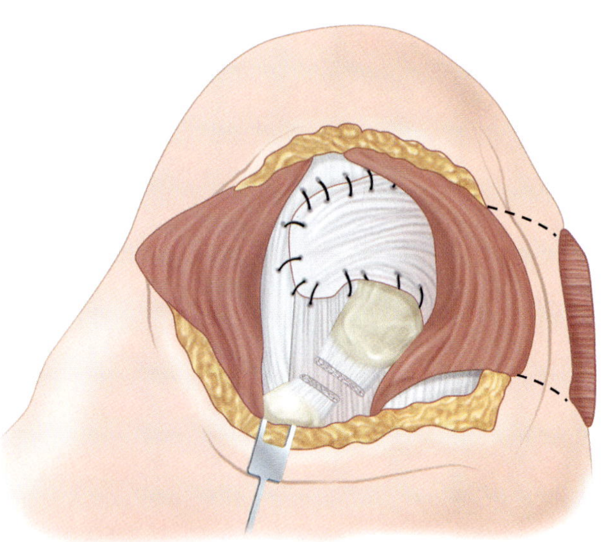

A B

FIGURE 32

- The tendon is attached to the upper border of the subscapularis with two or three nonabsorbable sutures in a horizontal mattress fashion (Fig. 32A and 32B). The lateral edge of the latissimus is sutured to the roughened area of the anatomic neck at the greater tuberosity with suture anchors.
- The wounds are closed routinely. The arm is immobilized in slight abduction, forward flexion, and external rotation.

Pitfalls

- *Introducing strenghtening before 12 weeks in any of these procedures, regardless of the size of tear, is fraught with the likelihood that the repair will pull apart.*

Postoperative Care and Expected Outcomes

- The dressing is changed after 24-72 hours. Passive forward elevation and external rotation to neutral in a supine position is begun at this time. The patient must be educated that this is a purely passive exercise.
- Range of passive forward flexion is slowly increased over the next 4-6 weeks. External rotation can be graduated to no more than 10-15° beyond neutral at the most.
- A shoulder immobilizer is used at all times except during these exercises for 6 weeks. With the latissimus transfer, the above-described position of immobilization is maintained in a brace when not exercising and the arm is not brought into extension, adduction, or internal rotation for 6 weeks.

- Active and assisted motion can be commenced after 6 weeks and srengthening at 3 months.
- Outcomes
  - Repair of small and medium-sized tears is successful in relieving pain, recovering function, and remaining structurally intact regardless of the repair technique.
  - With larger tears, pain relief and function after repair remain good but there is a lower likelihood that they will remain structurally intact.

Evidence

Birmingham PM, Neviaser RJ. Outcome of latissimus dorsi transfer as a salvage procedure for failed rotator cuff repair with loss of elevation. J Shoulder Elbow Surg. 2008;17:871-4.

Eighteen patients, referred from an outside institution with massive, irreparable rotator cuff tears and loss of elevation, were treated with a latissimus dorsi tendon transfer as a salvage procedure for failed prior attempted rotator cuff repair. Clinical outcomes were measured by the American Shoulder and Elbow Surgeons (ASES) score, pain level, and active range of motion. The average postoperative ASES score was 61, an increase from 43 preoperatively ($p = .05$)*. Active elevation improved to an average of 137° compared to 56° preoperatively* ($p < .001$)*. The average postoperative pain level was 22, down from 59* ($p = .001$)*, and the average postoperative active external rotation at the side was 45°, improved from 31°* ($p < .001$)*. Latissimus transfer, as a salvage procedure for failed rotator cuff repair with loss of elevation, allows for significant return of active elevation and function with minimal postoperative pain. (Level IV evidence)*

Cofield RH. Subscapularis muscle transposition for repair of chronic rotator cuff tears. Surg Gynecol Obstet. 1982;154:667-72.

Subscapularis transposition into a supraspinatus or supraspinatus and infraspinatus rotator cuff defect has been overlooked as a method of tendon repair. The surgical technique for this type of repair is described. Postoperatively, the extremity is supported in a position that does not allow stress to be placed on a repair until healing has occurred. Generally, physical therapy is begun early and continued for many months. Satisfactory relief of pain was achieved in 22 of 26 patients. Active abduction in the plane of the scapula averaged 120° for patients with rotator cuffs repair and prosthetic replacement and 130° for those with rotator cuff repair alone. Twelve patients gained more than 30° active abduction, and four lost this amount of motion or greater. In two patients, the repair was completely disrupted during the acute postoperative period. Twenty-five of the 26 patients were satisfied with the surgical procedure. This type of repair seems to be a secure repair, bring healthy tendon tissue into an area of tendon degeneration and loss of tissue substance. As such, it satisfies the basic surgical principles of achieving repair with healthy tissue that is not under tension. The results compare favorably with those reported in the literature on rotator cuff repair and further suggest that this technique is an acceptable alternative for repairing large or massive rotator cuff tears that have tendon substance loss. (Level IV evidence)

Cooper DL, O'Brien SJ, Warren RF. Supporting layers of the glenohumeral joint. An anatomic study. Clin Orthop. 1993;289:144-55.

Through dissection of 15 fresh frozen and two embalmed shoulders, the authors defined four tissue layers supporting the glenohumeral joint.

Gerber C, Vinh TS, Hertel R, Hess CW. Latissimus dorsi transfer for the treatment of massive tears of the rotator cuff: a preliminary report. Clin Orthop Relat Res. 1988;(232):51-61.

Symptomatic irreparable rotator cuff tears usually entail complete loss of the substance of the supraspinatus and infraspinatus tendons. Loss of external rotation control and cranial migration of the humeral head on attempted flexion or abduction of the shoulder are the functional hallmarks. Transfer of the latissimus dorsi tendon from the humeral shaft to the superolateral humeral head provides a large, vascularized tendon that can be used to close a massive cuff defect and that exerts an external rotation and head-depressing moment that allow more effective action of the deltoid muscle. This procedure was carried out in 14 patients without any significant complications. Pain relief and functional results in those four cases with a minimum follow-up period of 1 year (average, 14 months) compared favorably with alternative treatment methods. (Level IV evidence)

Karas SE, Giacello TL. Subcapularis transfer for reconstruction of massive tears of the rotator cuff. J Bone Joint Surg [Am]. 1996;78:239-45.

Twenty patients who had a massive tear (>5 cm) of the rotator cuff that was not amenable to direct tendon-to-bone or tendon-to-tendon repair had reconstruction consisting of transfer of the subscapularis tendon in conjunction with subacromial decompression. At a mean of 30 months (range, 23-70 months) after the operation, 17 of the patients were satisfied with the result. Nineteen patients reported a decrease in pain compared with preoperatively. However, nine patients had weakness and discomfort with prolonged or repetitive overhead activities, and two patients had lost active elevation of the shoulder despite substantial relief of pain. Subscapularis transfer is a useful adjunct in the operative treatment of massive tears of the rotator cuff; it facilitates the closure of larger defects that are not amenable to simpler, more traditional reconstructive techniques. However, because there is a risk of the procedure adversely affecting active elevation of the shoulder, it should be used with caution in patients who have full functional elevation preoperatively.

Neviaser JS. Ruptures of the rotator cuff: new concepts in the diagnosis and operative treatment for chronic tears. Arch Surg. 1971;102:483-5.

Ten patients with an average age of 57 years had a large to massive rotator cuff tear reconstructed with a free long head of the biceps tendon graft, when the defect could bt reduced with mobilization but not fully closed. Follow-up averaged 1 year. Nine of 10 patients had good pain relief and elevation of greater than 140°, and were satisfied with the outcome. (Level IV evidence)

Neviaser JS, Neviaser RJ, Neviaser TJ. The repair of chronic massive ruptures of the rotator cuff by use of a freeze dried rotator cuff graft. J Bone Joint Surg [Am]. 1978;60:681-4.

In 16 patients with massive tears of the rotator cuff, bridging of the defect with a freeze-dried graft of a rotator cuff from a cadaver produced a satisfactory repair in all cases. A good (elevation between 90° and 120°) or excellent (elevation over 120°) functional result was obtained in all but 2 patients, with a definite decrease or absence of nocturnal pain in all 16. The operative technique includes avoidance of a complete acromionectomy or detachment of the deltoid from the acromion. (Level IV evidence)

Neviaser RJ, Neviaser TJ. Major ruptures of the rotator cuff. In Watson M (ed). Practical Shoulder Surgery, Section V. London: Grune & Stratton, 1985:171-224.

This chapter provides the original detailed description of the subperiosteal elevation of the deltoid and the anterior-superior approach for open repair of the rotator cuff.

Neviaser RJ, Neviaser TJ. Transfer of the subscapularis and teres minor for massive defects of the rotator cuff. In Bayley I, Kessel L (eds). Shoulder Surgery. Heidelberg: Springer-Verlag, 1982:60-9.

Seventeen patients underwent transfer of the subscapularis and teres minor and were followed for 1-6 years. Preoperatively, 16 had elevation of less than 30° while postoperatovely, 12 had greater than 90°. Of the five poor results, three had deltoid damage from previous open surgery. This procedure is a satisfactory salvage alternative for irreparable massive tears with poor native motors, which preclude the use of a graft. (Level IV evidence)

PROCEDURE 5

Arthroscopic Repair of Massive Rotator Cuff Tears

Marc S. Kowalsky and Leesa M. Galatz

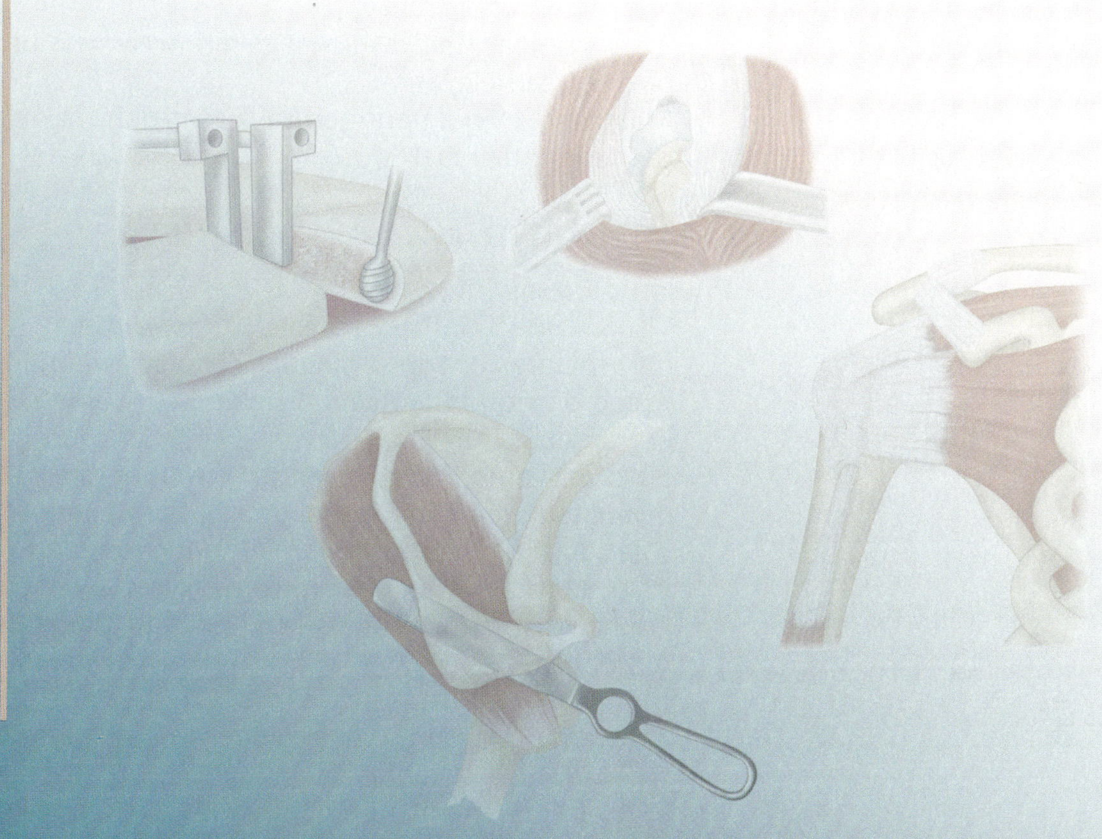

Pitfalls

- *Candidates for arthroscopic massive rotator cuff repair must have the ability to comply with a prolonged course of rehabilitation.*
- *Concomitant arthritis may indicate need for arthroplasty.*
- *Advanced atrophy and fatty change of rotator cuff musculature suggest irreparable tear.*
- *Rule out adhesive capsulitis.*

Controversies

- One should approach certain patients with caution, as advanced age, tobacco use, or certain systemic diseases may decrease likelihood of successful repair with healing and symptomatic relief (Galatz et al., 2004; Keener et al., 2010).
- Some surgeons have achieved effective pain relief and improved clinical outcomes with arthroscopic débridement, subacromial decompression, and biceps tenotomy, and offer this approach as an alternative, particularly when the reparability of a massive tear is in question (Boileau et al., 2007).

Indications

- Symptomatic, painful rotator cuff tear that does not respond to conservative modalities (nonsteroidal anti-inflammatory medication, physical therapy, and possible injections)
- Repairable rotator cuff tear as determined by careful evaluation of the characteristics of the tear on advanced imaging and intraoperative examination, including chronicity, size, retraction, muscle atrophy, and fatty degeneration
- An acute tear that results in severe weakness or loss of overhead elevation
- Massive tear in a younger (<60-year-old), high-demand individual

Examination/Imaging

Physical Examination

- Visual inspection may reveal atrophy of the infraspinatus or supraspinatus, scapular winging with range of motion indicating nerve injury, and shoulder asymmetry.
- Both active and passive range of motion are evaluated, including forward elevation, external rotation (ER) at the side, ER in abduction, and internal rotation/extension as measured by the most cephalad spinous process reached with the affected extremity.
- Manual strength testing is conducted.
  - External rotation with shoulder in slight internal rotation
  - "Thumbs-down" abduction with arms in scapular plane
- Certain findings indicate larger tears.
  - Lag sign with arm in maximal ER at the side—supraspinatus,infraspinatus
  - Hornblower's (strength in abduction and ER)—teres minor
  - Abdominal compression test—subscapularis
  - Lift-off test—subscapularis
- Provocative maneuvers are helpful to diagnose cuff-generated pain.
  - Neer and Hawkins signs, as well as the Jobe and drop arm signs
  - Provocative tests for pain from the long head of the biceps brachii, including Speed's and Yergason's tests

- The acromioclavicular joint must be assessed.
  - Tenderness to palpation
  - Pain with cross-body adduction

Treatment Options

- Nonoperative management
  - Nonsteroidal anti-inflammatory medications
  - Physical therapy
  - Possible corticosteroid injections
- Open rotator cuff repair
- Arthoscopically assisted mini-open rotator cuff repair
- Biceps tenotomy or tenodesis
- Subacromial decompression and débridement

Imaging Studies

- Radiographs
  - Anteroposterior (AP), true AP, scapular lateral, and axillary views are reviewed for acromioclavicular joint osteoarthritis, glenohumeral joint osteoarthritis, and acromial morphology.
  - Decreased acromiohumeral interval and/or proximal humeral migration of the humeral head in relation to the glenoid indicates large or chronic tear that may be irreparable (Keener et al., 2009).
- Magnetic resonance imaging is used to assess tear size and tendon involvement, tendon retraction, muscle quality and degree of degeneration, and glenohumeral joint pathology.
  - Degenerative labral and biceps lesions are common and not usually the primary source of pain.
  - Sagittal and coronal oblique T_2-weighted images are used to quantify the tear size and the degree of retraction, respectively (Fig. 1). A massive tear typically involves greater than 5 cm of the rotator cuff footprint, or at least two tendons.
  - Axial images are used to evaluate the subscapularis and long head of the biceps brachii.

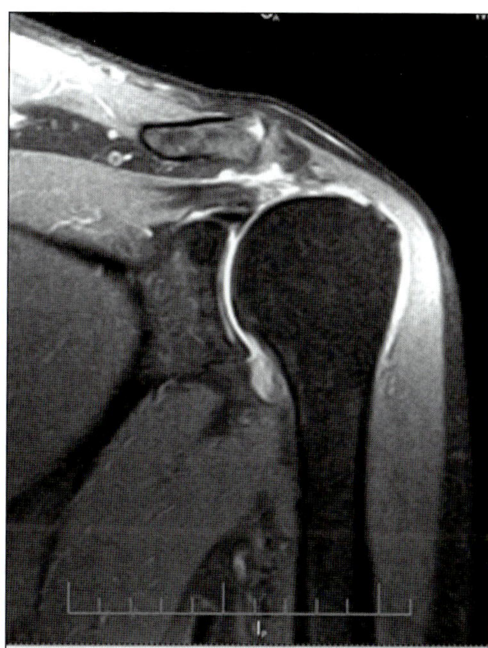

FIGURE 1

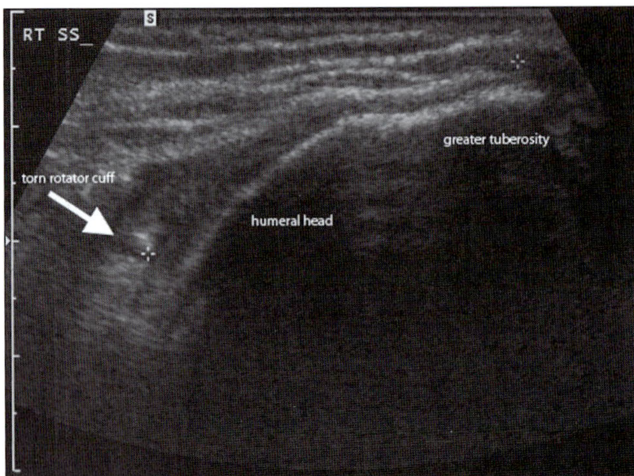

FIGURE 2

- Medial images of the sagittal T_1-weighted sequence are used to assess atrophy and fatty infiltration of the rotator cuff muscle bellies (Fuchs et al., 1999; Liem et al., 2007).

- Ultrasound has been proven to be a reliable modality for assessment of the rotator cuff (Fig. 2) (Teefey et al., 2004).
  - Ultrasonographer dependent
  - Very accurate for rotator cuff pathology
  - Not as useful for intra-articular biceps pathology

Surgical Anatomy

- The rotator cuff consists of the tendons of four muscles: the subscapularis anteriorly, the supraspinatus superiorly, and the infraspinatus and teres minor posteriorly. The rotator cuff muscles function in force couples, in which the deltoid counters the inferior rotator cuff (infraspinatus, teres minor, and subscapularis below the center of rotation), and the anterior rotator cuff (subscapularis) counters the posterior cuff (infraspinatus, teres minor) to maintain a centered humeral head relative to the glenoid.
- The rotator cable represents a crescenteric thickening of the tendon that inserts onto the greater tuberosity anteriorly and posteriorly. The function of this structure has been theorized to protect the relatively avascular zone of the rotator cuff tendon from stress during force transmission. Further, this structure preserves the coronal force couple even in the presence of an isolated supraspinatus tear by

transmitting force along the cable to the greater tuberosity.

- The rotator cuff insertion, or enthesis, consists of four zones: tendon, fibrocartilage, mineralized fibrocartilage, and bone. This continuous microstructure serves to distribute stress along the entire enthesis.
- Understanding of the anatomy of the rotator cuff footprint, and the contribution of each muscle, has evolved over time (Fig. 3) (Mochizuki et al., 2008).
  - According to the most current analysis thereof, the supraspinatus footprint is smaller than previously thought, representing a triangle with a medial-lateral length of 6.9 mm and an anterior-posterior length of 12.6 mm at its largest point adjacent to the humeral head articular surface.
  - The infraspinatus footprint has a trapezoidal shape, and measures 10.2 mm in medial-lateral length and 20.2-32.7 mm in anterior-posterior length.
  - The glenohumeral joint capsule inserts on the superior aspect of the greater tuberosity immediately adjacent to the humeral head articular surface, and has a medial-lateral footprint of 4.5 mm. As one moves posteriorly along the greater tuberosity, a bare area arises between the capsule and humeral head articular surface with no soft tissue attachments.

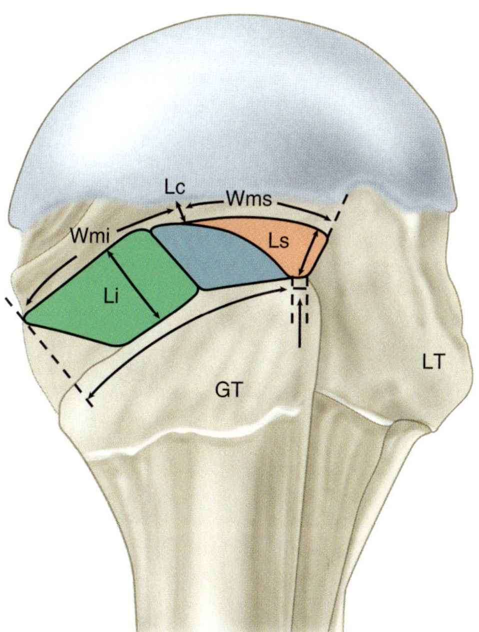

FIGURE 3

- The scapular spine serves as a landmark between the muscle bellies of the infraspinatus and supraspinatus, which can be used to determine the appropriate location for a posterior interval slide. Likewise, the coracoid serves as the landmark to determine the interval between the supraspinatus and subscapularis and can be helpful when an anterior interval slide is performed. Even when interval releases are not required, releasing the coracohumeral ligament, which originates on the coracoid and becomes confluent with the rotator interval tissue, is often necessary to adequately mobilize the rotator cuff for repair without tension.
- The rotator interval consists of the space and tissue between the upper border of the subscapularis and the anterior border of the supraspinatus. Soft tissues comprise the coracohumeral ligament and the superior glenohumeral ligament.
- The long head of the biceps tendon arises from the superior labrum at the supraglenoid tubercle and is intra-articular for approximately 2.8 cm before it exits the joint at the intertubercular groove. Normal anatomy of the superior and anterosuperior labrum is variable.
- The suprascapular nerve arises from the upper trunk of the brachial plexus and enters the supraspinatus fossa through the suprascapular notch, just medial to the coracoclavicular ligaments. It courses posteriorly approximately 1.5 cm medial to the superior glenoid rim, and enters the spinoglenoid notch to innervate the infraspinatus.
  - The nerve can be released arthroscopically. Its role in shoulder pain associated with rotator cuff tears is controversial.
  - This nerve should be protected inferior to the cuff during mobilization of retracted cuff tissue.
- The axillary nerve arises from the posterior cord of the brachial plexus. It courses inferior to the subscapularis and glenohumeral joint capsule as it travels posteriorly to innervate the deltoid and teres major and to provide sensation to the lateral arm.

Positioning

- Arthroscopic rotator cuff repair is performed in the beach chair or lateral decubitus position. The authors prefer beach chair.

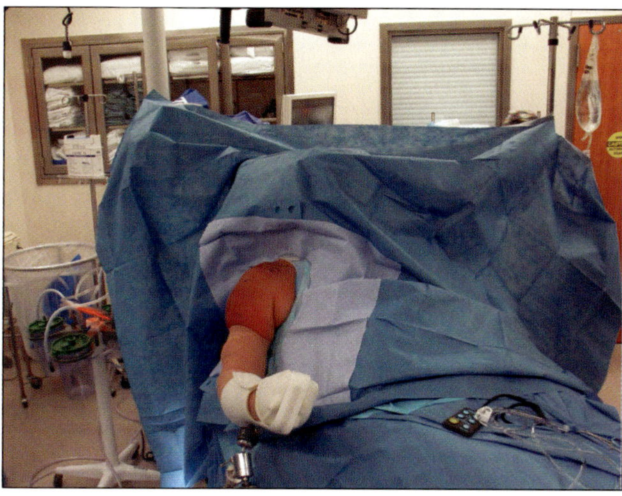

FIGURE 4

- The patient is placed in a sitting position 60° relative to the horizontal. The posterior shoulder must be adequately exposed to ensure proper access to the operative field (Fig. 4).
- The head is secured using a secure head positioner, maintaining the cervical spine in a neutral position.
- Using either a commercially available wedge or the operating table, the hips and knees are flexed appropriately to avoid undue tension on the neurovascular structures of the lower extremities.
- The contralateral extremity is secured to an armboard in a comfortable position. The ulnar nerve is padded.
- The table is angled approximately 45° away from the operative extremity to allow access to the posterior aspect of the shoulder.

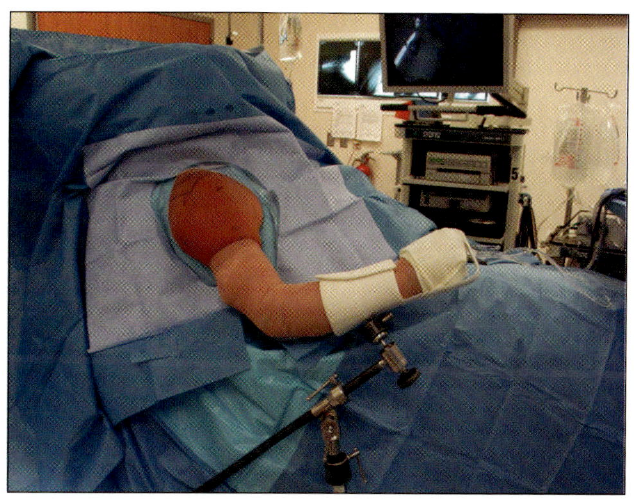

FIGURE 5

Pearls

- *Adequate exposure to both anterior and posterior shoulder is needed; the patient must be positioned as far as possible toward the operative side.*
- *A mechanical arm holder assists in holding the operative arm during the procedure and allows placement of traction on the arm to enlarge the subacromial space during repair (Fig. 5).*

Pitfalls

- *Inadequate exposure.*
- *Unstable cervical spine and head position.*
- *Inadequate padding of the contralateral arm and lower extremities.*
- *Some elderly patients may be at risk for a sudden drop in blood pressure while being positioned upright, so the back should be raised slowly with blood pressure monitoring.*

Equipment

- A commercially available extremity positioner
- Either a commercially available beach chair adapter, or an operating table that can accommodate the beach chair position

Controversies

- Some surgeons prefer to perform arthroscopic rotator cuff repair in the lateral decubitus position. This decision should be based primarily on surgeon experience and comfort.
- Increasing attention has been given to the relationship between the beach chair position and cerebral perfusion. The surgeon and anesthesiologist must assure that the patient's blood pressure resulting from elevation of the torso as well as hypotensive anesthesia remains within a safe range relative to the patient's baseline status.

Pearls

- *An accessory posterolateral portal on the lateral shoulder closer to the posterolateral corner of the acromion can be created to allow better visualization of the tear for tear pattern recognition. A 7-mm cannula can be inserted to ease movement of the arthroscope among portals.*
- *Percutaneous portals created along the anterolateral, lateral, and posterolateral borders of the acromion are created for insertion of anchors at the ideal angle.*
- *Percutaneous portals can also be used for antegrade suture-passing devices. These devices are helpful in retracted tears with tenuous tissue to allow suture placement as medial as possible.*

Portals/Exposures

- A posterior viewing portal is created 1-2 cm distal and 0.5-1 cm medial to the posterolateral corner of the acromion (Fig. 6).
  - If this portal is utilized exclusively for viewing, no cannula is necessary; however, if it will also be used as a working portal, then a 7-mm cannula can be inserted to ease movement of the arthroscope among portals.
- An anterolateral working portal is created 3 fingerbreadths distal to the lateral edge of the acromion, slightly anterior to the posterior edge of the acromioclavicular joint (Fig. 7).
  - A 7-mm cannula is inserted in this portal to allow insertion of instruments, including suture-passing devices.

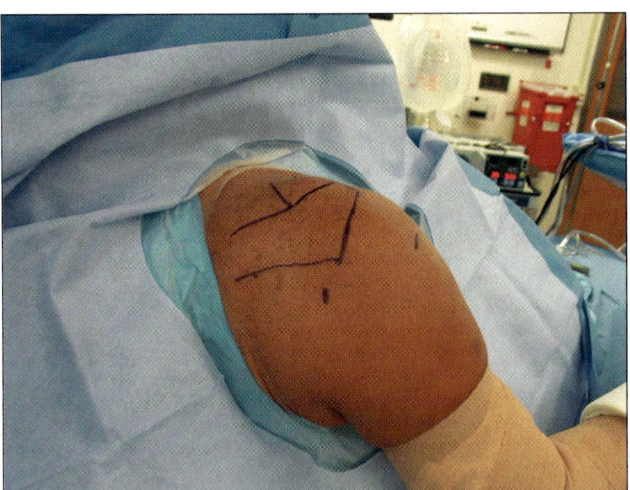

FIGURE 6

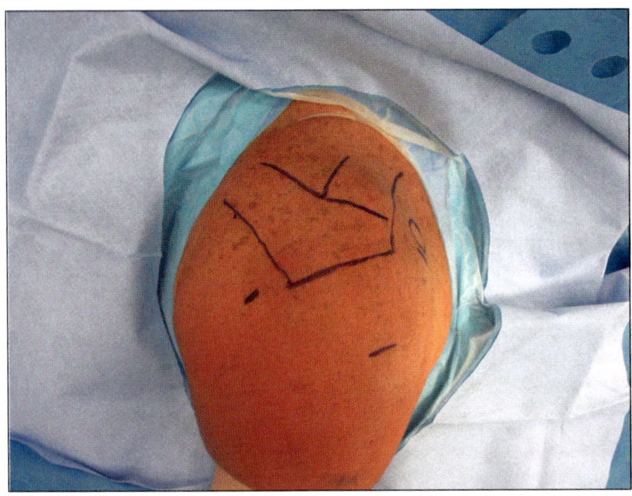

FIGURE 7

Pitfalls

- *The anterior and posterior portals should be placed sufficiently distal relative to the acromion to avoid caudal angulation of the cannulas as shoulder swelling increases.*
- *Particularly when using a posterior viewing portal exclusively, this portal should be placed sufficiently lateral to allow optimal visualization of the rotator cuff tear. Therefore, these authors advise creating this portal only slightly medial to the posterolateral acromial edge, rather than the traditional description of 1 cm medial to this landmark.*

Instrumentation

- 7-mm threaded cannulas for all working portals
- 5.5-mm cannula for the anterior shuttling portal

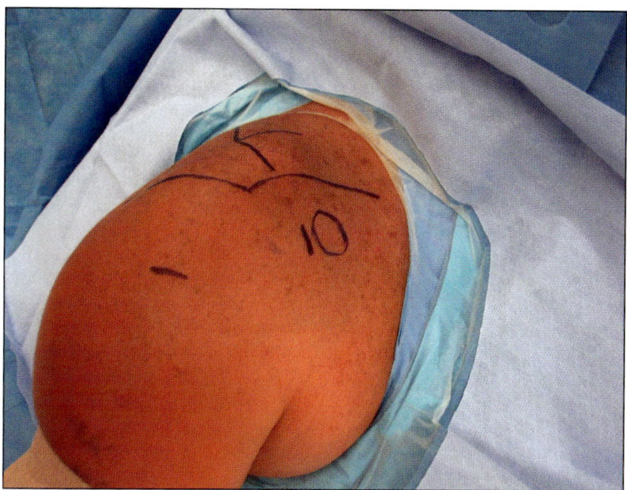

FIGURE 8

- A rotator interval portal is created immediately lateral to the coracoid process (Fig. 8).
  - This portal is utilized during the intra-articular examination. The cannula is redirected into the subacromial space to be used as a working portal during the rotator cuff repair.
  - If this portal is utilized exclusively for suture shuttling, a 5.5-mm cannula can be inserted; however, if it will also be used for suture passage, a 7-mm cannula can be inserted to allow insertion of suture-passing instruments.

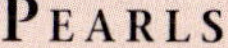

Pearls

- *Tears of the subscapularis are often missed and/or underappreciated.*

Pitfalls

- *Failure to identify and address concomitant long head of the biceps brachii tendon disease may lead to failed repair of a rotator cuff tear due to persistent postoperative pain.*

Procedure

Step 1

- Standard intra-articular diagnostic arthroscopy is first performed, with the arthroscope inserted through the posterior portal, and instruments inserted through the anterior rotator interval portal.
  - The long head of the biceps brachii tendon should be carefully examined for evidence of an unstable biceps origin, intrasubstance tearing, or instability in the bicipital groove. A biceps tenotomy or tenodesis may be indicated (Fig. 9).
- The subscapularis integrity is assessed to determine if repair is indicated (Fig. 10A and 10B).
- Other structures examined during intra-articular assessment include the undersurface of the cuff, the cartilaginous surfaces, labral tissue, and the inferior pouch. Their condition should be noted.
- The posterosuperior rotator cuff can be evaluated from the intra-articular perspective before proceeding

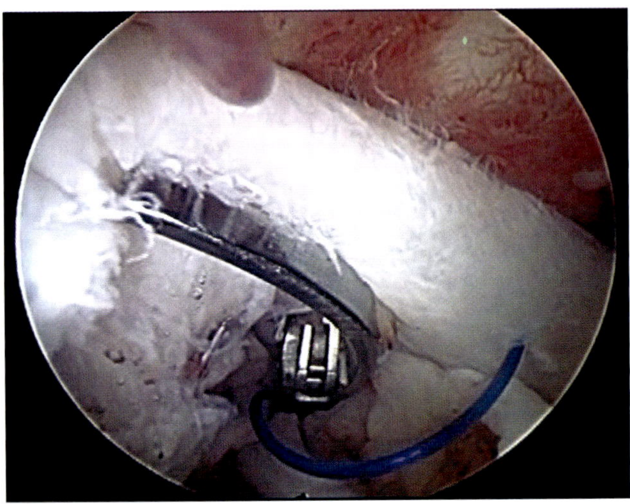

FIGURE 9

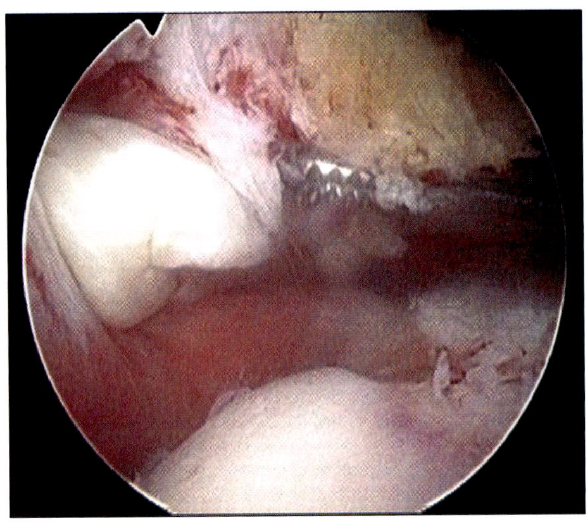

A

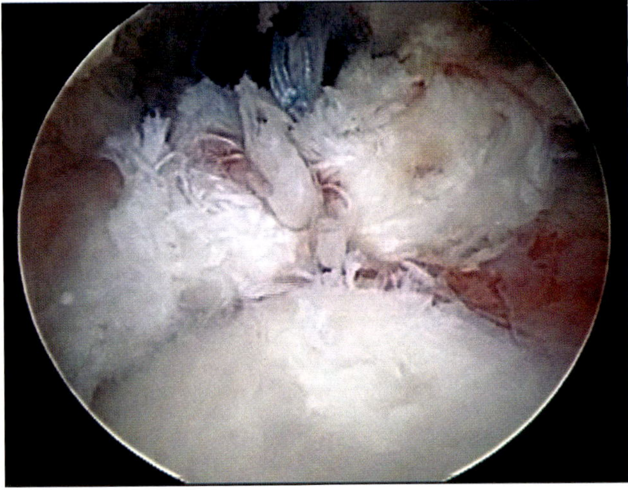

B

FIGURE 10

Controversies

- The decision to do a tenotomy or tenodess of the biceps is based on factors such as patient age, activity level, and body habitus. Older patients and those who will tolerate the cosmetic deformity well are treated with tenotomy. Young patients, or those who may be troubled by a cosmetic deformity, are instead treated with open tenodesis using screw fixation.

to the subacromial space (Fig. 11). This can provide valuable information about the degree of retraction, presence of delamination, and the status of the most posterior aspect of the rotator cuff.

Step 2

- The arthroscope is removed from the glenohumeral joint space and inserted into the subacromial space. Using slow deliberate movements, the bursa is swept in a medial-to-lateral direction from the underlying rotator cuff and overlying acromion.
- The anterolateral portal is created under direct visualization after spinal needle localization. The portal location should allow insertion of instruments parallel to the undersurface of the acromion for later

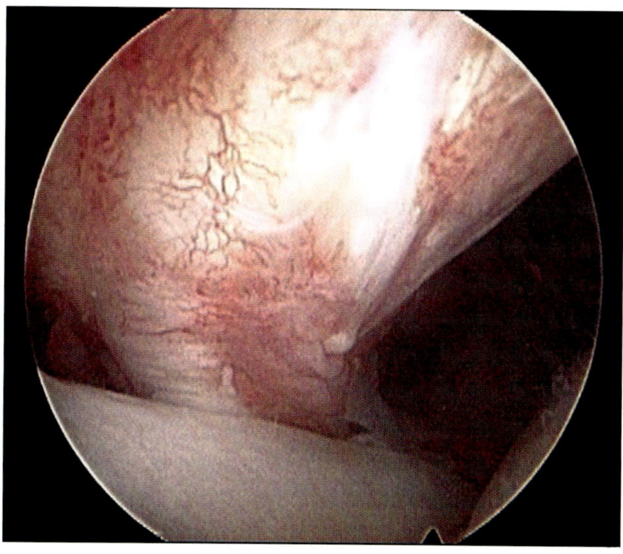

FIGURE 11

acromioplasty and allow access to the rotator cuff for suture passage. The cannula inserted through the anterior rotator interval portal is redirected into the subacromial space for later suture shuttling.

- A comprehensive bursectomy is performed using a combination of the arthroscopic shaver and thermoablation device. This is an exceedingly important step to assure visualization throughout the entire case, both medially for suture retrieval and laterally over the greater tuberosity for placement of lateral row anchors.
- Débridement of the rotator cuff tear is performed to define the tear edge, taking care to preserve as much tissue substance as possible (Fig. 12). The

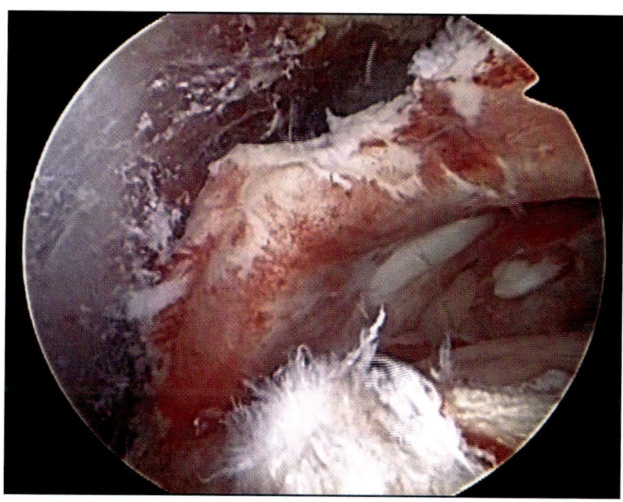

FIGURE 12

Pearls

- *Inserting the arthroscope into the anterolateral or accessory posterolateral viewing portal may aid in tear pattern recognition.*
- *Acromioplasty, if required, is reserved until after rotator cuff repair, as performing this step of the procedure, including takedown of the coracoacromial ligament, often allows escape of fluid into the deltoid and subcutaneous tissues, and may lead to excessive swelling.*

Pitfalls

- *Failure to recognize the tear pattern, and optimal method of reduction and repair of the torn tendon, may result in nonanatomic repair, which in turn will increase the likelihood of failure of the repair construct.*

Instrumentation/ Implantation

- 5.0-mm full-radius arthroscopic shaver
- Arthroscopic thermoablation device

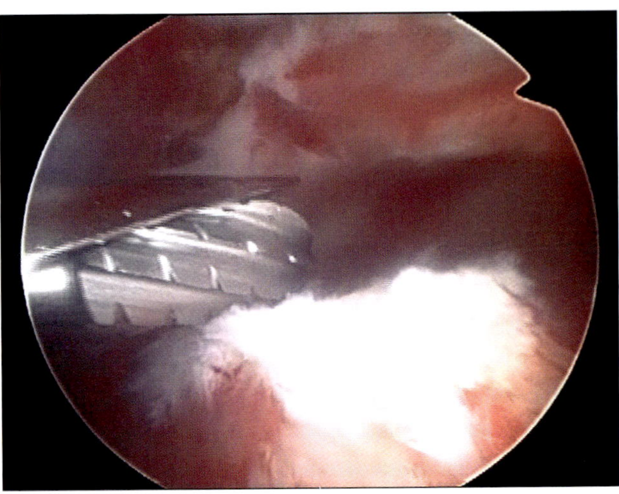

FIGURE 13

Controversies

- Some extol the virtues of posterior and anterior interval slides in order to enhance the mobility of a retracted massive rotator cuff tear. These authors feel that these techniques alter the biomechanical relationships of the individual rotator cuff tendons, and render the tissue difficult to manage during repair.

arthroscopic shaver and burr are also used to débride the rotator cuff footprint on the greater tuberosity to create a healing bed (Fig. 13).

- The rotator cuff tear is then carefully inspected to allow for recognition of the tear pattern. A tissue grasper can be inserted through the anterolateral portal to determine the optimal method of reducing the tear to its footprint, and to assess the degree of retraction and mobility of the tissue (Fig. 14). One must recognize if the tear is midsubstance in location. Identification of the myotendinous junction can also indicate the amount of residual tendon available for repair.
- If the tear cannot be reduced to its footprint without excessive tension, releases will be necessary.
  - Using the thermoablation device, the torn tendon can be released from the surrounding tissue on the

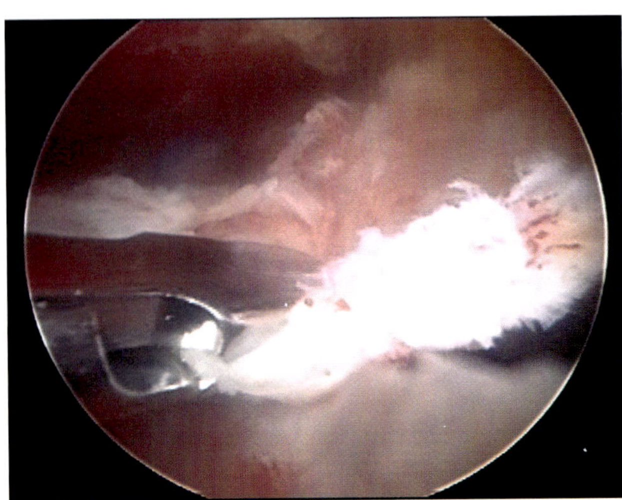

FIGURE 14

Pearls

- *The arm should be maximally adducted during anchor insertion to assure the ideal angle of insertion in the coronal plane.*
- *The arm can be internally and externally rotated to ease insertion of each anchor along the medial aspect of the tuberosity. For example, external rotation improves access to the anterior aspect of the tuberosity and internal rotation improves access to the posterior aspect of the tuberosity.*

Pitfalls

- *One must assure optimal depth of insertion of the suture anchors. Anchors that are inserted too deep may result in suture failure against cortical bone or repair construct elongation if the suture cuts through the cortical bone.*

Instrumentation/ Implantation

- An anchor specifically designed for rotator cuff repair is necessary to accommodate the soft and often osteopenic bone of the greater tuberosity. These anchors are larger and have broader threads compared to anchors designed for use in the glenoid.

glenoid and subacromial aspects. Care should be taken to maintain the device parallel to the tendon to avoid injury to the tissue. The tendon is released from adhesions in the subacromial space, especially at the base of the scapular spine. Adhesions can also occur between the cuff and the superior labrum.

- Release of the coracohumeral ligament is often very helpful in increasing mobility of the torn rotator cuff. The authors do not typically utilize posterior interval releases in the repair of massive rotator cuff tears.

- As the tear pattern dictates, margin convergence side-to-side suture repair may be necessary to translate the tendon edge laterally, closer to its footprint. This may further decrease the tension necessary to reduce the tendon to the greater tuberosity.

Step 3

- The rotator cuff tear and tuberosity should be inspected to determine the optimal number of medial-row anchors. Typically, two to three anchors are used along the medial row. These anchors are placed before insertion of the cannula into the anterolateral portal to avoid interference.
- A spinal needle is used to localize the percutaneous portal used for anchor insertion (Fig. 15). The starting point is typically along the lateral border of the acromion. This should allow anchor insertion at an angle of approximately 45° relative to the plane of the tuberosity.

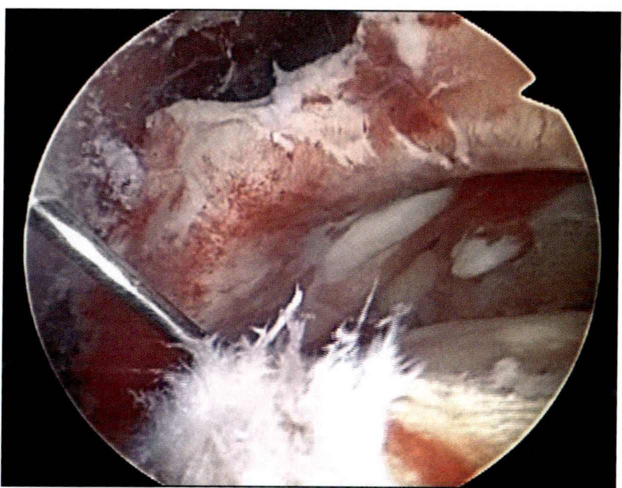

FIGURE 15

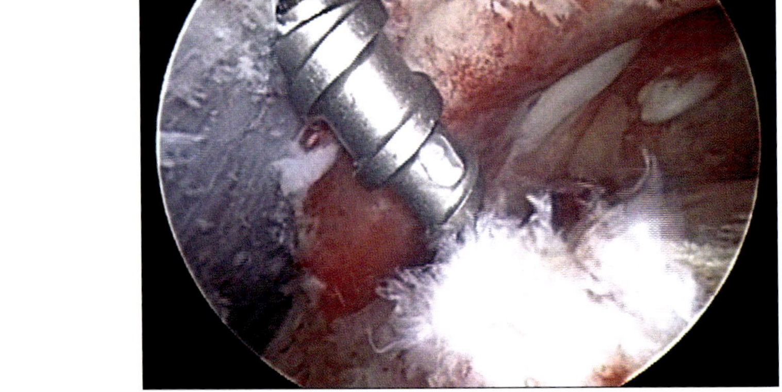

FIGURE 16

Controversies

- The authors prefer metallic anchors, although plastic and bioabsorbable anchors are available for rotator cuff repair. Metallic anchors have optimal resistance to pullout in poor-quality bone over time. They are visible on radiographs, should there be a need to localize them in the future. Bioabsorbable anchors often create a localized acidic environment resulting in lucency around the anchor and possible loosening.

- The knife is used to create a skin incision large enough to accommodate the suture anchor. A hemostat clamp is used to enlarge the path through the deltoid into the subacromial space.
- The first suture anchor is inserted, using a mallet to engage the threads of the anchor (Fig. 16). The anchor is inserted to a depth immediately beneath the cortical bone. Further, the orientation of the eyelet, as determined by a laser line on the inserter, should be perpendicular to the long axis of the tendon. This will allow the suture to slide more easily after passage in a horizontal mattress fashion.
- The inserter is removed, and traction on the sutures assures that the anchor is secure. The sutures are left in the percutaneous portal for later passage. The other anchors are then inserted in a similar manner through separate percutaneous portals (Fig. 17).

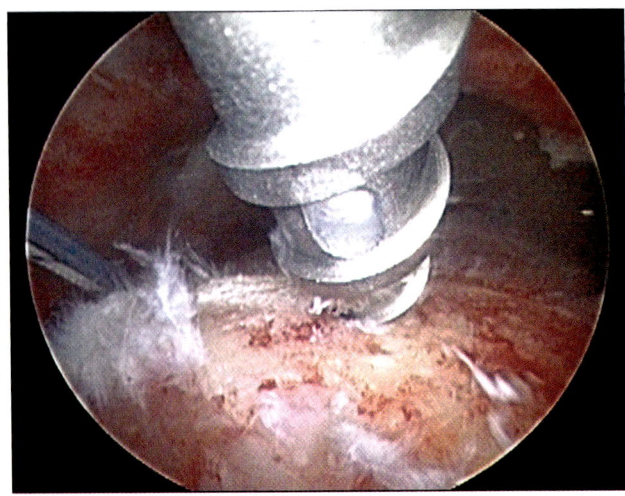

FIGURE 17

Pearls

- *Careful examination of the tear pattern, as discussed above, is exceedingly important in determining the optimal location for suture passage. The goal should always be reduction of the rotator cuff tendon to the greater tuberosity in as anatomic a position as possible.*
- *These authors typically park the passed suture limbs in the anterior cannula. Alternatively, these sutures can be retrieved through the percutaneous portal through which the anchor was inserted.*

Pitfalls

- *It is important to determine the orientation of the limbs of each suture through the anchor eyelet. The anterior limb should be retrieved and passed anteriorly to avoid crossing the limbs. Crossing suture limbs may inhibit sliding or result in suture abrasion against the eyelet.*

Step 4

- After all medial-row suture anchors have been placed, the 7.0-mm threaded cannula is inserted through the anterolateral portal. Sutures will be passed in a horizontal mattress fashion, working from anterior to posterior.
- The anterior-most suture limb of the first suture loaded through the anterior suture anchor is retrieved through the anterolateral portal using a suture grasper. Care is taken to avoid unloading the anchor while pulling this suture limb.
- A retrograde suture passing device (Scorpion) is used to pass each suture limb through the torn rotator cuff tendon (Fig. 18A and 18B). The suture limb is then retrieved through the anterior portal. This is repeated for each limb of each suture loaded through the anterior anchor.
- Care is taken to assure that enough substantial tendon tissue is captured with suture passage. If this cannot be achieved with the retrograde device, an antegrade device can be used from the Neviaser portal (Banana Lasso) (Fig. 19A and 19B). One must also assure that a sufficient bridge exists between the limbs of each suture to allow knot tying without cut-out of the suture through tendon. Once each of the sutures from a given anchor is passed through tendon and retrieved through the anterior portal, they are clamped together to avoid confusion and entanglement.
- This procedure is repeated for each of the sutures loaded through the remaining anchors of the medial

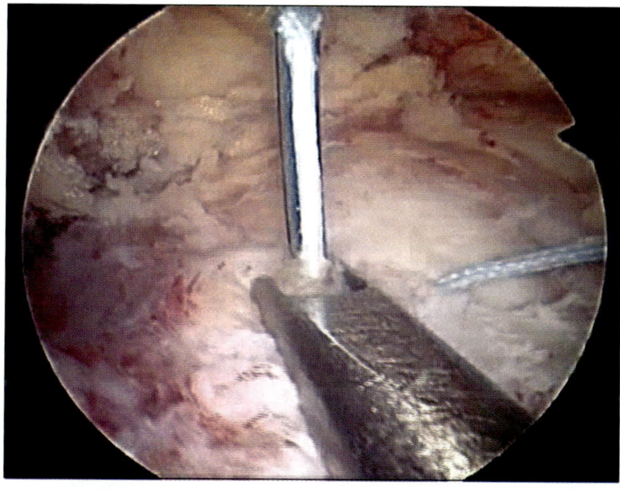

A

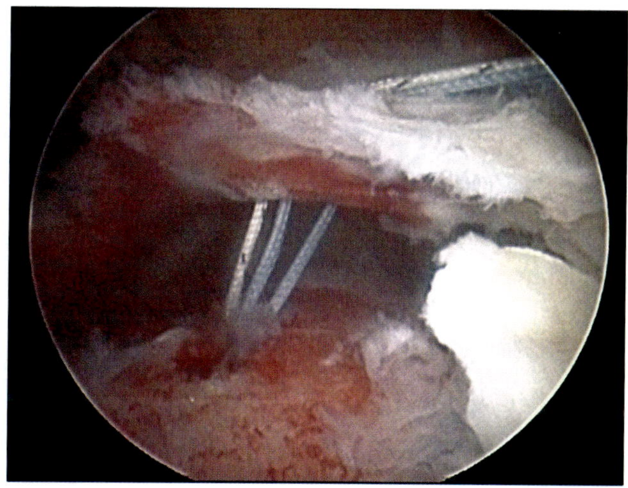

B

FIGURE 18

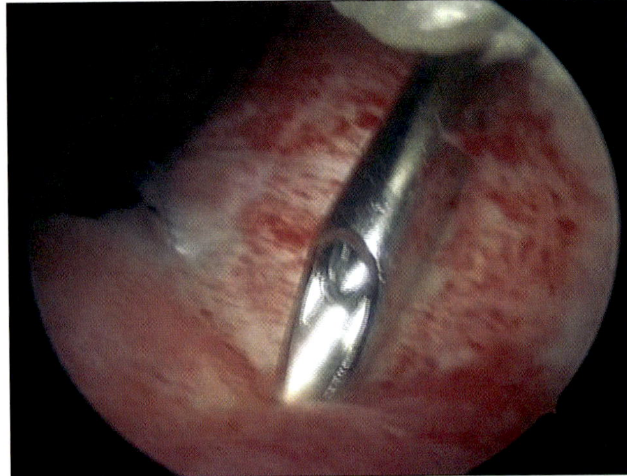

A

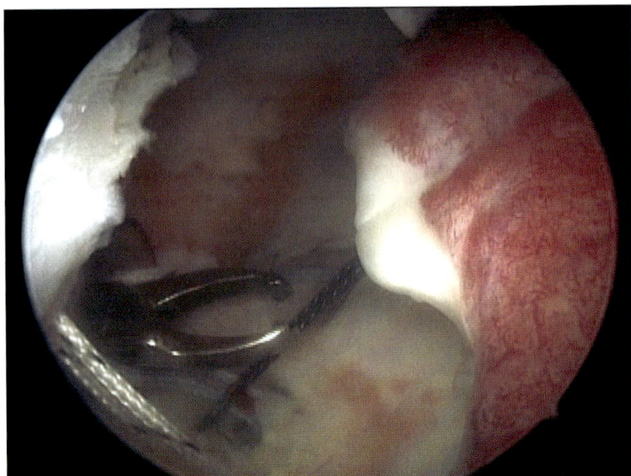

B

FIGURE 19

Instrumentation/ Implantation

- 7-mm threaded cannula
- Scorpion retrograde suture-passing device (Arthrex; Naples, FL)
- Banana Lasso antegrade suture-passing device (Arthrex; Naples, FL)
- Arthroscopic tissue grasper
- Arthroscopic suture grasper

row. All are retrieved through the anterior portal and clamped to separate the sutures of each anchors.

Step 5

- Once all suture limbs have been passed, sutures are tied beginning posteriorly.
    - The first pair of suture limbs is retrieved from the anterior portal through the anterolateral portal.
    - Sutures are tied using two half-hitch knots in the same direction to assure loop security, followed by three alternating half-hitch knots, alternating the post on the final throw, to achieve knot security (Fig. 20).
- After tying knots, the suture is retrieved through the percutaneous portal through which the anchor was previously placed for later placement of the lateral row anchors.

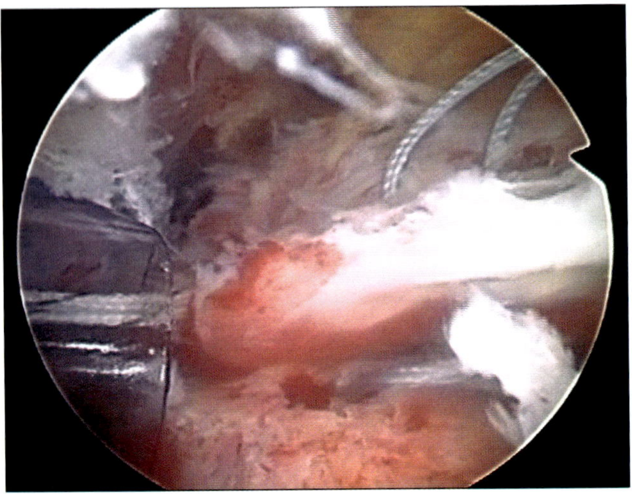

FIGURE 20

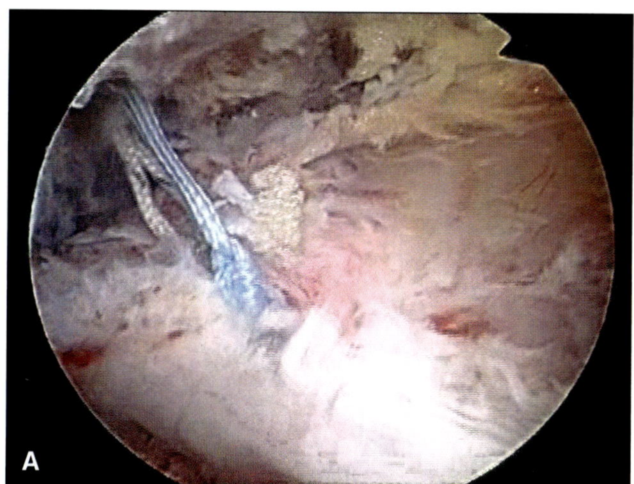

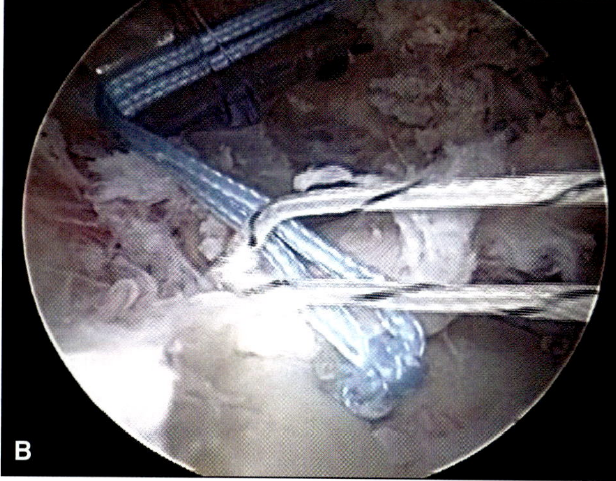

FIGURE 21

Instrumentation/ Implantation

- Arthroscopic suture grasper
- Arthroscopic knot pusher

Controversies

- The choice of knot is a matter of surgeon preference. These surgeons use two half-hitch knots in the same direction, followed by alternating half-hitches, alternating the post on the final throw.
- Alternatively, for the first knot, one can use a sliding knot such as the Tennessee Slider, or a sliding locking knot such as the Weston.

Pearls

- *Traction sutures can be placed in the torn rotator cuff and can be used to apply traction to the rotator cuff tendon, thus reducing the tendon prior to knot tying.*
- *The most posterior limb of the posterior sutures and the anterior limb of the anterior sutures should be chosen as the post to assure that the knots are placed posteriorly and anteriorly on the rotator cuff tendon.*
- *This divergence will assure, when placing the lateral row, that the suture configuration results in maximal surface area of compression of the tendon upon the footprint.*

Pitfalls

- *While secure knot tying is integral to assuring the strength of the repair construct, one must avoid abrading the suture, which may jeopardize the strength of the repair construct.*

- The remainder of the sutures are retrieved and tied through the anterolateral portal in sequence (Fig. 21A and 21B).

Step 6

- The authors use a transosseous-equivalent technique of repair. Once all sutures of the medial row have been tied, the lateral-row knotless suture anchors are placed. One suture limb from each of the medial-row anchors is retrieved through the anterolateral portal. The limbs are threaded through the eyelet of the knotless suture anchor (4.75-mm PEEK SwiveLock SP).

Pearls

- *The eyelet retention suture can be preserved and used to eliminate any residual "dog-ear" deformity by passing one limb through the tendon in either an antegrade or retrograde fashion. Otherwise, it can simply be removed and discarded.*

Pitfalls

- *The knotless suture anchor must be inserted to the appropriate depth.*
- *Inserting the anchor below cortical bone may jeopardize fixation, while inserting the anchor too proud may result in impingement within the subacromial space.*

Instrumentation/ Implantation

- 4.75-mm SwiveLock SP suture anchor (Arthrex; Naples, FL)
- Arthroscopic suture cutter

- The arm is brought into abduction to allow perpendicular placement of the anchor into the greater tuberosity. Just as the medial-row anchors are spaced equally along the medial aspect of the rotator cuff tear footprint, the lateral-row anchors should be spaced equally along the lateral aspect of the greater tuberosity, relative to the rotator cuff tear footprint. The arm can be rotated internally or externally to reveal the optimal location for anchor insertion.
- The thermoablation device is used to clear soft tissue from the lateral cortex in order to expose the bone for anchor insertion.
- The anchor is impacted using a mallet until the eyelet lies beneath the cortex. Preliminary tension is applied to the sutures to compress the torn rotator cuff tendon upon the footprint. The anchor is then impacted further until the tip of the anchor contacts the cortical bone. Final tension is applied to the sutures, and this tension is maintained. The anchor is then inserted by holding the thumb pad and rotating the handle until it is at the level of the cortical bone to ensure optimal fixation (Fig. 22). The eyelet retention suture is released, and the driver is removed. The suture limbs are then cut using an arthroscopic suture cutter.
- The rotator cuff repair should be examined both from the posterior and anterolateral portals, while internally and externally rotating the extremity (Fig. 23). The arthroscope may also be inserted into the glenohumeral joint space to examine the repair from the articular perspective.

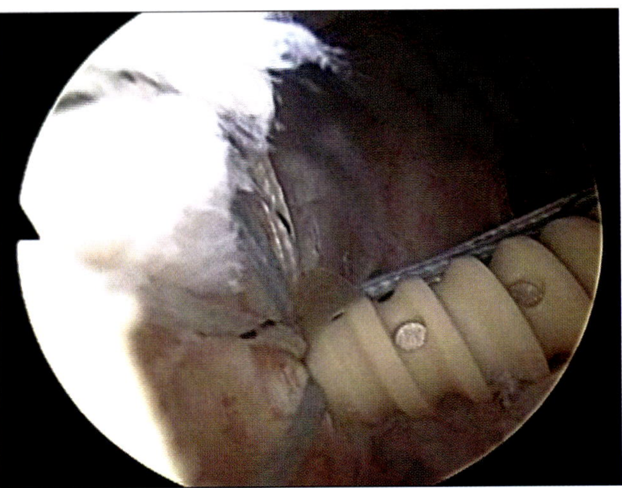

FIGURE 22

Controversies

- Controversy exists regarding single-row versus double-row repair. Double-row repairs have demonstrated enhanced biomechanical properties and restoration of the native footprint with compression of tendon to bone over a larger surface contact area.
- Effects of single-row versus double-row repair on healing and clinical outcome are varied and inconclusive, though improved postoperative structural integrity has been demonstrated with double-row techniques (Charousset et al., 2007; Park et al., 2008; Sugaya et al., 2005).
- Increased cost of double-row repair is a disadvantage.
- The authors prefer a double-row repair in younger patients in whom anatomic healing will likely have a greater effect on outcome and satisfaction.

Pearls

- *Avoid excessive bone removal.*
- *Protect the deltoid from injury.*

Pitfalls

- *Excessive bone removal, injury to the deltoid, and resection of the coracoacromial ligament could lead to iatrogenic anterior-superior instability.*
- *In the presence of an os acromiale, an acromioplasty is deferred to avoid destabilizing the fragment.*
- *If one is concerned about the security of the repair or likelihood of successful healing, one should consider deferring the acromioplasty to preserve the coracoacromial arch, which serves as a restraint to anterosuperior escape.*

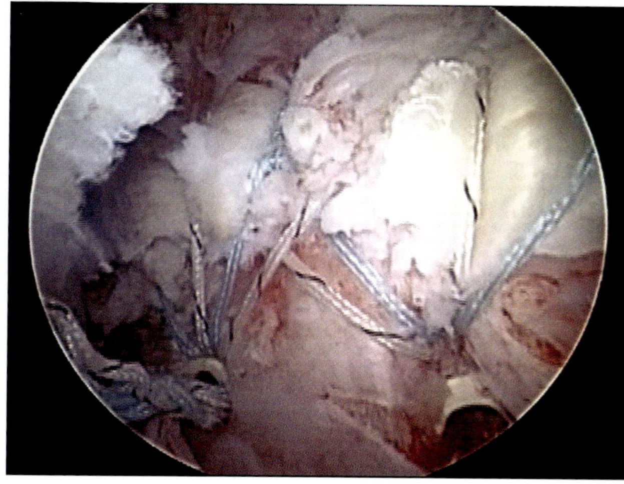

FIGURE 23

Step 7

- Once the repair is completed, attention is then turned to the acromioplasty. An acromioplasty is performed only in the presence of an acromial spur; it is not necessarily a routine part of the procedure.
- The borders of the acromion are defined using the thermoablation device. The acromial spur is exposed while taking care to preserve the deep deltoid fascia (Fig. 24).
- An acromioplasty is then performed using a 4.85-mm oval burr, removing only enough bone to reveal the native acromion, and to assure a flat undersurface (Fig. 25).
- The shaver is then used to complete the bursectomy, and to remove any loose osseous fragments from the acromioplasty.

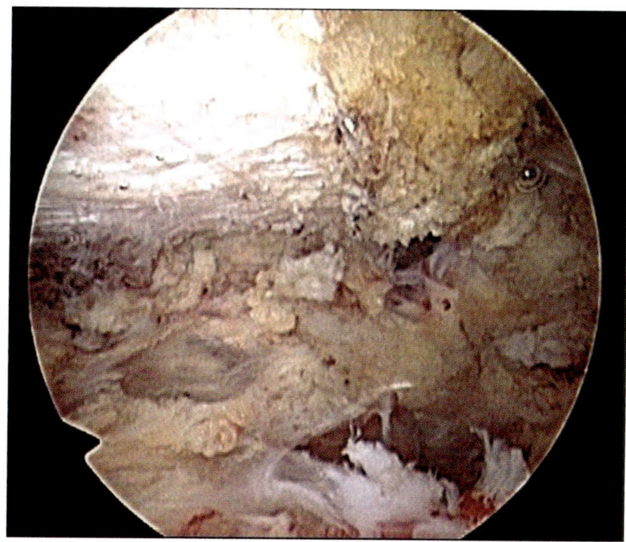

FIGURE 24

Instrumentation/ Implantation

- 4.85-mm arthroscopic burr
- 5.0-mm arthroscopic shaver

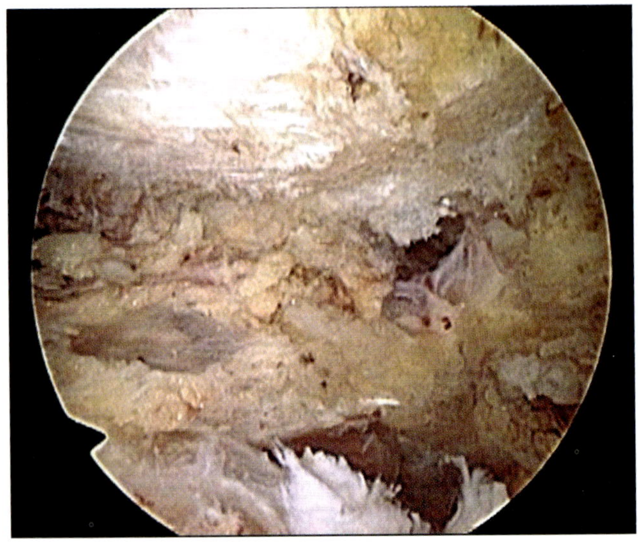

FIGURE 25

PEARLS

- *Adequate pain control is necessary to allow patients to progress with prescribed therapy.*
- *Cold therapy is useful in pain control and postoperative comfort.*

PITFALLS

- *Overly aggressive initial therapy may risk early repair failure.*

Controversies

- Conclusive evidence does not yet exist to support any specific rehabilitation protocol. Earlier protocols relied on early motion to avoid stiffness associated with open procedures.
- These authors have moved to a more conservative rehabilitation program in light of the low rate of healing after repair of massive rotator cuff tears. Further, stiffness may be less of a concern in the context of arthroscopic repair.

Postoperative Care and Expected Outcomes

- Patients who undergo massive rotator cuff repair are managed with a standard postoperative rehabilitation regimen:
  - Weeks 1-6: sling immobilization, waist-level activities of daily living, elbow/wrist/hand motion, no reaching/lifting/pulling/pushing.
  - Weeks 6-8: discontinue sling, begin passive range of motion (ROM)
  - Weeks 8-10: begin active-assisted ROM and active ROM
  - Weeks 10-12: begin progressive strengthening
- While healing rates of massive rotator cuff tears have been historically low, particularly in older patients with more aggressive rehabilitation, these patients are often still able to achieve favorable clinical outcomes (Galatz et al., 2004; Gerber et al., 2000; Harryman et al., 1991; Sugaya et al., 2007).
- Complications are rare with arthroscopic repair of massive rotator cuff tears. As discussed above, perhaps failure to heal is the most common complication. In addition, these patients may encounter stiffness, particularly when managed with a conservative rehabilitation regimen consisting of prolonged immobilization. Late stiffness can be treated with judicious use of corticosteroid injections and, in refractory cases, with arthroscopic lysis of adhesions.

Evidence

Boileau P, Baque F, Valerio L, Ahrens P, Chuinard C, Trojani C. Isolated arthroscopic biceps tenotomy or tenodesis improves symptoms in patients with massive irreparable rotator cuff tears. J Bone Joint Surg [Am]. 2007;89:747-57.

In this study, 68 patients who underwent arthroscopic biceps tenotomy or tenodesis for the treatment of massive irreparable rotator cuff tears were retrospectively reviewed at a minimum of 2 years after surgery; 78% of patients were satisfied. The mean Constant score improved from 46.3 to 66.5. There was no difference in outcome between the tenodesis and tenotomy groups. Cosmetic deformity occurred in 62% of patients, but none was symptomatic after tenotomy. Atrophic teres minor, pseudoparalysis, and severe cuff tear arthropathy were associated with worse clinical outcomes. (Level III evidence)

Charousset C, Grimberg J, Duranthon LD, Bellaiche L, Petrover D. Can a double-row anchorage technique improve tendon healing in arthroscopic rotator cuff repair? A prospective, nonrandomized, comparative study of double-row and single-row anchorage techniques with computed tomographic arthrography tendon healing assessment. Am J Sports Med. 2007;35:1247-53.

This prospective investigation compared patients who underwent arthroscopic single-row or double-row rotator cuff repair with minimum postoperative follow-up of 2 years using Constant scores, patient satisfaction, return to work, and postoperative computed tomography (CT) arthrogram to assess repair integrity at 6 months. There was no significant different in Constant scores between groups, with improvement in pain, activity, and strength in both groups. In addition, there was no difference in subjective satisfaction or return to work. While no statistically significant difference was detected in the incidence of "watertight" repairs on CT arthrogram (77.4% for double row, 60% for single row), there was a significantly higher incidence of "anatomic" footprint restoration in the double-row group. (Level II evidence)

Fuchs B, Weishaupt D, Zanetti M, Hodler J, Gerber C. Fatty degeneration of the muscles of the rotator cuff: assessment by computed tomography versus magnetic resonance imaging. J Shoulder Elbow Surg. 1999;8:599-605.

This study examined 41 patients undergoing shoulder surgery with CT and magnetic resonance imaging (MRI) to establish whether these methods were comparable in assessing rotator cuff fatty infiltration, and to establish a relationship between fatty infiltration and rotator cuff muscle atrophy. The study concluded that CT and MRI had excellent interobserver reliability, though the latter demonstrated superior reliability. The correlation between CT and MRI was fair to moderate. A relationship between fatty infiltration and atrophy was established.

Galatz LM, Ball CM, Teefey SA, Middleton WD, Yamaguchi K. The outcome and repair integrity of completely arthroscopically repaired large and massive rotator cuff tears. J Bone Joint Surg [Am]. 2004;86:219-24.

In this study, 18 patients who had complete arthroscopic repair of a tear measuring greater than 2 cm in the transverse dimension were evaluated at a minimum of 12 months and at 2 years after surgery. Seventeen of 18 patients demonstrated recurrent tears. Despite this lack of healing, clinical improvement was noted in certain patients at 12 months, including American Shoulder and Elbow Surgeons (ASES) scores greater than 90 points in 13 patients, improved functional outcome scores in 16, resolution of pain in 12, and improved motion with elevation above shoulder level in all 18. Clinical outcomes declined somewhat at 2 years, including ASES scores and forward elevation. (Level IV evidence)

Gerber C, Fuchs B, Hodler J. The results of repair of massive tears of the rotator cuff. J Bone Joint Surg [Am]. 2000;82:505-15.

This study prospectively evaluated 27 patients who underwent open repair of massive rotator cuff tears at a minimum of 2 years postoperatively with imaging and clinical evaluation. Overall, patients demonstrated improvement in the Constant score, range of motion, and pain; 63% of tendons demonstrated healing on final evaluation. Patients with recurrent tears demonstrated clinical improvement, albeit less than in those patients with intact repairs. Fatty infiltration was found to be irreversible, and muscle atrophy was only somewhat reversible, in intact supraspinatus repairs. (Level IV evidence)

Harryman DT 2nd, Mack LA, Wang KY, Jackins SE, Richardson ML, Matsen FA 3rd. Repairs of the rotator cuff: correlation of functional results with integrity of the cuff. J Bone Joint Surg [Am]. 1991;73:982-9.

In this study, 105 patients who underwent open rotator cuff repair were retrospectively reviewed at a minimum of 2 years postoperatively with imaging and clinical evaluation. Eighty percent of isolated supraspinatus tears successfully healed on ultrasound, whereas 50% of larger tears healed. Increased prevalence of recurrent tears was found in older patients and those who had undergone previous attempted repair. Most patients reported pain relief and satisfaction postoperatively, regardless of the status of the repair. However, patients with an intact repair demonstrated better function, range of motion, and strength.

Keener JD, Wei AS, Kim HM, et al. Revision arthroscopic rotator cuff repair: repair integrity and clinical outcome. J Bone Joint Surg [Am]. 2010;92:590-8.

This study retrospectively reviewed 21 patients who underwent revision arthroscopic rotator cuff repair at a minimum of 2 years after surgery. These patients demonstrated improvement in pain, Simple Shoulder Test scores, ASES scores, forward elevation, and external rotation. Forty-eight percent of patients demonstrated healing on postoperative ultrasound examination, including 70% of those with single-tendon tears and 27% of those with supraspinatus/infraspinatus tears. Patient age and number of torn tendons had a negative correlation with postoperative repair integrity. Those patients with intact repairs demonstrated higher Constant scores and improved scapular-plane elevation. (Level IV evidence)

Keener JD, Wei AS, Kim HM, Steger-May K, Yamaguchi K. Proximal humeral migration in shoulders with symptomatic and asymptomatic rotator cuff tears. J Bone Joint Surg [Am]. 2009;91:1405-13.

In this study, 117 patients with rotator cuff tears, both symptomatic and asymptomatic, were prospectively evaluated with plain radiographs and ultrasound. Proximal humeral migration was greater in symptomatic tears, as well as those tears that involved the infraspinatus. For symptomatic tears greater than 175 mm^2, pain and tear size have a significant effect on proximal migration. However, tear area was determined to be the most important predictor of proximal humeral migration. (Level II evidence)

Liem D, Lichtenberg S, Magosch P, Habermeyer P. Magnetic resonance imaging of arthroscopic supraspinatus tendon repair. J Bone Joint Surg [Am]. 2007;89:1770-6.

This study retrospectively reviewed 53 patients with isolated supraspinatus tears at a minimum of 24 months postoperatively. Overall, patients demonstrated improvement in the Constant score regardless of repair integrity. Seventy-five percent of patients demonstrated healing on final evaluation. Patients with recurrent tears demonstrated diminished abduction strength and decreased Constant scores. Preoperative fatty infiltration of grade 2 or more, supraspinatus atrophy, and age all were found to be associated with recurrent tears. Neither progression nor reversal of fatty infiltration or atrophy was observed in healed tears. However, recurrent tears demonstrated progression of both of these characteristics. (Level IV evidence)

Mochizuki T, Sugaya H, Uomizu M, et al. Humeral insertion of the supraspinatus and infraspinatus: new anatomical findings regarding the footprint of the rotator cuff. J Bone Joint Surg [Am]. 2008;90:962-9.

This cadaveric study of 113 shoulders sought to define the insertional footprint of the posterosuperior rotator cuff tendons, and discovered the footprint of the supraspinatus to be smaller, and that of the infraspinatus to be larger, than previously thought.

Park JY, Lhee SH, Choi JH, Park HK, Yu JW, Seo JB. Comparison of the clinical outcomes of single- and double-row repairs in rotator cuff tears. Am J Sports Med. 2008;36:1310-6.

This investigation compared patients who underwent single-row and double-row arthrosopic rotator cuff repair. These patients were evaluated at a minimum of 22 months with ASES and Constant scores, as well as a Shoulder Strength index. Overall, all outcomes improved in both groups, with no statistically significant difference between groups. However, when large and massive tears (>3 cm) were examined separately, the double-row group demonstrated superior results compared to the single-row group. (Level II evidence)

Sugaya H, Maeda K, Matsuki K, Moriishi J. Functional and structural outcome after arthroscopic full-thickness rotator cuff repair: single-row versus dual-row fixation. Arthroscopy. 2005;21:1307-16.

This investigation compared patients who underwent single-row and double-row arthroscopic rotator cuff repair. These patients were evaluated at a minimum of 2 years postoperatively with UCLA and ASES scores, as well as with MRI to assess structural integrity. Although all patients demonstrated improvement in outcome scores, with no statistically significant difference among groups, structural integrity did differ. Significantly more subjects in the single-row group demonstrated insufficient thickness and recurrent defects in the rotator cuff repair. Subjects with large to massive tears demonstrated a higher incidence of recurrent defects in the single-row group compared to the double-row group (44% versus 29%, respectively). (Level III evidence)

Sugaya H, Maeda K, Matsuki K, Moriishi J. Repair integrity and functional outcome after arthroscopic double-row rotator cuff repair: a prospective outcome study. J Bone Joint Surg [Am]. 2007;89:953-60.

In this study, 86 patients who underwent arthroscopic double-row rotator cuff repair were evaluated prospectively at a minimum of 2 years postoperatively. Overall, all clinical outcome scores, including JOA, UCLA, and ASES scores, improved on final evaluation. Eighty-three patients demonstrated healing on MRI, including 95% of small and medium tears and 60% of large and massive tears. Patients with a recurrent major defect demonstrated diminished outcome scores and strength, while those with a recurrent minor defect demonstrated no functional compromise. (Level IV evidence)

Teefey SA, Rubin DA, Middleton WD, Hildebolt CF, Leibold RA, Yamaguchi K. Detection and quantification of rotator cuff tears: comparison of ultrasonographic, magnetic resonance imaging, and arthroscopic findings in seventy-one consecutive cases. J Bone Joint Surg [Am]. 2004;86:708-16.

In this study, 71 patients who underwent shoulder arthroscopy were prospectively studied to examine the relative accuracy of ultrasound in evaluating the rotator cuff relative to MRI and arthroscopy. Ultrasound demonstrated accuracy comparable to MRI with regard to identifying a rotator cuff tear and distinguishing partial-thickness and full-thickness tears, as well as determining the dimensions of the tear. (Level I-1 evidence)

PROCEDURE 6

Operative Fixation of Symptomatic Os Acromiale

Neal C. Chen and Jon K. Sekiya

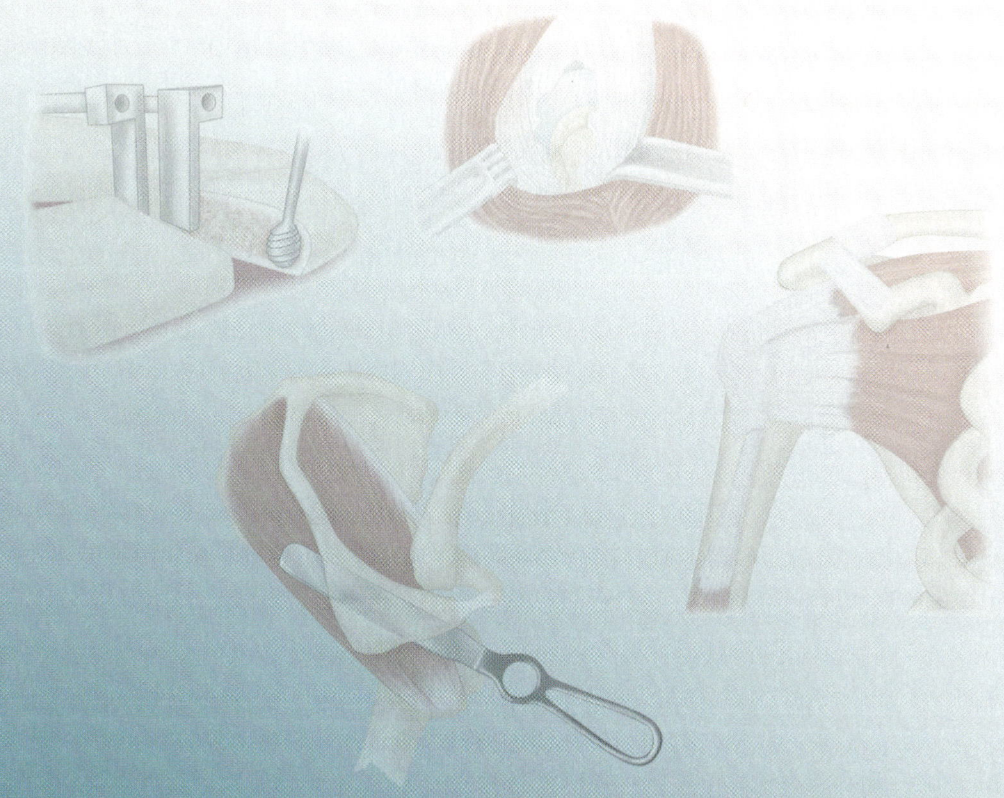

Figure 11 from Kurtz CA, Humble BJ, Rodosky MW, Sekiya JK. Symptomatic os acromiale. J Am Acad Orthop Surg. 2006;14:12–9.

PITFALLS

- *Asymptomatic os acromiale should not be treated operatively. It is important to prove that the os acromiale detected radiographically is the source of symptoms.*
- *Skeletal immaturity: The os acromiale may not fuse until up to age 25. If os acromiale is suspected, the contralateral shoulder should be examined radiographically. Anesthetic injection into the pseudarthrosis and bone scan and/or magnetic resonance imaging should be considered to help confirm the diagnosis.*
- *Caution should be taken with patients who are heavy smokers as they may have complications with arthrodesis.*

Controversies

- The role of os acromiale excision is unclear. Most authors agree that small fragments can be excised; however, it is controversial whether larger fragments can be excised without clinically noticeable deltoid dysfunction. There is considerable evidence that radical acromionectomy is problematic.
- There is limited evidence that arthroscopic decompression can be helpful in cases of a symptomatic os acromiale in patients with impingement symptoms but without tenderness at the os acromiale site.

Indications

- Three preconditions should be met prior to operative fixation of an os acromiale:
  - Os acromiale is associated with shoulder pain refractory to nonoperative treatment and tenderness at the pseudarthrosis site on examination.
  - Incomplete apophyseal fusion is documented radiographically or by other imaging study.
  - Gross instability is documented at the time of surgery. Gross instability without clinical signs is not a sufficient indication for operative intervention.

Examination/Imaging

- Tenderness over the os acromiale should be noted.
- Range of motion of the shoulder preoperatively should be noted.
- Impingement signs should be noted.
- Deltoid integrity and rotator cuff strength should be documented.
- An axillary lateral radiograph is the most important imaging study (Fig. 1A).
- Glenohumeral anteroposterior (Fig. 1B) and scapular Y views are also standard radiographs.
- An acromial profile view is helpful in identifying os acromiale if an axillary lateral view is not revealing and an os acromiale is still suspected.
- Magnetic resonance imaging (MRI) should be considered to evaluate concomitant shoulder pathology, as seen in the transverse MRI of os acromiale in Figure 2. Edema noted on MRI at the pseudarthrosis site provides correlative evidence that the os acromiale is symptomatic.
- Contralateral shoulder films may be helpful if the patient is skeletally immature.
- Bone scan may be a helpful adjunct to radiographs. If the third phase of the bone scan continues to localize to the os acromiale, it provides correlative evidence that the pseudarthrosis is symptomatic.

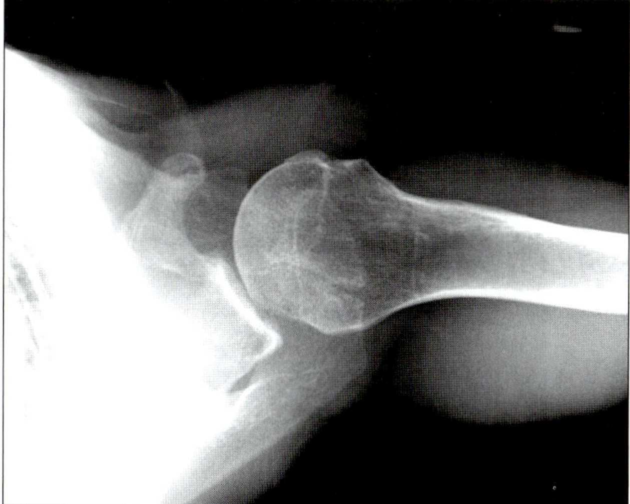

A

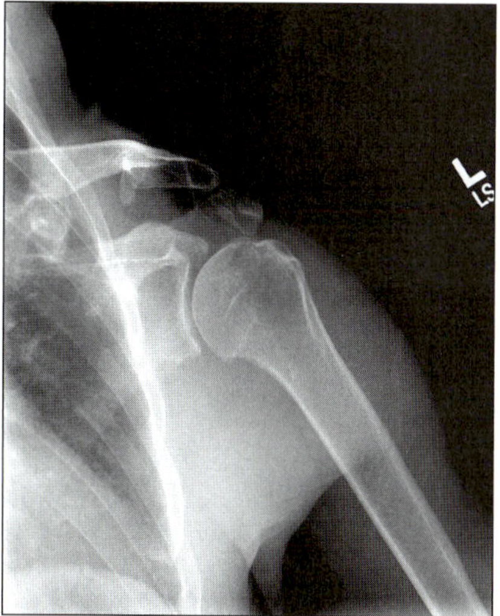

B

FIGURE 1

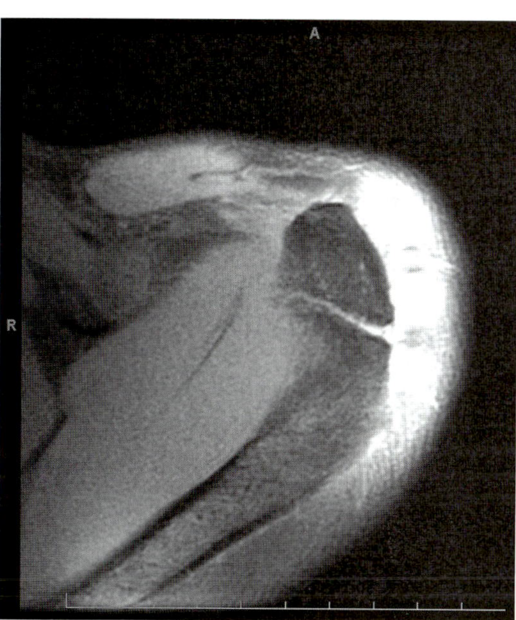

FIGURE 2

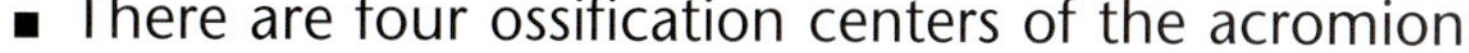

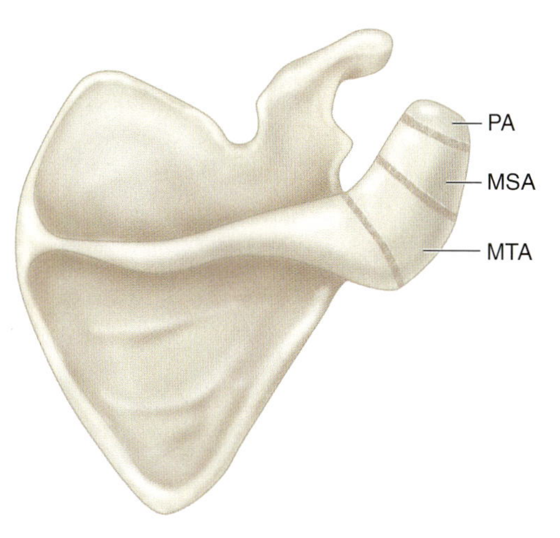

FIGURE 3

Surgical Anatomy

- There are four ossification centers of the acromion:
  - Preacromion
  - Mesoacromion
  - Meta-acromion
  - Basiacromion
- Three of these ossification centers, the preacromion (PA), the mesoacromion (MSA), and the meta-acromion (MTA), determine os acromiale (Fig. 3).
- The basiacromion fuses at approximately 12 years of age, while the pre-, meso-, and meta- acromion fuse at approximately 15 years of age. However, these ossifications centers may not fuse up to age 25.

Treatment Options

- Nonoperative treatment should be pursued initially including nonsteroidal anti-inflammatories and impingement protocol physical therapy.
- Corticosteroid injection may be helpful in treating symptoms as well as confirming the os acromiale as the source of the pain.
- Arthroscopic débridement has been reported as an alternative treatment to fusion in patients with only impingement signs and no tenderness over the os.

Pearls

- *The deltoid attachment to the acromion and os acromiale is preserved if possible to preserve blood supply to the bone fragments.*

Pitfalls

- *Avoid excessive detachment of the deltoid muscle. This will devascularize the os acromion as well as increase the risk of deltoid dehiscence.*

Positioning

- Surgery may be performed in either the beach chair or lateral decubitus position.
- If an autologous bone graft is to be used, access to a graft harvest site (iliac crest, proximal tibia, olecranon, etc.) should be considered when positioning.
- If fluoroscopy is being used, the position of the fluoroscope should be checked prior to preparation and draping to ensure that a proper image can be obtained.

Portals/Exposures

- If the subacromial space is being examined arthroscopically, instability of the os acromiale is identified. In Figure 4A, there is downward pressure on the tip of the acromion illustrating instability at the pseudarthrosis site.
- An anterosuperior exposure of the shoulder is made from the posterior acromion to approximately 1 cm lateral to the coracoid process.
- The pseudarthrosis site is localized using an 18-gauge spinal needle (Fig. 4B).
- Instability of the os acromiale is documented.
- The deltotrapezial fascia/acromial periosteum is incised in line with the pseudarthrosis. Figure 5 shows the saber skin incision within Langer's lines. An attempt to maintain the periosteal attachment to the remainder of the bony structures is preferred to preserve healing.

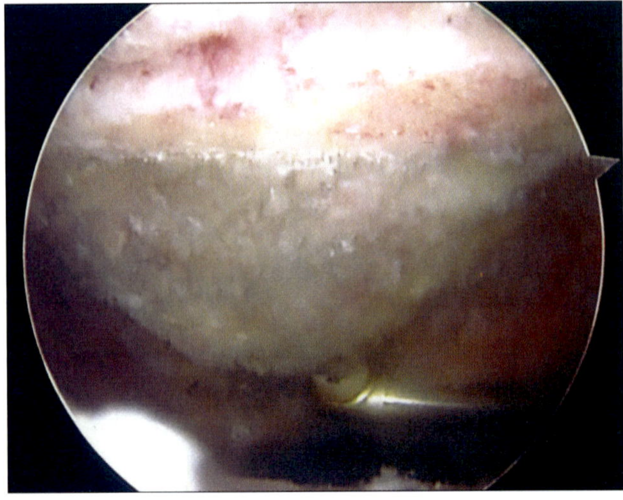

A

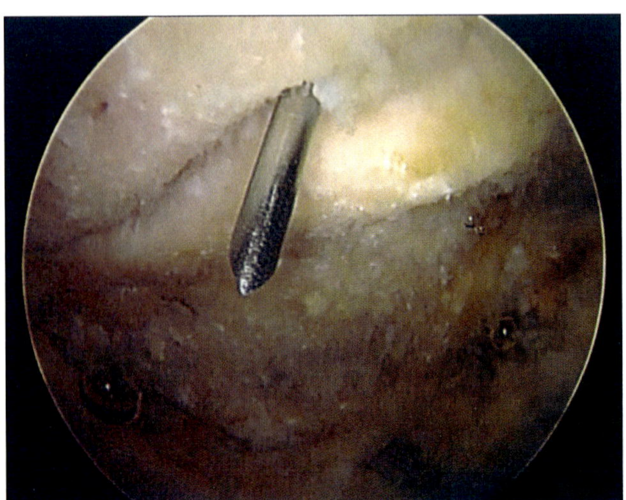

B

FIGURE 4

PEARLS

- *If necessary, a laminar spreader can be placed into the pseudarthrosis site to gain improved access (see Fig. 6).*

PITFALLS

- *Incomplete preparation can lead to failure of fusion.*

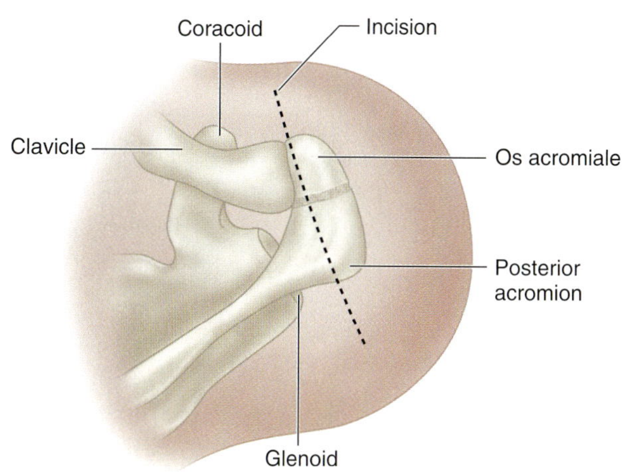

FIGURE 5

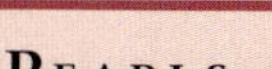

PEARLS

- *If using a tenaculum forceps, it may be helpful to make a small guide hole to avoid forceps slippage.*
- *A larger tenaculum from a pelvic fracture kit can be helpful. Dual tenaculum forceps may also be helpful to maintain reduction.*

PITFALLS

- *It is important to avoid malreduction with the provisional fixation.*
- *Provisional fixation should not be placed where definitive fixation needs to be placed.*

Procedure

STEP 1: PREPARATION OF THE PSEUDARTHROSIS

- The pseudarthrosis is prepared with a burr, rongeur, and curette (Fig. 6).
- The pseudarthrosis should be cleared until reaching bleeding, cancellous bone. The entire length and depth of the pseudarthrosis should be prepared.

STEP 2: BONE GRAFTING AND PROVISIONAL FIXATION

- Bone graft or bone substitute is packed into the pseudarthrosis site.
- The os acromiale is held using either a tenaculum forceps or Kirschner wires (K-wires) provisionally.
  - Guidewires for the cannulated screws may also be used for provisional fixation.
  - Figure 7 shows provisional fixation of the pseudarthrosis with a tenaculum forceps and guidewires for a cannulated screw.
- Arthroscopic viewing of the subacromial space can ensure fixation of the os in an optimal position.

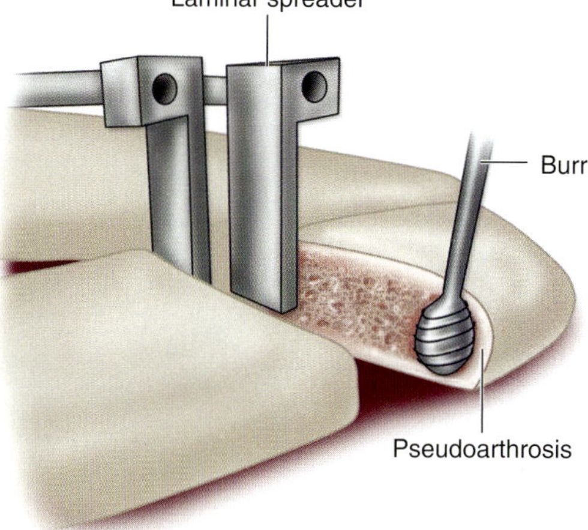

FIGURE 6

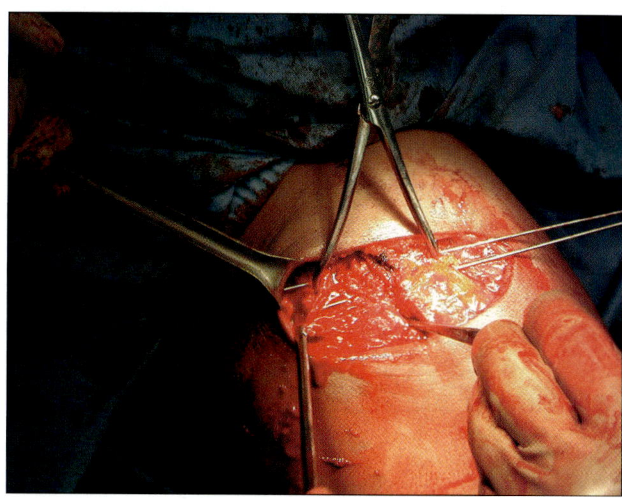

FIGURE 7

Instrumentation/ Implantation

- 0.062″ K-wires
- Tenaculum forceps
- Fluoroscopy

Pearls

- *If there is difficulty determining the depth that has been reamed, subtract the length of the first guidewire from that of a second guidewire.*

Pitfalls

- *A common mistake is to make the cannulated screws longer than the os acromiale–acromion construct. The tension band construct is neutralized and no compression is obtained when this occurs.*
- *A second error is to place cancellous screws with threads crossing the fracture site. This will also neutralize the tension band construct.*

Step 3: Cannulated Screw Placement

- Two 4.0-mm cannulated cancellous screw guidewires are placed perpendicular to the pseudarthrosis. The guidewires should pass through both cortices.
- A 2.5-mm reamer is used to over-ream the guidewires.
- The screws may be placed either anteriorly to posteriorly or posteriorly to anteriorly, as in Figure 8.
  - An advantage of posterior-to-anterior screw placement is less prominence of the screw heads anteriorly; however, it is important to note the length of the threaded portion of the screw relative to the length of the os. If the os is shorter than the length of the screw threads, the screw should be placed anterior to posterior.
- The screw length is measured. The screw should be shorter than the actual length of the acromion by at least 4 mm.
- A determination is made as to use of a long-threaded or short-threaded screw. The threads should not cross the pseudarthrosis site. This may be checked with fluoroscopy.

Step 4: Tension Band

- A strong nonabsorbable suture or an 18- or 20-gauge stainless steel wire is passed in a figure-of-8 configuration through the cancellous screws (Fig. 9).
  - If a nonabsorbable suture is used, this is tied down in standard fashion.
  - If a stainless steel wire is used, a large needle holder is used to tighten the wire and cut the wire end.

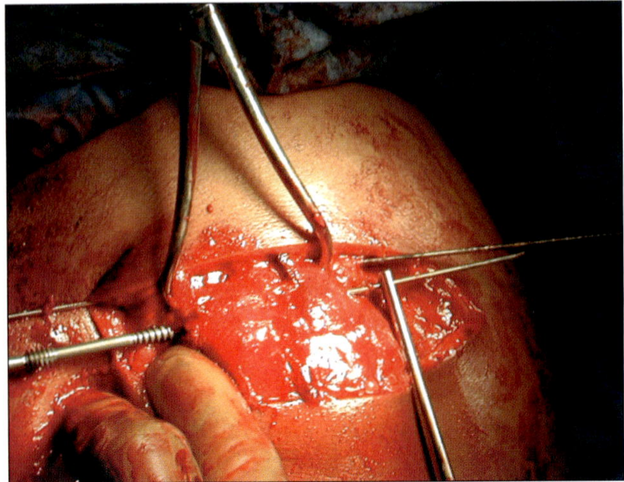

FIGURE 8

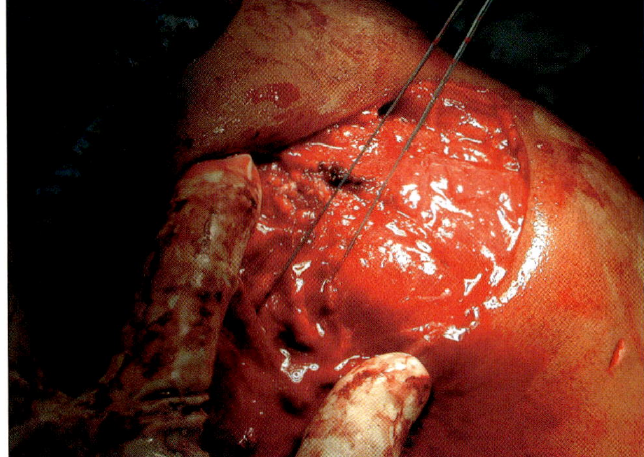

FIGURE 9

Instrumentation/ Implantation

- Synthes 4.0-mm cannulated stainless steel screw kit

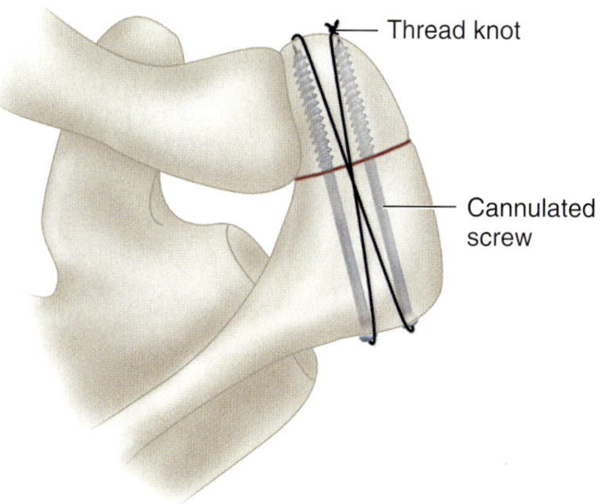

FIGURE 10

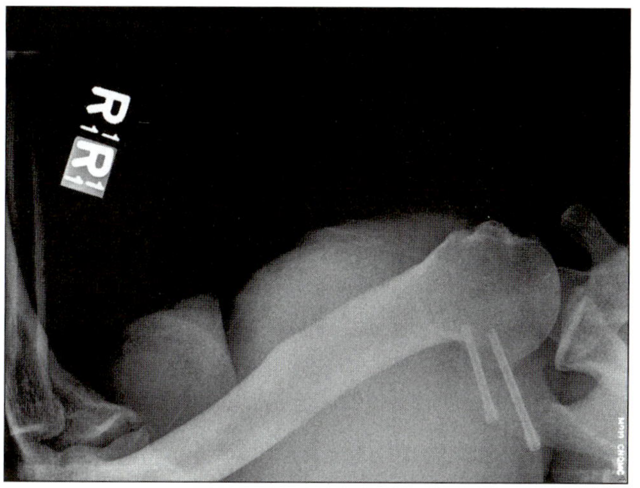

A

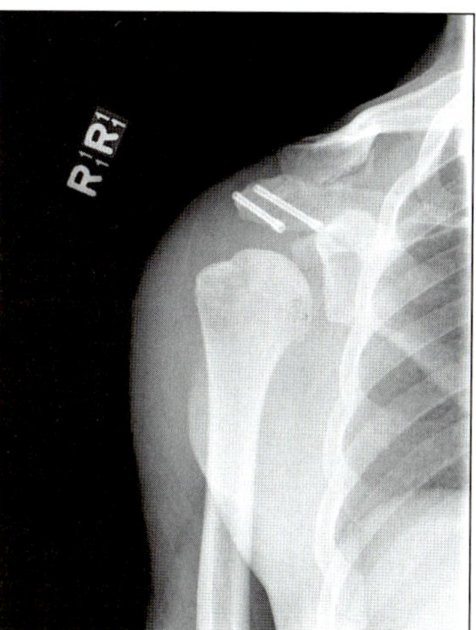

B

FIGURE 11

Pearls

- *The wire end can be twisted, cut, and buried into the posterior subcutaneous tissues or musculature as needed.*
- *An alternative to a single 18-gauge wire is to use paired 22- or 24-gauge wires. This construct is less prominent.*

Pitfalls

- *The wire and the screws must be made of the same alloy. Do not use a stainless steel wire with titanium screws.*

- Figure 10 shows the final tension band construct, which is seen in the postoperative radiographs in Figure 11A and 11B.

Postoperative Care and Expected Outcomes

- Postoperatively, the arm is maintained in a shoulder immobilizer for 6 weeks.
  - Active motion may be initiated at the end of this time, as the tension on the wire-screw construct should help compress the fusion site.
  - Overhead motion and heavy lifting should be avoided for 12 weeks.
- Radiographs should be obtained at 6-week intervals until healing is documented.

Instrumentation/ Implantation

- 18- or 20-gauge wire or strong #2 or #5 nonabsorbable suture

Pitfalls

- *Nonunion rates are relatively high. It is better to be conservative with motion initially.*
- *Hardware should not be removed for at least 1 year, if it is necessary.*
- *Complications after hardware removal include deltoid dehiscience and late fracture. Hardware removal should not be undertaken without consideration of these problems.*

Evidence

Edelson JG, Zuckerman J, Hershkovitz I. Os acromiale: anatomy and surgical implications. J Bone Joint Surg [Br]. 1993;74:551-5.

In this study of 270 cadaveric and archeological specimens, 22 os acromiale were identified (8.2%). There is limited evidence regarding the incidence of os acromiale. (Grade C recommendation)

Kurtz CA, Humble B, Rodosky MW, Sekiya JK. Symptomatic os acromiale. J Am Acad Orthop Surg. 2006;14:12-9.

The authors presented a general review of os acromiale, including natural history, indications, nonoperative and operative management, and clinical results.

Mudge MK, Wood VE, Frykman GK. Rotator cuff tears associated with os acromiale. J Bone Joint Surg [Am]. 1984;66:427-9.

This study documented eight patients with os acromiale with concomitant rotator cuff tear. It is unclear whether these claims of an association have statistical merit. (Grade C recommendation)

Neer CS II, Marberry TA. On the disadvantages of radical acromionectomy. J Bone Joint Surg [Am]. 1981;63:416-9.

This study documented 30 patients who underwent radical acromionectomy. Problems included persistent pain, cosmetic deformity, and decreased function. Reconstruction of the deltoid was not successful in general. (Grade C recommendation)

Peckett WRC, Gunther SB, Harper GD, Hughes JS, Sonnabend DH. Internal fixation of os acromiale: a series of 26 cases. J Shoulder Elbow Surg. 2004;13:381-5.

In this case series of 26 os acromiale treated with tension band fixation using a lag screw construct, there was a high rate of union (96%). (Grade C recommendation)

Warner JJ, Beim GM, Higgins L. The treatment of symptomatic os acromiale. J Bone Joint Surg [Am]. 1998;80:1320-6.

In this retrospective case-control series of os acromiale treated with tension band fixation with K-wires versus tension band fixation with a cannulated screw construct, the cannulated screw tension band construct had a higher union rate. (Grade B recommendation)

Wright RW, Heller MA, Quick DC, Buss DD. Arthroscopic decompression for impingement syndrome secondary to an unstable os acromiale. Arthroscopy. 2000;16:595-9.

In this case series of 12 patients with unstable os acromiale treated with arthroscopic acromioplasty, 11 patients had UCLA shoulder scores greater than 27. (Grade C recommendation)

SECTION I

SHOULDER

Arthritic Shoulder

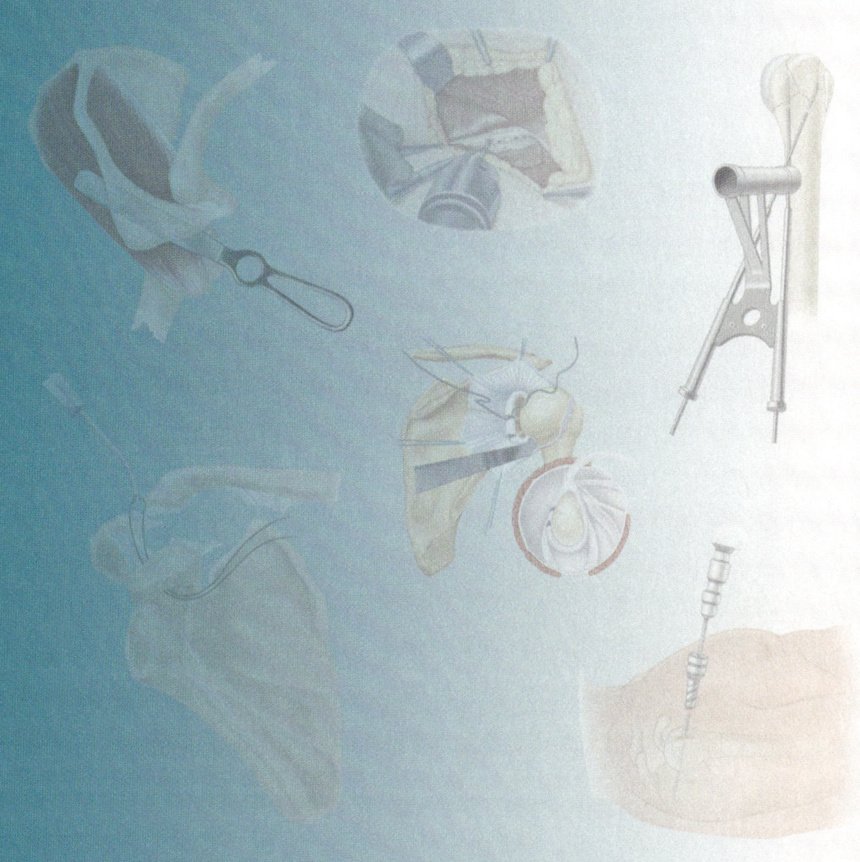

PROCEDURE 7

Humeral Head Resurfacing Arthroplasty

Ross A. Shumar and Lynn A. Crosby

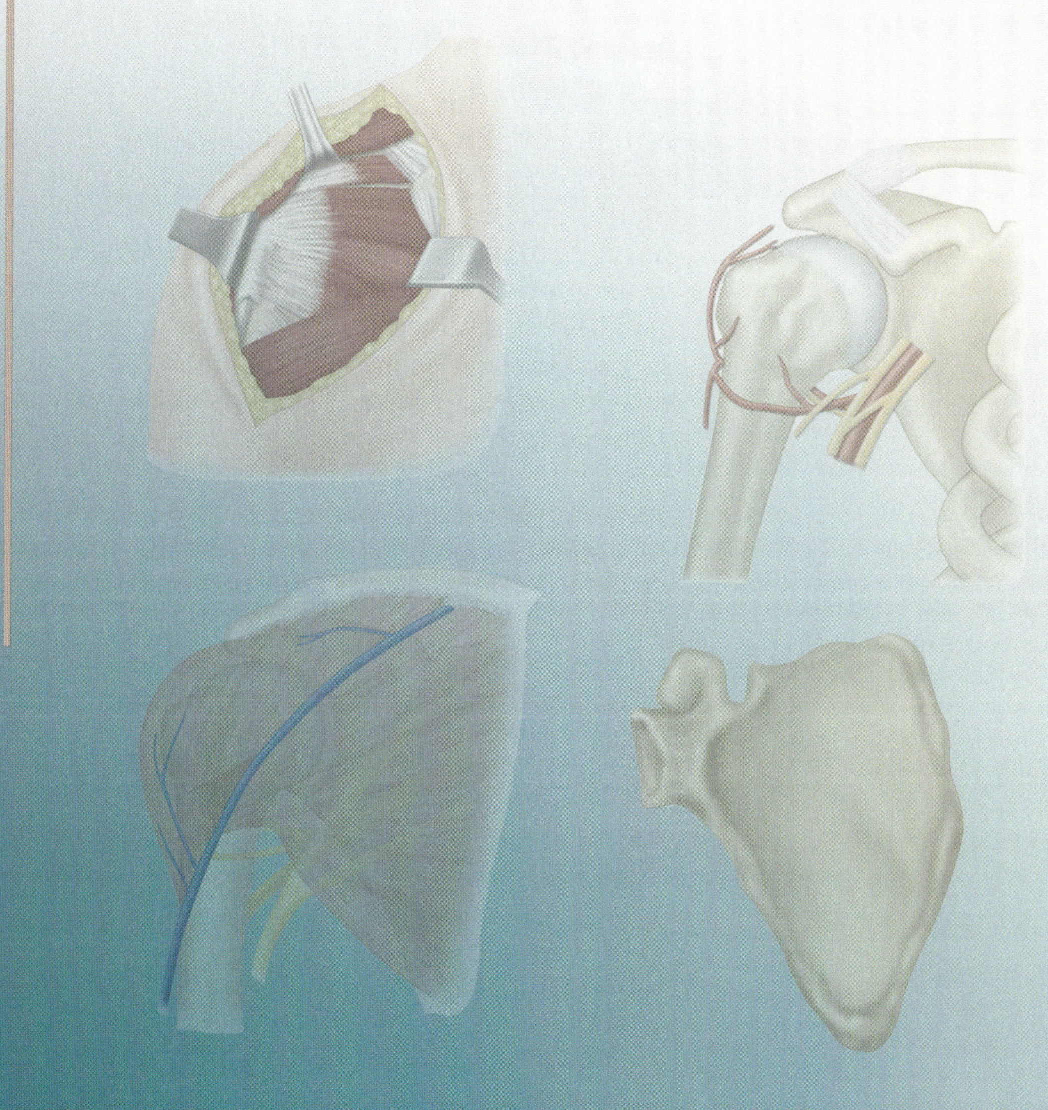

Pitfalls

- *Be cautious when addressing patients with bipolar arthritis as exposure of the glenoid can be difficult without removal of the humeral head.*
- *Osteonecrosis with significant collapse (>75%) may not allow adequate fixation of the resurfacing prosthesis, requiring conversion to a stemmed humeral component. Always have stemmed humeral components available during surgery.*
- *Humeral head resurfacing is relatively contraindicated in those patients with an irreparable rotator cuff tear or continued instability.*
- *Absolute contraindications include skeletal immaturity and active local or systemic infection.*

Controversies

- Glenoid arthritis—biologic glenoid resurfacing should be considered in the young patient with glenoid involvement
- Poor bone quality (osteoporosis)—when performing humeral head resurfacing in an osteoporotic patient, strongly consider cementing the prosthesis.

Treatment Options

- Stemmed hemiarthroplasty (monopolar or bipolar)
- Total shoulder arthroplasty
- Arthroscopic débridement
- Soft tissue interposition arthroplasty
- Arthrodesis
- Osteoarticular allograft

Indications

- Symptomatic glenohumeral arthritis in the younger patient, who is best served by a bone-preserving implant.
- Arthritis involving primarily the humeral head with a relatively normal glenoid and intact or reparable rotator cuff.
- Humeral head resurfacing may be indicated in those patients with posttraumatic arthritis, osteonecrosis, arthritis of instability, inflammatory arthritis, or humeral head fracture/nonunion/malunion.

Examination/Imaging

Physical Examination

- A thorough physical examination of the shoulder and cervical spine should be completed to exclude any other possible sources of pain. Both active and passive range of motion should be evaluated.
- In addition to the office examination, every patient should be examined under anesthesia prior to surgical incision. Contractures can be addressed through capsular release, and instability may require capsular reefing or reconstruction.
- Diagnostic injection of the acromioclavicular (AC) joint and/or subacromial space may be considered to evaluate the potential contribution of symptomatic AC joint arthritis and subacromial impingement to the overall clinical presentation. Procedures to address these problems (distal clavicle resection or subacromial decompression) can be completed at a single surgical setting.

Imaging Studies

- A complete series of radiographs (anteroposterior, axillary lateral, scapular Y, and internal rotation views) should be evaluated for both diagnostic (Fig. 1) and templating (Fig. 2) purposes.
  - Careful attention should be paid to glenoid version and erosion on the axillary view.
- A computed tomography scan should be considered to evaluate
  - Extent of subchondral collapse in osteonecrosis
  - Amount of humeral head involvement with a Hill-Sachs lesion
  - Glenoid bone stock with bony Bankart lesions
- In the patient with clinical evidence of a rotator cuff tear, a magnetic resonance imaging study should be obtained to determine the extent of tendon retraction and fatty infiltration. An irreparable cuff

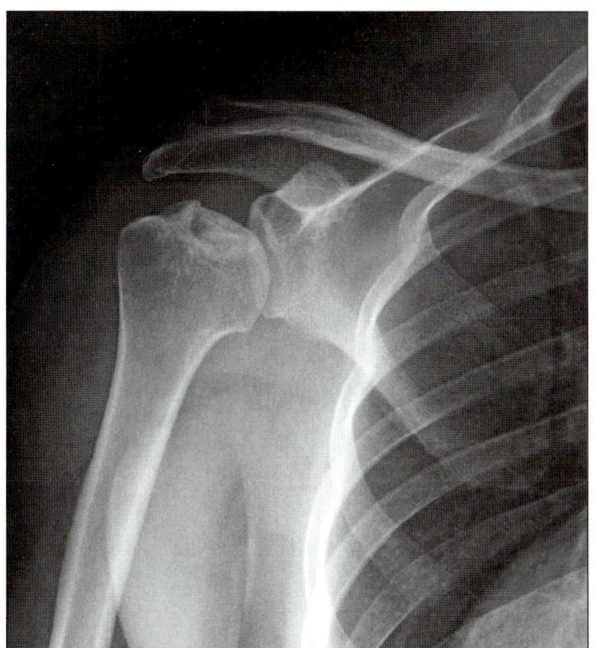

FIGURE 1

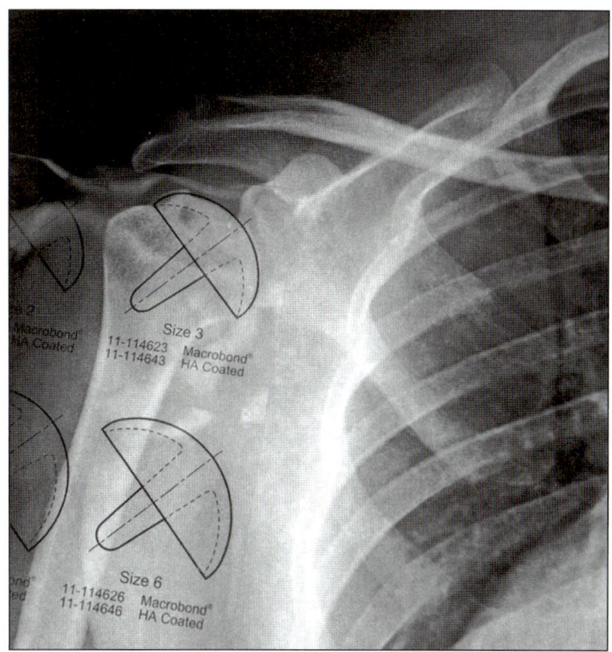

FIGURE 2

tear or significant fatty infiltration are relative contraindications to resurfacing arthroplasty.

Surgical Anatomy

- The surgeon should be familiar with the musculature (Fig. 3A), vasculature (Fig. 3B), and nerves (see Fig. 3B) in the area of the humeral head.
- Humeral alignment parameters
  - Humeral neck-shaft angle: 30–55 degrees
  - Humeral head retroversion: 0–55 degrees
  - Humeral head resurfacing makes no attempt to redefine these parameters and is focused on restoring the patient's natural alignment.

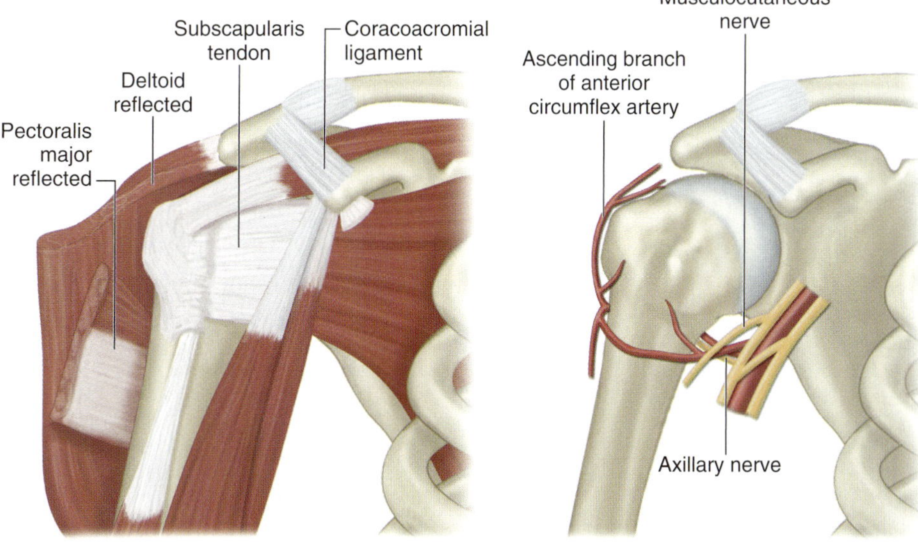

FIGURE 3 A B

Positioning

- The patient is positioned in the beach chair position with the arm draped free. The patient's torso should be inclined approximately 30–40° from horizontal.
- A head rest is used to maintain cervical alignment, and care is taken to assure stable positioning prior to draping.
- A side bolster is used along the chest wall to prevent shifting of the patient during surgery.
- The patient's hips are flexed to prevent the patient from sliding down the table, and the knees are flexed to take tension off the sciatic nerve.
- Adequate extension of the shoulder must be ensured to allow delivery of the humeral head through the deltopectoral interval. This requires a drop-back table.
- We prefer to suspend the patient's arm from a table outrigger and prep the arm out to the wrist.
- A sterile impervious stockinette is placed over the hand and wrapped with a self-adherent bandage up to the elbow.

Pearls

- *Take care to avoid "draping yourself out" by draping over to the medial border of the clavicle and up onto the side of the neck.*
- *Use an armholder or a sterile Mayo stand to support the arm during the procedure.*

Portals/Exposures

- A standard deltopectoral approach just lateral to the coracoid process is used.
- Once through the deltopectoral interval, the deltoid is mobilized and any bursal tissue excised.
- The inferior edge of the coracoacromial ligament is incised for additional superior exposure, but care must be taken not to release too much to prevent any future humeral head escape in the case of rotator cuff deficiency.
- The axillary nerve should be palpated at the inferior border of the subscapularis tendon and protected throughout the procedure.
- The surgeon should stay lateral to the conjoint tendon and limit excessive retraction to avoid injury to the musculocutaneous nerve.
- The ascending branch of the anterior circumflex artery is identified and ligated or coagulated to prevent excessive bleeding.
- The subscapularis tendon and capsule are taken down, leaving approximately a 1-cm cuff of tissue for later repair.

Pearls

- *Place tag sutures in the subscapularis tendon prior to fully releasing it to aid in tendon retraction and later repair.*

Controversies

- Exposure can also be accomplished through the anterosuperior Mackenzie approach. We advise against this exposure due to the risk of failure of repair, resulting in anterior deltoid insufficiency.

- After releasing the subscapularis tendon, an arthrotomy is performed beginning in the rotator interval and extending distally along the anatomic neck. The inferior capsule is released off the humeral neck by externally rotating the arm with care to avoid injury to the axillary nerve.

Procedure

Step 1: Preparation of Humeral Head

- The arm is extended and externally rotated to dislocated and deliver the humeral head into the operative field.
- Release of the inferior capsule off of the humeral neck is continued as needed for adequate exposure.
- Any osteophytes are excised to help clearly identify the anatomic neck.
- The head diameter, radius of curvature, and height are measured using the prosthesis-specific guide.
- The center of the humeral head is identified. This can be done in one of two ways. Both methods involve surgeon interpretation, as it is our experience that no guides fully cover the humeral head.
    - One method involves marking the most superior and inferior aspects of the humeral head and drawing a line between them. Then a line is drawn from the most anterior to the posterior aspect of the humeral head. The central point will be at the intersection of the two lines (Fig. 4).
    - The other method is to place the prosthesis-specific guide centered on the humeral head and drill the central guidewire.
- The guidewire is drilled through the lateral cortex for added stability.

Pearls

- *Complete the capsular release to the posterior inferior margin to help deliver the humeral head into the wound.*
- *Place a curved retractor along the superior margin of the antomic neck to protect the long head of the biceps and rotator cuff tendons.*
- *The concave reamer will bottom out when the central portion contacts the humeral head. Additional reaming can be performed after drilling for the central peg as this allows further seating of the reamer.*

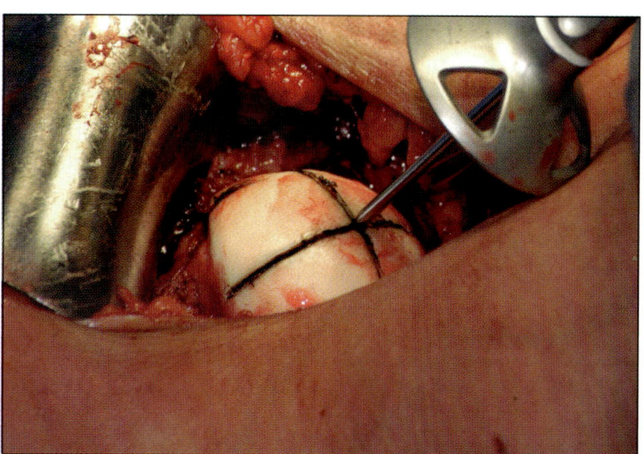

FIGURE 4

- The central peg is drilled (Fig. 5) and the head reamed (Fig. 6A–C) for the desired implant.

Step 2: Implant Trialing and Soft Tissue Balancing

- Adequate seating of the implant is ensured.
- Soft tissue tension is evaluated throughout the range of motion.
- The surgeon should avoid overstuffing the shoulder.

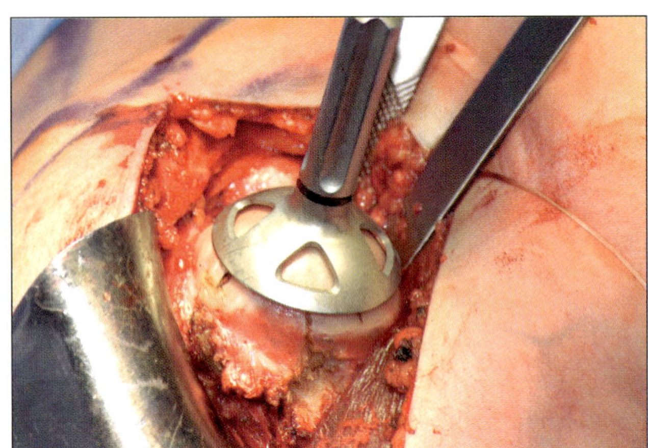

FIGURE 5

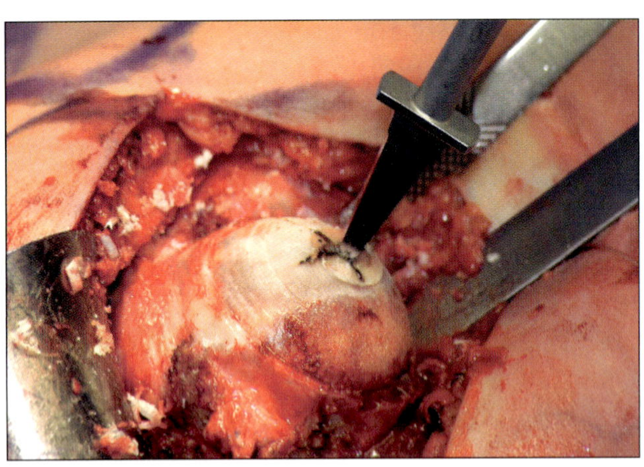

A

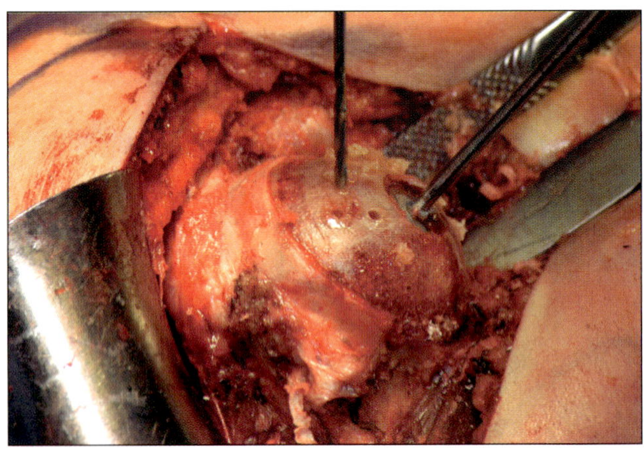

B

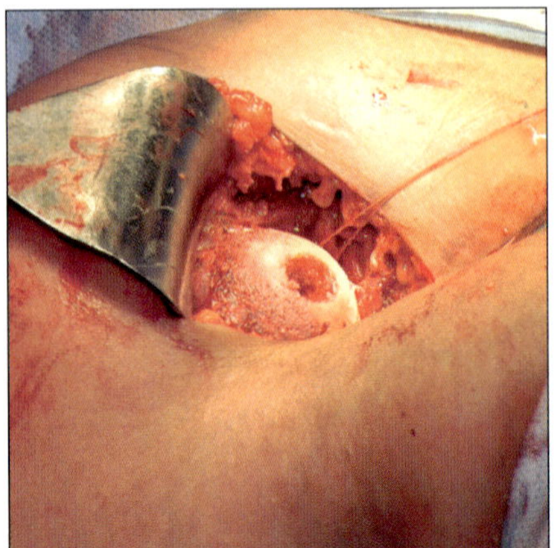

C

FIGURE 6

- The subscapularis tendon is reapproximated to its insertion while trialing to ensure external rotation to 30° without excessive tension. If the subscapularis does not have enough excursion, the surgeon should consider freeing adhesions from the anterior capsule and glenoid or reattching it to a more medial location on the lesser tuberosity or anterior neck with the use of suture anchors or bone tunnels.
- A posterior capsulotomy can aid with internal rotation contracture.

Step 3: Insertion of Component

- Any humeral head defects are bone grafted. Very little usable bone graft is retrieved from the reaming process, so the surgeon should consider using allograft when needed.
- If cementing in the face of sclerotic bone, placing drill holes to allow for cement interdigitation should be considered.
- The prosthesis is inserted with manual pressure as far as possible prior to fully seating it with a mallet (Fig. 7A and 7B).

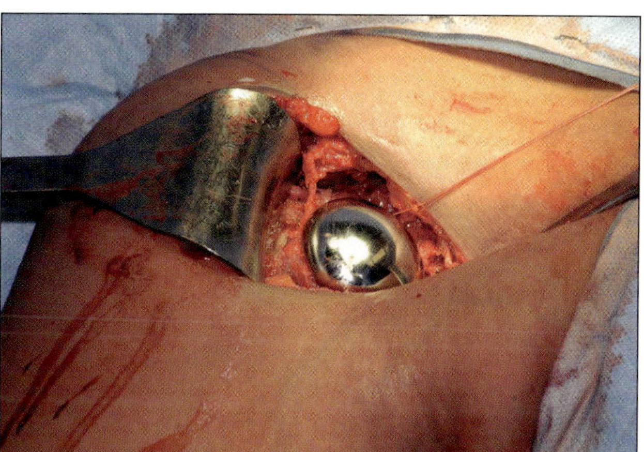

A

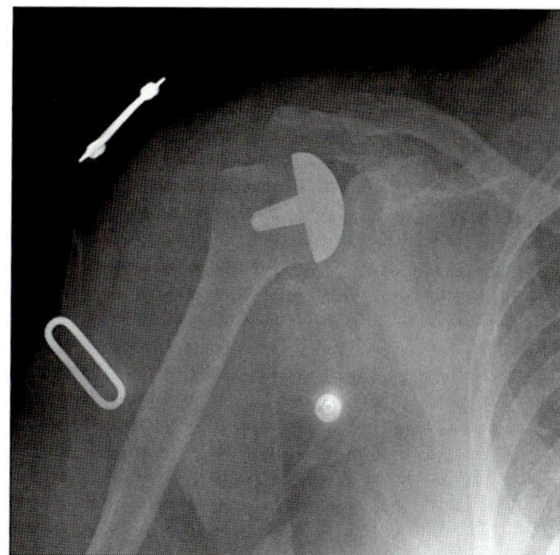

B

FIGURE 7

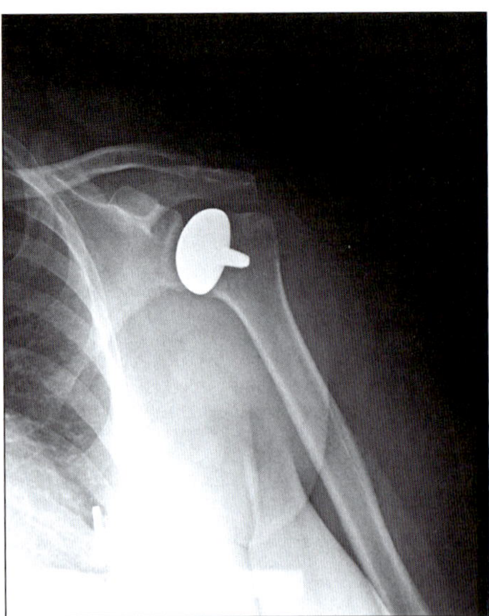

A

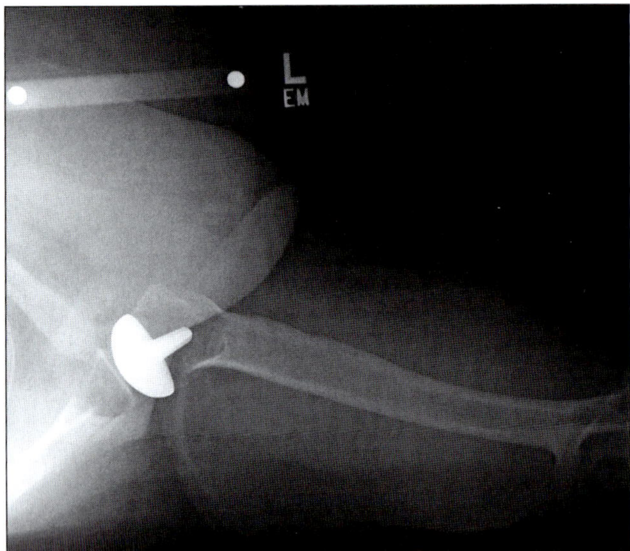

B

FIGURE 8

- Postoperative radiographs are obtained in the anteroposterior (Fig. 8A) and lateral (Fig. 8B) positions to check final prosthesis placement.

Step 4: Wound Closure

- Any necessary rotator cuff repair is performed at this time.
- The rotator interval is closed with absorbable suture.
- The subscapularis is repaired either to a cuff of soft tissue, through bone tunnels, or with the use of suture anchors as needed. If repairing the subscapularis tendon through bone tunnels or suture anchors, the surgeon should consider roughening the bony surface with a curette or burr to enhance tendon-to-bone healing.
- The deltopectoral interval is closed in interrupted fashion. We recommend using nonabsorbable suture to close the deltopectoral interval. This aids in identifying the interval in the case of revision surgery.
- Subcutaneous tissues are closed with 2-0 or 3-0 absorbable suture in interrupted fashion and skin is closed per surgeon preference.

Pearls

- *If a rotator cuff repair was performed, then the patient should follow standard rotator cuff repair postoperative rehabilitation guidelines.*

Postoperative Care and Expected Outcomes

- A sling or shoulder immobilizer is placed in the operating room.
- Passive range of motion, pendulum exercises, and deltoid isometrics are begun on the first postoperative day.

- An external rotation safe zone should be determined intraoperatively at the time of subscapularis tendon closure depending on its tension. Typical limits are between neutral and 30°.
- The patient should not be allowed to perform any active internal or external rotation prior to 6 weeks to protect the subscapularis tendon repair.
- Patients should be cautioned against pushing themselves up from a seated position as this requires forceful contraction of the subscapularis.
- The sling is discontinued at 4 weeks and resistance exercises begin after 6 weeks.
- With the exception of contact sports or heavy weight lifting, unrestricted activity is permitted at 8–10 weeks.
- Most patients reach full recovery by 9 months.
- Glenoid erosion is the primary mode of failure.
- In the case of progression of glenoid arthritis, revision total shoulder arthroplasty can be performed with satisfactory outcomes.

Evidence

Bailie DS, Llinas PJ, Ellenbecker TS. Cementless humeral resurfacing arthroplasty in active patients less than fifty-five years of age. J Bone Joint Surg [Am]. 2008;90:110-7.

This study suggested that resurfacing arthroplasty is a viable treatment option for younger patients (mean 42.3 years) without signs of implant loosening or glenoid wear in short-term follow-up (mean 38.1 months). (Level IV evidence)

Hattrup SJ. Revision total shoulder arthroplasty for painful humeral head replacement with glenoid arthrosis. J Shoulder Elbow Surg. 2009;18:220-24.

This study reviewed the results of 17 patients who had conversion of humeral hemiarthroplasty to total shoulder arthroplasty. There were seven excellent, five satisfactory, and five unsatisfactory results.

Kerr BJ, McCarty EC. Outcome of arthroscopic debridement is worse for patients with glenohumeral arthritis of both sides of the joint. Clin Orthop Relat Res. 2008;(466):34-638.

This study demonstrated that arthroscopic débridement can be effective in symptom management in young patients with arthritis. Patients with unipolar lesions had greater symptomatic relief than those with bipolar lesions. (Level IV evidence)

Krishnan SG, Nowinski RJ, Harrison D, Burkhead WZ. Humeral hemiarthroplasty with biologic resurfacing of the glenoid for glenohumeral arthritis: two to fifteen-year outcomes. J Bone Joint Surg [Am]. 2007;89:727-34.

This study showed that humeral head hemiarthroplasty with biologic resurfacing of the glenoid can provide pain relief similar to total shoulder arthroplasty and allow younger patients to maintain an active lifestyle without the risk of polyethylene wear.

Levy O, Copeland SA. Cementless surface replacement arthroplasty (Copeland CSRA) for osteoarthritis of the shoulder. J Shoulder Elbow Surg. 2004;13:266-71.

The authors reported on 79 CSRAs with a mean follow-up of 7.6 years. There were no cases of loosening of the humeral component, and 89.9% of patients reported feeling better or much better after surgery.

Nicholson GP, Goldstein JL, Romeo AA, Cole BJ, Hayden JK, Twigg LT, McCarty LP, Detterline AJ. Lateral meniscus allograft biologic glenoid arthroplasty in total shoulder arthroplasty for young shoulder with degenerative joint disease. J Shoulder Elbow Surg. 2007;16:S261-6.

The authors reported on 30 patient who underwent total shoulder arthroplasty with the use of lateral meniscus allograft instead of polyethylene for glenoid resurfacing. Patients had significant improvement in range of motion and validated shoulder scoring systems (ASES, SST, and VAS). Five of 30 (17%) had complications requiring additional surgery within the study period.

Pearl, ML. Proximal humeral anatomy in shoulder arthroplasty: implications for prosthetic design and surgical technique. J Shoulder Elbow Surg. 2005;14:S99-104.

This paper detailed the variability in proximal humeral anatomy, with a large range of normal anatomy.

Sperling JW, Cofield RH. Revision total shoulder arthroplasty for the treatment of glenoid arthrosis. J Bone Joint Surg [Am]. 1998;80:860-7.

The authors reviewed the results of 18 shoulders in 17 patients who had conversion of a hemiarthroplasty to total shoulder arthroplasty for glenoid arthrosis. Although most patients had improvement in pain and range of motion, several had decreased motion after revision surgery and 7 of 18 shoulders were rated as unsatisfactory according to a modification of the Neer rating system.

Sperling JW, Cofield RH, Rowland CM. Minimum fifteen-year follow-up of Neer hemiarthroplasty and total shoulder arthroplasty in patients aged fifty years or younger. J Shoulder Elbow Surg. 2004;13:604-13.

Long-term results of 114 patients (78 hemiarthroplasties and 36 total shoulder arthroplasties) were reviewed in this study. The estimated survival rates for total shoulder arthroplasty were 97% and 84% at 10 and 20 years, respectively. The estimated survival rates for hemiarthroplasty were 82% and 75% at 10 and 20 years, respectively. The most common failure mechanism for hemiarthroplasty was painful glenoid arthrosis. The authors cautioned against shoulder arthroplasty in the young patient.

PROCEDURE 8

Humeral Hemiarthroplasty with Biologic Glenoid Resurfacing

Eric D. Bava, Sumant G. Krishnan, Leah T. Cyran, and Wayne Z. Burkhead

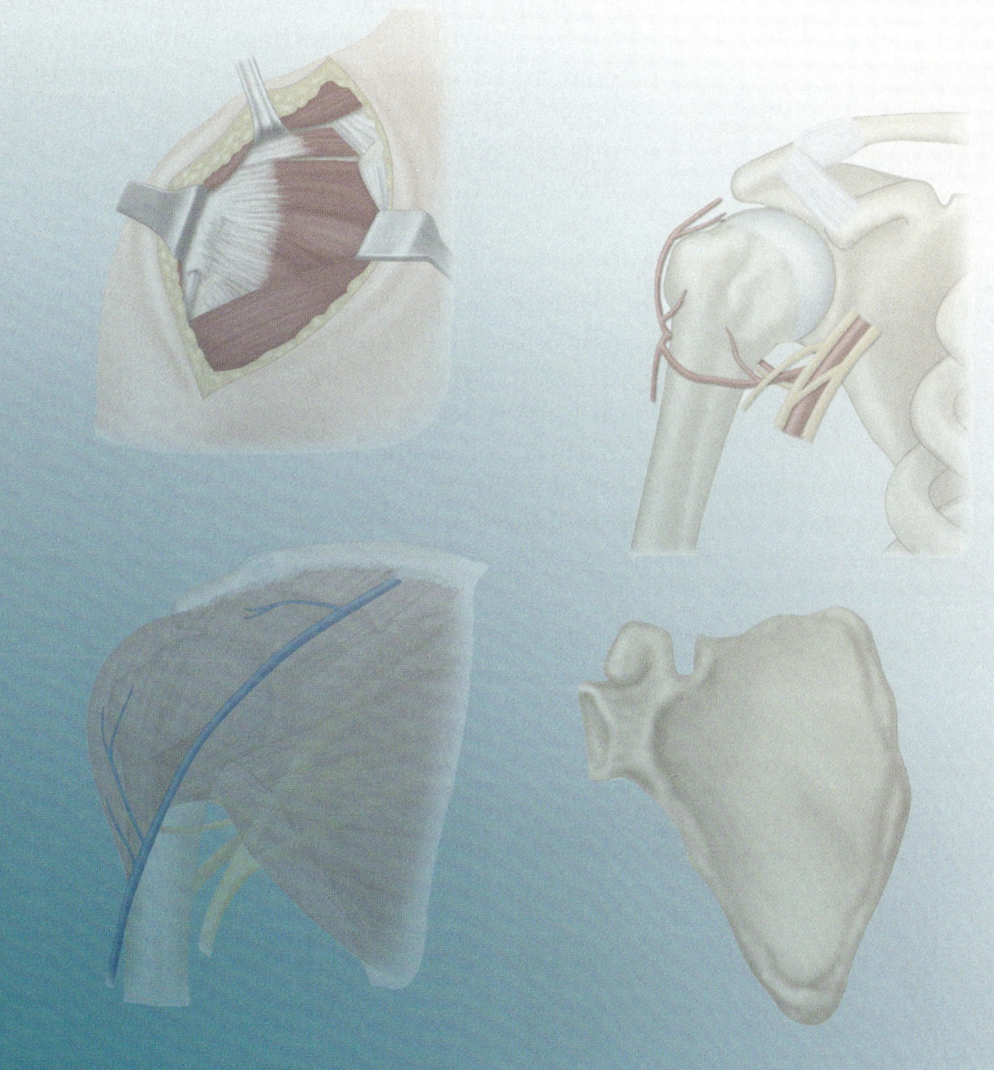

Indications

- Young patient (under 60 years of age) with an intact and functioning deltoid and rotator cuff
- Active individual or one who performs strenuous manual labor
- Primary glenohumeral arthritis, posttraumatic arthritis, or postoperative arthritis
- Revision of failed shoulder arthroplasty that requires glenoid resurfacing

Treatment Options

- Glenohumeral arthrodesis can provide satisfactory pain relief; however, this comes at the cost of a significant loss of motion and increased stress on the acromioclavicular joint and scapulothoracic musculature.
- Hemiarthroplasty is an option in younger patients; however, it has been shown to provide less pain relief and durability than total shoulder arthroplasty.
- Total shoulder arthroplasty with a conventional polyethylene glenoid component is often avoided because of concern about early glenoid component failure with accelerated loosening and wear.

Examination/Imaging

- A standard shoulder examination is performed. Motion of the glenohumeral joint often will elicit pain and crepitus. Rotator cuff strength testing is often normal; however, weakness may be exhibited due to pain.
- A diagnostic injection into the glenohumeral joint with 1% lidocaine can be used to predict pain relief following shoulder arthroplasty.
- Plain radiographs, including true anteroposterior (Fig. 1A) and axillary (Fig. 1B) views, are used to evaluate the severity of glenohumeral arthritis, including loss of joint space and presence of osteophytes. Radiographs can also help assess any bony deformity or glenoid wear and are used for preoperative planning and templating.
- Computed tomography (CT)
  - Axial (Fig. 2A) and coronal (Fig. 2B) CT images can be used to better evaluate any bony deformity present, including amount and pattern of glenoid wear and estimating glenoid bone stock.

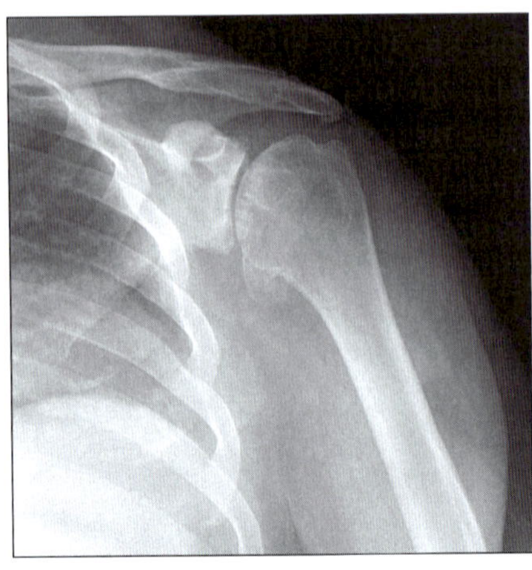

A

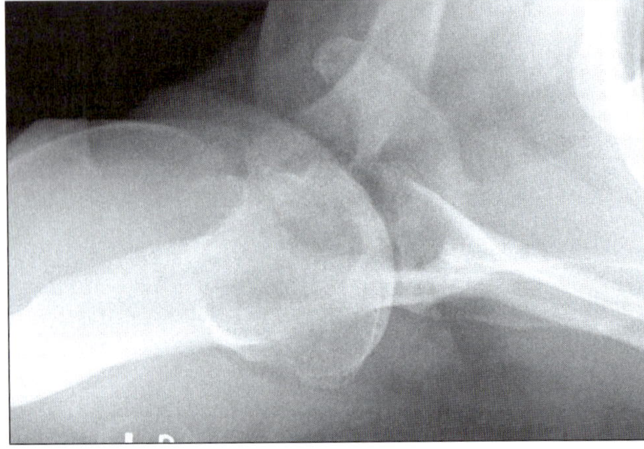

B

FIGURE 1

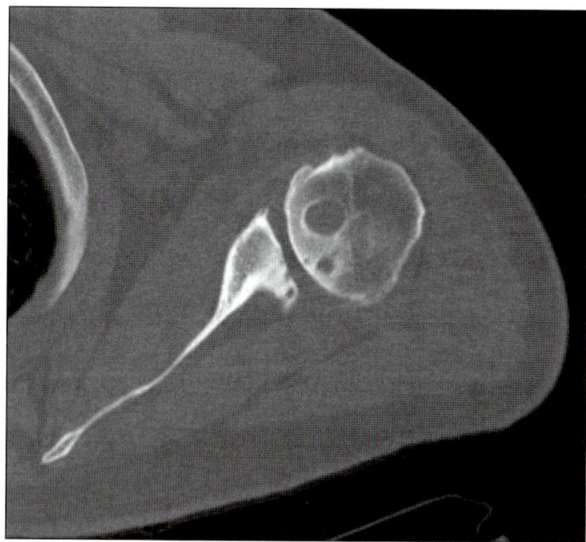

A

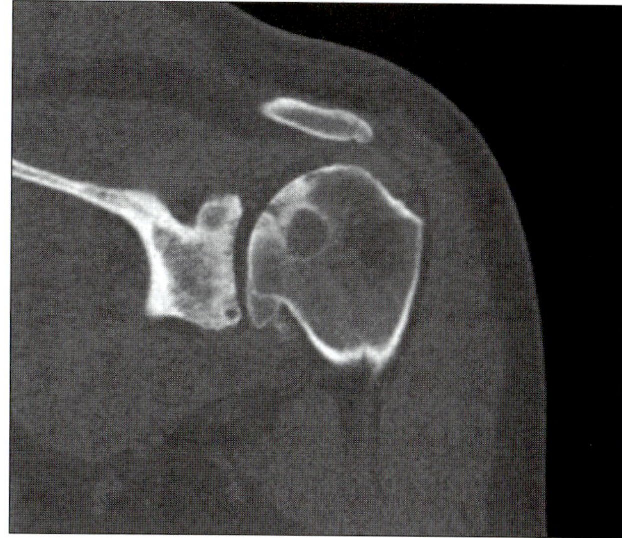

B

FIGURE 2

- CT with three-dimensional reconstructions is accurate for determining glenoid wear pattern (Fig. 3).
- Intra-articular contrast can be included with the CT examination to evaluate the integrity of the rotator cuff.

- In addition to the previous studies, either magnetic resonance imaging or ultrasound may be used to confirm rotator cuff integrity, but they are not necessary.

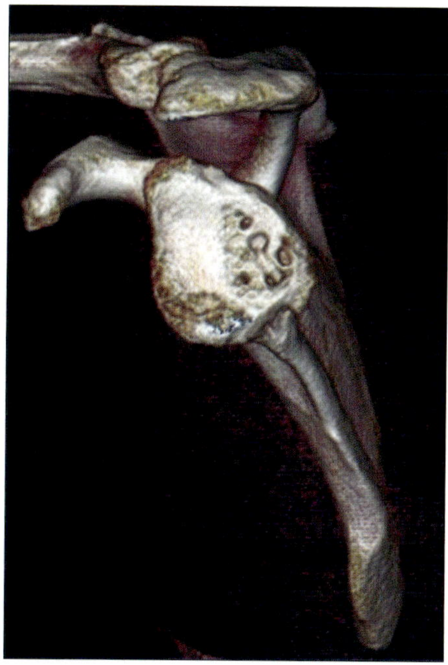

FIGURE 3

Surgical Anatomy

- Relevant bony landmarks of the proximal humerus include the humeral head, greater tuberosity, lesser tuberosity, bicipital groove, and humeral shaft (Fig. 4).
  - The greater tuberosity serves as a point of attachment for the supraspinatus, infraspinatus, and teres minor.
  - The lesser tuberosity is where the subscapularis attaches to the proximal humerus.
- Relevant bony landmarks of the scapula include the glenoid, supraglenoid tubercle, and coracoid process (Fig. 5).
  - The glenoid labrum is a fibrocartilaginous ringed structure attached to the rim of the glenoid.
- The cephalic vein and clavipectoral fascia are found within the deltopectoral interval, which is the internervous plane between the deltoid and pectoralis major muscles.
- The conjoined tendon attaches to the tip of the coracoid process and lies deep to the pectoralis major.
- The axillary nerve crosses the subscapularis muscle belly, running from superomedial to inferolateral, and then runs near the inferior capsule of the glenohumeral joint.

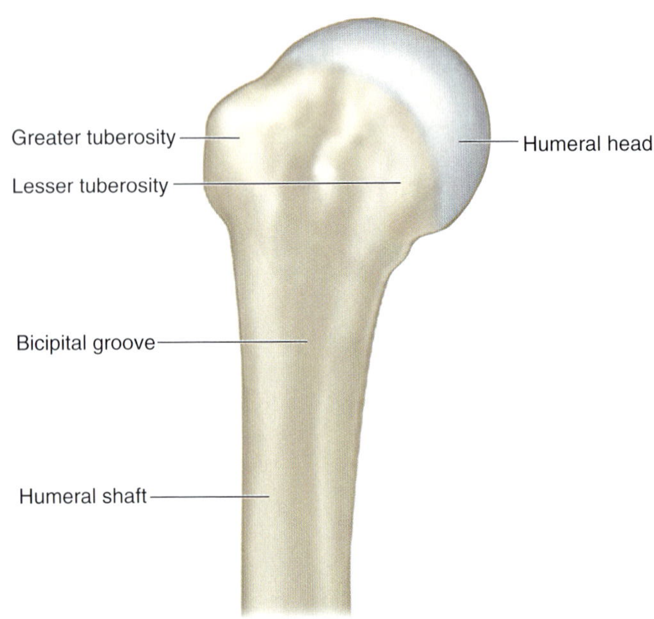

FIGURE 4

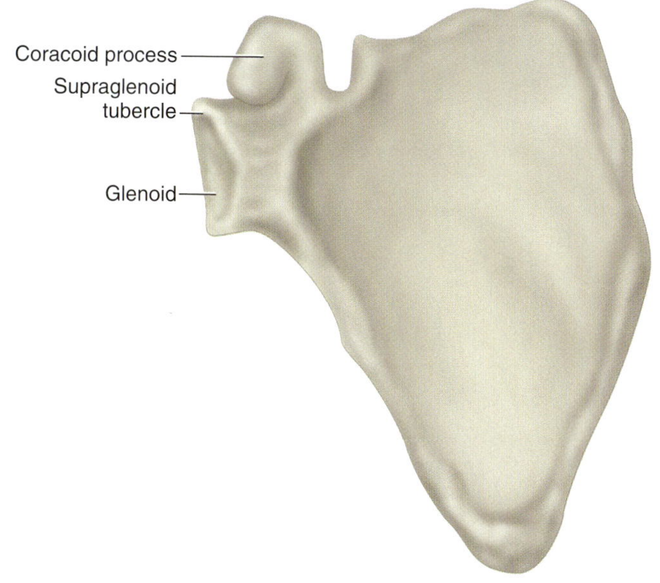

FIGURE 5

- The tendon of the long head of the biceps runs within the bicipital groove and attaches to the glenoid at the supraglenoid tubercle.
- The long axis of the humeral shaft can be found proximally at a point 5–13 mm (avg. 9 mm) posterior to the bicipital groove.

Pearls

- *Use of a head positioning device (see Fig. 7) allows the shoulder girdle and neck to be clear of the operating table and facilitates the use of fluoroscopy if desired.*

Pitfalls

- *Inadequate positioning can create significant difficulty with surgical exposure, bone preparation, and implant position, especially with respect to the glenoid.*

Positioning

- A modified beach chair semi-supine position is used (Fig. 6).
  - The patient is placed on a beanbag in order to stabilize him or her on the operating table.

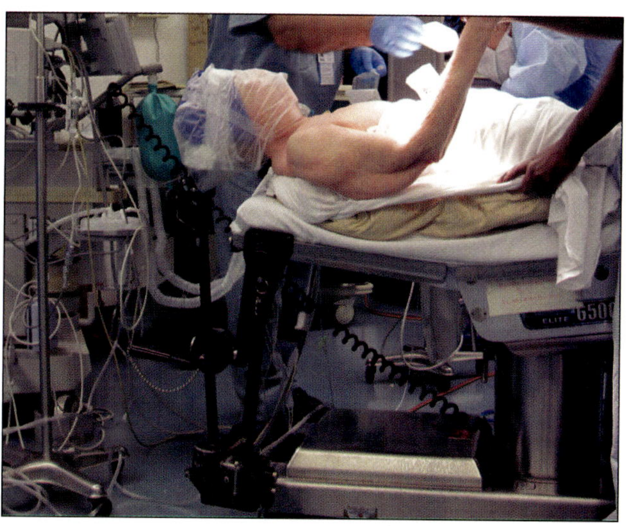

FIGURE 6

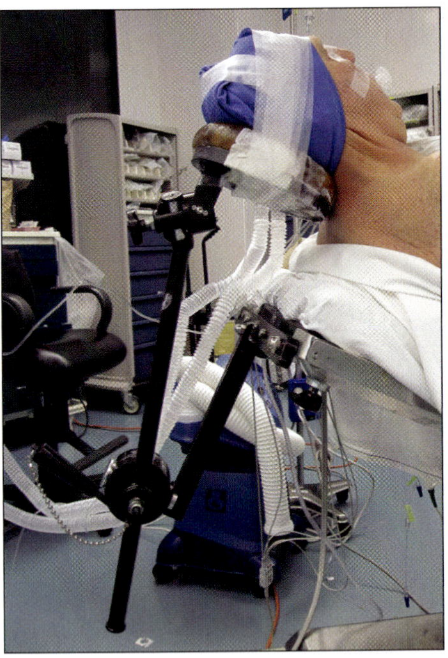

FIGURE 7

Equipment

- *Beanbag, size #30*
- *McConnell head positioning device (Greenville, TX)*

Controversies

- Concern exists regarding possible cerebrovascular events with beach chair positioning; with the modified semi-supine position the patient's head is minimally elevated.

Pearls

- *Retracting the cephalic vein medially helps to prevent injury to the vein by instruments used later in the procedure.*

Pitfalls

- *Skin incisions made too far laterally can lead to injury to the deltoid and prevent adequate visualization.*

  - Pillows are placed under the knees to allow the knees to rest in a flexed position and avoid injury to the sciatic nerve.
  - The beanbag is placed along the inferomedial border of the scapula in order to stabilize the scapula.
  - The head of the bed is elevated 20°.
  - The contralateral upper extremity rests in the patient's lap with all bony prominences well padded.
  - The patient is secured to the operating table with a safety strap.
- The patient's head is secured using a head positioning device (Fig. 7).

Portals/Exposures

- Deltopectoral Approach
  - A 5-cm skin incision is made from the tip of the coracoid process extending distally and paralleling the cephalic vein (Fig. 8).
  - Dissection is continued through the subcutaneous tissue and clavipectoral fascia, retracting the cephalic vein and conjoined tendon medially.
  - The axillary nerve can then be identified crossing over the subscapularis and traveling in an inferolateral direction.

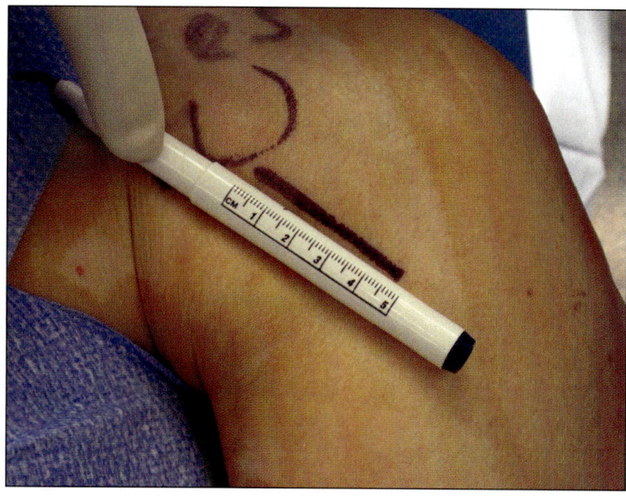

FIGURE 8

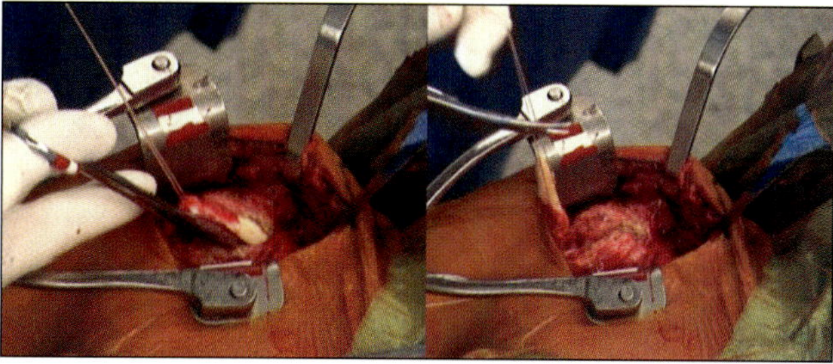

A B

FIGURE 9

Instrumentation

- Scalpel
- Electrocautery
- Forceps
- Hohmann retractors
- Self-retaining retractors (Gelpi and Kölbel retractors)
- Dissecting scissors
- Needle driver
- Suture

Pearls

- *The anterior-inferior joint capsule is divided to improve subscapularis excursion and glenohumeral joint motion.*

Pitfalls

- *Excessive dissection at the anterior aspect of the subscapularis runs the risk of neurologic injury and subscapularis denervation and should be avoided.*

- The tendon of the long head of the biceps is identified within the bicipital groove, tagged with a suture for tenodesis at a later time (Fig. 9A), and then detached from the supraglenoid tubercle (Fig. 9B).

Procedure

Step 1: Subscapularis Release with Lesser Tuberosity "Fleck" Osteotomy

- The superior, inferior, and lateral borders of the subscapularis are identified.
- A curved osteotome is used to release the subscapularis from the lesser tuberosity along with a small "fleck" of bone measuring 2 cm long, 1 cm wide, and 3–4 mm thick (Fig. 10).
- The subscapularis is detached from the proximal humerus along with the underlying joint capsule and then mobilized along the superior, inferior, and posterior aspects.

FIGURE 10

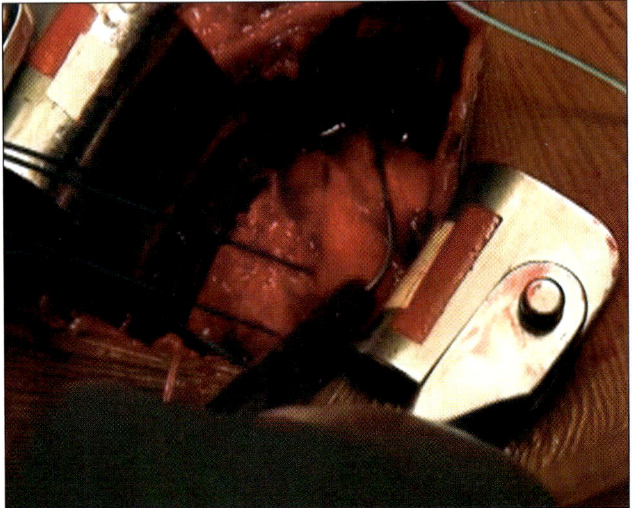

FIGURE 11

- Four heavy nonabsorbable sutures are placed through the subscapularis at the bone-tendon junction (Fig. 11).

Step 2: Humeral Osteotomy

- A Darrach retractor and Hohmann retractors are placed around the humeral head to expose the humeral head and deliver it out of the wound.
- A curved osteotome and rongeur are used to remove the ring of osteophytes around the inferior humeral head (Fig. 12).
- Once the osteophytes are removed, the true anatomic neck can be identified. An oscillating saw is used to perform the osteotomy of the humeral head (Fig. 13).

Instrumentation/ Implantation

- Curved osteotome
- Mallet
- Fukuda retractor
- Dissecting scissors
- Forceps
- Needle driver
- Four heavy nonabsorbable sutures

Pearls

- *Excellent exposure of the humeral head is necessary, including direct visualization of the posterior cuff insertion.*

Pitfalls

- *A careless osteotomy with the oscillating saw can risk detachment of the rotator cuff from the proximal humerus.*

Instrumentation/ Implantation

- Darrach retractor
- Hohmann retractors
- Curved osteotome
- Mallet
- Rongeur
- Oscillating saw

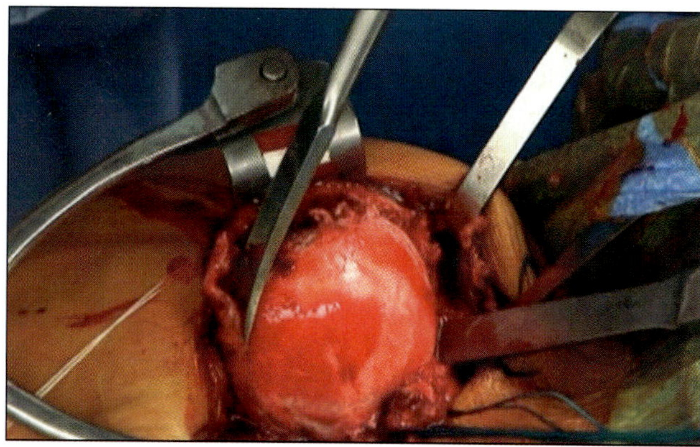

FIGURE 12

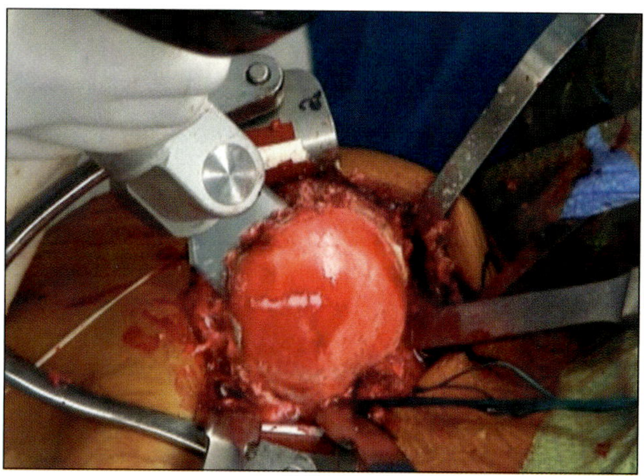

FIGURE 13

Step 3: Glenoid Surface Preparation and Suture Placement

- Glenoid Surface Preparation
  - All previous retractors are removed and a Darrach retractor is placed at the posterior-inferior aspect of the glenoid rim and is used to retract the proximal humerus posteriorly.
  - A Bankart retractor is placed at the anterior aspect of the glenoid rim and is used to retract the anterior capsule and subscapularis.
  - Additional Hohmann retractors can be placed at various locations around the glenoid rim to assist with visualization.
  - The anatomic center of the glenoid is determined and the centering drill is used to make a starter hole for reaming.
  - The glenoid is then reamed with sequentially larger sized motorized glenoid reamers until the appropriately sized reamer is used to ream the entire face of the glenoid (Fig. 14).

Pearls

- *Glenoid version can be corrected by reaming the glenoid surface perpendicular to the scapula. The initial starter hole must be drilled in line with the scapula to allow for this.*
- *Absorbable suture anchors are preferred over metal anchors because metal anchors may loosen and erode through the graft.*

Pitfalls

- *The glenoid labrum provides additional points of fixation for the graft and thus the labrum should not be excised.*

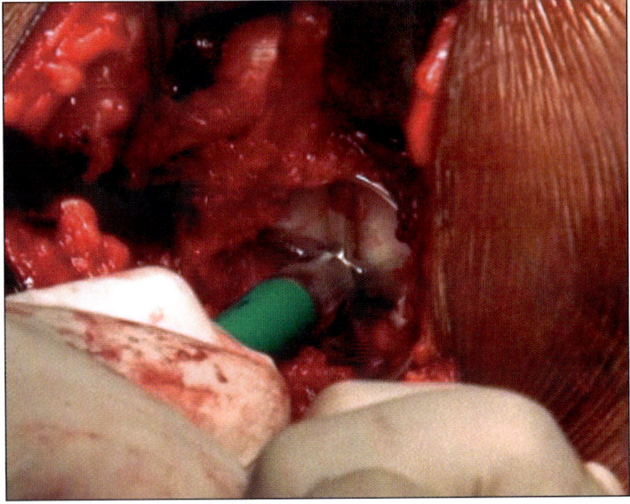

FIGURE 14

Instrumentation/ Implantation

- Darrach retractor
- Bankart retractor
- Hohmann retractors
- Drill
- Centering drill bit for reamer
- Glenoid reamers
- 2.0-mm drill bit
- Absorbable suture anchors
- 4 heavy nonabsorbable sutures
- Needle driver
- Forceps

  - The glenoid is reamed until the surface is decorticated and bleeding bone is exposed.
  - Several drill holes are made on the surface of the glenoid using a 2.0-mm drill bit.
- Suture Placement
  - Four double-loaded absorbable suture anchors are placed into the prepared glenoid surface in a cruciate pattern with an anchor at each position corresponding to the 3, 6, 9, and 12 o'clock positions (Fig. 15).
  - A heavy nonabsorbable suture is placed through the glenoid labrum midway between each suture anchor (Fig. 16).

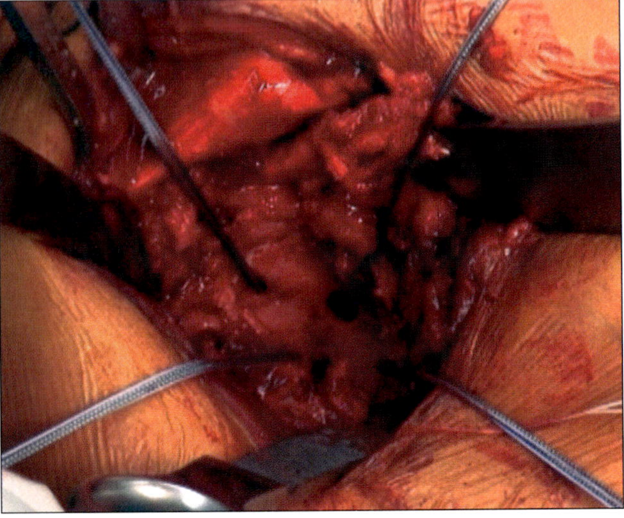

FIGURE 15

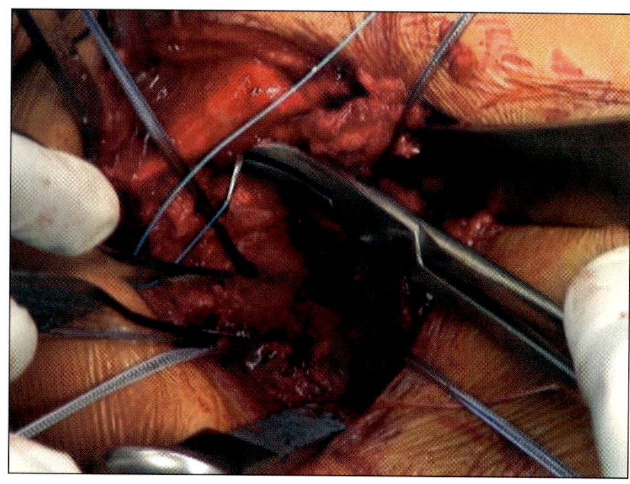

FIGURE 16

> **PEARLS**
>
> - *A trial glenoid component can be used as a guide for cutting the graft to the appropriate size.*

> ## Instrumentation/ Implantation
>
> - Graftjacket MaxForce Extreme (Wright Medical)
> - Dissecting scissors
> - Needle driver
> - Free needle
> - Forceps
> - Trial glenoid component

STEP 4: GRAFT PREPARATION AND FIXATION

- Graft Preparation
  - The human dermal allograft (Graftjacket) is allowed to thaw in normal saline while performing the glenoid preparation.
  - The graft is cut to the appropriate size and shape corresponding to the prepared glenoid surface using the trial glenoid component as a guide (Fig. 17A and 17B).
- Graft Fixation
  - All sutures from the suture anchors are passed through the graft at its periphery in a horizontal mattress suture fashion.
  - The sutures through the labrum are passed through the periphery of the graft in a simple suture fashion (Fig. 18).
  - As the sutures are tied, the graft is slid down the sutures until it rests on the glenoid surface. Once

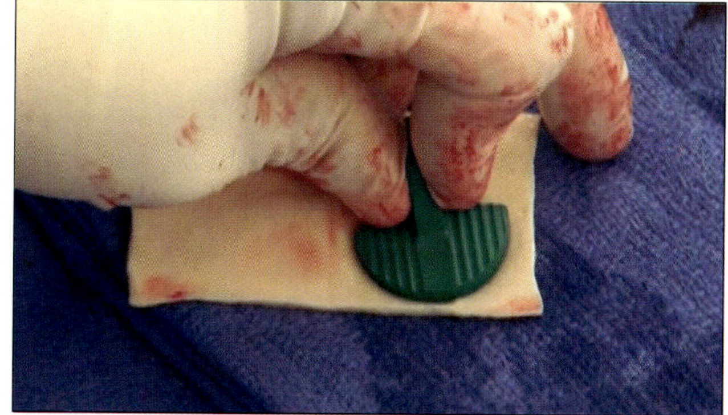

A

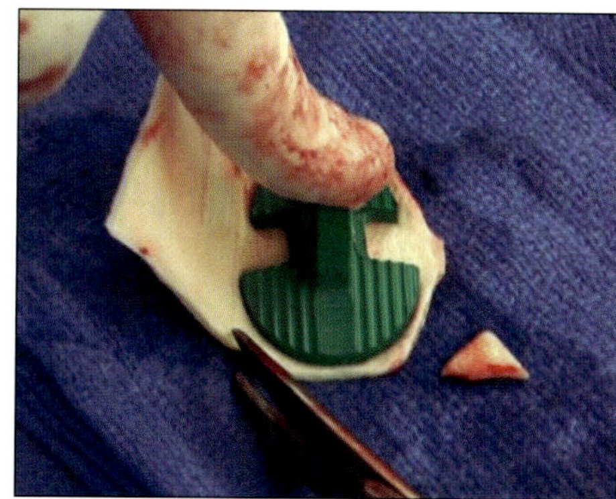

B

FIGURE 17

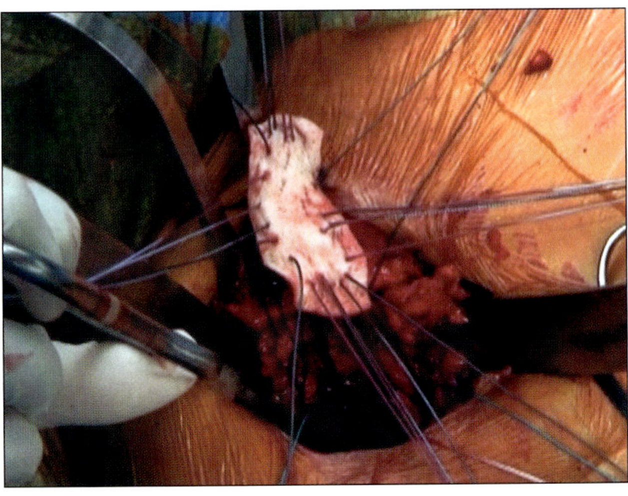

FIGURE 18

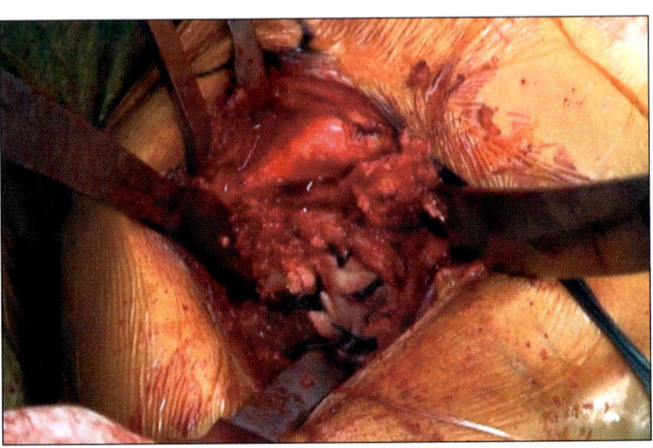

FIGURE 19

all of the sutures are tied, the graft is secured to the glenoid surface (Fig. 19).

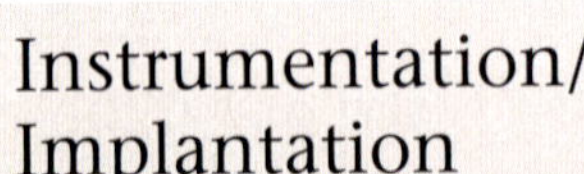

Instrumentation/ Implantation

- Darrach retractor
- Hohmann retractor
- Kölbel retractor
- Humeral reamers
- Humeral broaches
- Humeral trial components
- Drill
- Four heavy nonabsorbable sutures
- Needle driver
- Forceps
- Cement restrictor (possible)
- Cement (possible)
- Humeral prosthesis
- Mallet
- Impactor

Step 5: Humeral Preparation and Prosthesis Implantation

- Humeral Preparation
  - All previous retractors are removed, and the Kölbel retractor is used to retract the deltoid and conjoined tendon.
  - The proximal humerus is better visualized and delivered out of the wound by placing a Darrach retractor on the posterior aspect of the humeral head and a Hohmann retractor inferiorly.
  - Proximal humeral preparation is performed according to the humeral arthroplasty system being used. This would consist of reaming, broaching (Fig. 20), and trialing of the humeral stem (Fig. 21A) and humeral head (Fig. 21B) as is done typically for a shoulder hemiarthroplasty.

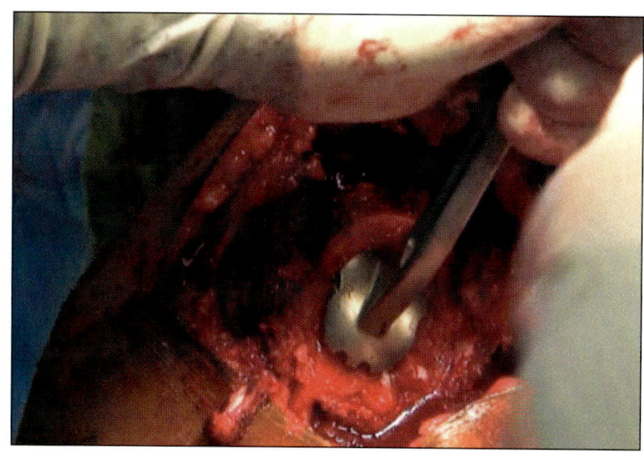

FIGURE 20

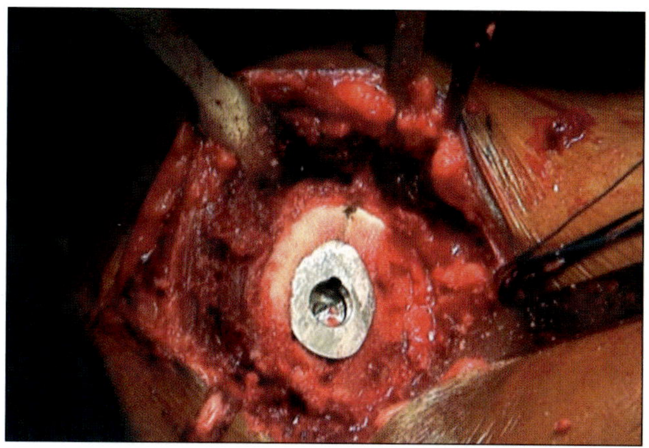

A

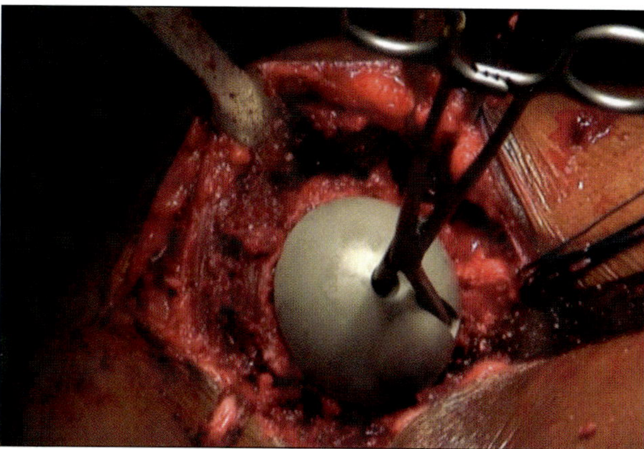

B

FIGURE 21

- Humeral Prosthesis Implantation
  - The trial is removed, and a drill is used to make four drill holes along the lesser tuberosity. A heavy nonabsorbable suture is placed through each transosseous hole (Fig. 22).
  - The final humeral prosthesis is impacted into position with an impactor and mallet (Fig. 23).

Pearls

- *Suture management can be achieved using surgical clamps on corresponding limbs of sutures.*

Step 6: Repair and Closure

- Dual-Row Subscapularis Repair
  - Both ends of the four transosseous sutures within the lesser tuberosity are passed through the tendinous portion of the subscapularis in a horizontal mattress fashion; this establishes the medial row of fixation (Fig. 24).
  - The four sutures placed through the subscapularis when it was released at the start of the procedure are now passed through the bone or soft tissue at the lateral aspect of the proximal humerus in a

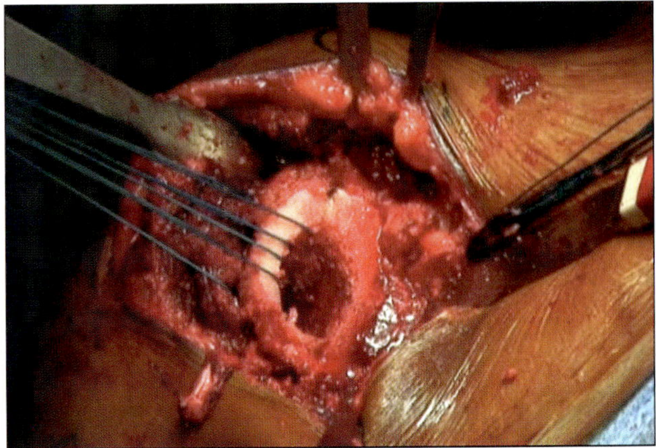

FIGURE 22

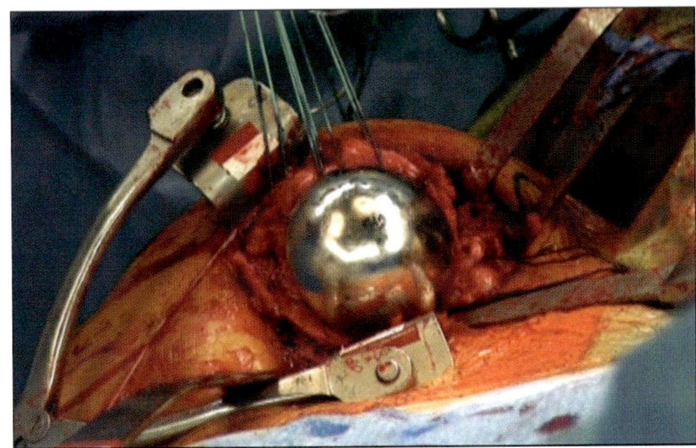

FIGURE 23

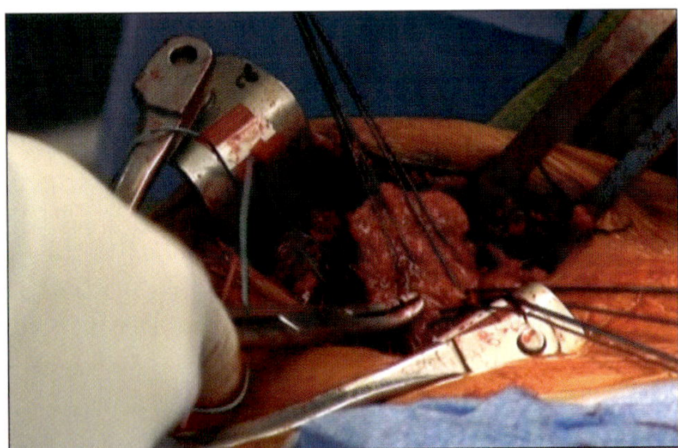

FIGURE 24

Instrumentation/ Implantation

- Needle driver
- Forceps
- Free needle
- Awl
- Heavy nonabsorbable suture

simple suture fashion; this establishes the lateral row of fixation.

- The subscapularis and attached bone "fleck" are reduced anatomically to the lesser tuberosity and held in place with an awl while all sutures are tied, securing the subscapularis to the lesser tuberosity.

■ Biceps Tenodesis
- The arm is positioned in 30° of external rotation and a heavy nonabsorbable suture is used to close the rotator interval.
- The biceps tendon is identified, the tag suture is removed, and a soft tissue biceps tenodesis is performed using a locking heavy nonabsorbable suture through the biceps tendon and through the rotator cuff tissue in the rotator interval.

■ Wound Closure
- The wound is irrigated copiously and adequate hemostasis is obtained.
- Standard wound closure is completed by closing the deltopectoral interval, subcutaneous tissues, and skin.
- A sterile dressing is applied and the upper extremity is placed in a sling.
- Final postoperative radiographs are obtained to confirm proper placement of the prosthesis (Fig. 25).

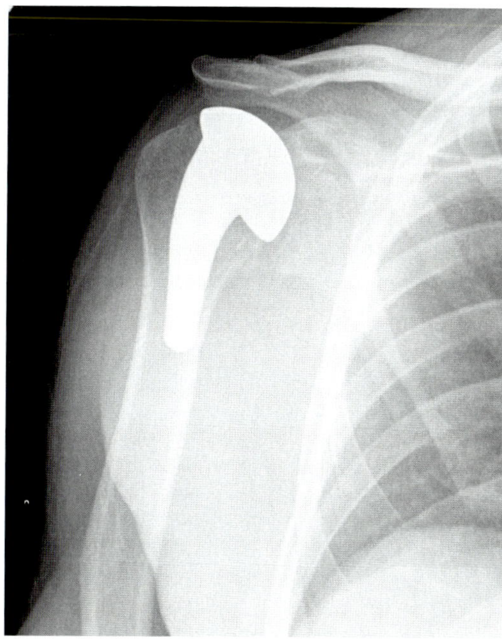

FIGURE 25

Pearls

- *Healing of the subscapularis can be confirmed with an axillary radiograph on which bony callus can be seen at the site of the "fleck" osteotomy.*

Pitfalls

- *Early resistance exercises or excessively forced motion can lead to failure of the subscapularis repair.*

Postoperative Care and Expected Outcomes

- Postoperative care is the same as conventional shoulder arthroplasty, with sling immobilization for the first 4 weeks and immediate passive motion exercises.
- Full active motion exercises are initiated at 4 weeks following surgery.
- Resistance and strengthening exercises can begin at 8 weeks after surgery.
- It is expected that the patient will be able to return to full unrestricted activity by 3–6 months after surgery.

Evidence

Krishnan SG, Reineck JR, Nowinski RJ, Harrison D, Burkhead WZ. Humeral hemiarthroplasty with biologic resurfacing of the glenoid for glenohumeral arthritis: surgical technique. J Bone Joint Surg [Am]. 2008;90(Suppl 2, Pt 1):9-19.

This paper provided a complete description of the previous surgical technique using an Achilles tendon allograft instead of Graftjacket for resurfacing of the glenoid.

Krishnan SG, Nowinski RJ, Harrison D, Burkhead WZ. Humeral hemiarthroplasty with biologic resurfacing of the glenoid for glenohumeral arthritis: two to fifteen-year outcomes. J Bone Joint Surg [Am]. 2007;89:727-34.

In this retrospective review, 36 shoulders that were treated with humeral hemiarthroplasty and soft tissue resurfacing of the glenoid were followed for at least 2 years after surgery. Outcome was based on radiographs and clinical parameters including pain, motion, and ASES scores. (Level IV evidence [case series])

Burkhead WZ, Hutton KS. Biologic resurfacing of the glenoid with hemiarthroplasty of the shoulder. J Shoulder Elbow Surg. 1995;4:263-70.

In this retrospective review, 6 patients were followed for 2 years after surgery that consisted of humeral hemiarthroplasty and soft tissue resurfacing of the glenoid. The original surgical technique described used anterior capsule or fascia lata autograft for the soft tissue resurfacing of the glenoid. (Level IV evidence [case series])

PROCEDURE 9

Total Shoulder Arthroplasty

Robert U. Hartzler, John W. Sperling, and Robert H. Cofield

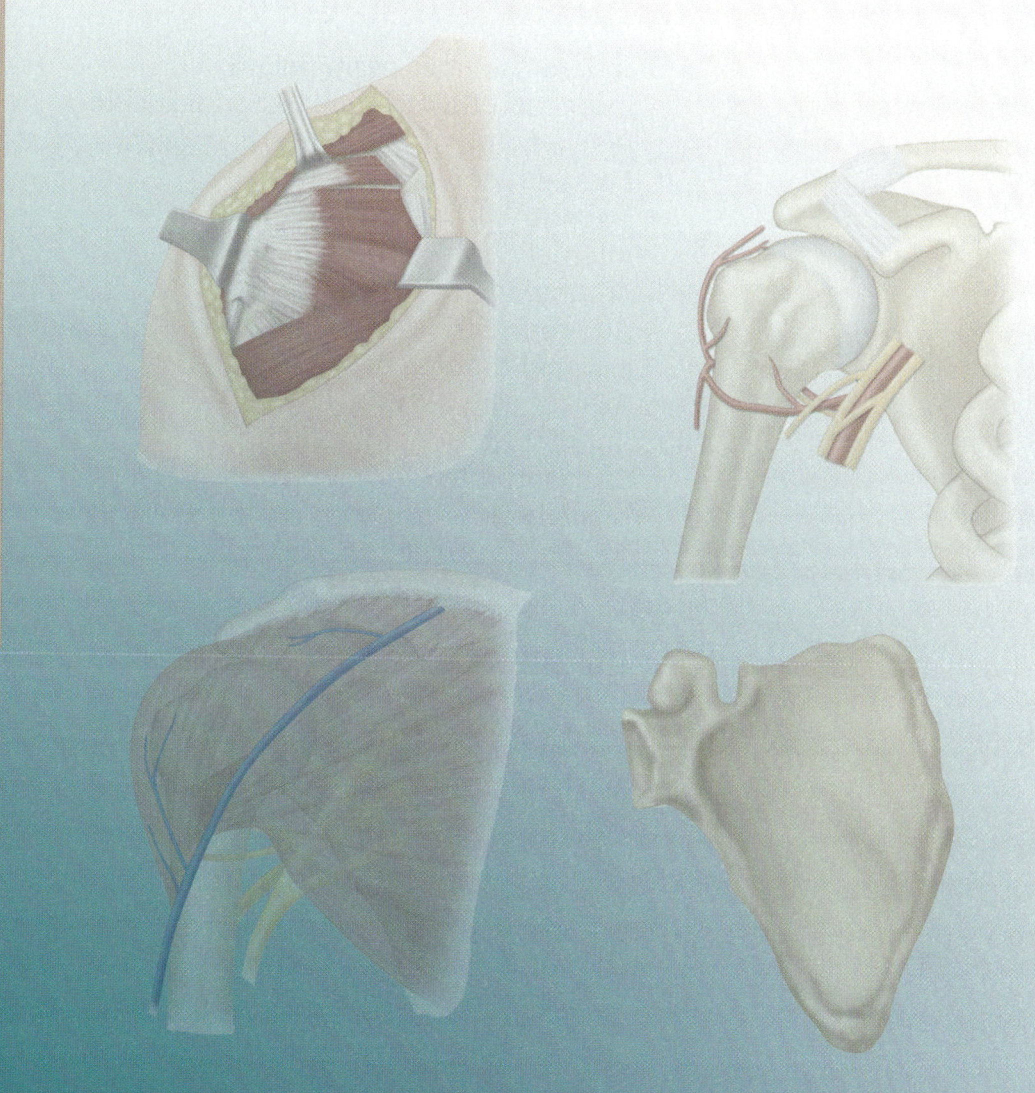

PITFALLS

- *Rotator cuff arthropathy*
- *Neuropathic joint*
- *Glenohumeral instability*
- *Active infection*
- *Massive glenoid bone loss*

Controversies

- Hemiarthroplasty for glenohumeral arthrosis has certain indications, but has been found to have less reliable pain relief and a high revision rate compared to TSA (Rispoli et al., 2006).

Treatment Options

- Nonoperative: pharmacotherapy viscosupplementation or steroid injections, activity modification, physical therapy.
- Hemiarthroplasty or reverse TSA is indicated for glenohumeral arthrosis from rotator cuff arthropathy.
- Hemiarthroplasty is indicated for joint arthrosis with massive glenoid bone loss.

Indications

- Total shoulder arthroplasty (TSA) is indicated for pain relief from glenohumeral arthrosis in patients willing to accept postoperative restrictions and comply with rehabilitation.
- Common etiologies include primary osteoarthritis, rheumatoid arthritis, and posttraumatic arthritis. Other causes include advanced humeral head osteonecrosis (with glenoid involvement) and capsulorrhaphy arthrosis.

Examination/Imaging

- Standard shoulder examination
  - Inspection for atrophy and prior incisions
  - Active range of motion with inspection of scapula
  - Passive range of motion
  - Strength in abduction, flexion, extension, and internal and external rotation
- Radiographs
  - Anteroposterior 40° oblique views in internal and external rotation
  - Axillary view (Fig. 1)
- Computed tomography (CT)
  - CT is indicated for preoperative planning when glenoid erosion is seen on the axillary radiograph to quantify bone loss and determine glenoid version and wear (Fig. 2).
  - Three-dimensional reconstructions of the humerus and glenoid are helpful for complex cases.

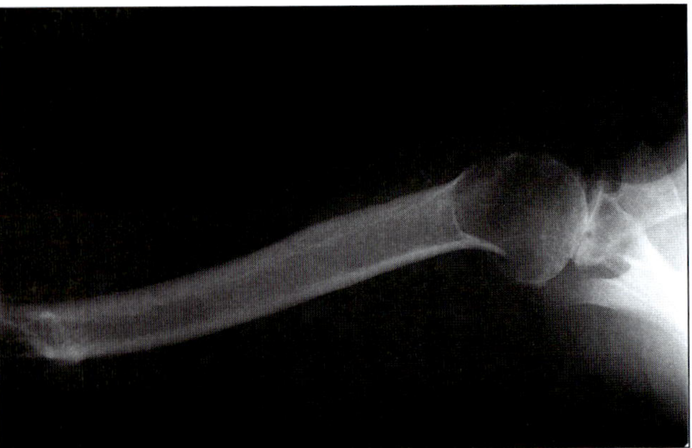

FIGURE 1

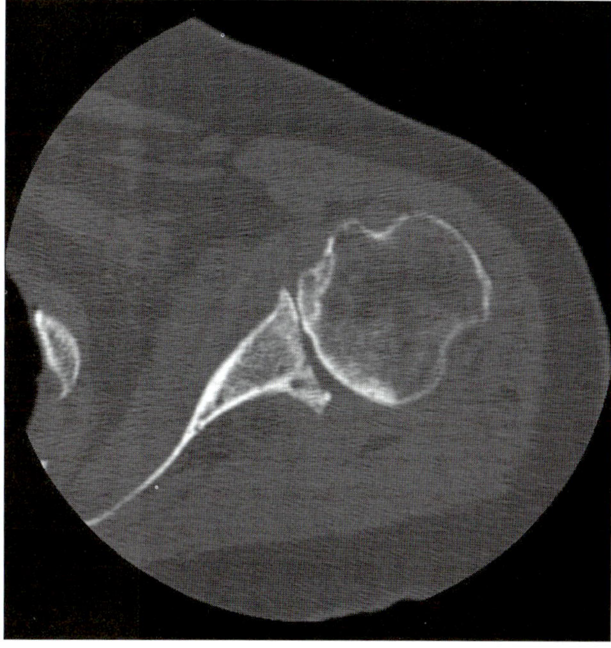

FIGURE 2

Surgical Anatomy

- Important external landmarks include the spine of the scapula, the anterior and lateral borders of the acromion and clavicle, and the coracoid process.
- Identify the proximal deltopectoral interval using the characteristic triangular infraclavicular fat pad (Fig. 3A). The cephalic vein is on the pectoralis major medially within the fat pad (Fig. 3B).
- The acromial and deltoid branches of the thoracoacromial artery will be cauterized during the exposure.

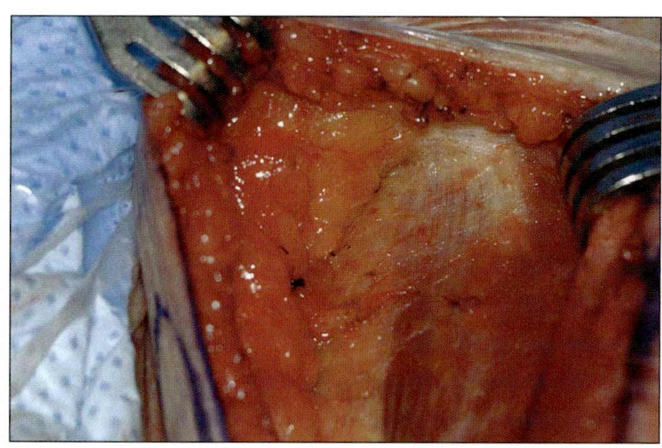

A

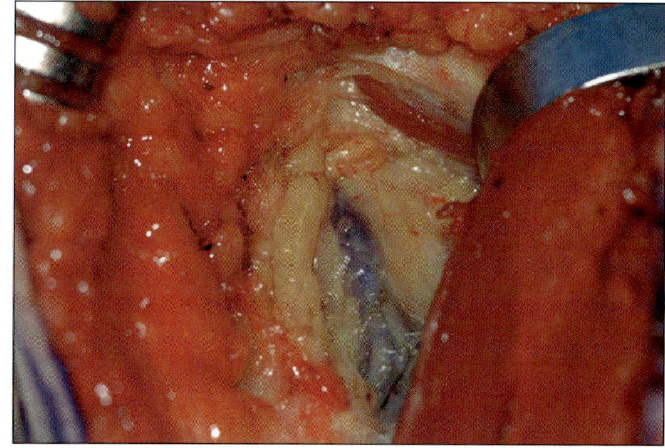

B

FIGURE 3

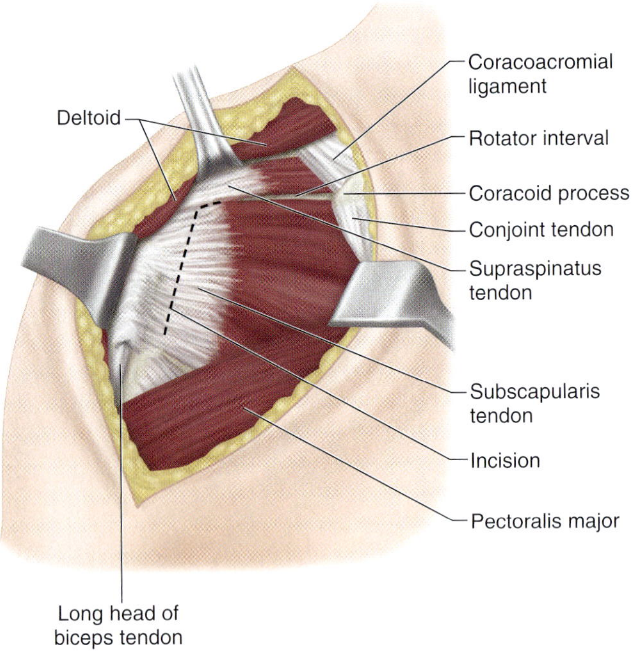

FIGURE 4

- The rotator interval is identified with the subscapularis tendon inferior (Fig. 4).

Positioning

- The patient is placed in the beach chair position with the waist at 45° and the legs at 30° (Fig. 5A and 5B).
- The operating table is airplaned away from the operative shoulder slightly.
- An examination under anesthesia is performed after positioning, documenting range of motion and stability.

PEARLS

- *Place a rolled up towel under the medial border of the ipsilateral scapula. Ensure scapular mobility by testing for easy passive motion.*

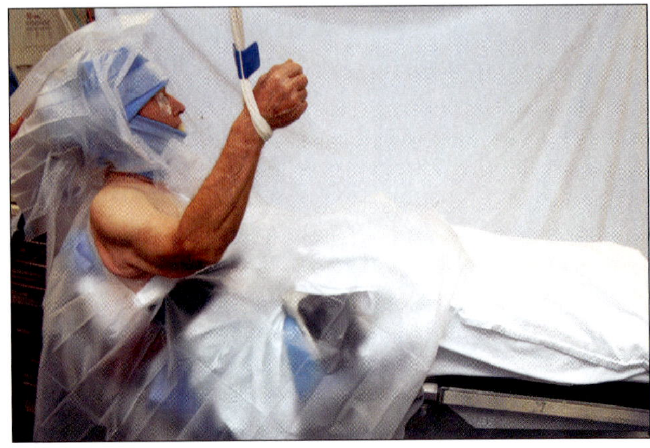

A

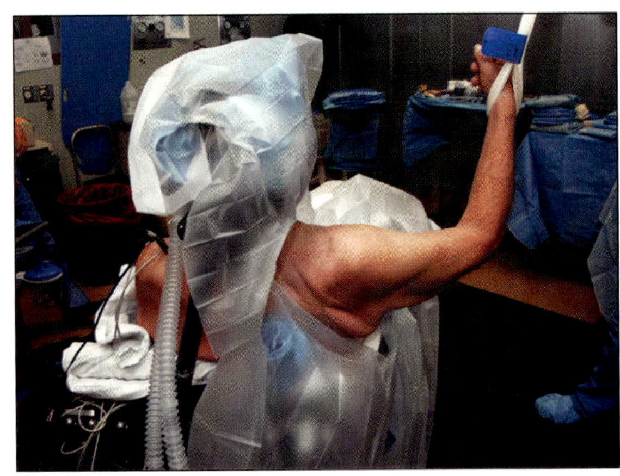

B

FIGURE 5

Equipment

- We use a draped and padded Mayo stand to aid in intraoperative positioning of the arm. Bring the stand in to achieve a stable position in abduction or flexion.

PEARLS

- *Develop the distal half of the deltopectoral interval with the arm at 30° abduction.*
- *During the inferior capsule release from bone, gradually externally rotate the arm in an adducted position to tension the capsule.*

PITFALLS

- *Use care while releasing scar at the coracoid base, as both axillary and musculocutaneous nerves are in close proximity.*
- *Protect the axillary nerve under direct visualization while releasing the inferior capsule directly from bone.*

Portals/Exposures

- The shoulder is exposed using a standard deltopectoral approach.
- The vertical incision passes 0.5–1 cm lateral to the coracoid process beginning at the anterior portion of the distal clavicle and extending about 15 cm (Fig. 6).
- The deltopectoral interval should be developed starting proximally at the infraclavicular fat pad. The cephalic vein remains on the pectoralis major medially.
- If necessary, the exposure can be extended by elevating periosteally the anterior portion of the deltoid insertion on the humerus or by mobilizing the deltoid origin from the clavicle.
- The clavipectoral fascia is incised starting proximally at the coracoacromial ligament and extending distally.
- The plane between the conjoined group and the subscapularis is identified. Any scar tissue at the base of the corocoid process is released.
- After release of any scar tissue in the subacromial space, the shoulder is reexamined.
- The rotator interval is identified. The release of the subscapularis–anterior capsule complex begins by extending the interval laterally while making sure to protect the long head of the biceps tendon.
- A marking stitch is placed into the superolateral corner of the incision (Fig. 7). The incision is carried inferiorly to complete the release after placing retention stitches into the subscapularis tendon.
- Our technique for release of the subscapularis tendon depends on passive external rotation (ER) under

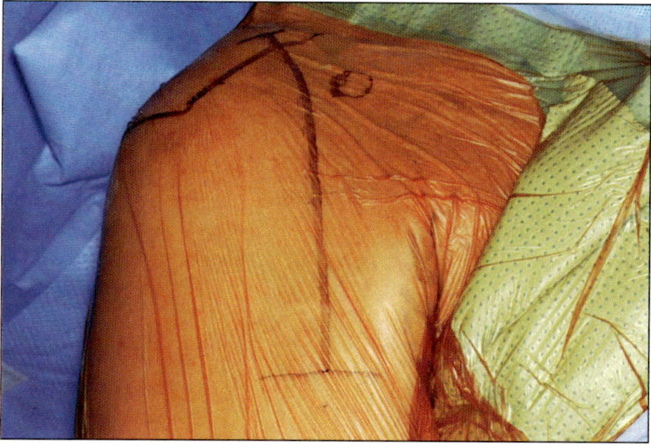

FIGURE 6

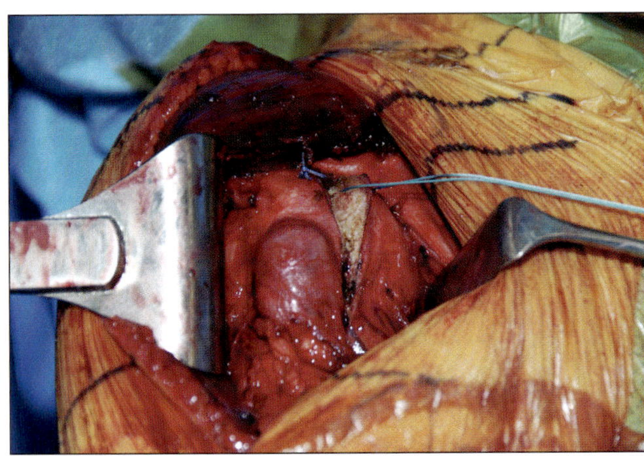

FIGURE 7

anesthesia. If the ER is less than 30°, the tendon is released directly from bone for later medialization. If the ER is greater than 30°, we cut through the tendon substance for later tendon-tendon repair.

- The shoulder capsule release is continued from bone inferiorly to the 8 o'clock position (left shoulder).

Controversies

- We retract the cephalic vein medially to reduce tension on the vessel and decrease risk for iatrogenic injury. Others leave it laterally, as the deltoid side has been shown to have more tributary vessels (Radkowski et al., 2006).
- Lesser tuberosity osteotomy has been advocated by some authors (Scalise et al., 2010).

Procedure

Step 1. Humeral Preparation

- The humeral head is dislocated by placing the arm in slight extension and adduction and then externally rotating the arm. Dislocation is assisted with an elevator placed along the posterior-inferior aspect of the humeral head (Fig. 8).
- Both sides of the rotator cuff are carefully inspected, as tears must be repaired prior to completion of the procedure.

Pearls

- *Use a drill or burr to gain access to the humeral canal, but prepare the humeral canal with hand reaming only.*

Pitfalls

- *Care must be taken not to place too much force on the humeral shaft to avoid fracture.*

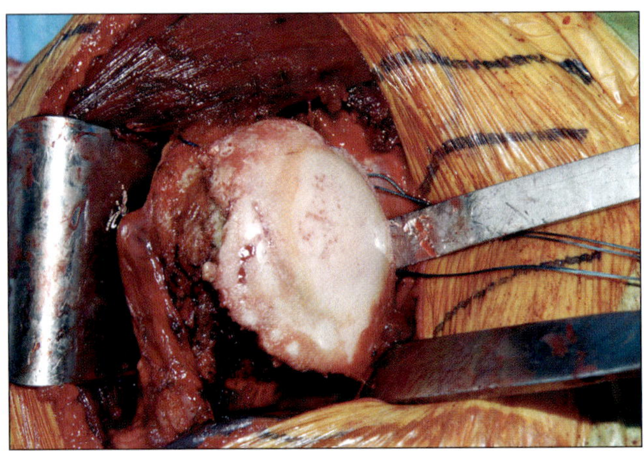

FIGURE 8

Instrumentation/ Implantation

- Darrach retractors are useful for protecting the soft tissues during the humeral head cut.

- After osteophyte removal, an entry hole is made in the superior aspect of the humeral head (Fig. 9). The entry hole is typically 1 cm posterior and 1 cm medial to the proximal bicipital groove.
- The humeral canal is then prepared with circular reamers, progressing in size until firm resistance is encountered (Fig. 10).
- A humeral resection guide is then placed with the cutting block 1 mm superior to the rotator cuff insertion.
  - The humerus is typically cut in 30–35 of retroversion (Fig. 11A; 30° retroversion shown).
  - The height of the cut in relation to the rotator cuff is confirmed (Fig. 11B).
- A trial humeral stem (Fig. 12; 30° retroversion shown) and trial head are placed.

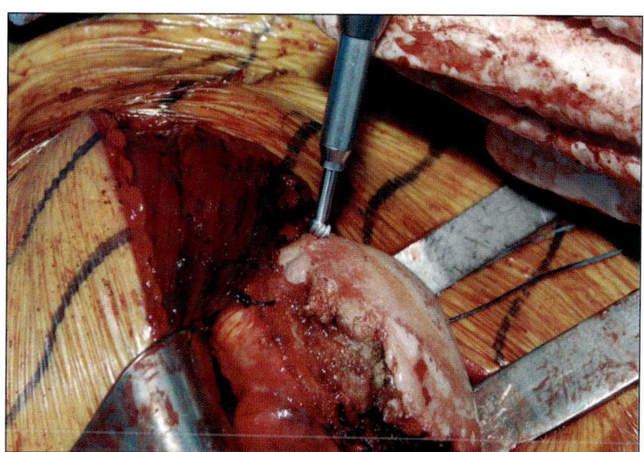

FIGURE 9

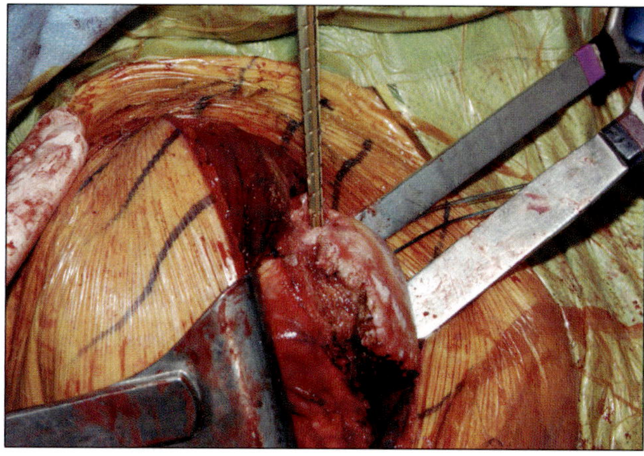

FIGURE 10

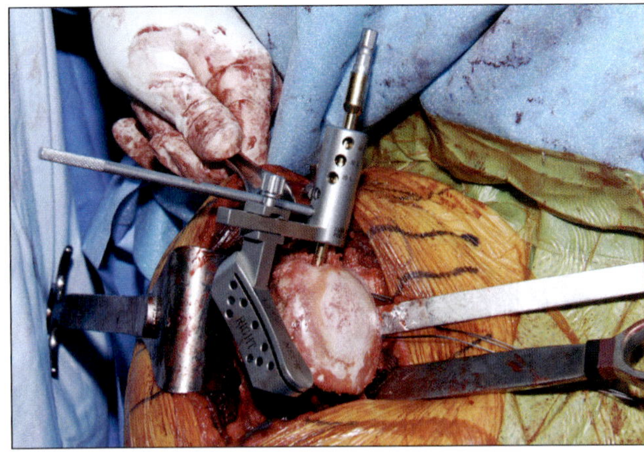

A

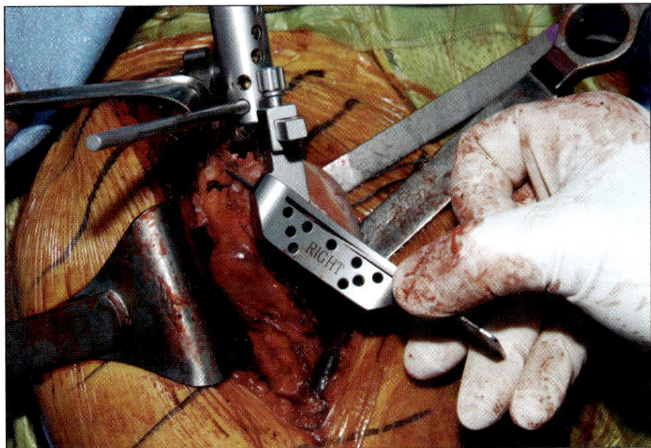

B

FIGURE 11

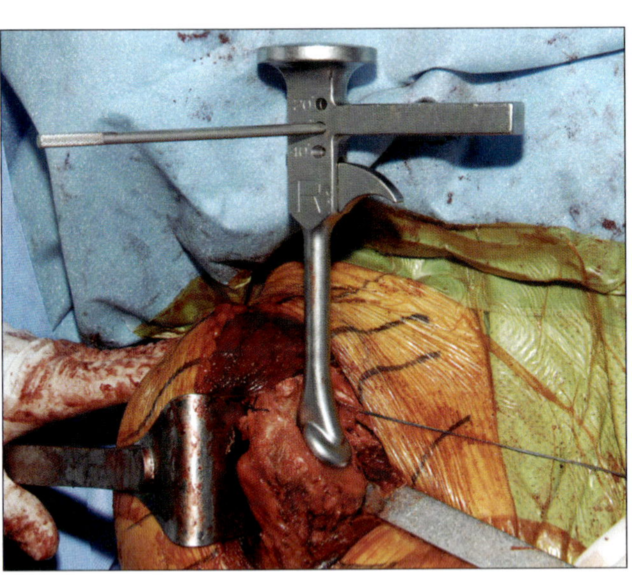

FIGURE 12

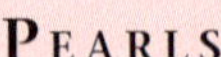

PEARLS

- *Typically in osteoarthritis, the glenoid is worn posteriorly. Therefore, glenoid reaming often must be directed anteriorly.*

PITFALLS

- *Common reasons for difficult glenoid exposure include insufficiencies in deltoid mobilization, capsular release, or humeral osteophyte removal, and an elevated humeral head cut.*
- *During cement polymerization, avoid pressure on the glenoid component with retractors.*

- Any osteophytes or metaphyseal bone extending beyond the extent of the trial head are trimmed (Fig. 13).
- Preliminary humeral head trialing is performed. See Step 3 below for our rules of thumb for trialing (Fig. 14).

STEP 2. GLENOID PROSTHETIC ARTHROPLASTY

- Keeping the trial humeral stem in place, the humerus is retracted posteriorly using a Fukuda retractor placed posterior to the glenoid rim. The arm is placed in 70–90° of abduction with slight flexion to expose the glenoid (Fig. 15).

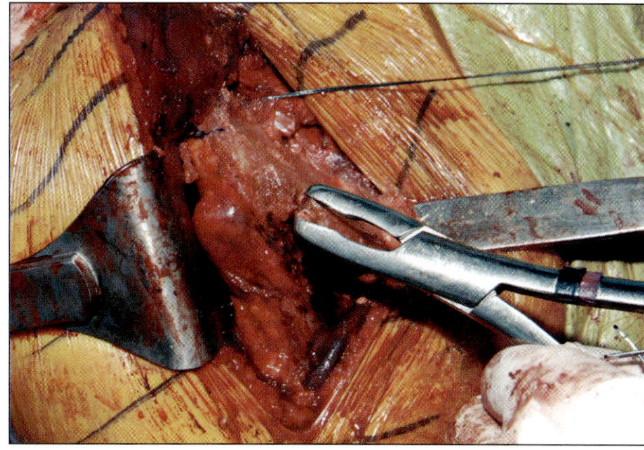

FIGURE 13

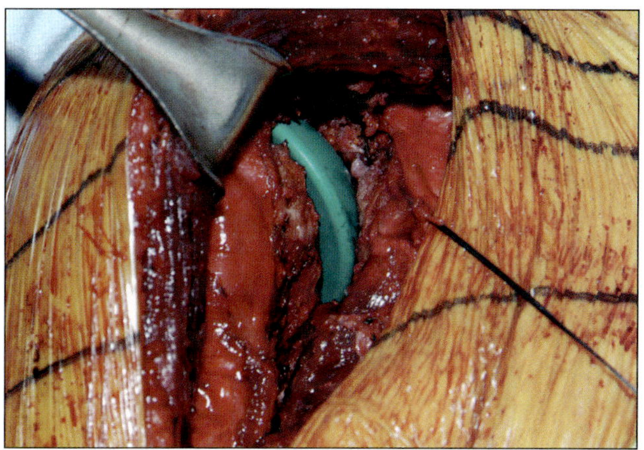

FIGURE 14

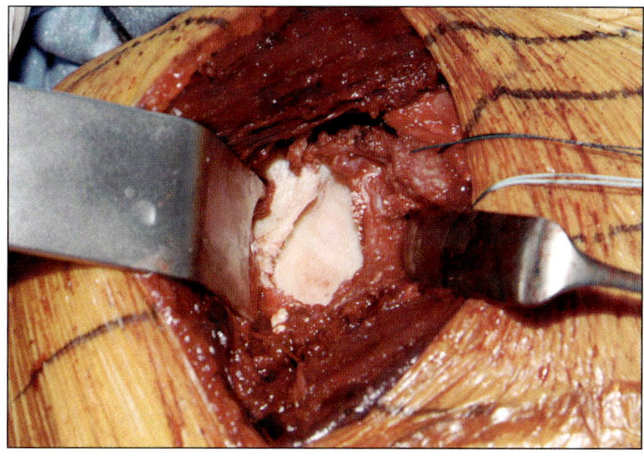

FIGURE 15

Instrumentation/ Implantation

- We prefer an all-polyethylene convex-backed glenoid. Surgeon preference dictates choice between a pegged versus a keeled component (Rahme et al., 2009).
- We reserve the use of a metal-backed glenoid for cases with significant glenoid bone deficiency (Tammachote et al., 2009).

- Excess synovium is removed and the glenoid labrum carefully excised circumferentially (Fig. 16).
- The anterior capsule is incised from the glenoid rim starting superiorly and extending anteroinferiorly to approximately the 8 o'clock (left shoulder) position (Fig. 17A).
- A second retractor (e.g., knee retractor) can then be repositioned at the anterior glenoid rim (Fig. 17B).
- The pattern of glenoid wear and version are determined. The anatomic center of the glenoid is marked (Fig. 18), taking care not to be misled by osteophytes. The CT scan, if available, should be reviewed.
- The glenoid component is sized.

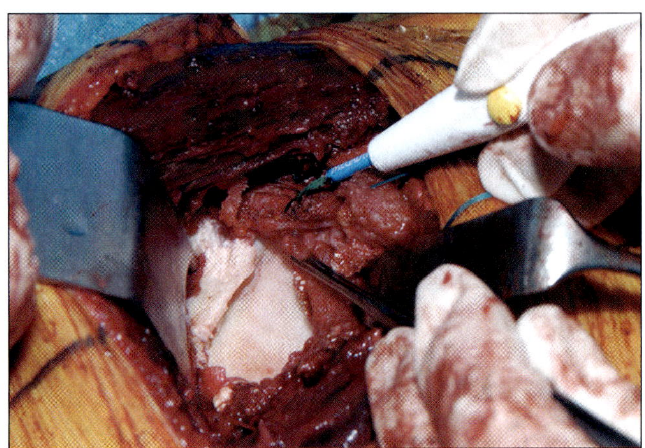

FIGURE 16

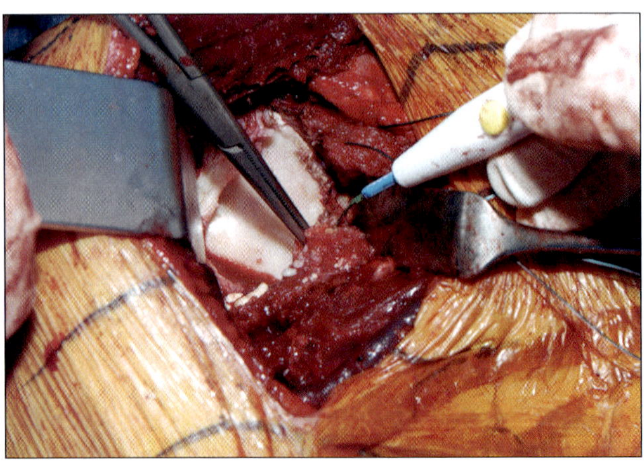

A

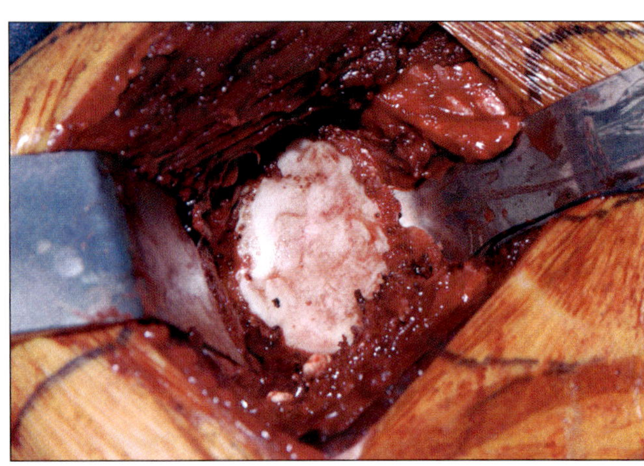

B

FIGURE 17

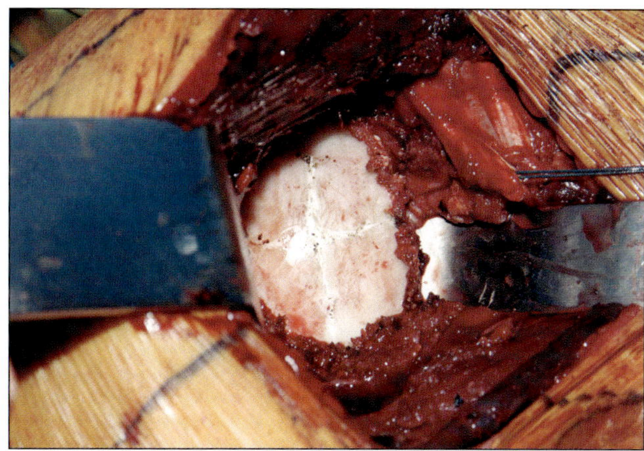

FIGURE 18

Controversies

- Instrumented rather than finger pressurization of cement has been shown to improve the cement mantle around polyethylene glenoid components (Nyffeler et al., 2006). Instrumented pressurization is recommended by some authors.

- The glenoid component has been implicated as the weak link in shoulder arthroplasty. Thus, considerable attention must be addressed to the details of glenoid preparation and cementing.
- Glenoid preparation
  - A centering hole is created with an awl or burr (Fig. 19). The position is checked with the guide, and the location altered if necessary.
  - Meticulous bone preparation must be performed. Instrumentation should be utilized to ream in an exacting and sequential manner (Fig. 20A), preserving some subchondral bone (Fig. 20B).
  - Depending on bone loss, the reaming may need to be directed toward one or more quadrants.
  - The glenoid is prepared to accept component keel or pegs. Using a drill guide (Fig. 21A), the peg

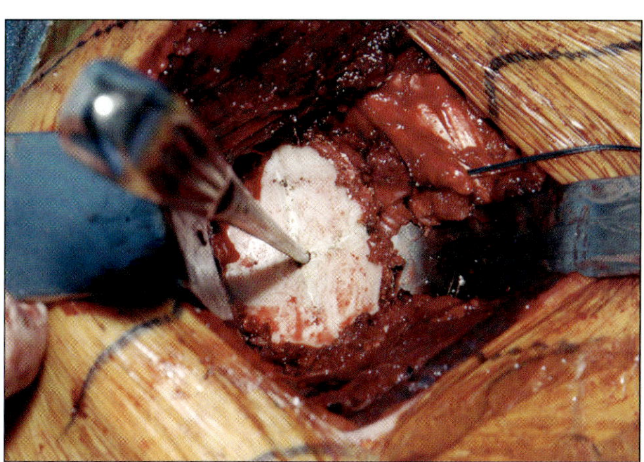

FIGURE 19

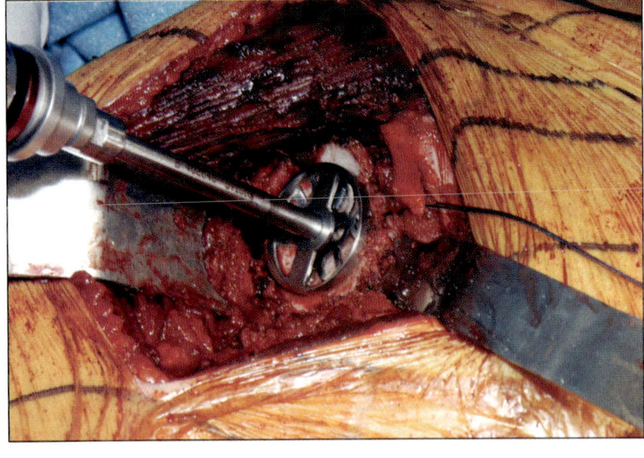

A

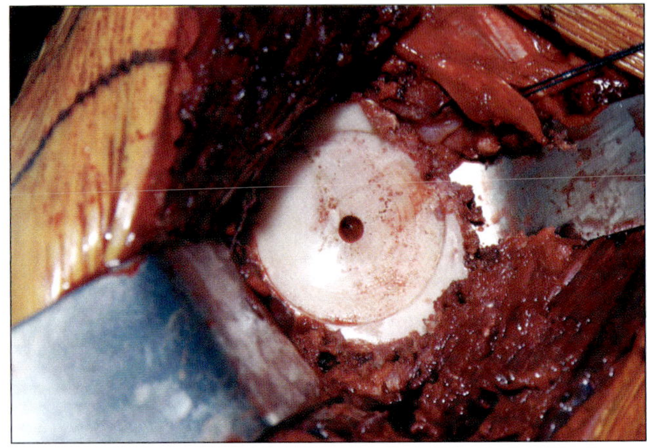

B

FIGURE 20

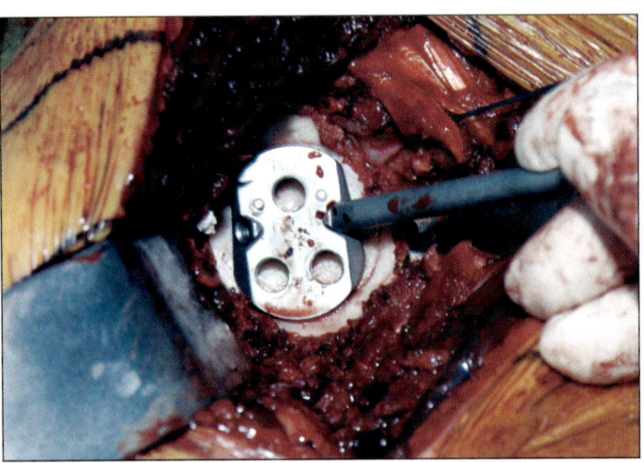

A

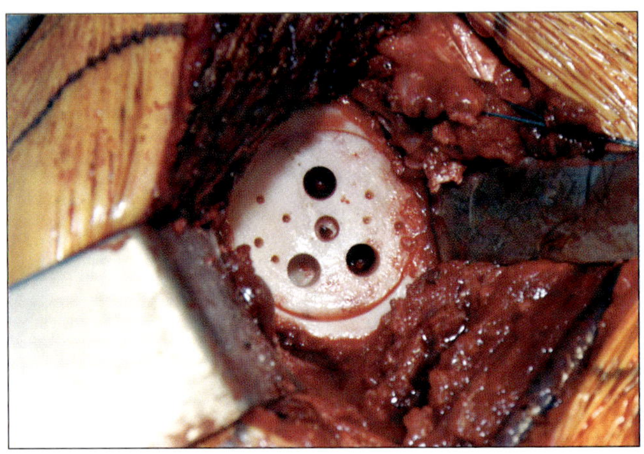

B

FIGURE 21

holes are drilled (Fig. 21B). The slot or columns are undercut with a burr to facilitate cement locking.
  - A trial glenoid is placed (Fig. 22).
- Glenoid cementation using third-generation techniques
  - The bone is washed with pulsatile lavage followed by careful, repetitive drying with sponges (Edwards et al., 2007; Mileti et al., 2004).
  - The bone cement is prepared using vacuum mixing to enhance its strength (Mileti et al., 2004).
  - The cement is placed in the columns or keel slot and finger-pressurized three times (Mileti et al., 2004).
  - The glenoid is impacted into the cement bed and held with an instrument while extra cement is removed.

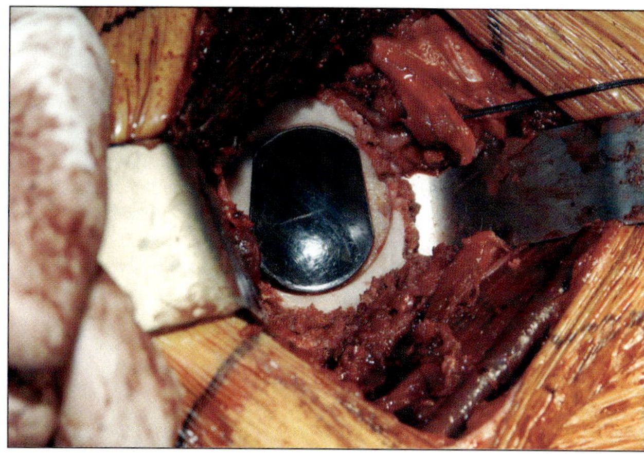

FIGURE 22

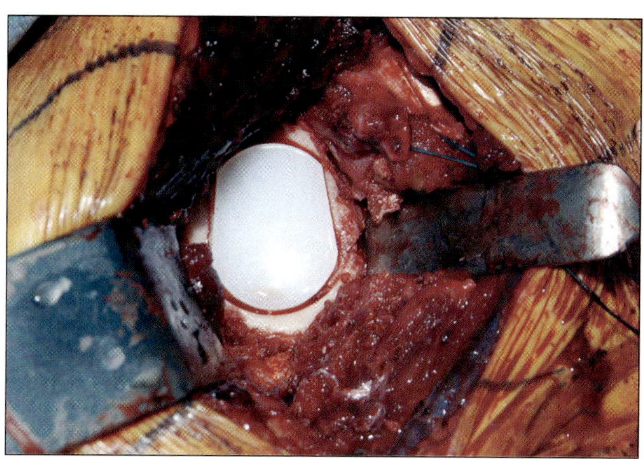

FIGURE 23

- Figure 23 shows the appearance of the final glenoid component.

Step 3. Soft Tissue Balancing and Completion of the Humerus

- Humeral drill holes and sutures are placed as needed for tendon repairs.
- The final humeral stem is impacted into place.
- Trial reductions and soft tissue balancing are performed, keeping in mind the need for both stability and motion (Fig. 24).
- Humeral head selection is based on patient size, capsular and rotator cuff laxity, and bone resection.
- Anterior capsule–subscapularis lengthening is often required to balance laxity in the posterior structures.

Pearls

- *If performing rotator cuff or subscapularis repairs with a tendon-to-bone construct, place multiple drill holes 5 mm apart prior to stem placement.*
- *Place the rotator interval stitches with the arm in external rotation prior to seating the final humeral head.*

Pitfalls

- *To avoid an oversized humeral head, check that the subscapularis repair will be tension free with the arm placed in the desired position of maximum rotation.*
- *Ensure that the rotator cuff is not tented superiorly.*

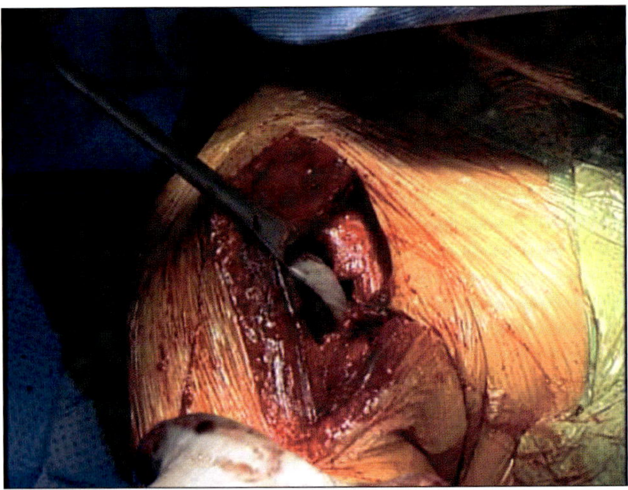
FIGURE 24

Instrumentation/ Implantation

- We prefer a modular humeral component with a proximal ingrowth stem.
- Have available a variety of humeral head sizes with the option for eccentric or offset components.

- At the final trialing, we use the following rules of thumb:
  - Humeral head should face opposite the glenoid in the neutral position.
  - Minimum of 90° of internal rotation and elevation of 150° using the superior rotator cuff to gauge soft tissue tension.
  - The humeral head should translate as follows: one half of the head exposes anteriorly with the arm in neutral, one quarter of the humeral head exposes inferiorly with the arm in 15–20° of abduction.
  - Subscapularis repair can be accomplished.
- The final humeral head is impacted into place (Fig. 25).

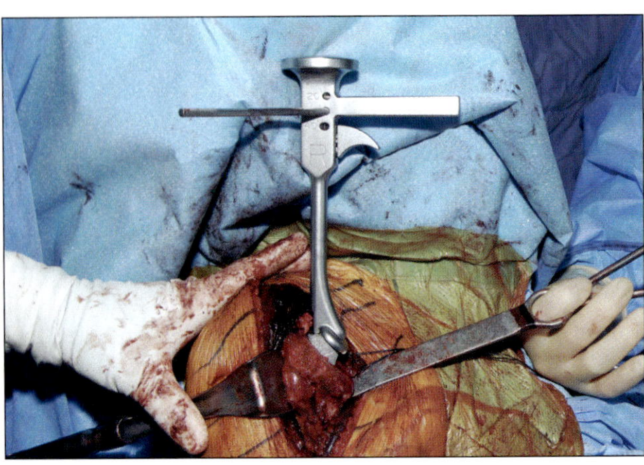
FIGURE 25

Controversies

- Cemented humeral components have been shown to have improved survivorship as compared with noncemented types (Cil et al., 2009). However, we prefer noncemented implants for primary TSA to balance long-term durability with ease of revision.

Pearls

- *Every 1-cm medial advancement of the subscapularis tendon results in a 20–30° gain of external rotation.*

Pitfalls

- *In our experience, many of the failures of the anterior repair are through the interval and do not include substantial disruption of the vertical portion. Therefore, secure repair of the rotator interval is crucial.*

Step 4. Arthrotomy and Soft Tissue Closure

- Closure begins by tying the rotator interval sutures. This should be performed with the arm in the desired degree of maximum external rotation.
- The subscapularis is repaired tendon-to-tendon or tendon-to-bone as indicated.
- After arthrotomy closure, the shoulder is taken through the final range of motion. translation of the humeral head is assessed anteriorly, posteriorly, and inferiorly. The amount of motion that can be achieved passively without stressing the repair is recorded, as this will guide postoperative rehabilitation.
- If necessary, the elevated deltoid attachments are repaired, and the wound is closed in layers in a standard fashion.

Postoperative Care and Expected Outcomes

- The patient is placed into a shoulder immobilizer postoperatively.
- On postoperative day 1, passive range-of-motion exercises are started using parameters determined during surgery.
- Pulley and wand exercises are incorporated into the rehabilitation program at 4–6 weeks postoperatively, with gentle isometric strengthening exercises following.
- Potential complications include, in order of decreasing frequency, component loosening, instability, rotator cuff tear, periprosthetic fracture, infection, component failure, and deltoid deficiency (Wirth and Rockwood, 1996).
- Patients can expect reliable pain relief and return of shoulder motion, as greater than 90% of patients have excellent or satisfactory short-term outcomes reported. TSA has long-term survivorship reported to be greater than 90% after 10 years (Adams et al., 2007).

Evidence

Adams JE, Sperling JW, Schleck CD, Harmsen WS, Cofield RH. Outcomes of shoulder arthroplasty in Olmsted County, Minnesota: a population-based study. Clin Orthop Relat Res. 2007;(455):176-82.

In this review of TSA and hemiarthroplasty done in a community population, outcomes compared favorably with those reported in the literature. The Neer ratings were excellent or satisfactory in 92% of TSAs at minimum 2-year follow-up. Survival was 96% at 10 years. (Level III evidence [retrospective review])

Cil A, Veillette CJ, Sanchez-Sotelo J, Sperling JW, Schleck CD, Cofield RH. Survivorship of the humeral component in shoulder arthroplasty. J Shoulder Elbow Surg. 2009.

At long-term follow-up of 10 years, cemented humeral components had a longer survival free of revision or removal (96.2% vs. 91.2%, HR, 0.37; 95% confidence interval, 0.18–0.76; p = .007). (Level III evidence [retrospective review])

Edwards TB, Sabonghy EP, Elkousy H, et al. Glenoid component insertion in total shoulder arthroplasty: comparison of three techniques for drying the glenoid before cementation. J Shoulder Elbow Surg. 2007;16:S107-10.

Using the outcome of immediate postoperative glenoid radiolucencies, no differences were detected between three drying techniques (including saline lavage and sponge drying). The other two methods cost 70 times that of sponge drying. (Level I evidence [prospective randomized trial])

Mileti J, Boardman ND 3rd, Sperling JW, Cofield RH, Torchia ME, O'Driscoll SW, Rowland CM. Radiographic analysis of polyethylene glenoid components using modern cementing techniques. J Shoulder Elbow Surg. 2004;13:492-8.

With modern techniques, including irrigation and drying of the cancellous bone of the glenoid keel, vacuum mixing of the cement to reduce porosity, and pressurization of the cement into the glenoid, 87% of patients had minimal or no immediate radiolucencies that could be attributed to poor surgical technique. (Level III evidence [retrospective review])

Nyffeler RW, Meyer D, Sheikh R, Koller BJ, Gerber C. The effect of cementing technique on structural fixation of pegged glenoid components in total shoulder arthroplasty. J Shoulder Elbow Surg. 2006;15:106-11.

Using micro-CT, six specimens were examined after receiving cemented polyethylene glenoid components. The three specimens undergoing instrumented pressurization of cement had 100% complete peg cement mantles, while three specimens undergoing finger pressurization of cement had a rate of 47% incomplete peg cement mantles. (anatomic study)

Radkowski CA, Richards RS, Pietrobon R, Moorman CT 3rd. An anatomic study of the cephalic vein in the deltopectoral shoulder approach. Clin Orthop Relat Res. 2006;(442):139-42.

In 40 fresh frozen cadaver specimens, the lateral tributary vessels significantly outnumbered medial vessels (2.8 ± 1.7 vs. 1.3 ± 1.1, p < .0001). Of the 38 specimens with a cephalic vein, 27 shoulders had more lateral feeder vessels versus 4 with more medial feeders (p < .0001). (anatomic study)

Rahme H, Mattsson P, Wikblad L, Nowak J, Larsson S. Stability of cemented in-line pegged glenoid compared with keeled glenoid components in total shoulder arthroplasty. J Bone Joint Surg [Am]. 2009;91:1965-72.

At a minimum follow-up of 2 years, no differences were found radiographically or clinically between pegged and keeled all-polyethylene cemented glenoid components. (Level I evidence [prospective randomized trial])

Rispoli DM, Sperling JW, Athwal GS, et al. Humeral head replacement for the treatment of osteoarthritis. J Bone Joint Surg [Am]. 2006;88:2637-44.

At minimum 5-year follow-up, 16 of 51 patients continued to experience moderate or severe pain. Nine of 51 underwent revision surgery for painful glenoid arthrosis. (Level III evidence [retrospective review])

Scalise JJ, Ciccone J, Iannotti JP. Clinical, radiographic, and ultrasonographic comparison of subscapuleris tenotomy and lesser tuberosity osteotomy for total shoulder arthroplasty. J Bone Joint Surg [Am]. 2010;92:1627-34.

In a short-term retrospective review, the authors found few abnormal tendons and higher postoperative shoulder scores in the lesser tuberosity osteotomy group. (Level III evidence)

Tammachote N, Sperling JW, Vathana T, Cofield RH, Harmsen WS, Schleck CD. Long-term results of cemented metal-backed glenoid components for osteoarthritis of the shoulder. J Bone Joint Surg [Am]. 2009;91:160-6.

At a minimum of 2 years of follow-up, 95 shoulders undergoing TSA with cemented metal-backed polyethylene glenoid components were reviewed. Pain relief and motion were satisfactory, as was stability. However, there was a high rate of periprosthetic glenoid lucency (83%). (Level III evidence [retrospective review])

Wirth MA, Rockwood CA, Jr. Complications of total shoulder-replacement arthroplasty. J Bone Joint Surg [Am]. 1996;78:603-16.

The authors reviewed 41 studies, 32 of which included unconstrained TSAs for a total of 1615 shoulders. Overall, duration of follow-up for these studies was short, with only eight studies having average follow-up greater than 4 years. Complications of TSA were as noted in Postoperative Care and Expected Outcomes. (Level III evidence [review of retrospective studies])

PROCEDURE 10

Rotator Cuff Tear Arthroplasty

Bryan Wall and Gilles Walch

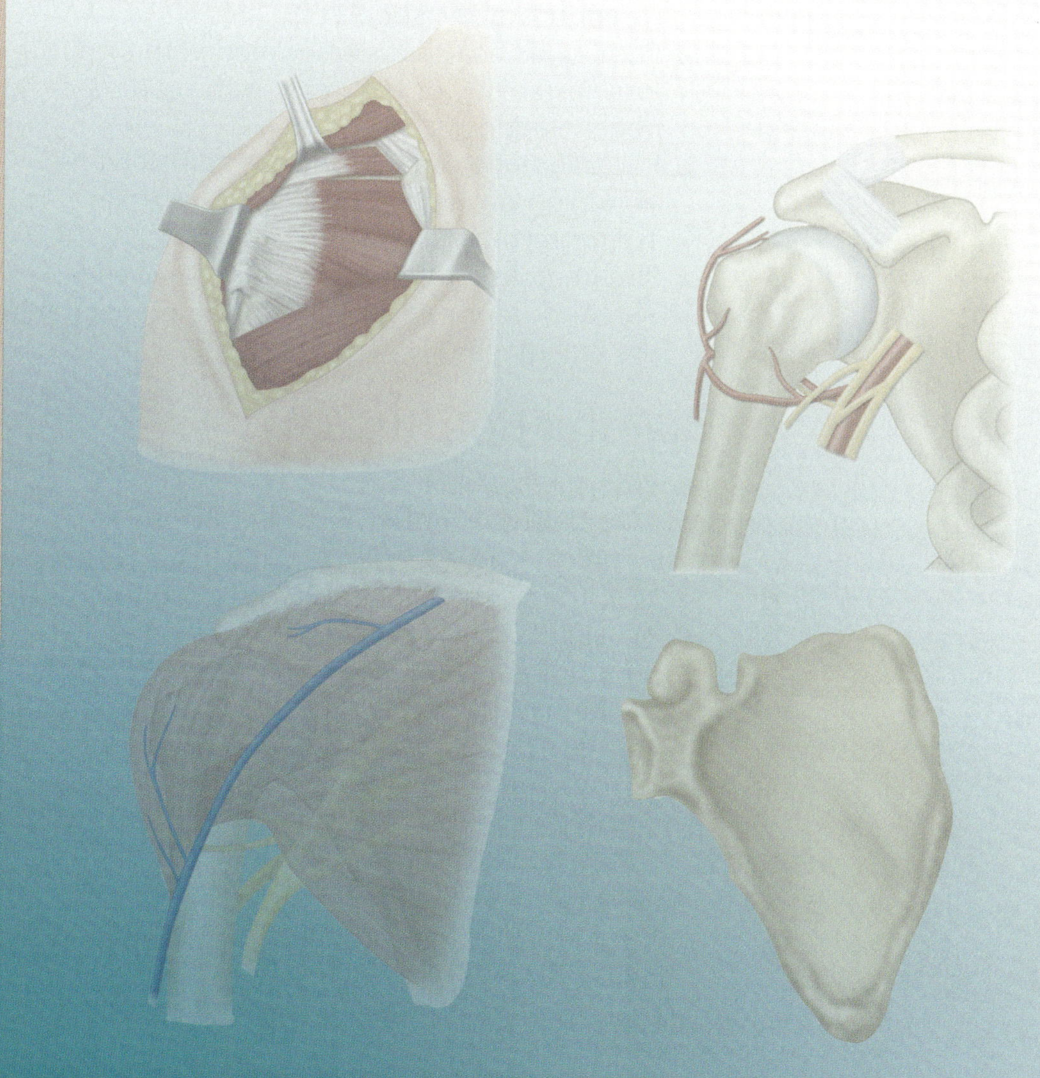

PITFALLS

- *The deltoid must be functioning. Reverse shoulder arthroplasty in patients with deltoid insufficiency can result in poor function and component instability.*
- *Glenoid bone stock must be adequate to support the glenosphere.*
- *The patient must have no significant infections.*

Controversies

- Younger, higher demand patients may develop eventual component loosening and should be approached cautiously.
- Patients with good elevation and intact coracoacromial arches have been suggested for hemiarthroplasty by some authors.

Treatment Options

- Arthrodesis may be considered for younger patients with high functional demands.
- Tendon transfers or biceps tenotomy may be appropriate for patients without significant glenohumeral changes.

Open Surgical Treatment

Indications

- Significant pain and dysfunction in older patients with irreparable cuff tears and degenerative glenohumeral changes
- Revision of failed total shoulder arthroplasty or hemiarthroplasty for loosening, instability, or bone loss
- Massive cuff tears without glenohumeral arthritis in patients with significant functional deficits (pseudoparalytic shoulder)
- Primary osteoarthritis associated with significant bone loss, instability, or cuff tears with grade 3 or 4 fatty degeneration
- Posttraumatic osteoarthritis with malunion or nonunion of the tuberosities
- Tumor reconstruction
- Rheumatoid arthritis with cuff insufficiency
- Three- or four-part fracture of the humeral head in the elderly patient

Examination/Imaging

- Physical examination
  - A positive Hornblower's sign or drop arm test can indicate the loss of the teres minor. The presence of the teres minor can affect prognosis as these patients tend to have better function postoperatively.
  - The belly press test and lift-off test are used to assess presence and function of the subscapularis. Subscapularis deficiency may be associated with increased incidence of instability and can alter postoperative rehabilitation protocols.
- Radiographs
  - Plain radiographs routinely include anteroposterior (AP) views in neutral rotation, internal rotation, and external rotation performed under fluoroscopic control in order to see the subacromial space and the glenohumeral joint properly. An axillary view and scapular Y view are also obtained.
    - Proximal humeral morphology is important to visualize in order to determine the starting point for the humeral cutting guide. Figure 1 shows an AP radiograph of a patient with cuff tear arthropathy demonstrating proximal humeral

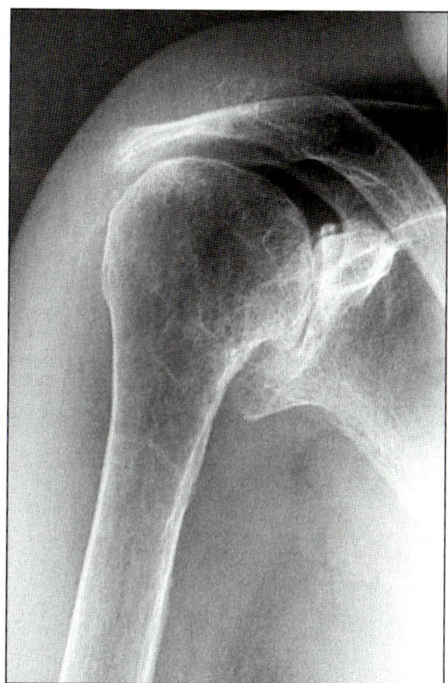

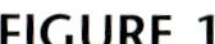
FIGURE 1

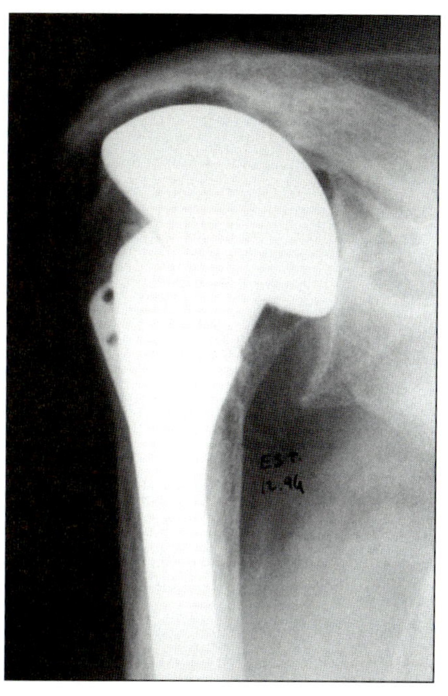

FIGURE 2

        migration and superior glenoid erosion. This is also critical for posttraumatic arthritis patients who may have malunited tuberosities.
        - Revision cases should have proximal humeral bone stock carefully evaluated to be certain that the humeral component can be appropriately secured. Figure 2 shows an AP radiograph of a failed hemiarthroplasty with proximal migration of the humeral component.
    - In cases of humeral bone deficiency or loss of bony landmarks, comparative scaled radiographs are helpful for restoring appropriate humeral length and deltoid tension.
- A computed tomographic arthrogram is useful for assessing glenoid bone loss, as well as rotator cuff status.
    - The glenoid frequently shows superior or posterior wear patterns. Significant bone loss may result in the need for grafting.
    - Fatty infiltration can be staged as described in the Goutallier classification.
    - The presence or absence of the subscapularis and teres minor can affect patient outcome, surgical technique, and postoperative rehabilitation.
- Magnetic resonance imaging (MRI) can also be used to evaluate the remaining cuff and glenoid bone stock. However, it can be more difficult to visualize glenoid morphology by MRI.

Surgical Anatomy

- The deltoid originates from the lateral clavicle and acromion, then inserts onto the humerus at the deltoid tuberosity (Fig. 3).
- The pectoralis major originates from the sternum and medial clavicle and inserts broadly at the proximal humerus.
- The cephalic vein runs in the deltopectoral interval (Fig. 4). It typically has more crossing branches connecting to the deltoid muscle.
- Neurovascular structures of the brachial plexus lie medial to the conjoint tendon.
- The axillary nerve is at risk along the inferior border of the subscapularis and the inferior glenoid. The nerve is routinely identified during the approach.
- The coracoacromial ligament attaches to the lateral tip of the coracoid and extends obliquely across the superior aspect of the surgical field.
- The biceps tendon is deep to the pectoralis major insertion. This tendon marks the lateral border of the subscapularis insertion.
- The anterior circumflex humeral vessels are a series of three vessels that run transversely across the humeral neck, deep to the pectoralis major and inferior to the subscapularis.

Pearls

- *Leaving the arm free allows for easy mobilization throughout the surgery and facilitates exposure.*
- *If positioned properly, the arm will frequently rest securely in the patient's lap with minimal effort during the approach.*

Pitfalls

- *Positioning the patient too medially on the table blocks arm motion and can make exposure of the proximal humerus and access to the humeral canal difficult.*

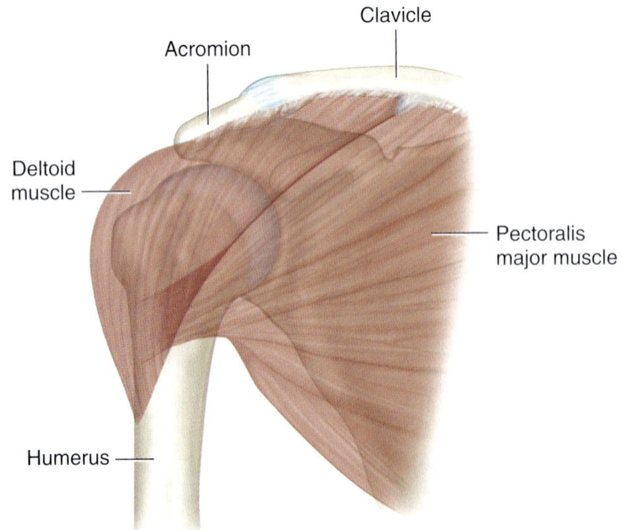

FIGURE 3

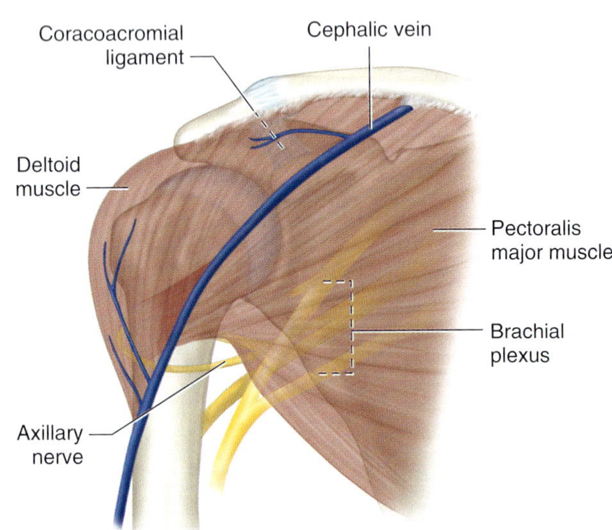

FIGURE 4

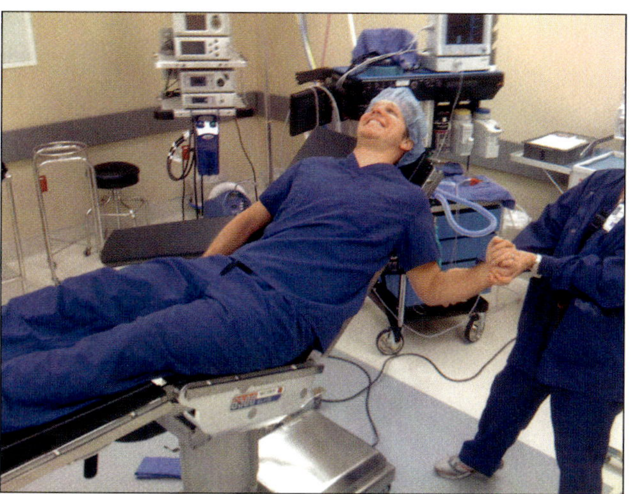
A

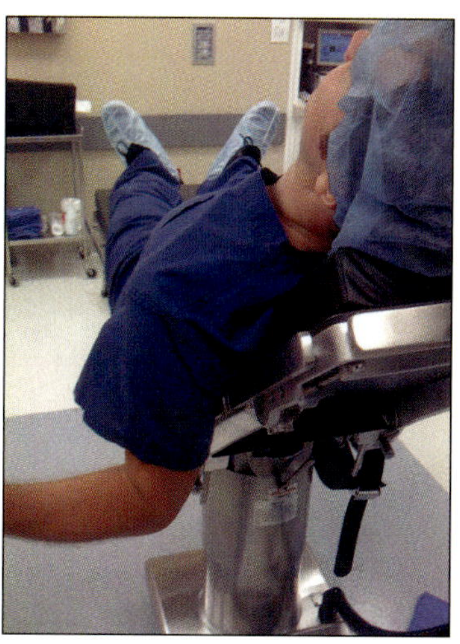
B

FIGURE 5

Positioning

- The beach chair position is used (Fig. 5A).
- The affected shoulder should be placed just lateral to the edge of the table (Fig. 5B).
- Positioning should allow for hyperextension of the humerus inferiorly and dislocation of the humeral head, allowing access to the humeral medullary canal.
- The shoulder is draped so that there is access to the lateral half of the clavicle anteriorly and the lateral half of the scapula posteriorly.

Pearls

- *In larger patients, a larger blunt hand-held retractor (Richardson) can be placed underneath the conjoint tendon to improve visualization. It is immediately exchanged for a smaller retractor to avoid neurovascular complications from prolonged retraction.*

Pitfalls

- *Inadequate release of the soft tissue attachments at the inferior glenoid will make posterior humeral head retraction and glenoid preparation difficult. This step is critical for appropriate glenoid exposure.*

Portals/Exposures

- The deltopectoral approach or the superolateral approach can be used. We prefer the deltopectorial approach for routine use for several reasons.
  - It is commonly used and familiar to most surgeons.
  - There is no need to take down any portion of the deltoid and risk injury.
  - The exposure is extensile and allows access to the entire humerus if necessary.
  - Positioning of the glenosphere inferiorly on the glenoid face is easier.
- For the deltopectoral approach, the incision starts at the coracoid process and extended distally and laterally, angled toward the midpoint of the humerus, for 10–15 cm. Revision cases require more extensive incisions to allow access to the proximal humeral diaphysis.

Controversies

- A superolateral approach can also be used. It may have a lower rate of postoperative dislocation.

- The deltopectoral interval is easiest to identify at its most superior and medial extent. Two small hand-held retractors are helpful in exposing this. One should be placed superiorly in the incision. The second can be placed at the superomedial part of the incision.
- The cephalic vein is left with the deltoid muscle, laterally. This minimizes bleeding.
- A Hohmann retractor is placed over the top of the coracoid process. Placing the arm in abduction and external rotation will help facilitate this.
- The arm is then returned to full adduction with minimal external rotation. The pectoralis major insertion is then identified and the superior 1–2 cm are released.
- The anterior circumflex humeral vessels will lie at the inferior border of the subscapularis just deep to the pectoralis major. These are ligated using two absorbable sutures. The vessels tend to be friable and may cause bleeding throughout the surgery if they are not ligated.
- The coracoacromial ligament is cut just lateral to the coracoid insertion. This will help facilitate glenoid exposure. The ligament is not needed when using a reverse shoulder prosthesis.
- The fascia from the lateral portion of the conjoint tendon is released and a small blunt retractor is placed underneath the conjoint tendon and coracobrachialis muscle. This exposes the underlying subscapularis muscle.
- Placing the arm in adduction, slight forward flexion, and neutral rotation removes tension from the conjoint tendon. After it is retracted, the axillary nerve can be seen just medial to the subscapularis.
- The biceps tendon is identified by putting the arm in abduction and internal rotation. It should be medial and deep to the pectoralis major insertion. If it is still intact, cutting transversely with a pair of scissors oriented perpendicular to the tendon usually allows easy entrance into the biceps sheath.
- The arm is kept in the same position, and the superior border of the subscapularis is identified behind the tip of the coracoid process.
- Two stay sutures are placed in the subscapularis, and the tendon is divided approximately 1.5 cm medial to its insertion on the lesser tuberosity. This should follow the anatomic neck of the humerus. The superior portion of the tendon is cut using a scalpel.

The inferior portion is cut using electrocautery to avoid excessive bleeding.

- A humeral head retractor is introduced into the joint. The head is retracted posteriorly.
- The subscapularis is released by performing a juxtaglenoid capsulotomy:
  - Identify the superior (semitubular) portion of the subscapularis tendon. Scissors are slid along the superior tendon edge, releasing any subcoracoid adhesions.
  - Starting superiorly, the deep surface of the muscle is bluntly dissected from the underlying capsule and middle glenohumeral ligament. Working inferiorly and medially to the glenoid rim, the middle glenohumeral ligament and capsule are released.
  - Previously transected muscle fibers of the inferior subscapularis can been seen in cross section. The inferior glenohumeral ligament and capsule are just deep to these fibers. They are dissected free and cut, working superiorly and medially back to the level of the glenoid.
- The subscapularis muscle is buried in the subscapularis fossa. A small sponge is placed on top to protect the muscle.
- A Kölbel retractor is put into the subscapularis fossa. This retracts the subscapularis muscle, conjoint tendon, and neurovascular structures.
- Release the inferior glenoid capsular attachments using electrocautery. This should be done past the 6 o'clock position, around to the 7 o'clock position in the right shoulder or the 5 o'clock position in the left shoulder. The release is done directly at the level of the bony attachment and extends medial to the glenoid rim for 2–3 mm.

Pearls

- *A minimal humeral head cut will preserve humeral length. This allows the prosthesis to be placed with maximal tension of the deltoid. Barring significant deformity, this cut level results in predictable tension across the final prosthesis.*

Pitfalls

- *Trial components should be removed from the proximal humerus after trialing. They can prevent proper posterior retraction of the humeral head and interfere with glenoid exposure.*

Controversies

- The appropriate retroversion of the humeral component is controversial. Recommendations typically range from 0° to 30°. To date, there is no consensus on proper placement.

Procedure

Step 1

- Remove the posterior humeral head retractor and dislocate the head anteriorly to expose it for humeral component preparation.
- A small, sharp Hohmann retractor is used to retract any remaining cuff tendon posteriorly.
- The biceps tendon is cut at the level of the glenoid insertion if it is still intact.
- The intramedullary humeral head cutting guide is inserted.
  - There is frequently osteonecrosis and deformity of the head, so preoperative radiographs are used to

help determine the starting point. Choose the starting point that gives the most direct in-line access to the medullary canal. This may differ significantly from patient to patient.

- The version of the humeral cutting guide is set to maximize the bony containment of the metaphyseal portion of the prosthesis.
- In Figure 6, an intramedullary humeral cutting guide has been placed and a minimal humeral head cut has been made.
- The thickness of the resection is only a few millimeters after the initial humeral head cut (Fig. 7).

■ The proximal humerus is reamed using a hemispherical power reamer.

- The flat, back edge of the reamer is oriented parallel to the plane of the humeral cut. During reaming, this relationship is maintained.
- Ream until the flat edge of the reamer is flush with the surrounding bone and parallel to the original proximal humeral cut (Fig. 8), unless there is significant pre-existing proximal bone loss.

■ The diaphysis is reamed using hand-held reamers. Trial components are used to evaluate proper humeral preparation and fit.

■ Trial components are removed in order to allow proper glenoid exposure and preparation.

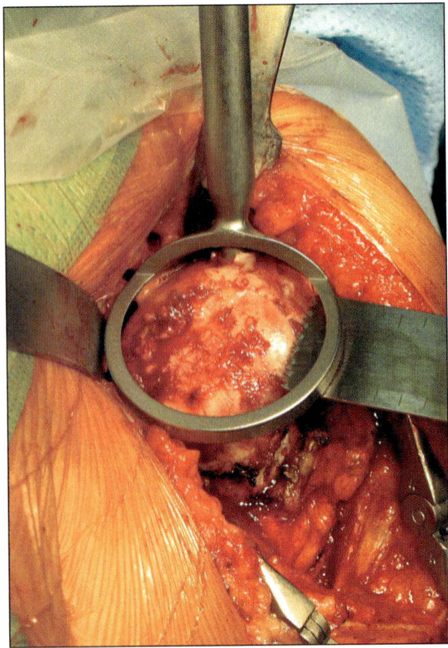

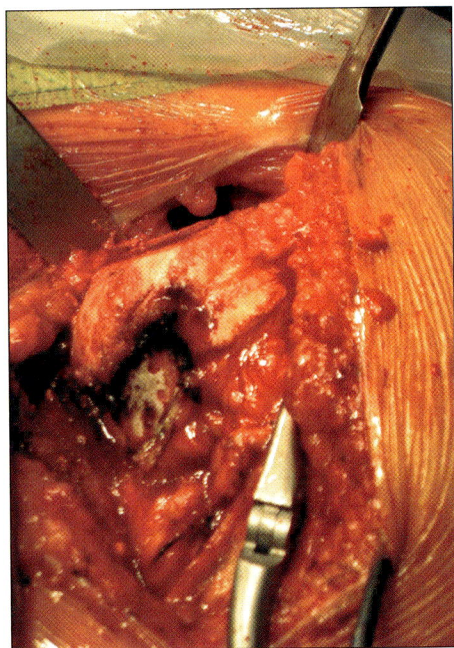

FIGURE 6

FIGURE 7

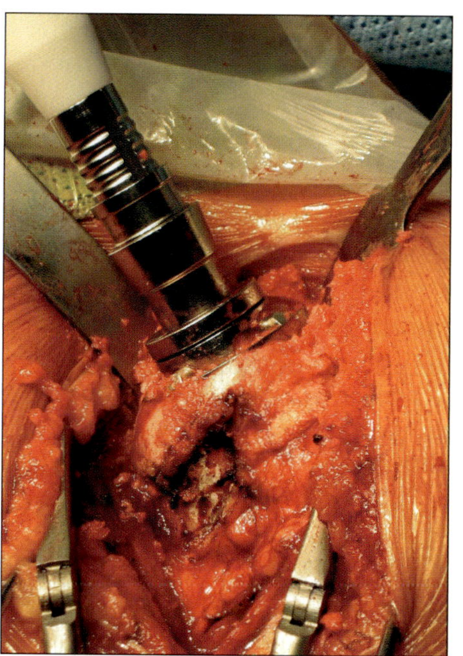

FIGURE 8

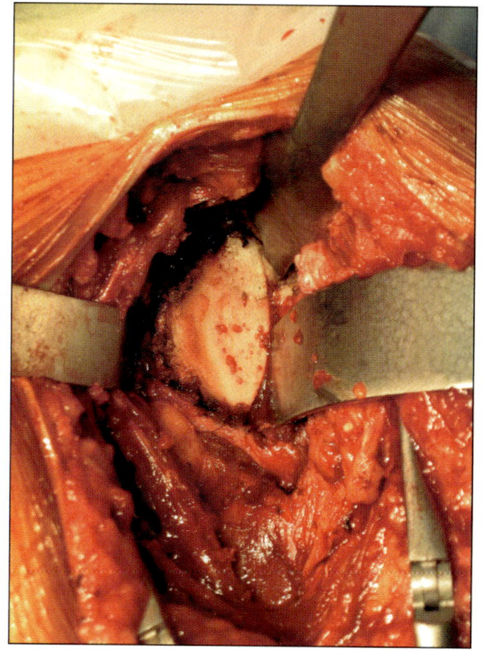

FIGURE 9

PEARLS

- *Trial components should be removed from the proximal humerus after trialing. They can prevent proper posterior retraction of the humeral head and interfere with glenoid exposure.*

PITFALLS

- *It is very important to avoid superior tilt of the glenosphere, as this can have a significant effect on implant forces and lead to early loosening.*

STEP 2

- Glenoid preparation begins by reinserting a humeral head retractor into the joint, and retracting the head posteriorly.
  - Adequate posterior retraction of the humeral head is critical. The reamer is the largest instrument used in glenoid preparation. Additional posterior or inferior retractors can be added as needed if soft tissue interferes with reaming and implantation.
  - The humeral head retractor will frequently fracture the anterior portion of the humeral metaphysis (controlled fracture). The fracture has no effect on prosthetic implantation or fixation and is only possible if the humeral trial component has been removed.
  - A small Hohmann retractor is placed over the top edge of the glenoid.
  - In Figure 9, a retractor is placed anteriorly in the subscapularis fossa. A second retractor is positioned around the posterior edge of the glenoid and is retracting the proximal humerus posteriorly. A third retractor is over the superior edge of the glenoid.
- The central peg-hole drill starting point should be several millimeters inferior to the center of the glenoid, in the midline. The component is placed as far inferiorly as possible without jeopardizing implant fixation. The component is placed with an inferior tilt of approximately 10°.

Instrumentation/ Implantation

- A selection of several different types of humeral head retractors is helpful if exposure proves difficult. Some manufactures have specialized retractors with cutouts to accommodate reamers and specially designed inferior retractors.

PEARLS

- *Screws can be angled into one of three major areas: the base of the coracoid, the scapular spine, and the scapular pillar.*

PITFALLS

- *Care must be taken to be sure that no soft tissue interferes with seating of the glenosphere. Proper retractor position will help avoid this problem.*

- The humeral head will push the reamer anteriorly, causing the central peg of the reamer to cut out of the pilot hole anteriorly, jeopardizing peg fixation. This same process can also produce excessive anteversion of the glenoid component.
- If the reamer is compressed tightly against the glenoid surface and started, a large amount of torque is created and this may result in fracture. The reamer should be started and then gradually pressed against the glenoid face, lessening the torque created and the risk of glenoid fracture.
- The glenoid is reamed using appropriately sized reamers.

STEP 3

- The glenoid baseplate is impacted using an insertion device and fixed in place with screws.
  - The implant in Figure 10 has compression holes in the anterior and posterior positions. The superior and inferior holes are for multidirectional locking screws.
  - Most implants feature fixed or multidirectional locking screws. When possible, two normal compression screws are first placed anteriorly and posteriorly, firmly securing the plate to the underlying glenoid bone.
  - These are followed by locking screws placed superiorly and inferiorly.
  - All screws are placed bicortically when possible.

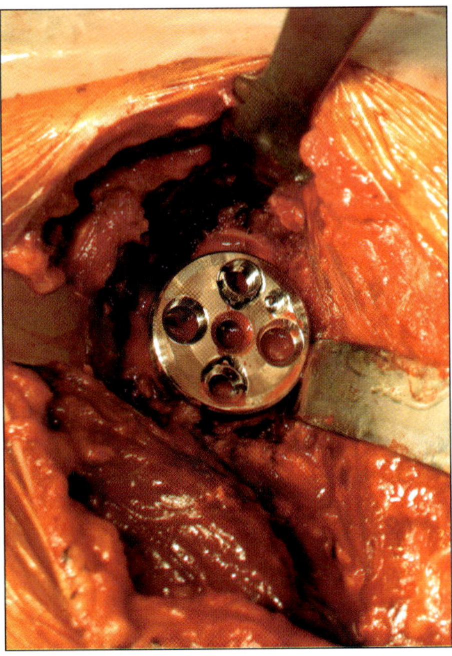

FIGURE 10

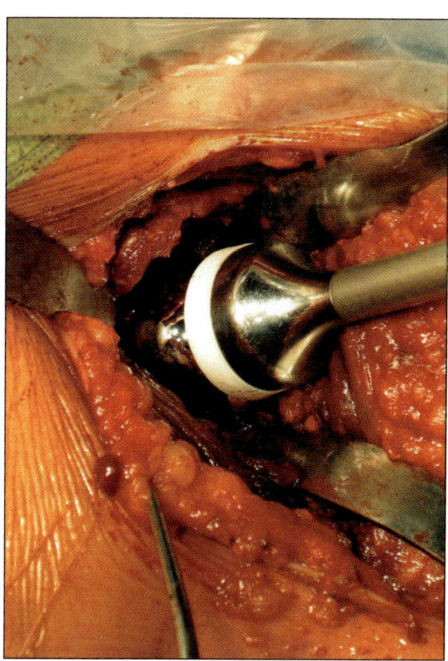

FIGURE 11

- The glenosphere is impacted on the baseplate (Fig. 11).

STEP 4

- The humeral head retractor is removed and the humeral head is dislocated anteriorly.
- Three transosseous nonabsorbable sutures are passed in order to reattach the subscapularis later if there was sufficient subscapularis remaining.
- The humeral prosthesis is implanted using the retroversion guide to replicate the version that was created with the original humeral cut.
- Trial components are available to test implant stability. Once the appropriate thickness of polyethylene liner is selected, it is impacted into the humeral component.
- Pulling in-line traction on the arm and pushing posteriorly on the humerus reduce the prosthesis. If this is not possible due to excessive deltoid tension, changing the position of the arm is sometimes helpful. As the humeral component lies anterior to the glenoid, placement of the arm in internal rotation will decrease the profile of the humeral cup that the glenoid must clear in order to properly reduce.

PEARLS

- *Trial components can be very difficult to remove once the shoulder is reduced. If a minimal head cut is made, a 6-mm polyethylene cup is frequently adequate to ensure proper implant tension.*

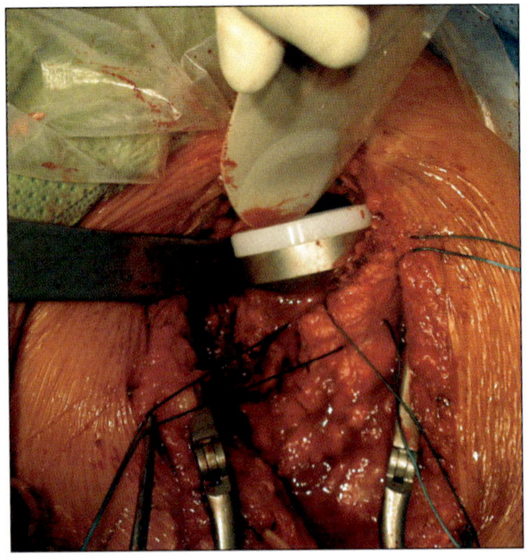

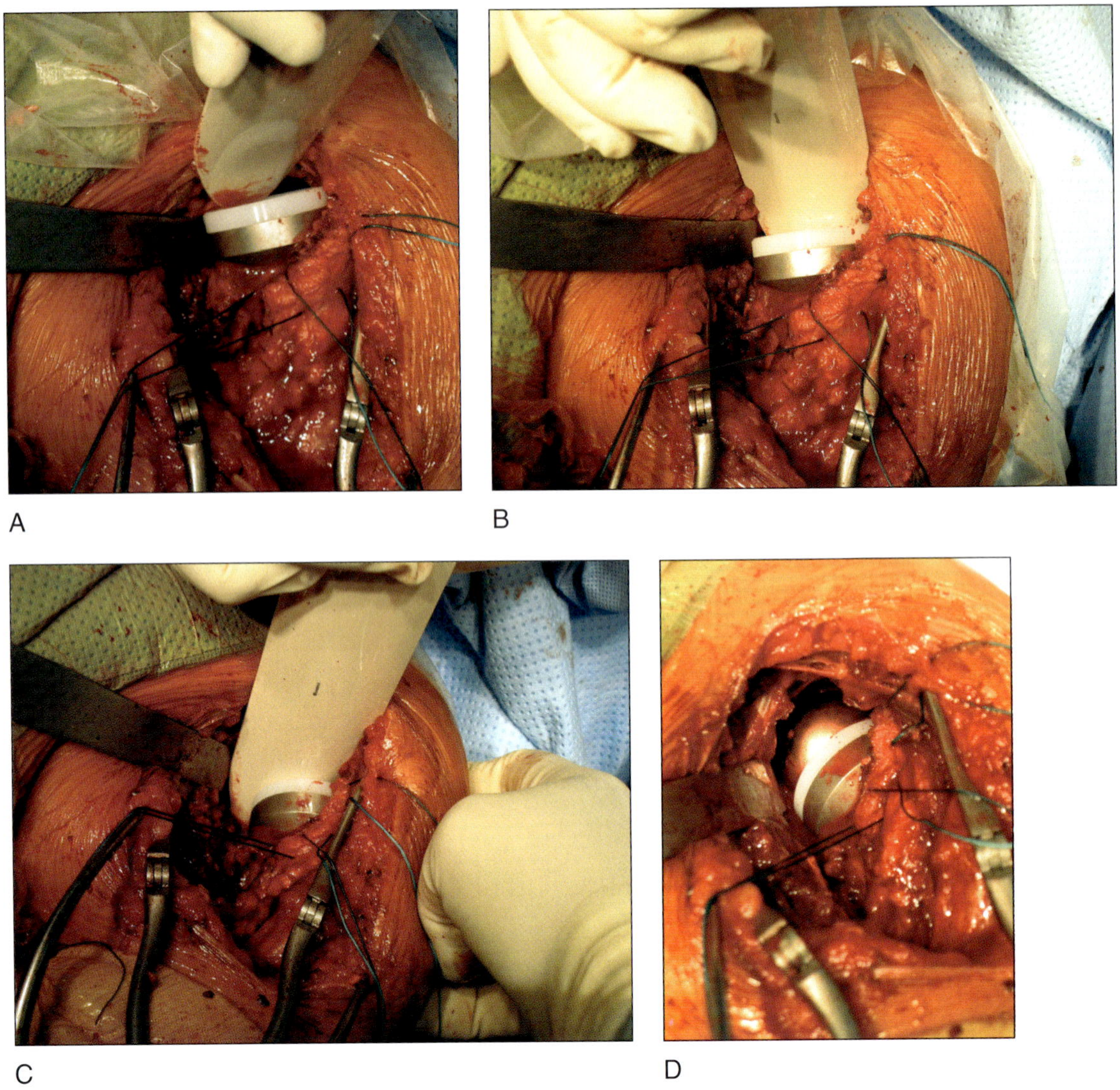

A

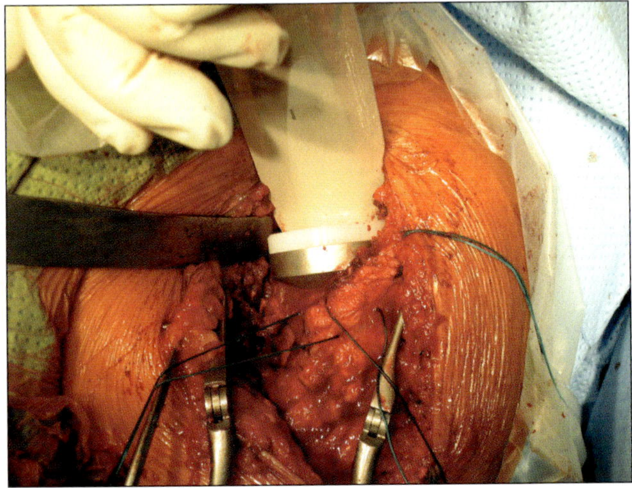

B

C

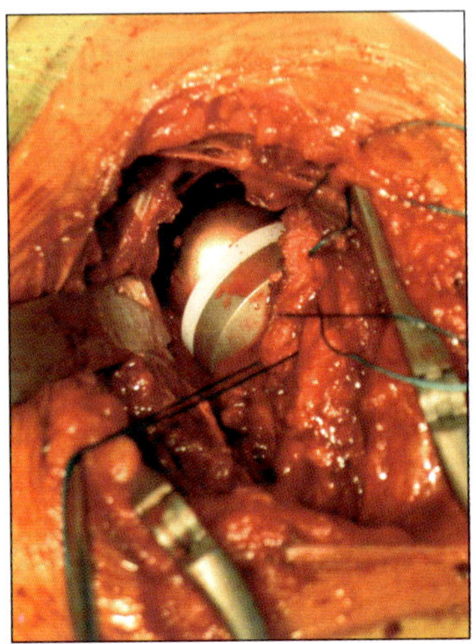

D

FIGURE 12

Instrumentation/ Implantation

- Several manufacturers now have instruments specifically designed for the purpose of reducing the prosthesis in cases in which the reduction is difficult.

- A wide, flat instrument, such as an osteotome, can be used as a skid to reduce the prosthesis. This is placed between the glenosphere and the humeral cup (Fig. 12A). The instrument is used to lever the humeral component laterally, clearing the glenosphere (Fig. 12B). The humeral cup is then slid posteriorly, along the flat side of the instrument (Fig. 12C). Once the cup has cleared the glenoid, the instrument is removed while the humerus is held in place, allowing the prosthesis to reduce (Fig. 12D).
- After reduction, the shoulder is taken through a range of motion to ensure that there is no significant impingement.
- The polyethylene liner is changed to a thicker size if there is any pistoning between the humeral and glenoid components. A modular spacer can be used if the thickest liner is already in place.

- The subscapularis is then reattached using the transosseous sutures that were passed previously. If the external rotation is significantly reduced by the tension on the subscapularis, the muscle can be released and allowed to retract free.
- The wound is closed over a drain using absorbable deep and skin sutures. The deltopectoral interval is not routinely closed.

PEARLS

- *Early motion should be avoided in revision cases and in patients with a deficient subscapularis. These patients may be left in a simple sling with range of motion for only the fingers, wrist, and elbow.*

Complications

- Common postoperative complications include:
  - Instability
  - Infection
  - Hematoma
  - Glenoid component loosening
  - Humeral component loosening
  - Scapular spine fracture
  - Humeral fracture

Postoperative Care and Expected Outcomes

- Postoperative immobilization consists of a simple sling in internal rotation for 1 month.
- Passive range-of-motion and pendulum exercises are begun immediately.
- The sling is discarded and the patient is allowed activity as tolerated at 1 month postoperatively.
- Hydrotherapy is started as soon as possible if available (usually 2 weeks postoperatively).
- Patient outcomes are influenced by the reason for reverse shoulder arthroplasty and other preoperative factors.
  - Revision cases will generally have poorer results with higher rates of complication.
  - Typical patients will see significant gains in range of motion for active elevation.
  - Improvement of external rotation is better for patients with an intact teres minor.
  - Pain levels should be significantly improved.

Evidence

Boileau P, Chuinard C, Roussanne Y, Neyton L, Trojani C. Modified latissimus dorsi and teres major transfer through a single delto-pectoral approach for external rotation deficit of the shoulder: as an isolated procedure or with a reverse arthroplasty. J Shoulder Elbow Surg. 2007;16:671-82.

This study demonstrated that the use of a modified latissimus dorsi and teres major transfer, along with a reverse shoulder arthroplasty, is possible using a single incision technique. It may improve both active elevation and external rotation in patients with teres minor deficits. (Level IV evidence)

Edwards TB, Williams MD, Labriola JE, Elkousy HA, Gartsman GM, O'Connor DP. Subscapularis insufficiency and the risk of shoulder dislocation after reverse shoulder arthroplasty. J Shoulder Elbow Surg. 2009;18:892-6.

This study suggested that reverse total shoulder arthroplasty in the face of an irreparable subscapularis tendon results in a statistically significant risk for postoperative dislocation. (Level IV evidence)

Humphrey CS, Kelly JD 2nd, Norris TR. Optimizing glenosphere position and fixation in reverse shoulder arthroplasty, Part Two: the three-column concept. J Shoulder Elbow Surg. 2008;17:595-601.

The authors described the three major columns of scapular bone that may be utilized for baseplate fixation. These are the base of coracoid, the spine, and the pillar, and they will allow for optimal initial fixation of the glenosphere.

Lévigne C, Boileau P, Favard L, Garaud P, Molé D, Sirveaux F, Walch G. Scapular notching in reverse shoulder arthroplasty. J Shoulder Elbow Surg. 2008;17:925-35.

This study showed that positioning of the glenoid baseplate influences rates of scapular notching. High positioning of the baseplate and superior tilting are associated with higher rates of notching. (Level III evidence)

Wall B, Nové-Josserand L, O'Connor DP, Edwards TB, Walch G. Reverse total shoulder arthroplasty: a review of results according to etiology. J Bone Joint Surg [Am]. 2007;89:1476-85.

The results of this study supported the use of reverse shoulder arthroplasty for complex shoulder disorders from multiple etiologies. This includes patients with cuff tear arthropathy, massive cuff tears, posttraumatic arthritis, and revision cases. (Level II evidence)

PROCEDURE 11

Open Unconstrained Revision Shoulder Arthroplasty

David M. Lutton and Evan L. Flatow

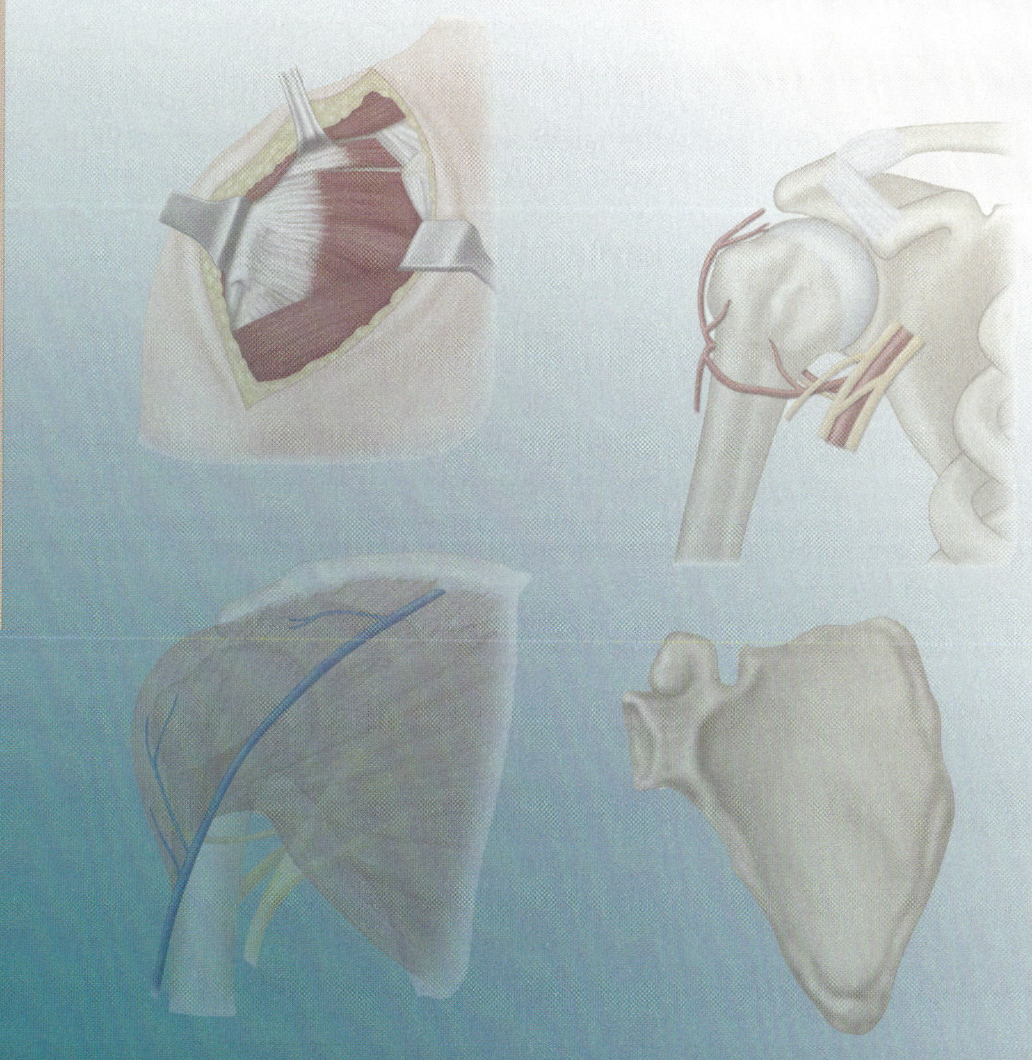

Work conducted at the Mount Sinai School of Medicine, New York, NY.
Figures 4 and 6 courtesy of Jessie McCarron, MD.
Figure 9A is reprinted with permission from Connor PM, Flatow EL. Surgical considerations of bony deficiency in total shoulder arthroplasty. In Warner JJP, Iannotti JP, Gerber C (eds). Complex and Revision Problems in Shoulder Surgery. Philadelphia: Lippincott-Raven, 1997:339-54.

Indications

- Open unconstrained revision shoulder arthroplasty is a difficult surgical challenge requiring a systematic approach to achieve an optimal outcome. This procedure focuses on the revision open surgical techniques for several etiologies:
  - Glenoid arthrosis after humeral head resurfacing (HHR)
  - Postoperative instability after HHR or total shoulder arthroplasty (TSA) (tendon rupture/malpositioned components)
  - Failed open reduction and internal fixation
  - Loosening (aseptic or septic)
  - Contracture/stiffness
- The first step in treatment is to identify the cause of the failed shoulder. All records, especially the original operative report, must be reviewed. Serial radiographs should be examined for progressive lucency or component migration.
  - It is important to always consider the possibility of infection. Night sweats, insidious gnawing pain, pain that never resolved after the index procedure, and pain at rest, as well as a history of postoperative drainage, are all suggestive of an infection. Fastidious organisms may lead to a benign physical examination but a history of pain and progressive stiffness (Coste et al., 2004).

Examination/Imaging

History

- Chief complaint: pain or loss of function?
- Onset of symptoms: traumatic or insidious?
- Prior operative reports are essential to provide the revision surgeon a roadmap to avoid predictable complications. Reports are reviewed to identify:
  - Previous vascular or neurologic injury.
  - Potential need for microsurgery to address nerve scarring.
  - The prosthesis, corresponding size, type of extractor needed, and the like.

Physical Examination

- Erythema, induration, or fluctuance
- Weakness, lag signs
- Instability
- Nerve injury
- Range of motion

PEARLS

- *Always examine for signs and symptoms of infection during the physical examination.*
- *Instruct the laboratory to culture glenohumeral joint aspiration specimens for 2 weeks, as fastidious organisms may require a longer culture than is normally completed. Literature is scant on the specific use of cell count with TSAs.*
- *MRI*
  - *Look for cuff integrity and muscle quality in the stiff shoulder. In the case of revision HHR, examine for glenoid version and bone stock. Some centers utilize specialized MRI sequences optimized for visualization even with a metal prosthesis (Sperling et al., 2002). Early identification of glenoid defects and version abnormalities is essential for surgical preparation.*
  - *Halo effect or tremendous synovitis is suggestive of infection.*

PITFALLS

- *Cultures have a high false-negative rate, even in the face of a clear infection.*

Basic Laboratory Evaluation

- Complete blood count with differential
- Erythrocyte sedimentation rate
- C-reactive protein
- Glenohumeral joint aspiration and/or tissue biopsy via arthroscopy may be used for identification of infection. Cultures have relatively low sensitivity rates due to a constellation of confounding variables, including fastidious organisms (*Propionibacterium acnes, Staphylococcus epidermidus*) (Sperling et al., 2001). The cell count is diagnostic if very high.

Plain Radiographs

- Anteroposterior (AP), true AP of the glenohumeral joint, scapular Y, and axillary views are obtained to look for malposition, lucency, and migration.
  - Both septic and aseptic loosening may lead to progressive erosions and lucency around implants.
  - Postoperative instability results in subluxation or dislocation on the axillary radiograph.
- In a previous HHR or TSR, humeral prosthesis malposition may be identified. Figure 1 is an example of a preoperative HHR requiring revision for malpositioned height. This places stress on the rotator cuff, and predisposes the tendons to rupture.
- In the posttraumatic shoulder, metaphyseal issues may be identified, including tuberosity nonunion or malunion. Diaphyseal issues present as fractures or loosening.
- Prosthetic glenoid failure is the result of loosening (septic or aseptic), catastrophic failure, or subsidence.

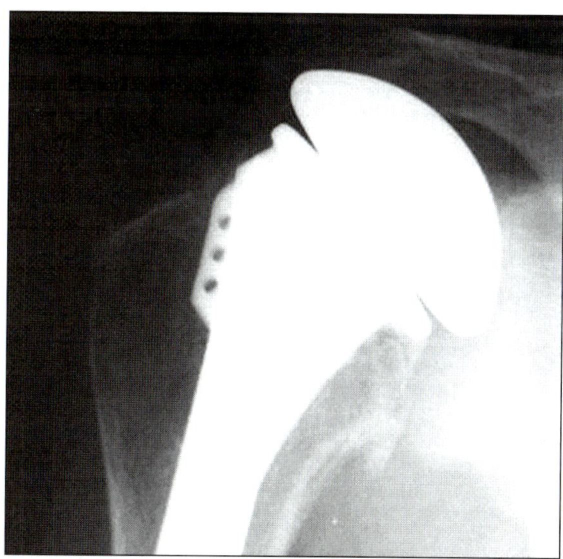

FIGURE 1

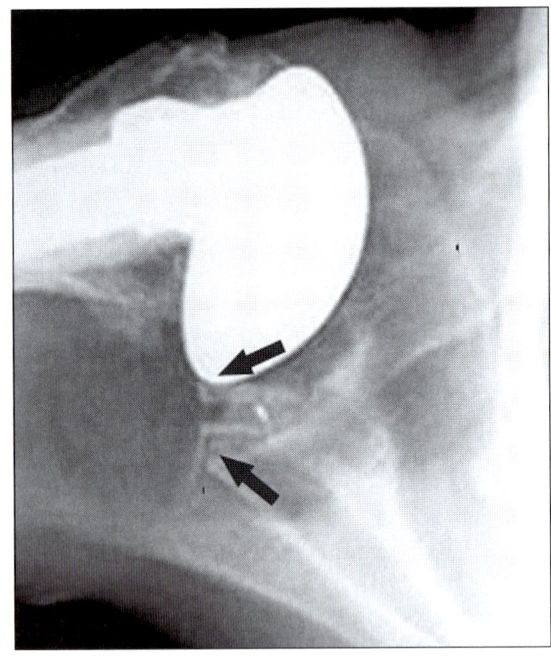

FIGURE 2

Treatment Options

- Isolated glenoid loosening in elderly patients or patients unwilling to undergo open revision is amenable to arthroscopic glenoid removal (O'Driscoll et al., 2005).
- Preoperative identification of severe posterior wear or significant humeral head posterior subluxation on MRI may require grafting, posterior plication, and immobilization in a gunslinger brace.
- In the infected shoulder, not all patients require reimplantation. Debilitated patients, severe bone loss, and cuff/soft tissue deficiency are all poor indications for reimplantation. Resection arthroplasty is an option with predictably good pain relief but poor function (Sperling et al., 2001).

  - The axillary radiograph in Figure 2 of a 60-year-old skier after a fall demonstrates a loose, free-floating glenoid in the shoulder. This illustrates glenoid loosening, but also the value of a quality axillary radiograph, as this is difficult to appreciate on an AP view. The *arrows* highlight a glenoid component that has dislocated out of the glenoid vault.
- Patients who have failed HHR often demonstrate glenoid arthrosis, seen as progressive joint space narrowing and glenoid wear.
- Arthrosis after a prior anterior instability repair demonstrates significant posterior glenoid erosion and an internal rotation contracture.

Imaging Studies

- Magnetic resonance imaging (MRI)
  - Noncontrast MRI allows for evaluation of glenoid version, bone stock, and rotator cuff muscle-tendon unit integrity. The MRI in Figure 3 shows a TSA with an intact supraspinatus and good-quality muscle.
  - Specialized MRI sequences can be helpful (Sperling et al., 2002).
- Combined technetium-99m and indium nuclear medicine scans can be used to evaluate for infection.
- Electromyography/nerve conduction velocity studies are used to evaluate nerve dysfunction.

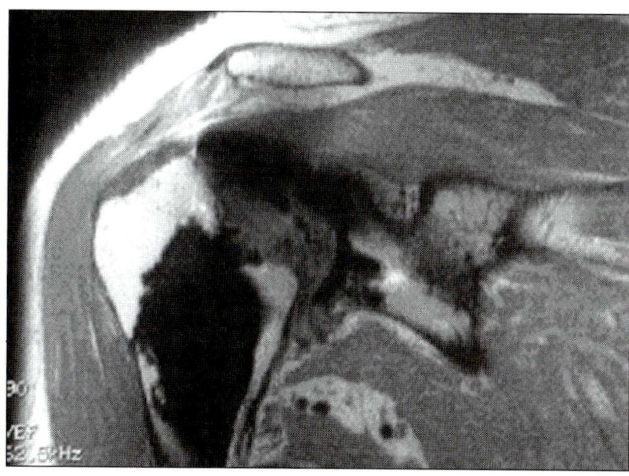

FIGURE 3

> **PEARLS**
>
> - *Position and drape the posterior shoulder free to allow for accessory incisions if necessary.*

Surgical Anatomy

- Albeit distorted, the surgical anatomy of revision unconstrained total shoulder arthroplasty is identical to that of the index procedure. This is addressed in Procedure 10.

Positioning

- Patients undergoing revision shoulder arthroplasty should be positioned in the beach chair position with 45° of hip flexion and 30° of knee flexion.
  - The head is cushioned in a padded holder with the neck in a neutral position in both the coronal and sagittal planes.
  - The contralateral arm is secured across the body.
  - Venodynes are placed on the calves to decrease the incidence of deep venous thrombosis.

Portals/Exposures

- Anesthesia
  - There are two basic anesthetic options: general anesthesia or a regional block with sedation, or both. We routinely use regional anesthesia with sedation.
  - Ideally, nonparalytic anesthesia should be used to assist in nerve protection during dissection or neurolysis, since use of electrocautery will locally stimulate nearby nerves and produce muscle activation.
- Two basic surgical approaches can be used for revision shoulder arthroplasty cases: the deltopectoral and anterosuperior approaches. This procedure

discusses the revision deltopectoral approach in detail.

- For the vast majority of revision shoulder arthroplasty cases (constrained or unconstrained), we utilize the extensile deltopectoral approach.
- Two situations arise for the use of an anterosuperior approach. If previously utilized (in the context of an intact subscapularis muscle tendon unit, minimal deformity, and a supple shoulder), exploiting this established interval is viable. Alternatively, if a previously implanted resurfacing cap is to be retained, the superior approach may provide adequate exposure to place a glenoid component.
- Additional posterior approaches may be used as needed for posterior adhesion releases and/or neurolysis.

Pearls

- *Successful revision unconstrained shoulder arthroplasty requires the humeral head to be centered on the glenoid. The cuff must be either intact or reparable to prevent the possibility for rapid glenoid loosening due to the "rocking horse" phenomenon and edge loading.*
- *The deltopectoral approach allows for preservation of the anterior deltoid, predictable exposure of the humerus and inferior glenoid, and tendon transfers if necessary.*

Pitfalls

- *During the subdeltoid release in revision cases, protect the axillary nerve, as it may be scarred to the humerus.*
- *Neurovascular structures may be scarred to the subscapularis and/or strap muscles. Delicate dissection is required to prevent injury.*

Deltopectoral Approach: Superficial

- The skin incision is begun just lateral to the coracoid, thereby minimizing retraction damage on the subcutaneous tissue. Previous incisions are incorporated if possible.
- Two self-retaining retractors are placed to retract the skin and develop cutaneous flaps medially and laterally.
- The cephalic vein is identified within the fat stripe between the deltoid and the pectoralis major. On index procedures, we mobilize the cephalic vein medially and suture ligate each of the medium-sized deltoid branches; however, scar may dictate the direction in which that vessel is taken in revision cases.
- If the interval is difficult to identify, the coracoid can be palpated within the proximal infraclavicular triangle formed by the lateral border of the pectoralis major, the medial clavicular insertion of the deltoid, and the clavicle. Using meticulous blunt dissection in concert with cautery, this plane is opened; once opened, the pectoralis tendon and deltoid tendon should be clearly evident (Fig. 4).

Deltopectoral Approach: Deep

- The deep dissection is begun on the metaphyseal-diaphyseal region of the humerus, developing the subdeltoid and subacromial spaces sharply with curved Mayo scissors or a Cobb elevator.
- The axillary nerve is protected on the undersurface of the deltoid, as it may be encased in scar as it wraps

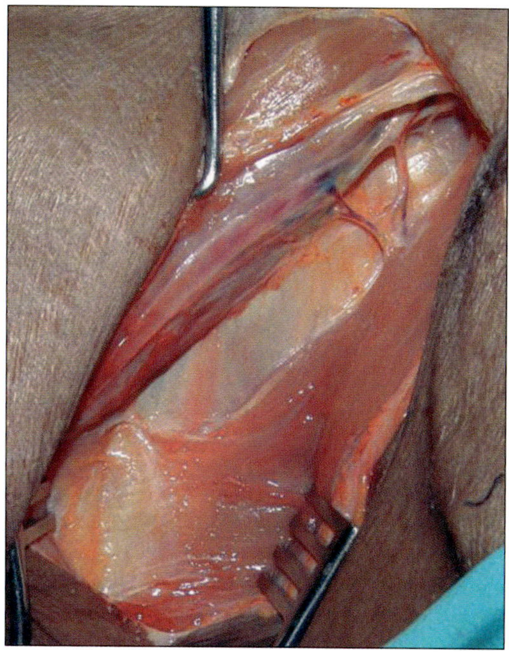

FIGURE 4

around the humerus approximately 5 cm distal to the acromion.

- The strap muscles/tendons are identified. Often, the pectoralis major muscle belly will be adherent to the conjoined tendon; this will need to be released to allow complete mobilization.
- The arm is slightly forward flexed to relieve tension on the tendons.
- The coracoid is palpated, and the sub–strap muscle interval is carefully opened. Remnant clavipectoral fascia may be present, and must be incised from the coracoid tip distally. The coracoacromial ligament is left intact as a secondary soft tissue restraint to anterosuperior translation of the humeral head.
- The strap muscles are often adherent to the underlying subscapularis.
- The axillary nerve is identified, and a "tug test" is performed.
  - Figure 5 shows a demonstration of a tug test on a cadaveric specimen (Flatow and Bigliani, 1992). The *arrows* point to the axillary nerve on either side of the humerus.
  - If the axillary nerve is deeply invested with scar, we perform a neurolysis (beyond the scope of this procedure).

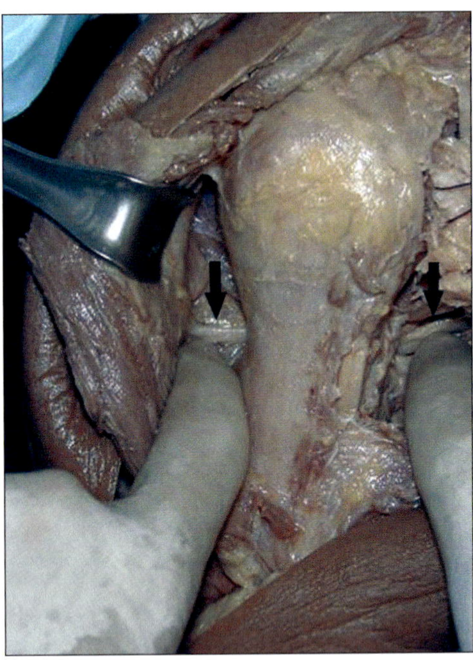

FIGURE 5

- A deep retractor is placed underneath the strap muscles for gentle medial retraction. Overzealous retraction can cause a musculocutaneous nerve palsy.
- If exposure remains limited, the superior 10 mm of the pectoralis major tendon can be released (rarely needed).

Pearls

- *Assume every revision case is for infection until the frozen section is negative for acute inflammation. If infection is a possibility, hold intravenous antibiotics until cultures are taken and sent to pathology.*
- *Identification of the coracoid is essential to safe dissection.*

Pitfalls

- *If the exact prosthesis type has not been verified, a malpositioned stem may be difficult to remove without the correct extractor, or a well-positioned stem may require unneccessary removal if appropriately mating heads and glenoids are not available.*
- *The surgeon must be prepared to address all forms of instability in the revision case. Uncorrected instability is usually disastrous.*

Procedure

Step 1: Surgical Approach

- Scenario 1: Revision after Fracture Fixation
  - If the revision procedure is indicated for a failed fracture fixation, then all hardware is removed, fibrous tissue is débrided, screw holes are curetted, and tissue is sent to pathology for culture and frozen section.
  - The wound is thoroughly irrigated.
- Scenario 2: Instability after Arthroplasty
  - Anterior instability after a hemiarthroplasty or TSA is often due to subscapularis failure. If the failure is acute, a subscapularis repair may be completed. The rolled edge of the subscapularis can be identified beneath the coracoid, along the glenoid margin. Dissection should be kept lateral to the coracoid to minimize risk to the neurovascular structures. Gentle traction is applied on sutures placed in the subscapularis and the tendon is gradually released off of the coracoid and glenoid

Instrumentation/ Implantation

- Open shoulder tray
- Saws and burrs
- Universal extractor
- Osteotomes drill
- Cement extractors
- Midas Rex
- Cement melter (ultrasound)
- Long-stemmed prosthesis, cables
- Antibiotic cement and cementation instruments

Pearls

- *Although we are advocates of a lesser tuberosity osteotomy for primary arthroplasty for osteoarthritis, for revision cases we routinely tenotomize the subscapularis tendon.*

Pitfalls

- *Z-lengthening of the subscapularis often results in poor subscapularis function.*

margin; this should allow for progressive mobilization of the tendon.

- Chronic anterior instability is addressed with two basic options: allograft reconstruction of the capsular ligaments or a subcoracoid pectoralis major transfer (Klepps et al., 2001). We generally prefer the latter. The use of a reverse prosthesis for severe cases of instability, especially in association with cuff loss, is beyond the scope of this procedure.
- Posterior instability may be due to either posterior cuff failure or, more commonly, excessive retroversion of the humeral head or glenoid.
- Inferior instability in the case of an intact axillary nerve is extremely uncommon, and usually caused by inadequate restoration of humeral height leading to deltoid laxity.
- Superior instability is usually due to rotator cuff insufficiency and is usually addressed by reverse TSA.

Step 2: Arthrotomy

- The subscapularis is demarcated.
  - An attempt is made to identify and suture ligate the leash of vessels normally coursing along the inferior border of the subscapularis; however, these may have been ligated during the index procedure. Identification of the anterior humeral circumflex vessels (Fig. 6, *arrow*) allow for

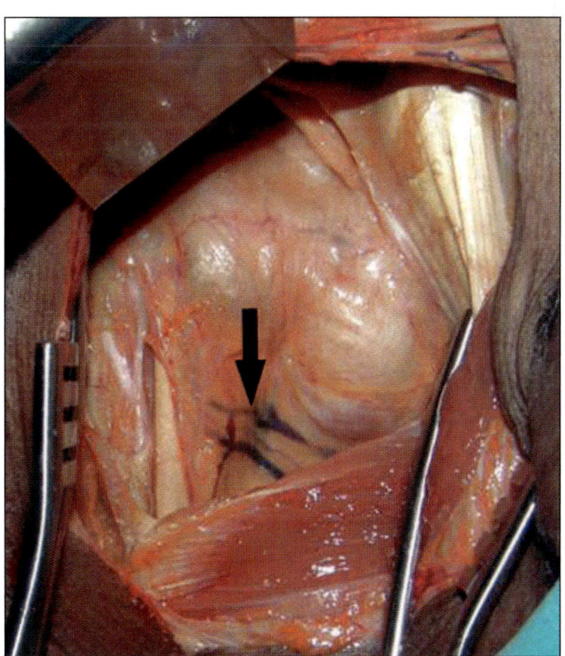

FIGURE 6

demarcation of the inferior border of the subscapularis tendon.
  - The lower border of the subscapularis is defined with the needle-tipped Bovie.
  - The bicipital groove and rotator interval are opened.
  - The biceps is tenotomized at the labrum if not previously completed; the biceps is tagged for later tenodesis to the pectoralis major tendon upon completion of the procedure.
  - Intra-articular tissue and fluid are sent for frozen and permanent section, and culture.
  - The arm is forward flexed and externally rotated. The axillary nerve is rechecked.
- The subscapularis tendon is tenotomized along with the joint capsule.
  - In the patient with external rotation past neutral, the subscapularis tendon is divided approximately 1 cm medial to its insertion to allow for a cuff of tissue for later repair, along with the subjacent capsule.
  - In patients with severe internal rotation contractures, we prefer to directly release the tendon from the lesser tuberosity to gain additional tendon length by repairing it more medially on the humeral neck.
  - Tagging stitches are placed into the free tendon.
- The anteroinferior glenohumeral ligaments are released from the humerus.
  - The soft tissues are sequentially stripped off of the humerus as it is progressively forward flexed and externally rotated.

Step 3: Humeral Head Inspection, Exposure, and Extraction

- The humeral head is dislocated.
  - The shoulder is extended while placing a posterior-to-anterior translation force on the humeral head. The arm is externally rotated to approximately 90°.
  - In concert with gentle abduction, a Browne deltoid retractor is placed to retract the deltoid. A Darrach retractor is placed along the neck of the prosthesis, followed by a second Darrach between the coracoid and the humerus. This delivers the humeral head or prosthesis into the center of the wound.

Pearls

- *As with primary open shoulder procedures, special care must be taken to preserve the deltoid muscle during humeral dislocation.*
- *Humeral prosthesis positioning should demonstrate 20–40° of retroversion and the articular surface should be 5–7 mm higher than the greater tuberosity.*

Pitfalls

- *During the anteroinferior glenohumeral ligament release, the axillary nerve is at risk. Recheck the location of the nerve, and liberally irrigate the wound to prevent thermal necrosis of the nerve from electrocautery use.*
- *Prevent scratching of the trunion of a retained humeral prosthesis to ensure a good morse tape fit.*

Pearls

- *It is crucial to understand the biomechanics of stem fixation. Regardless of fixation technique, micro-interdigitation exists between either the native bone–cement or native bone–prosthesis interface. Extraction requires disruption of this lock.*
- *Osteotomes follow the path of least resistance, and therefore must be used with great care not to skive off into the host bone, resulting in tremendous bone loss or fracture.*
- *Osteotomy has the goal of widening the space between the cement and host bone to unlock the micro-interdigitation preventing extraction.*
- *It is not necessary to remove all cement unless in the face of infection.*

- The humeral prosthesis is inspected for malposition and the head is removed.
  - The version and height of the humeral prosthesis are evaluated. If malpositioned, the stem may require revision in addition to head revision.
  - In the case of a prior modular humeral prosthesis, the tuning fork is used to remove the prosthetic head from the trunion of the stem.
  - The humeral stem is left in place to protect the humerus during retraction for glenoid exposure. If the stem is to be left, then skip to Step 4.

Step 4: Humeral Extraction

- The proximal humerus is re-dislocated with the previously described technique. If the shoulder is being revised for infection, the humeral prosthesis must be extracted. In the aseptic scenario, the humeral prosthesis is assessed for loosening.
  - All soft tissue is circumferentially removed from around the prosthesis and cement.
  - The prosthesis-specific or universal extractor is placed on the humerus.
  - The extractor handle is gently struck to evaluate for micro-motion; if none exists, then the humeral prosthesis may be retained if it is in good position and infection is not the cause of failure.
- The humeral stem is extracted (if necessary).
  - A universal (or implant-specific) extractor may be used with a slap hammer to remove a poorly fixated prosthesis (Fig. 7A).

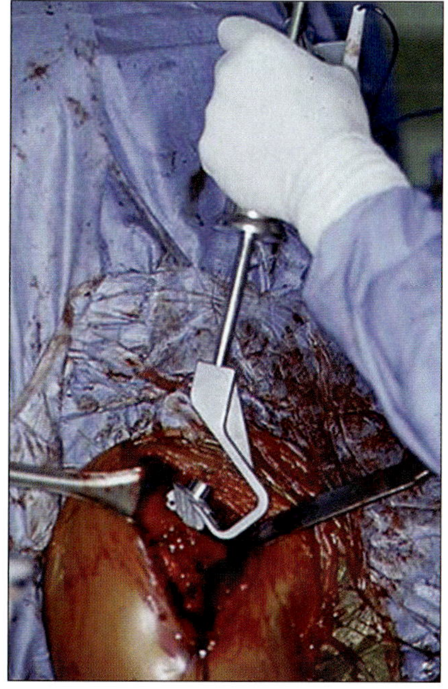

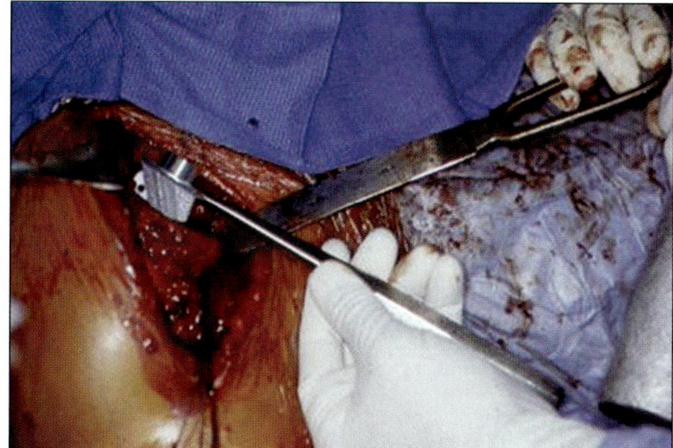

FIGURE 7 A B

PITFALLS

- *HHR revision with posterior glenoid wear and static subluxation (see Fig. 7) predisposes the patient to postoperative posterior instability.*
- *Direct, forcible extraction can be dangerous with a well-fixed ingrown stem, as it may cause a fracture and/or bone loss.*

- Alternatively, a tamp may be placed under the medial lip of the humeral prosthesis and impacted (Fig. 7B). A small gap between the prosthesis and the native humeral bone must be present to use this technique; a simple rongeur or burr can be used to create this space.
- If the humeral component does not loosen, the flexible osteotomes are used to free the cement-bone interdigitation. The osteotomes should only be used to the level of the metaphyseal-diaphyseal junction to minimize the potential for tuberosity fracture.
- Once the stem is maximally loosened, an attempt should be made to explant it with a tamp or extractor.
- If the prosthesis is still well fixed, then removal will require an osteotomy.
- The incision is extended distally, to an extensile anterior approach to the humerus.
- A controlled osteotomy is created, just posterior to the bicipital groove. It should extend distally between the pectoralis major and the deltoid insertion, and end several centimeters proximal to the prosthetic tip, with predrilling to prevent fracture propagation. A simple longitudinal osteotomy may be sufficient for extraction of the component; however, if not, a cortical window must be opened.
- Transverse cuts are made at the proximal and distal extents of the osteotomy, approximately one third of the circumference of the humeral shaft.
- A wide osteotome or elevator is placed within the longitudinal osteotomy and gently twisted to open the window off of a posteriorly based hinge.
- Later reconstruction with allograft and two to three cables can provide an excellent reconstruction. Figure 8 shows a reconstruction of the humeral shaft after an osteotomy repaired with cerclage wires.

- Cement extraction
  - As much cement is extracted as possible. Cement extractors, ultrasound, and a Midas Rex with a long burr are useful.
  - If the shoulder is being revised for infection, all cement should be removed.

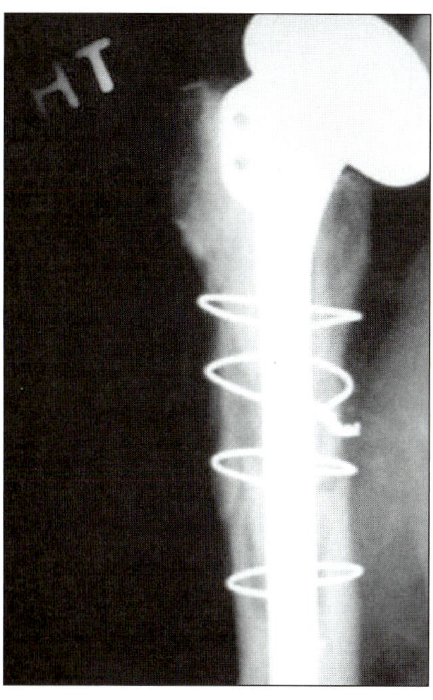

FIGURE 8

> **Pitfalls**
>
> - *Nagda et al. (2007) have described the importance of intermittent relaxation of the brachial plexus and axillary nerve. This should be completed several times during the procedure; it is important to remove all instruments and place the arm in a neutral position.*

Step 5: Glenoid Exposure, Inspection, and Extraction

- The glenoid is exposed.
  - The arm is abducted and placed in slight flexion and external rotation.
  - A Fukuda retractor is placed posterior to the glenoid rim to retract the humerus posterolaterally.
- The subscapularis is released.
  - The subscapularis tendon is released from the underlying capsule and any scar or remnant of the coracohumeral ligament. Superomedial dissection along the anterior border of the muscle should be avoided to prevent injury to the small subscapular nerves.
  - Once released, a gentle tug on the tagging stitches should elicit a bounce of the muscle. The subscapularis may now be tucked medially, and a spiked glenoid retractor placed along the anterior glenoid neck.
- The capsulotomy is completed.
  - The Fukuda retractor is used to lever the humeral head posterolaterally to place the inferior capsule on stretch.
  - The inferior capsulectomy is continued off of the inferior glenoid neck; extreme care must be utilized, as the axillary nerve passes directly under the capsule and glenoid rim at this level.

- Several situations may arise that dictate differential capsular release or plication.
- Scenario 1: HHR revision with a centered humeral head and typical glenoid wear
  - An anteroinferior release is completed.
- Scenario 2: HHR revision with significant posterior glenoid wear and static posterior subluxation on the axillary radiograph
  - Undercorrection of glenoid version can lead to posterior instability (Fig. 9A), as seen in the radiograph in Figure 9B. Excessive humeral retroversion can also result in posterior instability (Fig. 9C).
  - Release is limited to an anteroinferior release.
  - The posterior capsular redundancy may require posterior capsular plication and postoperative immobilization in a gunslinger brace.

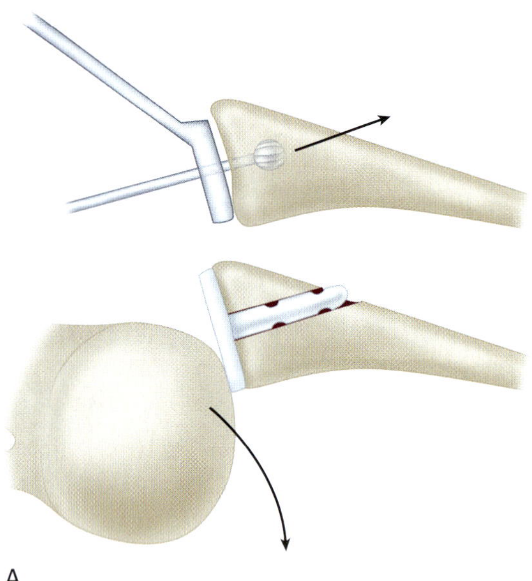

A

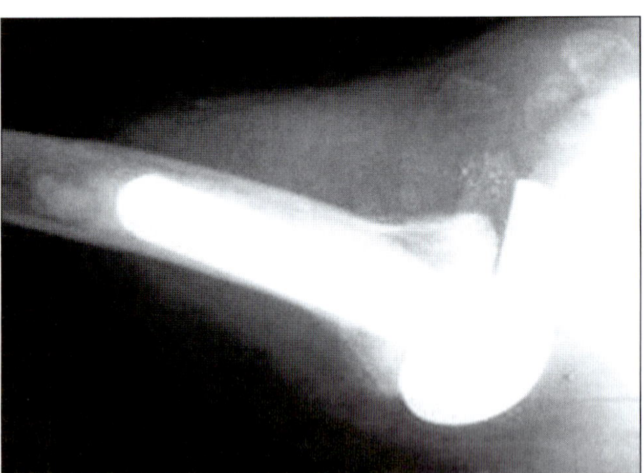

B

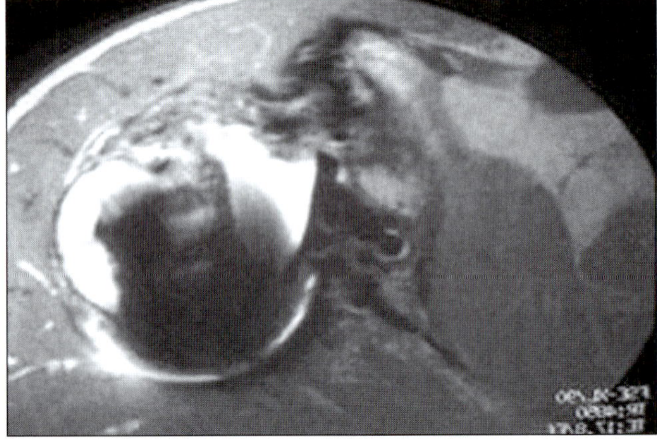

C

FIGURE 9

- Scenario 3: posttraumatic arthrosis and avascular necrosis
  - These two conditions often present with global capsular tightening, requiring a pan-capsular release.
  - Posterior capsular release is facilitated by removal of the Fukuda retractor and retraction with a bone hook.

- The glenoid is examined.
  - HHR, post-capsulorraphy revision, and fracture revisions have now been converted into a standard primary procedure, and the surgeon may proceed with the standard primary surgical technique.
  - In a revision TSA, the glenoid component should be examined. Often, the glenoid component is sufficiently loose that it will be easily removed with a Kocher clamp. If the glenoid component is sufficiently loose, worn, malpositioned, or infected, then it must be revised.
- The glenoid component is removed.
  - Similar to a humeral component, the glenoid component is loosened with an osteotome, being careful not to skive into the native bone to minimize bone loss (Fig. 10A and 10B).
  - A thin osteotome is placed at the interface between the glenoid component and the underlying bone and impacted. The pegs or keel of a plastic or trabecular metal glenoid component may be cut to aid in extraction. Retained pegs, posts, or cement can be burred out.

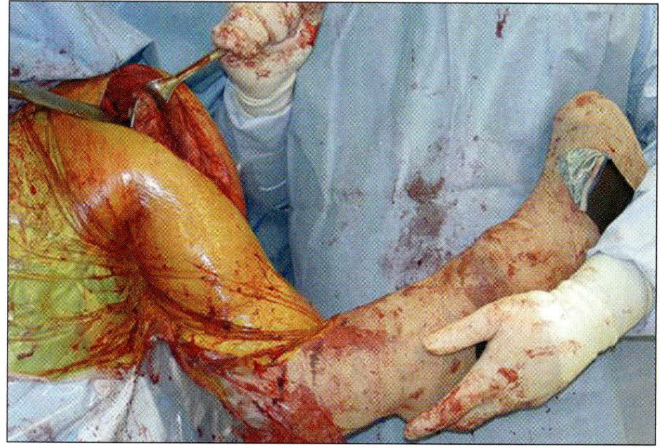

A

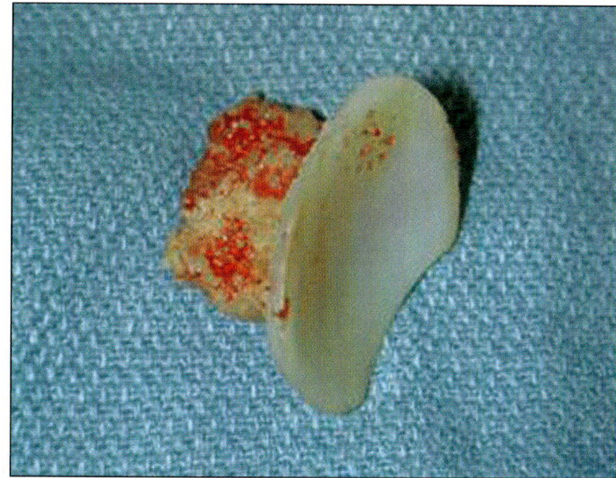

B

FIGURE 10

Pearls

- *Glenoid revision can be the most challenging portion of the revision arthroplasty.*
- *Determine whether posterior plication will be required to restore soft tissue balance. This can be completed with a purse-string technique or via plication through suture anchors.*
- *The cement used for fixation should be normal to higher viscosity cement; this will aid in forcing the remaining blood and fat out of the trabeculae (see Fig. 11).*
- *Although we do not routinely use a vent hole, some surgeons advocate drilling a coracoid hole to allow for theoretically improved evacuation of marrow and blood from the glenoid vault.*
- *The revision glenoid component may need an extra-long peg (10–15 mm longer than the standard) to achieve purchase.*

Pitfalls

- *Stable glenoid fixation requires the pegs/keel to be implanted into host bone.*

Step 6: Glenoid Revision

- In the aseptic revision, the anatomy is assessed to plan for the glenoid revision.
  - The glenoid is examined for bony defects and version. Glenoid defects are stratified into "contained" and "uncontained" defects.
  - Contained defects are those that have cortical containment and are amenable to impaction grafting and cementation. Cancellous graft is impacted into the defect; as the glenoid will provide a lateral wall, this does not require supplemental fixation.
  - Uncontained defects lack an anterior or posterior wall, and the goal is to convert the glenoid to a contained defect with cortical graft. These defects will require supplemental fixation to minimize loosening rates; screws and bioabsorbable implants are available. Norris et al. (2007) have described an elegant technique of one-stage grafting using tricortical iliac crest graft.
- The glenoid version is re-established.
  - A burr or reamer is used to re-establish a neutral glenoid version if adequate glenoid bone stock exists.
  - If the glenoid can be successfully grafted such that the new component can be fixed into native bone, then a new glenoid component may be implanted.
  - If the glenoid pegs or keel cannot be seated in native bone, then the procedure is staged: the glenoid is grafted and a humeral prosthesis is implanted with the plan to resurface the glenoid at a later date.
- Posterior plication is performed (if necessary)
  - Redundant posterior capsule may need plication.
  - If required, we place two to three suture anchors at the posterior glenoid rim prior to implantation of the new glenoid component.
  - Alternatively, a purse-string suture may be placed after glenoid implantation.
- The new glenoid component is implanted.
  - Fully cemented fixation requires cortical containment with abundant clean trabecular bone. Either native bone or native bone and graft can serve as the trabecular framework. Pulsatile lavage or pressurized gas is used to remove the fat from within the bone. The cement is impacted into the bone to achieve a good peg/keel-cement interface, with no cement mantle on the back of the

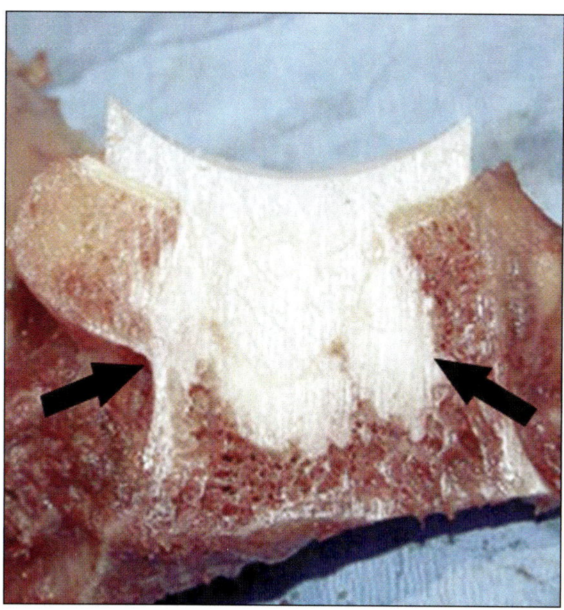

FIGURE 11

Pearls

- *A cement restrictor may be used if the canal is large enough to accept the implant. This is important in the rheumatoid patient, who may require an elbow replacement at a later date.*
- *Proper cementation technique requires sufficient trabeculae to allow interdigitation with the cement.*
- *A well-balanced shoulder arthroplasty demonstrates 60° of internal rotation of the arm elevated in the coronal plane, 50% posterior subluxation of the humeral head on the posterior drawer test, 140° of elevation, and 40° of external rotation fo the adducted arm with the subscapularis reapproximated.*

Pitfalls

- *The subscapularis repair must be secure, and postoperative external rotation limited by the motion easily obtained at surgery without stressing the repair. A subscapularis pull-off can degrade the results of revision.*

glenoid. Good cementation technique results in interdigitation and deep penetration of the cement into the bone (Fig. 11).

- Some newer designs reduce cement use and have some ingrowth potential. Press-fitting such a glenoid requires minimal to no bone defect. The vault should be filled with morcellized graft, and the implant rigidly anchored in native bone.

▪ Once the new glenoid component has been implanted, the Fukuda retractor is gently removed without levering on the glenoid, and the humeral head is re-dislocated.

Step 7: Humeral Revision

▪ In a revision for infection, an antibiotic-impregnated spacer is implanted.
  - A cement spacer is created using a Rush rod or Steinmann pin as a rigid core, and coated circumferentially with antibiotic cement.
  - The cement stem is mated with a ball of humeral cement (often the rubber top of the bulb suction provides an effective mold) while it is still soft.
  - The cement prosthesis is fine-tuned with a burr.
  - The antibiotic-impregnated cement spacer is implanted, the subscapularis loosely repaired and the biceps tenodesed, and the shoulder is closed. All sutures should be resorbable monofilament to decrease the risk of persistent infection.

- Aseptic humeral reimplantation
  - Scenario 1: malunited articular fracture fragment
    - If the revision is for a malunited articular fracture, two options arise: HHR or cementing a low-profile/thin humeral stem in slight varus or valgus.
  - Scenario 2: HHR and TSA revision
    - The humerus is examined to decide whether grafting will be required. A capacious humerus with only cortical bone remaining may require impaction grafting. Impaction grafting fills the canal with dense trabecular bone and is followed by cementation of a new humeral prosthesis.
    - Three types of humeral stem fixation may be employed: cement, press-fit, and bony ingrowth. In elderly patients, we exclusively revise with antibiotic-impregnated cement. Bony ingrowth is an option that we often use for younger patients.
    - Prior to cementation, a same-size trial is placed into the humerus to ensure that the final cemented prosthesis will fit.
    - The trial is removed, and the revision prosthesis cemented in the proper retroversion.
    - The head is trialed again. Eccentric modular heads placed with maximal offset posteriorly can tension the posterior soft tissue and decrease the incidence of posterior instability.
    - The final head is impacted onto the trunion.
    - The subscapularis is reattached using Krakow sutures through bone tunnels tied over a small plate or EndoButton (Smith and Nephew, Memphis, TN).
    - A lateral rotator interval closure is completed with the shoulder in maximal external rotation.
    - The external rotation limit is reassessed to guide the physical therapist as to the limit for postoperative external rotation.

Step 8: Closure

- Closure after a revision shoulder arthroplasty mirrors that of a primary arthroplasty.
  - Hemostasis is achieved.
  - A medium-sized closed-circuit drain is placed.
  - The deltopectoral interval is loosely closed.
  - The dermis is closed with buried interrupted stitches and a subcuticular closure is performed.

  - Dressings are applied and the arm is placed in a sling.
- A true AP view of the glenohumeral joint should be obtained in the operating room to allow critical postoperative assessment.

Postoperative Care and Expected Outcomes

- Postoperatively, patients are admitted to the hospital, where they recover for approximately 48 hours. Physical therapy begins on postoperative day 1, but varies with etiology of revision.
  - For the patient not requiring posterior capsular plication, phase I stretches are initiated, with the endpoints and limitations dictated by intraoperative findings. We use passive elevation in the scapular plane, external rotation with a stick, pulleys, and pendulums. Active internal rotation is prohibited for 6 weeks after the procedure; however, passive internal rotation is allowed to the chest. Patients are allowed to use their affected arm for their activities of daily living as long as they adhere to the aforementioned limitations.
  - In the revision case for instability, limitations are based upon preventing stress on the capsulotendinous repairs.
  - Posterior plication requires immobilization in a gunslinger brace and elevation only in the plane of the brace in neutral or slight external rotation.
  - Regardless of etiology, hand, wrist, and elbow range of motion should be instituted to prevent contracture.
- Patients are seen in the office at 2 weeks after the procedure to examine the wound and ensure strict adherence to physical and occupational therapy. Patients again are seen at the 6-week mark to evaluate range of motion, and to begin active exercises. Phase II and III stretching exercises are begun, with the addition of gentle strengthening. Patients are seen at the 12-week mark to continue strengthening and range-of-motion exercises. Follow-up visits are then scheduled for 6 months, 1 year, and 2 years, and then on a multiyear basis.

Evidence

Coste JS, et al. The management of infection in arthroplasty of the shoulder. J Bone Joint Surg [Br]. 2004;86:65-9.

(Level IV evidence)

Debeer P, Plasschaert H, Stuyck J. Resection arthroplasty of the infected shoulder: a salvage procedure for the elderly patient. Acta Orthop Belg. 2006;72:126-30.

(Level IV evidence)

Flatow EL, Bigliani LU. Tips of the trade. Locating and protecting the axillary nerve in shoulder surgery: the tug test. Orthop Rev. 1992;21:503-5.

(Level IV evidence)

Klepps SJ, Goldfarb C, Flatow E, Galatz LM, Yamaguchi K. Anatomic evaluation of the subcoracoid pectoralis major transfer in human cadavers. J Shoulder Elbow Surg. 2001;10:453-9.

(Level IV evidence)

Nagda SH, et al. Neer Award 2005: Peripheral nerve function during shoulder arthroplasty using intraoperative nerve monitoring. J Shoulder Elbow Surg. 2007;16(3, Suppl 1):S2-8.

(Level IV evidence)

Norris TR, Kelly JDI, Humphrey CS. Management of glenoid bone defects in revision shoulder arthroplasty: a new application of the reverse total shoulder prosthesis. Tech Shoulder Elbow Surg. 2007;8:37-46.

(Level IV evidence)

O'Driscoll SW, Petrie RS, Torchia ME. Arthroscopic removal of the glenoid component for failed total shoulder arthroplasty: a report of five cases. J Bone Joint Surg [Am]. 2005;87:858-63.

(Level IV evidence)

Sperling JW, et al. Infection after shoulder arthroplasty. Clin Orthop Relat Res. 2001;(382):206-16.

(Level IV evidence)

Sperling JW, et al. Magnetic resonance imaging of painful shoulder arthroplasty. J Shoulder Elbow Surg. 2002;11:315-21.

SECTION I

SHOULDER
Instability

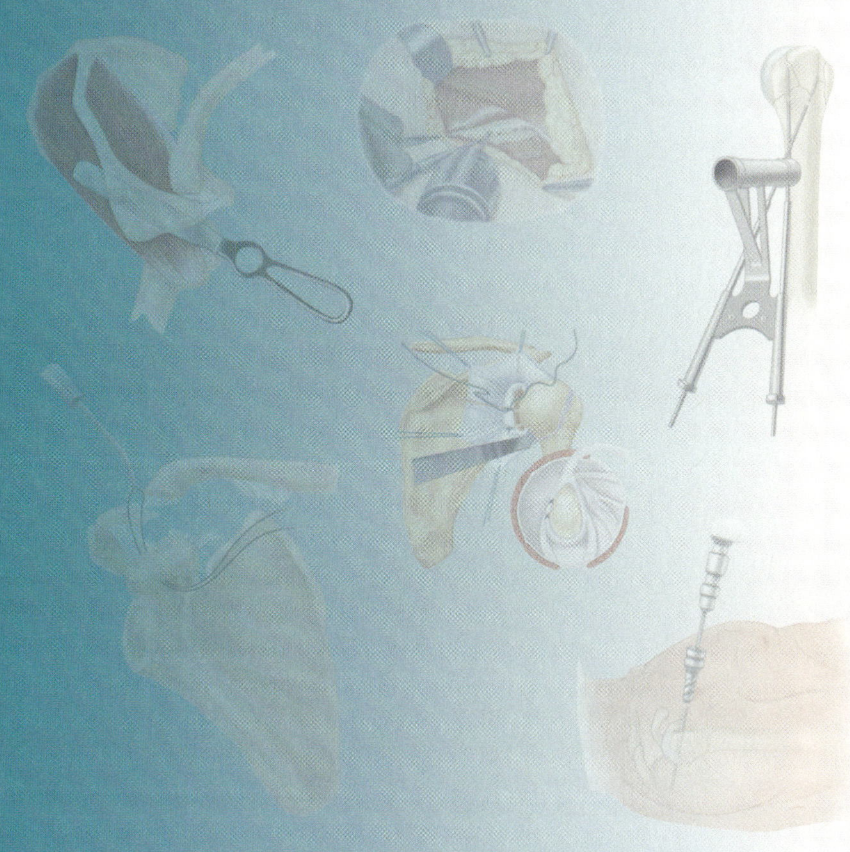

PROCEDURE 12

Arthroscopic Treatment of Traumatic Anterior Instability of the Shoulder

Matthew Denkers and Robert Hollinshead

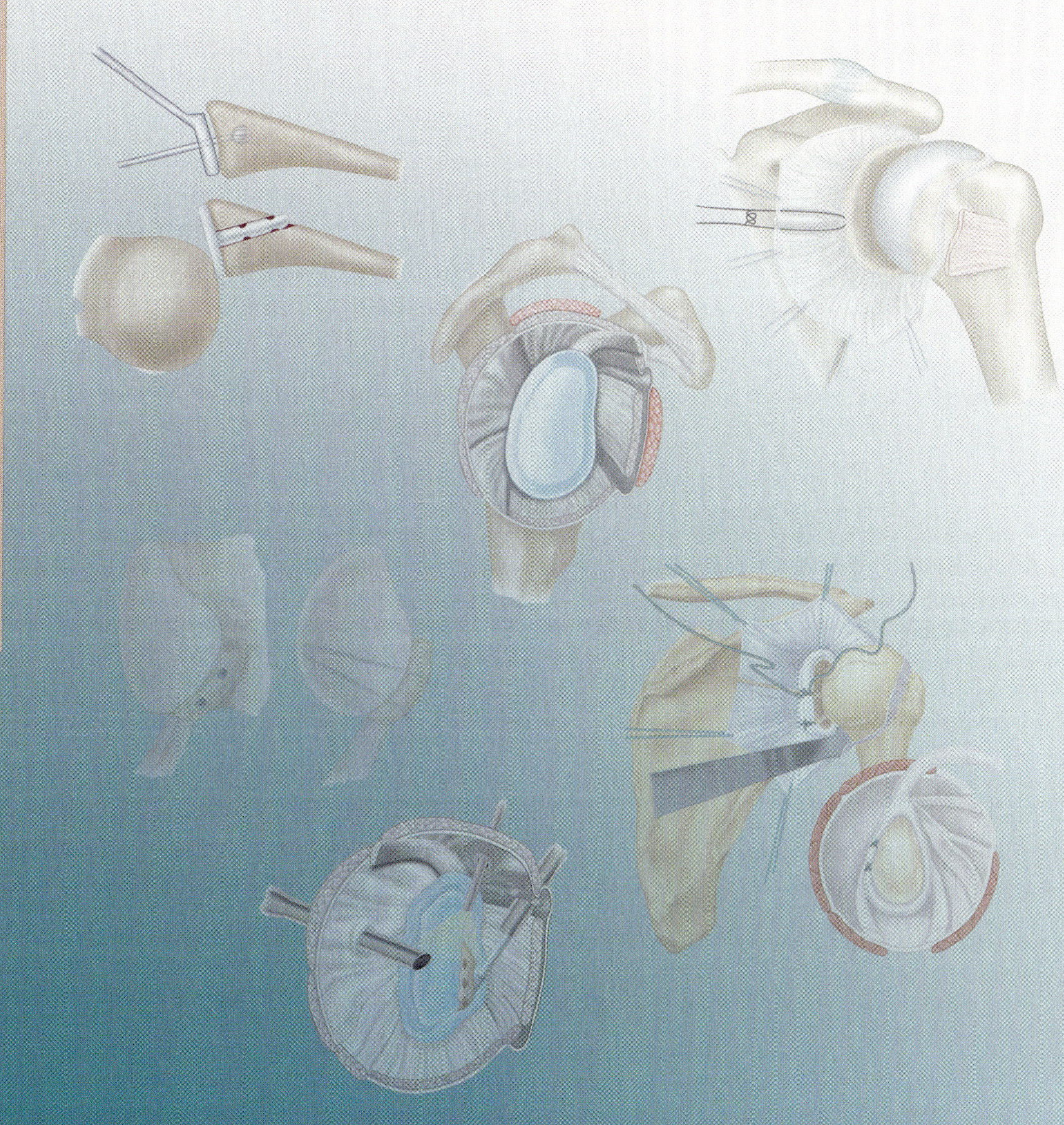

Pitfalls

- *Atraumatic multidirectional instability is experienced by patients with underlying generalized ligamentous laxity. Surgical intervention is reserved for patients that fail initial nonoperative treatment, including patient education focusing on strengthening of the dynamic stabilizers of the glenohumeral joint as well as the scapular stabilizers to compensate for lax ligamentous constraints.*
- *Patients with significant glenoid bone loss (i.e., >25% anterior glenoid) may require an open coracoid transfer or bone-grafting procedure (Burkhart and DeBeer, 2000).*

Controversies

- Based on their risk of recurrence, younger patients (Kirkley, 1999) or high-level athletes may benefit from repair after their first episode of anterior instability, whereas older patients should be addressed when the instability is recurrent.
- Contact athletes are involved in activities placing them at higher risk for recurrence, leading some to advocate that an open procedure be the repair of choice.
- Patients requiring revision anterior stabilization may be considered for an open procedure given that the initial procedure has failed.
- If a large engaging Hill-Sachs lesion contributes to the instability and needs to be addressed, an open procedure may be considered.

Indications

- Traumatic anterior shoulder instability in patients willing to participate postoperatively in progressive rehabilitation

Examination/Imaging

- In addition to the standard shoulder examination for instability, which would include translation findings and apprehension signs (anterior, inferior, and posterior), it is important to evaluate the entire shoulder for the injuries known to accompany instability, such as a superior labrum anterior-posterior (SLAP) tear, long head of the biceps involvement, and rotator cuff tear.
- A complete neurovascular examination of the extremity should be performed as well to detect a concomitant injury, with an axillary nerve injury being most commonly associated with anterior glenohumeral dislocation.

Imaging Studies

- Plain radiographs of the shoulder should be obtained, including the standard three views (anteroposterior, trans-scapular, and axillary), to assess the presence of bony pathology.
  - Hill-Sachs lesions (Fig. 1)
  - Bony Bankart lesion (Fig. 2)
- Special views (i.e., Stryker notch, West Point axillary) may be obtained for further assessment.

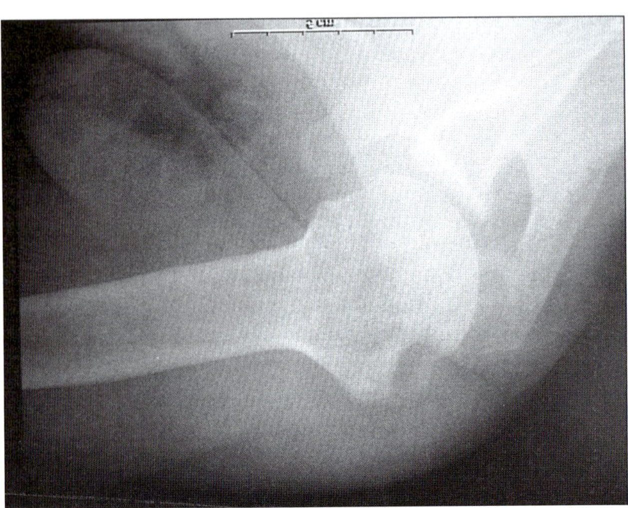

FIGURE 1

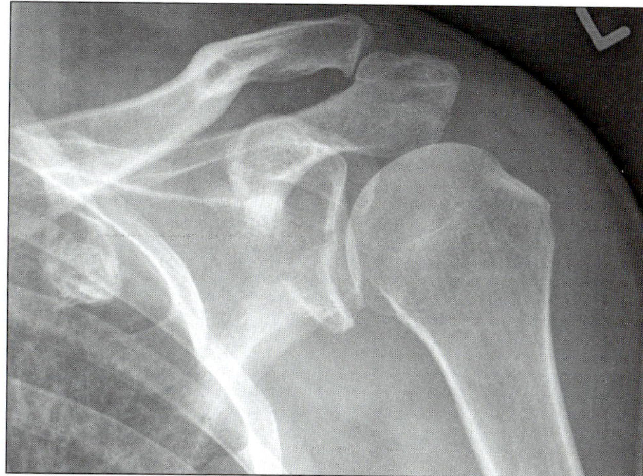

FIGURE 2

- Computed tomography, especially with three-dimensional reconstructions, can demonstrate the presence and extent of humeral or glenoid bony lesions, which may alter the surgical planning and necessitate an open procedure.
- Magnetic resonance imaging may be helpful to evaluate associated pathology (e.g., rotator cuff tear, cartilaginous lesions, SLAP tear) if the patient has ongoing pain or weakness between episodes of instability or if the patient is a first-time dislocator at an older age and subject to a higher incidence of rotator cuff tear occurring with anterior dislocation (Neviaser et al., 1993).
- A magnetic resonance arthrogram (Fig. 3) is not routinely used as, once a decision to operate is made

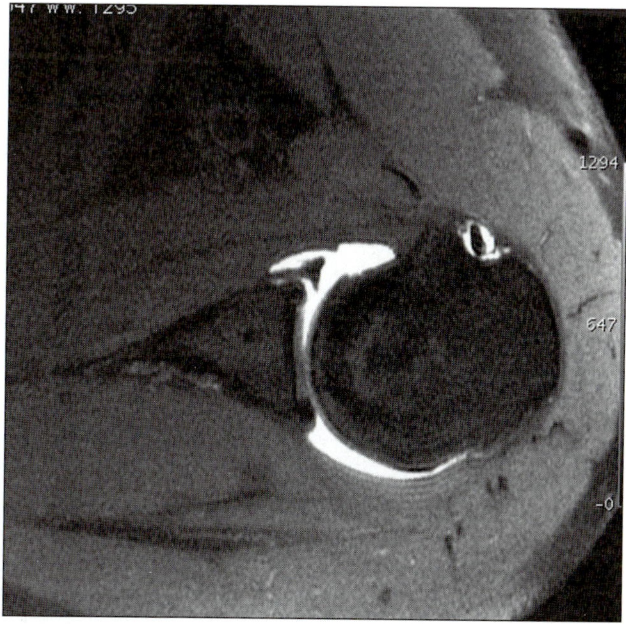

FIGURE 3

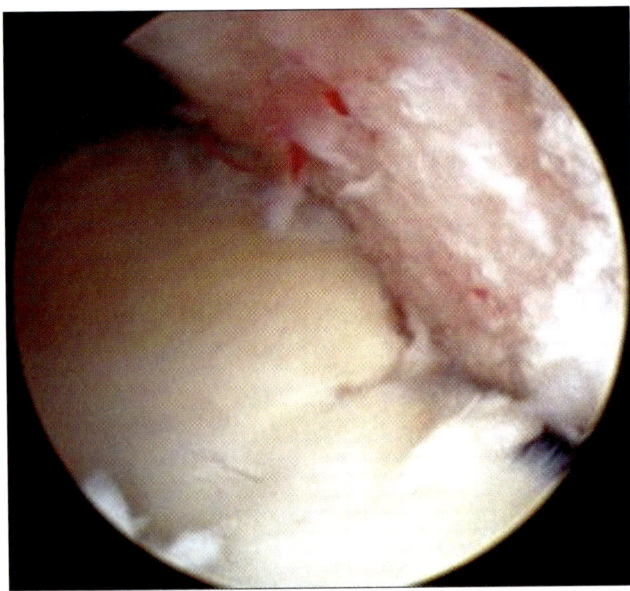

FIGURE 4

Treatment Options

- Nonoperative treatment with external rotation bracing has been described as being successful in the treatment of first-time dislocators (Itoi et al., 2007).
- Open surgical repair has been the gold standard for anterior instability until recently challenged by the results of skillful arthroscopic repair as arthroscopic techniques improve (Mohtadi, 2005; Lenters et al., 2007).

on a clinical basis, all labral and capsular pathology can be confirmed and treated at the time of the arthroscopic procedure.

- Arthroscopy remains the "gold standard" as a diagnostic modality for shoulder instability and associated conditions. It allows inspection and probing of unstable labrum, glenoid, and humeral head bony lesions; patulous ligaments and capsule, associated tendon tears; and whether Hill-Sachs lesions are engaging (Fig. 4) or not.

Surgical Anatomy

- Glenoid labrum and glenohumeral capsule and ligaments (Fig. 5)
  - Anterior-inferior glenohumeral ligament—the main static restraint to anterior translation in the at-risk position of abduction–external rotation
  - Middle glenohumeral ligament—be aware of the normal variant Buford complex (Fig. 6) and focally absent labrum
  - Superior glenohumeral ligament
- The glenoid is normally pear shaped, with the bare area indicating its center. An inverted-pear shape (Fig. 7) indicates significant (i.e., >25%) anterior-inferior bony loss as the result of either a bony Bankart lesion or erosion (Lo et al., 2004).
- The humeral head has a bare area just medial to the insertion of the infraspinatus into the greater

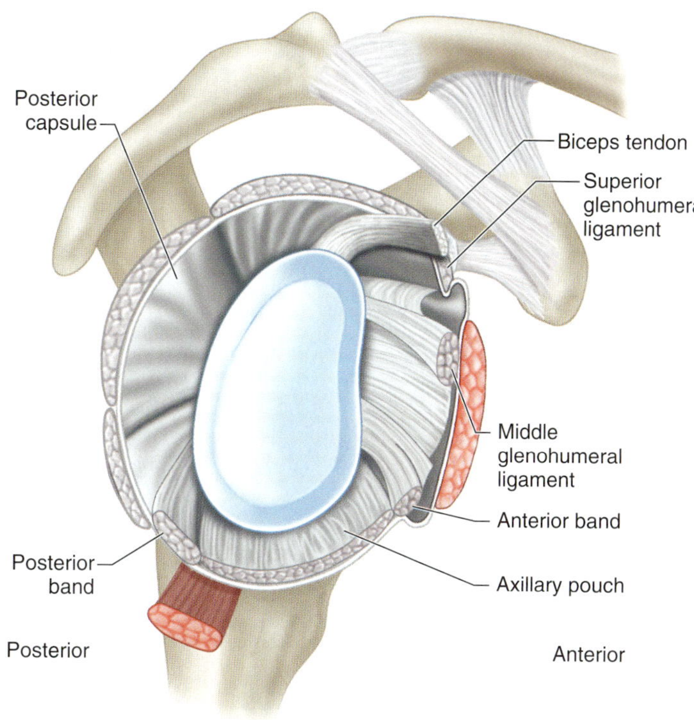

FIGURE 5

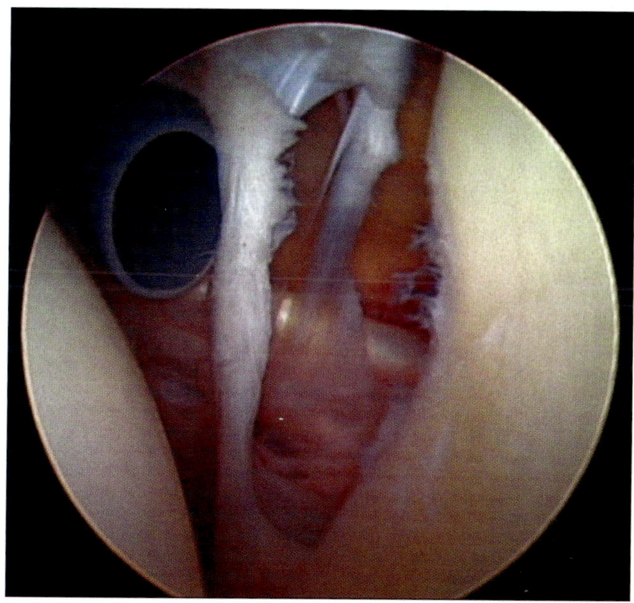

FIGURE 6

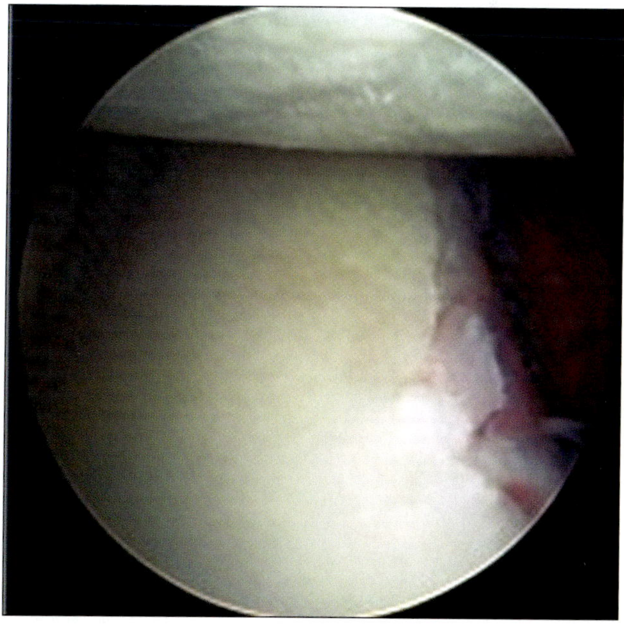

FIGURE 7

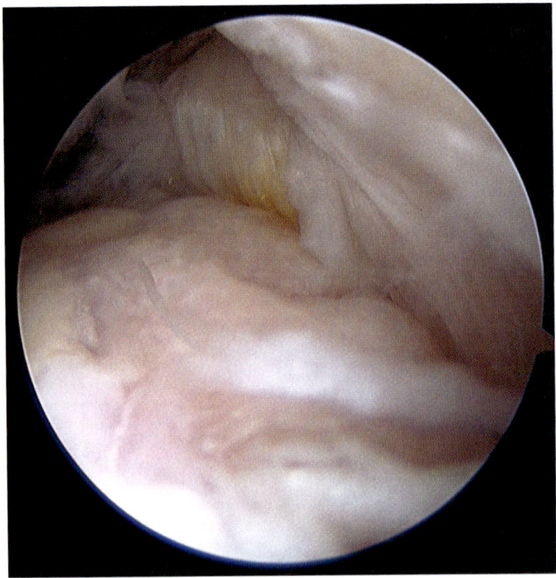

A

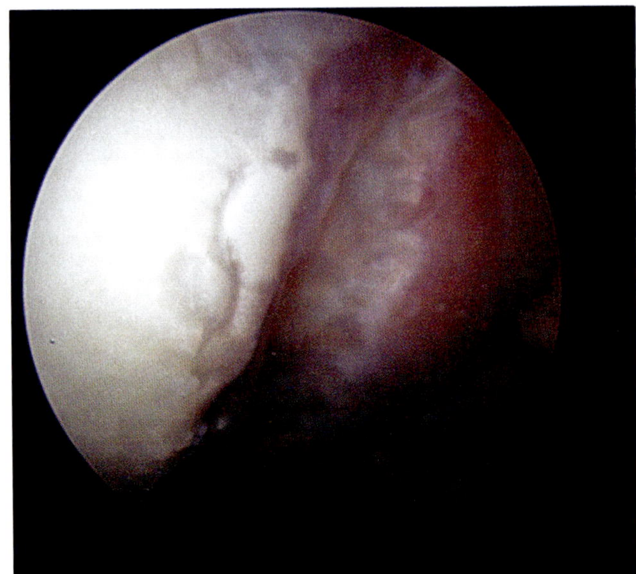

B

FIGURE 8

Pearls

- *The patient should be placed as upright as possible to facilitate exposure.*
- *Anterior and posterior portal exposure are essential. In the beach chair position, the shoulder must be well lateral to the edge of the bed in order to freely access the posterior portal.*
- *The head should be maintained in a neutral position and traction on the arm avoided to prevent injury to the brachial plexus.*

tuberosity (Fig. 8A), which should be discerned from a Hill-Sachs lesion (Fig. 8B).

- Axillary nerve and brachial plexus
  - The axillary nerve travels on the underside of the inferior capsule or pouch of the joint.
  - The brachial plexus should not be encountered with liberation of the medialized labral lesion unless passing medial to the coracoid.

Positioning

- The patient may be placed in the upright beach chair position (Fig. 9).

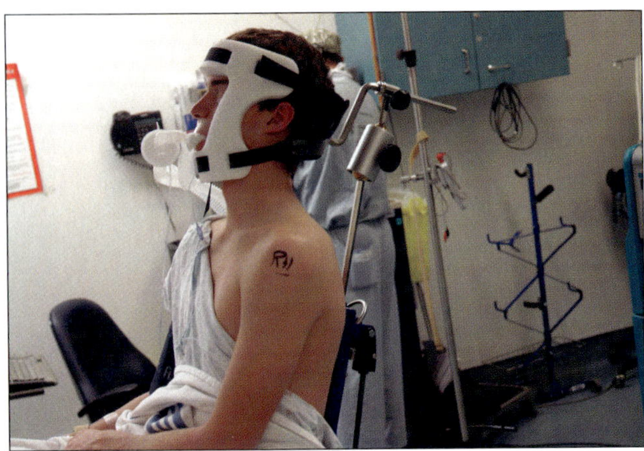

FIGURE 9

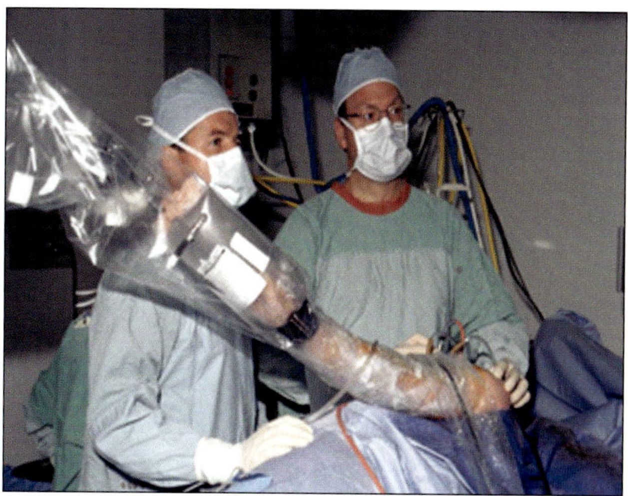

FIGURE 10

■ With the patient supine on the bed, the axis of rotation at the patient's hips should lie even with or just superior to the break in the bed such that, when the bed is transitioned to the upright beach chair position, a stable upright position is assumed instead of inducing lumbar lordosis and a less comfortable slouched position.

■ As the patient is gently elevated from the supine to the upright position, the head should be stabilized, but not rigidly secured to the bed to avoid a cervical traction injury. Once upright, the face mask should be applied with the head in a neutral position, avoiding cervical traction, flexion, or extension.

Pitfalls

- *Care should be taken to protect and remain cognizant of the airway and eyes beneath the drapes as instrumentation through the anterior portal often comes in close proximity.*
- *Cerebral hypotension (and in some rare instances cerebral infarction) can occur secondary to anesthesia-induced hypotension and failure to recognize the significant orthostatic gradient that exists in the upright position when the blood pressure cuff is placed on the calf. Patient and positioning factors must be accounted for and the blood pressure carefully monitored (Papadonikolakis et al., 2008).*

Equipment

- Specialized tables allow for easy upright beach chair positioning and support, as well as providing better access to the posterior portal with removable panels.
- Pneumatic or weighted rope-and-pulley dynamic arm positioners can secure the arm in different positions as well as provide longitudinal and lateral traction, freeing the surgical assistant from these duties.

Controversies

- There are advocates of both upright beach chair and lateral decubitus positioning. Many find the upright position offers a more anatomic vertical position of the glenoid, which is more easily correlated to the arthroscopic image. Proponents of the lateral position suggest it allows more comfortable instrumentation of the inferior aspect of the glenohumeral joint and easier visualization through an anterosuperolateral portal, thus freeing both the anterior and posterior portals for instrumentation (Fig. 10).

Pearls

- *The pull-back maneuver is performed by the assistant by using his or her arm as a lever between the thorax and humerus of the patient (Fig. 14). This provides lateral and posterior distraction to enhance the view of the anteroinferior glenoid and labrum.*

Pitfalls

- *As the case progresses and extra-articular soft tissue swelling ensues, the portal sites at the skin will be moved laterally and superiorly from their original position. Therefore, consider erring medially and inferiorly when initially placing the posterior portal.*

Instrumentation

- #11 scalpel
- 18-gauge spinal needle
- For the anterior portal, insert either a small cannula with sharp trocar or a switching stick initially, then switch to a large cannula inserted over a dilator.

Portals/Exposures

- Two-portal technique (Fig. 11)
  - A posterior viewing portal is placed two fingerbreadths medial and one thumbwidth down from the posterolateral corner of the acromion at the soft spot.
  - An anterior working portal is placed just superior to the subscapularis tendon using an "outside-in" technique by localizing with a spinal needle under arthroscopic visualization (Fig. 12A and 12B). Proper placement is critical to ensure the appropriate angle of approach and adequate access to the inferior glenoid for anchor placement.
- An optional anterosuperolateral viewing portal (Fig. 13A–C) can be used to provide an "en-face" view of

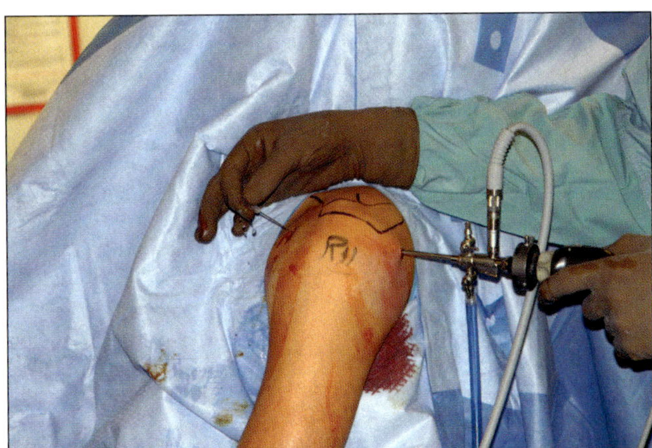

FIGURE 11

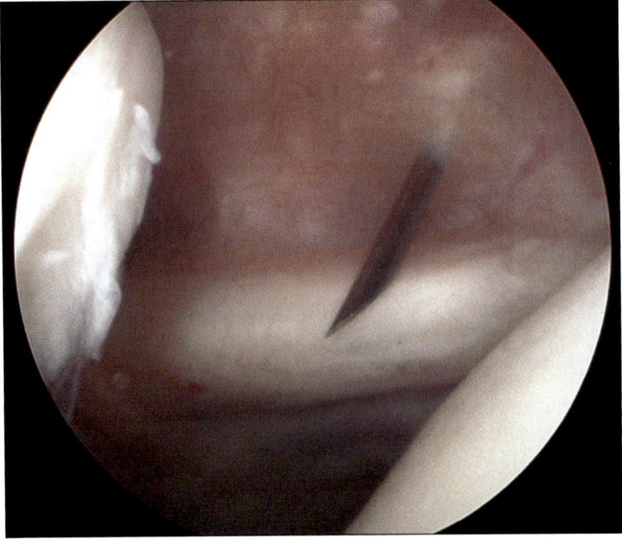

A

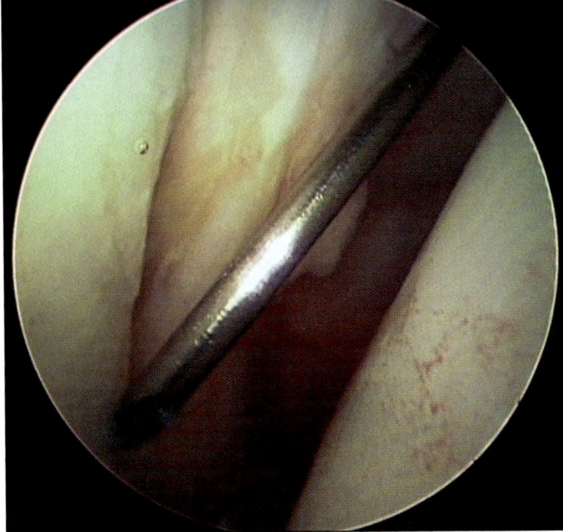

B

FIGURE 12

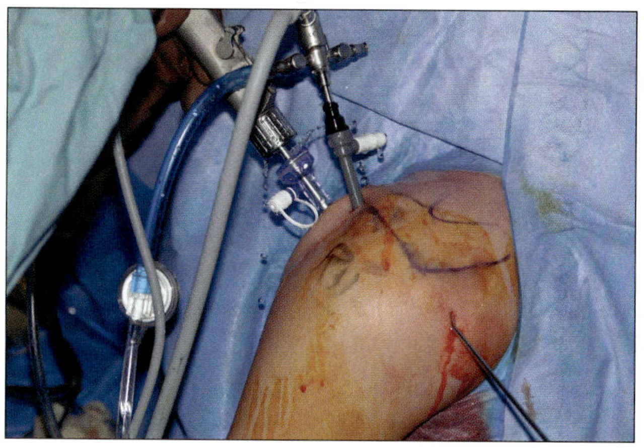
A

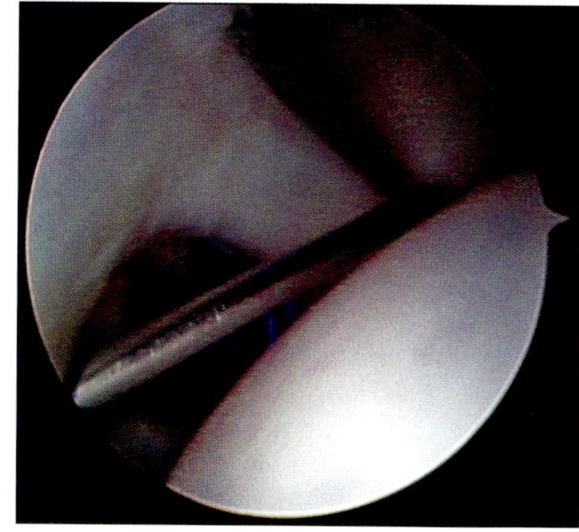
B

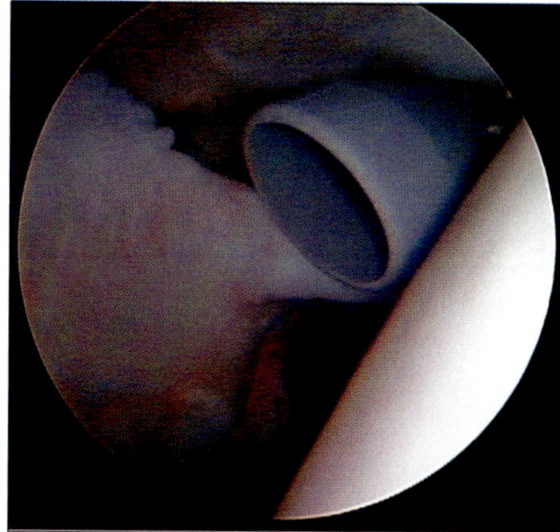
C

FIGURE 13

Controversies

- An inferior-anterior or trans-subscapularis portal is rarely necessary, but provides a more direct line of approach to the inferior glenoid for secure anchor placement, avoiding skiving of the drill or cutout of the anchor.

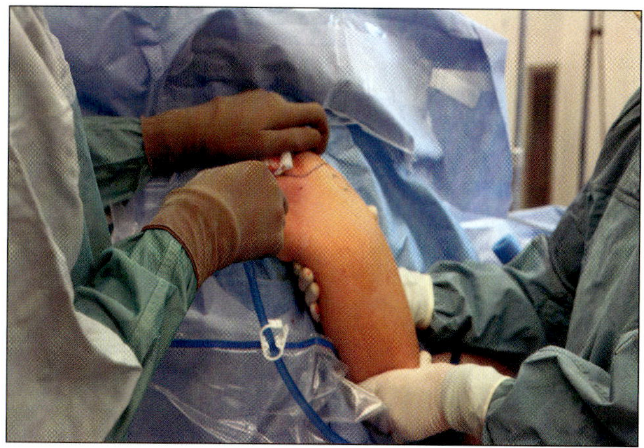

FIGURE 14

the glenoid and improved visualization of the anterior-inferior glenoid and medialized labrum, as well as making both the posterior and anterior portals available for instrumentation.

Pearls

- *Examination under anesthesia should be performed to assess the stability of the shoulder, as important information regarding overall laxity and direction of instability can alter intraoperative decisions. Care must be taken to perform the tests gently to avoid frank dislocation as intra-articular bleeding may be caused, which may impede the subsequent arthroscopy.*

Pitfalls

- *ALPSA lesions are easily missed and mistaken for attrition of the labrum. Consider using a 70° arthroscope posteriorly or visualizing through the anterior or anterosuperolateral portal to see medially on the glenoid neck.*
- *Be sure to detect pan-labral defects leading to combined instability.*
- *Rule out bone loss, capsular laxity, or multidirectional instability as this may dictate a change in surgical technique.*

Procedure

Step 1: Diagnostic Arthroscopy

- Diagnostic arthroscopy is performed to define pathology.
  - Labral Bankart lesion (Fig. 15A and 15B)
  - Bony Bankart lesion (Fig. 16)—need to assess amount of glenoid bone loss due to erosion or a detached bone fragment with the labrum
  - Anterior labroligamentous periosteal sleeve avulsion (ALPSA) (Fig. 17A and 17B, from the posterior and the anterior viewing portal, respectively) with the anterior labrum medialized and adherent to the anterior glenoid neck (Fig. 17C), requiring diligent mobilization (Neviaser, 1993)
  - Hill-Sachs lesion—need to assess size and whether it is "engaging" the anterior edge of the glenoid in the functional position of abduction–external rotation.

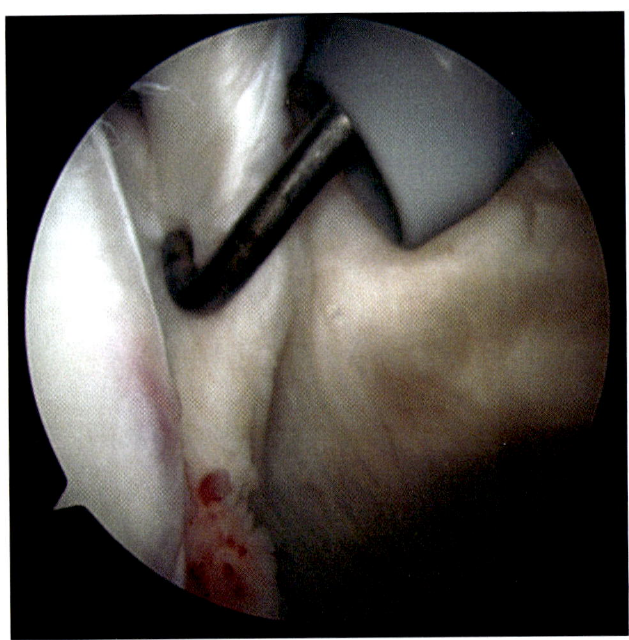

A

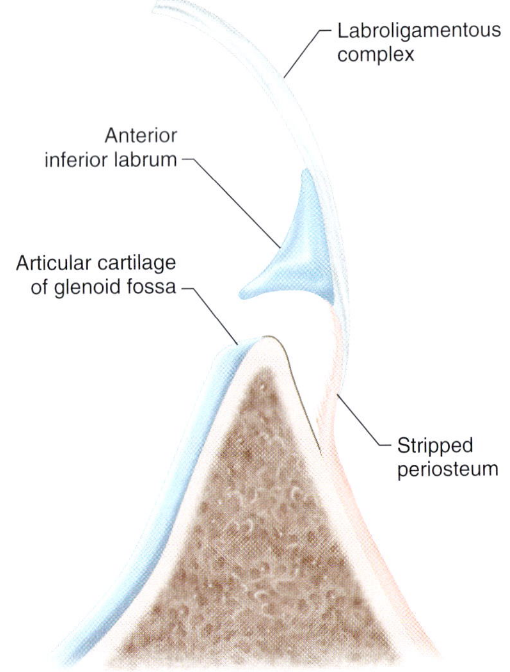

B

FIGURE 15

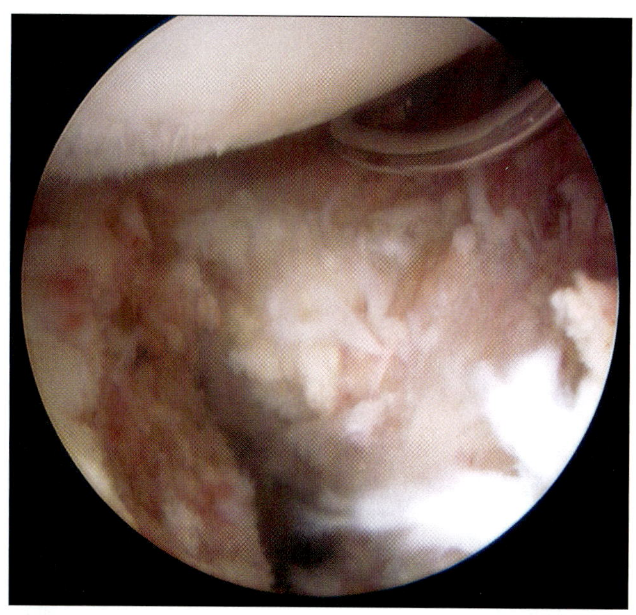

FIGURE 16

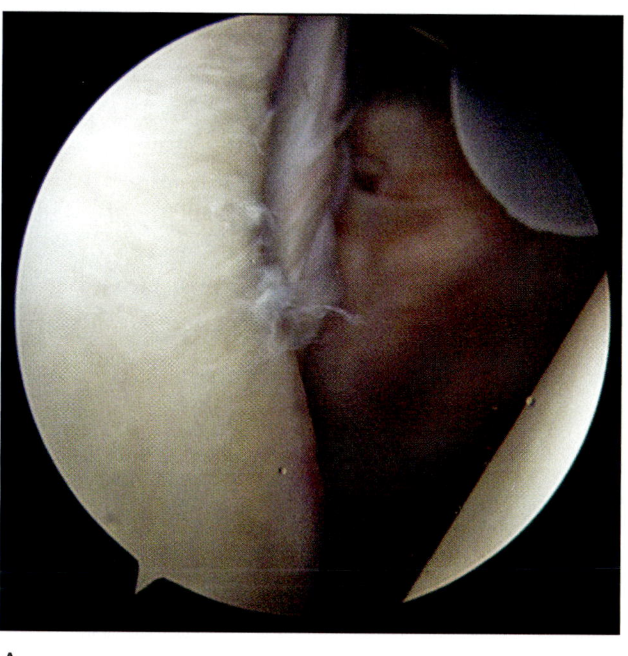

A

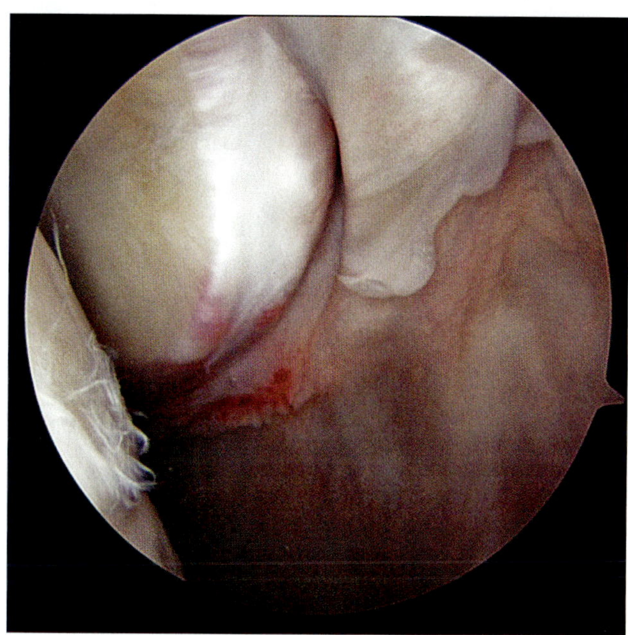

B

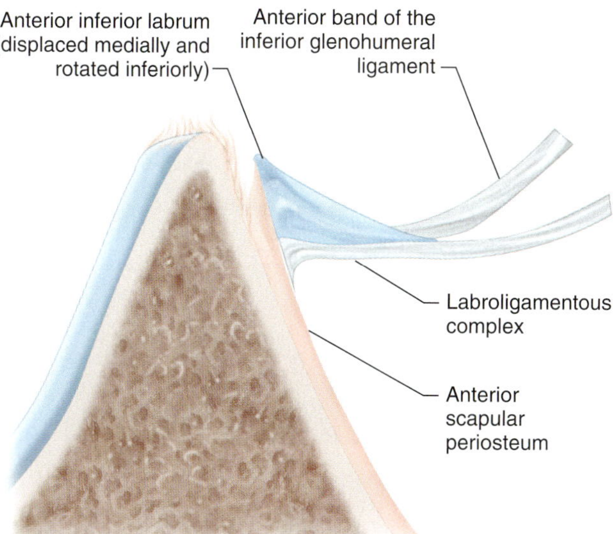

C

FIGURE 17

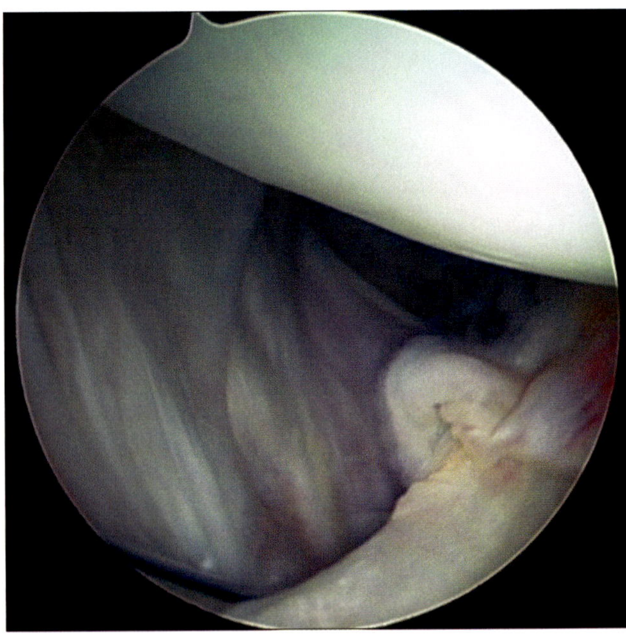

FIGURE 18

Instrumentation/ Implantation

- 30° and 70° arthroscope
- Hook probe

Controversies

- Excessive laxity or multidirectional instability may require rotator interval closure or posterior capsular plication.

- Humeral avulsion of the glenohumeral ligament (Fig. 18)—needs to be recognized as this may contribute to anterior instability (Wolf et al., 1995)
- Labral defects posteriorly or SLAP tear
- Anterior-inferior glenohumeral ligament (AIGHL), medial glenohumeral ligament (MGHL), or inferior pouch laxity (Fig. 19)

Step 2: Labral and Glenoid Preparation

- "Prep" work is critical and may take almost as long as the actual repair.

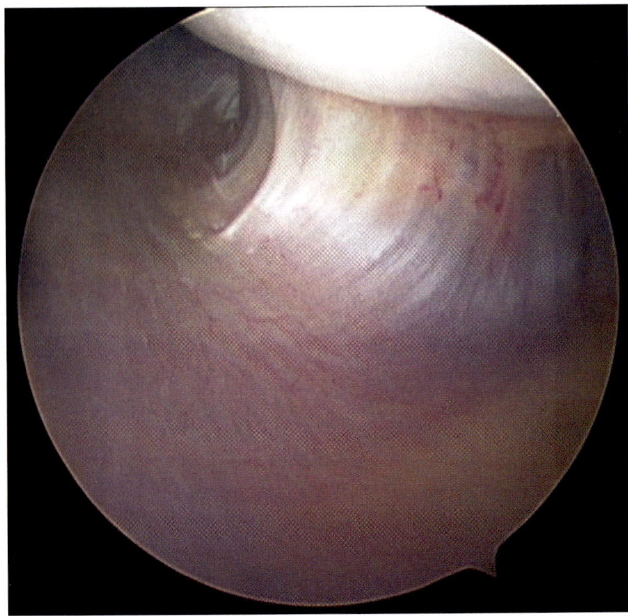

FIGURE 19

Pearls

- *It is essential to liberally mobilize the labrum such that it "floats up" to the glenoid edge so that the ensuing repair is not under tension.*
- *ALPSA lesions can be difficult to mobilize. A visual key that ensures adequate liberation of the labrum is seeing subscapularis fibers in the interval created between the glenoid and the labrum.*
- *The polished backside of the Bankart rasp can be used as a mirror to visualize the adequacy of the glenoid bone preparation when viewing from a posterior portal (Fig. 22).*

Pitfalls

- *The labrum may be attenuated or macerated, so take care to avoid transecting the labrum when freeing it with the Bankart rasp.*
- *Débride any chondral injury at the anterior-inferior aspect of the glenoid.*

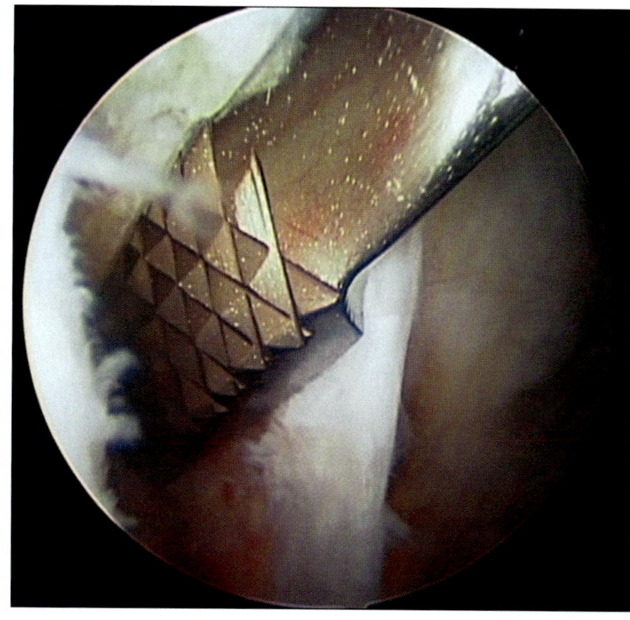

FIGURE 20

- After identifying the labral lesion, the labrum should be freed from the underlying glenoid neck. The Bankart rasp is most useful for initial labral mobilization (Fig. 20) but can be followed by an oscillating shaver in the interval between the labrum and glenoid.
- Once the labrum is free, there is a space in which to prepare the glenoid bony bed. Using a rasp, shaver, or burr, the glenoid bed is débrided at the chondral interface (Fig. 21A) down to a fresh bleeding bone surface (Fig. 21B).

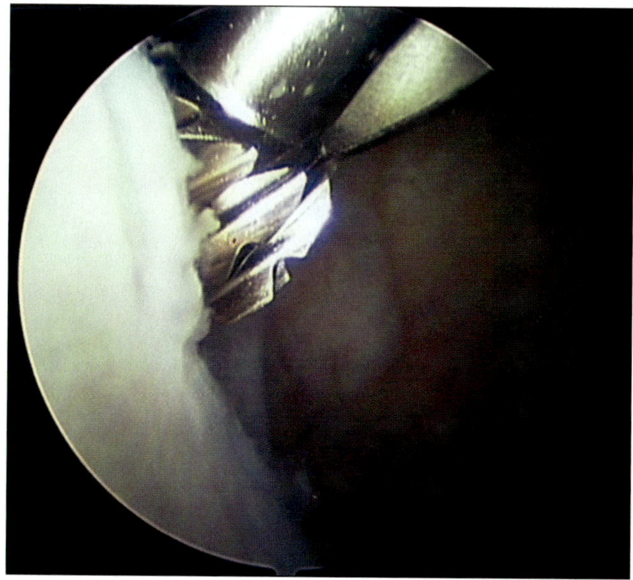

A

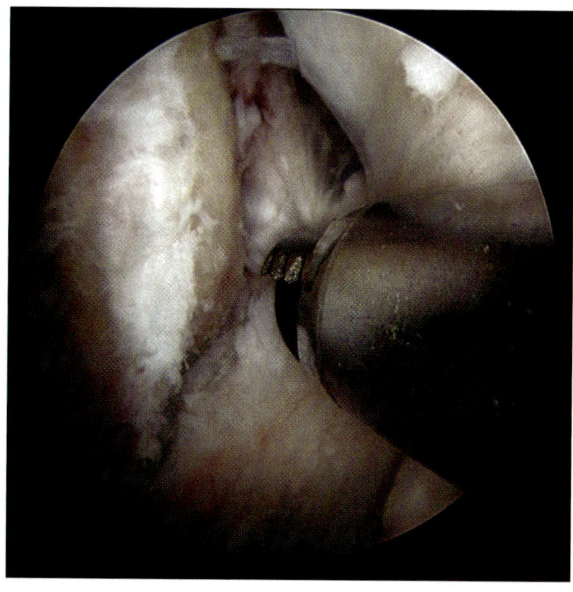

B

FIGURE 21

Instrumentation/ Implantation

- Bankart rasp/Liberator
- Motorized oscillating shaver
- Small spherical or rounded burr for final bone bed preparation

Controversies

- Some advocate débriding the chondral surface 2 mm onto the glenoid face, while others only débride to the chondral interface, but still place the anchors 2 mm onto the face.

Instrumentation/ Implantation

- "Screw-in" or "push-in" anchor
- Corresponding awl, drill, or tap
- "Suture-first, push-in, flip" implant (preferred by authors)

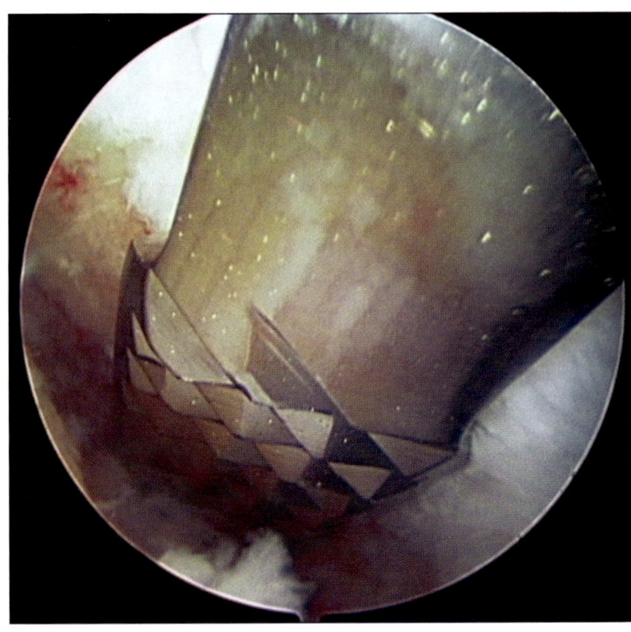

FIGURE 22

Step 3: Anchor Placement

- It is important to place anchors just over the glenoid articular margin as this will help to re-create the soft tissue "medial bumper."
- Anchor placement is usually below the equator of the glenoid and in an inferior-to-superior direction (Fig. 23A and 23B).

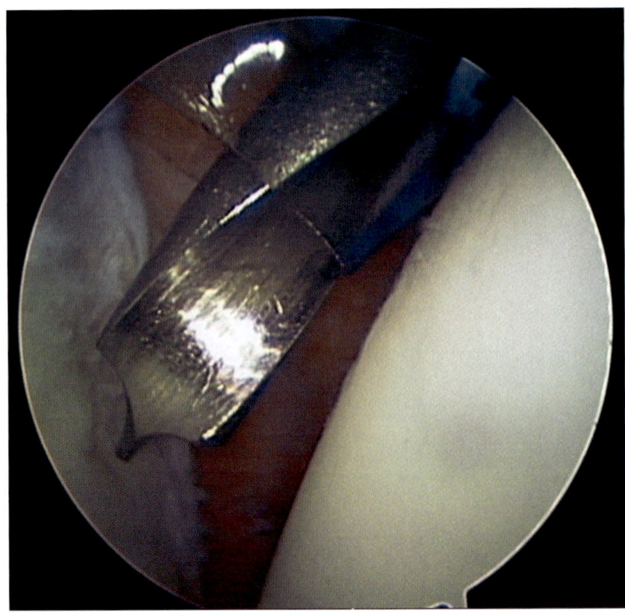

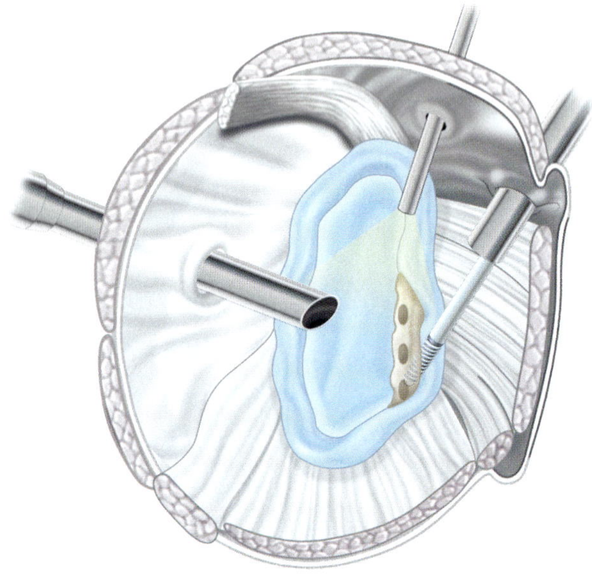

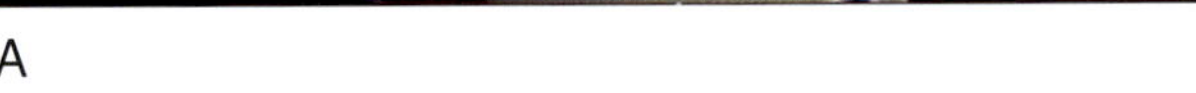

A

B

FIGURE 23

Pearls

- *With the anchor-first technique, anchors can be double-loaded, providing insurance sutures that can be used if needed.*
- *In addition to the pull-back maneuver, the cannulated anchor drill guide may be used to increase the angle of anchor placement in two planes by levering against the soft tissues inferior to the anterior cannula and against the humeral head posteriorly to gain an appropriate line of approach to the glenoid face.*

Pitfalls

- *Placing an anchor on the glenoid neck medial to the rim will fail to re-create the medial soft tissue bumper and may lead to unsatisfactory results.*
- *Placing anchors too close together can cause loss of anchor purchase and a cavitary bony defect.*
- *Anchor cutout may be solved by reinserting a larger anchor or selecting a new anchor site.*
- *In the event of suture or tissue failure with the anchor remaining in situ, it may be possible to stack a second anchor in the original hole with good pullout strength.*

Controversies

- Implant technology continues to evolve, providing many different implant options:
  - Absorbable versus nonabsorbable materials
  - Screw-in versus push-in, flip anchor
  - Anchor-first versus suture-first technique
  - Knot versus knotless

- Sufficient anchors are used to ensure adequate stabilization (usually two to five).

Step 4: Suture Placement and Knot Tying

- As with the anchor placement, sutures are passed in an inferior-to-superior sequence.
- Anterograde, retrograde, or shuttling suture passage can be performed, with shuttling being the authors' preference.
- Deciding on the amount of AIGHL to capture along with the labrum should be based on several factors (amount of initial external rotation, tissue quality, occupation, activities, etc.), which will help determine the amount of desirable postoperative external rotation.
- The authors prefer a suture-first technique.
  - A suture-passing hook is placed through the labrum (Fig. 24A and 24B).
  - After the suture has been passed around the labrum and retrieved out the anterior cannula (Fig. 25A–D), a "push-in, flip" anchor is loaded on the

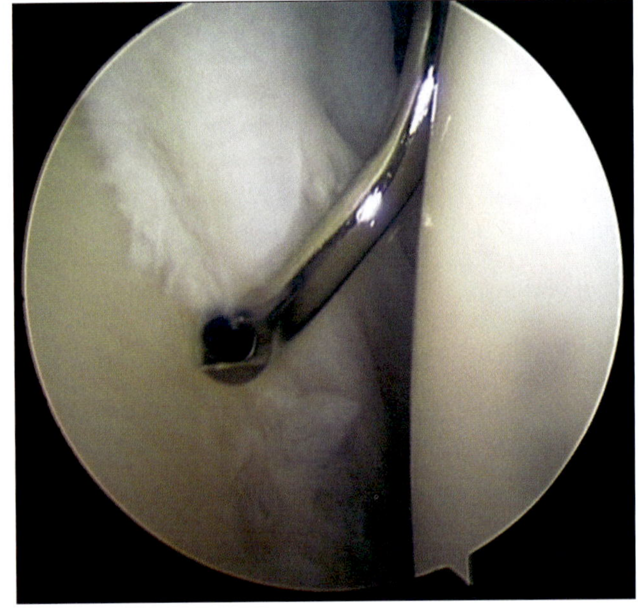

A

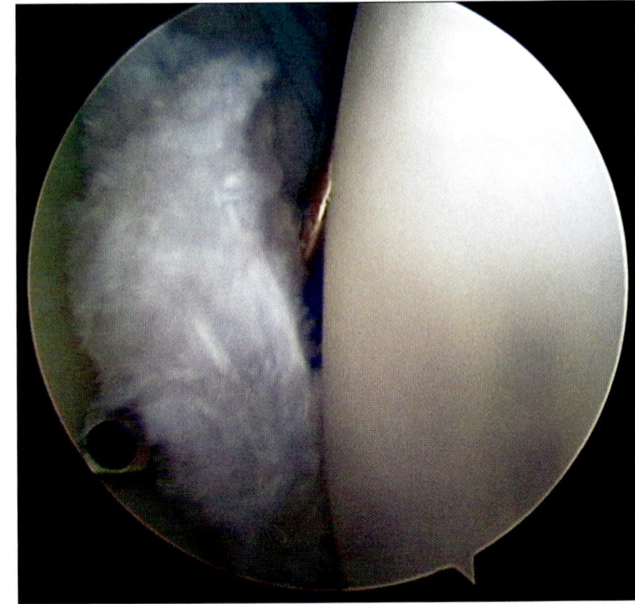

B

FIGURE 24

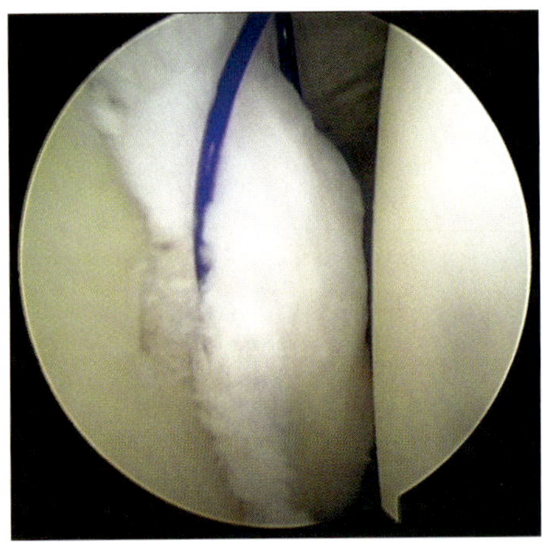

A

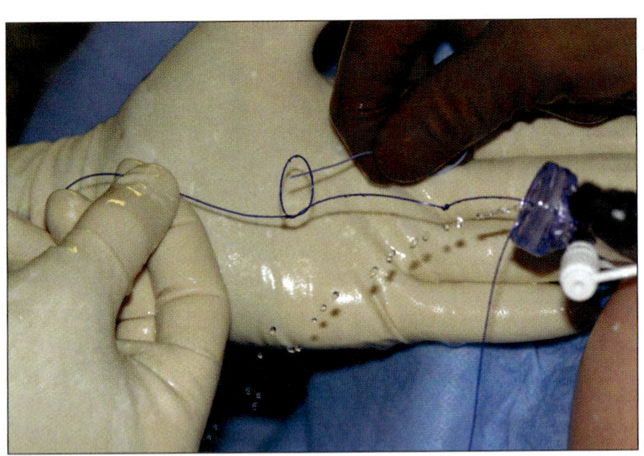

B

C

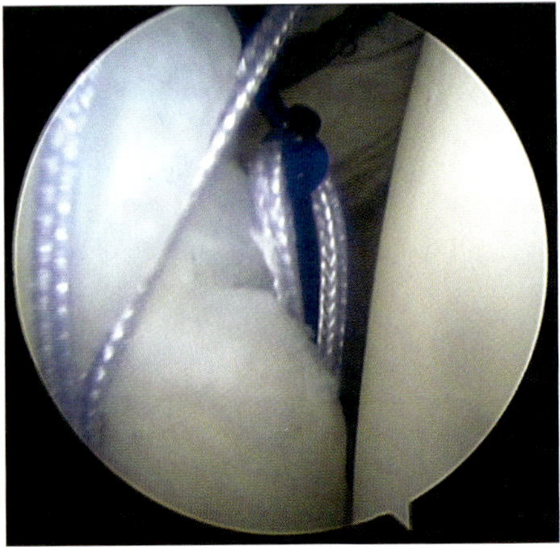

D

FIGURE 25

Pearls

- *If using a hooked suture-passing device, choose a right hook for a right anterior shoulder and vice versa.*
- *Suture placement should be just inferior to the anchor placement in the anchor-first technique or to the pilot hole in the suture-first technique in order to obtain an inferior-superior capsular shift.*
- *A traction stitch can allow for easier and more accurate passage of the definitive suture for the inferior anchor to accomplish the inferior-superior shift.*
- *It may be easier to pass subsequent sutures if the previous suture remains untied, allowing the interval between the labrum and glenoid to remain open and more amenable to suture passage.*
- *If using an anterosuperolateral portal for visualization and the anterior portal for instrumentation, the posterior portal can be used for suture management.*
- *If having difficulty with a hooked suture-passing device, consider switching to an anterograde suture passer.*

Pitfalls

- *The labrum may be poorly defined, macerated, or absent. This requires passing the suture through the remaining attenuated anterior capsule and possibly the MGHL, taking care to preserve the desired amount of external rotation.*
- *Caution should be used to prevent excessive restriction of external rotation. Beyond the most inferior anchor, the amount of external rotation should be evaluated following the tying of each subsequent suture to ensure that excessive restriction of external rotation does not occur. In the event of overtightening, the most superior sutures should be repassed.*
- *Both limbs of the suture must be retrieved together through the cannula to avoid a loop, twist, or "soft tissue bridge."*

deep suture limb and inserted into the previously drilled anchor hole (Fig. 26A and 26B).

- The anchor inserter is sharply removed and the suture limbs tensioned to flip the anchor and test purchase.
- A sliding knot (authors' preference is the SMC knot) is tied externally (Fig. 27A and 27B) with the superficial suture limb as the post and passed down the cannula to approximate the labrum to the anchor site (Fig. 28A and 28B). The knot is locked and then secured with two to three reversing half-hitches on alternate posts.

Instrumentation/ Implantation

- Suture-passing instrument: anterograde, retrograde, shuttling
- Suture retriever
- Single-hole knot pusher
- Arthroscopic suture scissor

Controversies

- Amount of external rotation restriction
- Suture-first versus anchor-first technique
- Static knot versus sliding knot

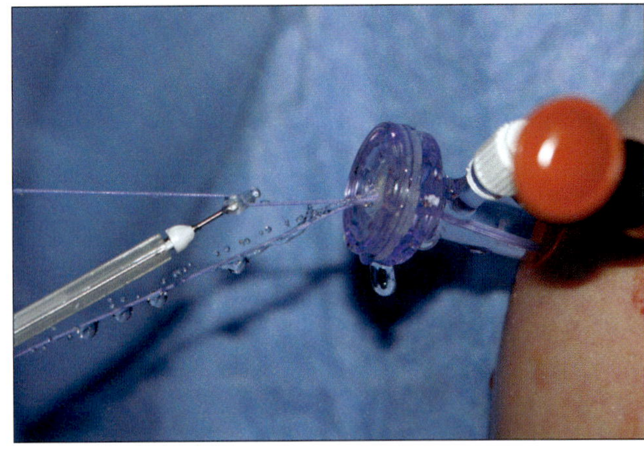
A

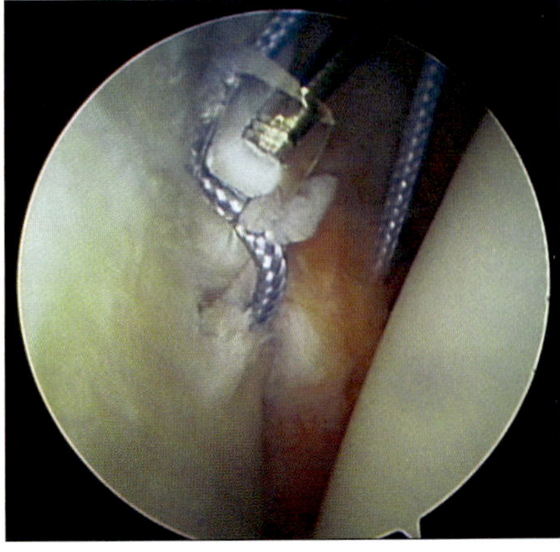
B

FIGURE 26

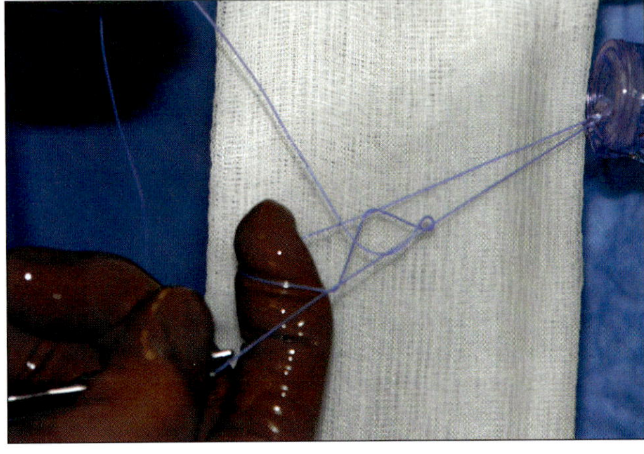
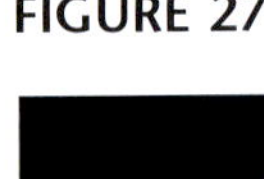
A

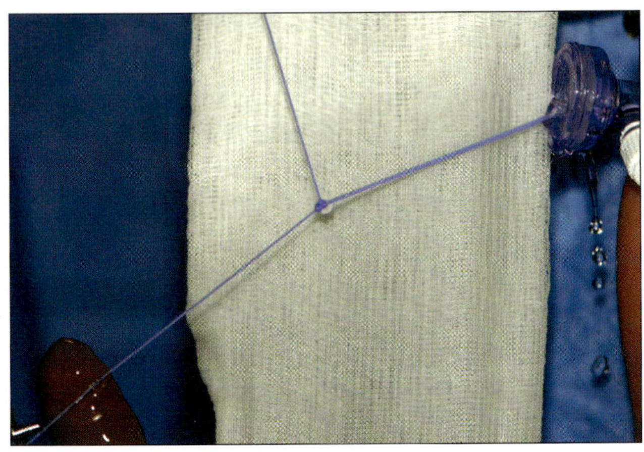
B

FIGURE 27

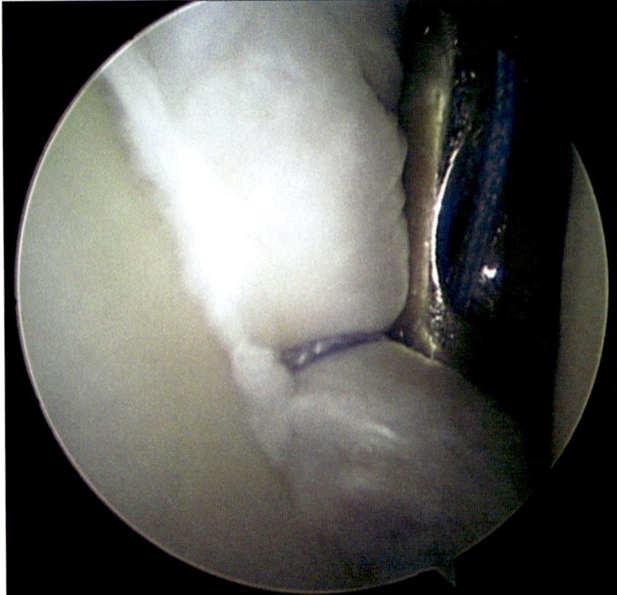
A

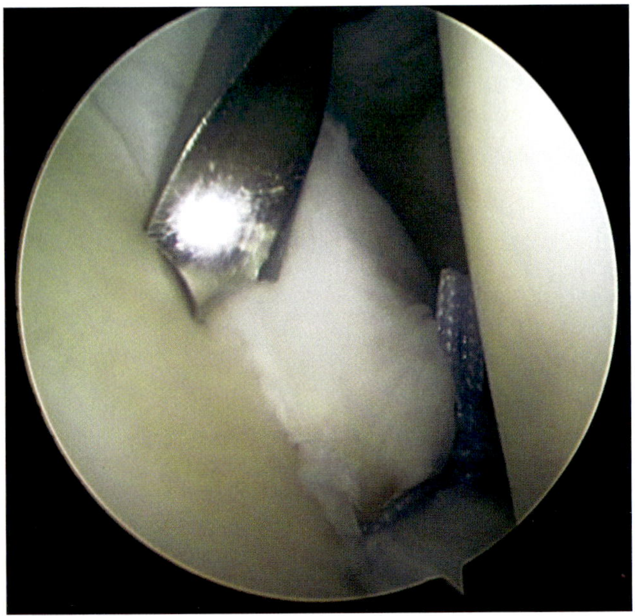
B

FIGURE 28

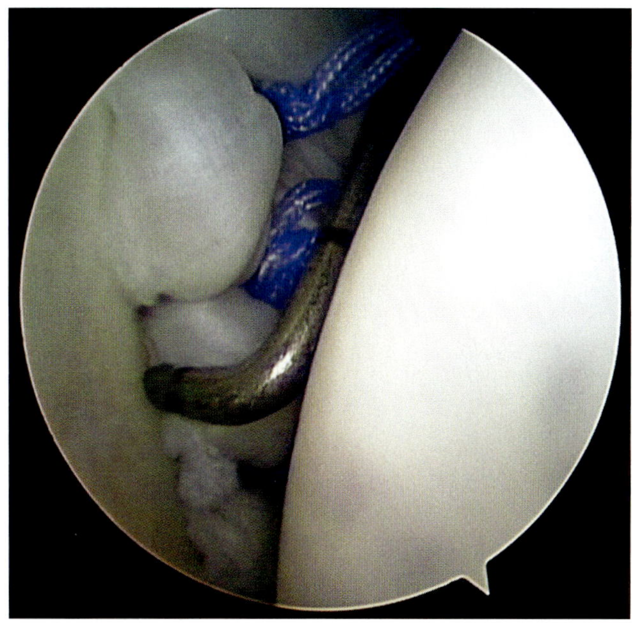

FIGURE 29

Pearls

- *If inferior or posterior-inferior laxity remains, consider a rotator interval closure as an adjunct. This is rarely required in cases of traumatic anterior instability.*

- The next anchor site is drilled and the process repeated.

Step 5: Final Assessment

- The labral repair is probed for stability (Fig. 29).
- The surgeon should assess whether the humeral head has recentered on the glenoid from its preoperative anteriorly translated position.
- External rotation is performed under arthroscopic visualization to define the safe zone and establish postoperative restrictions.

Pearls

- *Expect good return of overall function, strength, and stability by 3 months, but a 2-year instability recurrence rate of up to 10%, often as the result of a new traumatic event.*

Pitfalls

- *If the immobilization period is too prolonged, patients may experience unwanted restriction of their range of motion; however, early cessation of immobilization carries the risk of recurrent instability or disruption of the repair.*
- *Returning to high-risk activities (i.e., football, hockey, snowboarding, waterskiing) carries with it increased risk of recurrence.*

Postoperative Care and Expected Outcomes

- Strict postoperative immobilization in a shoulder immobilizer is used for the first 2 weeks.
- Range-of-motion (ROM) exercises should be performed for the ipsilateral elbow, wrist, and hand.
- Gentle shoulder pendulum exercises are added at week 2–3.
- A progressive rehabilitation ROM and strengthening program is begun at week 4–5.
- Return to sport-specific activities is permitted at 3 months if rehabilitation has progressed satisfactorily.
- Return to contact sport or high-risk activities is permitted at 6 months.

Evidence

Burkhart SS, De Beer JF. Traumatic glenohumeral bone defects and their relationship to failure of arthroscopic Bankart repairs: significance of the inverted-pear glenoid and the humeral engaging Hill-Sachs lesions. Arthroscopy. 2000;16:677-94.

This case series of 194 patients with an average 27 month follow-up identifies a higher rate of recurrence of instability following arthroscopic stabilization in those patients with the characteristic glenohumeral bone defects. (Level IV evidence)

Itoi E, Hatakeyama Y, Sato T, et al. Immobilization in external rotation after shoulder dislocation reduces the risk of recurrence. A randomized controlled trial. J Bone Joint Surg [Am]. 2007;89:2124-31.

The authors randomized 198 patients to immobilization in external rotation or internal rotation after traumatic anterior shoulder dislocation with recurrence of instability as the primary outcome. Bias leading to differences in compliance between treatment groups downgraded this non-blinded, randomized clinical trial. (Level II evidence)

Kirkley A, Griffin S, Richards C, et al. Prospective randomized clinical trial comparing the effectiveness of immediate arthroscopic stabilization versus immobilization and rehabilitation in first traumatic anterior dislocations of the shoulder. Arthroscopy. 1999;15:507-14.

This study randomizes 40 young patients following their index traumatic anterior dislocation to either non-operative care or arthroscopic stabilization with rate of redislocation and disease-specific quality of life scores as the primary outcomes. (Level I evidence)

Lenters TR, Franta AK, Wolf FM, et al. Arthroscopic compared with open repairs for recurrent anterior shoulder instability. A systematic review and meta-analysis of the literature. J Bone Joint Surg [Am]. 2007;89:244-54.

This meta-analysis reviews 18 primary studies of varying quality comparing open shoulder stabilization with arthroscopic repair of varying technique. (Level II evidence [based on quality of primary studies])

Lo IKY, Parten PM, Burkhart SS. The inverted pear glenoid: an indicator of significant glenoid bone loss. Arthroscopy. 2004;20:169-74.

In this case series, glenoid bone lesions were quantified in both patients and cadaveric specimens, to objectify the inverted pear shape of affected glenoids. (Level IV evidence)

Mohtadi NG, Bitar IJ, Sasyniuk TM, et al. Arthroscopic versus open repair for traumatic anterior shoulder instability: a meta-analysis. Arthroscopy. 2005;21(6):652-8.

The authors successfully conduct a meta-analysis of eleven primary studies of varying quality and differing arthroscopic technique. (Level III evidence [based on quality of primary studies])

Neviaser RJ, Neviaser TJ, Neviaser JS. Anterior dislocation of the shoulder and rotator cuff rupture. Clin Orthop Relat Res. 1993;291:103-6.

The authors identified a series of 37 patients over the age of 40 with rotator cuff tears after primary traumatic anterior dislocation. The significance of the contribution of the rotator cuff tear to recurrent instability is explored. (Level IV evidence)

Neviaser TJ. The anterior labroligamentous periosteal sleeve avulsion lesion: a cause of anterior instability of the shoulder. Arthroscopy. 1993;9:17-21.

In this case series, the anatomic features and significance of an ALPSA lesion is described as well as its response to surgical repair. (Level IV evidence)

Papadonikolakis A, Wiesler ER, Olympio MA, Poehling GG. Avoiding catastrophic complications of stroke and death related to shoulder surgery in the sitting position. Arthroscopy. 2008;24:481-2.

These authors review the potential complications involved with upright patient positioning in shoulder surgery and make recommendations for precautionary measures. (Level V evidence)

Wolf EM, Cheng JC, Dickson K. Humeral avulsion of glenohumeral ligaments as a cause of anterior shoulder instability. Arthroscopy. 1995;11:600-7.

This study successfully identifies and describes the HAGL lesion as a cause of recurrent anterior instability. The authors go into detail for each of the six patients identified with the lesion and both the open and arthroscopic repairs performed. (Level IV evidence)

PROCEDURE 13

Open Treatment of Anterior-Inferior Multidirectional Instability of the Shoulder

Katie B. Vadasdi, Chad J. Marion, and Louis U. Bigliani

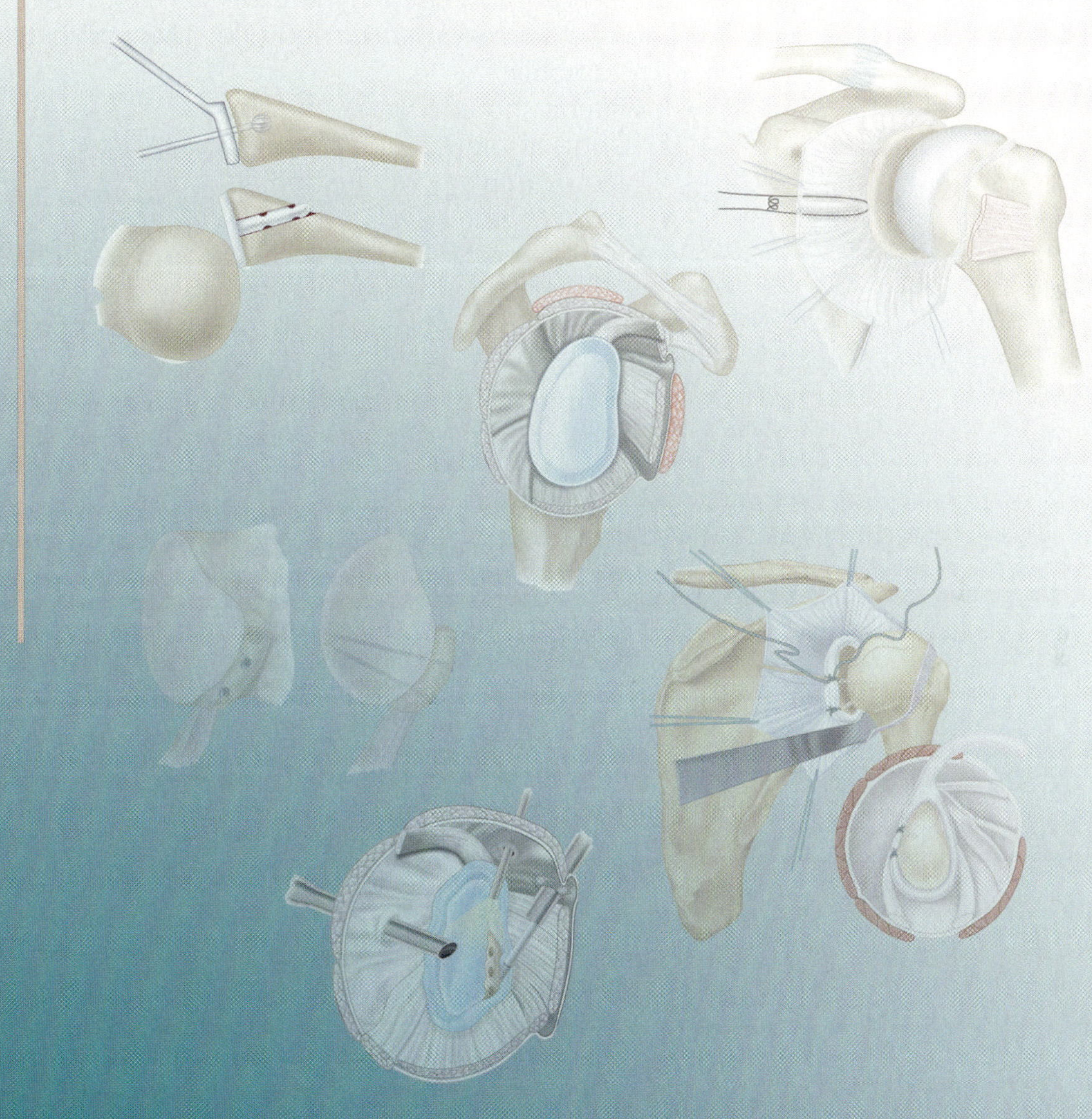

Figures courtesy of Louis U. Bigliani, MD.

PITFALLS

- *Compromised results in voluntary dislocators*
- *Patients who are unable or unwilling to complete postoperative physical therapy program*

Controversies

- Voluntary instability
- Active infection
- Paralysis or nerve damage

Treatment Options

- Nonoperative management: physical therapy
- Arthroscopic stabilization
- Open stabilization: anterior-inferior capsular shift

Indications

- Persistent pain and disability due to instability despite adequate nonoperative management
- Favored for revision cases or instability in presence of bony deficit

Examination/Imaging

- Examine the contralateral shoulder for the patient's normal shoulder range of motion and laxity
- Generalized ligamentous laxity: test for elbow and metacarpophalangeal hyperextension (Fig. 1A), thumb-to-forearm abduction (Fig. 1B), and patella hypermobility.
- Ipsilateral shoulder:
  - Range-of-motion and motor examination
  - Neurovascular examination
  - Provocative tests:
    - Load-and-Shift Test—Axially load the humeral head in the glenoid and translate the head anteriorly and posteriorly (anterior and posterior instability).
    - Anterior Apprehension or Crank Test—Abduct the arm to 90° and externally rotate with anterior force on the humeral head, producing apprehension if positive (anterior instability).
    - Relocation Test—Place posteriorly directed force on the humeral head following the anterior apprehension test, with relief of symptoms (anterior instability).
    - Posterior Stress Test—Place posterior force with arm flexed to 90° and internally rotated, with pain or subluxation (posterior instability).
    - Sulcus Sign—Inferior traction on arm (inferior instability). Persistent sulcus in external rotation suggests a deficient rotator interval.
- Imaging
  - Radiographs: anteroposterior (AP), lateral, and axillary; AP in internal rotation (Hill-Sachs lesion); Stryker notch view (Hill-Sachs lesion); West Point axillary (glenoid rim deficits)
  - Computed tomography: glenoid and humeral head defects
  - Magnetic resonance imaging (MRI) arthrography: labral, rotator cuff, and capsular pathology. Figure 2 shows an MRI arthrogram demonstrating a patulous inferior capsule.

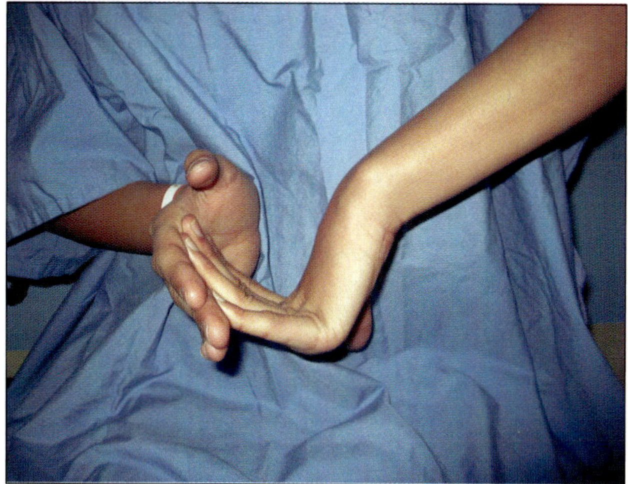

A

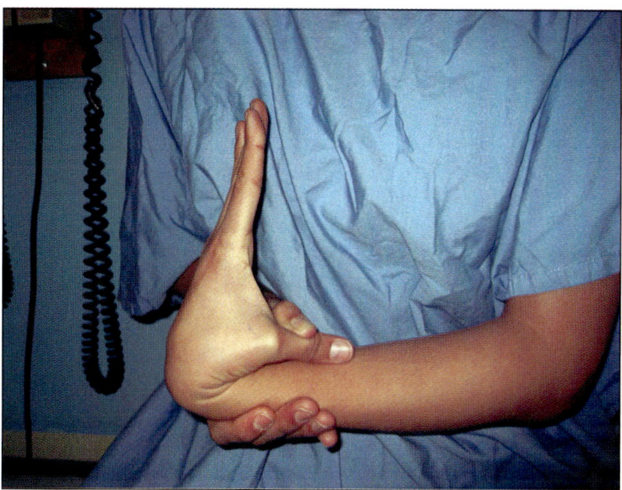

B

FIGURE 1

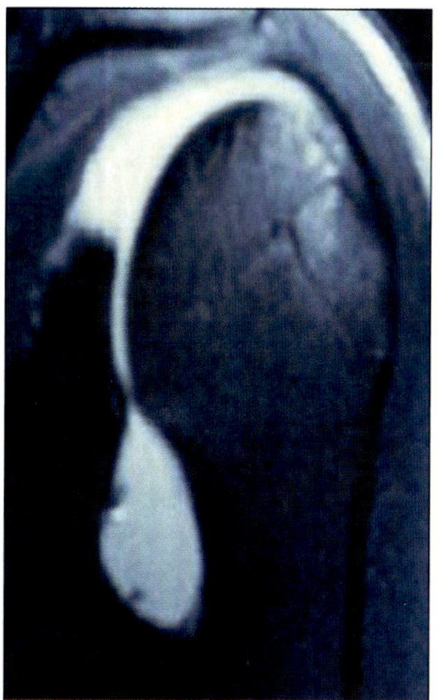

FIGURE 2

PEARLS

- *Examination under anesthesia should be performed to confirm office examination findings.*

PITFALLS

- *Keep the arm and humeral head out of extension by placing a bump on the arm board. This will reduce tension on the anterior structures.*

Equipment

- Short arm board

PEARLS

- *Avoid excessive medial retraction of the strap muscles to prevent injury to the musculocutaneous nerve.*

Controversies

- Axillary incision is more cosmetic than deltopectoral.

Surgical Anatomy

- Deltopectoral interval
  - Cephalic vein must be identified in this interval and protected medially or laterally throughout the case
- Subscapularis superior border is identified with the rotator interval, and the inferior border is identified with the anterior humeral circumflex artery and veins.
- The inferior aspect of the subscapularis and capsule are distinct; they are confluent superiorly. The inferior capsule has two layers of attachment on the humeral neck.

Positioning

- The patient is placed in the beach chair position with the head elevated to 30°.
- The ipsilateral arm is prepped and draped free.
- An ipsilateral arm board with a bump is used to prevent humeral head extension.

Portals/Exposures

- An anterior axillary incision approximately 6 cm in length is made in the axillary fold, starting approximately 3 cm inferior to the coracoid (Fig. 3).
- Deltopectoral exposure:
  - The deltopectoral interval is identified and developed.
  - The cephalic vein is taken laterally with the deltoid (Fig. 4).
  - The superior 0.5–1 cm of the pectoralis major insertion is released and tagged if more inferior exposure is required.
- The rotator interval and coracoid are identified.
- The clavopectoral fascia is incised just lateral to the strap muscles.
- A wedge is excised from the anterior aspect of the coracoacromial ligament for enhanced superior exposure (Fig. 5).
- The interval between the strap muscles and subscapularis medially and the deltoid and the rotator cuff laterally is developed.
- The superior border of the subscapularis muscle is identified with the rotator interval. The inferior border of the subscapularis is identified with the anterior circumflex humeral artery and veins, which are coagulated.
- The subscapularis tendon is incised 1 cm medial to its insertion on the lesser tuberosity (Fig. 6).

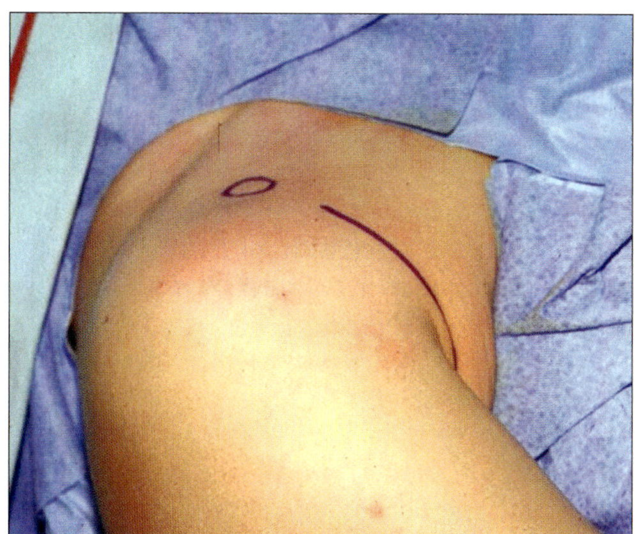

FIGURE 3

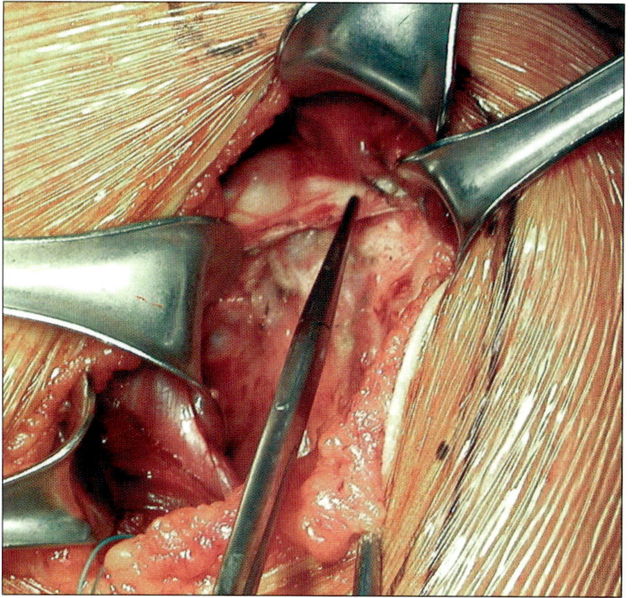

FIGURE 5

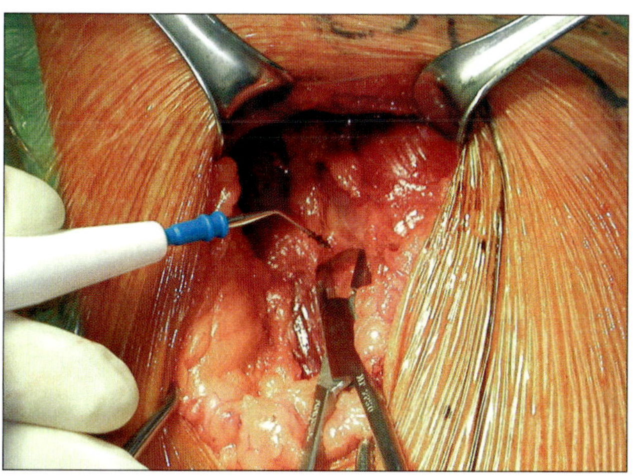

FIGURE 4

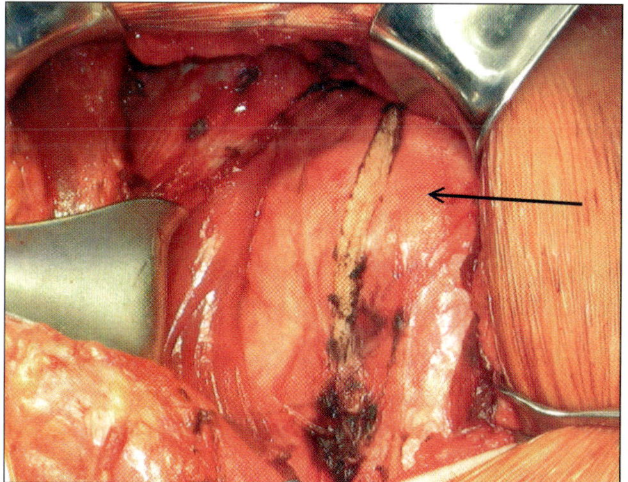

FIGURE 6

Pearls

- *Protect the axillary nerve during the release with arm adduction and external rotation.*
- *The amount of capsular release depends upon the pathology: anterior instability versus multidirectional instability.*
- *Release both inferior layers of capsule from the humeral neck.*

Procedure

Step 1: Capsular Release

- The subscapularis is separated from the capsule using blunt dissection (Fig. 7; see Video 1).
  - The inferior aspect of the subscapularis and capsule are distinct structures. They are confluent superiorly (Fig. 8, *dotted arrow*). The *solid arrow* in Figure 8 points to the deep side of the subscapularis. Separation is started by defining the plane inferiorly where the two are distinct structures (see Fig. 8, *dashed arrow*). Sharp dissection is used to continue superiorly where the two are confluent.
  - Tagging sutures are placed in the free edge of the subscapularis for traction to aid in separation.
- The axillary nerve is identified with the "tug test" and by placing the arm in adduction and external rotation, and is protected during release of the subscapularis.
- A tagging suture is placed in the superior aspect of the capsule to aid in closure. The capsule is incised 5 mm medial to the scubscapularis stump (Fig. 9). Beginning at the rotator interval and proceeding inferiorly, the capsule is released off the humeral neck. Tagging sutures are placed in the free edge of the capsule (Fig. 10).
- The inferior capsule has two layers of attachment on the humeral neck (Fig. 11, *arrows*). Adequate release of both inferior attachments of the capsule to the humeral neck must be ensured.
- The extent of the capsular release depends on the degree of instability. In the case of anterior instability, the anterior capsule is released. In the presence of multidirectional instability, the anterior and inferior capsule are released.
- To assess the capsular release, the surgeon places a finger into the pouch and pulls superior traction on the capsular tagging sutures (Fig. 12, *1*). If adequate release has been performed, the pouch will be obliterated and the surgeon's finger will be forced out of the pouch (Fig. 12, *2*).
- Any remaining subscapularis muscle is released from the capsule to allow for maximum shift.

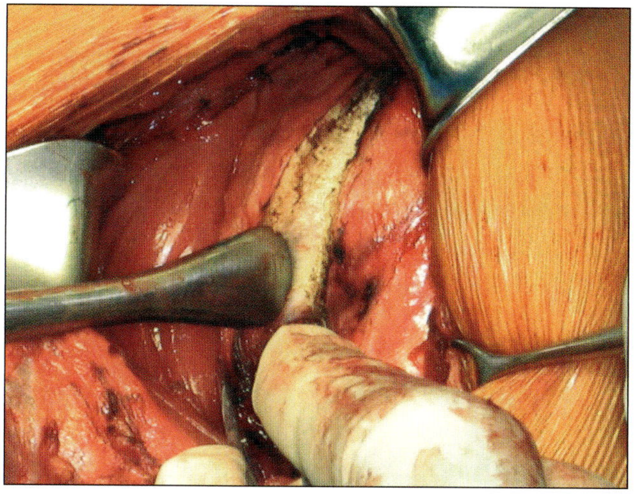

FIGURE 7

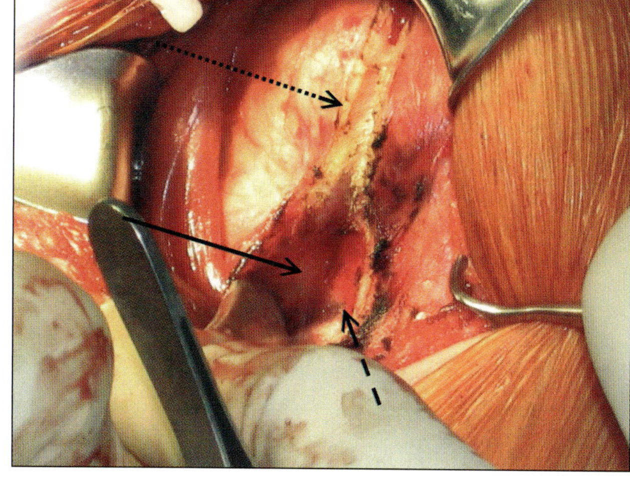

FIGURE 8

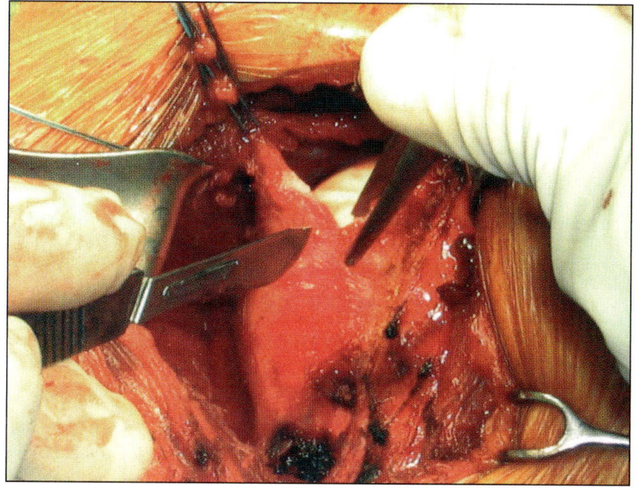

FIGURE 9

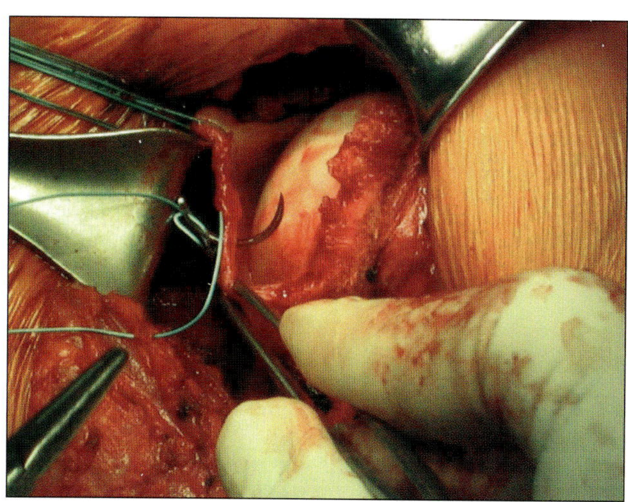

FIGURE 10

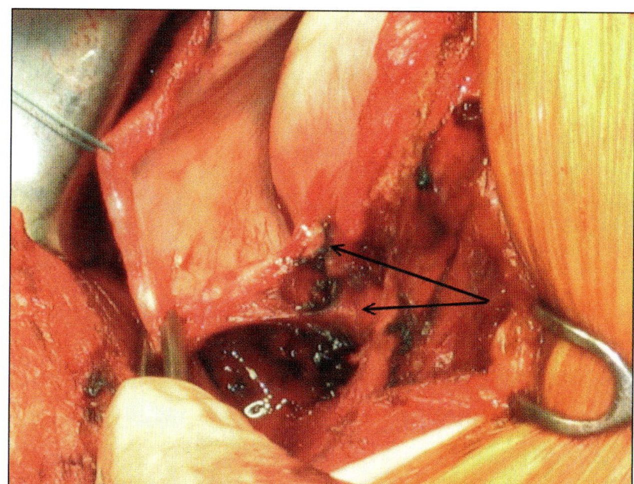

FIGURE 11

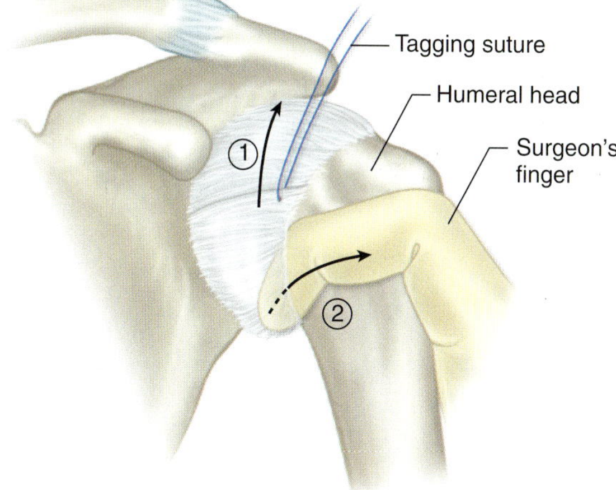

FIGURE 12

Pitfalls

- *Do not place the suture anchors or tunnels too far medial on the glenoid as that would not provide an adequate buttress.*

Pearls

- *Begin the shift with the inferior aspect of the capsule to ensure reduction of the inferior pouch.*
- *Ensure that the the inferior capsule is reattached superiorly to maximize the shift.*

Pitfalls

- *Take caution to prevent overtightening the capsule, especially in overhead athletes.*

Step 2: Glenoid Exposure

- A Fukuda retractor is placed in the glenohumeral joint to move the humeral head posteriorly and allow for inspection of the glenoid and labrum.
- If there is a Bankart lesion, it should be repaired at this time with either suture anchors or tunnels.
- If there is capsular redundancy with an attenuated labrum, a "barrel stitch" may be placed (Fig. 13A and 13B).
  - The stitch is passed from the external aspect of the capsule to the internal aspect superiorly and then from internal to external inferiorly (see Video 3). The knot is then tied on the external aspect of the capsule.
  - The crimping stitch creates an anterior bolster (Fig. 14A and 14B).
- If there is a significant inferior pouch, a horizontal incision is made between the middle and inferior glenohumeral ligaments to allow for an overlapped repair.

Step 3: Capsular Shift

- The arm is placed in 20–30° of abduction and 20–30° of external rotation for the shift. More abduction and external rotation are used in overhead athletes and less is used in the presence of a large Hill-Sachs lesion or bony Bankart lesion.
- The inferior aspect of the capsule is tensioned superiorly and reattached to the capsular cuff on the humerus (Fig. 15A and 15B).
- The subscapularis is repaired anatomically (Fig. 16).
  - If a horizontal incision was made in the capsule, the superior capsule is now repaired to the inferior

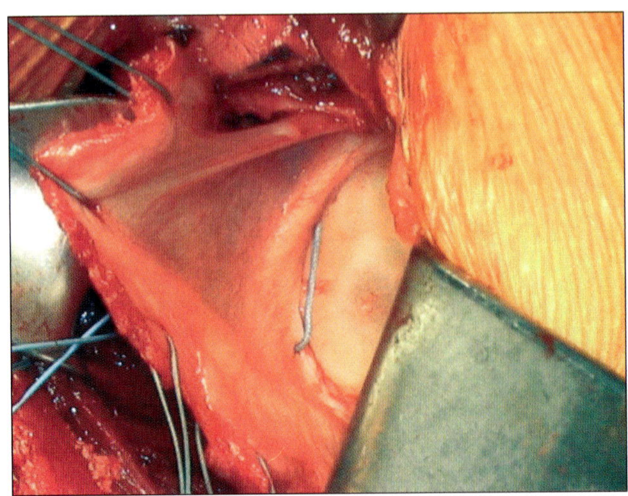

A

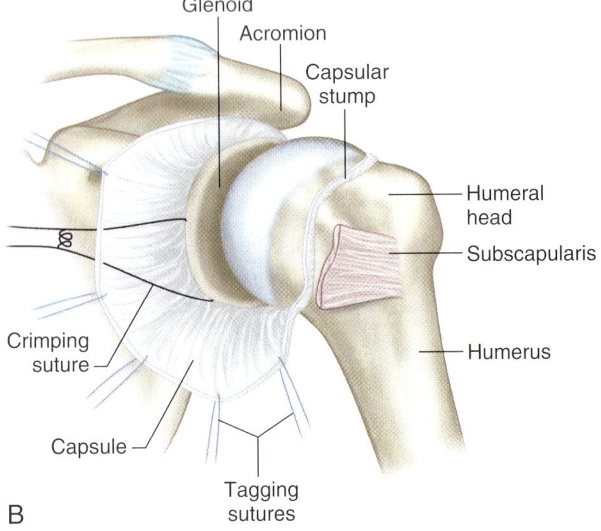

B

FIGURE 13

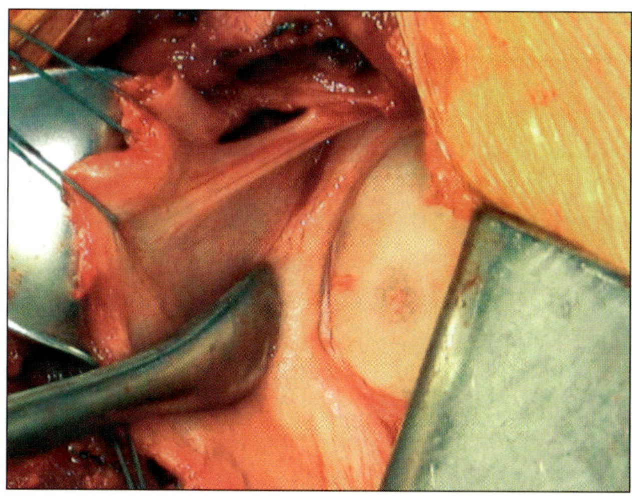
A

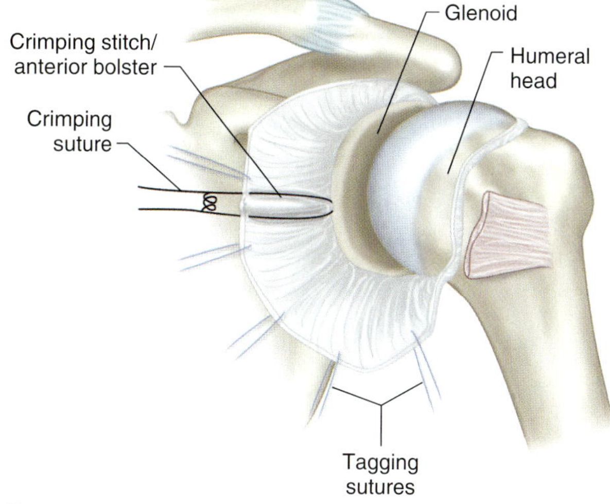

B

FIGURE 14

capsular limb with overlap to further reduce capsular redundancy (Fig. 17).

- The superior limb is then reattached to the capsular cuff on the humerus.

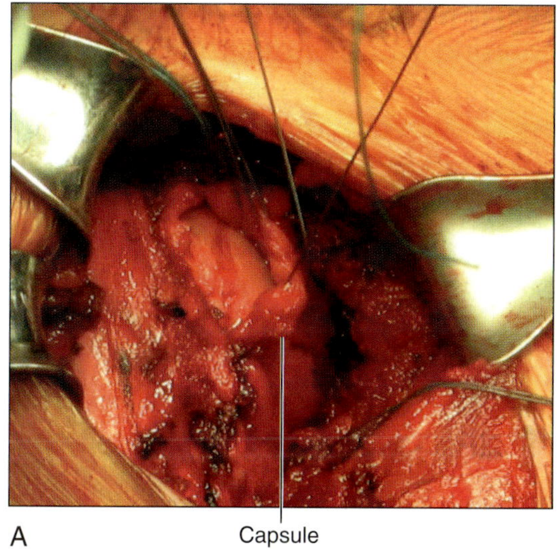

A

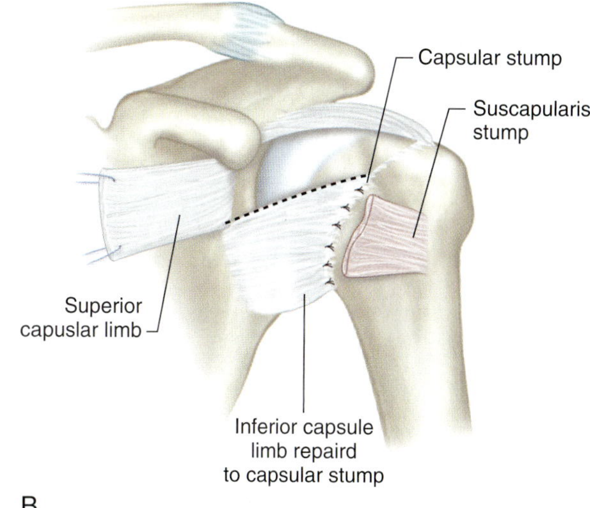

B

FIGURE 15

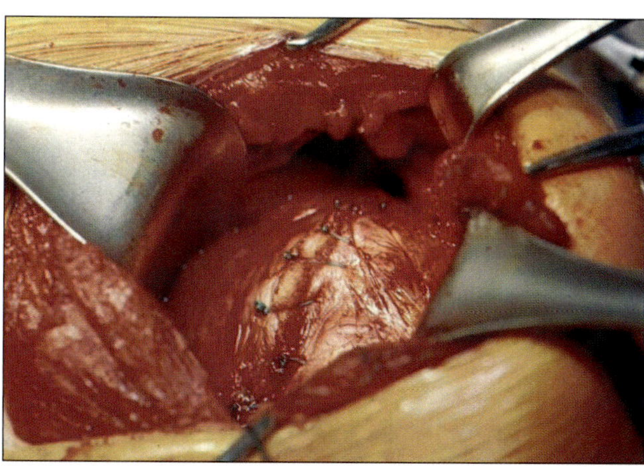

FIGURE 16

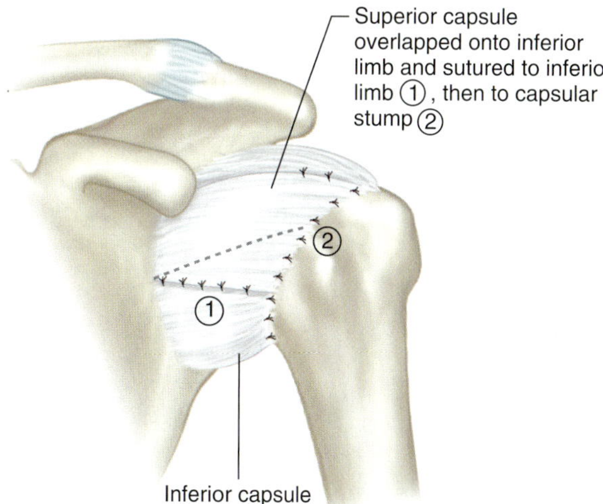

FIGURE 17

- The rotator interval is only repaired if the sulcus sign remained positive in external rotation.

STEP 4: CLOSURE

- The subscapularis tendon is repaired anatomically.
- The pectoralis major tendon insertion is reattached if it was released during the exposure.
- The deltopectoral interval is reapproximated with nonabsorbable simple sutures.
- The subcutaneous layer is closed with simple absorbable sutures. The skin is closed with a running absorbable subcuticular suture.
- A sterile dressing is placed over the wound.

PEARLS

- *Postoperative range-of-motion limits should be determined intraoperatively based on the quality of tissue and repair.*
- *Postoperative rehabilitation should be monitored carefully to prevent compromise of the repair while obtaining progressive range of motion.*

PITFALLS

- *Postoperative range of motion must be balanced with protection of the repair to allow complete healing. If exercises are advanced too quickly, the repair and patient outcome can be compromised.*

Postoperative Care and Expected Outcomes

- The patient is placed in a padded sling in the operating room. The patient is protected in the sling for 6 weeks postoperatively.
- Physical therapy exercises are initiated within 10 days, starting with pendulums.
- Passive range of motion is initiated at 10 days. From 10 days to 2 weeks, the usual forward flexion and external rotation are 100° and 15°, respectively.
- From 2 to 4 weeks, range of motion is generally increased to 140° of forward flexion and 30° of external rotation. Gentle resistive exercises are generally initiated at this time.
- From 4 to 6 weeks, range of motion is generally increased to 165° of forward flexion and 40° of external rotation. Resistive exercises are increased.
- From 6 weeks on, terminal forward flexion is achieved along with increased external rotation.
- At 3 months, terminal external rotation is achieved.

Evidence

Ahmad CS, Freehill MQ, Blaine TA, et al. Anteromedial capsular redundancy and labral deficiency in shoulder instability. Am J Sports Med. 2003;31:247-52.

In this study, 49% of patients treated with anterior-inferior shift also demonstrated anteromedial capsular redundancy and were treated with a concomitant anterior crimping stitch. Patients with anteromedial capsular redundancy treated with a crimping barrel stitch had longer duration of preoperative symptoms and a greater number of dislocations, but they had outcomes similar to those without redundancy. (Level IV evidence)

Bankart A. The pathology and treatment of recurrent dislocation of the shoulder. Br Med J. 1938;26:23-9.

The author provided an anatomic description of the "essential" lesion as an avulsion of the anterior-inferior glenoid labrum with its attached inferior glenohumeral ligament and its association with recurrent shoulder instability. (Level IV evidence)

Bigliani LU, Kelkar R, Flatow EL, Pollock RG, Mow VC. Glenohumeral stability: biomechanical properties of passive and active stabilizers. Clin Orthop Relat Res. 1996;(330):13-30.

This biomechanical study demonstrated the viscoelastic properties of the inferior glenohumeral ligament in tension, supporting the role of the anterior inferior capsule as the primary static anterior stabilizer of the glenohumeral joint. Anterior instability can be the result of injury to the inferior glenohumeral ligament in its substance (capsular redundancy) or at its insertion (Bankart lesion), and both should be assessed and addressed in the surgical management.

Bigliani LU, Kurzweil PR, Schwartzbach CC, et al. Inferior capsular shift procedure for anterior-inferior shoulder instability in athletes. Am J Sports Med. 1994;22:578-84.

In this study of anterior-inferior capsular shift in patients with anterior-inferior instability, 94% had good or excellent results and 75% returned to their previous activity level. Only 2% redislocated. (Level IV evidence)

Levine WN, Flatow EL. The pathophysiology of shoulder instability. Am J Sports Med. 2000;28:910-7.

This review of the pathoanatomy of shoulder instability supported the primary causative injury as detachment of the labrum with subsequent loss of tension of the glenohumeral ligaments. Thus techniques addressing only the labrum and not the capsule have higher failure rates.

Neer CS 2nd, Foster CR. Inferior capsular shift for involuntary inferior and multidirectional instability of the shoulder: a preliminary report. J Bone Joint Surg [Am]. 1980;62:897-908.

In this study of 36 patients treated with inferior capsular shift for unvoluntary multidirectional instability of the shoulder, 29 of 45 shoulders had not had previous surgery for instability. Thirty-two shoulders were followed for more than 1 year and 17 shoulders were followed for more than 2 years; only 1 had unsatisfactory results. (Level IV evidence)

Pollock RG, Owens JM, Flatow EL, Bigliani LU. Operative results of the inferior capsular shift procedure for multidirectional instability of the shoulder. J Bone Joint Surg [Am]. 2000;82:919-28.

In this study of 49 shoulders treated with an inferior capsular shift procedure, with an average follow-up of 61 months, 94% showed excellent or good, and 6% fair or poor results. At the time of follow-up, 96% of the shoulders were stable, 92% had ability to perform strenuous activity, and return to sport was possible in 86%. (Level IV evidence)

Townley CO. The capsular mechanism in recurrent dislocation of the shoulder. J Bone Joint Surg [Am]. 1950;32:370-80.

The author presented an anatomic description, based on surgical cases and anatomic dissections, of capsular lengthening and separation of the medial attachment of the capsule from the anterior glenoid as the primary causes for recurrent shoulder dislocation. Of 26 shoulders treated with surgical management, none redislocated. A total of 19 shoulders were followed up for 6 to 24 months; 17 showed excellent or good and 2 fair results. (Level IV evidence)

PROCEDURE 14

Arthroscopic Treatment of Anterior-Inferior Multidirectional Instability of the Shoulder

Maxwell C. Park and James E. Tibone

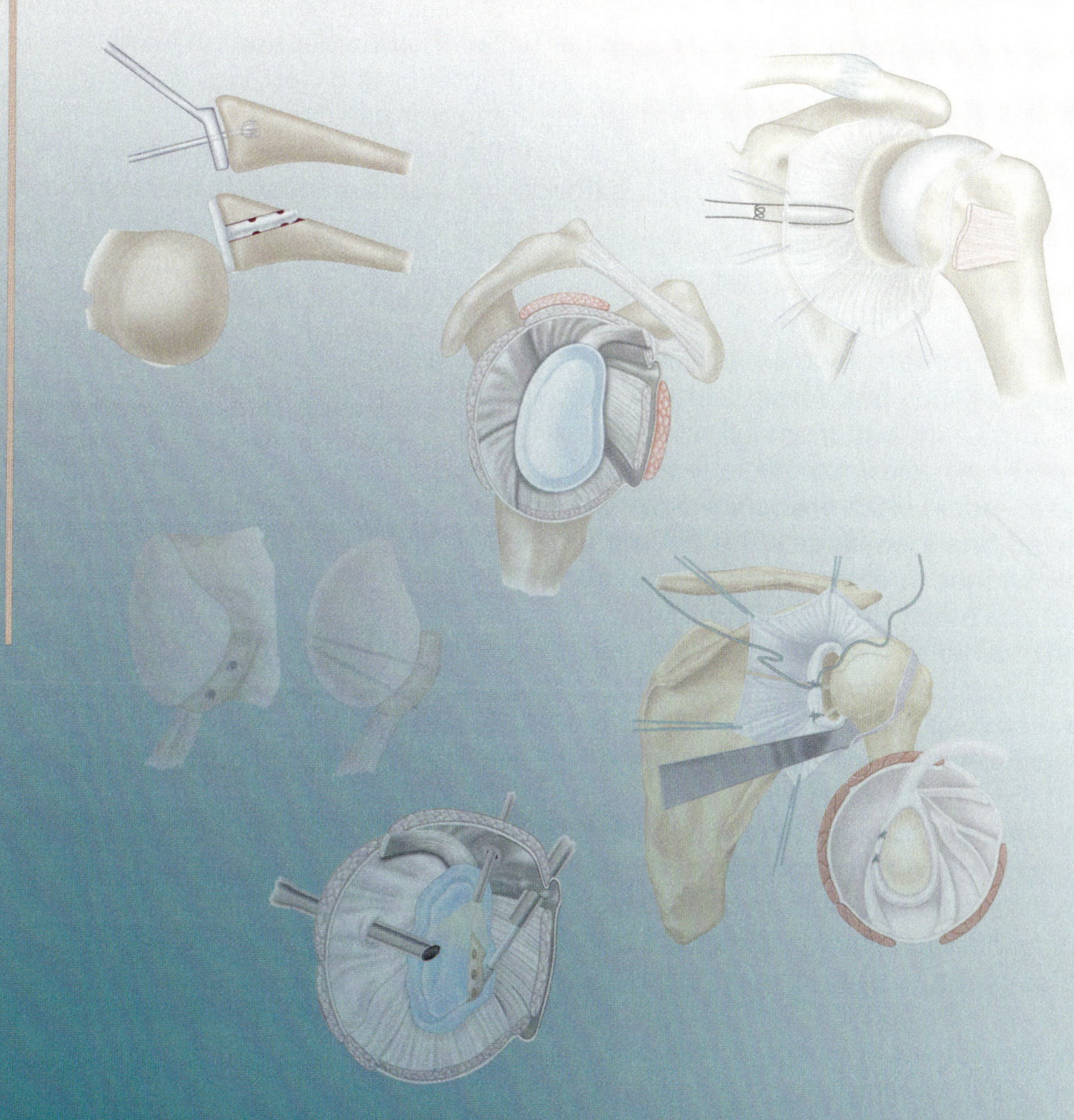

Pitfalls

- *Voluntary instability*
- *Missed posterior instability*
- *Other concomitant injuries (e.g., superior labral lesions, partial- or full-thickness rotator cuff tears)*

Treatment Options

- Supervised physical therapy of the rotator cuff and scapular stabilizers
- Open inferior capsular shift (humeral or glenoid based)—may be preferable in the revision setting

Indications

- Recurrent symptoms of apprehension or instability in a patient who has failed nonoperative treatment.

Examination/Imaging

- Standard examination includes measuring passive range-of-motion, and assessing for generalized ligamentous laxity (including contralateral joints).
  - Compensatory scapular winging should be noted by careful inspection.
  - During instability testing, a distinction should be made between apprehension and pain.
  - Standard anterior and posterior load-and-shift tests should be performed.
  - Sulcus testing with arm adducted (>2 cm is pathognomonic) is mandatory for gauging inferior laxity; Figure 1 shows a positive sulcus test (*arrow*). Sulcus testing with external rotation is also performed to assess the rotator interval—if there is no decrease in the sulcus distance, then the rotator interval is considered pathologic.
- Plain radiographs should include anteroposterior (AP), AP with internal rotation, lateral, and axillary (e.g., West Point) views.
- If osseous defects are suspected, consider obtaining a computed tomography scan to characterize the extent of injury.
- A magnetic resonance imaging arthrogram should be obtained to assess for concomitant soft tissue injury (e.g., rotator cuff tears, biceps pathology, "hidden" lesions of the biceps).

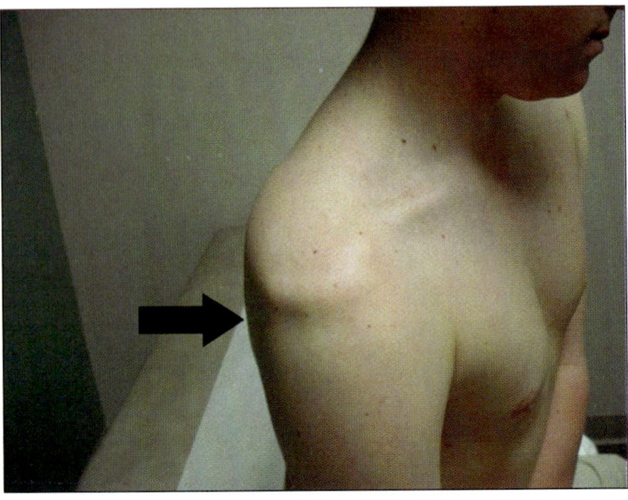

FIGURE 1

Surgical Anatomy

- The rotator interval is delimited by the supraspinatus and subscapularis tendons, and consists of the coracohumeral ligament superficially, and the superior glenohumeral ligament on the articular side.
  - A widened rotator interval can be assessed by arthroscopic inspection. The superior glenohumeral ligament will appear capacious with respect to its distance from the biceps tendon, and often will reside superior and posterior to the tendon itself.
  - Note the widened space between the superior glenohumeral ligament (*arrow*) and the proximal biceps tendon (*B*) in Figure 2.
- The inferior glenohumeral ligament complex has a broad attachment site, through the labrum, on the inferior glenoid.
  - In most cases, thickened "bands" are present delimiting the anterior and posterior extents of the ligament complex.
  - As seen in Figure 3, the inferior glenohumeral ligament (IGHL) typically lacks the appearance of a labral "bumper" (*arrows*), and falls away medially into redundant voluminous capsular tissue (H, humeral head; G, glenoid).
- The axillary neurovascular structures are deep to the inferior glenohumeral ligament complex.

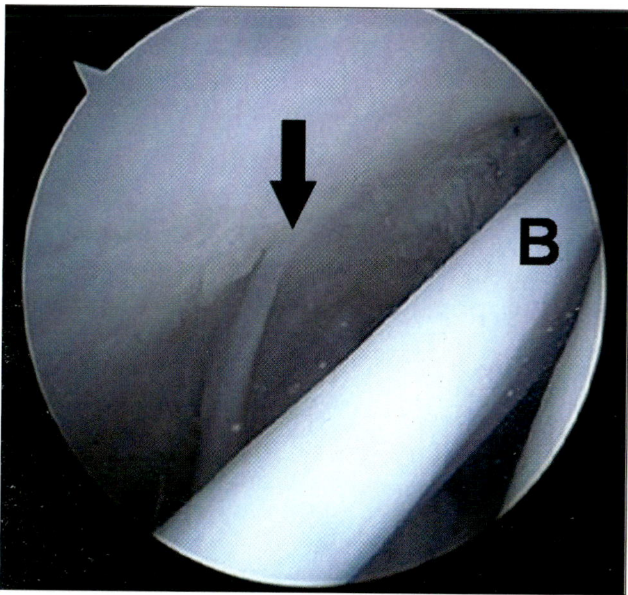

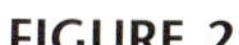
FIGURE 2

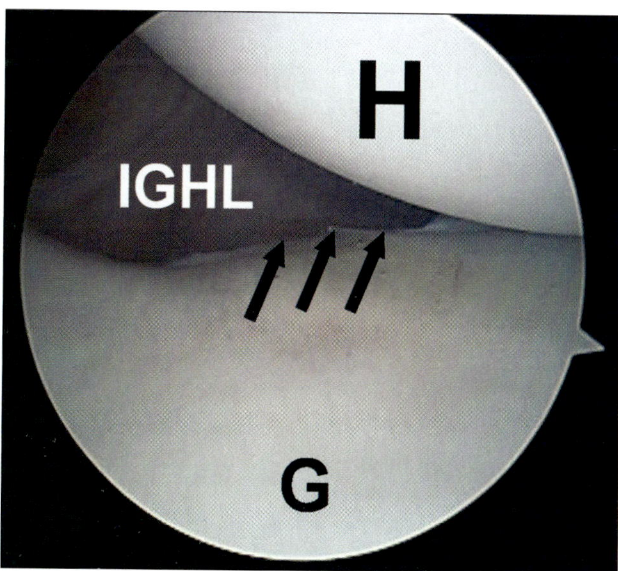

FIGURE 3

PEARLS

- *Folded towels placed in the axilla can provide lateral translational displacement of the humerus away from the glenoid, and may be helpful for visualization depending on the size of the patient.*

PITFALLS

- *Do not drape out the coracoid, as this may limit anterior portal placements.*

Equipment

- 30° arthroscope
- Four 7-mm cannulas (5-mm cannulas may be used for the anterosuperior and posterior portals)

Positioning

- The patient is placed in a standard lateral position with the arm in 30° of abduction.
- The operative extremity is placed in balanced traction using 10–15 pounds.
- In Figure 4, the right upper extremity is depicted with the patient in the lateral decubitus position. The arthroscope is in the posterior portal (*arrow*). The anterior portals are lateral to the coracoid process (*black dot*). (AS, anterosuperior portal; AI, anteroinferior portal.)

Portals/Exposures

- A standard posterior portal is used to access the glenohumeral joint superior on the glenoid.
- An anterosuperior (AS) portal is established using needle localization. A needle targets the rotator interval superiorly, above the level of the superior glenohumeral ligament, in expectation of potential rotator interval closure.
- An anteroinferior (AI) portal is then established, again using needle localization superior to the subscapularis tendon.
  - Figure 5A is an external view of the AS and AI portals lateral to the coracoid process (*arrow*). (A, acromion; C, clavicle)
  - Figure 5B is an intra-articular view of the AS and AI portals on either side of a widened rotator interval at the level of the superior glenohumeral ligament (*arrow*). (B, proximal biceps tendon; G, glenoid.)
- For posterior plications, a posteroinferior (PI) portal is created using needle localization directed through the capsule at the level of the posterior glenohumeral ligament. On the skin, the PI portal is placed lateral relative to the standard posterior portal.
- Figure 6 is an external view of all required portals for a right shoulder. (AI, anteroinferior; AS, anterosuperior; PI, posteroinferior; P, posterior)

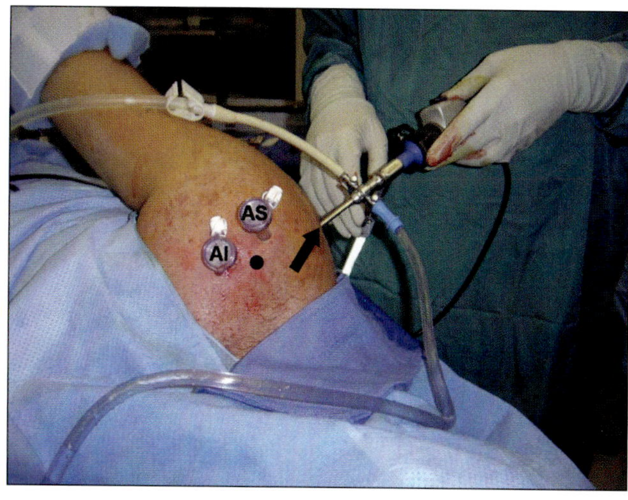

FIGURE 4

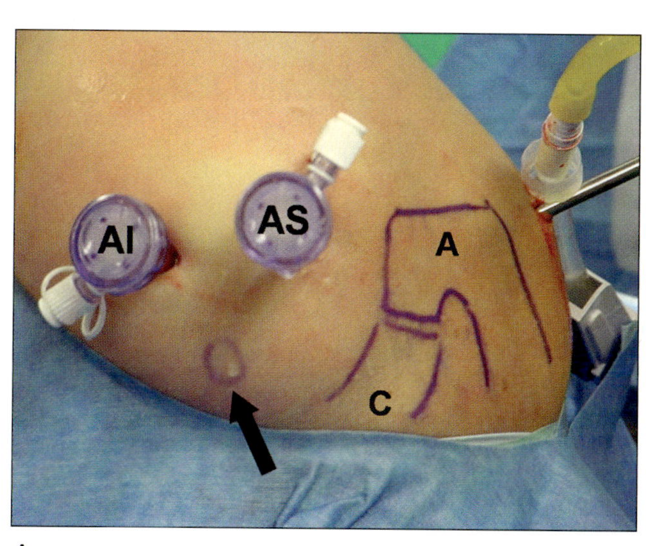

A

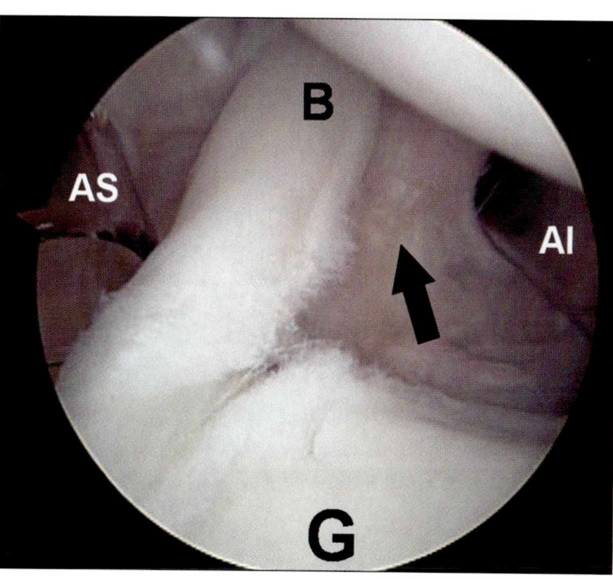

B

FIGURE 5

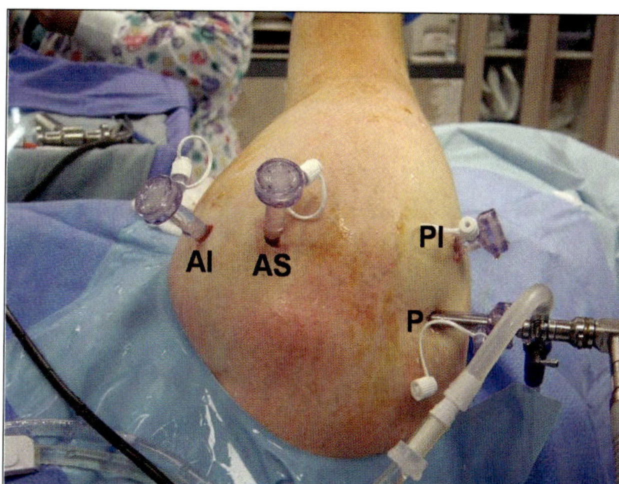

FIGURE 6

Procedure

Step 1

- Examination under anesthesia is performed (anterior and posterior load-and-shift test, sulcus sign testing).
- The arthroscope is introduced through the posterior portal (superior on the glenoid). The "drive-through" sign is normally positive in this setting, with the arthroscope easily advancing to the anteroinferior glenoid.
- An AS portal is established at the level of the superior glenohumeral ligament using needle localization.
  - The needle is localized to target the superior aspect of the rotator interval at the level of the superior glenohumeral ligament (Fig. 7; H, humeral head; B, proximal biceps tendon).
  - A cannula is placed through the targeted area (Fig. 8).
- A probe is introduced and diagnostic arthroscopy is performed, assessing additional soft tissue structures including the rotator cuff, biceps, and superior labrum.
- Using needle localization, an AI portal is established superior to the subscapularis tendon (Fig. 9, *S*), trial-positioning for access to the inferior glenoid.
- A cannula is then passed through the targeted area (Fig. 10).

Pearls

- *Note that the arthroscope can be placed in the AS portal during the anterior plication, with suture management through the posterior portal, should visualization be difficult; however, with a capacious joint with a positive drive-through sign, this is typically not the case.*

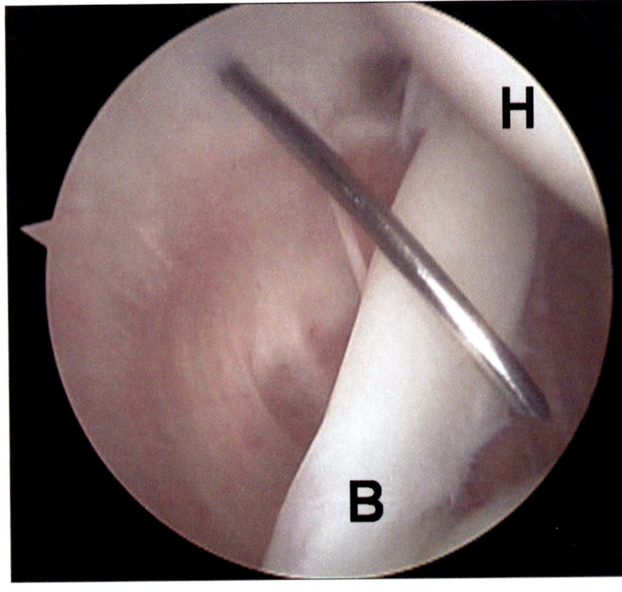

FIGURE 7

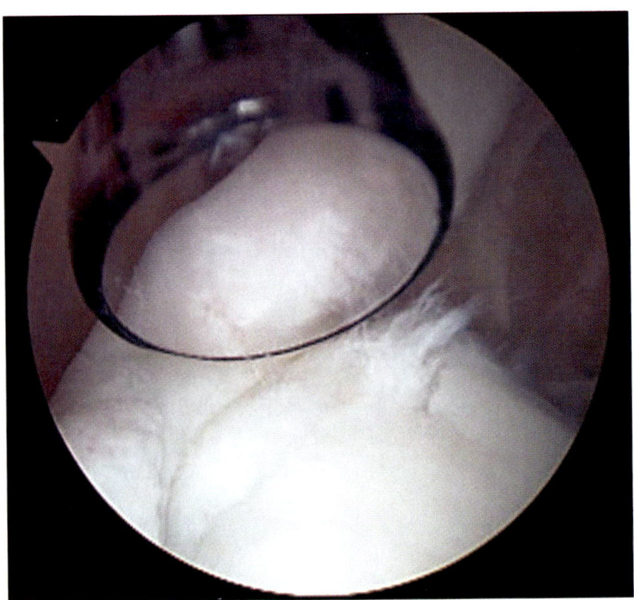

FIGURE 8

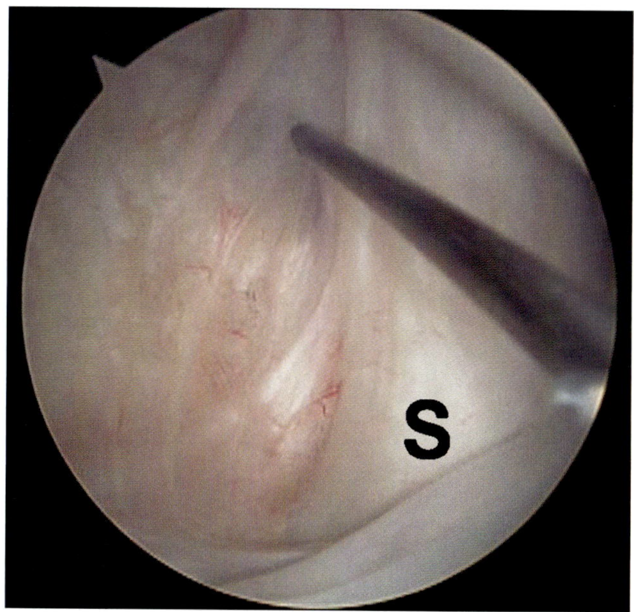

FIGURE 9

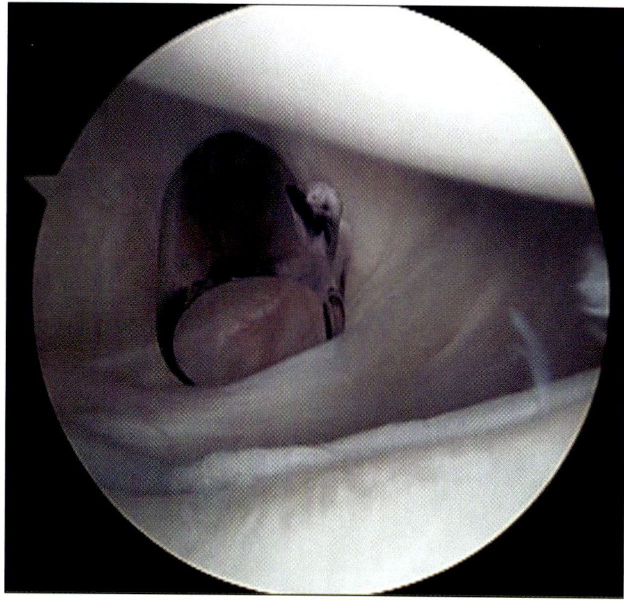

FIGURE 10

Instrumentation/ Implantation

- Suture shuttling device (e.g., 45° and 90° SutureLasso and BirdBeak suture grasper; Arthrex, Inc.)
- Anchors
- Crochet hook or "crab claw" device
- Knot pusher

Step 2: Anterior Capsulorrhaphy

- Plications are performed through the AI portal, with suture shuttles through the AS portal.
  - The anchors are placed at approximately the 3:30–4 o'clock and 5 o'clock positions—the first anchor is placed at the most inferior position (Fig. 11A and 11B).

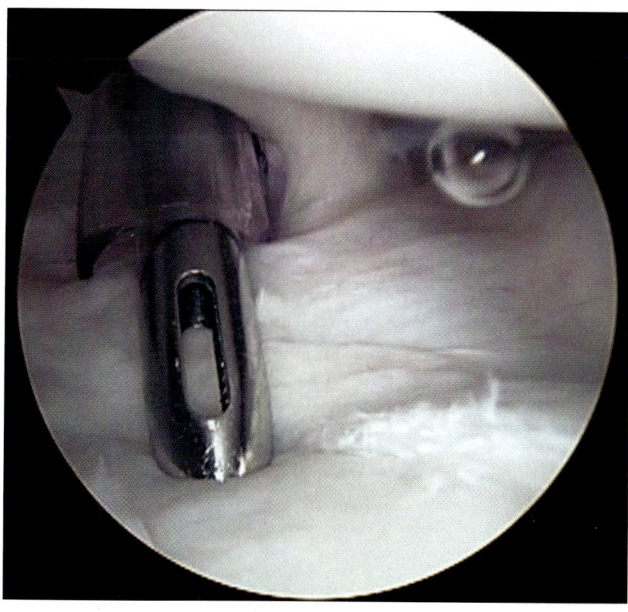

A

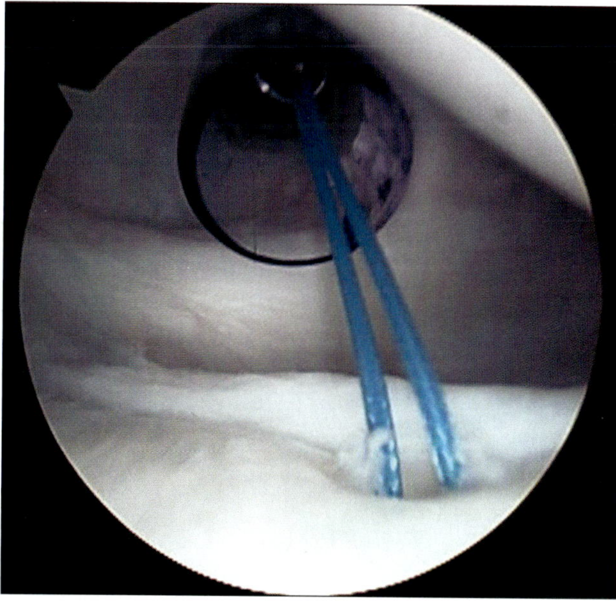

B

FIGURE 11

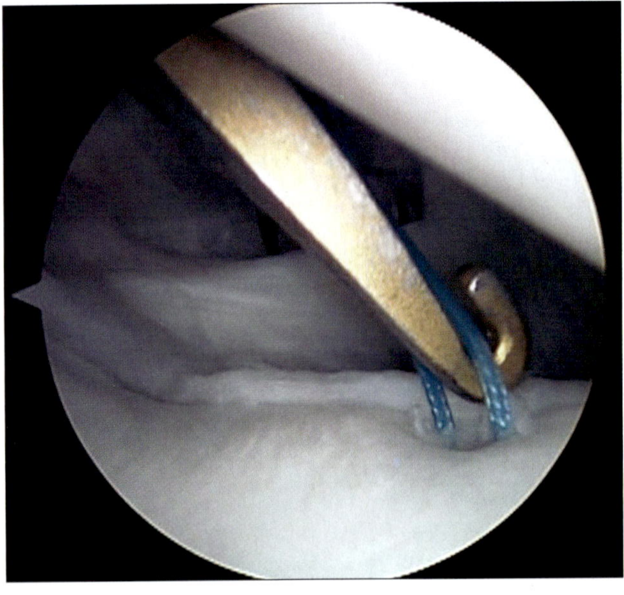
A

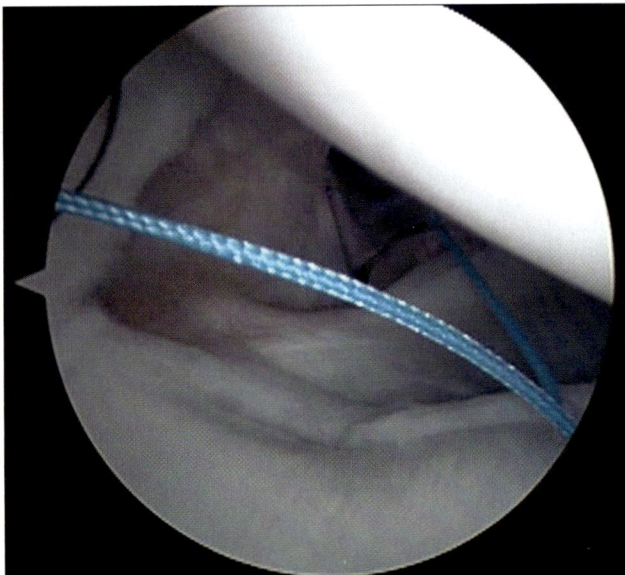
B

FIGURE 12

- A crochet hook is used to capture the more lateral suture limb (Fig. 12A), and is brought through the AS portal (Fig. 12B).

■ A suture-passing device is placed via the AI portal to capture the anterior IGHL (Fig. 13A and 13B).

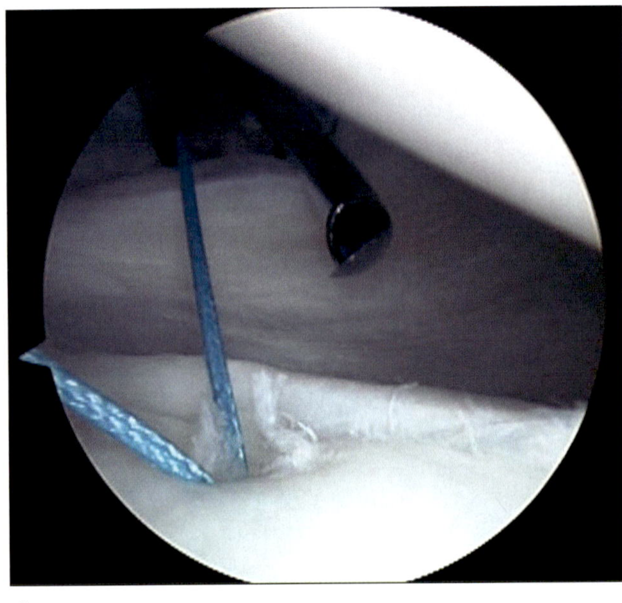
A

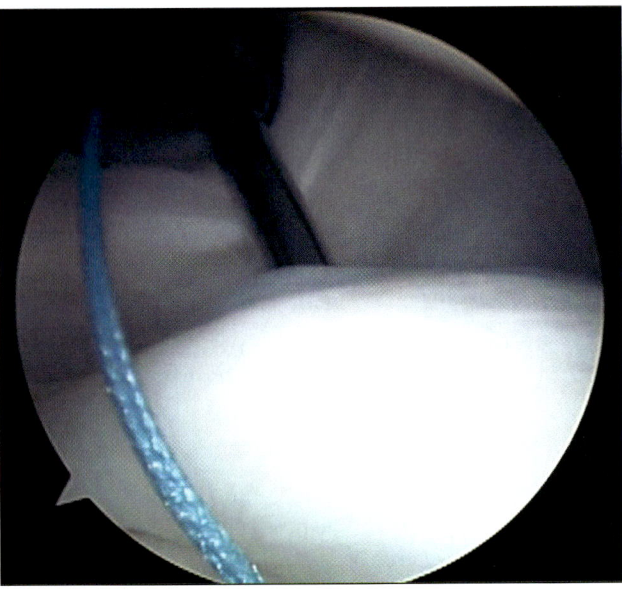
B

FIGURE 13

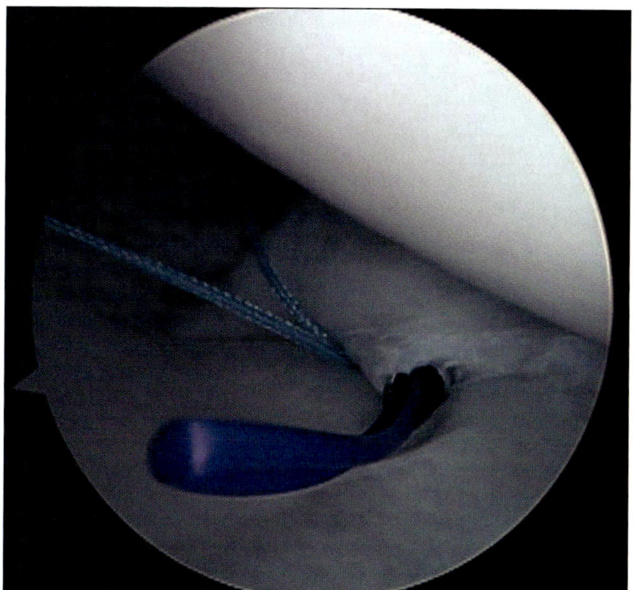
FIGURE 14

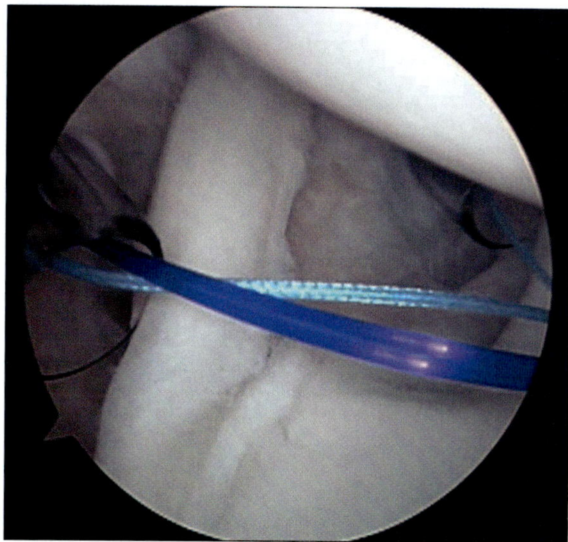
FIGURE 15

- The device is passed inferior and medial so that the plication is advanced superior and lateral to the corresponding anchor (Fig. 14).
- The suture-shuttling loop is brought through the AS portal (Fig. 15).

- After loading the suture limb through the shuttling loop outside the AS portal, the suture is shuttled through the AI portal (Fig. 16). Using this limb as the "post," standard arthroscopic knot tying is performed (Fig. 17).

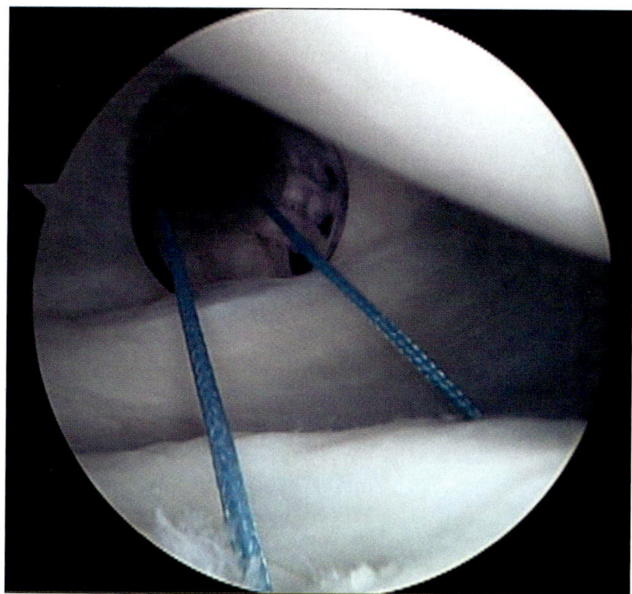
FIGURE 16

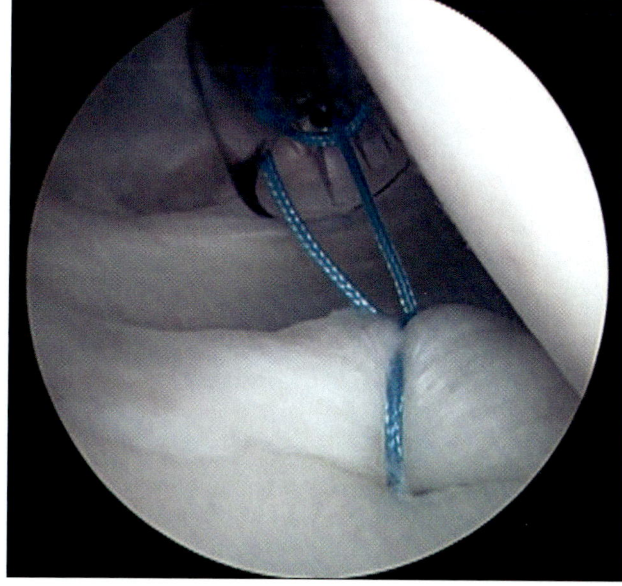
FIGURE 17

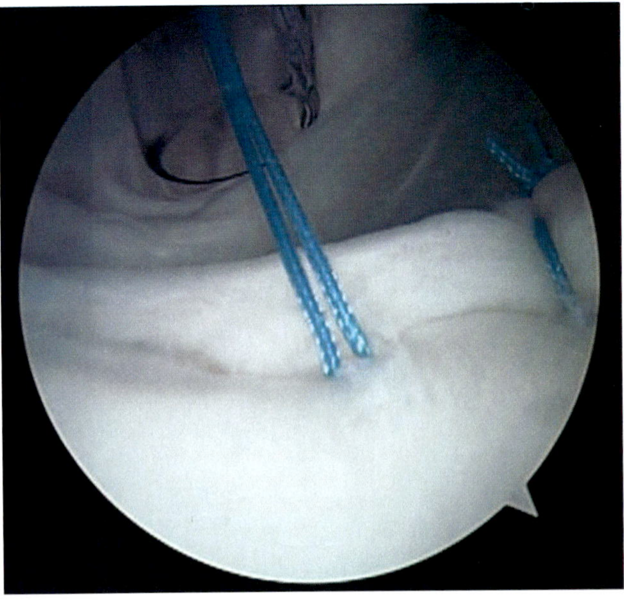

FIGURE 18

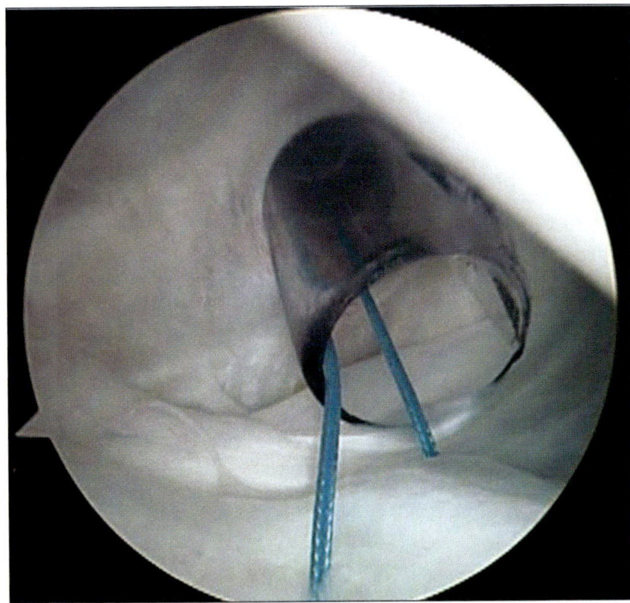

FIGURE 19

- A second anchor is placed to augment the anterior-inferior capsulorrhaphy at approximately the 3:30–4 o'clock position (Fig. 18).
  - Again, the lateral limb is shuttled through a relatively inferior and medial position through the capsule (in order to advance the capsule superior and lateral to the anchor) (Fig. 19).
  - Standard arthroscopic knot tying is performed. Figures 20A and 20B show the resulting anterior-inferior capsulorrhaphy as viewed from the P and AS portals, respectively.

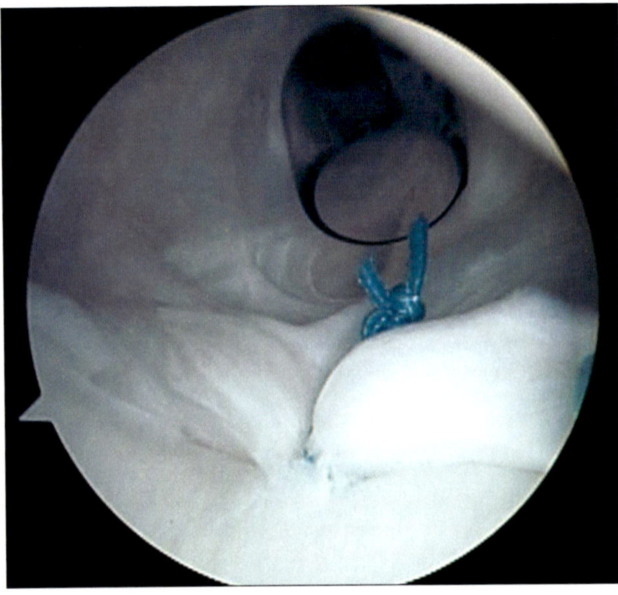

A

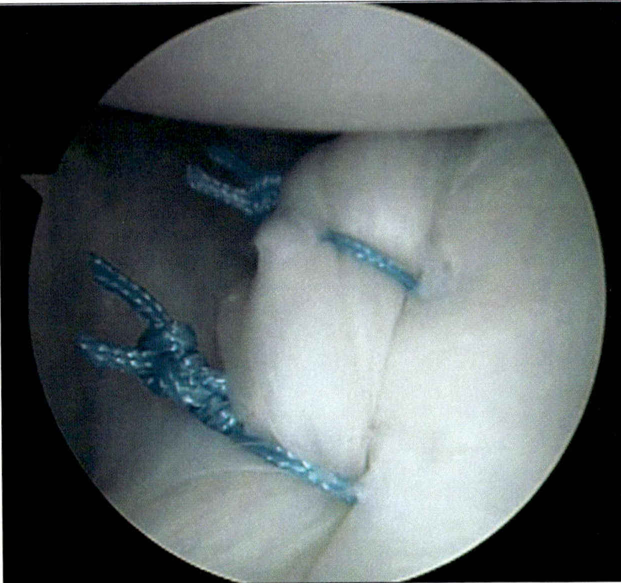

B

FIGURE 20

Step 3: Posterior Capsulorrhaphy

- For the posterior plications, the arthroscope is then introduced through the AS portal.
- The PI portal is established at the level of the posterior IGHL with the expectation of advancing the ligament to a relatively superior and lateral position toward the suture anchors.
  - Needle localization is preferred, as seen in Figure 21, where the needle is targeting the posterior IGHL near the 7 o'clock position.
  - Figure 22 is an external view showing needle localization for the PI portal (*arrow*). (P, posterior portal.)

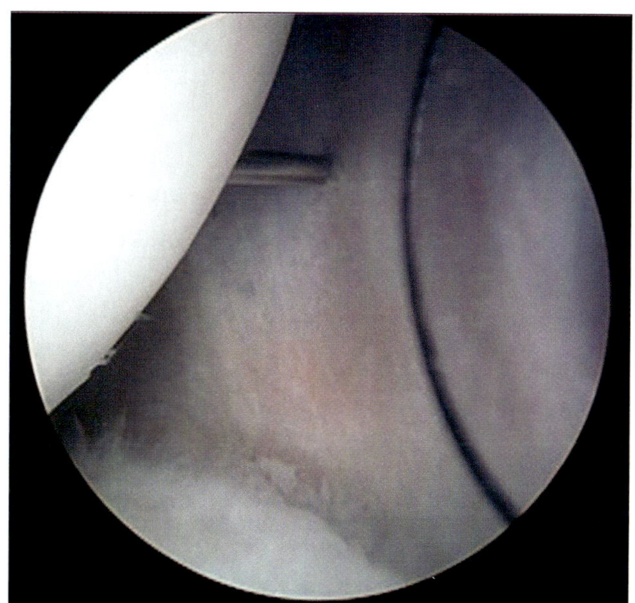

FIGURE 21

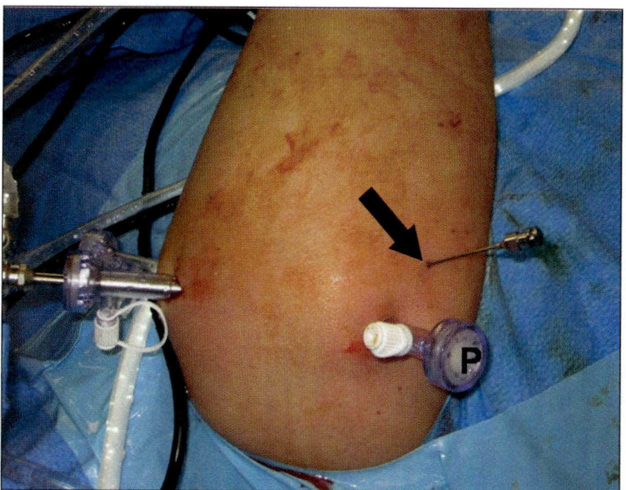

FIGURE 22

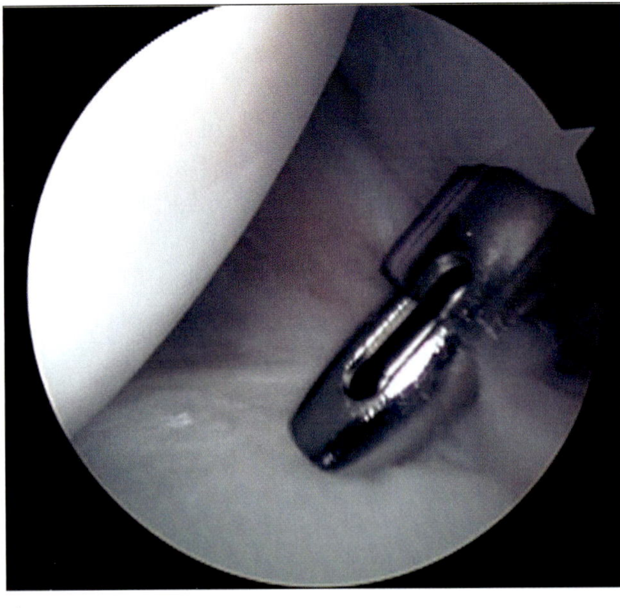
A

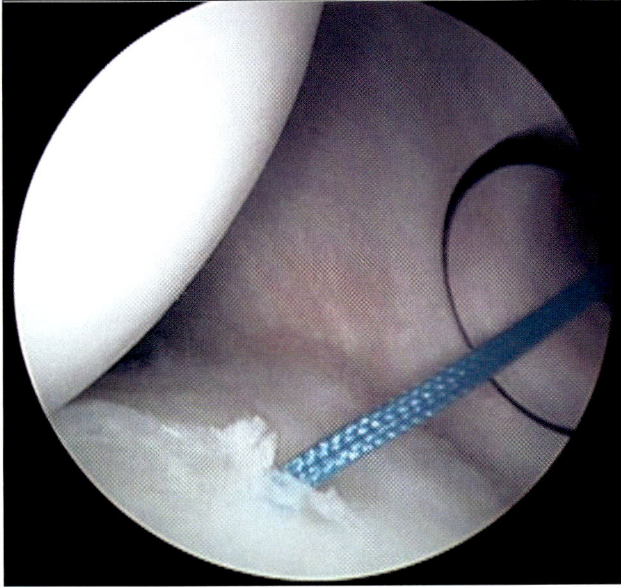
B

FIGURE 23

- Plications are performed via the PI portal with anchor placements at the 7 o'clock and 8–8:30 positions. The first anchor is placed at the more inferior position (Fig. 23A and 23B).
- The posterior two plications are performed similarly relative to the anterior two plications (using the same suture-passing and suture-shuttling devices through similar corresponding cannulas); this balances the inferior capsulorrhaphy (Fig. 24A and 24B).

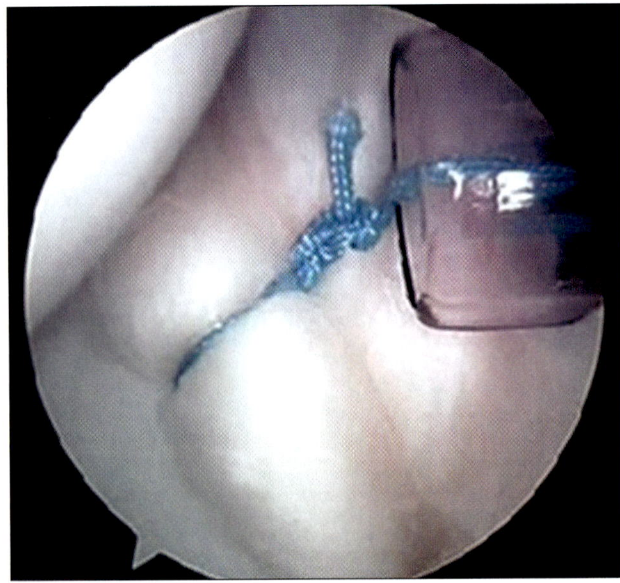
A

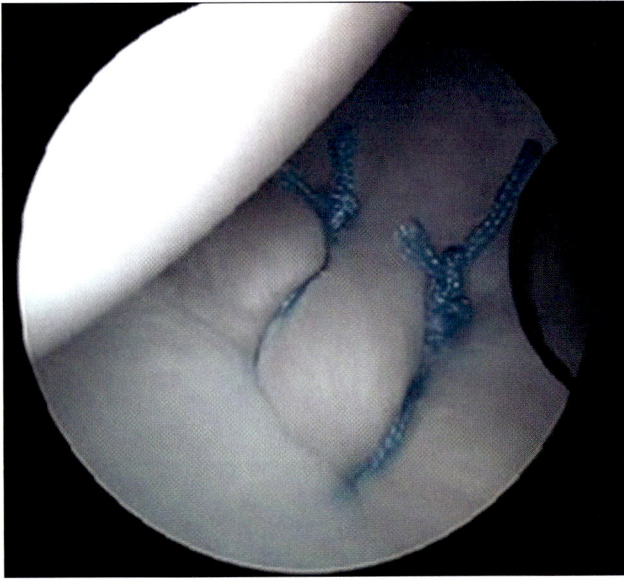
B

FIGURE 24

Pearls

- *If the tissue appears and feels weak a nonsliding knot is preferred, as this can be less traumatic.*

Step 4: Rotator Interval Closure

- For the rotator interval closure, the arthroscope is reintroduced through the posterior portal.
- Rotator interval plication is performed through the AS portal without an anchor, plicating the superior glenohumeral ligament (SGHL) and middle glenohumeral ligament (MGHL) to each other.
  - A suture-passing device is utilized to perform a "side-to-side" repair of the interval.
    - Figure 25 shows rotator interval closure with a side-to-side plication between the SGHL and MGHL.
    - In Figure 26, note that the middle glenohumeral ligament has been advanced to a glenoid anchor prior to rotator interval closure.
  - Suture shuttles can be taken through the AI or PI portals.

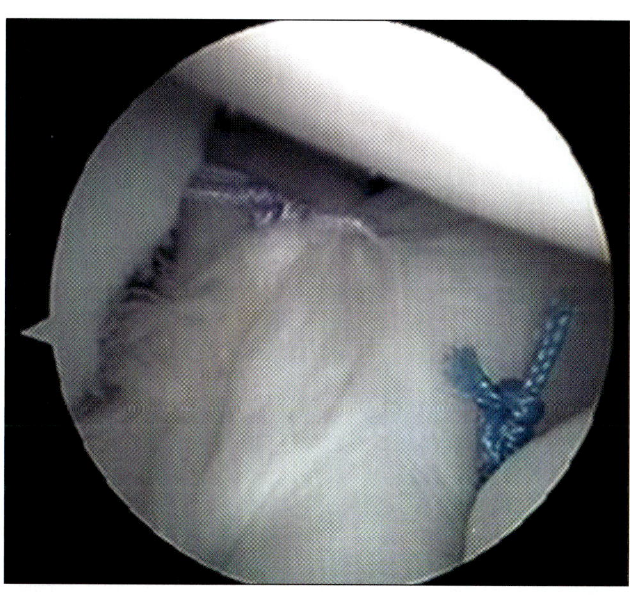

FIGURE 25

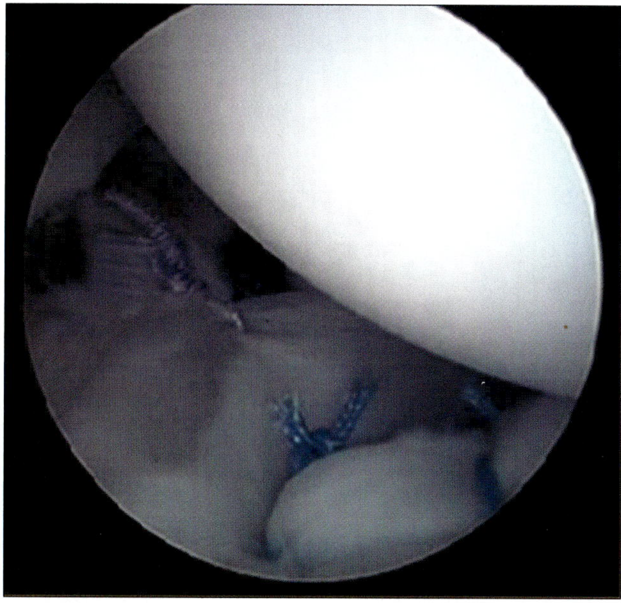

FIGURE 26

- Alternative method for rotator interval closure
  - A suture-passing device is utilized through the AI portal to capture the MGHL (Fig. 27). The now-shuttled suture limb is retrieved with a crochet hook (Fig. 28A and 28B).
  - A suture passer that directly captures suture (e.g., BirdBeak device) is then passed through the SGHL (Fig. 29). A knot pusher brings the suture limb to the direct-passer device (Fig. 30), and the suture is brought back through the SGHL.
  - A crochet hook is used to bring the now-shuttled suture limb through the AI portal (Fig. 31). The rotator interval plication is then ready for standard arthroscopic knot tying (Fig. 32).

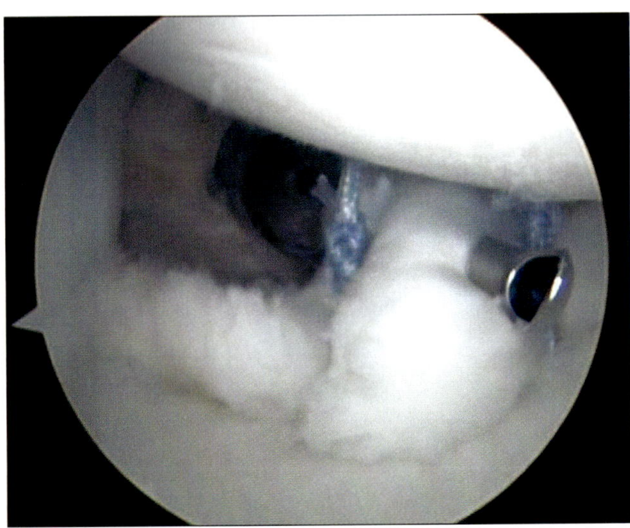

FIGURE 27

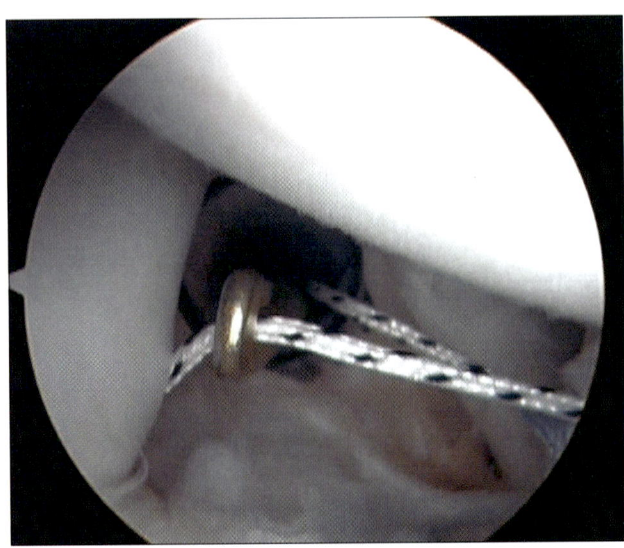

A

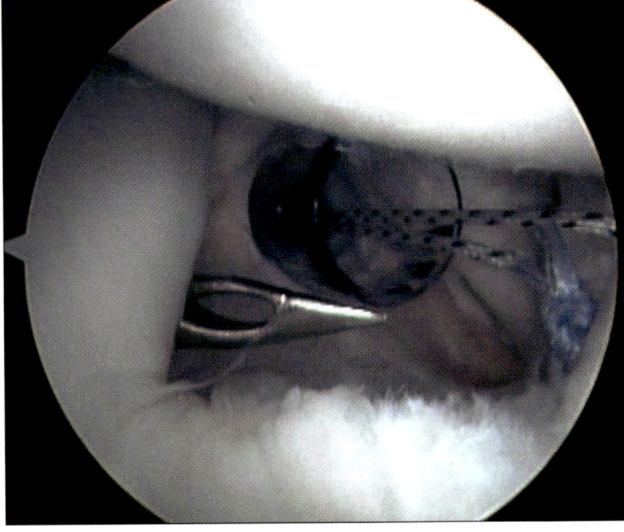

B

FIGURE 28

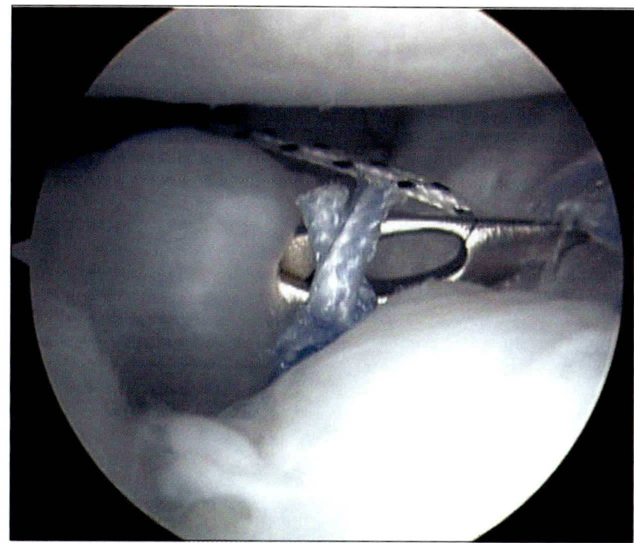

FIGURE 29

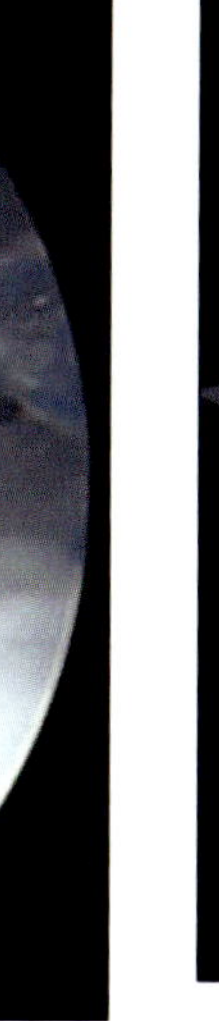

FIGURE 30

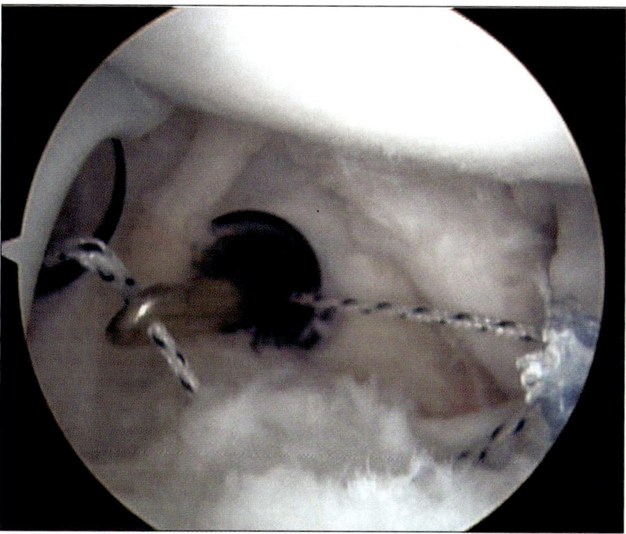

FIGURE 31

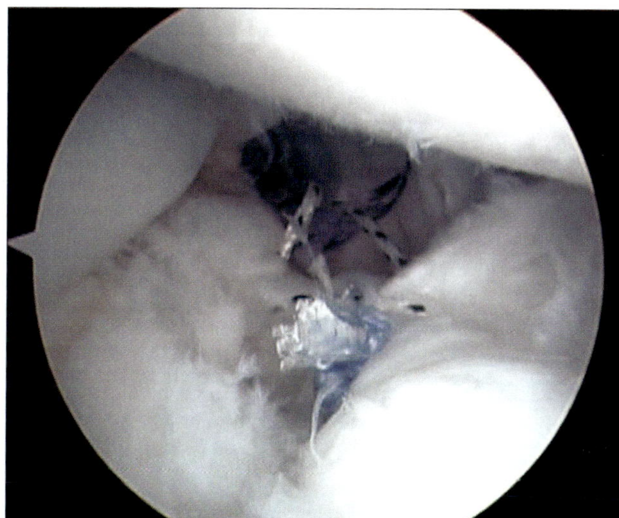

FIGURE 32

Postoperative Care and Expected Outcomes

- Immobilize the shoulder for 6 weeks.
  - No passive stretching is permitted from 6 to 12 weeks postoperatively. Progressive resistive exercises may be initiated from 6 to 12 weeks, with the goal of achieving symmetric range of motion by 6 months.
  - No sports participation is allowed for at least 6 months (better to wait 12 months); participation can then resume in the setting of a graded activity or sports-specific conditioning program.

- The number of studies reporting results after arthroscopic capsulorrhaphy for anteroinferior multidirectional instability is relatively low. The results have been favorable, with high rates of satisfaction and return to sport. Additional studies are required to help improve patient selection and determine the optimal amount of plication necessary with techniques that are reproducible.

Evidence

Alpert JM, Verma H, Wysocki R, et al. Arthroscopic treatment of multidirectional shoulder instability with minimum 270 labral repair: minimum 2-year follow-up. Arthroscopy. 2008;24:704-11.

The authors, in this retrospective case series, sought to analyze the results of arthroscopic stabilization with labral repair in patients with multidirectional instability and frank labral tear. Thirteen patients met criteria for review. Most patients (85%) had good results with a minimum 2-year follow-up. Two patients had a recurrence (15%) (subluxation or dislocation). The authors stated that the indications for rotator interval closure are still evolving. (Level IV evidence)

Cohen SB, Wiley W, Goradia VK, et al. Anterior capsulorrhaphy: an in vitro comparison of volume reduction. Arthroscopic plication versus open capsular shift. Arthroscopy. 2005;21:659-64.

The authors compared capsular volume reduction after arthroscopic plication and open lateral shift in a cadaver study. There were 7 shoulders in the plication group, and 8 shoulders in the shift group. The plication group used 3 anchors per specimen. Volume reduction was 22.8% in the plication group, and was 49.9% in the shift group. The authors recommended open lateral-based capsular shift for patients with multi-directional instability in which a larger shift is required. However, the amount of reduction necessary to eliminate instability in this setting remains unknown.

Gartsman GM, Roddey TS, Hammerman SM. Arthroscopic treatment of bidirectional glenohumeral instability: two- to five-year follow-up. J Shoulder Elbow Surg. 2001;10:28-36.

The purpose of this study was to evaluate the results of patients undergoing arthroscopic treatment for bidirectional (inferior with either anterior or posterior components) glenohumeral instability. Fifty-four patients were evaluated with minimum 2-year follow-up. Forty-nine patients (91%) rated a good to excellent result, with 40 patients returning to sports—ten (25%) returned to a lower level, however. Some patients were treated with thermal capsulorrhaphy, and rotator interval closure. Additional injuries were frequently encountered within the shoulder. The study was prospective, but without patient randomization or investigator masking. (Level IV evidence)

Tauro JC. Arthroscopic inferior capsular split and advancement for anterior and inferior shoulder instability: technique and results at 2- and 5-year follow-up. Arthroscopy. 2000;16:451-6.

This author prospectively evaluated 34 patients undergoing arthroscopic treatment for anterior-inferior instability. The first 5 patients were treated with transglenoid suture fixation—the remaining with suture anchors. The average Bankart score was 91.6 (range, 40-100). In 30 patients there were no recurrences, subluxations or dislocations. Twenty-eight patients were able to return to sports or work, with 21 of these patients returning to their pre-injury level. (Level IV evidence)

Treacy SH, Savoie FH 3rd, Field LD. Arthroscopic treatment of multidirectional instability. J Shoulder Elbow Surg. 1999;8:345-50.

The authors retrospectively reviewed 25 patients who were treated for multidirectional instability of the shoulder with an arthroscopic transglenoid technique. With a minimum 2-year follow-up, the average Bankart score was 95 (range 50-100). Twenty-one (88%) patients had a satisfactory Neer score. Three patients had episodes of recurrent instability after capsulorrhaphy. Pre-operatively, all patients initially had a history of atraumatic instability, although eleven patients had acute traumatic episodes superimposed on their pre-existing multidirectional symptoms. (Level IV evidence)

PROCEDURE 15

Anterior Glenohumeral Instability Associated with Glenoid or Humeral Bone Deficiency

Kristofer J. Jones, Christopher C. Dodson, and Russell F. Warren

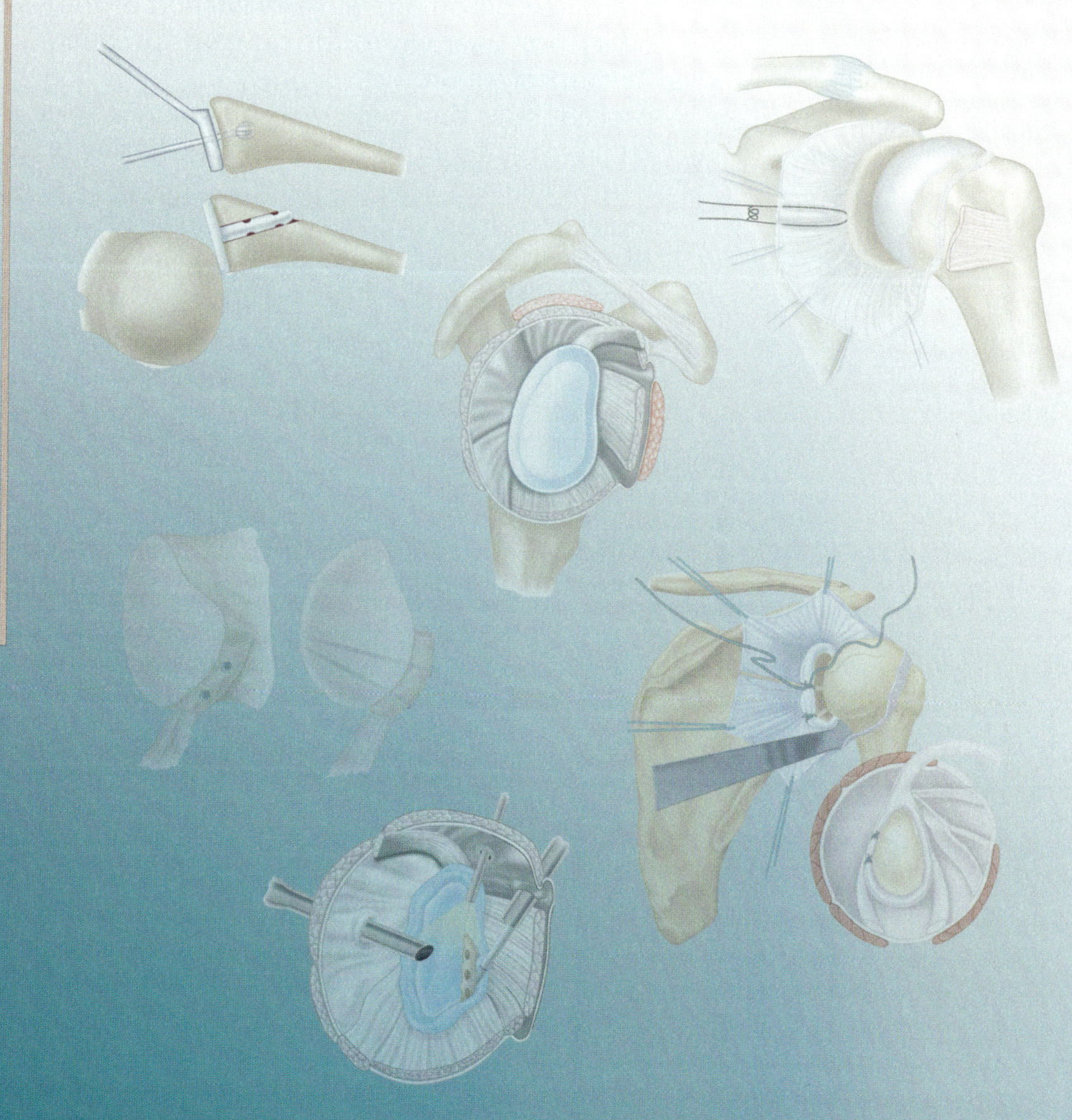

The Latarjet Procedure

Indications

- The goal of any surgical approach utilized to treat anterior glenohumeral instability is to restore joint stability while preserving both glenohumeral motion and strength to facilitate return to functional activities.
- Reconstructive procedures utilized to address bone loss associated with anterior glenohumeral intstability are based on preoperative evaluation of the osseous deficiency localized to the humerus or glenoid.
- At our institution, we routinely use the Latarjet procedure as our surgical technique of choice for recurrent anterior glenohumeral instability associated with significant osseous defects. The specific indications for this procedure include treatment of recurrent anterior instability associated with anteroinferior and anterior glenoid bone loss greater than 21% and 25%, respectively (Bigliani et al., 1998; Itoi et al., 2000; Yamamoto et al., 2009). Application of a coracoid graft restores the glenoid depth and width and creates a dynamic reinforcement of the inferior capsule with the conjoined tendon. This procedure is also effective for patients with an engaging Hill-Sachs lesion, as the reconstruction extends the glenoid arc, thereby preventing engagement of the humeral lesion.

Examination/Imaging

- Initial examination should be directed toward determining the direction of instability (anterior, inferior, posterior, or multidirectional). Clinical findings of instability are important in establishing a diagnosis; however, it is often difficult to ascertain whether bony defects are a contributing factor on routine examination.
- Provocative tests
  - The apprehension test is the classic provocative test for anterior instability. The relocation test is an extension of this clinical examination, as it was developed to increase the specificity of the apprehension test for cases of subtle anterior instability.

Pitfalls

- *While nonanatomic reconstructions such as the Latarjet procedure are largely successful in treating recurrent instability, they do not address additional pathologic lesions contributing to anterior instability, such as Bankart lesions, superior labrum anterior-posterior (SLAP) lesions, or anterior capsular deficiency.*
- *The Latarjet procedure is contraindicated in any patient who demonstrates instability associated with a tear or insufficiency of the subscapularis muscle.*

Controversies

- Long-term studies have demonstrated varying degrees of loss of external rotation in patients undergoing the Latarjet procedure. Significant scar formation within the subscapularis muscle can occur as a result of surgical dissection, ultimately leading to decreased tendon excursion and subsequent loss of external rotation. External rotation is an essential motion within the overhead throwing cycle, leading some authors to question the role of this procedure in overhead athletes.

Treatment Options

- Nonoperative approaches to recurrent anterior shoulder instability can be utilized in elderly or low-demand patients with humeral head or anteroinferior osseous defects measuring less than 20% if they are able to perform activities of daily living.
- Despite advances in arthroscopic stabilization procedures, there are some contraindications to arthroscopic treatment, including substantial glenoid or humeral bone defects that require osseous reconstruction, capsular deficiency, or irreparable rotator cuff deficiencies (Millett et al., 2005).

  - The load-and-shift test can be utilized to assess the competence of the anterior band of the glenohumeral ligament and quantify the degree of anterior instability. When performing this test intraoperatively, it is possible to experience a locked dislocation, which is consistent with a large osseous deficiency.
  - The sulcus sign determines the presence of inferior instability, and the jerk test can be used to assess the patient for posterior instability. The sulcus sign demonstrates a large gap between the humeral head and the undersurface of the acromion when longitudinal traction is placed on the humeral shaft (Fig. 1). This sign is thought to be pathognomonic of multidirectional instability.
- Plain radiographs
  - In most cases, glenoid and humeral bone defects can be detected with standard radiographic imaging. Anteroposterior (AP), internal rotation AP, and Stryker notch views (Fig. 2, *arrow*) can be utilized to evaluate patients for Hill-Sachs lesions (anterolateral impression defects of the humerus).
  - The West Point axillary view provides complete visualization of any bony defects localized to the anteroinferior glenoid rim.

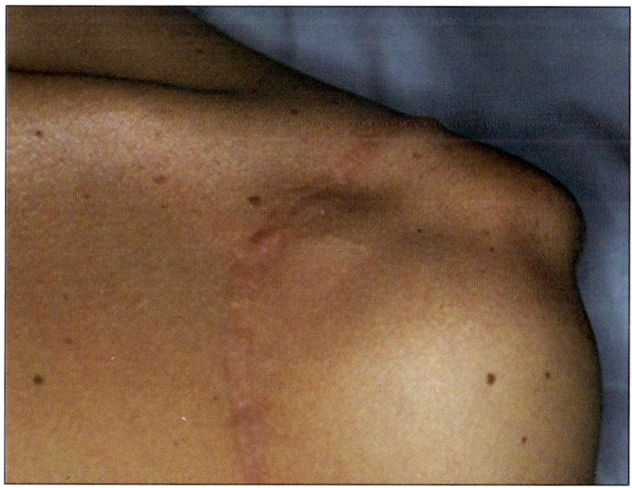

FIGURE 1

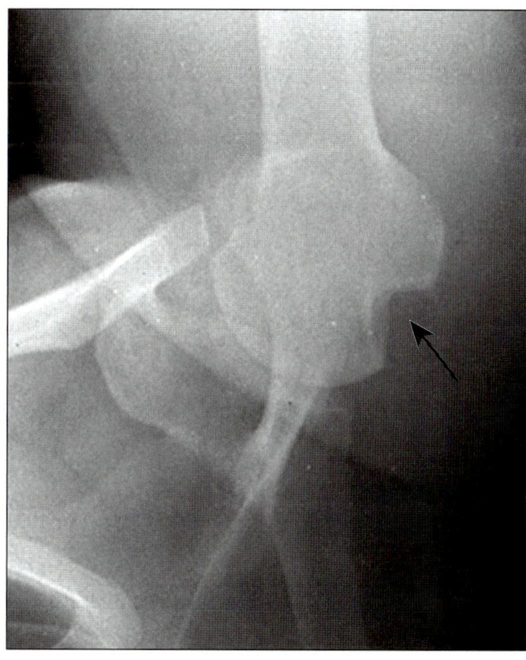

FIGURE 2

Treatment Options—cont'd

- In addition to the Latarjet procedure, which is detailed in this chapter, the Bristow procedure is an alternative coracoid process transferring procedure that can be used to address anterior instability in patients with bony defects of the inferior glenoid exceeding 20% of the glenoid diameter, or engaging humeral head deficits (Helfet, 1958).
- Shoulder arthroplasty or arthrodesis is a viable surgical option for patients with instability associated with degenerative arthritis of the glenohumeral joint.

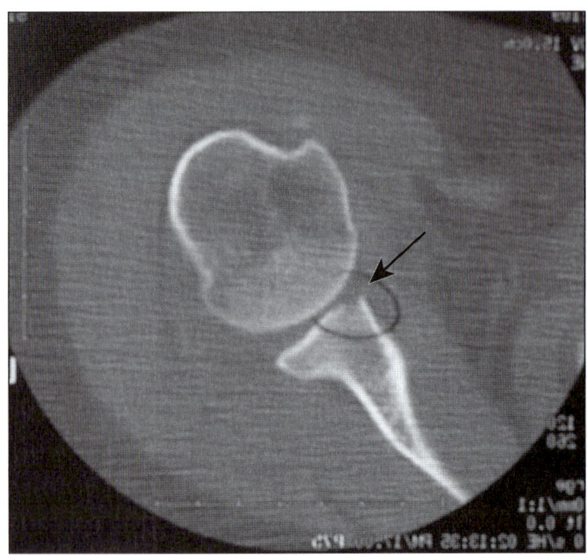

FIGURE 3

- Computed tomography (CT) scans with and without three-dimensional reconstruction are helpful when accurate quantification of glenoid or humeral bone loss is necessary for preoperative planning. The axial CT scan in Figure 3 demonstrates an osseous deficiency of the anterior glenoid with associated humeral head subluxation (*arrow*).
- Magnetic resonance imaging (MRI) aids in the assessment of labral tears, chondral defects, capsular laxity, and associated injuries to the rotator cuff. It is important to note that traumatic shoulder instability in older individuals can be associated with disruptions of the rotator cuff (particularly the subscapularis) (Neviaser et al., 1993; Neviaser and Neviaser, 1995), and any findings on physical examination consistent with rotator cuff pathology should be further evaluated with MRI.

Surgical Anatomy

- The coracoid process is an osseous structure that arises from the superior border of the head of the scapula, projecting forward and curving laterally. The coracoid process is located directly below the lateral fourth of the clavicle, connected to its undersurface by the coracoclavicular ligament.
  - The coracoid process serves as the attachment site for several muscles. The pectoralis minor is attached to the superior aspect of the coracoid.

The coracobrachialis is attached to the tip of the process on the medial side, and the short head of the biceps is attached to the tip of the process on the lateral side. Together, the tendinous attachments of the coracobrachialis and the short head of the biceps form the conjoined tendon.

- The coracoacromial and coracohumeral ligaments are attached to the lateral border of the coracoid as they arise from the acromion and humerus, respectively.

- The glenoid labrum is a fibrocartilaginous structure that surrounds the glenoid fossa and functions to deepen the glenoid cavity, thereby caudal to stabilization of the glenohumeral joint.
- A fibrous capsule envelops the glenohumeral joint and attaches to the medial side of the glenoid outside the margins of the glenoid labrum. The capsule is attached to the anatomic neck of the humerus as it extends laterally. The rotator cuff tendons (supraspinatus, infraspinatus, teres minor, and subscapularis) partially function to reinforce and functionally support the fibrous capsule.
- The subscapularis muscle arises from the anterior surface of the scapula and attaches as a broad tendon to the lesser tuberosity of the humerus and the front of the articular capsule. Anatomically, it forms a significant portion of the posterior axillary wall.

Positioning

- The patient is placed in the modified beach chair position for the Latarjet procedure. The primary advantage of this position is the ease with which an initial diagnostic arthroscopy can be followed with the open surgical approach, precluding the need to reposition the patient when converting procedures.
- Utilizing a standard operating room table and a triangular foam pillow with beveled ends, the patient is placed in a 45° lateral position. The table is flexed at the hips, with the head of the table elevated 30°. The foot of the bed is lowered approximately 10–15°. The arm can be flexed, abducted, and easily rotated in this position.

Equipment

- Standard operating table
- Large foam pillow with beveled ends

PEARLS

- *Research has demonstrated that the average anterior-posterior diameter of the inferior glenoid measures 23 mm (Burkhart et al., 2002). The amount of glenoid bone loss is determined by identifying the bare spot, which lies in the center of this measurement.*
- *As shown in Figure 6, a probe can be used to determine the distance from the anterior (A) and posterior (B) glenoid margins to the bare spot. Comparing these two measurements will allow the surgeon to quantify the percentage of anterior bone loss.*

Portals/Exposures

- Diagnostic arthroscopy is performed utilizing the standard anterior, posterior, and anterosuperior shoulder portals to identify and quantify bony deficiencies, as well as address concomitant pathologic lesions that may be contributing to instability.
  - Anterior superficial landmarks: acromion, clavicle, acromioclavicular joint, coracoid process
  - Posterior superficial landmarks: posterior acromion, spine of scapula
- The standard posterior portal is made in the "soft spot," located 2–3 cm inferior and 1 cm medial to the posterolateral corner of the acromion. This "soft spot" represents the interval between the infraspinatus and teres minor. The axillary nerve is at risk if portal placement is too inferior, and the suprascapular nerve and artery can be damaged if the portal placement is too far superior and medial.
- The anterosuperior portal is created after the posterior portal, using the posteriorly placed arthroscope for visual assistance. This portal is created 1 cm lateral and 1 cm superior to the coracoid process.
- Glenoid defects are easily visualized through the anterosuperior portal. Figure 4 is an arthroscopic view demonstrating a large osseous defect of the anterior glenoid (*arrow*).

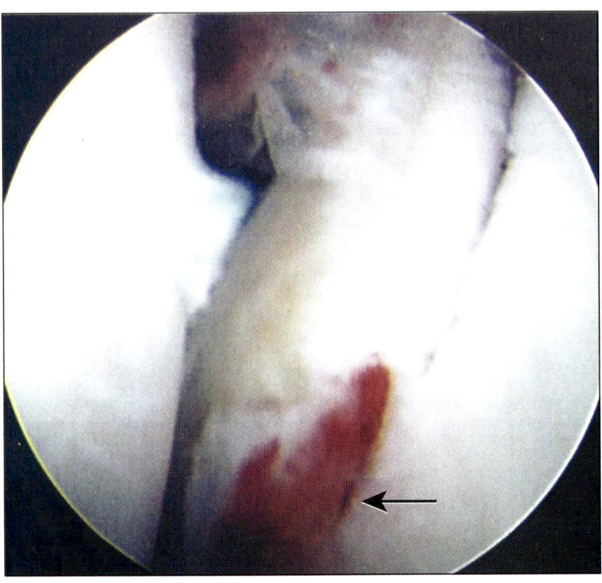

FIGURE 4

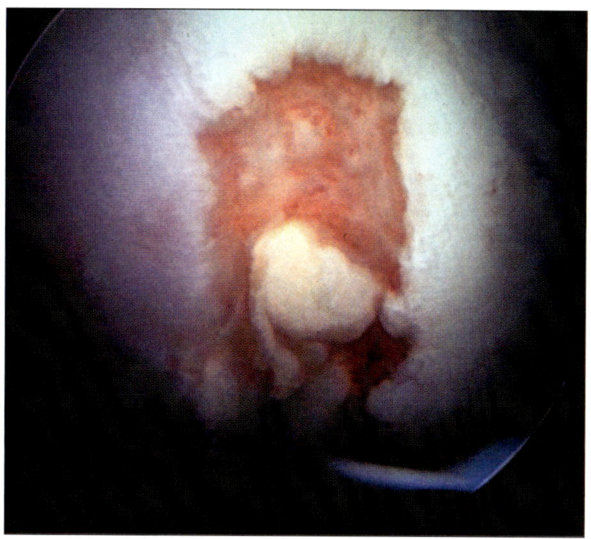

A

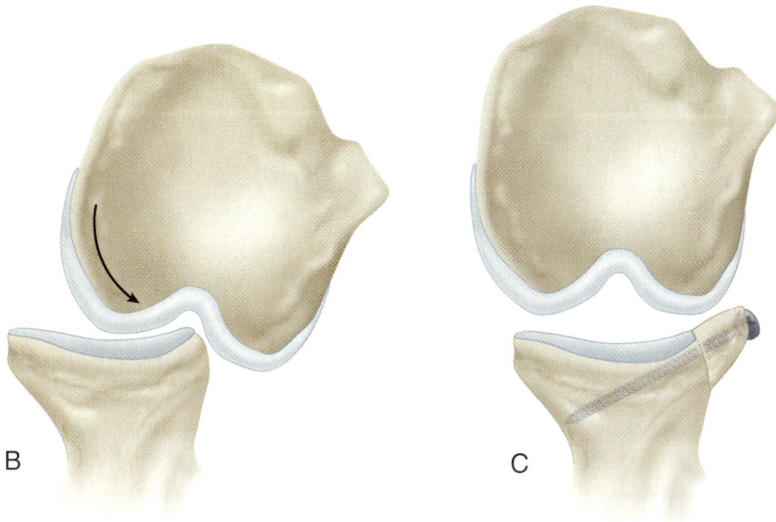

B C

FIGURE 5

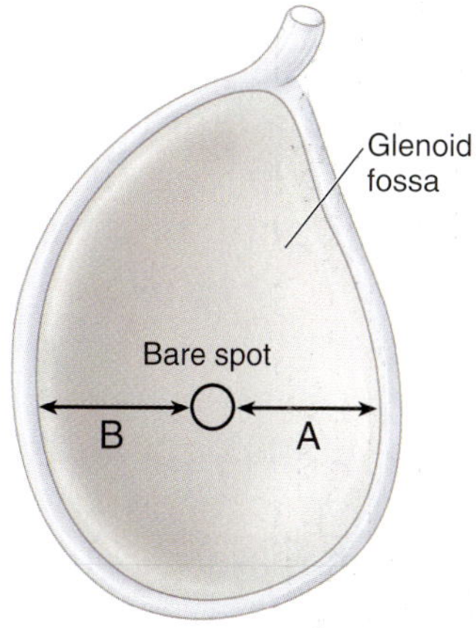

Total diameter = Avg 23mm

FIGURE 6

- In order to evaluate large Hill-Sachs lesions (Fig. 5A), the posterior and anterosuperior portals can be used to observe whether the humeral head defect engages the glenoid rim (Fig. 5B, *arrow*) in the "90–90" position (90° of abduction and 90° of external rotation).
- Application of a coracoid graft will extend the glenoid arc to prevent the humeral head from engaging the glenoid rim (Fig. 5C).

▪ A standard deltopectoral approach is used to perform the Latarjet procedure following diagnostic arthroscopy.

Pearls

- *It is important to sharply dissect the medial margin of the coracoid process and obtain full exposure prior to performing the coracoid osteotomy, as this medial surface will later be approximated to the anterior glenoid neck.*

Pearls

- *The osteotomy should be made between the pectoralis minor insertion and the attachment of the coracoclavicular ligaments. It is important to ensure that the coracoclavicular ligaments are left intact to avoid destabilizing the acromioclavicular joint.*
- *We prefer to obtain at least 2–3 cm of coracoid graft for later attachment to the glenoid neck.*
- *The conjoined tendon remains attached to the coracoid throughout this procedure, thereby preserving the vascular supply to the graft (vascularized graft).*

Pitfalls

- *It is important to adequately expose and protect the musculocutaneous nerve prior to obtaining the coracoid graft. Adequate mobilization of the graft is important to avoid stretch injury of the musculocutaneous nerve, which traverses the coracobrachialis muscle just distal to the coracoid attachment.*

Procedure

Step 1

- The incision is marked with a skin marker, and the skin is locally injected with lidocaine and 1% epinephrine.
- Utilizing a standard deltopectoral approach to the shoulder, a 6- to 8-cm skin incision is extended from the tip of the coracoid process inferiorly to the axillary fold. The cephalic vein is carefully dissected free and retracted laterally in order to preserve the vascular branches to the deltoid.
- The incision is carried down to the level of the clavicopectoral fascia, which is incised and bluntly dissected to expose the coracoid process at its base where the coracoclavicular ligaments insert. The pectoralis minor is sharply reflected from the medial aspect of the coracoid process, and the coracoacromial ligament is released from the lateral margin of the process to facilitate exposure.

Step 2

- After exposing the medial aspect of the coracoid process, it is carefully osteotomized at its base immediately distal to the insertion of the coracoclavicular ligaments using a small oscillating saw with deep, blunt retractors placed inferiorly and medially to protect medial neurovascular structures.
- Using a high-speed burr, a small area of bleeding cancellous bone is prepared on the medial coracoid surface to facilitate graft consolidation when attached to the anterior glenoid rim.

Step 3

- Following preparation of the graft, exposure of the glenohumeral joint is performed through an L-shaped dissection of the subscapularis muscle. The superior half of the muscle is detached distally and dissected from the underlying anterior capsule. Tagging sutures are placed in this portion of the muscle, which is reflected medially to facilitate adequate exposure.
- The inferior aspect of the subscapularis is subsequently elevated from the underlying anterior capsule. A vertical capsular incision is made approximately 1 cm lateral to the margin of the glenoid rim to develop a robust capsular flap for later capsulolabral repair.

Instrumentation/ Implantation

- As an alternative to the small oscillating saw, a sharp 0.75-inch osteotome can be utilized to perform the coracoid osteotomy. When using the osteotome, one must take great care to avoid fracture of the glenoid or scapula. The osteotome should be angled in a medial-to-lateral direction to avoid damage to medial neurovascular structures.

Pearls

- *A split in the subscapularis muscle can be utilized to expose the glenohumeral joint, thereby avoiding the need to repair the muscle and preserving the integrity of the tendinous attachment.*
- *If an L-shaped dissection is used to expose the joint, the inferior aspect of the subscapularis must be preserved to facilitate early active external rotation during the postoperative period.*

Step 4

- The fibrous capsule is subperiosteally elevated from the anterior glenoid neck to reveal the osseous deficiency (Fig. 7). The glenoid neck and rim are then decorticated with a high-speed burr in order to create a bleeding recipient bone bed for graft fixation. It is important to ensure that the recipient site is cleared of all fibrous tissue to avoid potential graft nonunion.
- Three suture anchors are inserted at the 3, 4, and 5 o'clock positions along the glenoid rim for later reattachment of the capsulolabral tissue.
- Using guidewires for 4.0-mm cannulated screws, the coracoid graft is provisionally fixed to the glenoid rim with the bleeding medial surface placed flush along the decorticated anterior inferior glenoid neck. The coracoid tip is oriented to point inferiorly so that the curved contour of the graft parallels the shape of the native glenoid rim. The high-speed burr can be used to contour the graft and ensure a proper fit.
- Once satisfactory orientation and fit is achieved, the graft is secured with two 4.0-mm cannulated screws that are placed superiorly and inferiorly (Fig. 8A and 8B). Note that the coracoid graft restores the "pear shape" of the glenoid by increasing its inferior diameter (Fig. 8C).

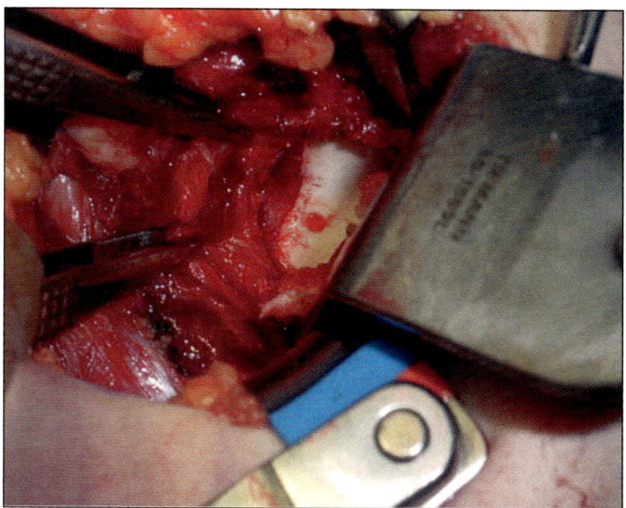

FIGURE 7

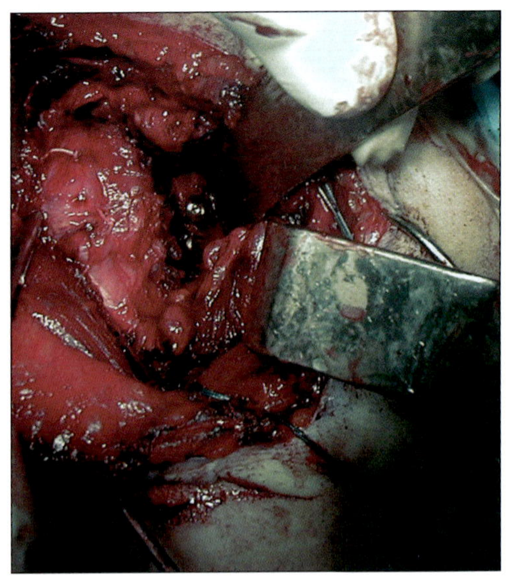
A

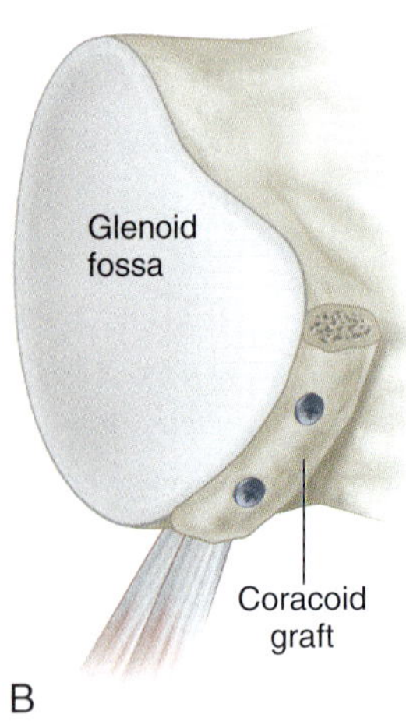

B

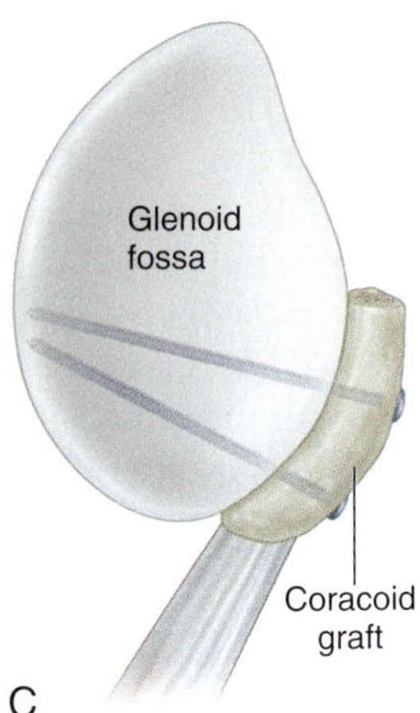

C

FIGURE 8

Step 5

- The reflected capsular flap is repaired to the native glenoid rim utilizing the previously inserted suture anchors. Next, the subscapularis is reapproximated to the lateral tendinous insertion that was preserved during the initial exposure using nonabsorbable sutures.
- The wound is copiously irrigated and all bleeding is controlled. The deltopectoral interval is not typically closed; however, the deep dermal and cutaneous fascial layers require closure with absorbable sutures.
- The patient is placed in a padded shoulder immobilizer.

Pearls

- *The superior and inferior coracoid holes are drilled in a bicortical fashion. When drilling the superior hole, the drill should exit the posterior glenoid below the spinoglenoid notch in order to avoid iatrogenic injury to the suprascapular nerve.*
- *Care should be taken when inserting the screws, as overtightening the cannulated screws can fracture the graft.*

Postoperative Care and Expected Outcomes

- The padded shoulder immobilizer is worn for the first 2 weeks postoperatively. Immediate shoulder motion is encouraged, as the immobilizer may be removed three times daily to begin passive external range-of-motion exercises to neutral with supervised physical therapy.
- Passive overhead motion is initiated 2 weeks postoperatively after the shoulder immobilizer is discontinued.
- At 6 weeks postoperatively, external rotation stretching and resisted shoulder motion is initiated.

Pitfalls

- *Significant medial displacement of the graft may lead to recurrent dislocation, as the graft fails to extend the articular arc of the glenoid. Lateral overhang of the graft acts as a "bone block" during glenohumeral motion and can lead to early pain and osteoarthritis (Burkhart and De Beer, 2000).*

Pitfalls

- *Repair of the subscapularis muscle should permit adequate excursion of the muscle around the transferred coracoid graft and conjoined tendon in order to preserve external rotation.*

- Patients are permitted to lift weights within the lesser arc of shoulder motion at 3 months and can expect to return to full athletic activities (including contact sports) at 6 months.
- Standard AP and internal rotation AP views of the shoulder are obtained during interval follow-up to monitor osseous union at the graft site (Fig. 9).
- Long-term follow-up studies investigating functional outcomes of patients treated with the Latarjet procedure for recurrent anterior glenohumeral instability have shown promising results with regard to recurrent dislocation.
  - In a study by Allain et al. (1998), the authors found that there were no recurrent dislocations in 52 shoulders treated with the Latarjet procedure at an average follow-up of 14.3 years. However, the same study demonstrated osteoarthritic changes of the operative shoulder in 34 patients (58%). While the majority of patients only had signs of grade I arthritis, the authors emphasized avoiding lateral fixation of the coracoid on the glenoid rim to prevent this potential complication.

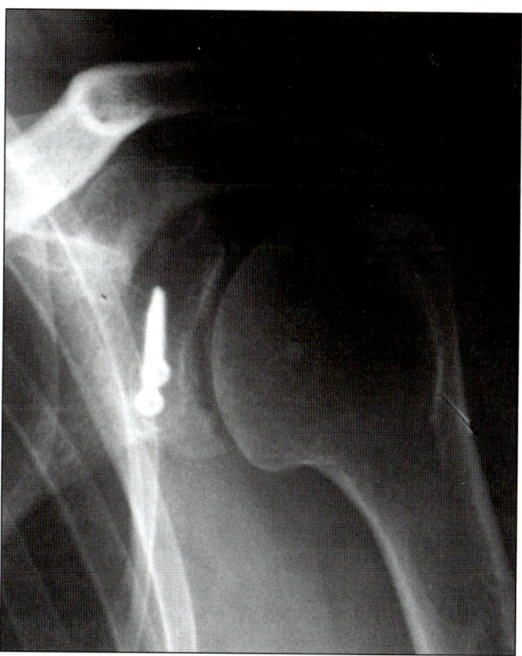

FIGURE 9

Evidence

Allain J, Goutallier D, Glorion C. Long-term results of the Latarjet procedure for the treatment of anterior instability of the shoulder. J Bone Joint Surg [Am]. 1998;80:841-52.

Paper addresses long term results of using the Laterjet procedure for treating patients with anterior instability. (Level IV evidence)

Bigliani LU, Newton PM, Steinmann SP, Connor PM, McLlveen SJ. Glenoid rim lesions associated with recurrent anterior dislocation of the shoulder. Am J Sports Med. 1998;26:41-5.

This article addresses how anterior bone loss can cause shoulder instability and discusses treatment. (Level IV evidence)

Burkhart SS, De Beer JF. Traumatic glenohumeral bone defects and their relationship to failure of arthroscopic Bankart repairs: significance of the inverted-pear glenoid and the humeral engaging Hill-Sachs lesion. Arthroscopy. 2000;16:677-94.

This article describes the significance of glenoid morphology and how it can cause shoulder instability. (Level IV evidence)

Burkhart SS, Debeer JF, Tehrany AM, Parten PM. Quantifying glenoid bone loss arthroscopically in shoulder instability. Arthroscopy. 2002;18:488-91.

Paper discusses a method of evaluating glenoid bone loss arthroscopically. (Level V evidence)

Helfet AJ. Coracoid transplantation for recurring dislocation of the shoulder. J Bone Joint Surg [Br]. 1958;40:198-202.

Technical paper discussing using the coracoid as a bone block in patients with shoulder instability. (Level IV evidence)

Itoi E, Lee SB, Berglund LJ, Berge LL, An KN. The effect of a glenoid defect on anteroinferior stability of the shoulder after Bankart repair: a cadaveric study. J Bone Joint Surg [Am]. 2000;82:35-46.

Cadaveric study evaluating the role of glenoid bone loss after Bankart repair.

Millett PJ, Clavert P, Warner JJ. Open operative treatment for anterior shoulder instability: when and why? J Bone Joint Surg [Am]. 2005;87:419-32.

Good review article of open treatment options for shoulder instability. (Level V evidence)

Neviaser RJ, Neviaser TJ, Neviaser JS. Anterior dislocation of the shoulder and rotator cuff rupture. Clin Orthop Relat Res. 1993;(291):103-6.

Case series of patients with anterior shoulder dislocations who had concomitant rotator cuff injuries (Level IV evidence)

Neviaser RJ, Neviaser TJ. Recurrent instability of the shoulder with onset after age 40. J Shoulder Elbow Surg. 1995;(4):416-18.

Yamamoto N, Itoi E, Abe H, Kikuchi K, Seki N, Minagawa H, Tuoheti Y. Effect of an anterior glenoid defect on anterior shoulder stability: a cadaveric study. Am J Sports Med. 2009;37(5):949-54.

Cadaveric study looking at anterior glenoid bone loss and how it affects shoulder instability.

PROCEDURE 16

Open Treatment of Posterior-Inferior Multidirectional Shoulder Instability

George M. McCluskey III

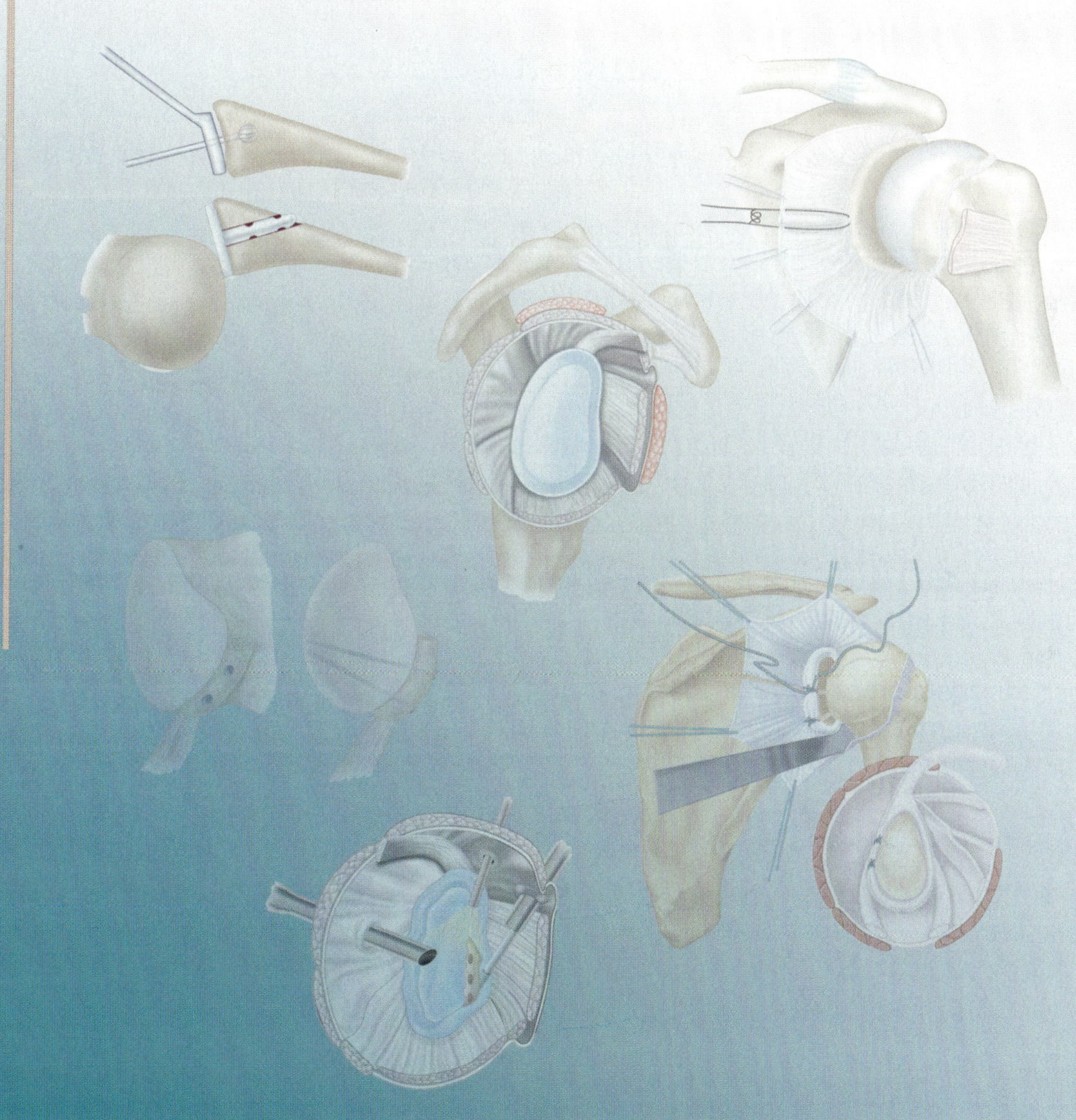

PITFALLS

- *Avoid operating on patients with Ehler-Danlos syndrome or Marfan syndrome.*
- *Avoid operating on patients who voluntarily dislocate the shoulder using selective muscular contractions with the affected arm at the side.*
- *Avoid operating on patients with certain psychological disorders.*

Indications

- Symptomatic posterior or posterior-inferior instability that has not responded to a comprehensive, nonoperative treatment program after 3–6 months.
- Symptomatic multidirectional instability with a predominant posterior-inferior component that has not responded to an operative treatment program after at least 6 months.
- Persistent posterior displacement of the humeral head relative to the glenoid (nonconcentric reduction) after attempted reduction.

Examination/Imaging

Physical Examination

- Always examine both shoulders for comparison because multidirectional instability often occurs bilaterally.
- Confirm the primary direction of symptomatic multidirectional instability with provocative instability and translational tests, such as the anterior and posterior apprehension tests, relocation test, jerk test, pivot-shift test, and load-and-shift test.
- A circumduction maneuver with the arm in the forward-flexed, internally rotated, and adducted position often elicits a "clunking" sensation.
- The shoulders should be evaluated for the sulcus sign, measuring the arms in neutral position and in external rotation for comparison.
- The patient should always be instructed to voluntarily dislocate the shoulder to differentiate between muscular (habitual) and positional dislocation.
- The patient with scapular winging must have a thorough neurologic examination to differentiate between primary scapular winging and compensatory, or secondary, scapular winging due to posterior multidirectional instability.

PITFALLS

- *Most patients with symptomatic multidirectional instability of the shoulder have hyperlaxity in both shoulders. It is critical to determine clinically that the patient has symptoms with translation of the humeral head on the glenoid rather than just asymptomatic excessive translation of the humeral head on the glenoid, as seen in a hyperlax joint.*

Imaging Studies

- Plain radiographs
  - True anteroposterior, axillary, and scapular Y views.
  - The shoulder is evaluated for a reverse Hill-Sachs lesion of the humeral head, excessive glenoid retroversion, a Bennett lesion, and a reverse bony Bankart lesion.

Treatment Options

- Nonoperative treatment
- Avoidance of provocative activities
- Dynamic stabilization of the scapulothoracic joint
- Strengthening exercises for the rotator cuff, deltoid, and scapula stabilizers
- Biofeedback and proprioceptive therapy
- Arthroscopic posterior capsulorrhaphy with pan-capsular plication with or without posterior Bankart or labral repair
- Occasional closure of a pathologically enlarged rotator interval
- Combined arthroscopic and open repair for a patient with a rotator interval lesion, superior labral tear, and/or anterior capsulolabral injury in addition to the posterior capsulolabral disorder
- Open posterior bone block combined with posterior-inferior capsular shift in patients with a glenoid rim defect or excessive glenoid retroversion
- Open posterior capsular reconstruction with an Achilles tendon allograft augmentation for posterior soft tissue deficiency, particularly in a patient having a revision procedure

- Magnetic resonance imaging
  - Best accomplished with gadolinium.
  - Used to evaluate for a patulous, loose capsule; a posterior Bankart lesion; and a posterior capsular tear.
- Computed tomography
  - Best test to evaluate the amount of glenoid retroversion and the size of a reverse Hill-Sachs lesion of the humeral head.

Surgical Anatomy

- The middle third and posterior third of the deltoid are demonstrated in Figure 1. The posterior third of the deltoid muscle originates along the lateral third of the scapular spine and the posterior portion of the acromion and inserts on the deltoid tuberosity. The middle third of the deltoid arises from the lateral portion of the acromion. The deltoid inserts at the deltoid tuberosity along the lateral humerus.
- The posterior rotator cuff comprises the infraspinatus and teres minor muscles. The infraspinatus muscle is a bipennate muscle with a fat stripe or a raphe that divides this muscle longitudinally into top and bottom portions. This raphe is often confused with the interval between the infraspinatus and teres minor muscles. The infraspinatus and teres minor

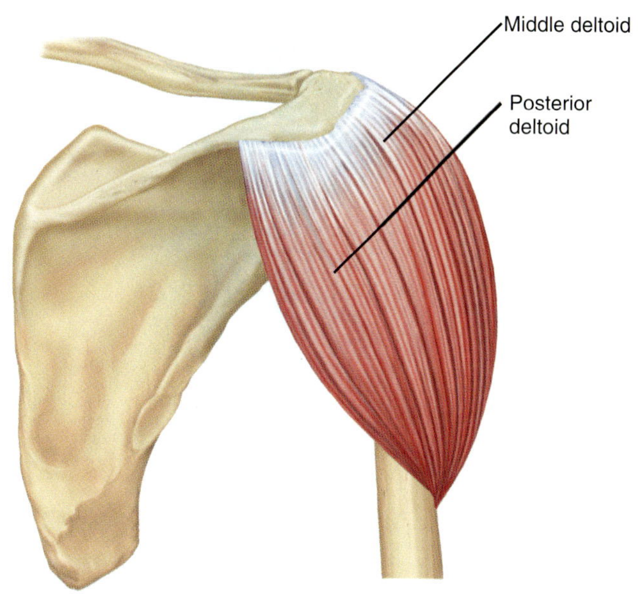

FIGURE 1

muscles are often difficult to distinguish from each other (Fig. 2).

- The larger infraspinatus muscle originates on the infraspinatus fossa of the scapula and inserts along the posterior facet of the greater tuberosity of the humerus.
- The teres minor is a smaller muscle located inferior to the infraspinatus that originates on the lateral aspect of the scapula and inserts just below the infraspinatus along the inferior portion of the greater tuberosity.

- The quadrangular space contains the axillary nerve and the posterior humeral circumflex artery. It is bounded by the teres minor, teres major, long head of the triceps, and the surgical neck of the humerus (Fig. 3).

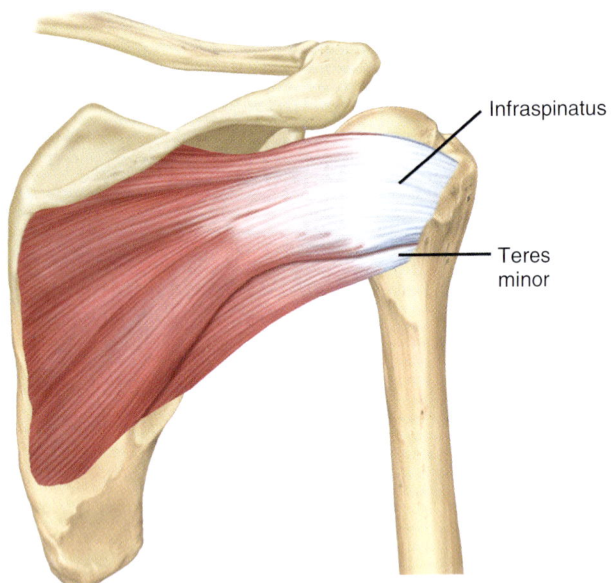

FIGURE 2

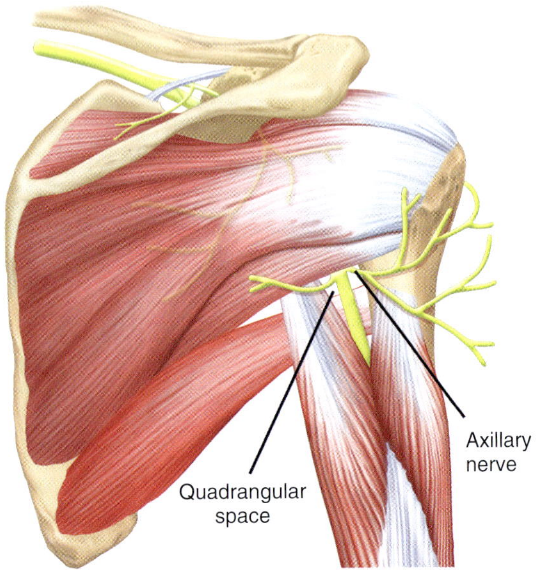

FIGURE 3

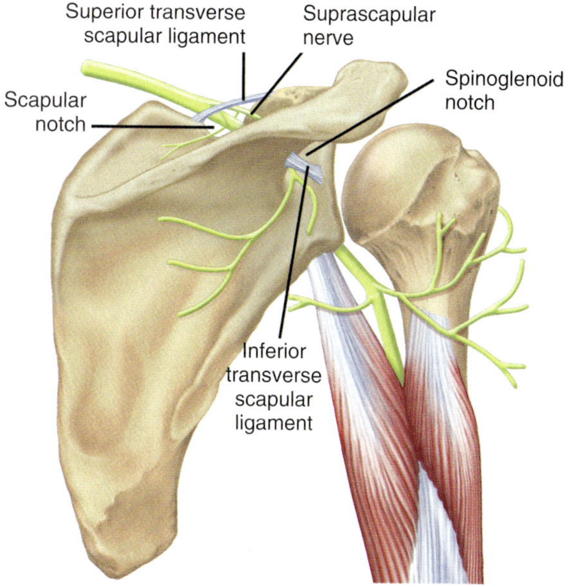

FIGURE 4

- The suprascapular nerve originates from the upper trunk of the brachial plexus and courses under the transverse scapular ligament and the scapular notch medial to the base of the coracoid (Fig. 4). It supplies the supraspinatus muscle before making a sharp turn around the scapula neck and traveling through the spinoglenoid notch to supply branches to the infraspinatus muscle. This nerve can be injured when medial retractors are used to retract the infraspinatus muscle, as the nerve is located 1.5–2.5 cm from the midposterior glenoid rim.
- Unlike the anterior capsule, the posterior capsule has no important glenohumeral ligaments with the exception of the posterior band of the inferior glenohumeral ligament, which is often small and indistinct. The capsule is thin and blends in with the deep portion of the infraspinatus tendon as it attaches to the posterior portion of the greater tuberosity.
- The axillary nerve is primarily at risk for injury during surgery as it enters the quadrangular space below the teres minor and divides into (1) a posterior trunk that innervates the teres minor and posterior deltoid and (2) an anterior trunk that travels along the deep portion of the middle third and anterior third of the deltoid muscle approximately 3–5 cm below the lateral edge of the acromion.

PEARLS

- *The operative arm is draped for full exposure of the anterior and posterior shoulder and scapula. The arm can be easily moved in various positions for retraction, exposure, and capsular tensioning during the procedure.*

PITFALLS

- *Some nerves are at particular risk of injury from excessive pressure when the lateral decubitus positioning technique is used. The ulnar nerve in the nonoperative arm is at risk because the arm and the elbow are generally in a sustained flexed position. In addition, the peroneal nerve in the leg that is against the operating table is at risk, so the leg should be padded to prevent injury.*

Positioning

- Both shoulders are examined under anesthesia before positioning to reconfirm the presence of instability patterns.
- The patient is placed in the lateral decubitus position and in slight reverse Trendelenburg position with the operative extremity up and the arm draped free (Fig. 5A). Figure 5B demonstrates the posterior axillary incision that would be used for this procedure.
  - The patient lies on a beanbag that, when inflated, molds and conforms to the patient from the midthorax to the midthigh.
  - An axillary roll is placed under the flexed, nonoperative extremity to protect the brachial plexus.
  - The head and neck are stabilized and protected with foam cushions, and protective goggles are placed on the eyes.
  - All pressure areas, including the ulnar nerve and peroneal nerve of the nonoperative upper and lower extremities, the feet, and ankles, are padded.
  - A pillow is placed between the legs.
  - Safety straps should be placed over the patient, and stabilizing side braces secured to the operating

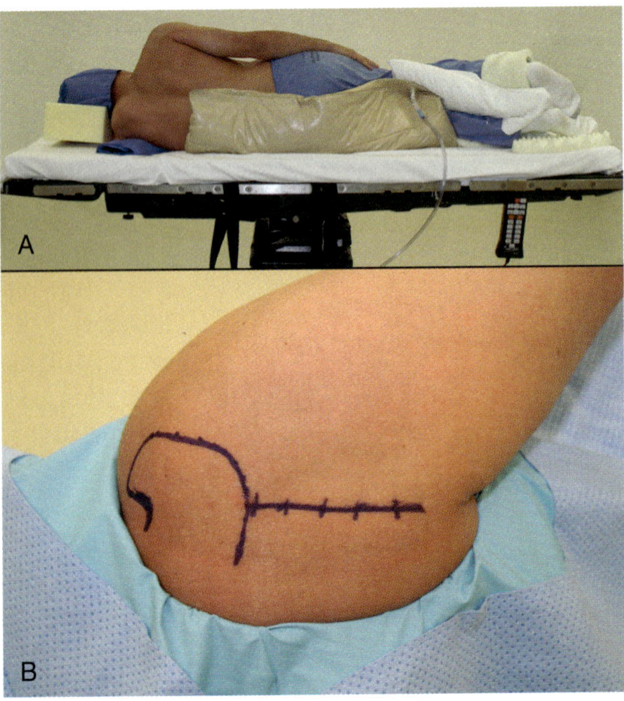

FIGURE 5

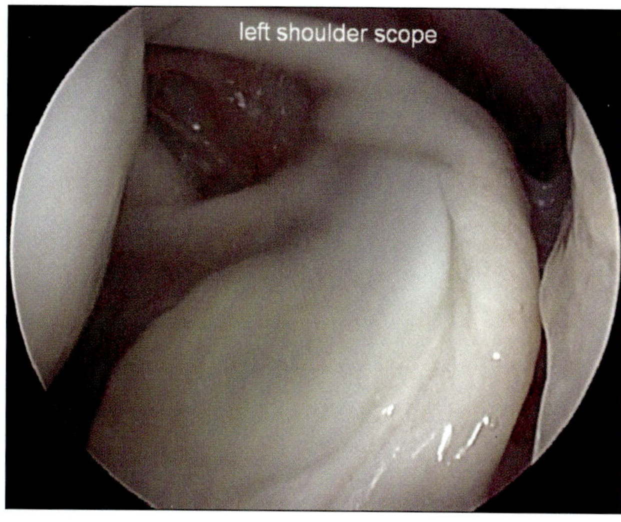

FIGURE 6

  - table and placed to support the beanbag and hold the patient in position in case the bag deflates during the procedure.
  - A warming blanket is placed over the patient when positioning is completed.
- Diagnostic arthroscopy from the lateral decubitis position is easily performed after positioning and draping and before making the incision for the open procedure. This allows the surgeon to inspect the glenohumeral joint and, when needed, to perform an arthroscopic repair before the open posterior repair. The arthroscopic view of a left shoulder with the camera in the posterior portion of the joint seen in Figure 6 demonstrates the voluminous capsule with a positive "drive-through" sign inferiorly.

Portals/Exposures

- A vertical 6- to 8-inch posterior incision is made beginning at the midposterior acromion and extending to the posterior axillary crease. The incision incorporates the posterior arthroscopy portal and is centered over the glenohumeral joint (Fig. 7).
- Subcutaneous dissection is made to create flaps about 5.0 cm (2 inches) around the circumference of the skin incision to enhance the exposure of the posterior deltoid.
- Deltoid split
  - The posterior deltoid split is made in line with its fibers beginning at the posterior-lateral angle of

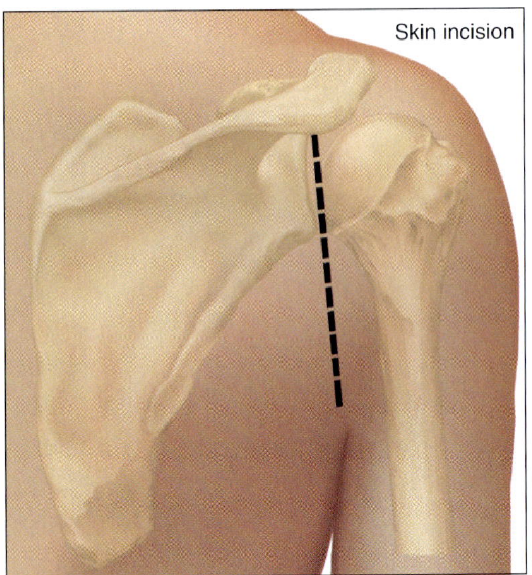

FIGURE 7

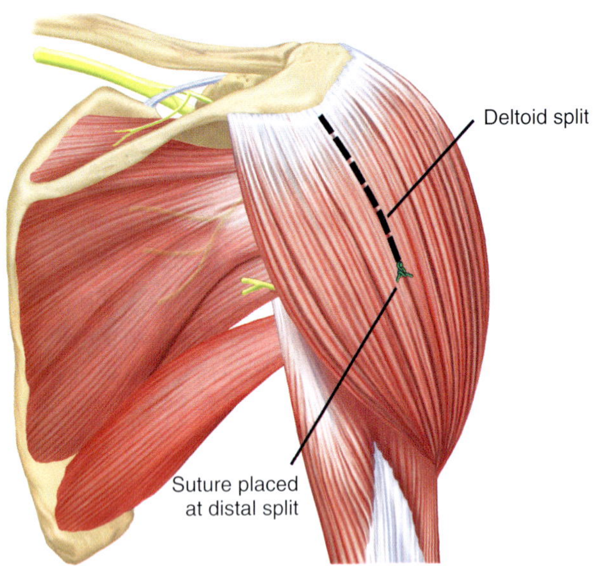

FIGURE 8

the acromion and extending approximately 4 cm (Fig. 8).

- A suture is placed at the distal extent of the deltoid split to prevent propagation of the split and to prevent injury to the anterior branch of the axillary nerve coursing along the deep surface of the deltoid.
- Retractors are placed in the deltoid split to expose the underlying infraspinatus tendon (Fig. 9).

■ The underlying infraspinatus muscle is identified. The intramuscular interval between the supraspinatus and the infraspinatus tendons is developed proximally,

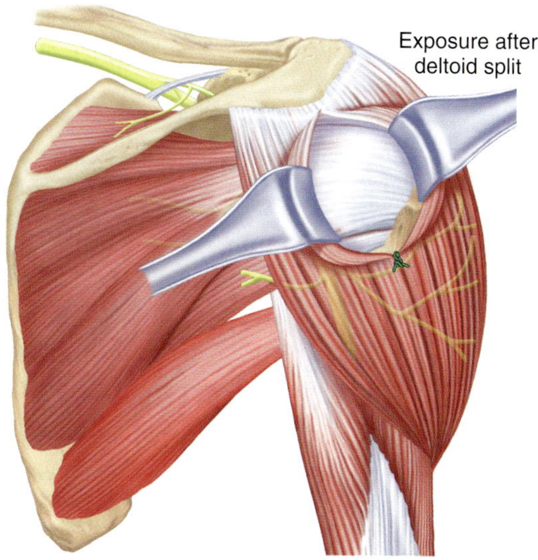

FIGURE 9

and the interval between the infraspinatus and teres minor is developed inferiorly (Fig. 10: *SS*, supraspinatus; *IS*, infraspinatus; *TMi*, teres minor).

- A vertical incision is made in the infraspinatus tendon 1 cm medial to its attachment at the posterior facet of the greater tuberosity. A combination of blunt and sharp dissections are used to carefully develop a plane of dissection between the deep portion of the infraspinatus tendon and muscle and the underlying capsule. Tagging sutures are placed in the infraspinatus tendon, which is dissected free from the

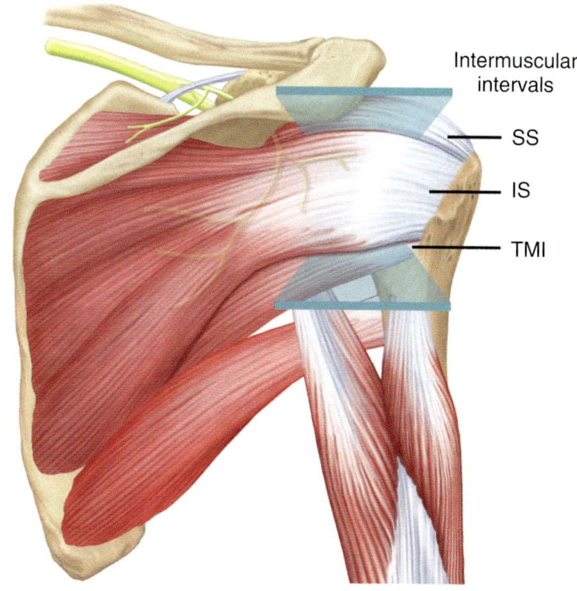

FIGURE 10

Pearls

- *The skin incision is made in Langer's lines to improve the cosmesis of the incision and decrease the chance for a thickened, scarred incision.*
- *With gentle retraction of the deltoid, the rotator cuff and capsule can be better visualized through the incision with rotation of the humerus.*
- *By placing the arm in 20–30° of internal rotation during the dissection of the infraspinatus tendon and muscle from the posterior capsule, the capsule will have some tension, and the plane of dissection can be developed more easily and with less risk of capsular violation or tear.*
- *A blunt elevator can be used to gently dissect the infraspinatus muscle and tendon from the inferior portion of the capsule.*

Pitfalls

- *Vertical release of the infraspinatus tendon from the greater tuberosity must be made so that adequate tissue is present on the medial and lateral sides for secure tendon-to-tendon repair and the completion of the capsular shift procedure.*
- *To prevent restriction of internal rotation, the infraspinatus tendon should be repaired anatomically and should not be shortened.*

underlying redundant capsule and reflected medially (Fig. 11).

Exposure Alternatives

- In some cases, the deltoid origin may be released from its acromial attachment at the proximal portion of the deltoid split for about 1 cm medial and about 1 cm lateral off the posterior-lateral angle of the acromion to improve exposure (Fig. 12).
- For more experienced shoulder surgeons, the midportion of the infraspinatus can be split from the glenoid rim to the insertion on the posterior facet of

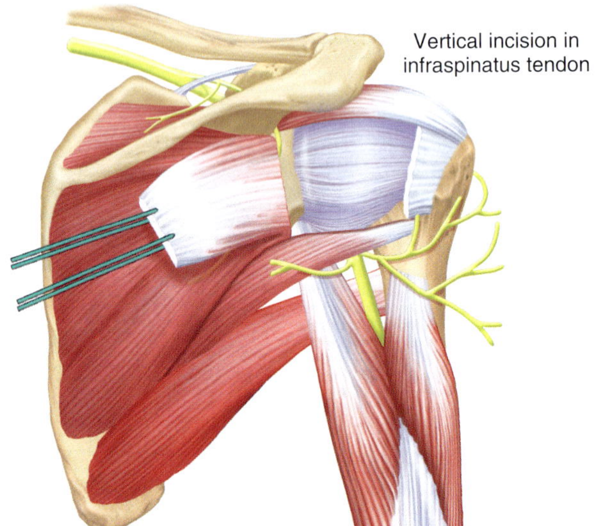

FIGURE 11

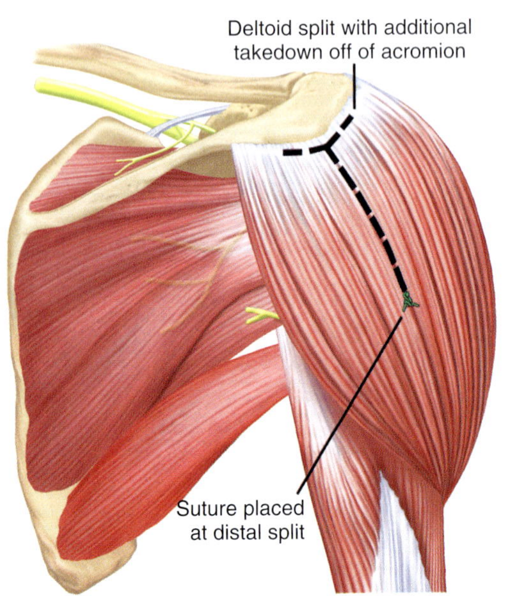

FIGURE 12

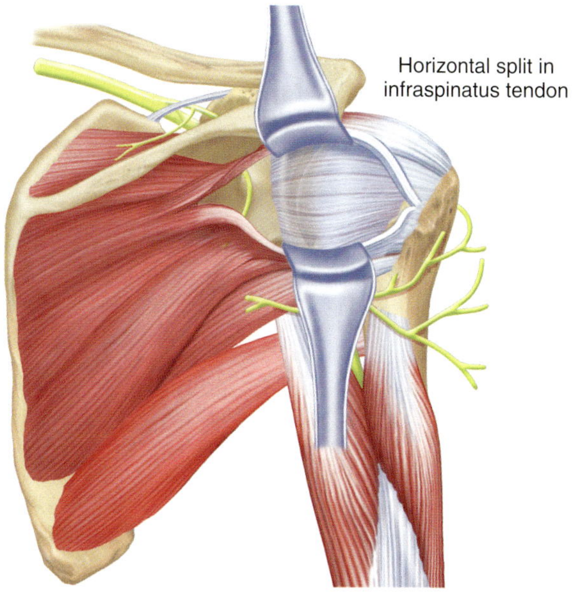

FIGURE 13

the greater tuberosity longitudinally without releasing the tendon from its insertion into the posterior facet of the tuberosity using the vertical incision (Fig. 13). Retractors are then placed to expose the underlying capsule.

Procedure

Step 1

- After adequate exposure has been achieved, the capsule is sharply incised vertically from superior to inferior 1 cm from its attachment to the humeral neck (Fig. 14), leaving a small cuff of tissue laterally to which it can be sewn at the completion of the capsular shift.
  - A blunt retractor is placed above the teres minor and pulled inferiorly to protect the axillary nerve and the posterior circumflex artery located in the quadrangular space below the teres minor.
  - This laterally based capsular incision is extended down inferiorly and with appropriate retraction and positioning of the arm, and this split is carried into the anterior-inferior quadrant.
- When releasing the capsule from the posterior-inferior and inferior humeral neck, the arm should be slightly extended and internally rotated.
  - A blunt Darrach retractor can be placed inside the capsule and around the humeral neck of the glenoid, staying inside the capsule. The retractor is

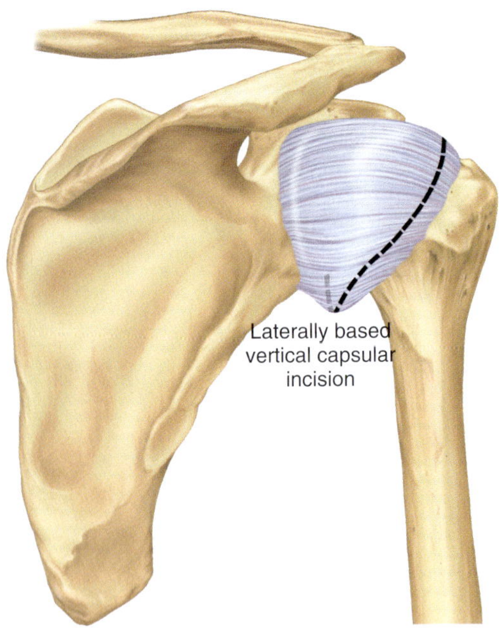

FIGURE 14

then pulled gently in a medial direction to provide good exposure of the capsule for release from the humeral neck inferiorly to the 6 o'clock position and around to the anterior-inferior quadrant of the joint (Fig. 15). This ensures that adequate mobilization and shift of the capsule can be performed.

- This inferior release is accomplished from inside the capsule with Bovie electrocautery, or a knife can be used to sharply release the capsule from the bone with the knife blade angled toward the bone to protect the neurovascular structures.

- Tagging sutures are placed in the released edge of the capsule after the vertical release has been performed (Fig. 16). These sutures assist in the development of the superior and inferior capsular flaps.
- Next, the capsule is divided transversely from lateral to medial at the midglenoid level. This creates a lateral-based T-shaped capsulotomy with superior

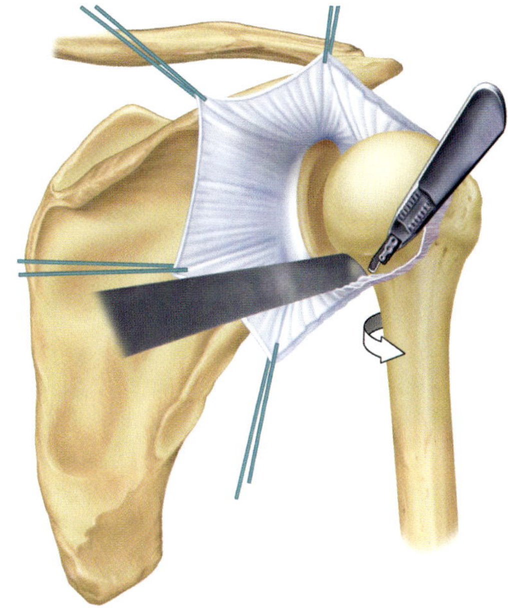

FIGURE 15

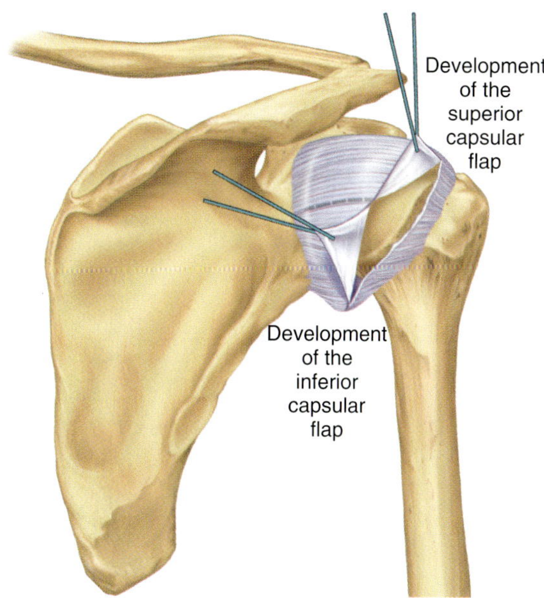

FIGURE 16

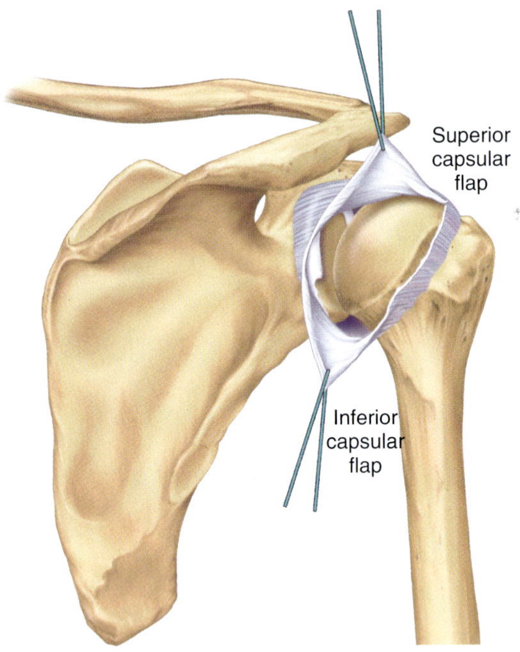

FIGURE 17

and inferior capsular flaps (Fig. 17). The medial extent of the capsular incision extends to the glenoid rim.

STEP 2

- The glenohumeral joint is inspected for posterior capsulolabral injury, glenoid and humeral articular surface injuries, and loose bodies. The diagnostic arthroscopy accomplished at the beginning of the procedure gives the surgeon a better opportunity to determine the status of the joint and any other conditions that may be present.
- If a reverse Bankart lesion or posterior capsulolabral injury is present, it is repaired with suture anchors properly placed along the prepared posterior glenoid rim (Fig. 18). Passage of the sutures through the labral capsular complex is performed in a routine manner.

STEP 3

- The capsular shift is performed after the surgeon determines the amount of capsular laxity that must be eliminated. With the patient's arm in 10° of external rotation, neutral flexion and extension, and 10° of abduction, the surgeon places his or her index finger inside the capsule along the humeral neck and pulls the inferior capsular flap superiorly and laterally

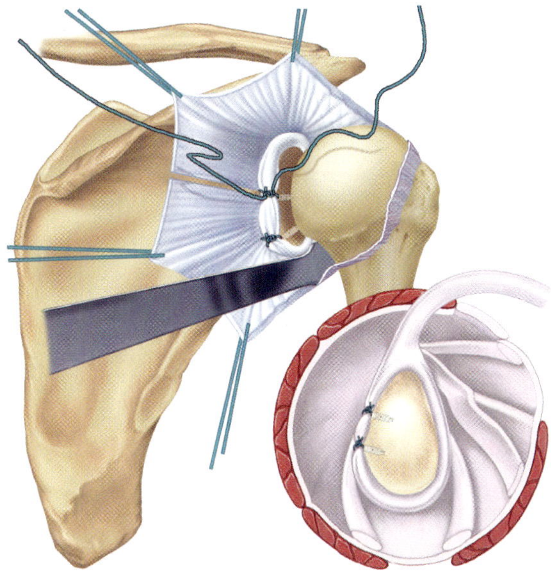

FIGURE 18

toward the capsular reattachment site. The tension created in the inferior capsular flap pushes the surgeon's finger out of the inferior recess as the capsule redundancy is eliminated.

- With the arm maintained in 10° of external rotation, 10° of abduction, and neutral flexion-extension, the superior capsular flap is shifted in an inferior and lateral direction and sutured with nonabsorbable sutures to the lateral capsular tissue that is attached to the humeral neck (Fig. 19).

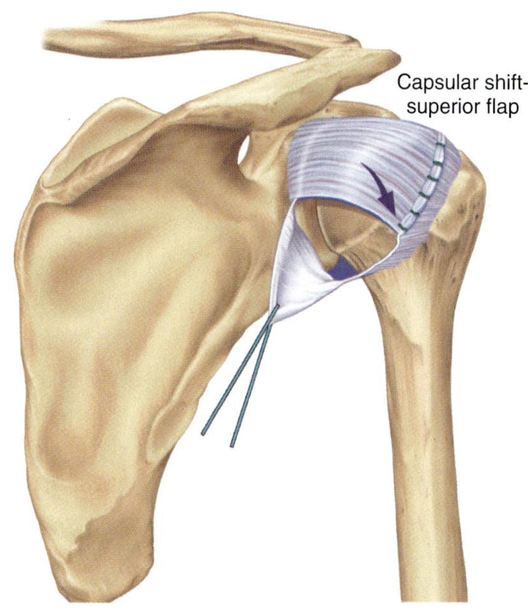

FIGURE 19

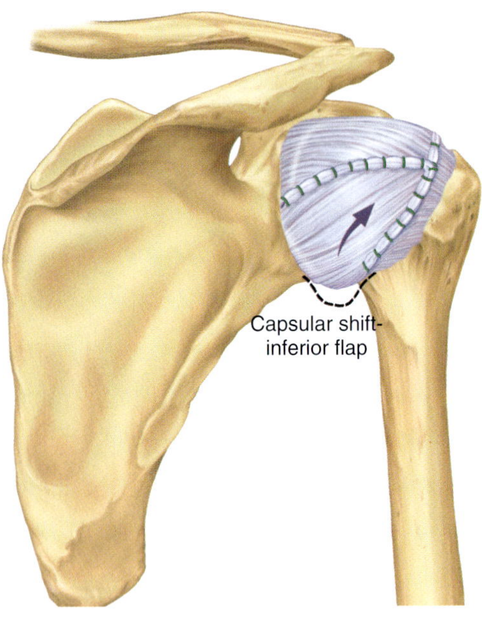

FIGURE 20

- With the arm maintained in a similar position, the inferior capsular flap is shifted superiorly and laterally to the lateral capsular edge of tissue over the capsular flap that was shifted superiorly (Fig. 20) and sutured to the lateral capsular tissue remaining on the humerus. This shift should properly tension the inferior capsule and remove the capsular redundancy that was present initially along the posterior-inferior, inferior, and anterior-inferior quadrants of the glenohumeral joint.
- Sutures are also placed horizontally to secure the inferior and superior flaps to each other.

Step 4

- With the arm maintained in neutral position for abduction, flexion-extension, and rotation, the infraspinatus tendon is sutured to the lateral portion of tendon that remains attached to the greater tuberosity and humerus (Fig. 21). Approximately five to eight single, interrupted, nonabsorbable #1 sutures are used for this repair.
- The deltoid split is repaired side to side with absorbable #1 or #0 sutures (Fig. 22). If the proximal deltoid was released along the posterior acromion, transosseous sutures are used to repair the deltoid origin back to the acromion.

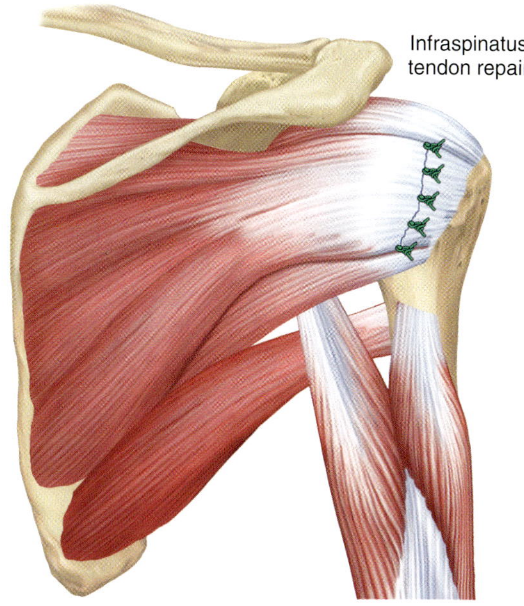

FIGURE 21

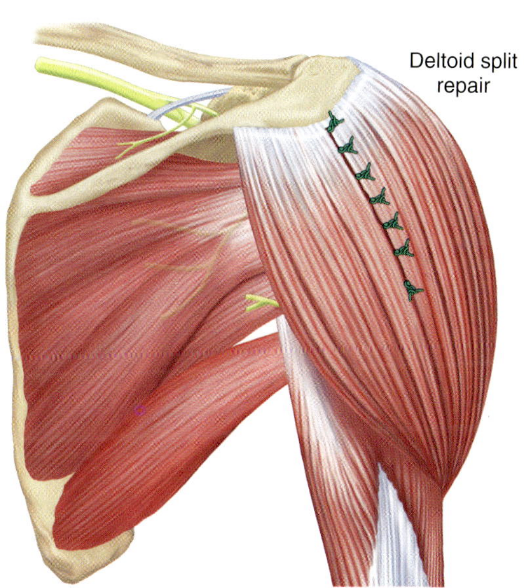

FIGURE 22

Procedure Alternatives

- Instead of a laterally based capsular shift, the surgeon may choose to perform the T-capsular shift on the glenoid or medial side of the joint (Fig. 23A).
- Additionally, an H-capsular shift can be made; the surgeon uses a medial and lateral vertical capsular incision connected by a horizontal capsular incision at the midglenoid region (Fig. 23B).

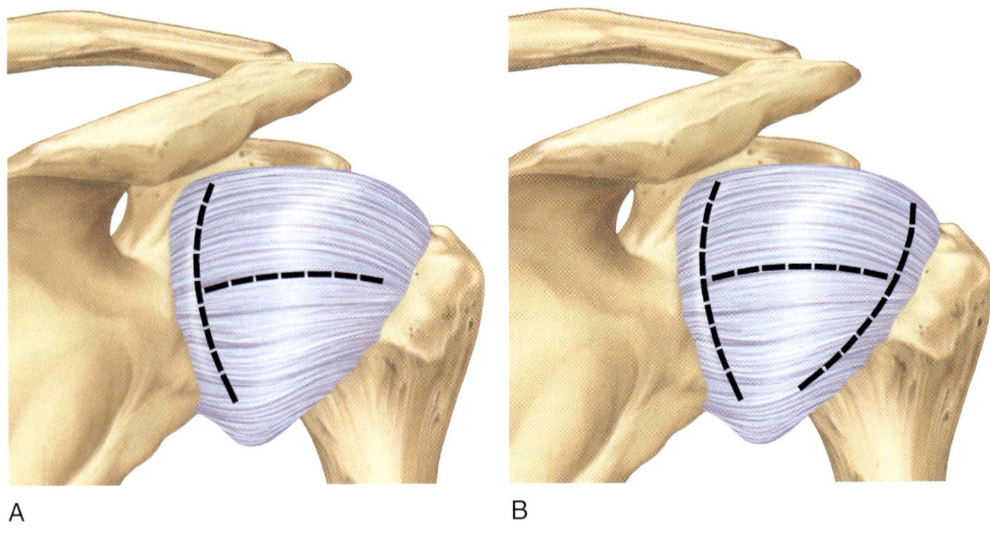

FIGURE 23

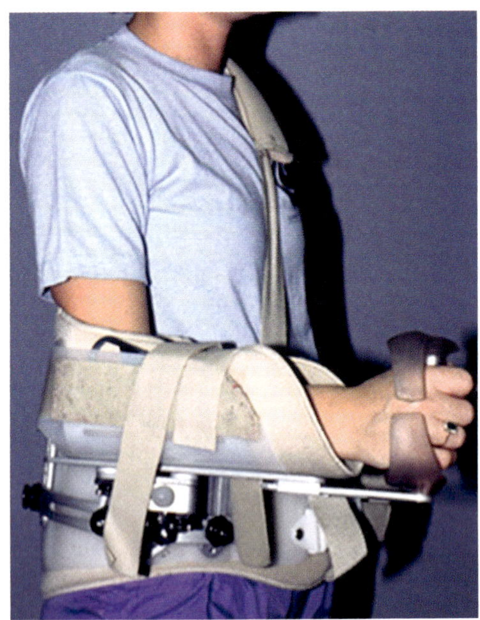

FIGURE 24

Pitfalls

- *In the early postoperative period, the provocative position of forward flexion, internal rotation, and adduction must be avoided for 6 weeks.*

Postoperative Care and Expected Outcomes

- A postoperative gunslinger brace is used for 6 weeks after surgery to maintain the arm in neutral rotation, neutral flexion-extension, and 10° of abduction (Fig. 24). The patient transitions from the brace to a sling at 6–8 weeks, after which time the arm does not need to be supported.

Complications

- Recurrent instability of the glenohumeral joint is the most common complication after open posterior capsular shift for multidirectional stability.
- Neurovascular injuries, including injuries to the axillary and suprascapular nerves, can occur; however, the surgeon should avoid injuring these structures through careful dissection technique, adequate knowledge of the surgical anatomy, and careful retraction of the deltoid and infraspinatus during the procedure.
- Postoperative stiffness or arthrofibrosis from overtightening the joint or from scar tissue and adhesion formation is unusual in patients with multidirectional instability and joint hyperlaxity. If present, it may lead to long-term degeneration of the glenohumeral joint.
- Infection.

- Postoperative day 1 through postoperative week 6
  - Passive forward elevation from the brace and the scapular plane to a maximum of 120° and passive external rotation to a maximum of 60° is started. Internal rotation should be limited to 25° across the chest. Internal rotation behind the torso should not be performed.
  - Elbow, wrist, and hand exercises and scapular shrugs are started on postoperative day 1.
- Postoperative weeks 6–12
  - Submaximal isometric strengthening exercises are begun.
  - Advanced passive and active-assisted range-of-motion exercises in all planes are begun to achieve full range of motion by postoperative week 9.
  - Active range-of-motion and strengthening exercises are begun starting at waist level and progressing overhead as tolerated.
- Postoperative week 12
  - Advanced strengthening exercises are begun, except those that involve large posteriorly directed forces.
- Postoperative month 6
  - Return to sports and other activities that require moderate to large posteriorly directed forces to the shoulder is allowed.

Evidence

Bigliani LU, Pollock RG, McIlveen SJ, Endrizzi DP, Flatow EL. Shift of the posteroinferior aspect of the capsule for recurrent posterior glenohumeral instability. J Bone Joint Surg [Am]. 1995;77:1011-20.

The researchers evaluated the outcome of 35 shoulders in 34 patients treated with superior shift of the posterior-inferior aspect of the capsule because of recurrent posterior glenohumeral subluxation and dislocation. A successful result was achieved in 23 of 24 shoulders undergoing initial repair. An unsatisfactory result was achieved in shoulders in which stabilization had already been attempted. (Case series)

Fronek J, Warren RF, Bowen M. Posterior subluxation of the glenohumeral joint. J Bone Joint Surg [Am]. 1989;71:205-16.

The results of this study revealed that nonoperative treatment with an intensive muscle-strengthening program should be used to treat patients with less severe symptoms of posterior subluxation of the glenohumeral joint. Posterior capsulorrhaphy should be used to treat patients who do not improve with nonoperative treatment or whose symptoms are severely disabling. (Case series)

Fuchs B, Jost B, Gerber C. Posterior-inferior capsular shift for the treatment of recurrent, voluntary posterior subluxation of the shoulder. J Bone Joint Surg [Am]. 2000;82:16-25.

This study revealed that, overall, operative correction of recurrent posterior subluxation in a consecutive series of 26 shoulders in 24 patients yielded satisfactory intermediate-term clinical results. (Case series)

Hawkins RJ, Janda DH. Posterior instability of the glenohumeral joint: a technique of repair. Am J Sports Med. 1996;24:275-8.

This study showed that patients who had posterior capsulotendinous tensioning procedures to treat recurrent posterior glenohumeral instability had improvements in pain and range of motion after surgery. However, four patients had minimal disability with activities of daily living, six had shoulder fatigue with occupational activities, and four had difficulty participating in sports activities. (Case series)

Misamore GW, Facibene WA. Posterior capsulorrhaphy for the treatment of traumatic recurrent posterior subluxations of the shoulder in athletes. J Shoulder Elbow Surg. 2000;9:403-8.

The study revealed that posterior capsulorrhaphy provided good or excellent results in 13 of 14 athletes with traumatic, unidirectional posterior subluxation. (Case series)

Murrell GA, Warren RF. The surgical treatment of posterior shoulder instability. Clin Sports Med. 1995;14:903-15.

In their review of the literature, the authors found that posterior shoulder instability was treated most successfully and most commonly with procedures involving reattachment of labral detachment and posterior capsular plication through a posterior approach. (Review)

Neer CS 2nd, Foster CR. Inferior capsular shift for involuntary inferior and multidirectional instability of the shoulder: a preliminary report. J Bone Joint Surg [Am]. 1980;62:897-908.

This study showed that the inferior capsular shift procedure satisfactorily corrected multidirectional instability of the shoulder through a single incision without damaging the articular surface. Seventeen of 40 shoulders were followed for more than 2 years. (Case series)

Pollock RG, Bigliani LU. Recurrent posterior shoulder instability: diagnosis and treatment. Clin Orthop Relat Res. 1993;(291):85-96.

This review revealed that a careful history and physical examination were the keys to making the diagnosis of recurrent posterior shoulder instability, and that there was no consensus on operative treatment. The authors reported that their most common finding was capsular laxity and that they preferred to treat it through a posterior-inferior capsular shift procedure, augmenting the repair with a posterior bone block in unusual cases. (Review)

Robinson CM, Aderinto J. Recurrent posterior shoulder instability. J Bone Joint Surg [Am]. 2005;87:883-92.

In this review, the authors reported that lesion-specific procedures to treat recurrent posterior shoulder instability provided better clinical results compared with nonanatomic techniques. (Review)

Tibone JE, Bradley JP. The treatment of posterior subluxation in athletes. Clin Orthop Relat Res. 1993;(291):124-37.

In this study, the authors reported that the operative treatment options varied and the results were not ideal for the small group of athletes who could not perform their sports after nonoperative treatment of recurrent posterior subluxation. The 40 athletes treated with posterior capsulorrhaphy had a 40% failure rate, with most failures related to ligamentous laxity and unrecognized multidirectional instability. Athletes competing at the highest levels had the worst results. (Case series)

Wolf BR, Strickland S, Williams RJ, Allen AA, Altchek DW, Warren RF. Open posterior stabilization for recurrent posterior glenohumeral instability. J Shoulder Elbow Surg. 2005;14:157-64.

This study revealed that open posterior shoulder stabilization reliably treated posterior instability without causing arthritic changes. Patients who had chondral defects at surgery and patients more than 37 years of age at surgery had poorer satisfaction and outcome scores compared with other patients. (Case series)

PROCEDURE 17

Arthroscopic Treatment of Posterior-Inferior Multidirectional Instability of the Shoulder

Chad J. Marion, Katie B. Vadasdi, and Christopher S. Ahmad

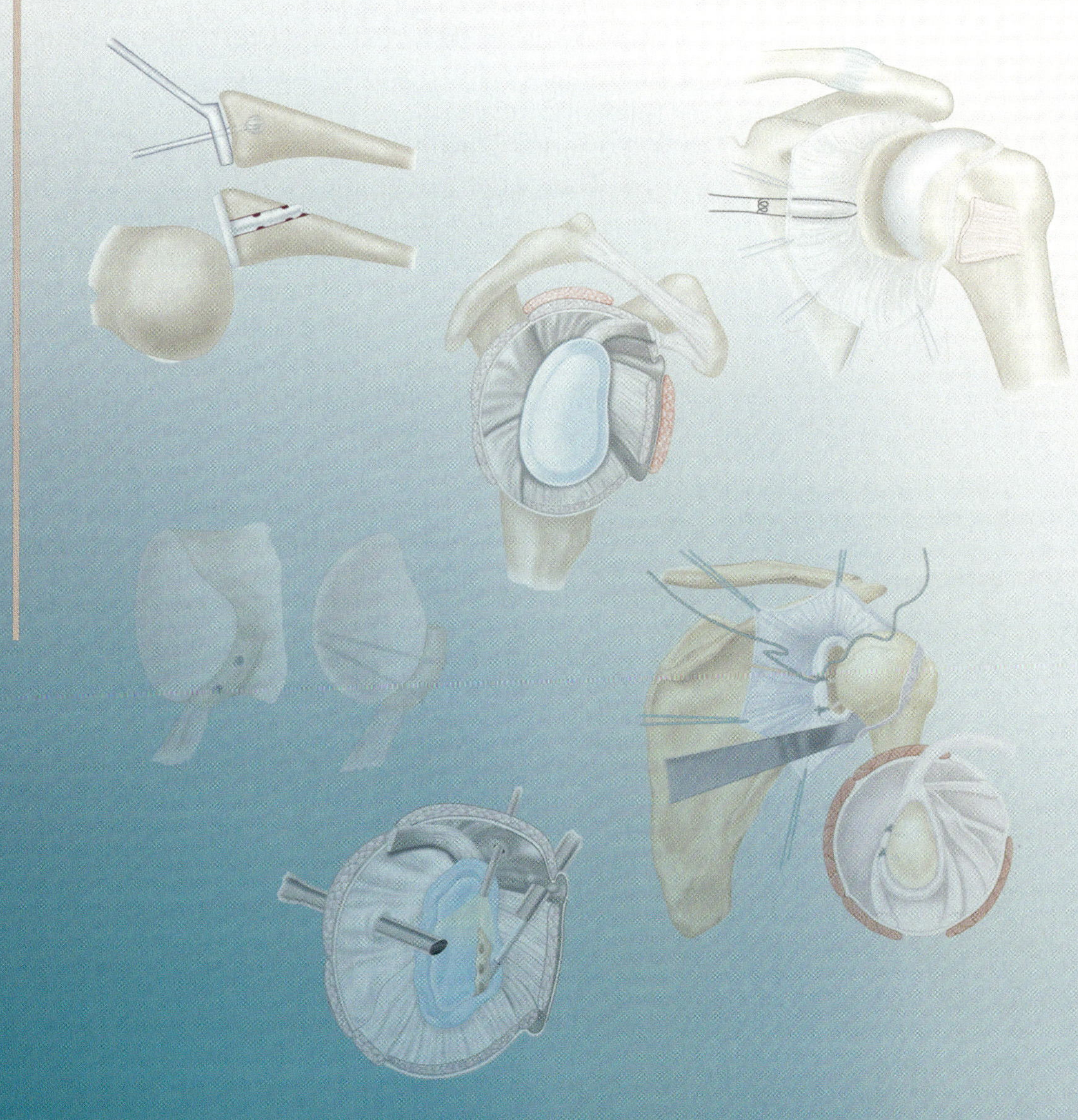

Figure 2 courtesy of Christopher S. Ahmad, MD.

Pitfalls

- *Patients who do not complete an adequate program of physical therapy*
- *Patients unwilling or unable to participate in postoperative physical therapy*
- *Voluntary dislocators with psychiatric disorders*

Controversies

- An increased risk of failure has been demonstrated historically in patients who are voluntary dislocators, as well as those with connective tissue disorders and hyperlaxity; however, successful results can be achieved in appropriately chosen individuals.

Indications

- Persistent shoulder pain, instability, or paresthesias refractory to nonoperative management

Examination/Imaging

Physical Examination

- Global tests for general ligamentous laxity include thumb abduction with palmar-flexed wrist (Fig. 1A), finger metacarpophalangeal hyperextension, and elbow hyperextension (Fig. 1B).
- Provocative tests for anterior instability include the apprehension test, relocation test, and release test.
- Examination for posterior instability includes the following tests:
  - Posterior drawer test
    - The patient is supine with the examiner standing level to the shoulder. For a left shoulder, the examiner grasps the patient's proximal forearm with the left hand, flexes the elbow to 120°, and positions the shoulder in 80–120° of abduction and 20° of forward flexion. The examiner holds the scapula with the right hand with the index and middle fingers on the scapular spine; the thumb lies directly lateral to the coracoid process so that the ulnar aspect of his or her thumb remains in contact with the coracoid while performing the test.
    - With the left hand, the examiner slightly rotates the upper arm medially and flexes it to about 80°; during this maneuver, the thumb of his or her right hand translates the humerus posteriorly. The posterior displacement can be appreciated as the examiner's thumb slides along the lateral aspect of the coracoid process.
  - Posterior load-and-shift test
    - The patient is seated with the examiner behind and on the side of the shoulder to be tested. For a right shoulder, the examiner's left hand is used to grasp and stabilize the scapula. Then his or her right hand grasps the proximal humerus, applies a medial force to center the humeral head relative to the glenoid, and then applies a posteriorly directed force, noting the amount of translation of the humeral head on the glenoid.
    - Translation is graded as 0 if there is minimal translation, +1 if the humeral head rides up on the posterior glenoid rim, +2 if the humeral head rides over the glenoid rim but reduces

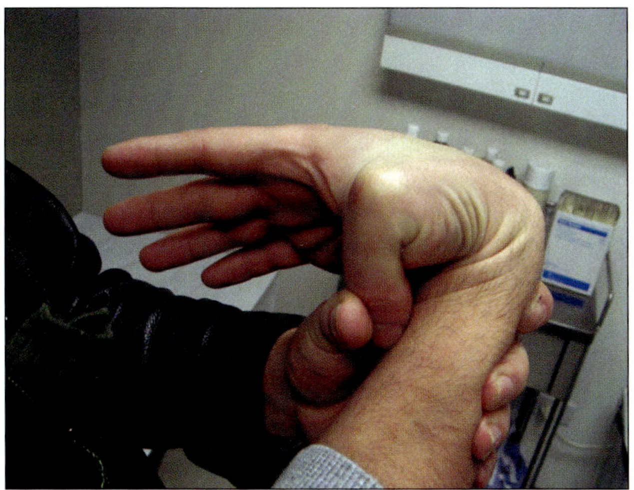

A

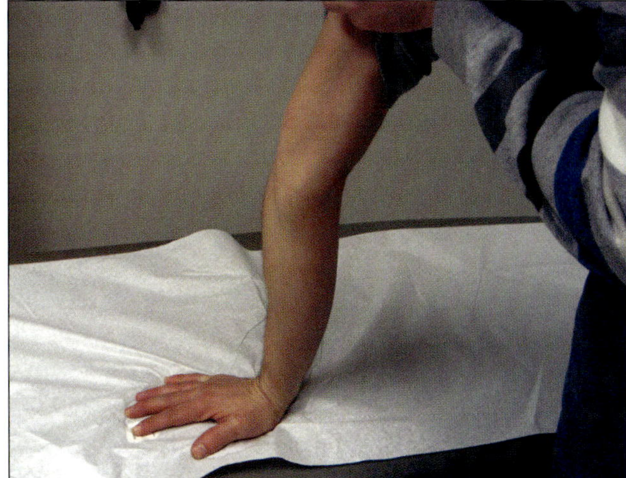

B

FIGURE 1

when the force is removed, and +3 if the humeral head dislocates posteriorly and remains dislocated when the posteriorly applied force is removed.

- Modified posterior load-and-shift test—The patient is supine with the tested shoulder on the edge of the table in neutral rotation. An axial force is applied at the elbow to concentrically reduce the humeral head, and then a posteriorly directed force is applied in varying degrees of rotation and elevation, grading the translation in the same manner as the posterior load-and-shift test.
- Posterior stress test—The patient lies supine and the arm is flexed to 90° and internally rotated. An axial load is applied to the humerus with one of the examiner's hands while the other hand is placed on the back of the shoulder to stabilize it. A positive test results in palpable or observable subluxation of the humeral head over the glenoid rim.
- Jerk test—The patient sits upright and the arm is flexed 90° and internally rotated, and the elbow is flexed 90°. An axial load is applied to the arm, with the other arm supporting the posterior shoulder, and then the arm is extended. A positive test is indicated when there is a sudden jerk as the glenohumeral joint is reduced from a posteriorly dislocated or subluxed humeral head.

- The sulcus test is performed with the patient seated as an inferiorly directed force is applied to the elbow.

The sulcus, or gap between the greater tuberosity and acromion, is visualized and measured in centimeters. A value greater than 2 cm suggests multidirectional instability (MDI). Failure to reduce in external rotation suggests rotator interval insufficiency, while a sulcus that does not decrease in abduction suggests redundancy of the inferior pouch.

Imaging Studies

- Plain radiographs
  - Glenohumeral anteroposterior views with the arm in internal and external rotation, as well as scapular Y and axillary views, should be obtained.
  - Radiographs are often normal but should be evaluated for humeral head or glenoid defects, wear, or reactive bone.
  - Glenoid retroversion should also be measured and, when excessive, the need for a bony procedure such as an opening wedge osteotomy may be indicated.
- Magnetic resonance imaging (MRI)
  - MRI arthrography offers excellent visualization of the labrum, glenohumeral ligaments, and rotator cuff.
    - Figure 2A is an axial plane MRI arthrogram demonstrating posterior labral detachment (*arrow*).
    - Figure 2B is an MRI arthrogram demonstrating a patulous capsule in a patient with MDI.
- Labral detachment and/or capsular redundancy are the most frequent findings in MDI and posterior instability; however, the MRI arthrogram may be completely normal.

Examination Under Anesthesia

- Examination under anesthesia (EUA) is 100% sensitive and 93% specific in determining the direction of shoulder laxity (Cofield et al., 1993).
- Findings of increased glenohumeral translation during EUA should be compared to the contralateral shoulder and should be combined with the history and physical as it does not always imply instability.

Treatment Options

- Nonoperative treatment with a course of physical therapy is the initial management of both MDI and posterior instability and may follow a period of treatment with immobilization and nonsteroidal anti-inflammatory drugs if there is significant pain.
- Open inferior capsular shift, bone grafting, or bone transfer have been described for posterior instability and are the treatment of choice if significant bony defects exist that contribute to instability.
- Arthroscopic treatment has decreased operative morbidity, and current techniques produce clinical results equal to open techniques.
- Arthroscopic techniques include multiple portals and a percutaneous technique. We prefer the percutaneous technique to minimize morbidity to the rotator interval and rotator cuff while facilitating improved anchor placement and suture passing.

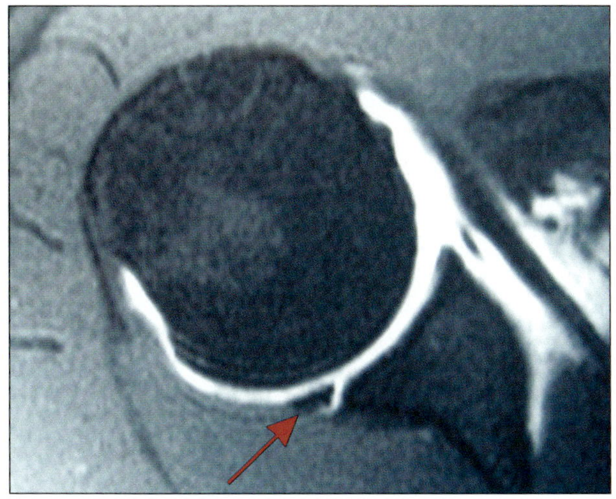

A

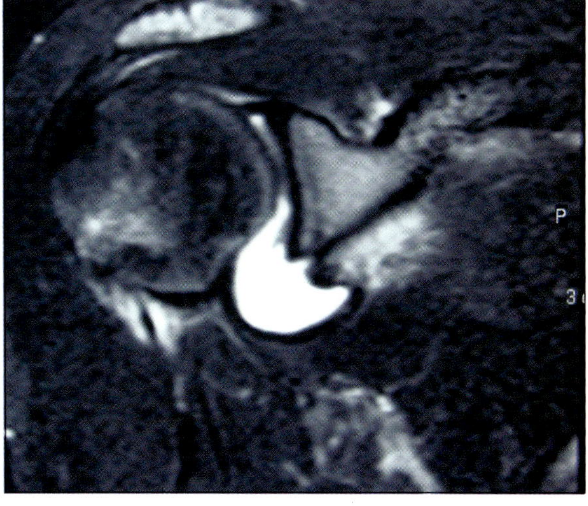

B

FIGURE 2

Surgical Anatomy

- Relevant structures during arthroscopic treatment of MDI include the labrum, superior glenohumeral ligament, middle glenohumeral ligament, subscapularis, supraspinatus, biceps tendon, and rotator interval, as seen in the sagittal view of a right shoulder in Figure 3, as well as the axillary nerve.
- MDI typically involves a large, patulous inferior capsular pouch with wide rotator interval, while posterior instability typically involves posterior labral tears (see Fig. 2A) and a patulous posterior capsule.

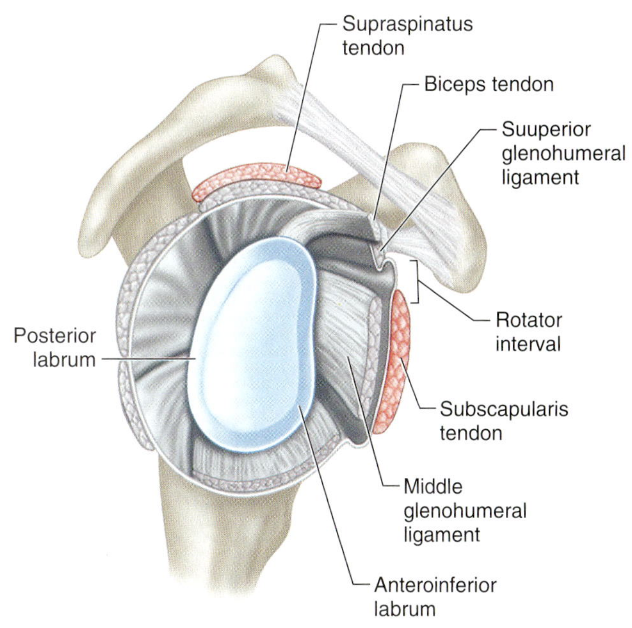

FIGURE 3

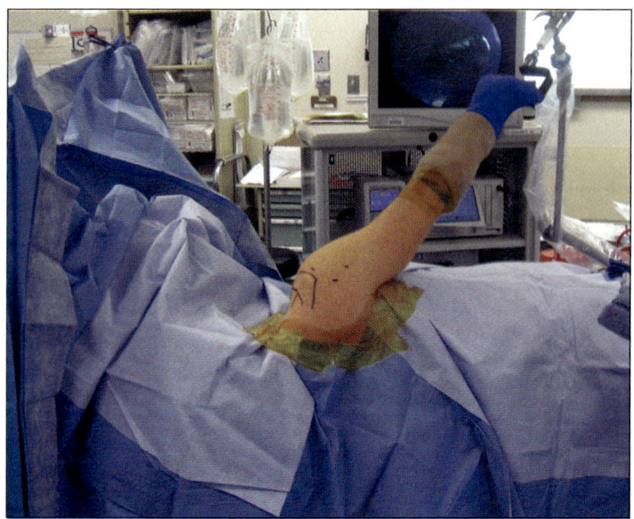

FIGURE 4

Pearls

- *A bump in the axilla of the operative shoulder creates improved working space in the glenohumeral joint by displacing the humeral head away from the glenoid.*
- *Patient positioning should allow the surgeon to stand at the patient's head to facilitate easy access to the posterior aspect of the shoulder while the camera is placed in the anterior aspect.*

Pitfalls

- *Overdistraction on the arm should be avoided as it can lead to brachial plexus injury. Typically 10 lbs of distraction is safe and sufficient.*

Equipment

- Hydraulic (see Fig. 4) or weight-suspension lateral positioning equipment allows movement in all planes as well as rotation and tension.

Positioning

- The lateral decubitus or beach chair position may be used based on surgeon preference.
- We prefer the lateral decubitus position with traction (Fig. 4) because of improved global visualization and access to the anterior, posterior, and inferior labrum and capsule.
- The patient is positioned with a beanbag, padding all bony prominences and using an axillary roll.
- The bed is positioned in 15° of reverse Trendelenberg and tilted approximately 10° posteriorly to position the glenoid parallel to the floor.
- The arm is placed in traction in 40° of abduction and 10° of forward elevation.

Portals/Exposures

- Mark out the traditional landmarks, including the acromion, clavicle, and coracoid.
- The posterior viewing portal (Fig. 5, *A*) is made 2 cm inferior to the posterolateral corner of the acromion. This is slightly lateral to the classic portal, allowing better visualization and instrumentation of the posterior labrum.
- The anterior portal (see Fig. 5, *B*) is placed using direct visualization through the rotator interval. Precise placement is achieved by using a spinal needle as a preliminary probe to access the labrum and glenoid.

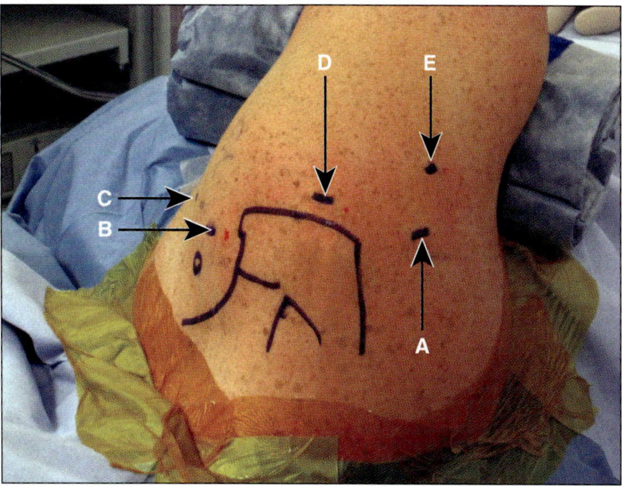

FIGURE 5

Controversies

- Beach chair versus lateral decubitus position

Pearls

- *The posterior viewing portal should be made more lateral than usual to facilitate viewing and instrumentation of the posterior capsulolabral complex.*
- *Exact percutaneous portal placement is determined using a spinal needle as a preliminary guide.*
- *Appropriate placement of the cannulas is imperative and can be tested by visualizing the entry point in the interval using a spinal needle as a probe and judging the best "angle of attack" on the labrum.*
- *If the posterior portal is not ideal for posterior labral work, it should be re-established under direct visualization from the anterior portal.*

- Percutaneous access to the anterior, superior, and posterior labrum is created at three locations:
  - The anteroinferior portal (see Fig. 5, *C*), approximately 3 cm inferior and 2 cm lateral to the coracoid
  - The Wilmington portal (see Fig. 5, *D*), just off and in the posterior third of the acromion
  - The posteroinferior portal (see Fig. 5, *E*), just inferior and lateral to the posterior viewing portal

Procedure

Step 1

- The posterior viewing portal is established and a diagnostic arthroscopy is performed.
  - Special attention is paid to the anterior, superior, and inferior labrum as well as any articular-side rotator cuff tears.
  - Often with MDI the humeral head will sublux inferiorly, and a "drive-through" sign will be present.
- A spinal needle is introduced through the interval and used as a probe to confirm appropriate access to the anteroinferior and superior labrum.
- An incision is made and a cannula is placed in the interval. A probe is introduced through the cannula and used to assess the integrity of the labral attachment to the glenoid.

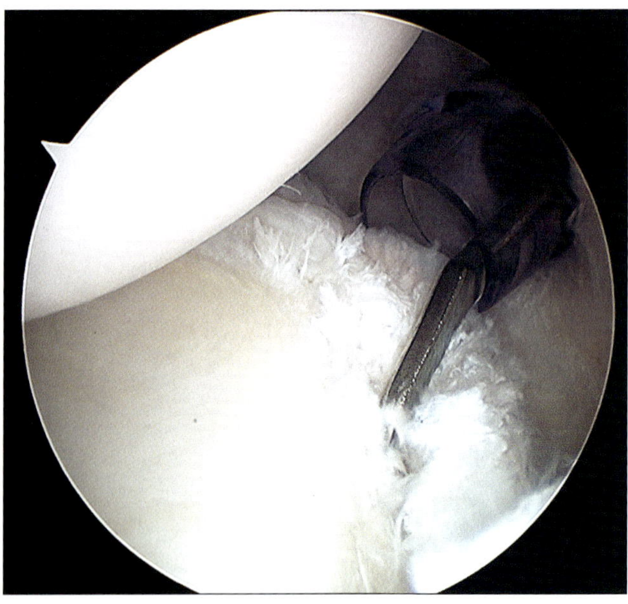

FIGURE 6

- Next, the arthroscope is placed into the anterior cannula to assess the posterior capsulolabral complex and the anterior-inferior glenoid bony architecture, and to identify anterior labral periosteal sleeve avulsion lesions. Figure 6 shows a posterior labral tear visualized from the anterior viewing portal.
- While the arthroscope is in the anterior portal, a 7-mm cannula is introduced over a switching stick in the posterior portal.

PITFALLS

- *Care should be taken while making the anteroinferior percutaneous portal as deviation into the axilla with instruments places neurovascular structures at risk.*

Step 2

- All labral tissues deemed necessary for repair in Step 1 are mobilized and the glenoid surfaces adjacent to the labrum are abraded to enhance healing.
  - An arthroscopic elevator (Fig. 6) is used to fully elevate and mobilize the torn labrum from the glenoid neck so that it can be mobilized back to anatomic position (see Video 1), and to abrade the glenoid neck (Fig. 7).
  - Next a motorized shaver is introduced through the cannula to débride the glenoid neck (Fig. 8; see Video 3).
- Figure 9 shows a posterior labrum mobilized from a medial scarred position and ready for repair.

PEARLS

- *The entire labrum should be probed for avulsions or tears and an overall plan determined prior to beginning the repair.*
- *The posterior labrum should be evaluated from the anterior portal.*

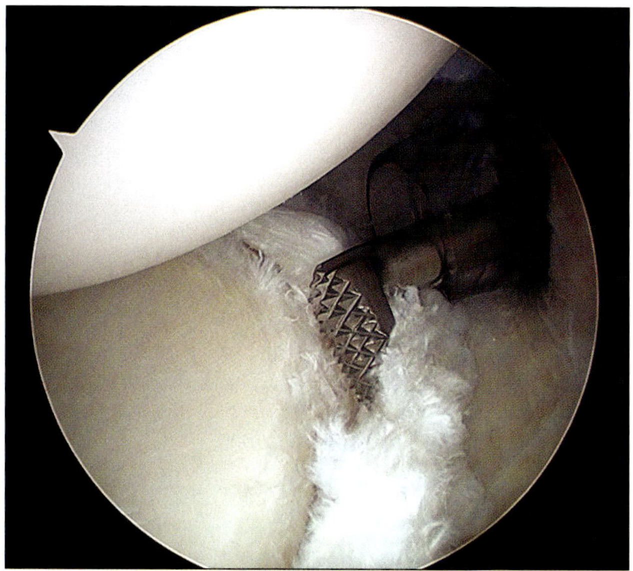

FIGURE 7

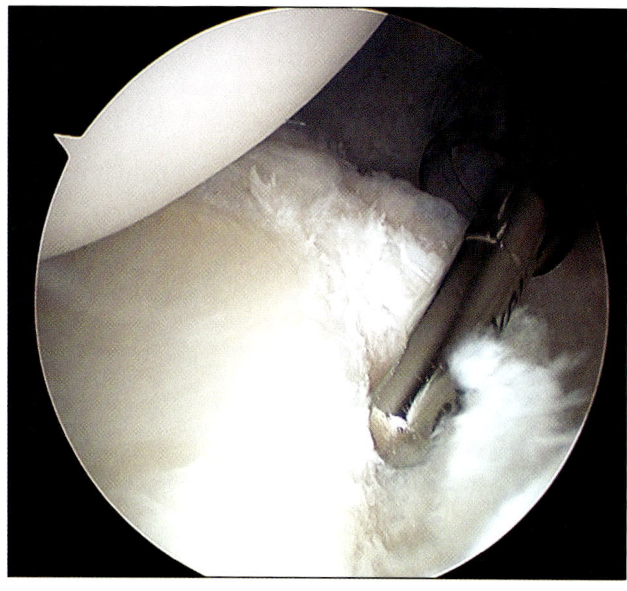

FIGURE 8

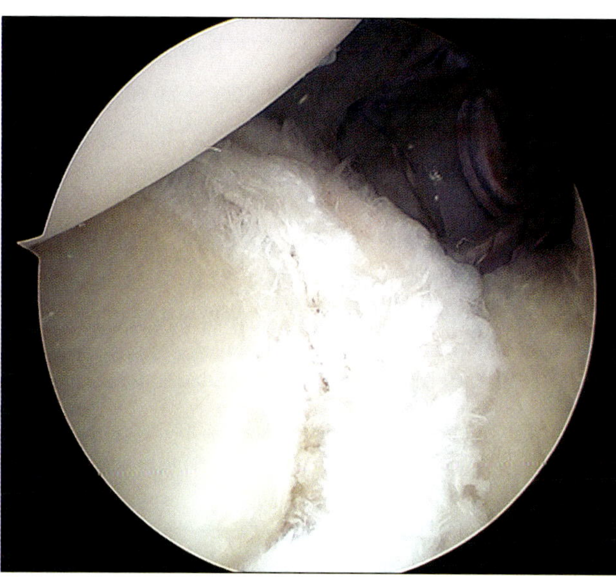

FIGURE 9

PEARLS

- *Typically the anterior labrum is worked on by viewing from the posterior portal and instrumenting through the anterior portal; conversely, for posterior work viewing is from the anterior portal and instrumenting from the posterior portal.*

STEP 3

- The posterior suture anchors are now placed and sutures passed. Our preferred technique is percutaneous placement of suture anchors and suture passing.
  - A spinal needle is introduced approximately 3 cm inferior and 1 cm lateral to the posterolateral acromion and adjusted as needed to allow optimal placement of anchors onto the glenoid rim.
  - A 3-mm stab incision is made and a 3-mm drill guide with a blunt tip is introduced through the posterior capsule under direct visualization from the anterior portal (see Video 4).

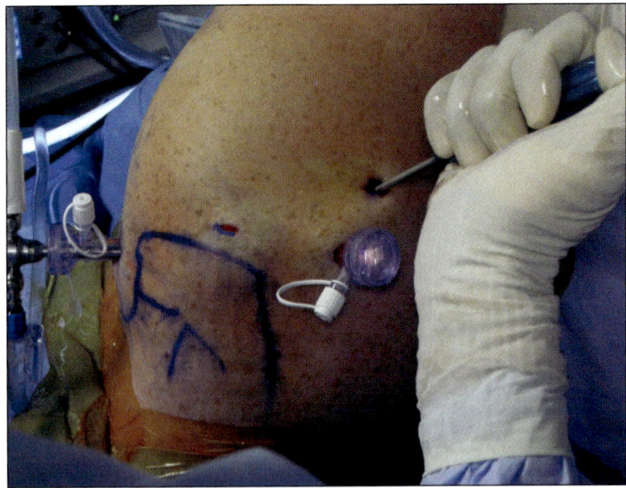

A

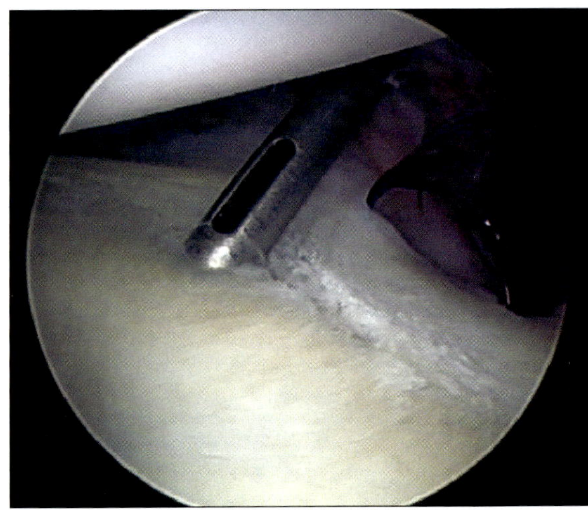

B

FIGURE 10

Instrumentation/ Implantation

- We prefer to use a 4.0-mm shaver inside the glenoid joint.
- A 90° "boot" rasp frequently allows excellent access to the posteroinferior labrum (see Fig. 7 and Video 2).

Pearls

- *The sequence of repair should be:*
  - *First, placement of posterior suture anchors and suture passage*
  - *Second, placement of anterior suture anchors, anterior suture passage, and anterior knot tying*
  - *Third, posterior knot tying*
  - *Fourth, rotator interval closure if the interval is found to be incompetent*

- Figure 10A shows the percutaneous placement of a drill guide and the angle necessary for anchor penetration into the glenoid neck.
- Figure 10B shows an arthroscopic view of drill guide placement for the most inferior anchor placement.
- The blunt trochar is removed, and the drill guide positioned on the margin of the articular surface.
- The hole is drilled through the guide and a 2.4-mm anchor placed. Anchor security is checked with a tug on the sutures (see Video 5).
- The suture limb closest to the labrum is retrieved out of the posterior cannula (see Video 6).
- A curved suture passer is introduced through the same percutaneous hole made by the drill guide in the posterior capsule (Fig. 11).

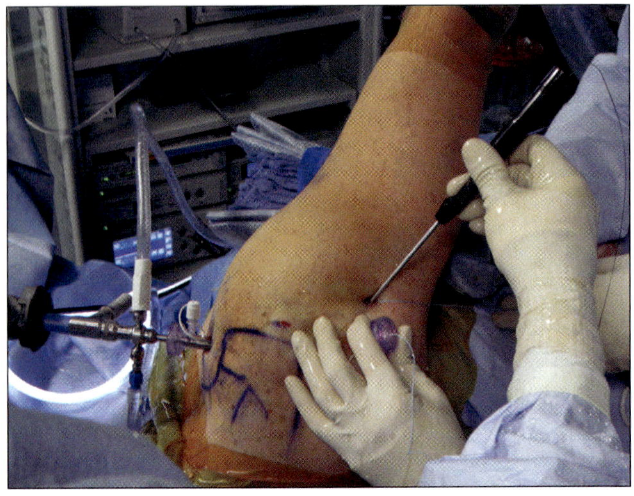

FIGURE 11

- If tissue imbrication is desired, the suture passer is passed into and out of the capsule roughly 1 cm posteroinferior to the anchor and then penetrates the labrum at the level of the suture anchor.
  - This "pinch-tuck" maneuver helps achieve a "south-to-north" shift of the capsule.
- The wire shuttle is advanced into the joint and retrieved out of the posterior cannula. Figure 12 shows the suture passer entering through the posterior capsular rent, penetrating the inferior capsule, and skiving under the labrum at the level of the suture anchor, and the wire being retrieved through the posterior cannula (see Video 7).
- The suture is shuttled by passing the suture through the loop outside the cannula and then retrieving the wire out the percutaneous working site (see Video 8). Figure 13 shows sutures exiting through the percutaneous posterolateral portal after passage through the capsule and labrum.

- Anchors should be placed and sutures passed from most inferior (6 o'clock) to superior and be spaced 5 to 8 mm apart.

Instrumentation/ Implantation

- We prefer to use 2.4-mm bioabsorbable anchors in the glenoid.
- 7.0-mm clear cannulas are preferred for ease of suture grasping and tying.
- A nonserrated loop grasper is used to retrieve sutures and the wire shuttle.

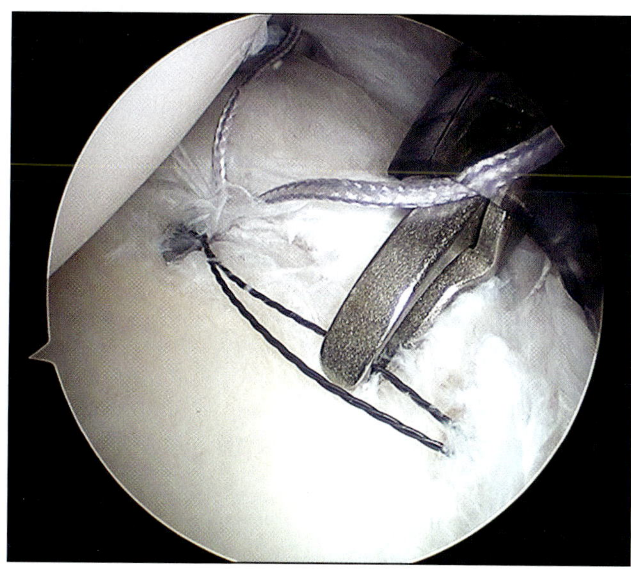

FIGURE 12

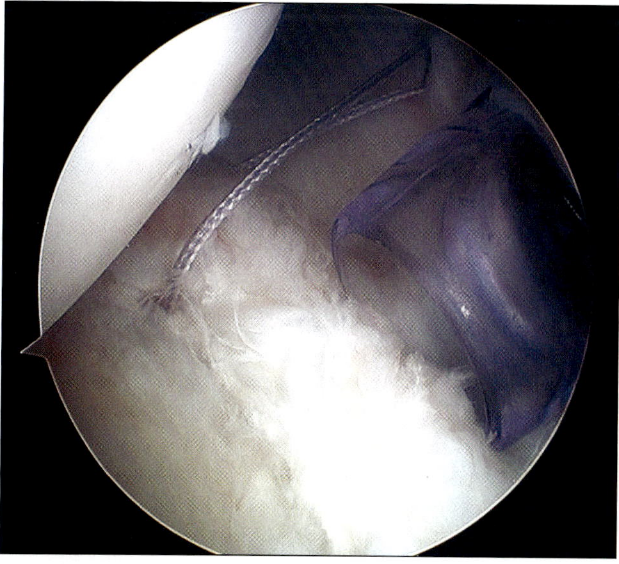

FIGURE 13

Controversies

- A nonpercutaneous method is available using an accessory posterolateral cannula. However, we find that the percutaneous method is less traumatic to the soft tissues and allows more precise placement of suture anchors and suture passing.

Pitfalls

- *A blunt trochar should be used through the anteroinferior percutaneous portal and care taken to avoid entering the axilla as the deep neurovascular structures can be injured.*

- Arthroscopic knot tying is done using the suture limb passed through the tissue as the post to position the labrum up onto the glenoid and keep the knot away from the articular surface (see Video 9). Figure 14 shows a second suture anchor ready for knot tying. Note that the posterior capsulolabral "bumper" is already improved after tying the first suture anchor.
- In the setting of MDI, the sutures are left in the percutaneous portal untied to optimize visualization and working room on the anterior structures.
  - If the labrum is robust and attached to the glenoid rim, capsular plication to the labrum without using an anchor may be performed.
- In the setting of isolated posterior instability, we tie the sutures from inferior to superior. Sutures are retrieved out of the posterior cannula and tied.
- The number of suture anchors depends on the extent of the pathology found, and placement of anchors continues until the labrum can be probed and is secure.

Step 4

- In the setting of MDI, the anterior suture anchors are now placed, and sutures are passed and subsequently tied, progressing inferior to superior.
  - The arthroscope is placed back into the posterior cannula and used for anterior structure visualization.
  - Again, we prefer a percutaneous technique for anterior suture anchor placement and suture passing.
  - A spinal needle is introduced approximately 4 cm inferior and slightly lateral to the anterior cannula and used to identify the ideal angle to place the most anteroinferior anchor, which typically is located at the 5–6 o'clock position on a right shoulder.
  - A 3-mm stab incision is made and the 3-mm drill guide with a blunt trochar is introduced through the subscapularus tendon and capsule and placed on the face of the glenoid rim.
  - The drill is used through the guide and an anchor is placed as previously described.
  - The suture closest to the labrum is retrieved through the anterior cannula, and subsequently a suture passer is introduced through the same small defect in the anterior capsule created by the anchor drill guide.
  - The suture passer enters the capsulolabral complex inferior to the anchor and pierces between the

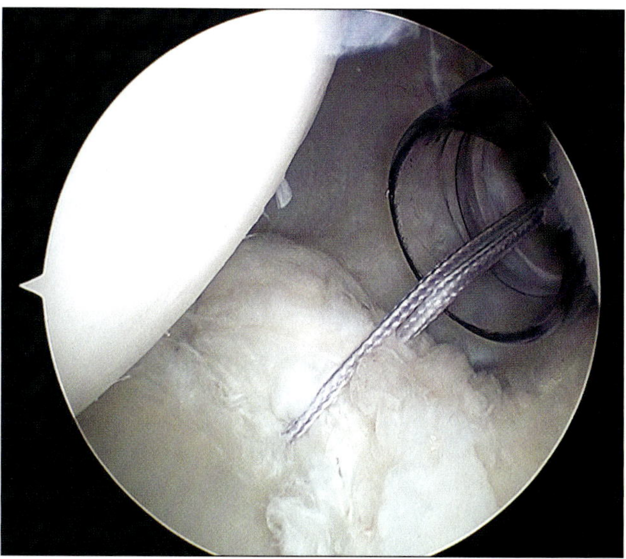

FIGURE 14

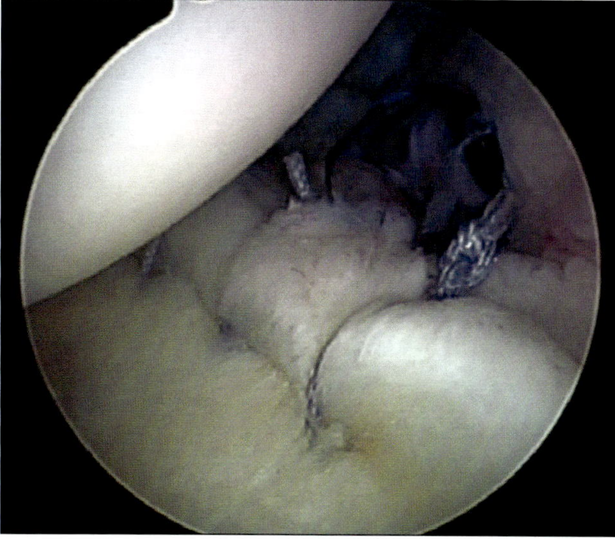

FIGURE 15

labrum and glenoid rim just inferior to or at the location of the anchor to achieve a superior shift.
- The shuttling wire is passed under the labrum and retrieved out of the anterior cannula. The suture is passed through the shuttle loop, and subsequently pulled out of the anteroinferior percutaneous portal with the suture-passing device.
- The sutures are then retrieved through the anterior cannula and tied. As with the posterior anchors, the post used in tying is always the suture passed through the labrum, to place the knot away from the articular surface.

■ The sutures are cut and the same steps are repeated progressing superiorly using the same percutaneous incision, typically ending with three or four total anchors.

Step 5

■ The arthroscope is then placed back into the anterior portal and the posterior knots are tied and cut from inferior to superior if not done previously (Fig. 15).

Step 6

■ The rotator interval is inspected by viewing through the posterior portal. If wide and also with a sulcus sign that does not reduce with external rotation, rotator interval closure may be elected.

■ A rasp is placed through the anterior portal and used to abrade the interval tissue.

■ A long monofilament suture is placed through the superior border of the subscapularis tendon or

Pearls

- *The SGHL can be found adjacent to the supraspinatus tendon.*
- *A second suture can be placed in the same manner if necessary.*

Pitfalls

- *External rotation should be assessed at the conclusion to ensure that the closure did not overconstrict motion.*

middle glenohumeral ligament (MGHL) using a suture-passing device, with the wire removed via the anterior cannula.

- The anterior cannula is then withdrawn to just outside the capsule and a penetrating suture grasper is placed through it, passing through the superior glenohumeral ligament (SGHL) 1 cm medial to the humeral insertion of the supraspinatus tendon.
- The penetrating suture grasper then retrieves the suture limb and pulls it out of the cannula. Figure 16 shows a penetrating suture grasper passed through the SGHL and retrieving the monofilament suture already passed through the MGHL.
- At this point, the monofilament suture can be tied and cut with the arm in external rotation, or a braided nonabsorbable suture can be tied to the monofilament and shuttled through the interval, at which point it is tied and cut.
  - Figure 17 shows a braided nonabsorbable suture passed through the interval prior to tying.
  - Figure 18 shows the rotator interval closed after tying the suture.

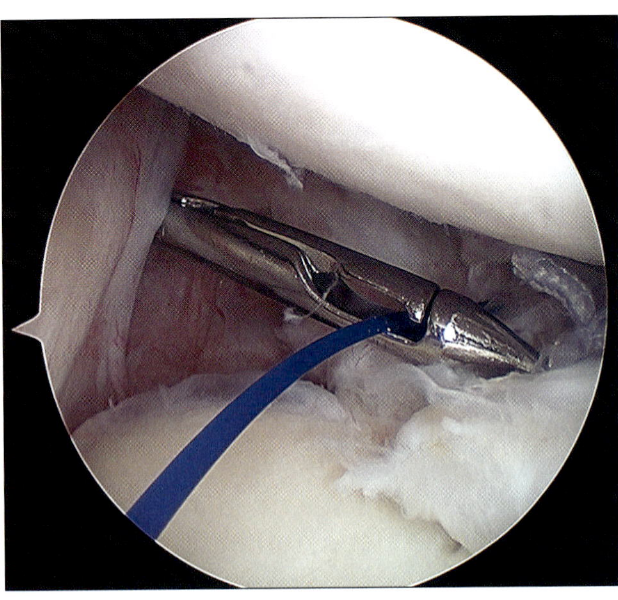

FIGURE 16

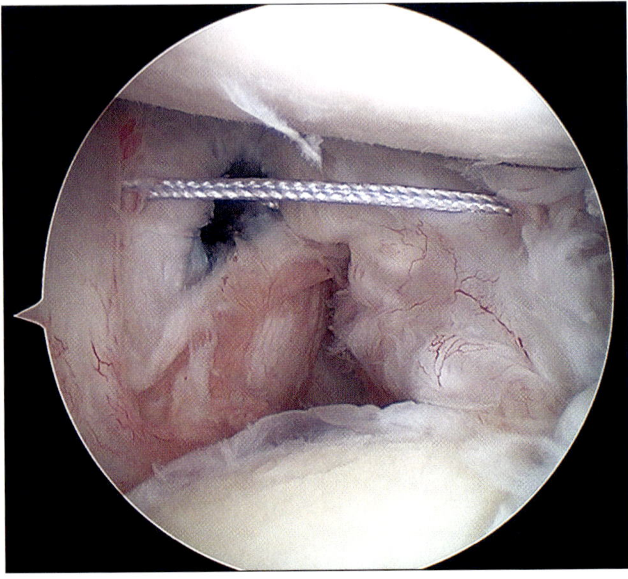

FIGURE 17

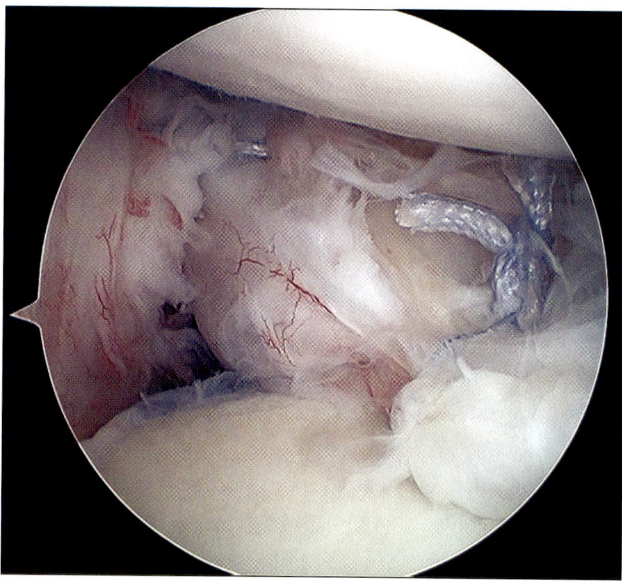

FIGURE 18

Postoperative Care and Expected Outcomes

- Immobilization in a sling with the arm in abduction and neutral to slight external rotation is recommended postoperatively for 3–6 weeks for posterior instability and 6 weeks for MDI patients.
- The patient comes out of the sling daily for elbow, wrist, and hand exercises only.
- At 3 weeks, gentle rotational exercises are begun with rotation limits that are extended at the 6-week mark.
- After 6 weeks, progressive strengthening exercises may begin.
- The patient should expect full strength and range of motion by 6 months, at which time he or she may return to full sports participation.
- External rotation exercises and strength should be emphasized and continued for patients with posterior instability.
- Potential complications include stiffness should the patient not be diligent in the physical therapy program or failure of the repair if the patient is active too early and is not compliant with the postoperative restrictions.

Evidence

Bradley JP, Baker CL 3rd, Kline AJ, et al. Arthroscopic capsulolabral reconstruction for posterior instability of the shoulder: a prospective study of 100 shoulders. Am J Sports Med. 2006;34:1061-71.

The authors reported 89% return to sport at 27 months, and 89% with good or excellent results, in their group of 71 shoulders that were treated with arthroscopic capsulolabral reconstruction for recurrent posterior shoulder instability.

Cofield RH, Nessler JP, Weinstabl R. Diagnosis of shoulder instability by examination under anesthesia. Clin Orthop Relat Res. 1993; Jun (291): 45-53.

D'Alessandro DF, Bradley JP, Fleischli JE, et al. Prospective evaluation of thermal capsulorraphy for shoulder instability: indications and results, two- to five-year follow-up. Am J Sports Med. 2004;32:21-33.

In this report on 84 shoulders treated for shoulder instability with thermal capsulorraphy, the average follow-up was 38 months. Overall results were excellent in 33 participants (39%), satisfactory in 20 (24%), and unsatisfactory in 31 (37%).

Duncan R, Savoie FH 3rd. Arthroscopic inferior capsular shift for multidirectional instability of the shoulder: a preliminary report. Arthroscopy. 1993;9:24-7.

This is the first reported series of 10 patients treated arthroscopically for MDI. All patients had a satisfactory result according to Neer criteria at 1 to 3 years postoperatively and an average Rowe score of 90 (range, 75-95).

Gartsman GM, Roddey TS, Hammerman SM. Arthroscopic treatment of multidirectional glenohumeral instability: 2- to 5-year follow-up. Arthroscopy. 2001;17:236-43.

The authors presented results in a series of 47 shoulders with MDI treated with suture anchors, capsular plication, and rotator interval closure with mean follow-up of 35 months. Postoperatively, 94% were rated good or excellent, with a 2% recurrence rate. Average passive external rotation was 88.2°, with 85% returning to desired level of sports participation.

Lichtenberg S, Habermeyer P, Magosch P, et al. Arthroscopic treatment of posterior shoulder instability. Op Orthop Traumatol. 2007;19:115-32.

In this prospective study of 11 shoulders, labral pathology was treated by mobilization and suture anchor fixation as well as capsular plication. The overall Rowe score was 95/100 at 33 months, with one traumatic redislocation and another patient with recurrent subluxations.

McIntyre LF, Caspari RB, Savoie FH 3rd. The arthroscopic treatment of multidirectional shoulder instability: two-year results of a multiple suture technique. Arthroscopy. 1997;13:418-25.

The authors reported on an arthroscopic capsular shift in 19 shoulders with a mean follow-up of 34 months. They found excellent or good results in 95% of patients with no loss of motion, 5% recurrence rate, and 89% of athletes returning to their previous level of performance.

Treacy SH, Savoie FH 3rd, Field LD. Arthroscopic treatment of multidirectional instability. J Shoulder Elbow Surg. 1999;8:345-50.

In this report on 25 shoulders with a 60-month follow-up, 88% had a satisfactory result according to Neer criteria, with a 12% recurrence rate; 96% had full range of motion; and none experienced loss of external rotation.

PROCEDURE 18

Open Bankart Procedure for Recurrent Anterior Shoulder Dislocation

Peter S. Vezeridis and Bertram Zarins

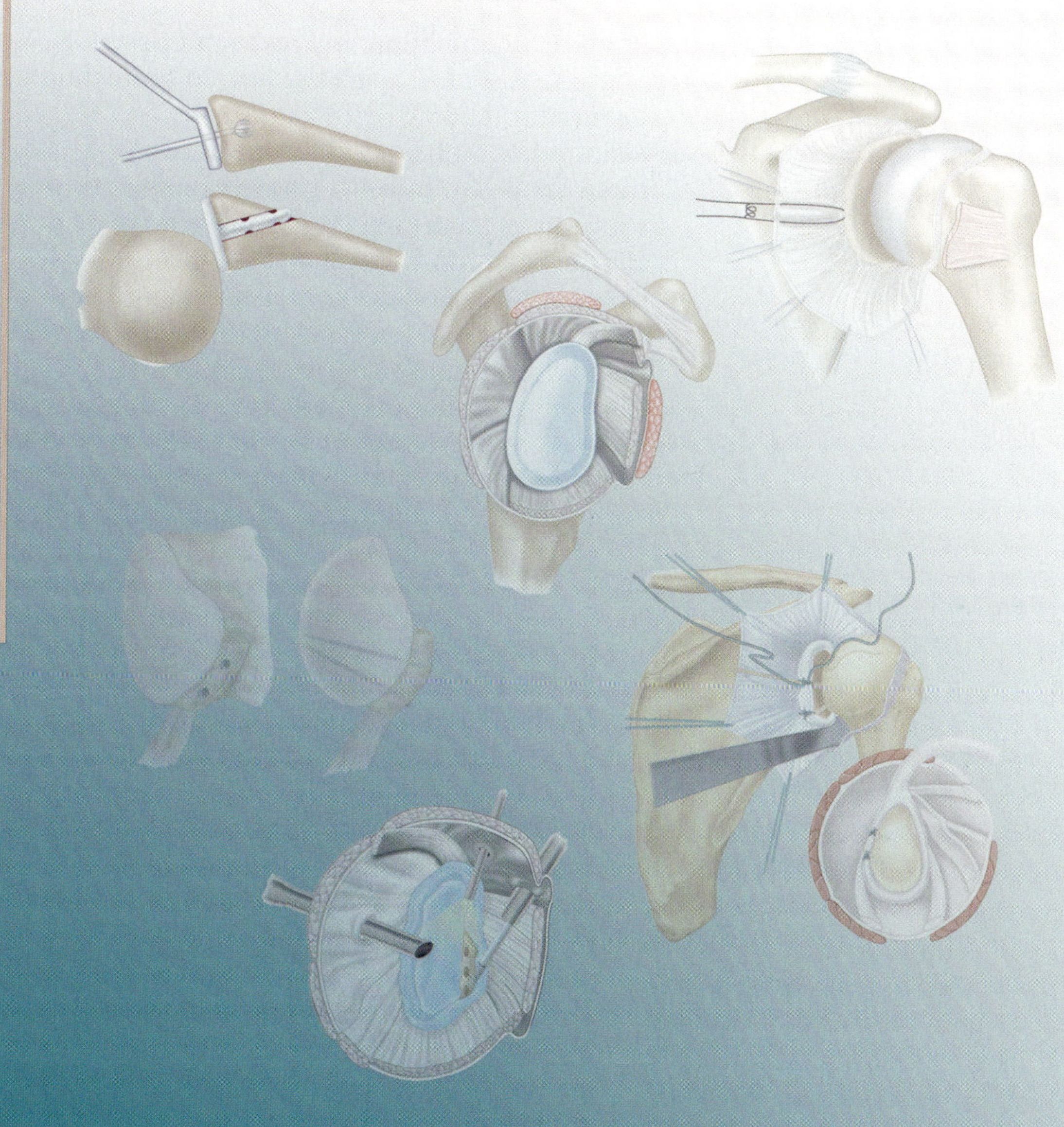

PITFALLS

- *A large fracture of the anterior glenoid rim might also need a bone graft.*
- *An altered surgical field, especially after a failed Bristow-type procedure, makes exposure difficult.*

Controversies

- The open Bankart procedure has been the "gold standard" for surgical stabilization of the glenohumeral joint, but arthroscopic repairs have become easier to perform and have success rates similar to those of open surgery.

Treatment Options

- Arthroscopic Bankart repair is usually the procedure of choice, but if there is insufficient capsular or labral tissue to repair, then open repair might give a better result.
- An open Bristow or Latarjet procedure may be indicated if there is large bone loss of the anterior glenoid rim.

Indications

- Recurrent anterior glenohumeral dislocation that cannot be repaired arthroscopically because of factors such as
  - Deficient anterior capsule
  - Fracture of the anterior glenoid rim
  - Failed prior arthroscopic or open Bankart repair
  - Failed prior open surgery if a Bankart lesion was not addressed

Examination/Imaging

- Physical examination will reveal a positive apprehension test with the arm in abduction and external rotation.
- Plain radiographs: an anteroposterior or axillary view often shows an indistinct anterior glenoid rim, suggesting fracture (bony Bankart lesion) and/or a Hill-Sachs lesion of the humeral head.
- Computed tomography scan with contrast will show avulsion of the anterior glenoid labrum from the glenoid rim (Bankart lesion) (Fig. 1).
- Magnetic resonance imaging with contrast will demonstrate avulsion of the anterior glenoid labrum from the glenoid rim (Bankart lesion) with the capsule retracted onto the glenoid neck (Fig. 2).

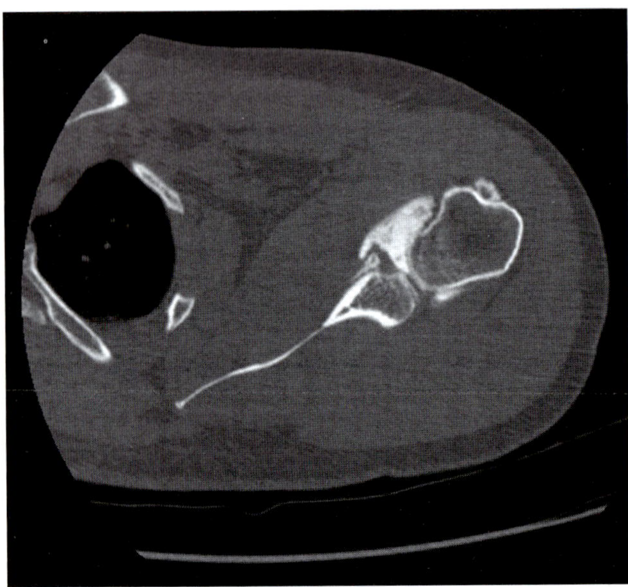

FIGURE 1

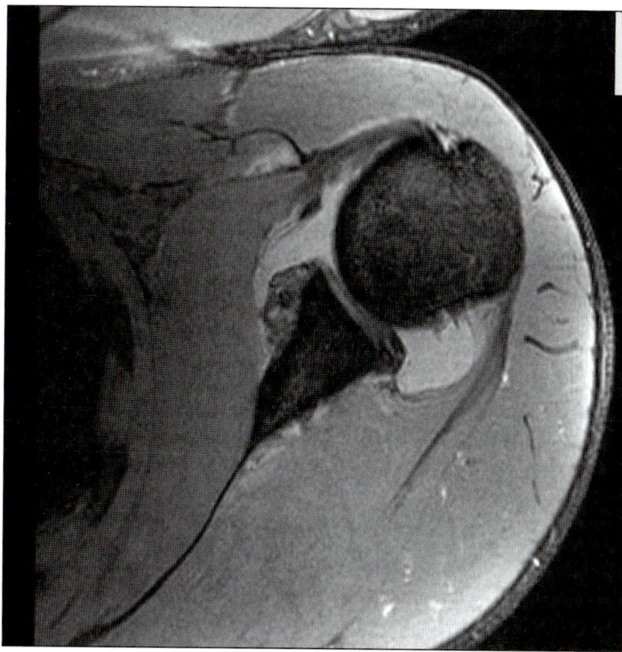

FIGURE 2

- Arthroscopy will show an absent or insufficient anterior shoulder capsule (avulsed anterior glenohumeral ligaments). In Figure 3, an arthroscopic view of the shoulder of the patient in Figure 2 shows an absent anterior shoulder capsule. Arthroscopic repair would have been difficult, and an open Bankart procedure was done to stabilize the shoulder.

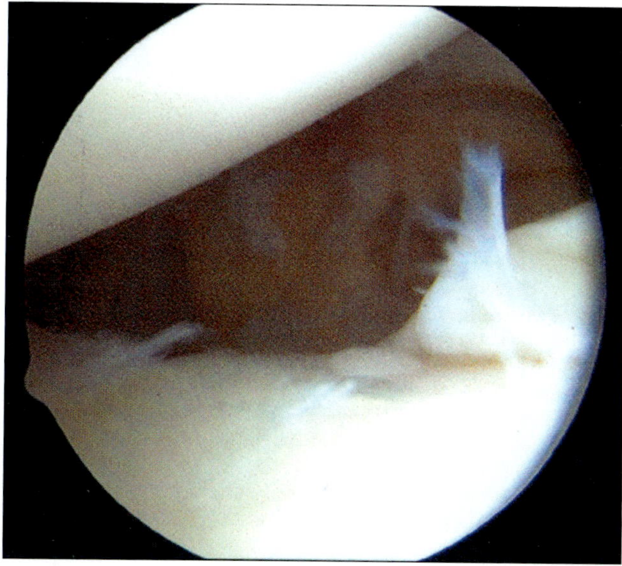

FIGURE 3

PEARLS

- *Rotating the armboard up toward the patient's head so it is next to the OR table will allow the patient's elbow to rest on the armboard and will allow the surgeon to stand next to the OR table.*

PITFALLS

- *Do not put a sandbag or other padding under the scapula. This padding will push upward on the humeral head, making exposure difficult.*

Surgical Anatomy

- The cephalic vein is retracted laterally with the deltoid muscle when developing the deltopectoral interval.
- The musculocutaneous nerve lies medial to the conjoined tendon and may be at risk if dissection is carried out medial to the conjoined tendon or if excess force is applied to the conjoined tendon with a retractor.
- The axillary nerve is located a short distance inferior to the 6 o'clock position of the glenoid rim.
- A leash of vessels marks the inferior border of the subscapularis tendon.
- The subscapularis tendon and capsule fuse into one layer at their insertion onto the humerus. Sharp dissection is needed to separate the two, but care needs to be taken maintain the proper thickness of each.

Positioning

- The patient is positioned supine and flat.
- No extra padding is placed under the scapula.
- An armboard is attached to the operating room (OR) table at the level of the patient's elbow.
- A bolster is placed on the armboard under the elbow to elevate the arm and allow the humeral head to drop posteriorly (Fig. 4).

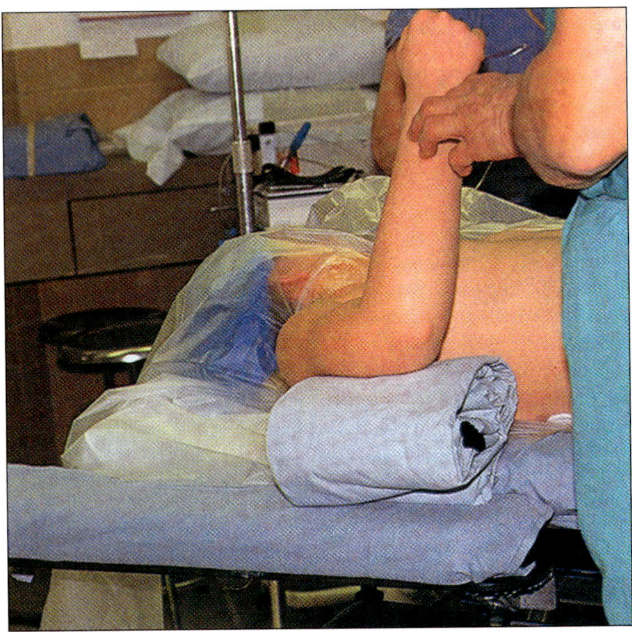

FIGURE 4

PEARLS

- *Mark the anterior axillary fold with a skin marker and make cross marks (to facilitate lining up the skin edges during closure) before applying a Steri-drape.*
- *Wrap the Steri-drape all the way around the shoulder (including the axilla) to allow the shoulder to be moved freely during the procedure.*
- *The incision can be made toward the axilla for a better cosmetic result.*
- *The cephalic vein is the guide to the deltopectoral interval.*
- *When looking for the lateral edge of the conjoined tendon, look for the thin edge of the coracobrachialis muscle lateral to the tendon.*

PITFALLS

- *When dissecting skin flaps, stay in the superficial fascial layer. If you see muscle, you have gone too deep and are through the deep fascial layer.*
- *When dissecting deep in the deltopectoral groove and looking for the conjoined tendon, the tendency is to go too far medially. Avoid this urge and stay lateral to the coracoid process.*
- *The lateral edge of the conjoined tendon is muscular (coracobrachialis muscle), not tendinous. If a muscle deep in the deltopectoral area is running vertically, it is probably the coracobrachialis (if it is not the deltoid or pectoralis muscle). Do not dissect between the coracobrachialis and conjoined tendon.*
- *Be sure you have complete muscle relaxation throughout the operation. The muscle paralysis often wears off halfway through the repair.*

Portals/Exposures

- The axillary fold is located by adducting the arm, and the fold is marked with a skin marker. Cross marks are made to facilitate lining up the skin edges during closure, and then a Steri-drape is applied (Fig. 5; left shoulder is seen in illustrations).
- The skin incision is made in line with the anterior axillary fold.
- Skin flaps are dissected, staying within the superficial fascia layer.
- Dissection is continued within the superficial facial layer, leaving the deep fascial layer intact. A line of fat deep to the superficial facial layer marks the deltopectoral interval (Fig. 6; note forceps).

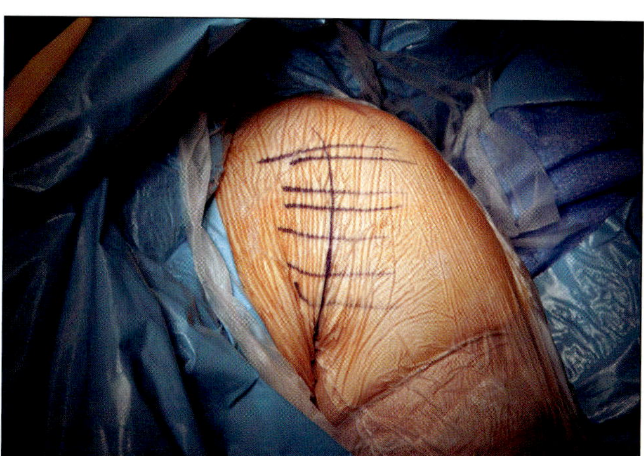

FIGURE 5

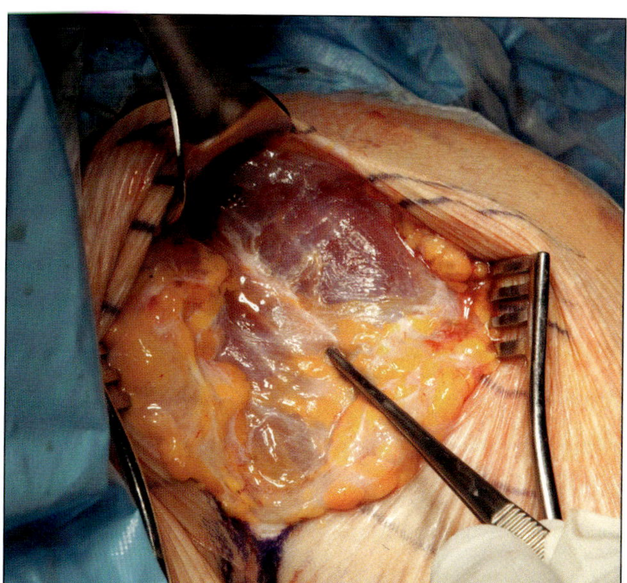

FIGURE 6

Instrumentation

- Head light
- Kölbel self-retaining retractor (Link, USA)
- Rowe single-spike retractor (Kirwan, USA)
- Curved spike (to make holes in the glenoid rim) and mallet
- #5 Mayo needles (smooth, trochar)
- #2 Orthocord or FiberWire sutures

- The deep fascia is incised in line with the fat. This is the deltopectoral interval.
- The deltopectoral interval is dissected using sharp dissection initially to find the interval, then using blunt dissection. The cephalic vein is identified and retracted laterally (toward the right in Fig. 7) with the deltoid muscle as the deltopectoral interval is developed. In Figure 7, note the forceps pushing the pectoralis major muscle medially, revealing the cephalic vein.
- A Kölbel self-retaining retractor is inserted to retract the deltoid muscle with the cephalic vein laterally (toward the right in Fig. 8) and the pectoralis major muscle medially (toward the left in Fig. 8).
- The lateral border of the conjoined tendon is identified (note forceps in Fig. 8; the conjoined tendon is to the left of the forceps), and retracted medially (toward the left in Fig. 8) with the pectoralis major muscle by repositioning the Kölbel retractor blade under the conjoined tendon.

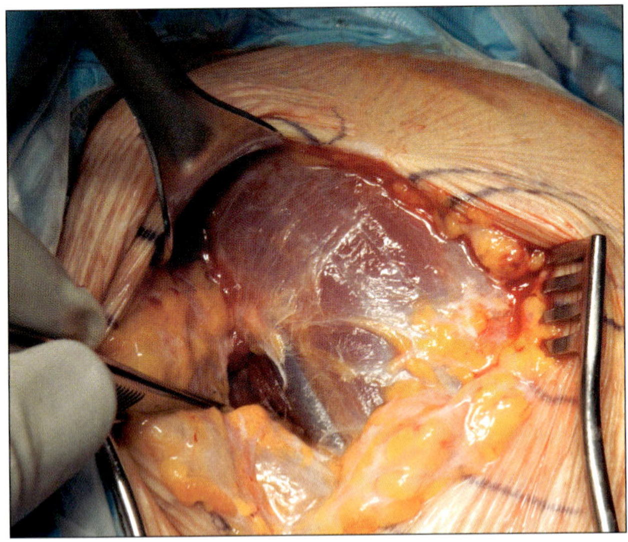

FIGURE 7

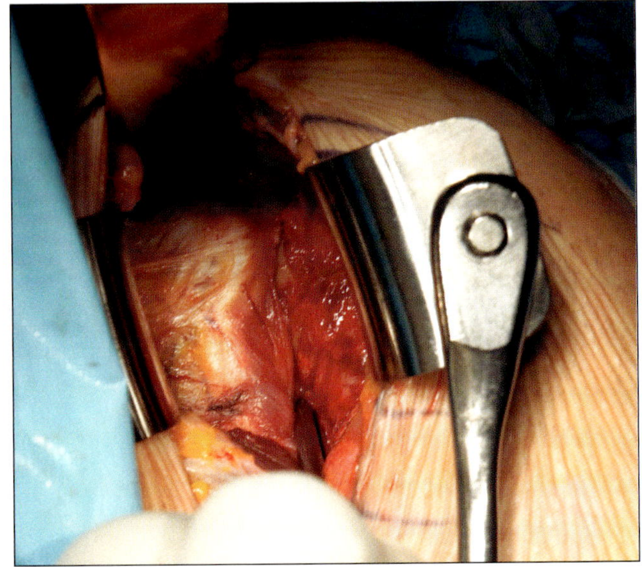

FIGURE 8

Pearls

- *When dissecting the subscapularis tendon, use a #15 blade on a long handle and have suction and cautery close by. This is meticulous dissection.*
- *Look at the direction of the fibers of the subscapularis tendon as you dissect. The fibers are oriented transversely. When the fibers lose their transverse orientation, you have reached the capsule—stay at this level and do not dissect deeper.*
- *If you need more exposure of the inferior capsule, extend the vertical incision in the subscapularis tendon distally, converting it to a T-shaped incision.*

Procedure

Step 1

- There is a normal interval between the anterior border of the supraspinatus tendon and the superior border of the subscapularis tendon. This interval allows the two structures to pass on either side of the coracoid process with normal shoulder motion.
- This interval can be enlarged (torn) when the humeral head dislocates anteroinferiorly (Fig. 9). The superior portion of the capsule (at the superior edge of the subscapularis tendon) is palpated for an interval tear. In Figure 9, note the forceps pointing toward the rotator cuff interval. An angled Gelpi retractor has been placed in the interval for exposure.
- If a tear of the rotator interval is palpated (i.e., if the interval extends laterally to the humeral head), it is closed with one or two figure-of-8 sutures using 0 Vicryl or similar suture material (Fig. 10). The interval should not be repaired too far medially.
- A vertical incision is made through the subscapularis tendon, halfway between the bicipital groove and the insertion of the subscapularis tendon into the humerus (see Fig. 10). The incision is extended distally to dissect sharply through three quarters of the subscapularis tendon but not through the

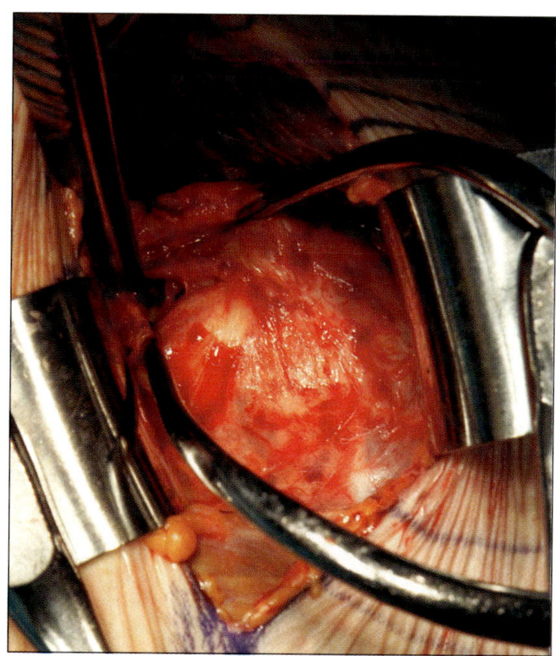

FIGURE 9

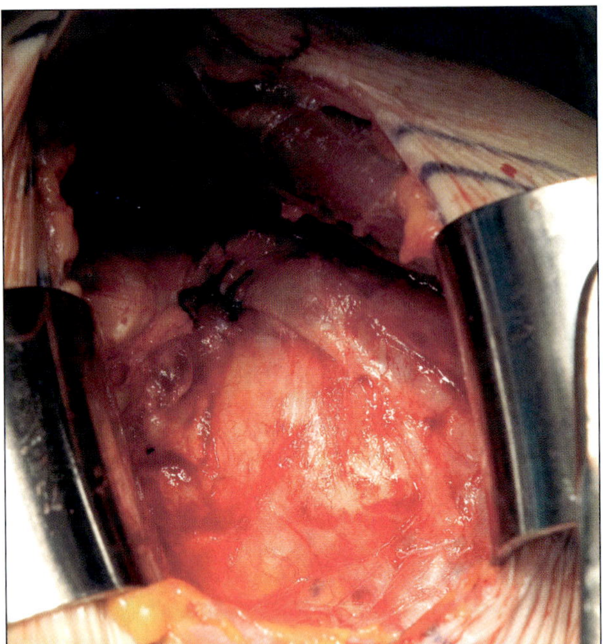

FIGURE 10

underlying shoulder capsule. This is about one-half the thickness of the fused tendon and capsule. This is converted to an L-shaped incision by extending the dissection horizontally at the junction of the upper three quarters of the subscapularis tendon and the lower one quarter (Fig. 11).

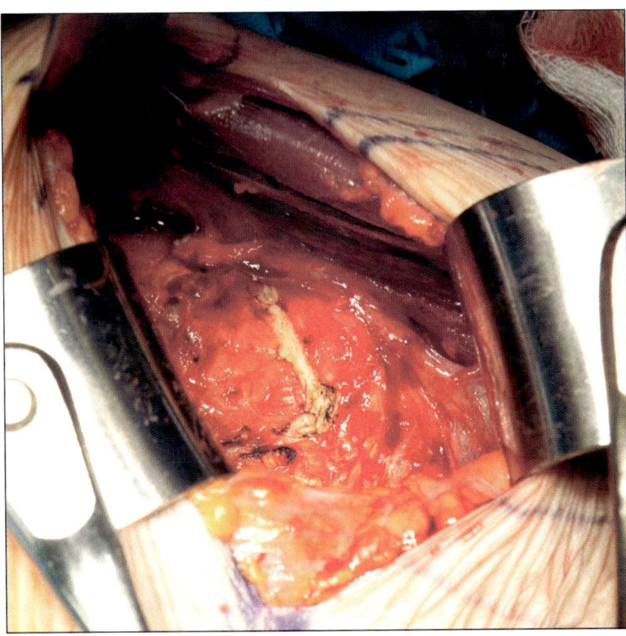

FIGURE 11

Pitfalls

- *When dissecting the subscapularis tendon from the anterior capsule, if you dissect too deeply and go through the capsule, suture the opening in the capsule and continue the dissection more superficially.*
- *An interval normally exists between the superior border of the subscapularis and anterior border of supraspinatus tendon. This interval allows the supraspinatus tendon to pass above and the subscapularis tendon to pass below the coracoid process when the arm is elevated with overhead shoulder motions. Closing this normal interval will limit shoulder motion. Only an enlargement of this interval (i.e., a tear) that extends laterally to the humeral head is abnormal and should be closed.*

  - The subscapularis tendon and capsule fuse laterally at the insertion. The subscapularis tendon will have transverse orientation of fibers, whereas the capsule has a homogeneous appearance.
  - Medially, the two structures can be easily separated close to the glenoid rim. The glenoid rim can be palpated through the capsule.
- Sharp dissection using a #15 knife blade is used to divide the subscapularis tendon from the underlying anterior shoulder capsule (see Fig. 11). The dissection becomes easier as it is carried medially and the subscapularis tendon is no longer adherent to the capsule.
- The anterior rim of the glenoid is palpated deep to the capsule.
- Using a Cobb elevator, the remaining subscapularis muscle is freed from the capsule.
- Dissection is continued between the remaining one quarter of the subscapularis tendon and capsule inferiorly toward the axillary pouch.
- A single-spike retractor is inserted under the subscapularis tendon that has been dissected free medially from the underlying shoulder capsule (Fig. 12).

Step 2

- A transverse incision is made in the midportion of the anterior capsule (i.e., at the equator of the

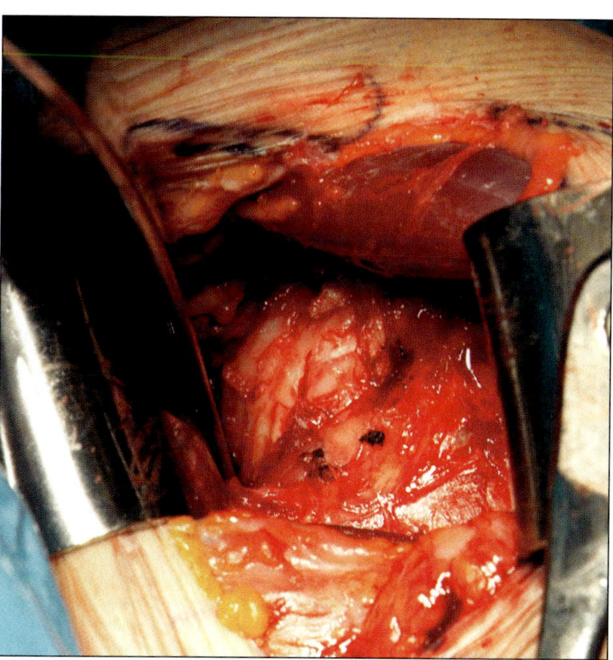

FIGURE 12

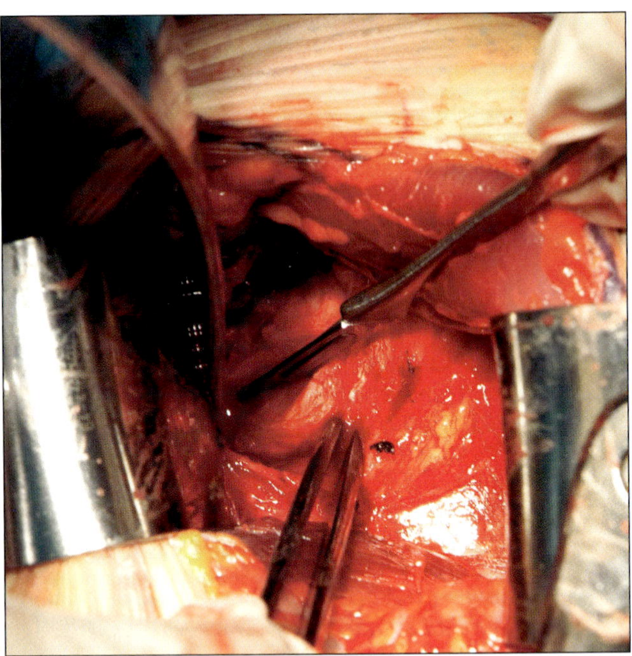

FIGURE 13

glenohumeral joint) and extended medially, until it reaches 0.5 cm from the glenoid rim (Fig. 13).

- The transverse incision is converted into a T-shaped incision by making a vertical incision through the capsule 0.5 cm lateral to the glenoid rim, leaving a 5-mm rim of shoulder capsule attached the glenoid rim.
- The corners of the T-shaped incision are tagged with 0 Vicryl or similar suture so they can be retracted and identified later (Fig. 14). The free ends are snapped with right-angle clamps.

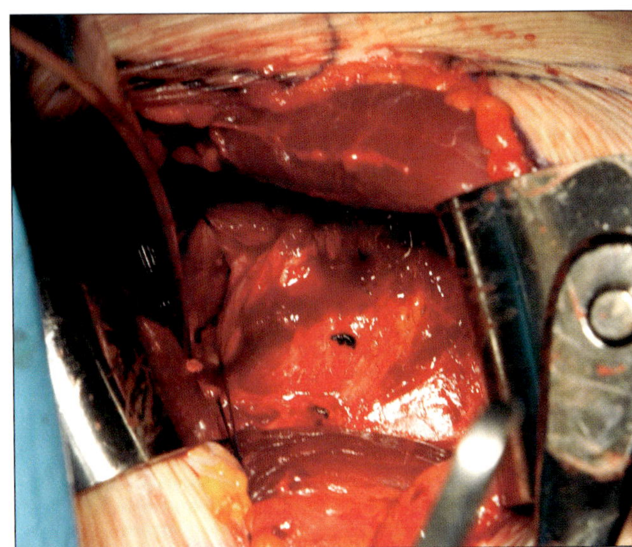

FIGURE 14

- A humeral head retractor (Fukuda or Rowe humeral head retractor) is inserted, and the humeral head retracted laterally to expose the glenohumeral joint (Fig. 15).
- The single-spike retractor is repositioned to be placed under the detached anterior glenoid labrum, and used to lift it up the detached labrum and shoulder capsule (Fig. 16). In Figure 16, note the sutures that are retracting the corners of the capsule. The single-spike retractor retracts the medial flap of capsule medially, exposing the glenoid rim.

STEP 3

- The anterior glenoid rim (the Bankart lesion) is scraped with a Cobb elevator down to bleeding bone.

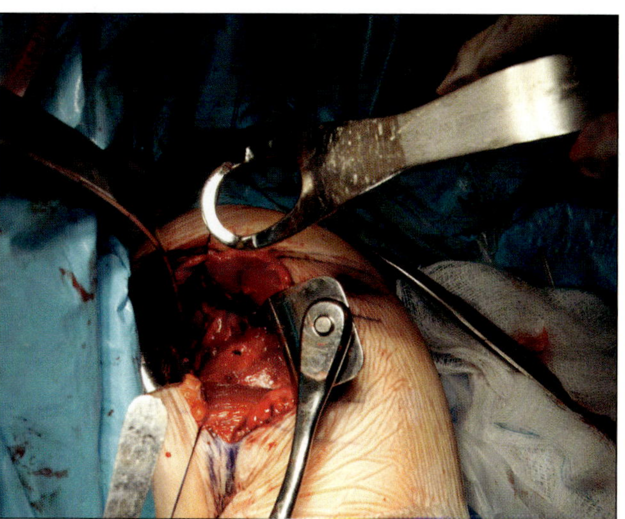

FIGURE 15

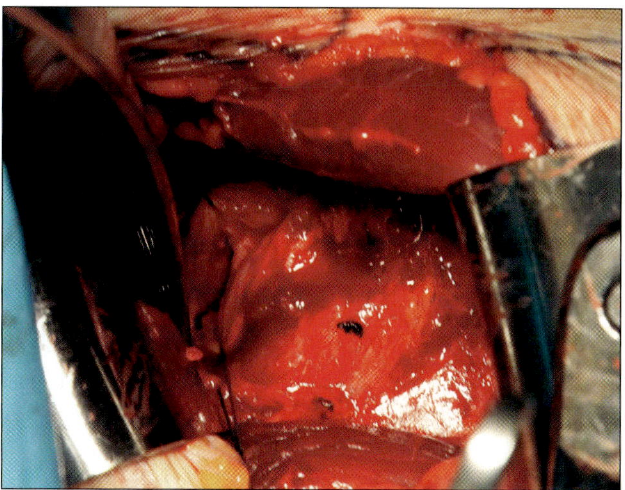

FIGURE 16

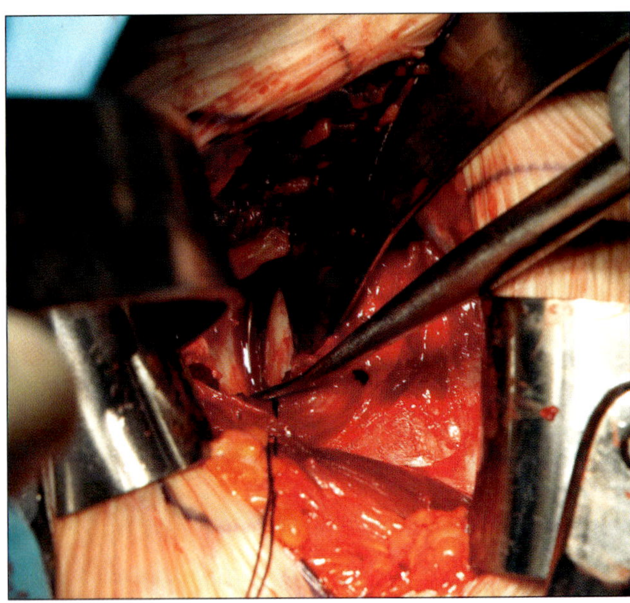

FIGURE 17

- Three holes (curved tunnels) are made in the anterior glenoid rim with a curved spike at the 2, 4, and 6 o'clock positions for the right shoulder (or 10, 8, and 6 o'clock positions for the left shoulder) (Fig. 17).
- A strand of #2 FiberWire or Orthocord is passed through each hole with curved needles, and hemostats are snapped onto the free ends of the sutures.
  - A small, strong, tapered needle (such as a #5 Mayo needle) is used to pass the sutures through the curved tunnels that have been made through the anterior glenoid rim (Fig. 18A).
  - Figure 18B demonstrates sutures retracting two corners of the capsule laterally (the humeral head retractor has been omitted) and three sutures passing through bone tunnels made in the anterior glenoid rim medially. (In Figure 18 and subsequent illustrations, the holes [curved tunnels] are marked A, B, and C [top to bottom] for identification purposes, and the corresponding two sutures that pass through each tunnel are marked A and A′, B and B′, and C and C′.)

Step 4

- The humeral head retractor is removed.
- The right-angle clamps that were used to tag the corners of the incision in the capsule are retrieved.
- Pulling on the lower right-angle clamp will deliver the lower flap of capsule into view.

Pearls

- *Incising the capsule transversely first allows one to look inside the glenohumeral joint to judge the distance from the glenoid rim.*
- *Use unique clamps (such as right-angle clamps) to tag sutures that have been placed to mark and retract the corners of the T-shaped capsular incision for easier identification later.*

Pitfalls

- *Do not make the vertical incision too close to the glenoid rim; otherwise, there will be no medial flap of capsule to reinforce the repair.*
- *Do not make the vertical incision too far from the glenoid rim; otherwise, the shoulder will lose external rotation after the capsule is reattached to the glenoid rim.*

Instrumentation/ Implantation

- A Fukuda or Rowe humeral head retractor is needed to expose the joint.

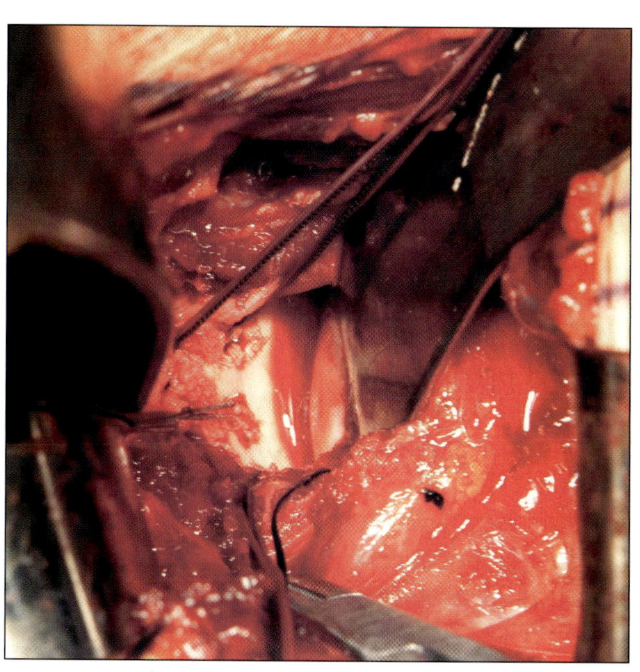

A

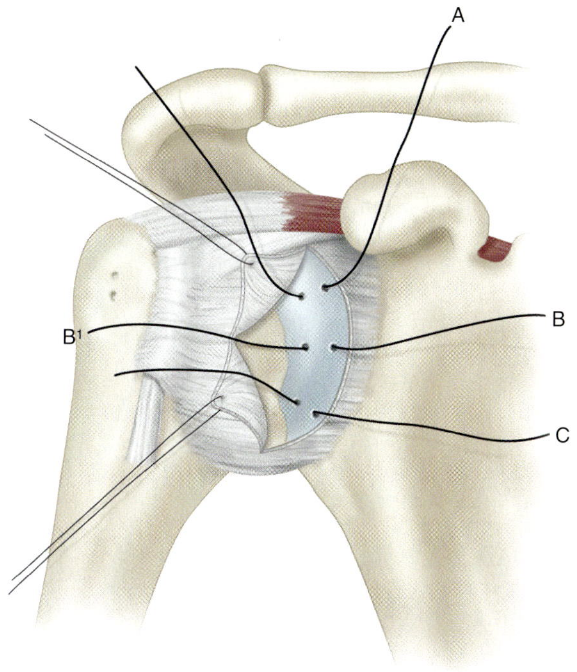

B

FIGURE 18

- The suture that passes through the most inferior tunnel (C) is passed through the free edge of the inferior capsule as distally as possible (at the 6 o'clock position).
- The suture that passes through the middle tunnel (B) is passed through the corner of the lower flap of capsule.
- Each of the sutures (C and B) is tied separately. In Figure 19, the lower two sutures (B and C) have

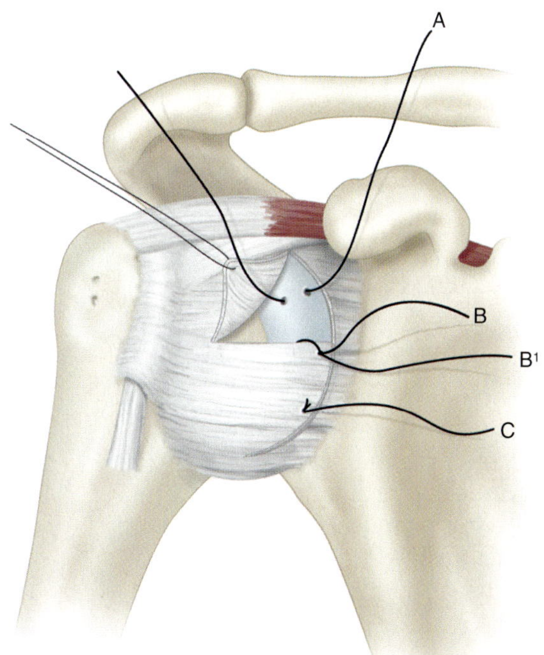

FIGURE 19

Pearls

- *When making the holes in the glenoid rim, first perforate the cortex of the anterior glenoid neck with a small scaphoid gouge. The curved spike is used to deepen and complete the hole, working from the glenoid neck side and the articular side, respectively, until the tunnels meet.*
- *Try to position the most inferior hole as close as possible to the 6 o'clock position.*
- *Instead of using a single strand of a strong suture, such as #2 Orthocord or FiberWire, two strands of weaker suture material, such as 0 Vicryl, can be used. The extra strand is for increased strength and for backup in case the first strand breaks when tied.*

Pitfalls

- *If the holes in the anterior glenoid rim are too close to the edge, they might break through the edge. If the holes are too far from the edge, it will be difficult to pass a needle thought the tunnel.*
- *The bone is somewhat weak at the 6 o'clock position, so care must be taken not to break through.*

Instrumentation/ Implantation

- A curved hand awl and/or a tenaculum can be used to complete the tunnel in the anterior glenoid rim.
- Mark the hemostats that are snapped to the sutures that pass through the bone tunnels (A, B, C) so they can easily be distinguished.

been passed through the inferior flap of capsule and tied. Only one strand of suture (C) has been cut after it has been tied, leaving the other strand long for later use.

- The suture that passes through the middle tunnel and has been tied (B) is passed through the corner of the upper flap of capsule.
- The suture that goes through the most superior tunnel (A) is passed through the free edge of the superior capsule as proximally as possible (at the 11 or 1 o'clock position).
- Sutures B and A are tied, thus overlapping the superior flap of capsule over the previously secured inferior flap (Fig. 20). One strand of suture A is cut. The capsule has now been secured to the anterior glenoid rim in an overlapped manner.
- Four strands of previously tied sutures that were left long remain (A, B, B′, and C). These are now used to overlap the medial flap of capsule over the repair to reinforce the repair (Fig. 21).
- The four sutures are passed through the medial flap of capsule (that is attached to the glenoid neck) and suture A is tied to B and suture B′ to C. The repair is now complete (Fig. 22).
- The transverse capsule incision is closed with interrupted 0 Vicryl figure-of-8 sutures.
- The subscapularis tendon to is reattached its insertion using 0 Vicryl figure-of-8 sutures (Fig. 23).

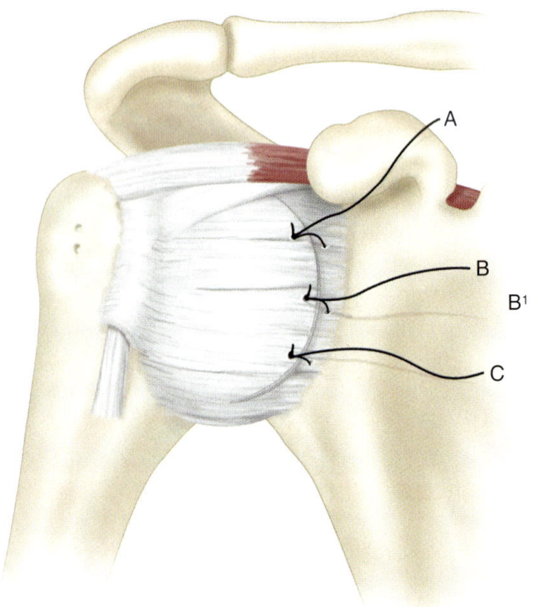

FIGURE 20

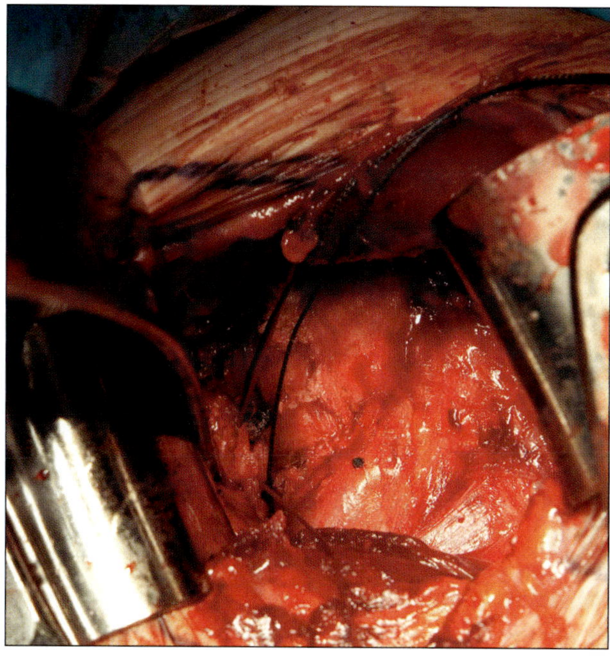

FIGURE 21

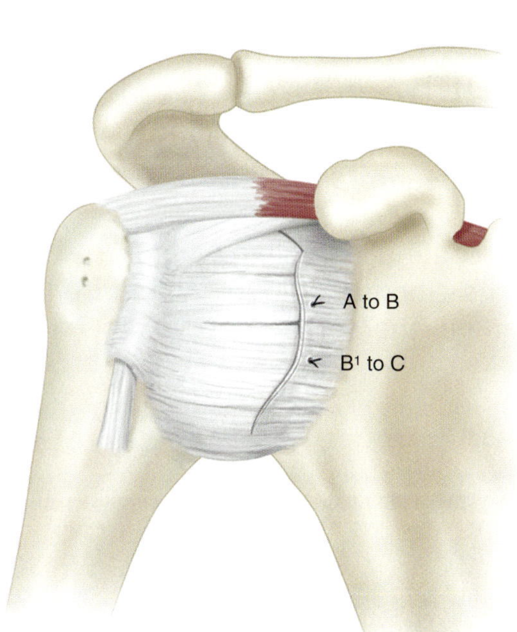

FIGURE 22

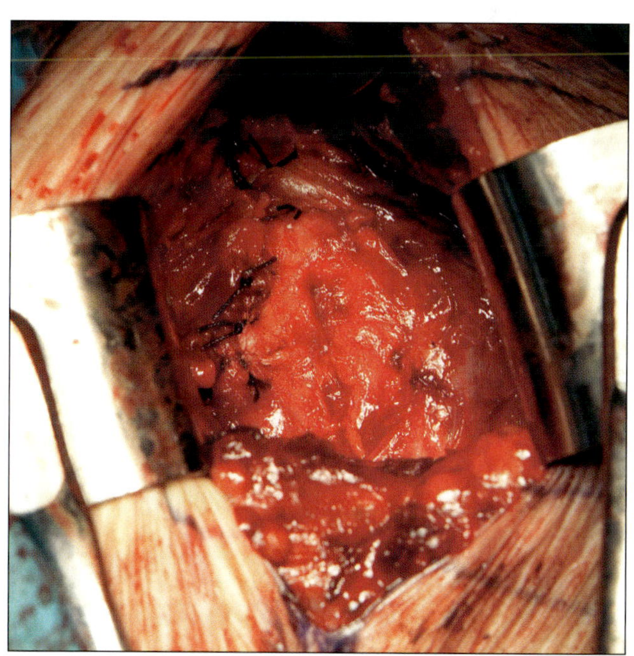

FIGURE 23

Controversies

- Instead of making tunnels through the bone of the anterior glenoid rim, suture anchors can be used to secure the sutures to the bone. Although putting in anchors is easier than making tunnels, the anchors give only spot fixation of the capsule after the sutures are tied compared to a wider surface area of fixation when tunnels are used. The author's experience was a higher failure rate when anchors were used compared to when bone tunnels were used.

Pearls

- *Place the arm into internal rotation when tying the capsular repair sutures.*

Instrumentation/ Implantation

- If the needle that is wedged onto the FiberWire or Orthocord is not the correct size to pass through the curved tunnel, use a #5 Mayo needle (small, smooth, strong trochar needle).

Controversies

- A pair of sutures, such as 0 Vicryl, can be used through each hole in the glenoid rim instead of using one strong suture (#2 Orthocord or FiberWire) in each tunnel.
- Closing the rotator cuff interval will limit shoulder motion and should be done judiciously—only close a tear and not a normal interval (i.e., close only an enlargement of the normally present interval).

Pearls

- *Early motion is permitted as long as the arm is kept in front of the body.*

- The deep fascial layer is repaired at the deltopectoral interval.
- The wound is closed in layers.

Postoperative Care and Expected Outcomes

- A sling is applied.
- Pendulum motion is begun on the first or second postoperative day.
- The patient can discontinue the sling when comfortable, but the elbow should be kept in front of the coronal plane of the body for approximately 6 weeks.

Evidence

Bottoni CR, Smith EL, Berkowitz MJ, Towle RB, Moore JH. Arthroscopic versus open shoulder stabilization for recurrent anterior instability: a prospective randomized clinical trial. Am J Sports Med. 2006;34:1730-7.

This prospective randomized controlled trial compared 29 patients who underwent open Bankart repair with suture anchors and 32 patients treated with arthroscopic Bankart repair. At a mean 32-month follow-up, there was no significant difference between the groups with respect to failures; however, patients treated with open Bankart stabilization experienced greater mean loss of shoulder motion. Subjective evaluations were equal in both groups. The authors concluded that open and arthroscopic Bankart repair provide comparable clinical outcomes. (Level I evidence)

Fabbriciani C, Milano G, Demontis A, Fadda S, Ziranu F, Mulas PD. Arthroscopic versus open treatment of Bankart lesion of the shoulder: a prospective randomized study. Arthroscopy. 2004;20:456-62.

This prospective randomized controlled trial compared 30 patients treated with an open Bankart procedure and 30 patients treated with arthroscopic Bankart repair. All repairs used metallic suture anchors. At 2 years' follow-up, no treatment failures occurred in either group, and Rowe and Constant scores were similar between groups. Patients treated with open repair were found to have greater loss of range of motion. (Level I evidence)

Freedman KB, Smith AP, Romeo AA, Cole BJ, Bach BR Jr. Open Bankart repair versus arthroscopic repair with transglenoid sutures or bioabsorbable tacks for recurrent anterior instability of the shoulder: a meta-analysis. Am J Sports Med. 2004;32:1520-7.

This meta-analysis of six studies compared open Bankart repair with arthroscopic repair using transglenoid sutures, bioabsorbable tacks, or suture anchors. There was a higher rate of recurrence of instability with arthroscopic Bankart repair with transglenoid sutures or bioabsorbable tacks (20.3%) as compared to the open Bankart procedure (10.3%). A higher percentage of patients undergoing open repair (88%) had a good or excellent postoperative Rowe score as compared with patients undergoing arthroscopic repair (71%). (Level II evidence)

Hobby J, Griffin D, Dunbar M, Boileau P. Is arthroscopic surgery for stabilisation of chronic shoulder instability as effective as open surgery? A systematic review and meta-analysis of 62 studies including 3044 arthroscopic operations. J Bone Joint Surg [Br]. 2007;89:1188-96.

This meta-analysis of 62 studies found a significantly higher failure rate after arthroscopic Bankart stabilization using staples or transglenoid sutures as compared to open Bankart repair or arthroscopic Bankart repair using suture anchors or bioabsorbable tacks. Comparable rates of failure at 2 years' follow-up were found when open repair was compared to arthroscopic repair using suture anchors or bioabsorbable tacks. (Level I evidence)

Hovelius LK, Sandström BC, Rösmark DL, Saebö M, Sundgren KH, Malmqvist BG. Long-term results with the Bankart and Bristow-Latarjet procedures: recurrent shoulder instability and arthropathy. J Shoulder Elbow Surg. 2001;10:445-52.

This retrospective review evaluated 26 shoulders in 24 patients with a mean 17.5-year follow-up after open Bankart stabilization with transosseous sutures. One patient underwent revision surgery for recurrent instability, and no patients had a positive apprehension test. Seventeen patients were "very satisfied," seven patients were "satisfied," and one patient was "dissatisfied." The authors concluded that the results of their study are consistent with the opinion that open Bankart repair is the gold standard.

Lenters TR, Franta AK, Wolf FM, Leopold SS, Matsen FA 3rd. Arthroscopic compared with open repairs for recurrent anterior shoulder instability: a systematic review and meta-analysis of the literature. J Bone Joint Surg [Am]. 2007;89:244-54.

This meta-analysis of 18 studies found that open Bankart repair was more effective than arthroscopic procedures in preventing recurrent instability and in enabling patients to return to work and/or sports. Arthroscopic Bankart repairs resulted in better function as reflected by Rowe scores. (Level II evidence)

Pelet S, Jolles BM, Farron A. Bankart repair for recurrent anterior glenohumeral instability: results at twenty-nine years' follow-up. J Shoulder Elbow Surg. 2006;15:203-7.

Thirty patients treated with open Bankart repair with transosseous sutures were reviewed with a mean follow-up of 29 years. All patients recovered their preinjury activity level. Three patients (10%) had recurrence of dislocation, one of whom underwent reoperation. The authors concluded that reliable long-term glenohumeral stability can be expected after the open Bankart procedure.

Rhee YG, Ha JH, Cho NS. Anterior shoulder stabilization in collision athletes: arthroscopic versus open Bankart repair. Am J Sports Med. 2006;34:979-85.

In this cohort study, 48 shoulders in 46 collision athletes were treated with open Bankart transosseous stabilization (32 shoulders) or arthroscopic Bankart repair (16 shoulders). At an average follow-up of 72 months, the patients treated with arthroscopic repair had a higher failure rate (25%) as compared to patients undergoing open repair (12.5%). The authors recommended the open Bankart procedure for anterior shoulder instability in collision athletes.

Rowe CR, Patel D, Southmayd WW. The Bankart procedure: a long-term end-result study. J Bone Joint Surg [Am]. 1984;66:159-68.

Treatment of 145 shoulders with open Bankart repair using transosseous sutures found five recurrences (3.5%) at an average 6-year follow-up. Ninety-eight percent of patients rated their result good or excellent. The authors concluded that, for most patients treated with the open Bankart procedure, postoperative immobilization is not necessary, early return of motion and function can be expected, and resumption of athletic activities is possible.

Rowe CR, Zarins B, Ciullo JV. Recurrent anterior dislocation of the shoulder after surgical repair: apparent causes of failure and treatment. J Bone Joint Surg [Am]. 1984;66:159-68.

This case series examined 39 patients treated for recurrent anterior shoulder dislocation after unsuccessful surgical repair. Reoperation with an open Bankart repair using transosseous sutures was performed on 24 shoulders. At a minimum 2-year follow-up, 10 patients rated their result as excellent, 12 patients as good, and 2 patients as poor. The incidence of recurrent instability after reoperation was 8%.

SECTION I

SHOULDER
Biceps Tendon

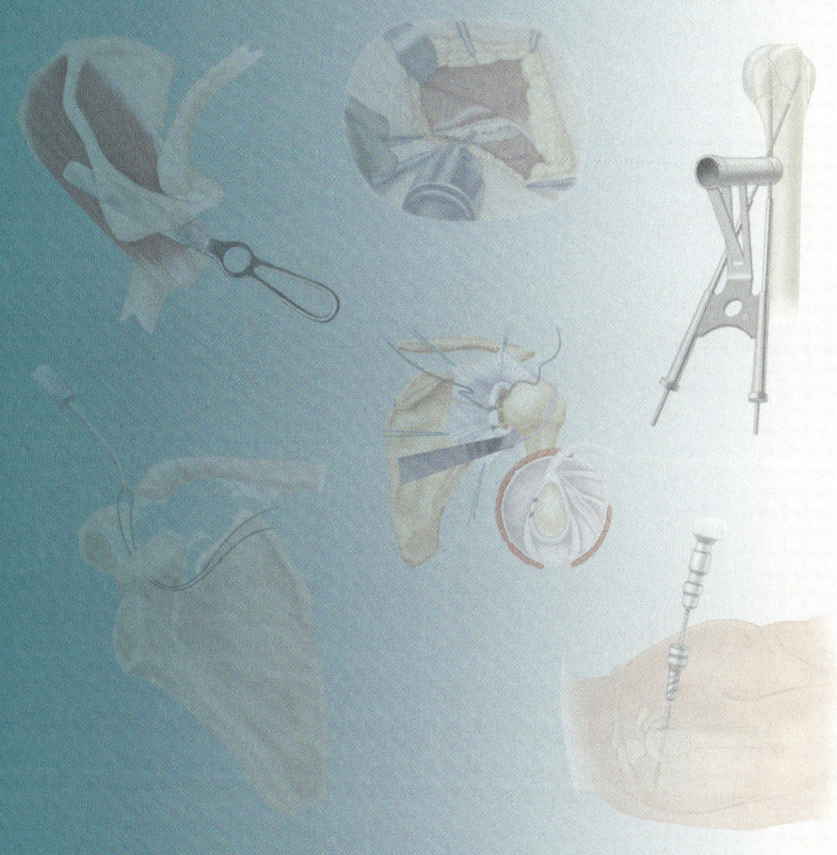

PROCEDURE 19

Mini-Open Biceps Tenodesis

Andrew S. Neviaser and Robert J. Neviaser

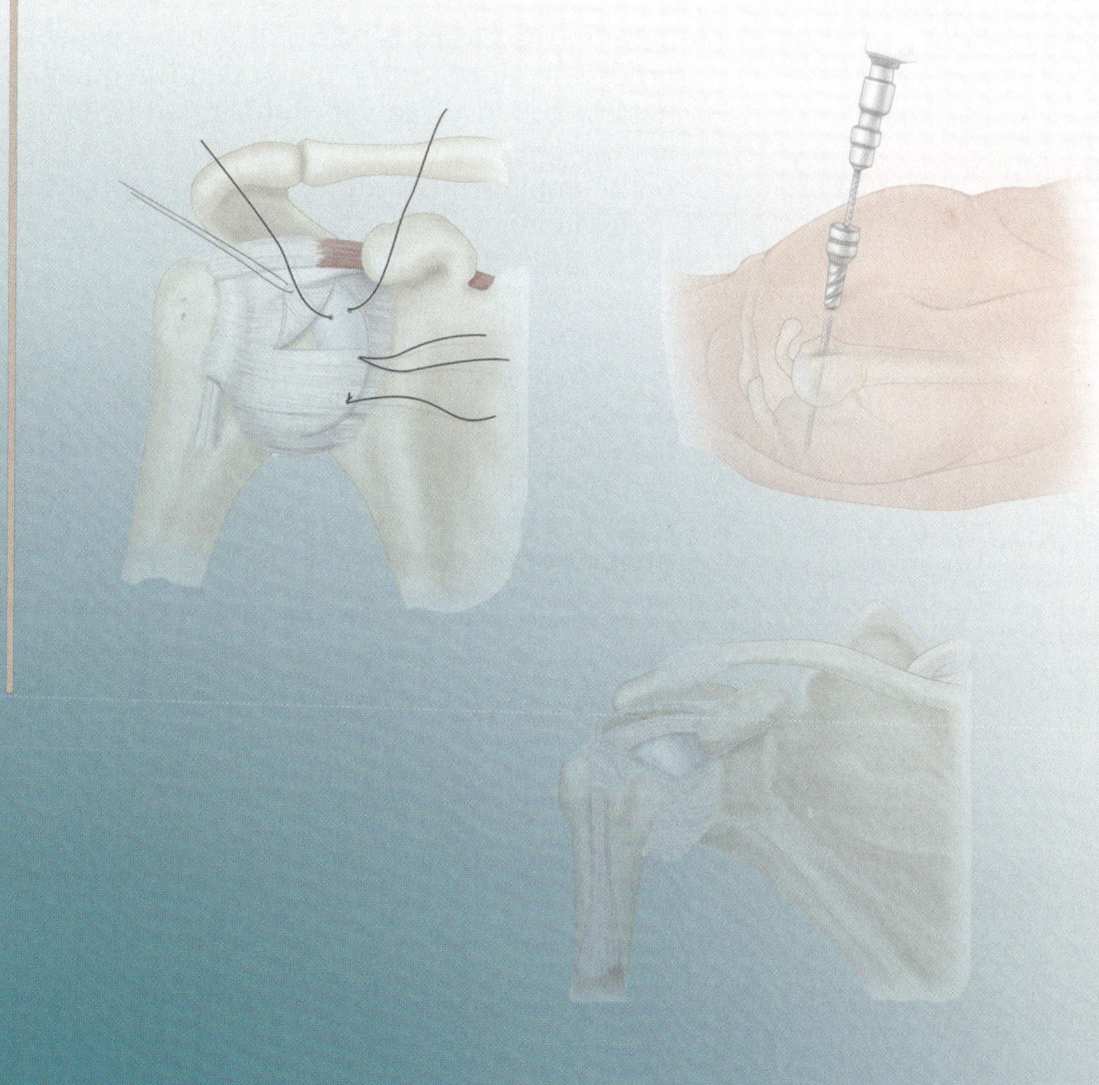

Pitfalls

- *Not recognizing that the long head of the biceps is an important component of the impingement process.*

Controversies

- Some feel that the long head of the biceps is a humeral head depressor; however, electromyographic studies have shown there is no activity in the biceps muscle when the elbow is not moving, confirming that it acts at the elbow, not the shoulder.

Indications

- Failure of nonoperative treatment as part of the impingement syndrome, including subacromial injection and therapeutic exercises for stretching and strenghtening of rotator cuff and biceps
- Biceps tendinitis or tenosynovitis
- Biceps subluxation/dislocation
- Biceps degeneration

Examination/Imaging

- Because the biceps is part of the impingement process, evaluating the rotator cuff is required. Rotator cuff involvement is implicated by the following tests:
  - The impingement sign: forcing the arm into elevation while stabilizing the scapula (Fig. 1A)
  - The palm-down abduction test: forcing the shoulder, in abduction and internal rotation, against the stabilized scapula (Fig. 1B)
- The biceps resistance test (Speed's sign) is performed by asking the patient to elevate the arm in the forward plane against resistance with the elbow extended (Fig. 2A). This combined with tenderness to palpation in the intertubercular or bicipital groove establishes the diagnosis (Fig. 2B).

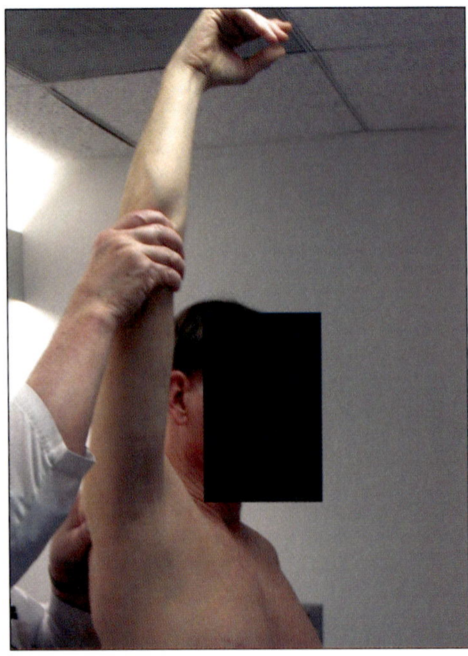

A

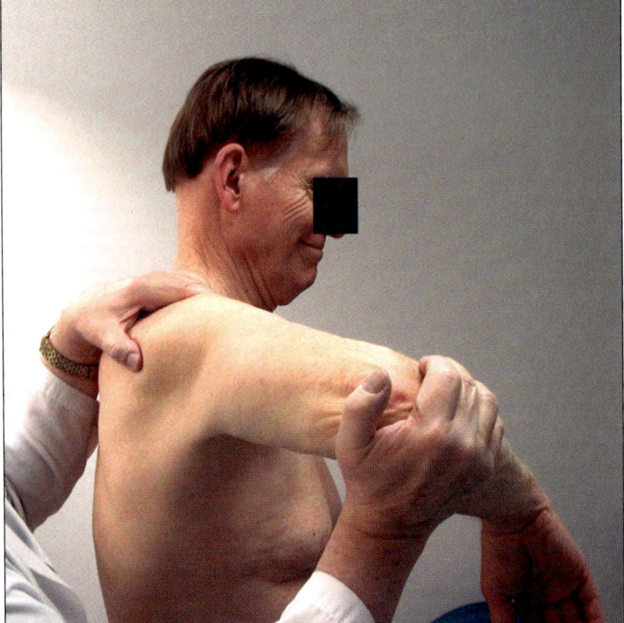

B

FIGURE 1

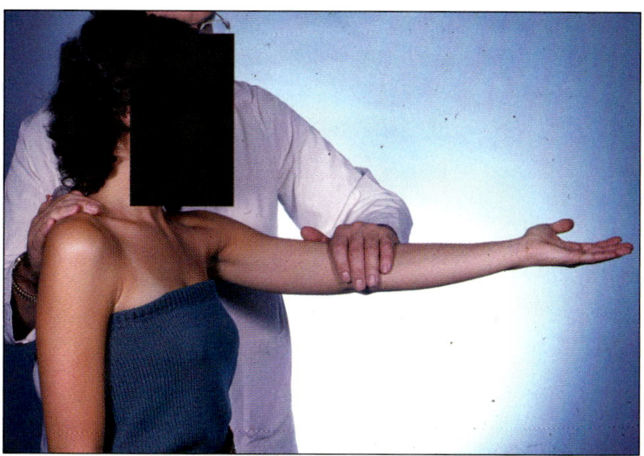

A

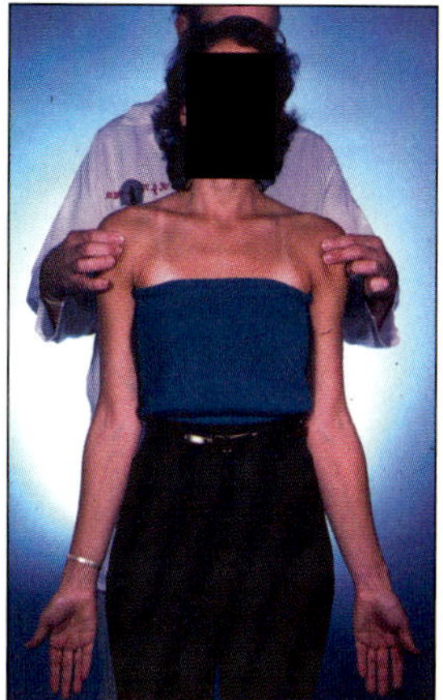

B

FIGURE 2

Treatment Options

- In addition to the nonoperative regimen outlined above, a biceps tenotomy can be performed. In comparing patients who had a tenotomy to those undergoing tenodesis, we found that tenotomy patients had a significantly higher rate of symptoms, including muscle cramping with elbow flexion and supination as well as an unsightly bulge in the arm (the Popeye sign) (Fig. 3). Tenotomy, therefore, is generally limited to sedentary, low-demand patients.

- Radiographs are not usually helpful but are taken to rule out other pathology.
- Magnetic resonance imaging is done to assess the lesions of the cuff but occasionally can show a subluxated/dislocated biceps on the axial cuts. However, biceps tendinitis is a clinical diagnosis rather than one based on imaging

Surgical Anatomy

- The biceps is a bipennate muscle. The short head originates on the coracoid process while the long head originates on the supraglenoid tubercle.
- The long head lies within the glenohumeral joint and passes underneath the tendon of the supraspinatus just posterior to the rotator interval.

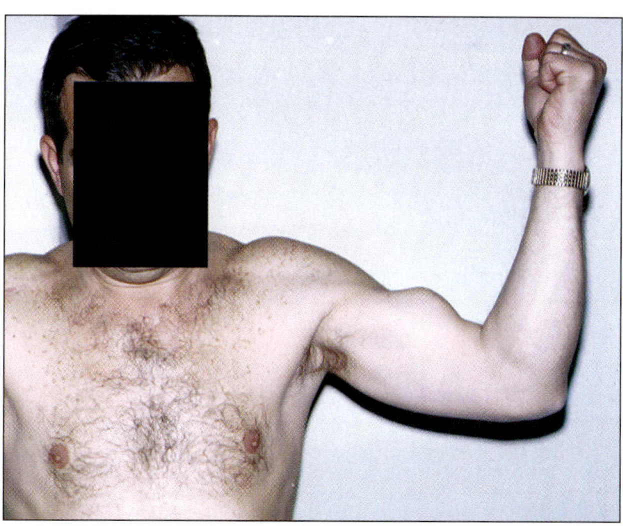

FIGURE 3

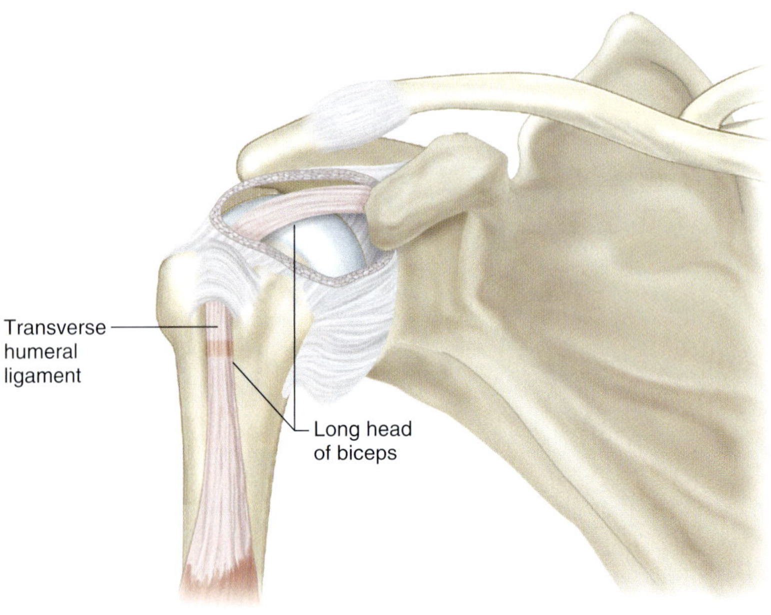

FIGURE 4

Pearls

- *Be sure to keep the posterior aspect of the shoulder and scapula adequately exposed because of the need to establish a posterior arthroscopic portal.*

Equipment

- An operating room table that allows the patient to be put in a sitting position and permits anterior and posterior access

- It exits the joint by passing through the intertubercular groove between the lesser and greater tuberosities of the humerus, where it lies beneath the transverse humeral ligament (Fig. 4).

Positioning

- The patient is placed in the sitting position with the arm draped free and the shoulder, most of the scapula, and upper part of the anterior chest exposed (Fig. 5A and 5B).
- The patient's head is secured in a headrest.

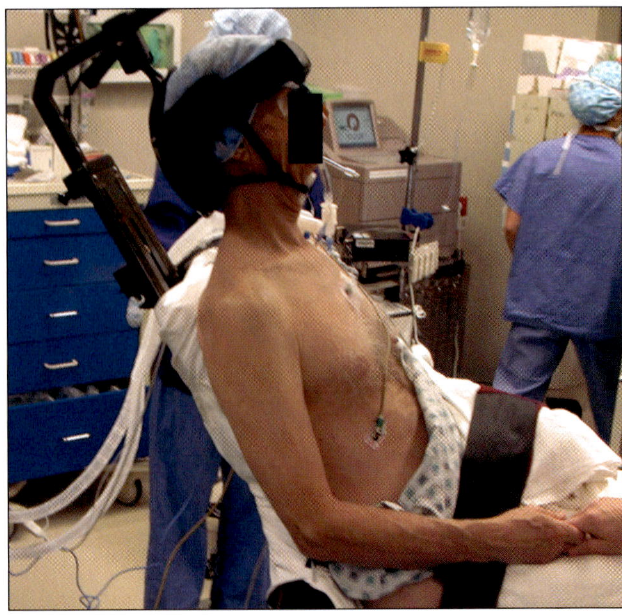

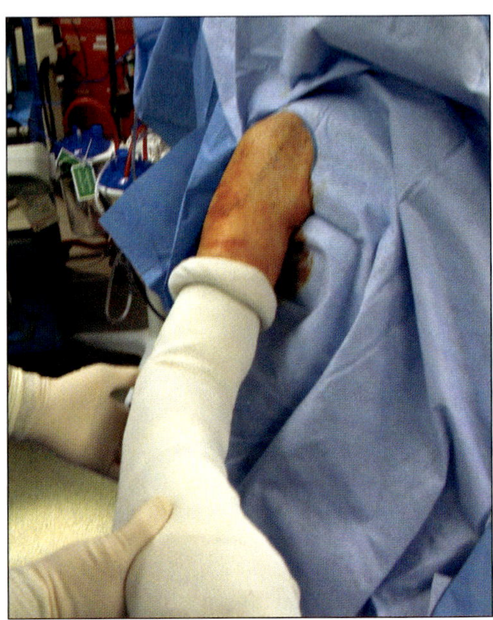

FIGURE 5 A B

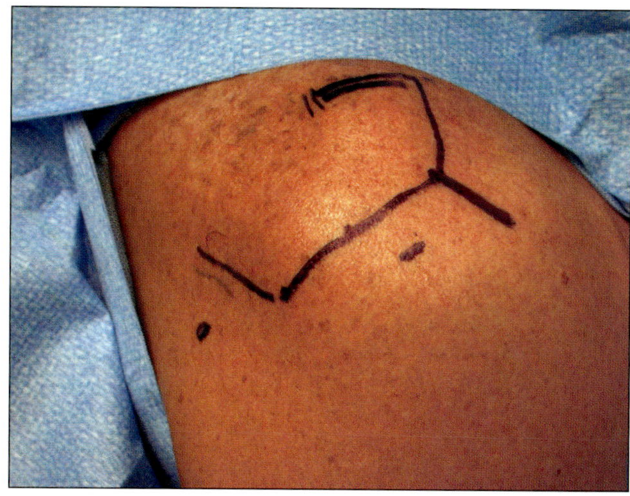

FIGURE 6

> **PEARLS**
>
> - *Making the mini-open incision too far laterally or medially can restrict access to the biceps tendon.*

Portals/Exposures

- Portals and the skin incision are marked (Fig. 6).
- Since the tenodesis is preceded by an arthroscopic decompression, a posterior viewing portal is established first.
- The anterior portal is established from the inside out.
- The lateral portal is in line with the posterior border of the clavicle at about the junction of the anterior and middle thirds of the acromion.
- A 1.5- to 2-cm vertical mini-open incision is made at the anterolateral corner of the acromion from the margin of the acromion distally.

> **PEARLS**
>
> - *Because the diagnosis of biceps tendinitis is a clinical one, the intra-articular portion may appear unremarkable. At other times, there are changes in this portion of the tendon (see Fig. 7).*

Procedure

STEP 1

- The joint is entered posteriorly with a cannula and blunt trochar.
- The arthroscope is inserted posteriorly into the joint and the joint inspected. Attention is directed to the intra-articular portion of the long head of the biceps (Fig. 7).
- A switching stick is placed through the cannula and out through the rotator interval to establish the anterior portal (Fig. 8A). The cannula containing the switching stick is advanced out of the skin, and another cannula is then passed over it into the joint (Fig. 8B).

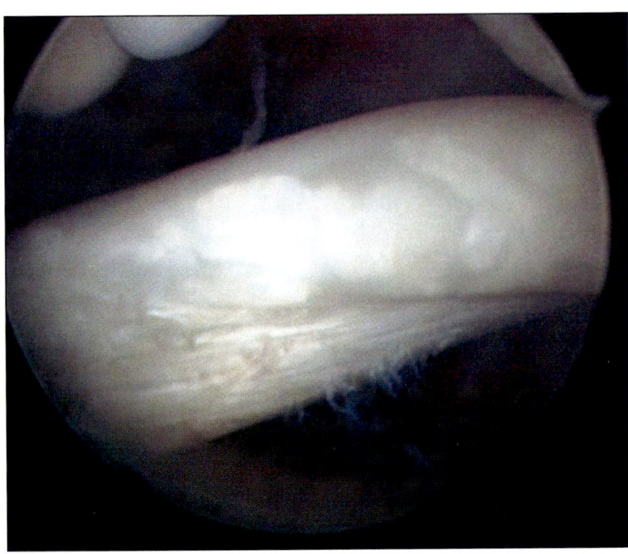

FIGURE 7

STEP 2

- A shaver is introduced through the anterior cannula and any fraying or other findings can be trimmed.
- The arthroscope is withdrawn from the joint, and the trochar replaces the camera in the cannula and is redirected into the subacromial space. The camera then replaces the trochar.
- A shaver is introduced through the lateral portal and the bursa is débrided enough to allow visualization of the undersurface of the acromion and the coracoacromial ligament.
- An arthoscopic decompression is performed as described elsewhere in this book (see Procedure 32). When this is completed, the arthroscope is replaced into the joint.

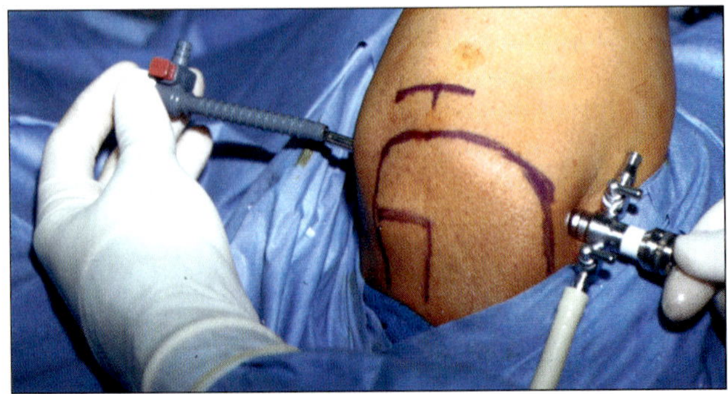

A

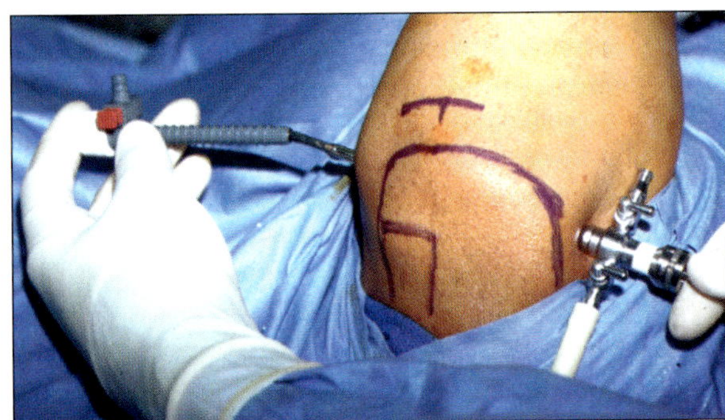

B

FIGURE 8

PEARLS

- *After placing the sutures through the transverse humeral ligament and the tendon, if there is any doubt about the security of the fixation, the vertical incision at the upper edge of the ligament can be done at this point and a clamp can be used to tug gently on the tendon before its release intraarticularly.*

PITFALLS

- *If the sutures in the ligament and tendon miss the tendon, it will retract into the arm upon its release from near its origin within the joint, effectively creating a tenotomy.*

STEP 3

- A mini-open incision of 1½–2 cm is made at the anterolateral corner of the acromion. The deltoid is split through its substance in line with its fibers via this incision. The deltoid is undermined on both sides of the split and the bursa incised, mobilized, and retracted with the deltoid.
- The tendon of the long head of the biceps is identified by palpation and visualization in the intertubercular groove under the transverse humeral ligament. Three figure-of-8, nonabsorbable, #1 sutures are passed through the transverse humeral ligament and the tendon (Fig. 9).
- Attention is then directed back intra-articularly via the arthroscope to the origin of the biceps at the supraglenoid tubercle. Using either an arthroscopic biter (Fig. 10A) or an arthroscopic cautery (Fig. 10B), the tendon is transected just distal to its origin.
- Returning to the mini-open incision, a vertical incision is made in the upper edge of the transverse

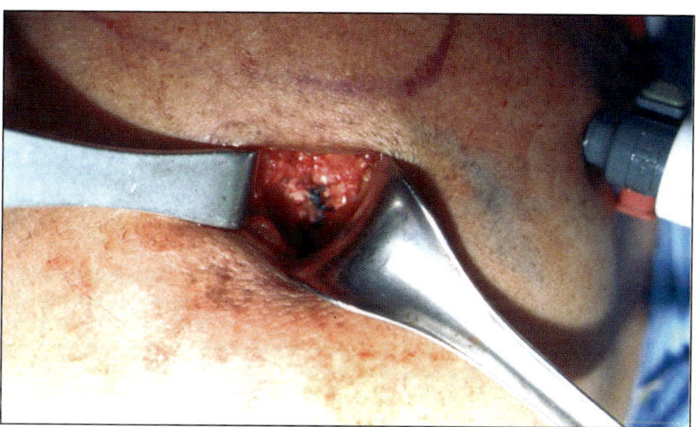

FIGURE 9

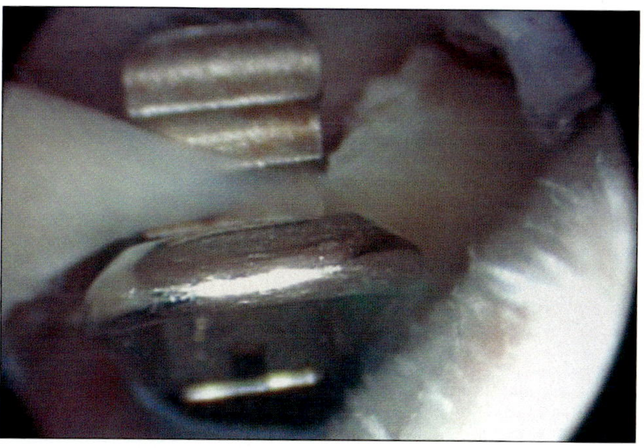

A

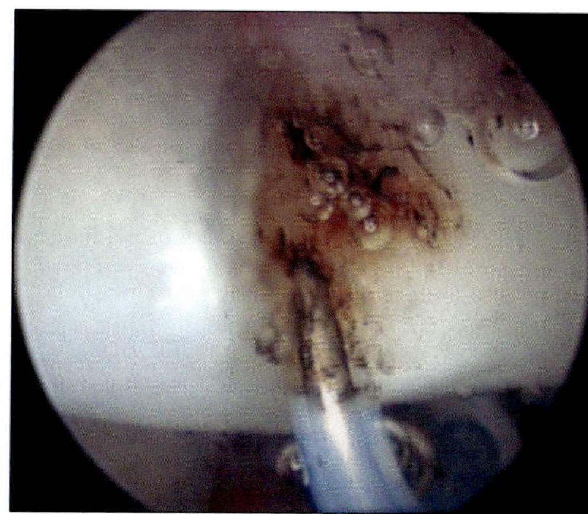

B

FIGURE 10

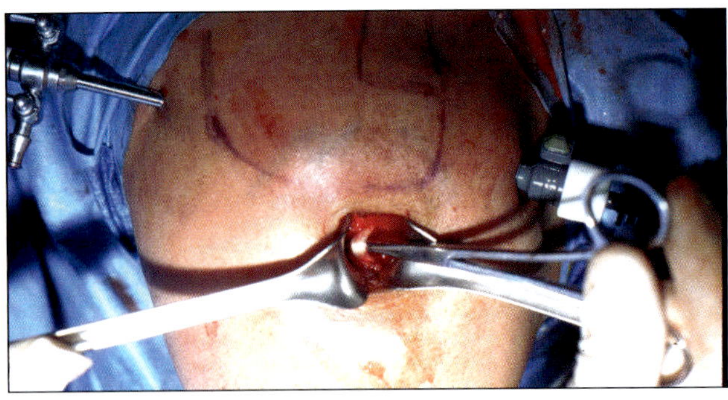
A

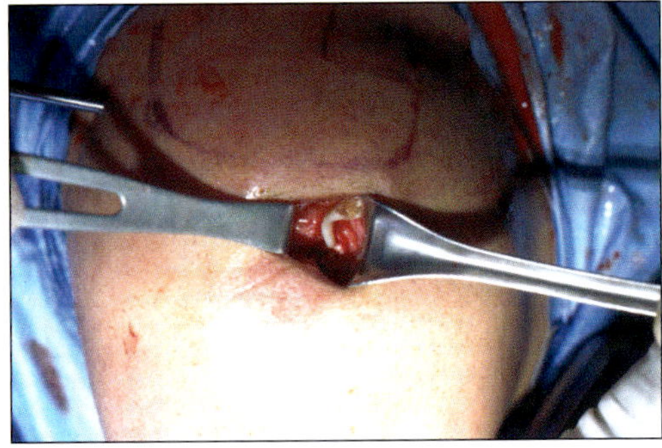
B

FIGURE 11

Controversies

- Some prefer to do a tenotomy rather than a tenodesis, but we have found that active people experience cramping in the biceps muscle with forceful use.

humeral ligament, just superior to the most proximal tenodesing suture (Fig. 11A). A curved clamp is introduced through this incision and looped around the biceps tendon to withdraw it from the joint (Fig. 11B). This piece of tendon is then resected.

- The deltoid split is repaired with two nonabsorbable sutures with the knots buried on the deep surface, and the skin over the split is closed with a subcuticular suture. The portals are closed with a single suture, and a sterile dressing is applied.

Pearls

- *Strengthening before 12 weeks has the significant risk of pulling out the tenodesis, effectively resulting in a tenotomy.*

Postoperative Care and Expected Outcomes

- The operative arm is placed in an immobilizer. After 2–3 days, the dressing is changed and passive exercises are started.
- While the patient is supine, the strap around the neck is undone, and using the other hand or with the assistance of someone else, the operative arm is passively elevated initially to 90° with the elbow extended (Fig. 12). In addition, with the elbow at

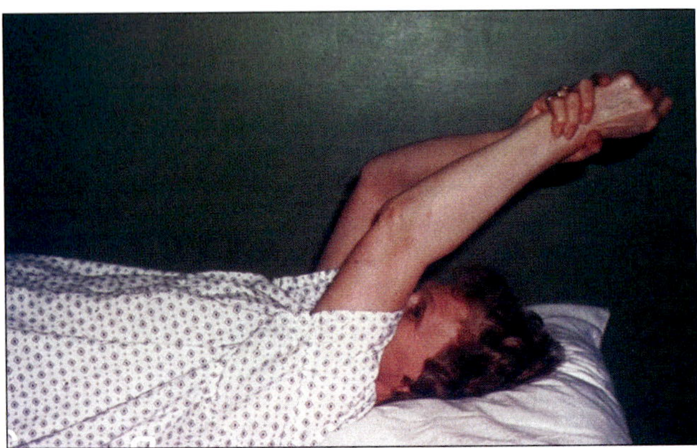

FIGURE 12

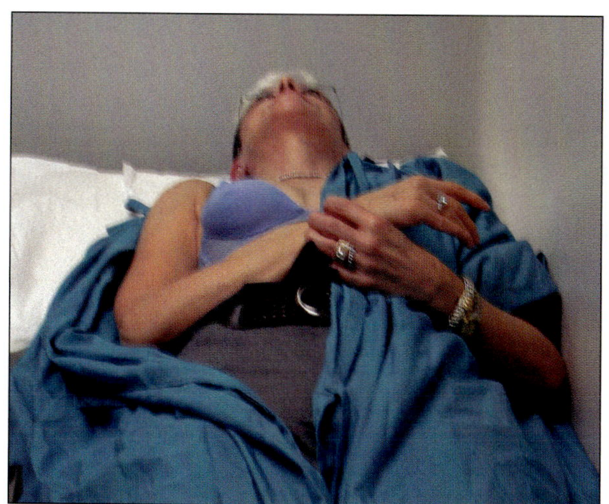

A

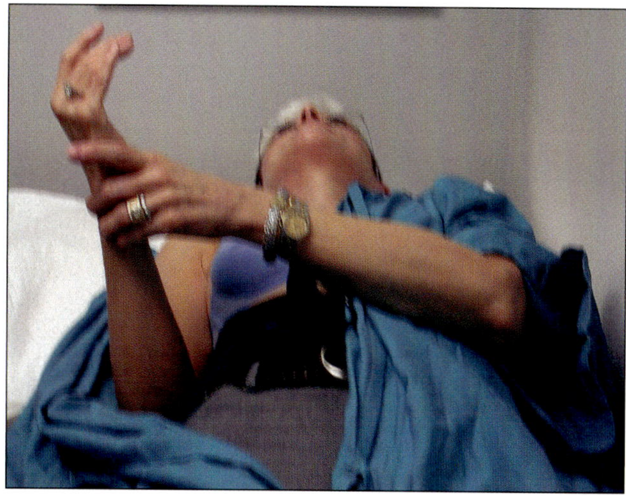

B

FIGURE 13

the side and flexed to 90°, the extremity is externally rotated (Fig. 13A and 13B). These exercises are repeated six to eight times during three sessions daily. Between exercise periods, the extremity is kept in the immobilizer.

- After 4 weeks, the immobilizer is discontinued and replaced by a simple sling for use outdoors and during sleep, and a formal rehabilitation/physical therapy program is begun. This phase is directed at regaining motion, and strengthening with weights, rubber bands, a UBE, or other machines is strictly avoided. Strengthening is added at 12 weeks.

Evidence

Neviaser TJ, Neviaser RJ, Neviaser JS, Neviaser JS. The four-in-one arthroplasty for the painful arc syndrome. Clin Orthop Relat Res. 1982;(163):107–12.

In this study, 89 patients with clinical signs of the painful arc syndrome were proven to have an associated biceps tenosynovitis by arthrography and at surgical treatment. The four-in-one arthroplasty consisted of 1) excision of the coracoacromial ligament, 2) acromioclavicular arthroplasty, 3) excision of the anterior-inferior area of the acromion process, and 4) transfer and tenodesis of the long head of the biceps. The operation decompressed the acromial arch and also eliminated the biceps tenosynovitis by tenodesis. Almost invariably, there was relief of pain within 4–5 months of postoperative rehabilitation, and at an average follow-up of 2–8 years. (Level IV evidence)

Post M, Benca P. Primary tendinitis of the long head of the biceps. Clin Orthop Relat Res. 1989;(246):117–25.

In this study, 17 patients with chronic painful shoulders who showed evidence of isolated bicipital tendinitis involving only the extracapsular, intertubercular portion of the long head of the biceps were chosen for surgical treatment when conservative treatment failed. The patients were thought to have primary bicipital tendinitis secondary to other shoulder pathologies. Thirteen patients had tenodeses and four patients had transfer of the long head of the biceps to the origin of the conjoined tendon. Overall, excellent and good results were noted in 94% of both groups of patients when the long head of the biceps was tenodesed or transferred. (Level IV evidence)

Wolf RS, Zheng N, Weichel D. Long head biceps tenotomy versus tenodesis: a cadaveric biomechanical analysis. Arthroscopy. 2005;21:182–5.

In a cadaver study, compared with tenodesis, biceps tenotomy resulted in a significant risk of distal long head of the biceps (LHB) tendon migration and significantly lower load to failure. Cyclic loads similar to those produced by gentle active range of motion without resistance resulted in failure in 40% of specimens tested after an average of 35 cycles. Based on these results, the authors recommended that LHB tenodesis be considered in any patient who may object to the cosmetic deformity and associated dysfunction produced by distal LHB tendon migration after tenotomy.

Yamaguchi K, Riew KD, Galatz LM, Syme JA, Neviaser RJ. Biceps activity during shoulder motion: an electromyographic analysis. Clin Orthop Relat Res. 1997;(336):122–9.

Electromyographic (EMG) responses in 44 shoulders from 30 subjects were examined. Fourteen shoulders from 13 patients had documented rotator cuff tears. The remaining volunteers had normal cuff integrity by history and examination. EMG responses were recorded from the long head of the biceps, brachioradialis (elbow control), and supraspinatus (shoulder control). Elbow-related biceps activity was minimized by using a brace locked in neutral forearm rotation and 100° of flexion. Analysis of normal and rotator cuff–deficient data was performed in a masked fashion and EMG activity normalized as a percentage of maximal muscle contraction during 10 shoulder motions based on the scapular plane. Normal shoulders in all ranges of active motion exhibited significant supraspinatus activity (20–50% maximum muscle contraction). The response followed patterns expected for a shoulder stabilizer. In contrast, in every normal shoulder, biceps and brachioradialis activity remained insignificant (1.7–3.6% maximum muscle contraction) and did not follow a patterned response. In patients with rotator cuff tears, biceps activity remained low (1.6–4.4% maximum muscle contraction). Given these findings, any function of the long head of the biceps in shoulder motion does not involve active contractions.

PROCEDURE 20

Arthroscopic Biceps Tenodesis

Pascal Boileau and Jason Old

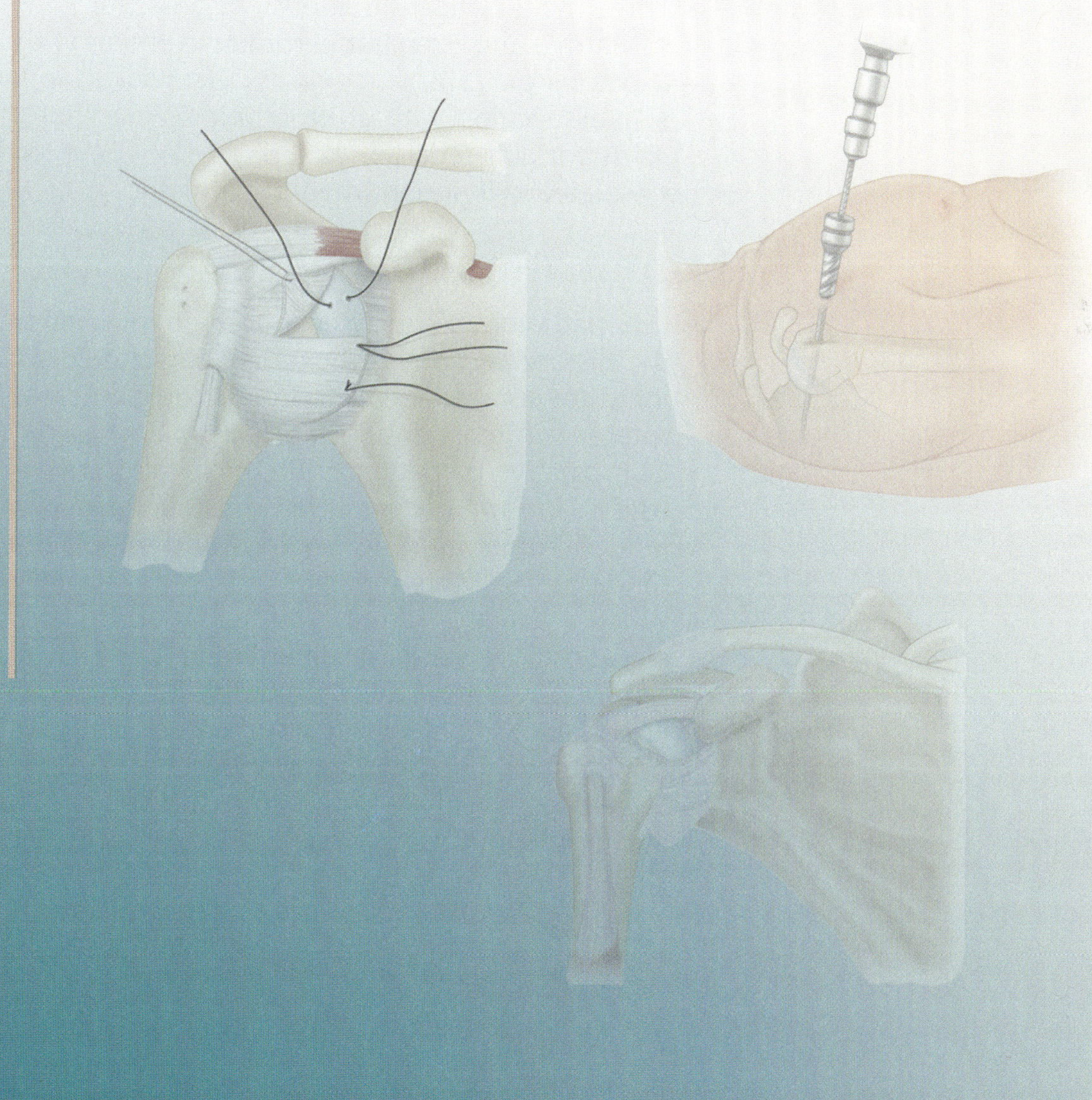

Pitfalls

- *True pseudoparalysis due to a massive rotator cuff tear that persists after rehabilitation is a contraindication to isolated biceps tenodesis. True pseudoparalysis may be differentiated from painful loss of elevation by using the "landing test."*
- *Very thin, frayed tendons in a state of pre-rupture should be treated with simple tenotomy.*

Controversies

- We perform arthroscopic tenodesis routinely in all cuff repairs.

Treatment Options

- Tenosynovitis may respond to rest, physiotherapy, and analgesia.
- Injections of steroid and local anesthetic have both a diagnostic and a therapeutic role, but should be placed in the bicipital groove under imaging guidance to improve accuracy.
- Many conditions of the LHB are mechanical and, when symptomatic, require surgical intervention.

Indications

- May be indicated in the treatment of pathology of the long head of the biceps tendon (LHB), including:
  - Tenosynovitis
  - Subluxations or dislocations
  - Entrapment of the LHB in the glenohumeral joint due to hypertrophy, producing the "hourglass biceps" (Fig. 1)
  - Type II or IV superior labrum anterior-posterior (SLAP) lesions
- Three main clinical situations are possible:
  - Massive and irreparable rotator cuff tear with pathologic LHB
  - In association with arthroscopic or mini-open rotator cuff repair
  - Isolated LHB lesion in young athletes

Examination/Imaging

- LHB pathology is rarely encountered in isolation, so the history and physical examination should also focus on commonly related pathologies such as rotator cuff tears and instability.
- Comparative palpation of the bicipital groove is often useful, and the groove is felt most easily in 10° of internal rotation. In dislocations of the LHB, the tenderness is more medial.
- When a patient presents with a loss of active elevation it is crucial to differentiate between true pseudoparalysis of the shoulder and painful loss of elevation. A shoulder with true pseudoparalysis is nonfunctional, exhibiting an ineffective shrug with attempted elevation of the arm, and will not respond to an isolated biceps procedure. A shoulder with

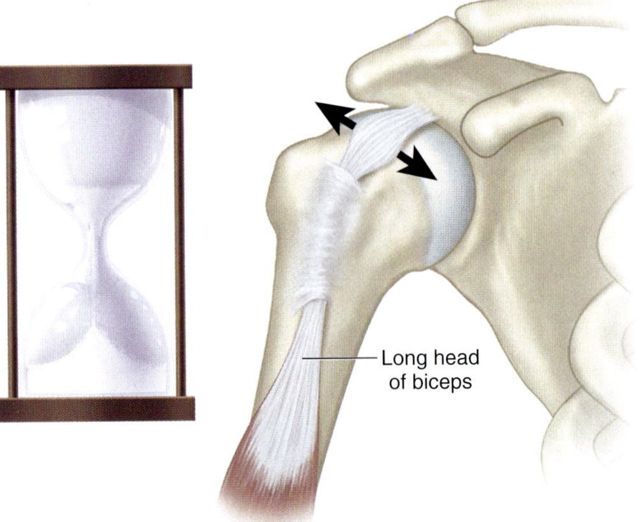

FIGURE 1

painful loss of elevation is functional but active elevation is limited because of pain and often responds well to a biceps tenotomy or tenodesis. Performing the "landing test" can help to differentiate between the 2 entities. The examiner passively places the arm just above the horizontal level (between 90° and 120°). A patient with true pseudoparalysis of the shoulder will not be able to actively maintain the arm in this position and it will fall down despite the patient's efforts.

- We also find Speed's test useful in diagnosing biceps pathology.
- Pain related to pathology of the LHB is located mainly at the anterior part of the shoulder, but pain may also be localized to the angle of the scapula posteriorly.
- Spontaneous rupture of the tendon is often accompanied by retraction of the tendon and the classic "Popeye" deformity. With subluxation or dislocation of the tendon, the muscle belly can appear attenuated, an appearance that we call a "false-Popeye" sign.
- The clinical sign of a hypertrophied and entrapped hourglass biceps is a limitation of the terminal 10–20° of active and passive elevation. There is no loss of rotation, and it should not be confused with a frozen shoulder.
- A standard series of radiographs should be obtained to rule in or out any associated abnormalities.
- We also find contrast studies (computed tomography [CT] arthrography, magnetic resonance imaging arthrography) very useful to assist in diagnosing pathology of the biceps tendon and rotator cuff before surgery. The CT arthrogram in Figure 2 demonstrates the LHB (*arrow*) dislocated in the substance of the subscapularis.

Surgical Anatomy

- The LHB originates on the glenoid labrum and supraglenoid tubercle.
- The bicipital groove runs vertically between the lesser and greater tuberosities and is oriented ~30° anterior to the plane of the glenoid when the humerus is in neutral rotation.
- The stability of the LHB in the bicipital groove depends on the biceps pulley (Fig. 3A), which has contributions from:
  - Superior glenohumeral ligament (SGHL)
  - Coracohumeral ligament (CHL)
  - Glenohumeral joint capsule

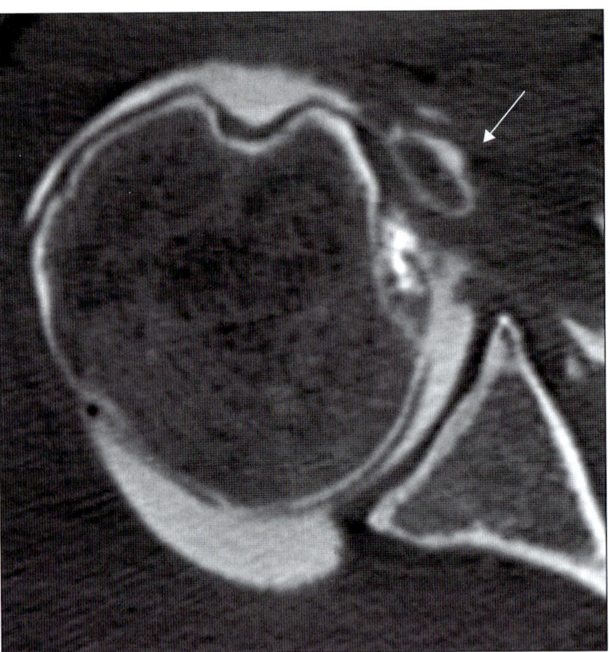

FIGURE 2

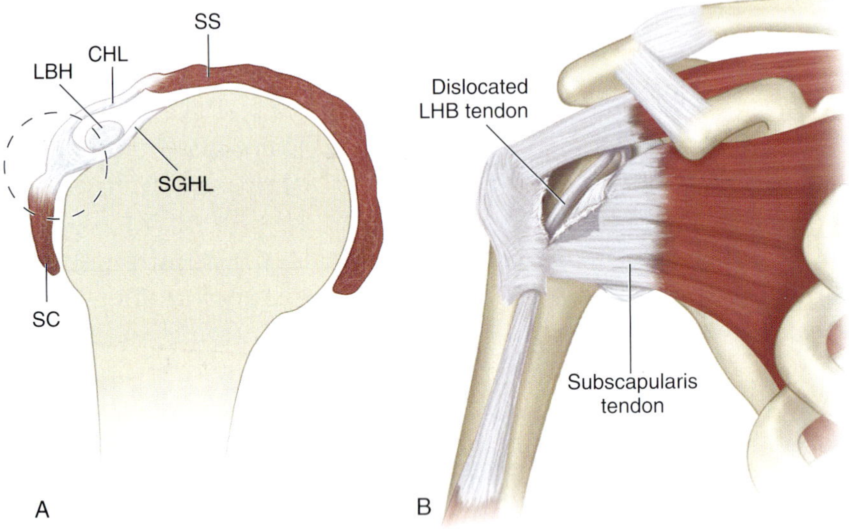

FIGURE 3

- Tendons of the subscapularis (SC) and supraspinatus (SS)

- The subscapularis is a major restraint to medial subluxation of the LHB. Full- or partial-thickness tearing of the subscapularis is pathognomonic of medial subluxation or dislocation of the LHB (Fig. 3B).
- The transverse humeral ligament does not play a major role in LHB stability.
- The anterior circumflex humeral artery and its dual venae comitantes, known as the "three sisters," cross the floor of the bicipital groove at the level of the distal margin of the subscapularis insertion, while its ascending branch runs along the lateral edge of the groove. These vessels should be preserved whenever possible.

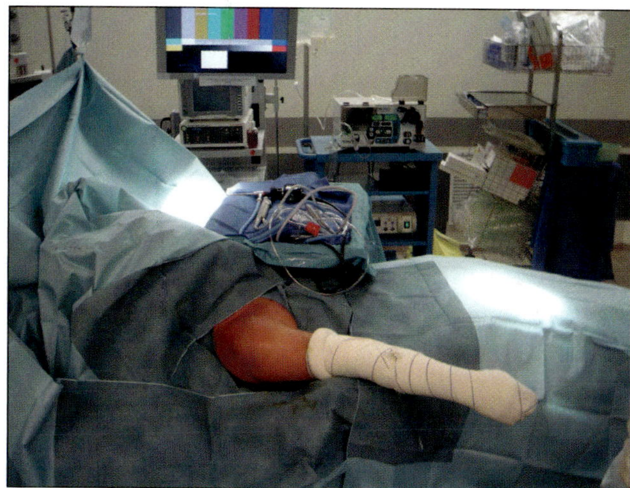
A

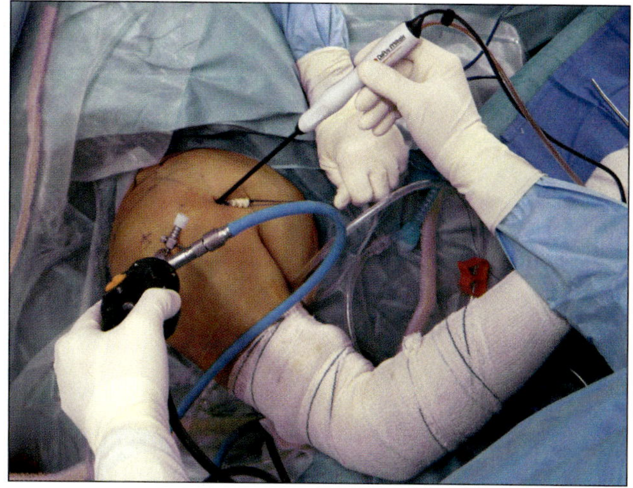
B

FIGURE 4

PEARLS

- *The position we describe has the following advantages:*
  - *Detensioning of the anterior deltoid fibers allows greater distention and easier visualization in the anterior subdeltoid space.*
  - *The ability to rotate and elevate the shoulder intraoperatively allows dynamic arthroscopic examination of the biceps and pulley system.*
  - *The ability to flex and extend the elbow intraoperatively allows the LHB to be tensioned or detensioned as needed, aiding in restoration of correct LHB tension and making the procedure technically easier.*

Positioning

- We perform this technique with the patient in a semi–beach chair position without traction (Fig. 4A).
- During the anterior extra-articular part of the procedure, the shoulder should be placed in approximately 30° of flexion, 30° of internal rotation, and 30° of abduction (arthrodesis position) (Fig. 4B).
- The elbow is placed on a support slightly above the shoulder, while the hand rests on a Mayo stand.

Portals/Exposures

- Bony landmarks and locations for the posterior, anteromedial, and anterolateral portals are drawn on the skin using the "two-finger rule" (Fig. 5).

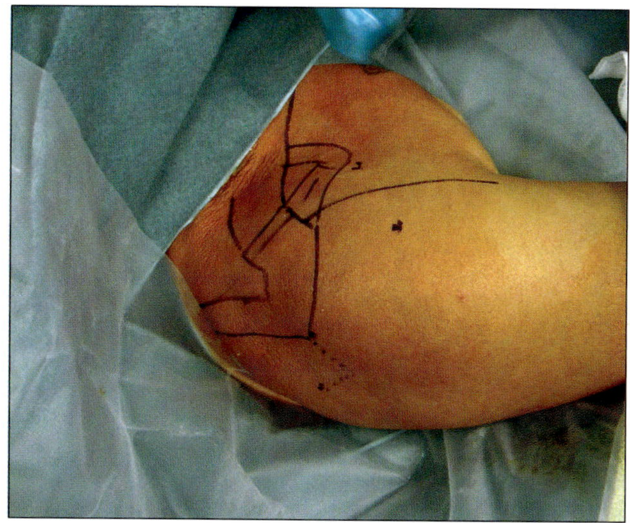

FIGURE 5

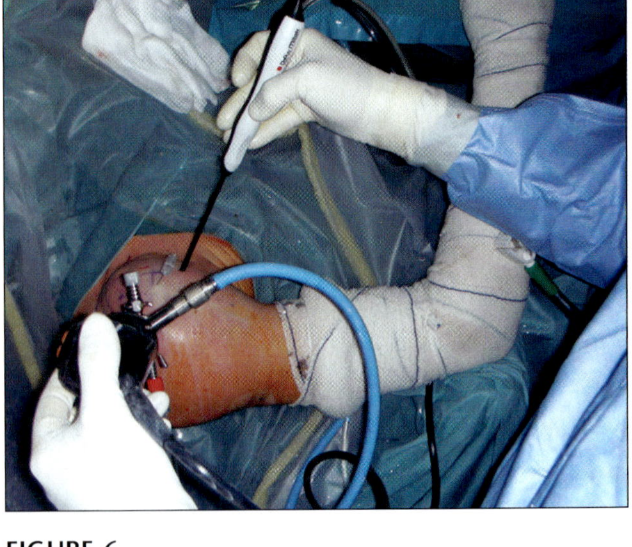

FIGURE 6

- The classic posterior portal is created 2 cm inferior and 2 cm medial to the posterolateral corner of the acromion.
- Two anterior portals (anterior and anterolateral) are created 1.5 cm on each side of the bicipital groove, 3 cm distal to the anterior corner of the acromion.
- The posterior and anterolateral portals are used as viewing portals and the anterior portal is used as a working portal. In the extra-articular portion of the procedure, the anteromedial portal is the working portal and the anterolateral portal is the viewing portal (Fig. 6).

Equipment

- The arm may be placed on a classic U-shaped knee support or a limb positioner such as the Spider arm positioner (Tenet Medical, Canada).

Controversies

- While the lateral position may be used for arthroscopic LHB tenodesis, we feel that it lacks the versatility of the beach chair position.

Procedure

Step 1: Glenohumeral Exploration and Tenotomy of the LHB

- A diagnostic arthroscopy of the glenohumeral joint is performed with the 30° arthroscope in the posterior portal.
- Dynamic examination of the biceps is then performed with the following tests:
  - Hourglass test—the shoulder is elevated in the scapular plane in neutral rotation with the elbow extended (Fig. 7A). In a positive hourglass test, the hypertrophic tendon fails to slide in the bicipital groove and buckles in the articulation, limiting elevation (Fig. 7B).

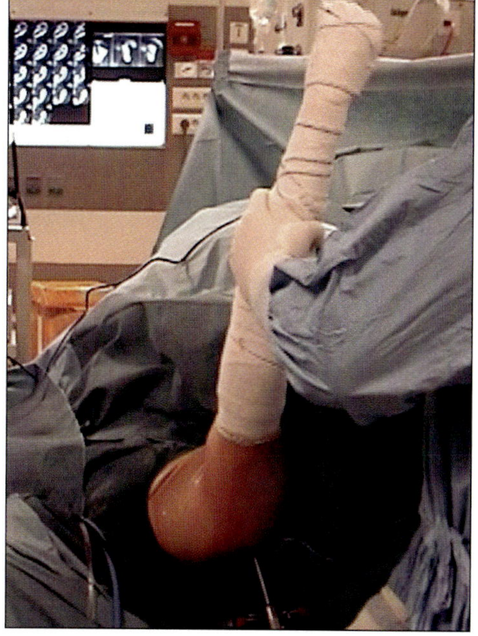

A

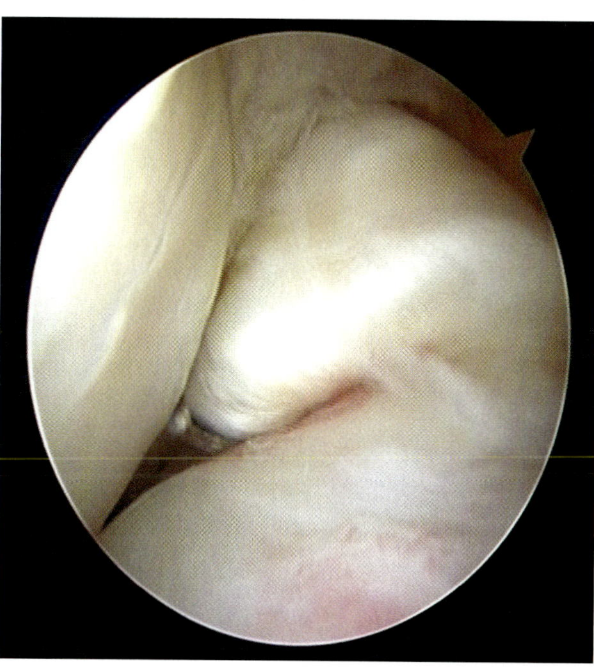

B

FIGURE 7

Pearls

- *To ensure enough space to work and triangulate, we use a "two-finger rule" when marking and establishing our portals. The anterior portals are located 2 fingerbreadths inferior to the anterior corner of the acromion, with 2 fingerbreadths between them (one fingerbreadth on either side of the LHB).*

Pitfalls

- *Avoid making the anterior portals too superior, as the subdeltoid space becomes closed down and the tissue is very vascular in this area and tends to bleed, reducing visibility.*

- Swinging test—the adducted shoulder is rotated internally and externally to look for instability of the LHB. Medial subluxation in external rotation indicates either a partial- or full-thickness tear of the subscapularis tendon, while lateral subluxation in external rotation indicates a tear of the suprapinatus that may be either partial articular-sided (partial articular-surface supraspinatus tendon avulsion, or PASTA lesion) or full thickness.

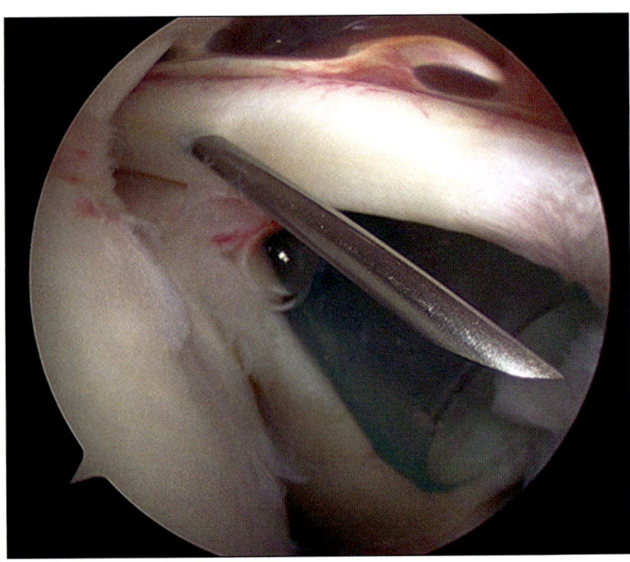

FIGURE 8

- An anterior portal is established using an inside-out technique, passing the trocar through the rotator interval, lateral to the coracoid process, 1 cm distal to it, and just above the subscapularis tendon.
- Biceps pathology is very often in the intertubercular groove portion, and it is important to draw this part of the biceps tendon into the joint with a probe.
- If a tenodesis is planned, the LHB is transfixed intra-articularly at its entrance into the groove with a spinal needle to avoid retraction out of the joint (Fig. 8). The tendon is then detached from its glenoid insertion using a scalpel, a punch, or electrocautery.
- If a simple tenotomy is planned, it is not necessary to place a needle and the tendon is allowed to retract out of the joint.

Pearls

- *An hourglass biceps tendon may not slide out of the joint with extension of the elbow and shoulder. In such cases of "autotenodesis," we simply resect the intra-articular portion of the LHB.*

Pitfalls

- *A dislocated LHB is sometimes mistaken for a ruptured tendon when it becomes encased in fibrous tissue medial to the glenoid and in front of the subscapularis. Care should be taken to expose the glenoid tubercle and base of the coracoid to avoid missing a dislocated biceps that will remain painful if neglected.*

Step 2: Identification and Opening of the Bicipital Groove

- The anterolateral portal is now created and the arthroscope is inserted here.
- The anterior cannula is removed and a blunt trocar is used to reorient the portal into the anterior subdeltoid space.
- A blunt trocar is used via the anteromedial cannula to palpate the "soft spot" corresponding to the bicipital groove, just medial to the lateral part of the greater tuberosity.
- The trocar is used to gently push the "cobwebs" of fibrous tissue off of the transverse ligament without disrupting the adjacent vessels.
- Visualization of the white fibers of the transverse ligament and of the ascending vessels on the lateral part of the groove also help to locate the bicipital groove.

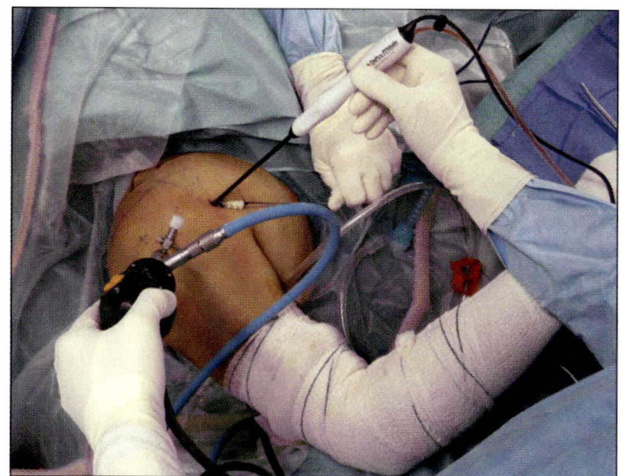
A

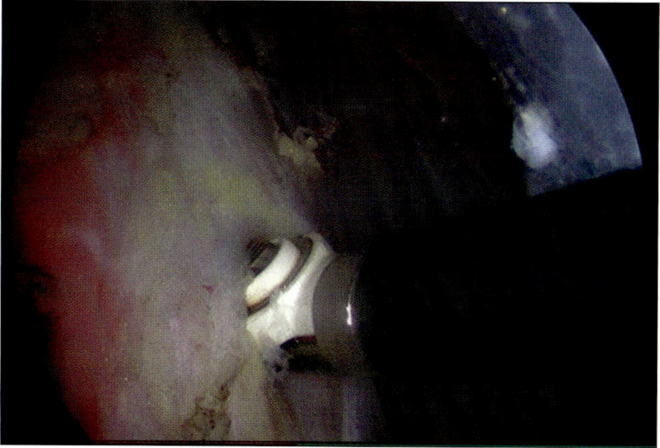
B

FIGURE 9

- With the arthroscope placed in the anterior subdeltoid space via the anterolateral portal, the bicipital groove is identified and opened with electrocautery (Fig. 9A). The bursa anterior to the bicipital groove is resected with either a motorized shaver or the Mitek VAPR device (Mitek Products, Sommerville, NJ) (Fig. 9B).
- The transverse humeral ligament is now opened in a longitudinal fashion, using a hook-tipped electrocautery because of the leash of vessels on either border of the groove.
- Once the groove is open, the LHB is probed and a careful synovectomy is performed using the shaver, freeing any possible adhesions.

Pearls

- *Care should be taken to avoid twisting the LHB during exteriorization.*

Pitfalls

- *Swelling of the shoulder due to fluid extravasation can make it difficult or impossible to exteriorize enough tendon. Fluid pressure should be kept under 30 mm Hg whenever possible. If other arthroscopic procedures are planned, the tenodesis should be performed first.*

Step 3: Biceps Exteriorization and Preparation

- Once the bicipital groove has been opened, the LHB is grasped, the spinal needle is removed, and the elbow is slowly extended. The biceps is then grasped by its most proximal end and exteriorized through the anteromedial portal (Fig. 10).

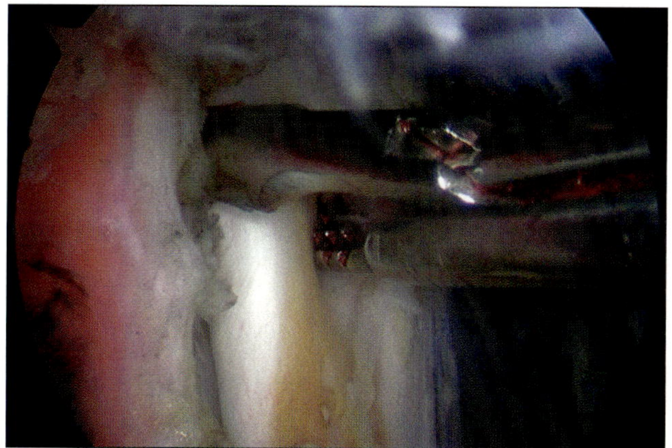

FIGURE 10

- Two atraumatic vascular clamps are used to grasp the LHB tendon progressively more distally to exteriorize as much tendon as possible (Fig. 11). About 4–5 cm of tendon should be exteriorized, which is facilitated by flexion of the elbow. A single clamp is then used to keep the tendon outside during tendon preparation.
- Any remaining synovium is removed, and if necessary the tendon is trimmed in the line of its fibers so that the diameter of the doubled tendon will be 8 mm.
- The tendon is now doubled over a #2 Ethibond suture (Ethicon, USA) and a #1 PDS suture (Ethicon, USA).
- The end of the tendon is doubled and sewn to its anterior face for a length of about 2 cm using a running baseball stitch with #1 absorbable suture (Vicryl, Ethicon, USA) (Fig. 12). A mark is made with ink on the base of the doubled tendon anteriorly.
    - The PDS suture is then tied at the end of the loop, with one end as long as possible and the other cut short. The PDS suture will later be used to guide the interference screw and screwdriver into the humeral socket.
    - The #2 Ethibond suture is left passing through the doubled tendon loop unsecured, as it will later be used to pull the tendon into the socket and subsequently removed after the tendon is fixed.
- The diameter of the double tendon is measured using an anterior cruciate ligament (ACL) graft sizer.
- The size of the double tendon determines the drill diameter needed to drill the humeral socket, and should be 7 or 8 mm.

Step 4: Drilling the Humeral Socket

- The bicipital groove is débrided of fibrous tissue with the shaver or the VAPR.
- Once the groove is adequately exposed, socket placement is planned. Optimal placement is approximately 10 mm below the top of the groove entrance to prevent any anterosuperior impingement with the acromial arch. In practice this is roughly halfway between the superior limit of the groove and the three sisters.
- A pilot hole for the humeral socket is made with an awl. A guidewire is placed in the bicipital groove approximately 1 cm below the entrance to the joint (Fig. 13A). The guidewire, oriented strictly perpendicular to the humerus and parallel to the lateral border of the acromion, is advanced until it engages the posterior cortex of the humerus (Fig. 13B).

Pearls

- *The ink mark on the anterior part of the doubled tendon guides both orientation and depth of insertion in the socket.*
- *The groove should be exposed from its entrance into the joint superiorly to the three sisters. To avoid bleeding, care must be taken not to disrupt the three sisters or the ascending vessels just medial and lateral to the groove.*

Pitfalls

- *The orientation of the socket should be carefully controlled, as it will determine the exit trajectory of the transhumeral Beath pin in the next step. It is theoretically possible to injure the axillary nerve if the pin exits too far inferiorly, though we have never experienced this complication.*

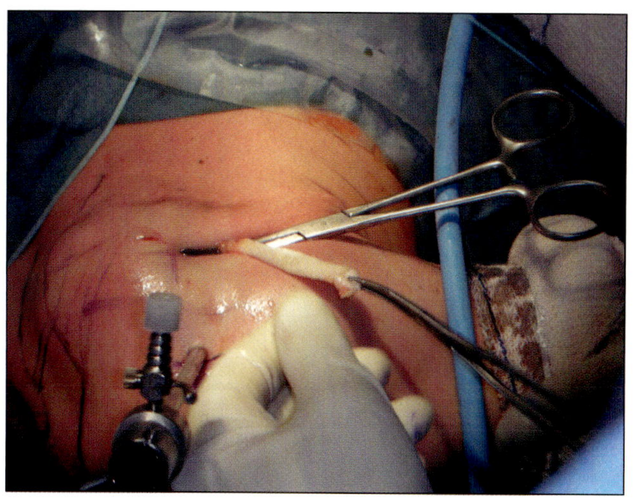

FIGURE 11

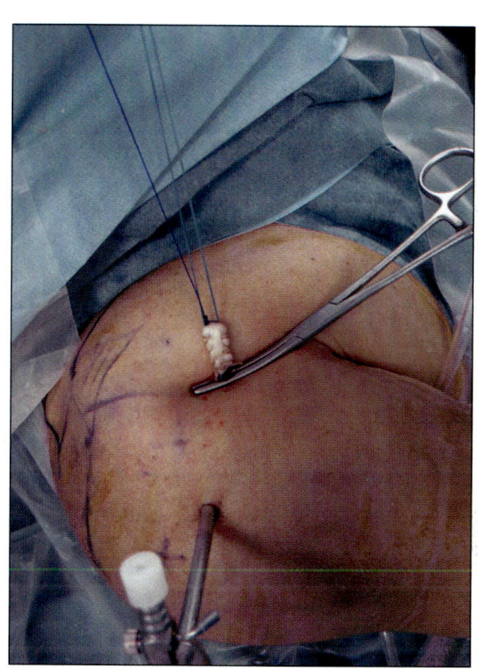

FIGURE 12

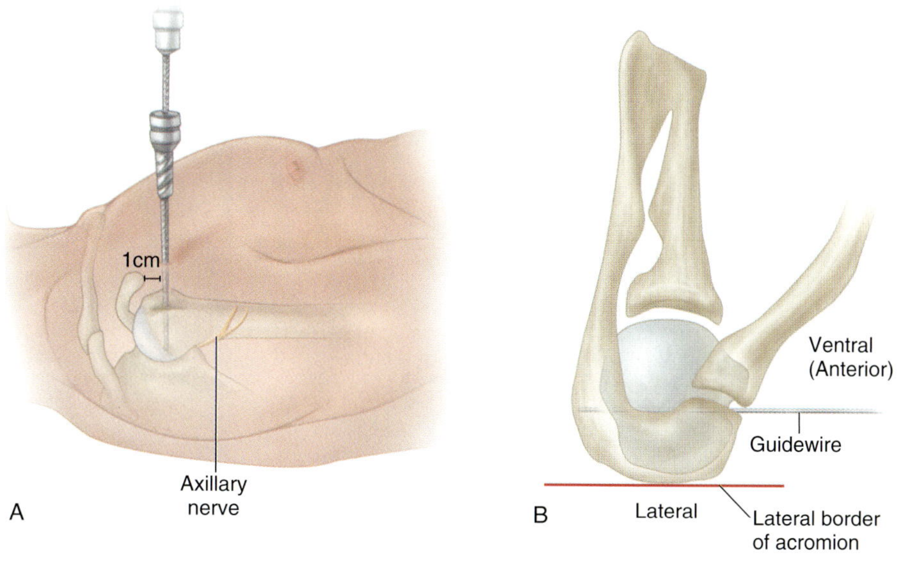

FIGURE 13

- The guidewire is then overdrilled with a 7- or 8-mm cannulated reamer (depending on the size of the doubled tendon) to a depth of 25 mm (Fig. 14A and 14B). The socket is then drilled perpendicular to the humerus and parallel to the acromion.
- After the reamer and drill bit are removed, the shaver, the VAPR, and a motorized burr are used via the anteromedial portal to chamfer smooth the edges of the socket entrance and remove bony debris and tissues that may contribute to tendon blocking and abrasion (Fig. 15).

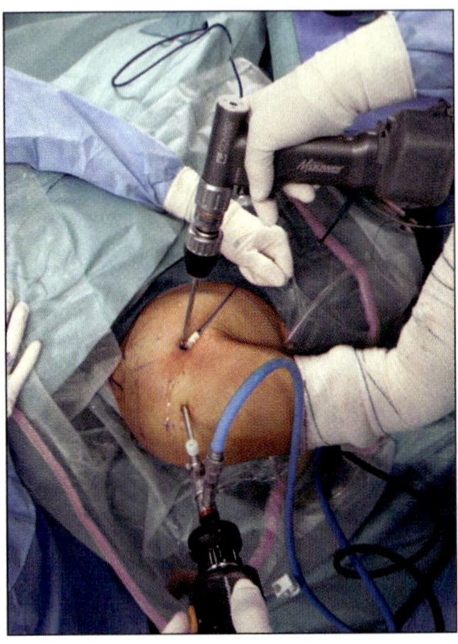

A

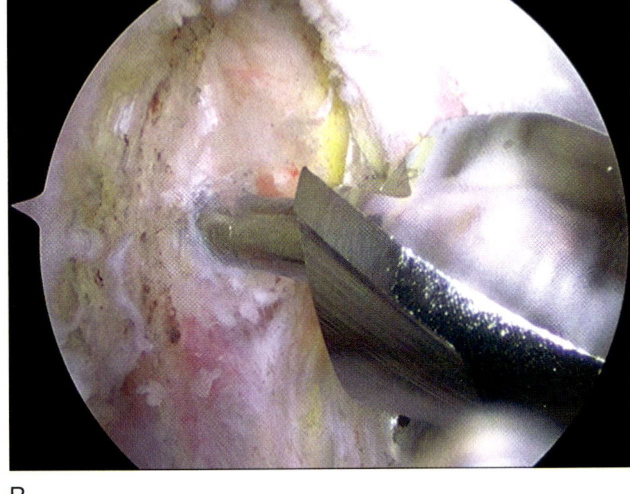

B

FIGURE 14

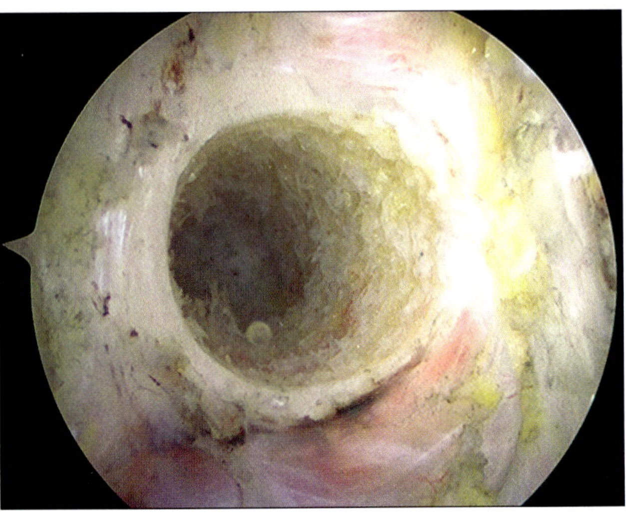

FIGURE 15

Instrumentation/ Implantation

- A Beath pin pull-through technique is used for tendon placement. Commonly used in ACL reconstruction, this pin has an eyelet on its trailing end and serves as a suture passer.

Step 5: Passing the Transhumeral Pin

- A Beath pin is placed through the anterior cannula into the humeral socket. In order to centralize the pin, we place the reamer in the socket in a reversed orientation, removing it once the pin has been advanced (Fig. 16).
- To avoid injury to the axillary nerve, the Beath pin should be strictly perpendicular to the humerus and parallel to the lateral border of the acromion.
  - The Beath pin is advanced through the posterior aspect of the humerus and used to pass the traction suture (Fig. 17).
  - The Beath pin is drilled until it exits the skin, which will be approximately 2 cm inferior and 2 cm medial the posterolateral border of the acromion.

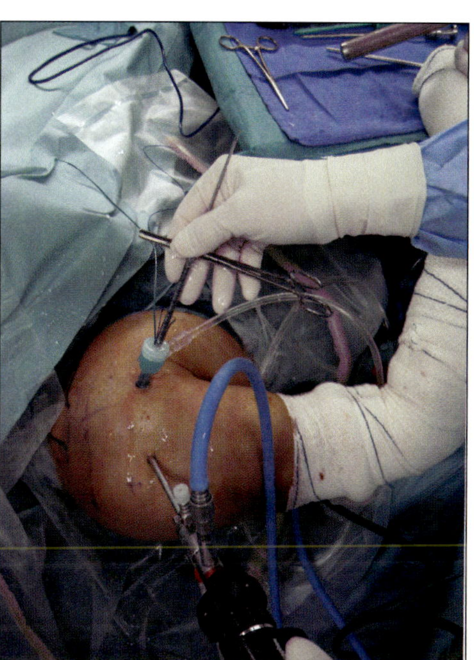

FIGURE 16

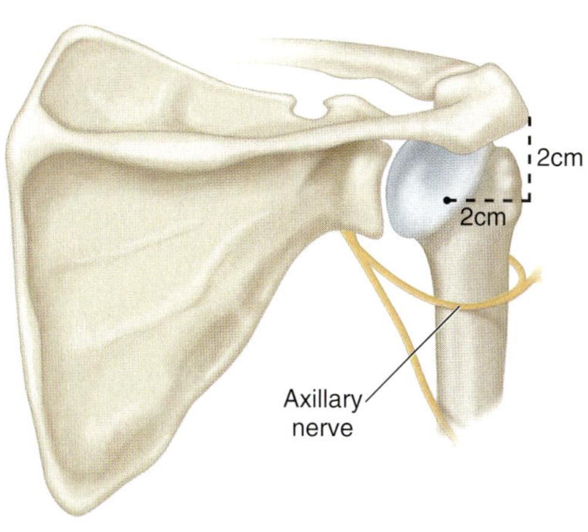

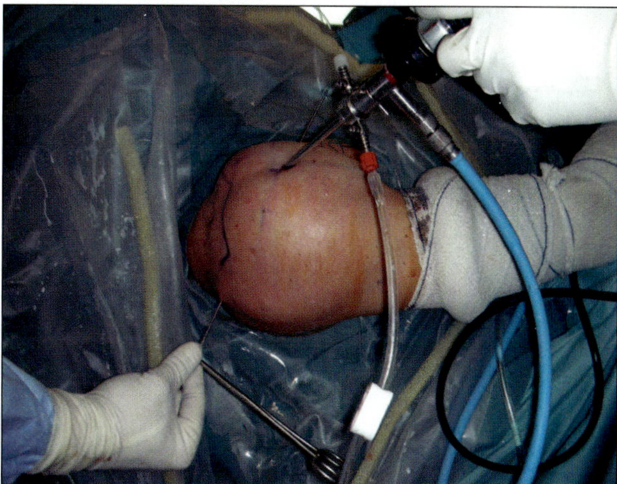

FIGURE 17 A B

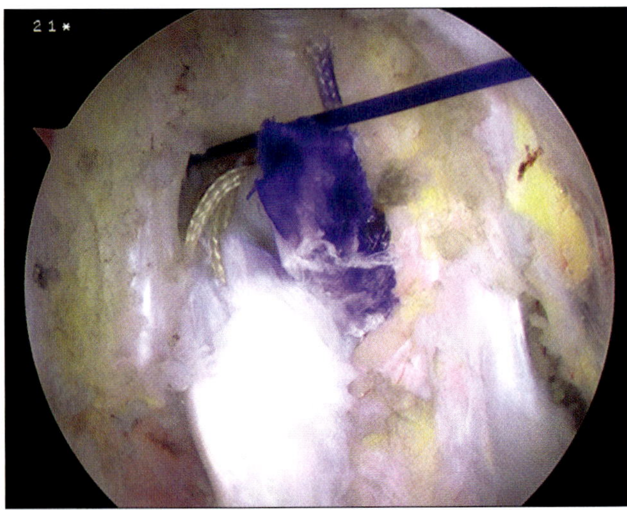

FIGURE 18

- Both ends of the Ethibond suture are threaded through the eyelet, and the pin and sutures are pulled through the humerus. The PDS suture is not passed posteriorly, as it will be used to guide the screw and screwdriver into the socket.
- The tendon is checked for twists, and if necessary it is reoriented with a probe or grasper.
- The Ethibond suture is used to pull the entire doubled loop of biceps tendon into the humeral socket (Fig. 18). The ink mark at the base of the doubled portion of the tendon is used to verify that the orientation and depth of insertion are correct. It should pass just inside the socket.

Instrumentation/ Implantation

- We use a bioabsorbable screw made of polylactic acid (PLA98) (Tenoscrew, Phusis; Tornier, USA). We like this screw because it is smooth so as not to damage the tendon, and slow-absorbing to minimize inflammation.

Step 6: Interference Screw Fixation

- The tendon is fixed in the socket using an 8.5 × 20-mm bioabsorbable interference screw. As a general rule, we use an interference screw that is 0.5 mm larger than the socket diameter.
- After removing the cannula, the screw is passed over the PDS suture and into the joint above the doubled tendon (Fig. 19). With the elbow still flexed to 90°, the screw is placed on the superior aspect of the tendon and advanced into the socket (Fig. 20).
- Once the tip of the screw is engaged between the tendon and the socket wall, the tendon is tensioned by extending the elbow. This prevents twisting and rotation of the tendon during screw placement.
- After complete insertion of the screw, the sutures are cut and removed. Tension and fixation are checked by probing the tendon in both flexion (Fig. 21A) and extension (Fig. 21B).

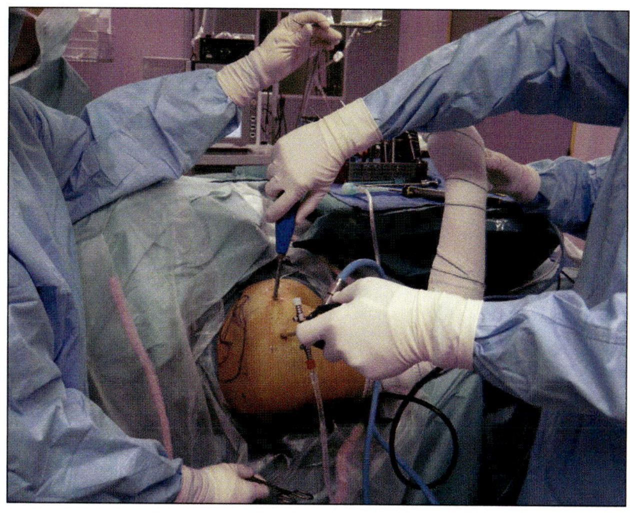

FIGURE 19

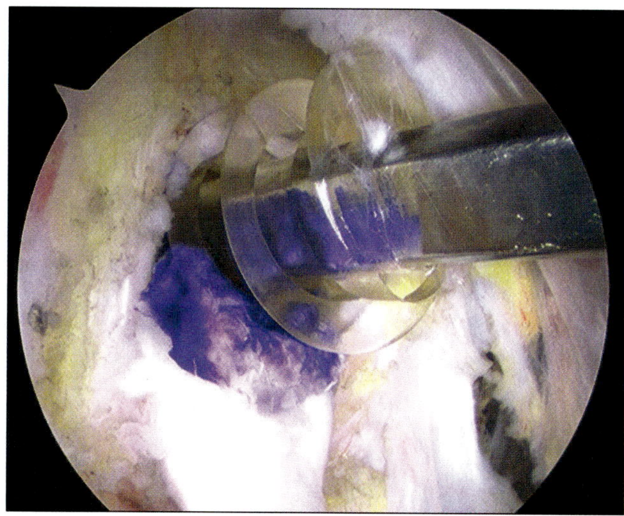

FIGURE 20

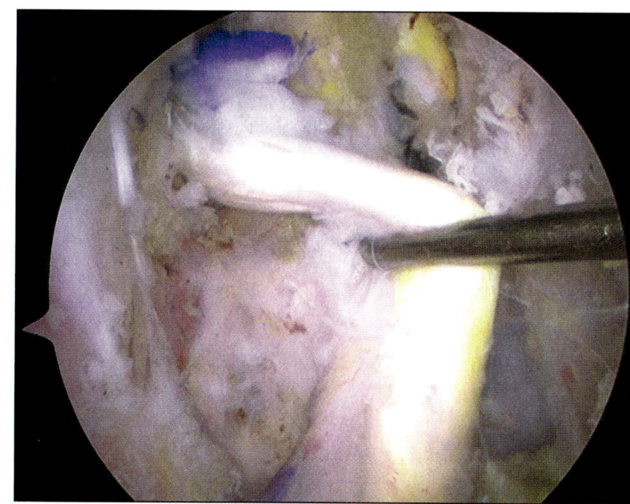

A

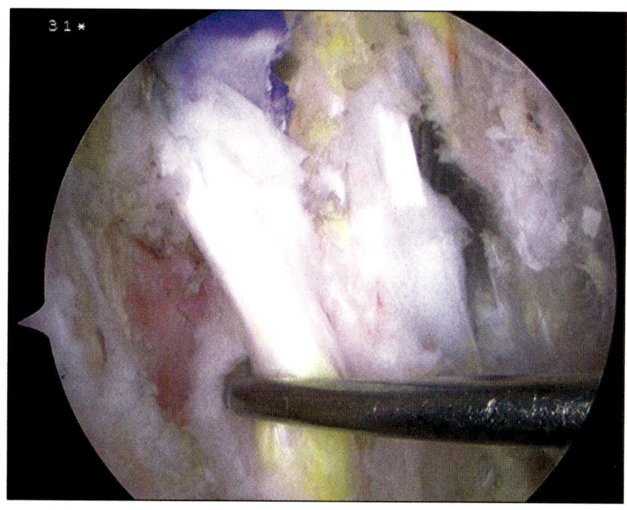

B

FIGURE 21

Postoperative Care and Expected Outcomes

- The arm is placed in a sling for comfort postoperatively.
- Pendular exercises are started immediately. Lifting is limited to less than 5 lbs, but the patient is encouraged to use the arm for activities of daily living as tolerated.

Evidence

Boileau P, Baque F, Valerio L, Ahrens P, Chuinard C, Trojani C. Isolated arthroscopic biceps tenotomy or tenodesis improves symptoms in patients with massive irreparable rotator cuff tears. J Bone Joint Surg [Am]. 2007;89:747-57.

In this retrospective series, 68 patients with irreparable rotator cuff tears were treated with arthroscopic bicpes tenotomy or tenodesis. At a mean follow-up of 35 months, 78% of patients were satisfied with the result. Mean Constant score improved from 46.3 to 66.5 points. There was no significant difference in outcome between the tenotomy and tenodesis groups. (Level IV evidence)

Walch G, Edwards TB, Boulahia A, Nove-Josserand L, Neyton L, Szabo I. Arthroscopic tenotomy of the long head of the biceps in the treatment of rotator cuff tears: clinical and radiographic results of 307 cases. J Shoulder Elbow Surg. 2005;14:238-46.

In this retrospective series, 307 patients with irreparable rotator cuff tears were treated with arthroscopic biceps tenotomy. At a mean follow-up of 57 months, 87% of patients were satisfied or very satisfied with the result. The mean Constant score improved from 48.4 to 67.6 points. Fatty infiltration of the rotator cuff had a negative influence on functional results. (Level IV evidence)

Walch G, Nove-Josserand L, Boileau P, Levigne C. Subluxations and dislocations of the tendon of the long head of the biceps. J Shoulder Elbow Surg. 1998;7:100-8.

In this retrospective series of 445 patients with rotator cuff tears, 71 patients (16%) were found to have medial displacement of the LHB (25 subluxations, 46 dislocations). In 69 cases (97%) there was an associated tear of the subscapularis tendon. (Level IV evidence)

PROCEDURE 21

SLAP Lesion: Arthroscopic Reconstruction of the Labrum and Biceps Anchor

Samuel A. Taylor, Mark C. Drakos, Jack T. Shonkwiler, and Stephen J. O'Brien

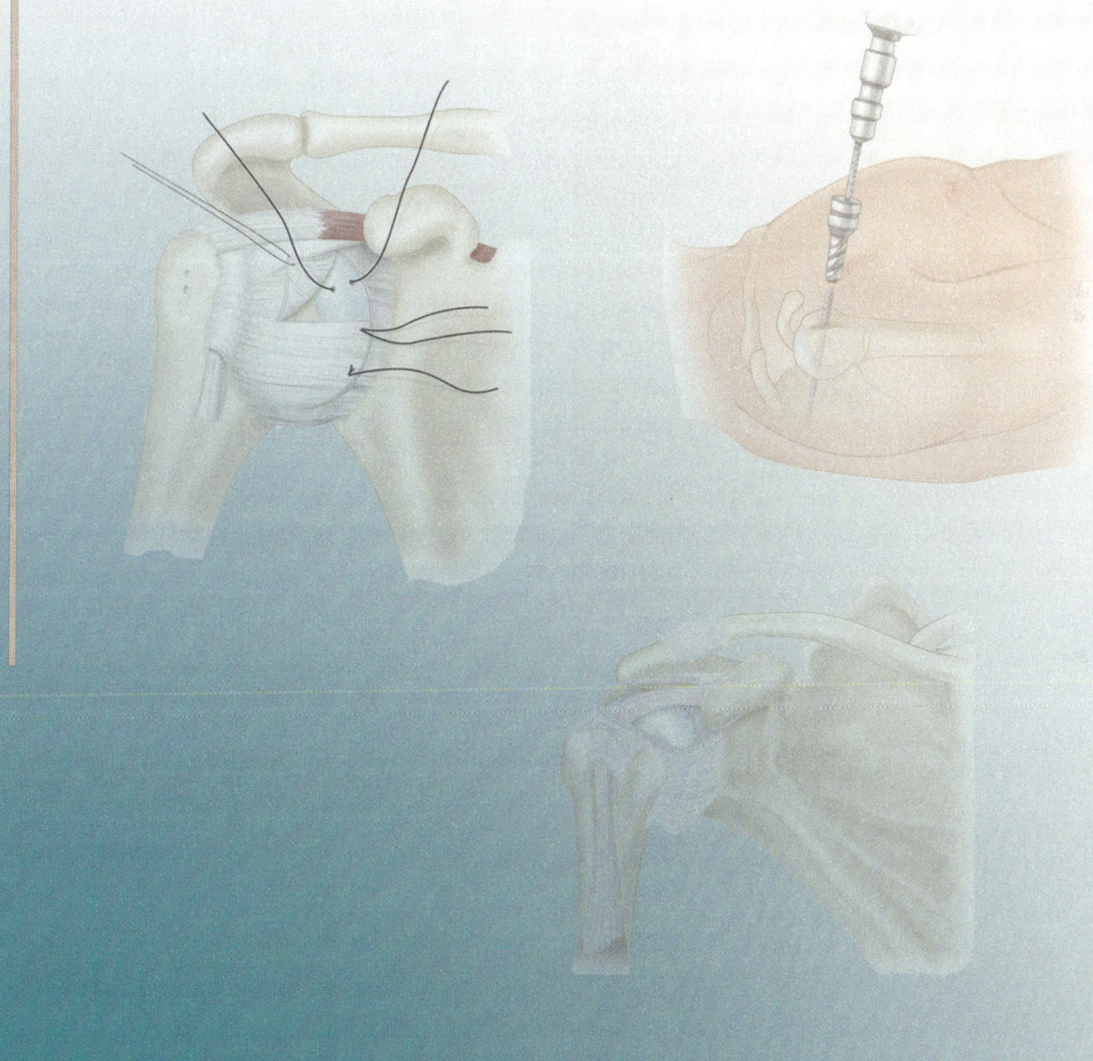

Figures 9, 13, 14, and 16–18 courtesy of Jack T. Shonkwiler.

PITFALLS

- *Concomitant pathology and other pain generators are frequent findings in patients with SLAP lesions (e.g., biceps lesions).*
- *Patients unable or unwilling to comply with an intensive postoperative physical therapy protocol may be suboptimal candidates for surgical intervention.*
- *Pause should be given in physiologically older individuals, as postoperative stiffness may be a common sequela.*

Indications

- Symptomatic lesion of the root of the biceps labrum complex recalcitrant to conservative measures in athletes and other high-functioning individuals who are willing to participate in a prolonged rehabilitation program

Examination/Imaging

- History may reveal a fall onto an abducted and forward-flexed arm, an acute traction injury, or repetitive microtrauma in an overhead athlete. Superior labrum anterior-posterior (SLAP) lesion symptoms may be variable and nonspecific and may include both mechanical symptoms (popping or clicking) with overhead activities and ill-defined pain from deep within or in the posterior shoulder.
- A thorough shoulder examination is crucial, as is maintenance of a broad differential diagnosis and sense of awareness. For example, weakness of external rotation may result from suprascapular nerve compression by a labral cyst, a common finding associated with labral tears (Fig. 1).
- Several clinical examination maneuvers have been described to expose SLAP lesions by stressing the biceps-labrum complex and thus display associated symptoms.

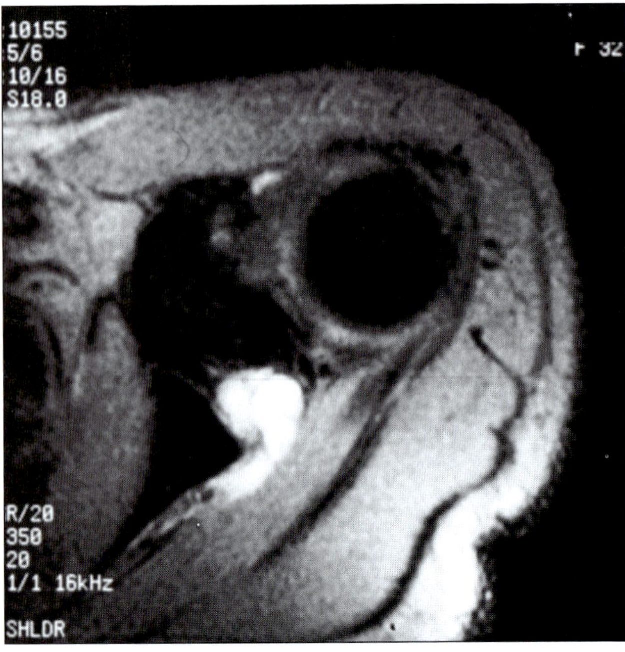

FIGURE 1

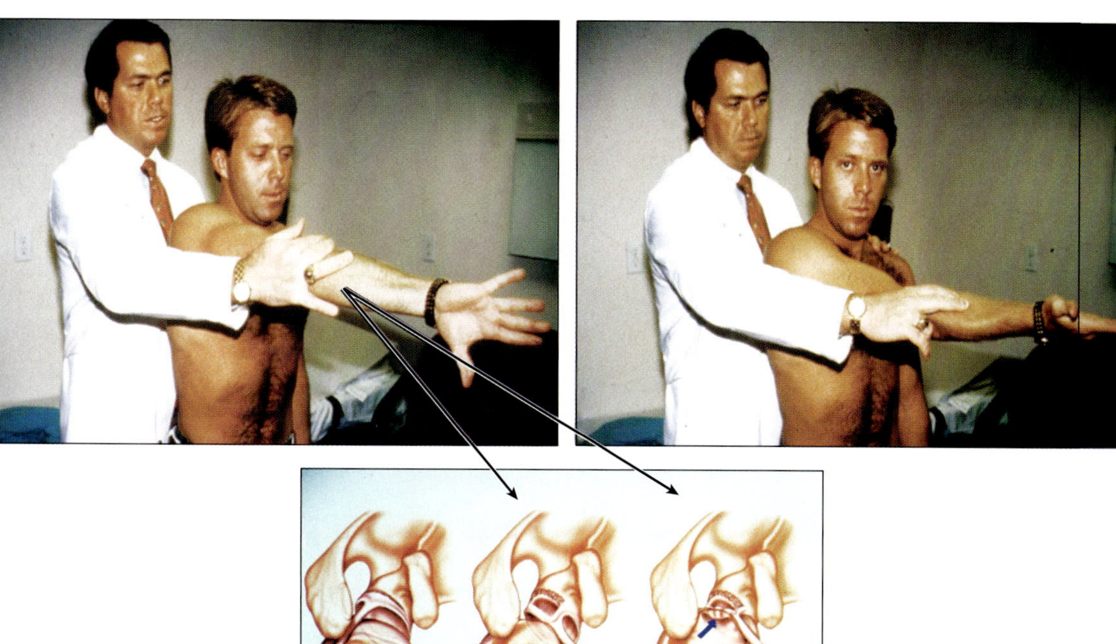

FIGURE 2

Controversies

- Clinical examination tools used to diagnose symptoms from SLAP lesions are often more sensitive than specific.
- The role of SLAP lesions as pain generators remains controversial, and they are frequently overdiagnosed.
- Arthroscopy is the most reliable method for diagnosis of SLAP lesions.
- Imaging findings must be correlated with clinical history and physical examination findings. Failure to do so can lead to an inaccurate treatment plan and patients who require chronic pain management and experience significant disability from sequelae such as adhesive capsulitis and reflex sympathetic dystrophy.

- Active compression test (O'Brien Sign)—The shoulder is forward flexed to 90° and adducted 10–15° with the elbow in full extension (Fig. 2). The examiner places downward force on the patient's arm, first in maximal internal rotation and then in maximal external rotation. Pain deep within the shoulder during the first action that is alleviated in maximal external rotation indicates a positive finding.
- Pain provocative test (Mimori)—From the seated position, the shoulder is abducted to 90–100° with the elbow in full extension. Similar to the O'Brien Sign, force is place on the fully pronated then supinated arm, with a positive test indicated by relief in the latter position.
- Compression rotation test (Andrews and Gidumal)—The shoulder is abducted to 90°, and the elbow also flexed to 90°. The examiner passively internally and externally rotates the humerus while axially loading the humeral head into the glenoid. Reproduction of pain or mechanical symptoms indicates a positive sign.

Treatment Options

- Physical therapy is often not helpful to treat SLAP lesions, but it may improve symptomatology from other associated diagnoses.
- Intra-articular injection is a powerful diagnostic *and* therapeutic tool.
- Activity restriction and rest may be helpful but may only be a temporizing measure.
- Surgical interventions are determined by the stability of the SLAP lesion. For an example, stable type I SLAP tears may be treated without fixation, utilizing labral débridement and/or superior glenoid decortication. An unstable SLAP lesion would require a fixation technique to restore normal anatomy.
- SLAP lesions often coexist with biceps pathology that may need to be addressed simultaneously. Surgical strategies may include biceps tenotomy, tenodesis, or transfer.

- Plain radiographs
  - Anteroposterior, lateral, and scapular Y views are obtained.
  - Radiographs are unrevealing in patients with isolated SLAP lesions but helpful in identifying concomitant shoulder pathology.
- Magnetic resonance imaging (MRI)
  - MRI is a very useful tool for evaluating the soft tissue structures about the glenohumeral joint, including labrum tears and SLAP lesions.
  - MRI arthrography is a more commonly used diagnostic tool for SLAP tears as it is less operator dependent.
- Shoulder arthroscopy is the "gold standard" for diagnosis and treatment of SLAP lesions. Indications for diagnostic arthroscopy include patients with (1) positive physical examination findings indicative of a SLAP tear with MRI correlation, or (2) chronic symptoms (>6 months) and positive physical findings for a SLAP lesion, with equivocal imaging data (e.g., large redundant labrum in the area of the sublabral foramen).
  - Static and dynamic arthroscopic examination is imperative. One should maintain a broad differential diagnosis and look for evidence of additional pain generators, including rotator cuff disease, arthritis, and biceps tendinopathy.
  - An arthroscopic active compression test, as described by O'Brien and colleagues, should be performed. To perform this test, the patient's shoulder is placed intraoperatively in the forward flexed (90°) and adducted (10–15°). Under direct intra-articular observation from the standard posterior portal, the arm is passively internally and externally rotated. In the setting of a SLAP lesion, the damaged anchor can be witnessed to displace inferiorly and medially. At times, arthroscopy may demonstrate an intact biceps anchor; however, during the arthroscopic active compression test, incarceration of the proximal long head of the biceps (Fig. 3A and 3B) may be visualized, elucidating the real etiology of the patient's symptoms.

Surgical Anatomy

- The superior labrum is a triangular fibrocartilaginous structure that encircles the glenoid surface. The

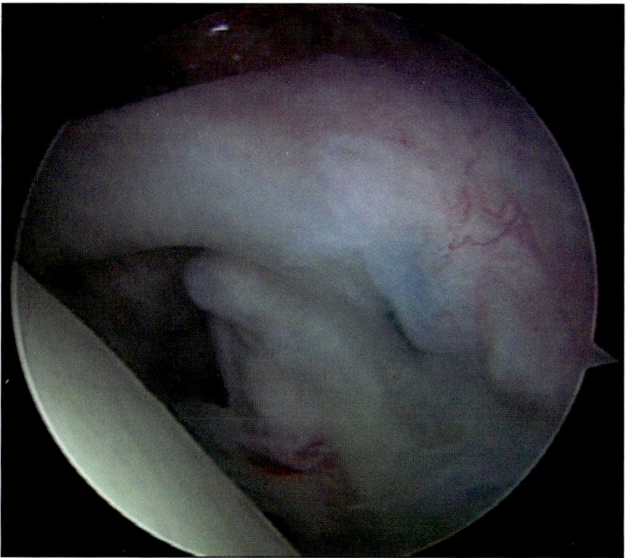

A

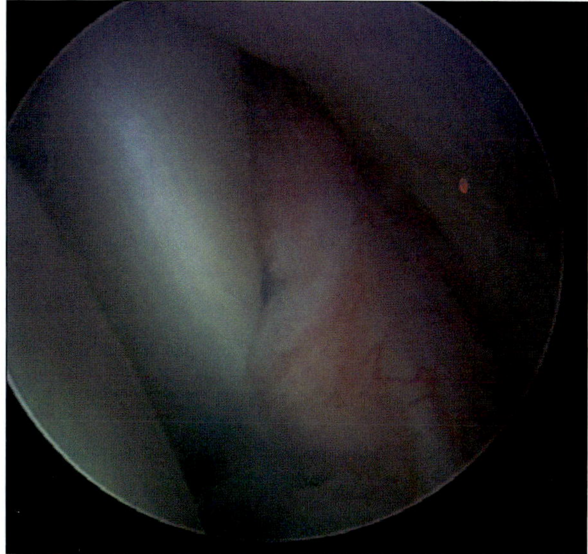

B

FIGURE 3

labrum functions to deepen the glenoid fossa to add stability to the humeral head (Fig. 4). As such, it is an important static stabilizer of the glenohumeral joint.

- The normal anchor of the biceps-labrum complex superiorly has tremendous anatomic variability. The biceps anchor may attach either to the superior labrum itself or the supraglenoid tubercle. In addition, there is significant variability in the anterosuperior labral attachment, such as the Buford complex or a sublabral foramen (see below).

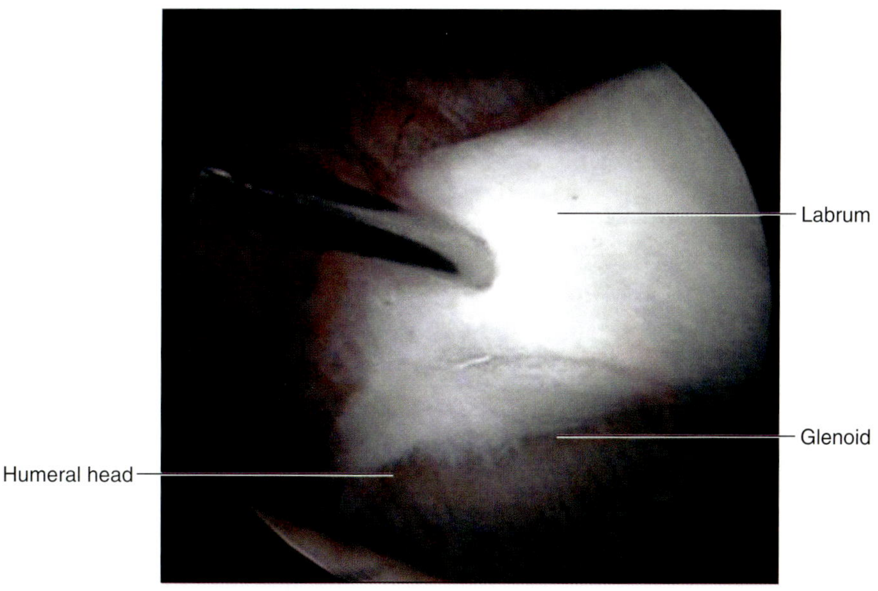

FIGURE 4

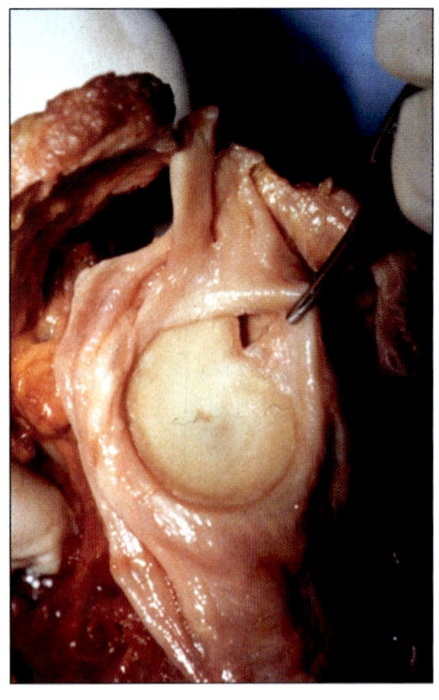
A

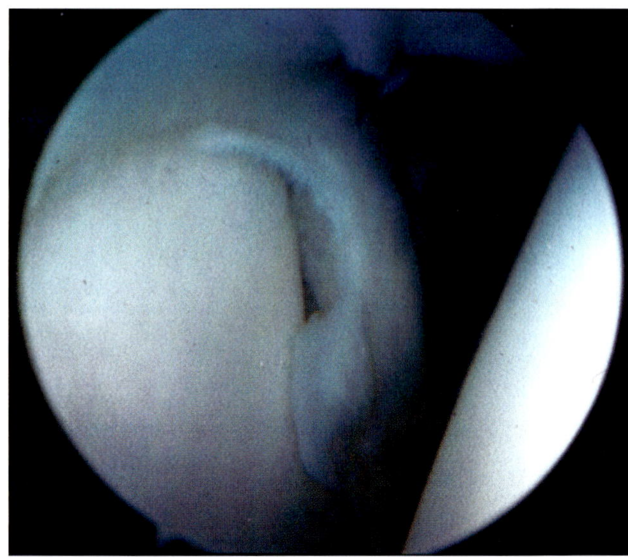
B

FIGURE 5

> **PEARLS**
>
> - *The beach chair position offers several unique advantages, including more anatomic positioning, greater comfort level of anesthesia and nursing staff, easy conversion to open procedure if necessary, and natural gravitational distraction of the glenohumeral joint.*

> **PITFALLS**
>
> - *Improperly addressing a normal biceps-labrum variant may result in an appreciable loss of external shoulder rotation, a frozen shoulder, and/or chronic pain.*

Equipment

- The effected upper extremity should be positioned during the surgery with any device that does not hinder movement of the arm during the surgery and allows multipositional maintenance.

- Clinically relevant biceps anchor anatomic variants:
  - Sublabral foramen
  - Sublabral foramen with cordlike middle glenohumeral ligament (MGHL) (Fig. 5A and 5B)
  - Absent anterosuperior labrum
  - Buford complex—cordlike MGHL with an absent anterosuperior labrum (Fig. 6A–C)
  - Variable biceps-labrum attachment to superior glenoid
- The intra-articular portion of the long head of the biceps tending is an underappreciated pain generator coexisting with SLAP lesions. *Failure to recognize and address biceps pathology may result in ongoing pain and disability* (e.g., incarcerating biceps tendon, biceps chondromalacia [Fig. 7]).

Positioning

- The patient may be placed in the lateral decubitus or beach chair position (our preference; Fig. 8), such that appropriate anterior and posterior portals may be freely accessed.

Portals/Exposures

- Appropriate portal placement facilitates repair, minimizes iatrogenic chondral defects, and reduces operative times. The surgeon should palpate and mark out the surface anatomy: clavicle, acromion, and coracoid.

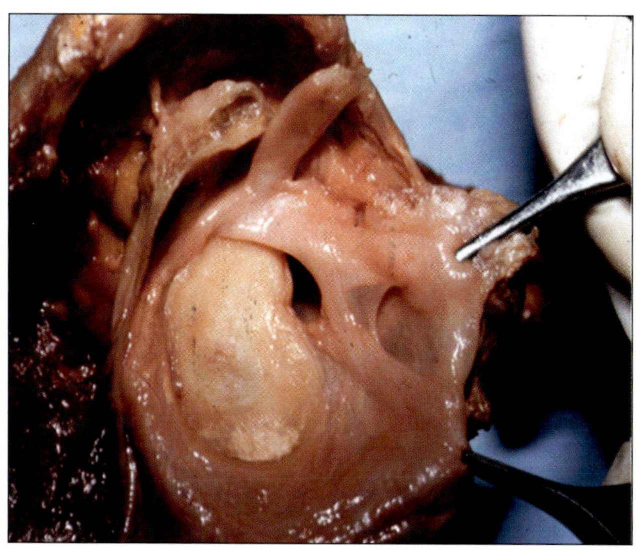

A

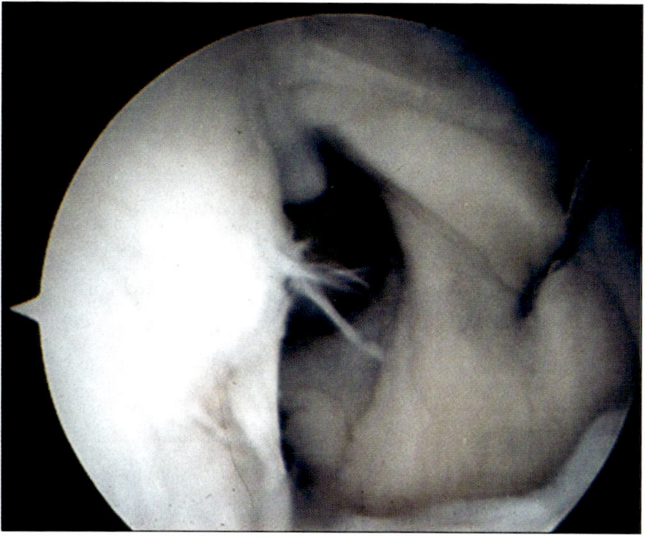

B

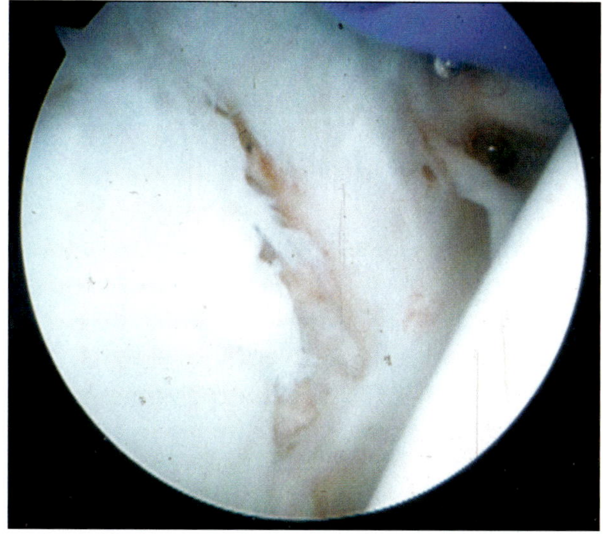

C

FIGURE 6

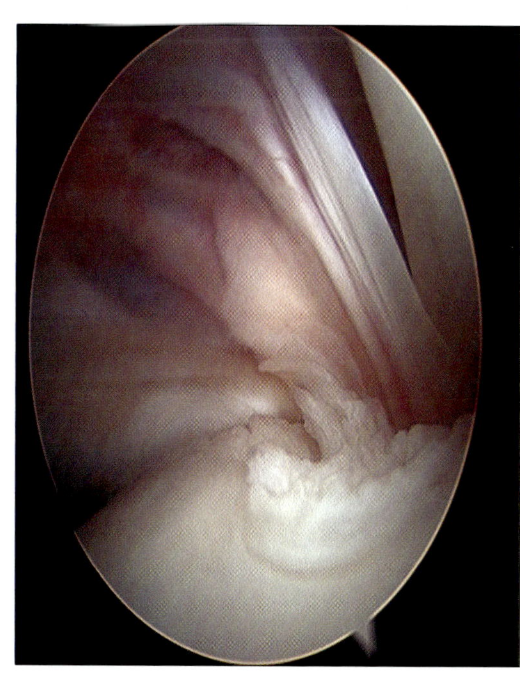

FIGURE 7

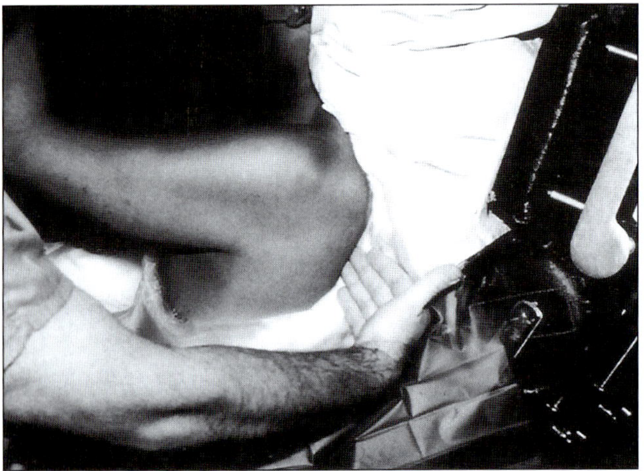

FIGURE 8

- The standard posterior portal (SPP) is created with a stab incision with a #11 scalpel. It should be made approximately 2 cm inferior and 1 cm medial to the posterolateral corner of the acromion. The glenohumeral joint is entered bluntly with an obturator (Fig. 9).
- "Twin" anterior portals (O'Brien)
  - An anterior superior portal (ASP) is placed under visualization, with spinal needle localization,

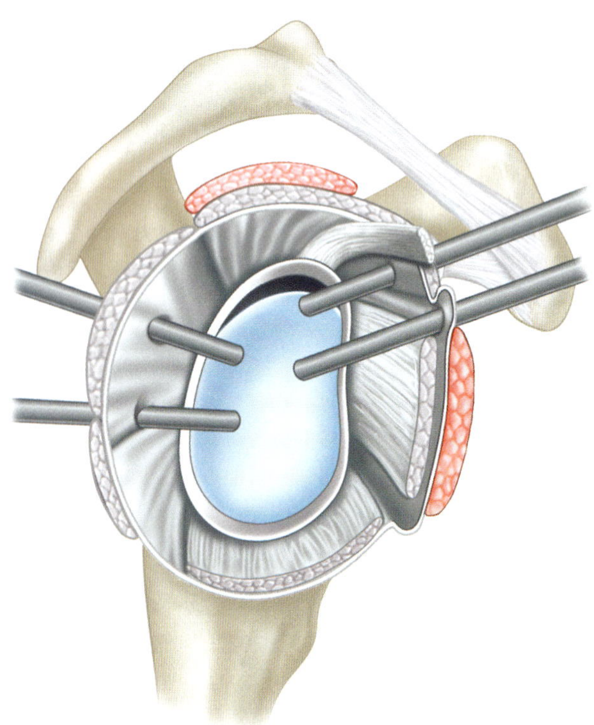

FIGURE 9

Pearls

- *If a portal is placed such that it is overcrowded or at a difficult angle, place an additional portal. Doing this will limit surgical time and optimize anchor placement.*
- *Maximizing the space between the twin anterior portals (anterosuperior and anteroinferior portals) improves portal versatility and facilitates repair.*

Pitfalls

- *Anterior portals placed too medially, laterally, or inferiorly may jeopardize the surgeon's ability to appropriately access the supraglenoid region.*

superior and lateral to the coracoid, and should enter the joint just superior to the biceps tendon in the rotator interval. Particular attention should be paid to placement of this portal, as it is the workhorse for suture anchor placement. Ideally, the vector of the portal should approach the supraglenoid tubercle at approximately 45° (see Fig. 9).
  - An anterior midglenoid portal (AMGP) is placed, with inside-out localization, 2 cm inferior to the ASP, within the rotator interval just superior the superior border of the subscapularis tendon (see Fig. 9).
- The trans–rotator cuff portal (O'Brien) is a powerful tool for addressing posterior extension of SLAP lesions. A spinal needle (Fig. 10) is used to localize the portal under direct visualization with the arthroscope. This assures an optimal approach angle to the posterosuperior labrum and minimizes rotator cuff trauma (see Fig. 9).
- Additional portals
  - The portal of Wilmington is located 1 cm anterior and 1 cm inferior to the posterolateral corner of the acromion.
  - The Neviaser portal (supraspinatus portal) is placed at the corner of the supraspinatus fossa under spinal needle localization.

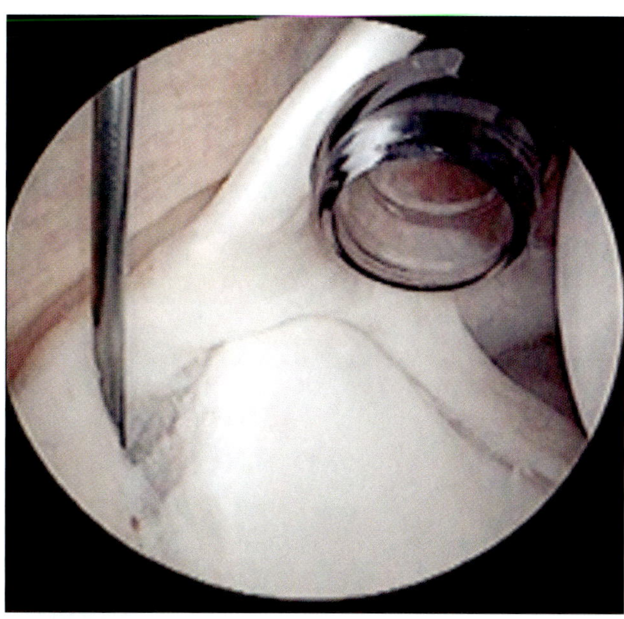

FIGURE 10

PEARLS

- *Particular attention should be paid to the intra-articular portion of the long head of the biceps tendon, as this segment is a clinically significant source of pathology and an active pain generator, both in conjunction with and independent of the biceps anchor.*

PITFALLS

- *Failure to address concomitant pathology leads to suboptimal patient satisfaction.*

Procedure

STEP 1

- A thorough diagnostic evaluation is imperative from both posterior and anterior and must include visualization of the inferior glenohumeral ligament complex, the labrum circumferentially, the rotator cuff insertion, the rotator interval, and any bony lesions that may be present, as well as the biceps anchor and the intra-articular portion of the long head of the biceps. The biceps anchor is most readily visualized from the posterior portal with anterior probing.
- An arthroscopic active compression test should be performed under direct posterior visualization with the arm in 90° of forward flexion and full elbow extension, followed by adduction of 10–15°, and finally internal rotation. The biceps tendon, anchor, and superior labrum are pulled inframedially. If an unstable SLAP lesion is present, the damaged labrum may become interposed between the glenoid and labrum. Biceps instability may result in incarceration of the biceps tendon within the articulation that is relieved with external rotation of the arm. Of note, this examination should be performed prior to any anterior portal placement that may alter biceps course or morphology.
- An assessment of instability is performed.
  - Dynamic translation—The surgeon should mechanically translate the humeral head anteriorly and posteriorly under direct arthroscopic visualization.
  - "Drive-through sign" (Fig. 11)—The arthroscopic drive-through sign is the ability to navigate the

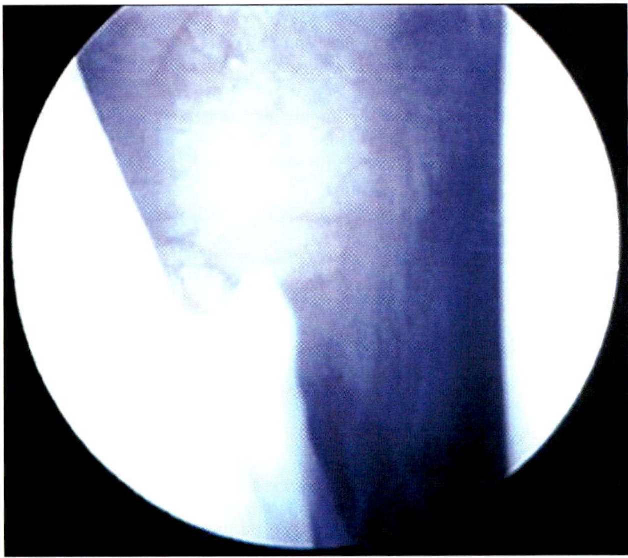

FIGURE 11

arthroscope from posterior to anterior in between the humeral head and the glenoid fossa at the level of the anterior band of the inferior glenohumeral ligament complex. This sign aids in the evaluation of glenohumeral laxity; it has been demonstrated to be a sensitive but not specific test for instability.
- A Bankart lesion, with or without bony attachment, occurs during anterior humeral head dislocation and is defined as a detachment of the anteroinferior glenoid labrum along with the anterior band of the inferior glenohumeral ligament complex. This lesion reduces tension in the anterior band and therefore the ligament's ability to retain the humeral head in the glenoid fossa.

Pearls

- *Stable SLAP lesions (types I and III) may be addressed with only débridement.*
- *Unstable SLAP lesions (types II and IV) must be reapproximated to their glenoid attachment (see Step 3).*

Pitfalls

- *Do not confuse normal anatomic variants with a pathologic SLAP tear.*

Step 2

- Normal anatomy must be differentiated from pathology.
- Lesions of the biceps anchor were first published by Andrews et al. (1985). Later Snyder et al. (1990) adeptly identified superior labral tears as a clinically significant entity and coined the term *superior labrum anterior-posterior (SLAP) tears* to classify these lesions. Other authors have added additional subcategorizations; however, the most clinically relevant part of any classification scheme is whether the biceps anchor is stable or unstable. The following represents Snyder's original classification scheme (Fig. 12).

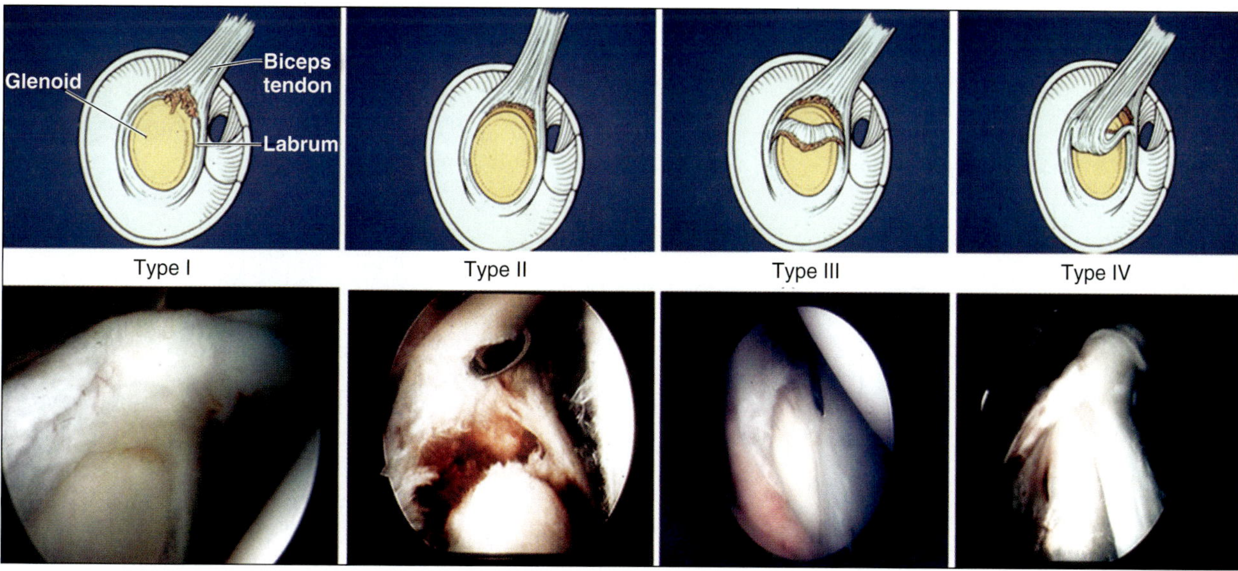

FIGURE 12

Pearls

- *A thorough dynamic assessment of the repaired biceps anchor should be performed, paying particular attention to positions that stress the repair. Such an assessment guides postoperative physical therapy progression and limitations on ROM.*
- *Placing the shaver in the SPP facilitates access to and débridement of the posterior aspect of the biceps anchor.*
- *After identifying an anchor site, maneuver your hand with the punch handle laterally and posteriorly to generate an entry site more perpendicular to the targeted bony surface of the superior glenoid (see Fig. 14).*

Pitfalls

- *An inaccurate approach angle or overaggressive manipulation with the punch can lead to damage of the articular surface or penetration into the glenoid neck, respectively.*
- *Use caution when repairing the anchor so as to not overtension or overconstrain the biceps anchor, which can lead to pain.*

- Type I (stable)—fraying of the superior labrum and limited degeneration. These lesions frequently represent a more chronic and repetitive mechanism. The clinical relevance of type I lesions is controversial. The biceps anchor remains intact.
- Type II (unstable)—detachment of the superior labrum and biceps anchor from the superior glenoid. These lesions are the most common type of SLAP tear and are amenable to surgical repair.
- Type III (stable)—bucket-handle labral detachment with an intact biceps anchor.
- Type IV (unstable)—bucket-handle labral detachment with involvement of the biceps attachment.

Step 3

- The sublabral fibrous tissue is débrided using a standard 4-mm shaver.
- The superior margin of the glenoid is decorticated below the biceps anchor to bleeding cancellous bone with either a ball-tipped burr or a shaver (Fig. 13).
- A suture anchor pilot hole is created using an arthroscopic punch through the ASP (Fig. 14).
- The number and placement of suture anchors are dictated by the desired repair.
  - Single-anchor, double-suture repair necessitates anchor placement directly below the biceps anchor such that the two attached sutures may be passed

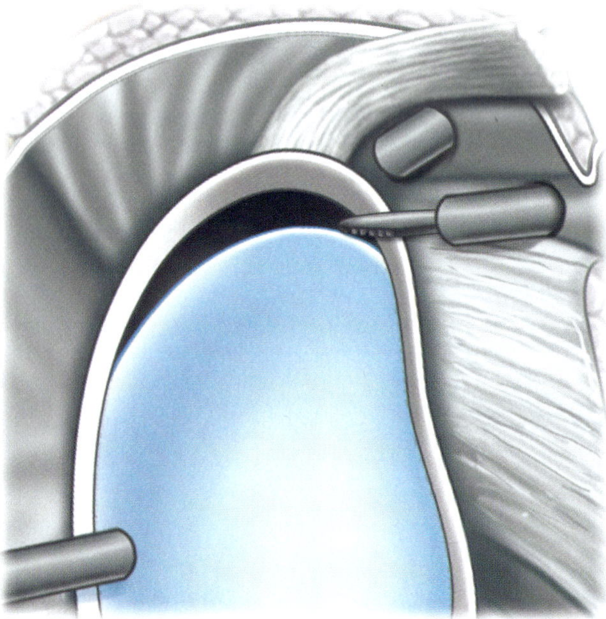

FIGURE 13

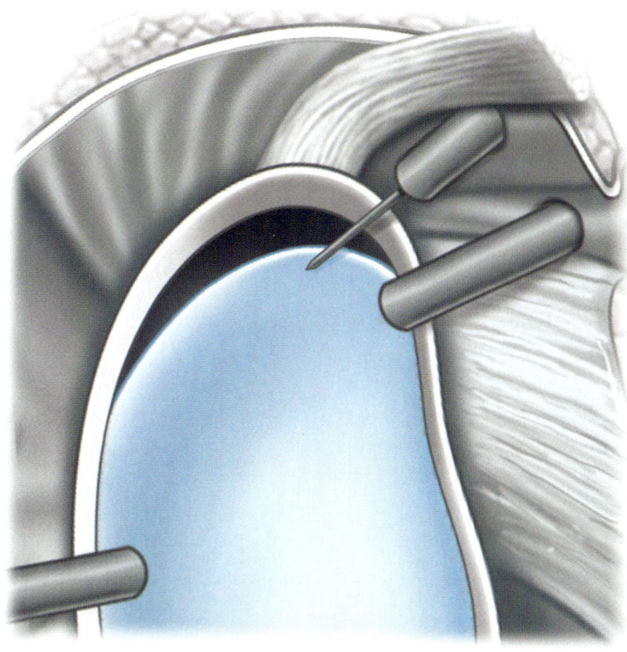

FIGURE 14

posterior (1) and anterior (1) to the biceps tendon origin point.

- For the double-anchor, double-suture repair using the trans–rotator cuff portal (our preferred method), anchor sites are just anterior (1) and just posterior (1) to the bicep tendon origin.
- Multiple suture anchor repair may be necessary for SLAP tears with asymmetric anterior or posterior extension. The trans–rotator cuff portal is particularly useful while addressing posterior extension of a SLAP tear. Figure 15A shows a large

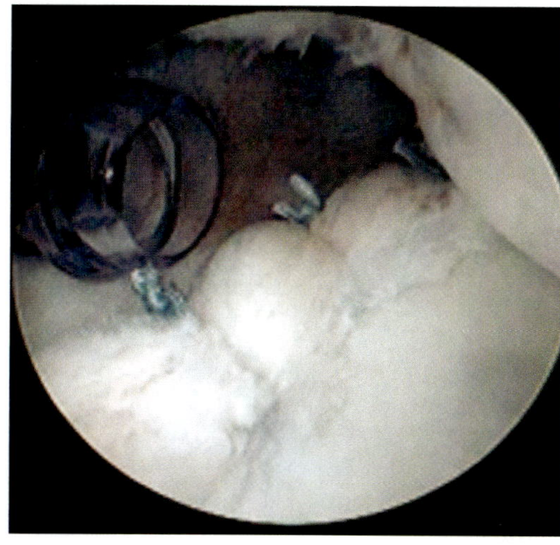

A

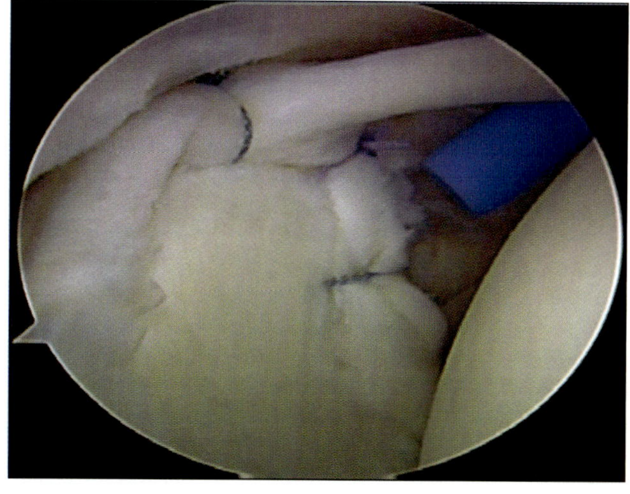

B

FIGURE 15

posterior extension of SLAP tear that was repaired using a trans–rotator cuff portal and three suture anchors (Fig. 15B).

- The desired suture anchor(s) are malleted/screwed into the pilot hole and seat anchor(s) to the appropriate depth.
- Anchor stability is tested with gentle tension on the attached sutures.
- Sutures are retrieved through the AMGP.
- A needle shuttle passer is passed though the biceps anchor from the ASP and the suture is retrieved though the AMGP. An additional needle shuttle passer is passed through the biceps anchor anteriorly and the suture retrieved though the AMGP.
  - Figure 16A shows suture passage in a single-anchor, double-suture repair.
  - Figure 16B shows suture passage in a double-anchor, double-suture repair using the trans–rotator cuff portal.
- Both limbs of the posterior suture are retrieved through the ASP, an arthroscopic sliding locking knot is tied using the translabral limb as a post, and any excess is cut.
  - Figure 17A shows the limbs of the posterior suture tied in a single-anchor, double-suture repair.

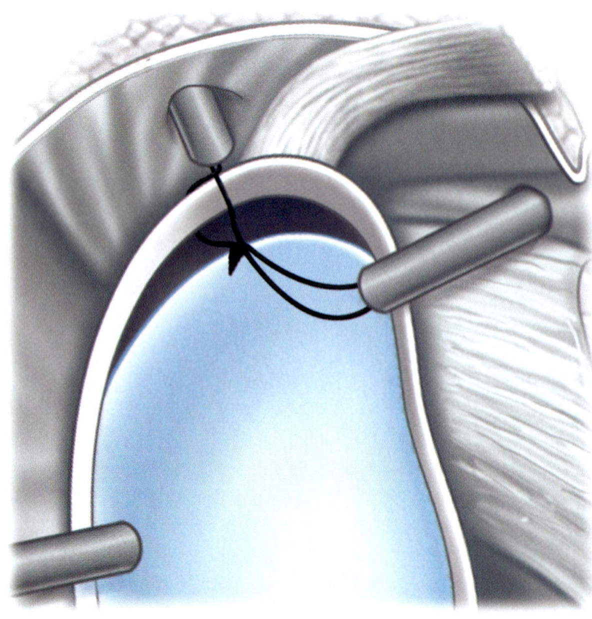

A

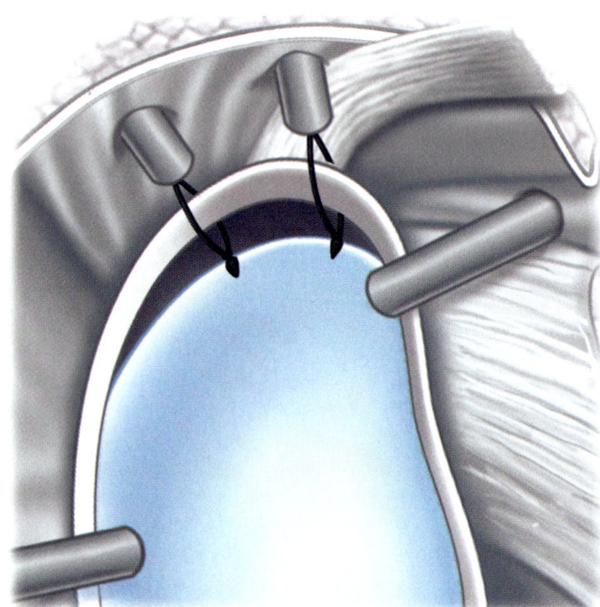

B

FIGURE 16

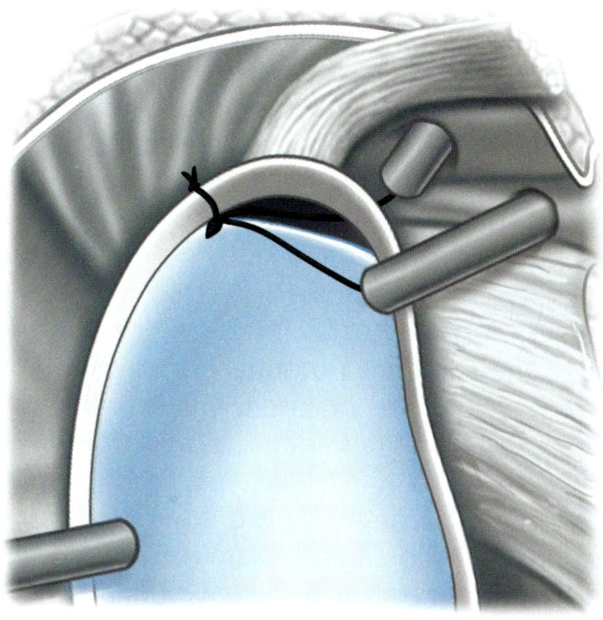
A

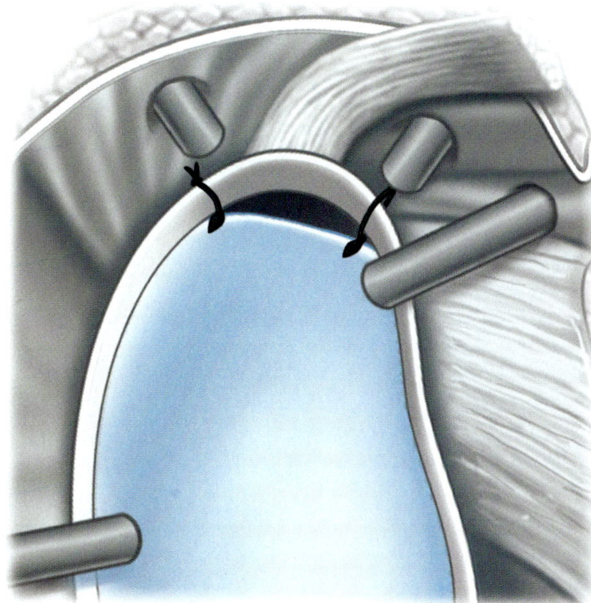
B

FIGURE 17

- Figure 17B shows the limbs of the posterior suture tied in a double-anchor, double-suture repair using the trans–rotator cuff portal.

- This procedure is repeated for the anterior suture, as shown in Figure 18A for a single-anchor, double-suture repair and in Figure 18B for a double-anchor,

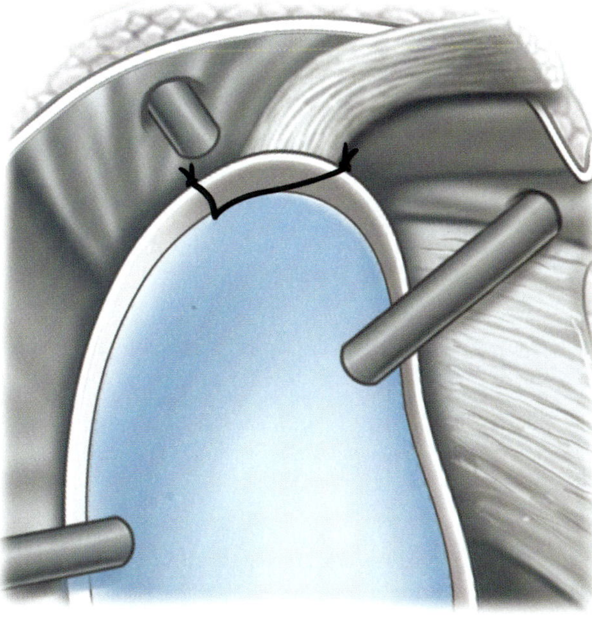
A

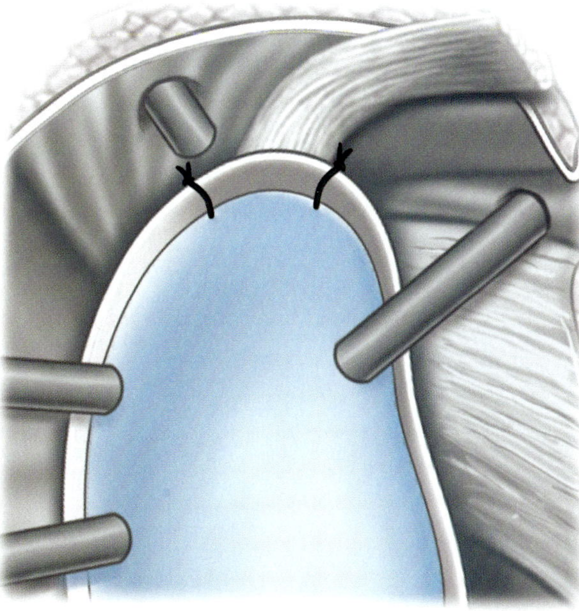
B

FIGURE 18

double-suture repair using the trans–rotator cuff portal.

- The repair is tested with an intra-articular probe.
- The shoulder is taken through the range of motion (ROM) under direct observation to determine stability of the repair and positions of vulnerability.

Pearls

- *During the passive ROM stage of rehabilitation, the patient should maintain sling immobilization between therapy sessions to allow appropriate scarring down of the repaired SLAP tear.*

Postoperative Care and Expected Outcomes

- In addition to the standard potential complications, specific adverse outcomes include implant pullout and migration, failure of repair, and synovial reaction.
- Postoperative return to activities is gradual and individualized, based on clinical examination and most importantly on final intraoperative dynamic arthroscopic evaluation.
- General guidelines may be thought of as follows:
  - Phase I (0–3 weeks)—Immediately postoperatively, patients are placed in a sling and allowed ROM of the fingers, wrist, and elbow only. Immobilization of the shoulder acutely minimizes pain, swelling, and inflammation.
  - Phase II (1–3 weeks)—Safe passive ROM and Codman exercises are initiated (as determined at time of surgery). The patient should refrain from external rotation of the abducted arm as this stresses the biceps anchor repair.
  - Phase III (3–6 weeks)—The sling is removed and ROM exercises are progressed as tolerated.
  - Phase IV (6–16 weeks)—The patient begins active ROM exercises and progresses to resistance activities.
  - Phase V (16+ weeks)—A progressive return to sport is begun.

Evidence

Andrews JR, Carson WG Jr, McLeod WD. Glenoid labrum tears related to the long head of the biceps. AJSM. 1985;13(5):337-41.

This is the original observational study, in 73 pitchers who underwent arthroscopy, describing pathology at the biceps labrum complex that would later be classified by Snyder as the SLAP lesion.

Cooper DE, Arnoczky SP, O'Brien SJ, Warren RF, DiCarlo E, Allen AA. Anatomy, histology, and vascularity of the glenoid labrum: an anatomical study. J Bone Joint Surg [Am].1992;74:46-52.

This cadaveric study offers anatomic and histologic insight into the glenoid labrum and biceps complex.

Jin W, Ryu KN, Kwon SH, Rhee YG, Yang DM. MR arthrography in the differential diagnosis of type II superior labral anteroposterior lesion and sublabral recess. AJR Am J Roentgenol. 2006;187:887-93.

This study evaluates the utility of MR arthrography in the differentiation between Type II SLAP lesions from sublabral recesses.

O'Brien SJ, Allen AA, Coleman SH, Drakos MC. The trans-rotator cuff approach to SLAP lesions: technical aspects for repair and a clinical follow-up of 31 patients at a minimum of 2 years. Arthroscopy. 2002;18:372-7.

This paper proposes the use of the trans-rotator approach to SLAP repair in 31 patients.

O'Brien SJ, Pagnani MJ, Fealy S, McGlynn SR, Wilson JB. The active compression test: a new and effective test for diagnosing labral tears and acromioclavicular joint abnormality. Am J Sports Med. 1998;26:610-3.

The authors present a new examination technique for evaluating patients with labral and AC pathology.

Snyder, SJ, Karzel RP, Del Pizzo W, Ferkel RD, Friedman MJ. SLAP lesions of the shoulder. Arthroscopy. 1990;6:274-9.

This landmark paper proposes the classification of superior labral lesions that has become know as SLAP.

Verma NN, Drakos M, O'Brien SJ. The arthroscopic active compression test. Arthroscopy. 2005;21:634.

This paper is the arthroscopic corollary to the O'Brien Sign, that allows direct visualization of biceps tendon incarceration within the glenohumeral joint.

Williams MM, Snyder SJ, Buford D Jr. The Buford complex—the "cord-like" middle glenohumeral ligament and absent anterosuperior labrum complex: a normal anatomic capsulolabral variant. Arthroscopy. 1994;10:586.

This study describes a normal anatomic variant.

PROCEDURE 22

Treatment of the Unstable Shoulder with Humeral Head Bone Loss

Anthony Miniaci and Robert G. Najarian

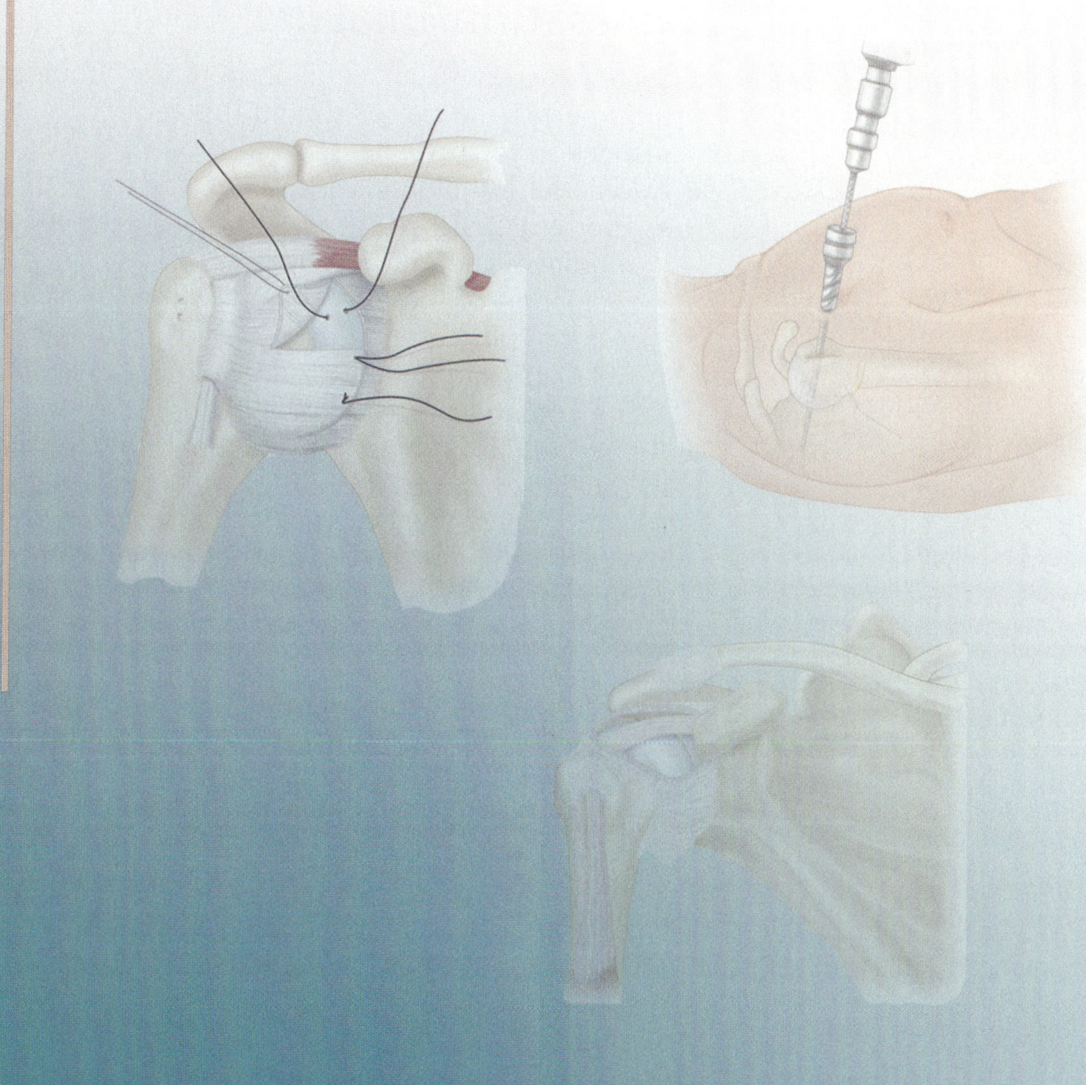

Pitfalls

- *Failure to recognize the contribution of a significant humeral head defect (in addition to the capsulolabral deficiency) in a patient with symptomatic anterior glenohumeral instability can result in continued shoulder instability if only the Bankart lesion is addressed at the primary operation.*
- *Contraindications include advanced glenohumeral arthrosis, an existing infection, unaddressed or irreparable rotator cuff deficiency.*

Controversies

- Large Hill-Sachs lesions that "fall into" the glenoid rim with the shoulder in a functional position of abduction and external rotation (i.e., "engaging" Hill-Sachs lesions), if they are identified prior to undergoing initial surgical treatment, can be addressed as part of the primary anterior stabilization procedure.
- Patients who are at a high risk of re-dislocation (e.g., epilepsy with recurrent anterior instability and large Hill-Sachs defects) may have their humeral head defect addressed at the primary operation.

Indications

- The indications for anatomic allograft reconstruction of humeral head defects are ongoing symptomatic anterior glenohumeral instability or painful clicking, catching, or popping in a patient with a large engaging Hill-Sachs lesion.
- This procedure is most commonly used as a secondary operation in patients who have failed previous soft tissue stabilization procedures.

Examination/Imaging

- Systematic physical examination of the shoulder with a humeral head defect should first focus on inspection for previous scars.
- Additional examination includes
  - Thorough assessment of active and passive shoulder range of motion
  - Evaluation of the integrity and strength of the rotator cuff, compared to the unaffected arm
  - Detailed examination for glenohumeral laxity in the anterior, posterior, and inferior directions
- An apprehension examination should be performed in multiple arm positions in patients with Hill-Sachs lesions. Patients with large Hill-Sachs lesions will typically exhibit apprehension with the arm in significantly less than 90° of abduction/90° of external rotation
- Plain radiographs
  - Anteroposterior (AP) (internal and external rotation), true AP of the glenohumeral joint, axillary lateral, and Stryker notch view of the involved shoulder
  - Plain radiographs will often significantly underestimate the size of the Hill-Sachs defect. Figure 1 shows AP (Fig. 1A) and axillary lateral (Fig. 1B) views of a large Hill-Sachs defect in a patient with a history of recurrent anterior shoulder dislocations.
- Computed tomography (CT)
  - All patients should have a preoperative axial CT imaging study to more fully define the bony architecture, morphology, and articular arc defect of the Hill-Sachs lesion.
  - Care must be taken when interpreting these axial studies since the plane of the Hill-Sachs defect is oblique to the plane of the axial image and

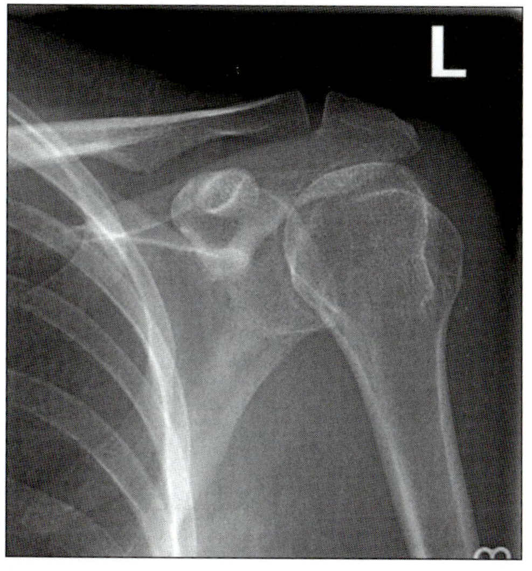

A

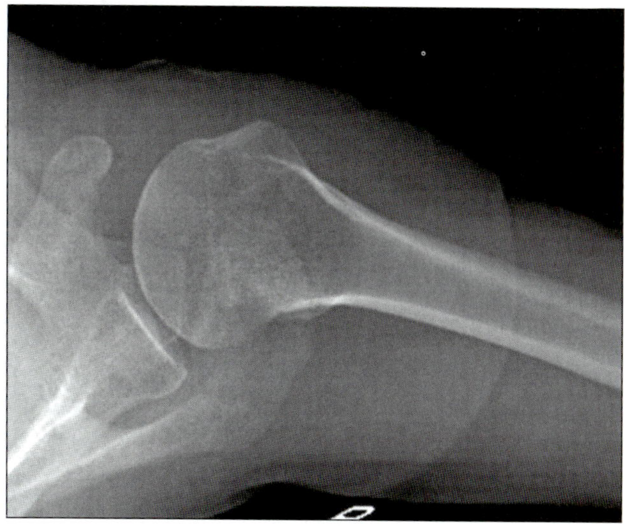

B

FIGURE 1

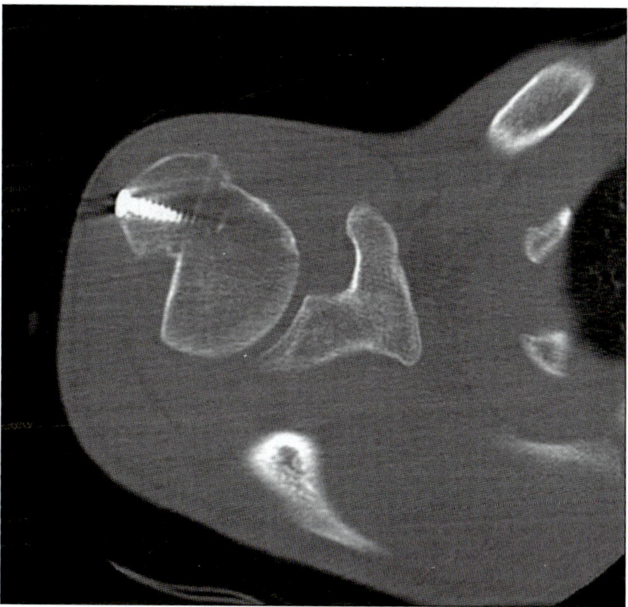

A

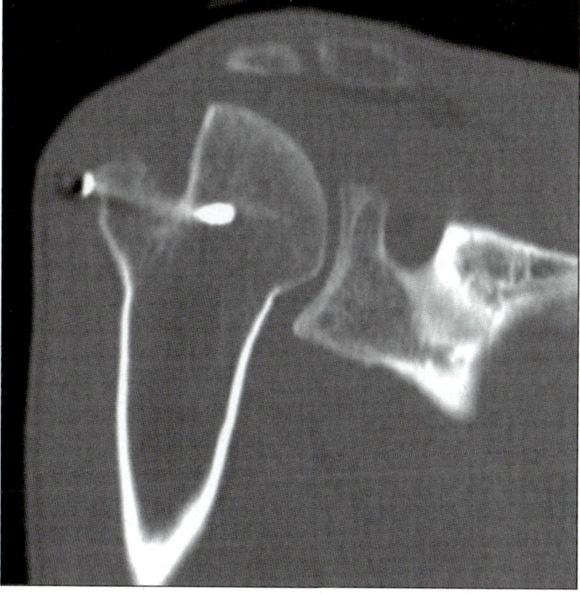

B

FIGURE 2

therefore the size of these defects can often be underestimated on axial cuts.

- Figure 2 shows axial (Fig. 2A) and coronal (Fig. 2B) CT images of a patient with recurrent anterior shoulder dislocations. There is a large engaging Hill-Sachs lesions seen in the posterosuperolateral humeral head. Note that the patient had a previous open reduction and internal fixation of a greater tuberosity fracture fixed with two screws, which are seen within the images.

Treatment Options

- Conventional guidelines suggest that nonoperative treatment can be undertaken for humeral head defects that involve less than 25% of the articular surface without clinical signs of glenohumeral instability.
- Surgical options for symptomatic engaging defects that involve 25–40% of the humeral head articular surface are quite varied in the literature. These include open anterior procedures, such as open capsular shift, designed to limit external rotation such that the humeral head defect is kept from engaging; rotational proximal humeral osteotomy; transfer of the infraspinatus into the defect to render the lesion essentially extra-articular or an arthroscopic remplissage; or filling in of the Hill-Sachs defect so that it can no longer engage, using either a corticocancellous iliac graft or a femoral head osteoarticular allograft. If the defect is severe (i.e., >45% or severe articular involvement), prosthetic replacement, using either hemiarthroplasty or a total shoulder arthroplasty is recommended, especially in the setting of chronic dislocations.

  - Three-dimensional CT reconstructions are a useful tool to aid in more clearly defining the size and location of the defect and to provide an estimation of the amount of articular surface involved.
- Magnetic resonance imaging (MRI)
  - MRI will aid in the assessment of associated soft tissue injury as well as provide details of the bony defect. Axial MRI can also be helpful in identifying not only the bony anatomy of a large Hill-Sachs defect, but the soft tissue pathology associated with anterior shoulder dislocations (Figs. 3 and 4).

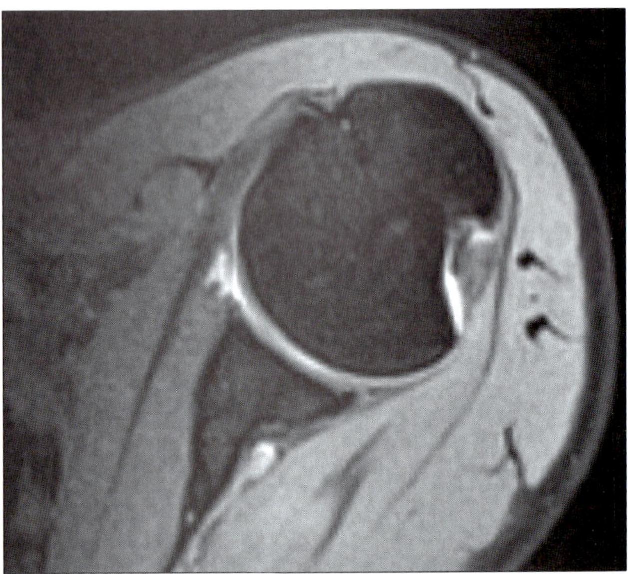

FIGURE 3

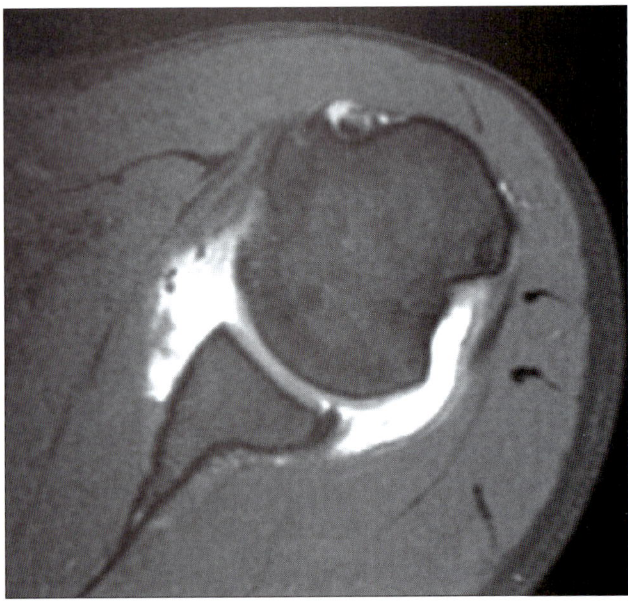

FIGURE 4

- Dynamic MRI with the arm in abduction and external rotation may be of value when attempting to determine the contribution of the bony defect with the shoulder in a position of instability.

- CT scan (standard or three-dimensional reconstruction) and/or MRI data are used preoperatively to determine the appropriate size of a humeral head allograft prior to allograft reconstruction. Plain radiographs with magnification markers can also be used.
- Appropriate sizing of a proximal humeral allograft requires a specific protocol to be arranged between the surgeon and the supplying tissue bank.

Surgical Anatomy

- An extended deltopectoral approach is used.
- Anatomic landmarks include
  - Anterior, lateral, and posterior borders of the acromion
  - Coracoid process
  - Distal clavicle
  - Acromioclavicular joint
  - Deltopectoral groove
- Superficial dissection
  - The cephalic vein is identified; it should be preserved if possible.
  - The internervous plane is between the deltoid muscle (axillary nerve) and the pectoralis major muscle (medial and lateral pectoral nerves).
  - Retraction of the pectoralis major medially and the deltoid laterally exposes the conjoined tendon.
- Deep dissection
  - The conjoined tendon is retracted medially, taking care to avoid injury to the musculocutaneous nerve. The nerve enters the body of the coracobrachialis medially, about 5–8 cm distal to the muscle's origin at the coracoid process.
  - A triad of the anterior humeral circumflex vessels traverse and help identify the inferior border of the subscapularis muscle.
  - The *axillary nerve* lies deep to the anterior humeral circumflex vessels and superficial to the subscapularis muscle at the level of the glenoid.
  - The subscapularis muscle tendon is transected vertically in its entirety, 0.5 cm medial to its insertion on the lesser tuberosity, and tagged with sutures for later repair.

Pearls

- *EUA will allow the surgeon to assess the degree and position of instability and to attempt to determine if a given humeral head defect "engages" the glenoid rim in a functional arm position. In turn, EUA will enable the surgeon to ensure that the maximal range of motion of the shoulder may be achieved with the given patient position and thus confirm the adequacy of the patient setup.*
- *When undertaking reconstruction of humeral head defects either with matched allograft or prosthetic resurfacing, some surgeons may elect to obtain intraoperative fluoroscopic images to judge the reconstruction. If so, the surgical team should ensure that adequate views will be acquired with the given patient position. To do so, it is recommended that the desired views be obtained with the fluoroscopic machine after patient setup and prior to prepping and draping of the patient.*

Pitfalls

- *Care must be taken to ensure that the entire involved extremity has been draped free, allowing for maximal range of motion of the shoulder as needed to address a given defect.*

  - The interval between the subscapularis and the anterior capsule is carefully developed using sharp dissection, continuing medial to the neck of the glenoid.
  - The inferior capsule is then further isolated using careful blunt dissection.
- Further detail regarding the approach to the humeral head chondral defect is described in the Portals/ Exposures section.

Positioning

- After the administration of general endotracheal anesthesia, the patient is positioned in the modified beach chair position with the head of the bed raised 30–45°.
- A bump is placed under the medial border of the scapula, and the involved upper extremity should be free to allow for maximal external rotation and extension as needed.
- An intrascalene block can be used and is a matter of surgeon preference.
- Examination under anesthesia (EUA) can be undertaken at this point.
- Diagnostic arthroscopy also may be undertaken prior to open intervention.
  - In Figure 5, diagnostic arthroscopy reveals chondral damage on the glenoid and an absence of the anteroinferior labrum in a patient with a history of recurrent anterior shoulder dislocations.

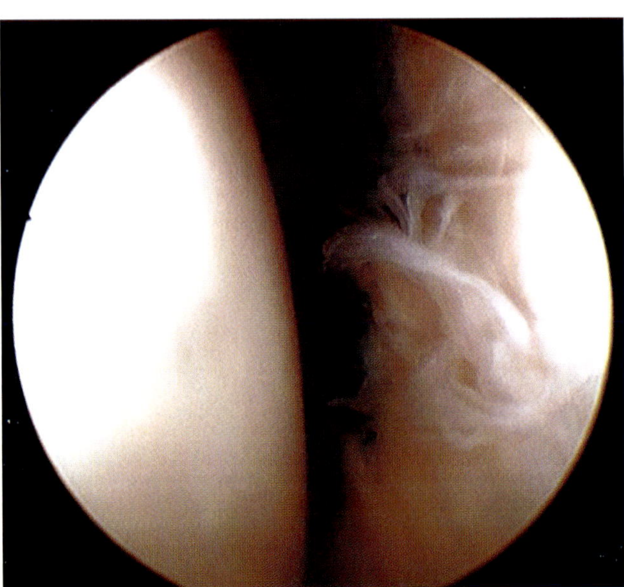

FIGURE 5

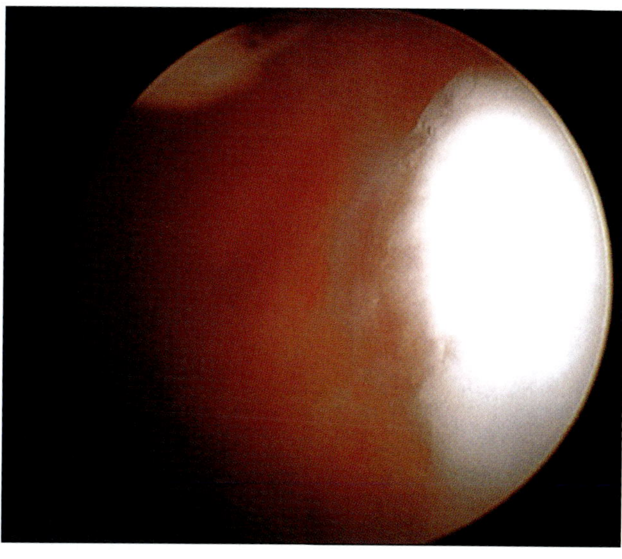

FIGURE 6

Controversies

- Diagnostic arthroscopy prior to open intervention is useful to assess the soft tissue and chondral injury, as well as the size, location, and "behavior" of the humeral head defect in various arm positions.

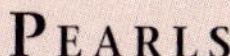

Pearls

- *The axillary nerve lies deep to the anterior humeral circumflex vessels and superficial to the subscapularis muscle at the level of the glenoid. If necessary, a rubber vessel loop can be used to protect or isolate the axillary nerve.*
- *It is important to separate the subscapularis and the capsule medial to the joint line in order to address a Bankart lesion if necessary.*
- *Unroofing the synovial expansion of the supraspinatus, which overlies the tendon of the long head of the biceps, will allow the humerus to be more fully externally rotated, allowing better visualization and access to the Hill-Sachs lesion.*

Pitfalls

- *Anterior-inferior capsular release from the anatomic neck of the humerus is an important step to obtain adequate exposure. Take care to release the capsule directly off of bone in order to minimize risk to the axillary nerve.*

- The large Hill-Sachs lesion evident in Figure 6 is seen to "engage" the anteroinferior glenoid rim with the arm placed in 90° of abduction and 90° of external rotation.

Portals/Exposures

- After appropriate positioning of the patient in the beach chair position, an extended deltopectoral approach is utilized.
- An incision of approximately 6–10 cm in line with the deltopectoral groove is made, extending from the tip of the coracoid and directed distally.
- The deltopectoral interval is developed and the cephalic vein is taken laterally. Lateral retraction of the cephalic vein is preferred because it helps preserve venous outflow from the deltoid. If the cephalic vein is injured during the approach, it should be tied off before proceeding with the deep dissection.
- The deltoid and pectoralis major muscles are retracted using a blunt, multipronged self-retaining retractor.
- The lateral border of the conjoined tendon is identified and gently retracted medially to expose the underlying subscapularis muscle. A blunt retractor placed under the conjoined tendon will facilitate exposure while minimizing risk to the musculocutaneous nerve.

Controversies

- The anterior capsule and the subscapularis can be left together and elevated as one complex; however, we find it simpler and easier to expose the humeral head and repair the capsulolabral structures separately.
- It has been recently described by some authors that patients with recurrent anterior instability and large humeral head defects can be addressed first arthroscopically (Bankart lesion), and then via a limited posterior approach to the humeral head to address the Hill-Sachs defect (Kropf and Sekiya, 2007). For allograft reconstruction of humeral head defects, we feel that the deltopectoral approach is still the "gold standard" and most familiar approach.

- The bursa atop the subscapularis muscle insertion is identified and removed. The anterior humeral circumflex vessels, which define the inferior aspect of the subscapularis tendon, are located. A 90° clamp can be used to isolate the vessels, and suture ligation of these vessels can be undertaken if needed.
- Tag sutures are placed in the lateral aspect of the subscapularis tendon to help retract the tendon and for definitive repair at the conclusion of the procedure. The entire tendon is transected vertically 0.5–1 cm medial to its insertion onto the lesser tuberosity. As the subscapularis tendon is released, external rotation of the humerus will help minimize the risk of injury to the axillary nerve at this point.
- Using sharp dissection, the interval between the subscapularis and the anterior capsule is then carefully developed, continuing medial to the neck of the glenoid. The inferior capsule is then further isolated using careful blunt dissection with a medium Cobb elevator.
- A laterally based capsulotomy is made with the vertical limb in line with the subscapularis incision and continuing superiorly.
- The anterior-inferior capsule is then released off of the surgical neck of the humerus with intra-articular dissection using a periosteal elevator.
- A humeral head retractor (i.e., Fukuda) is placed into the glenohumeral joint to allow inspection of the glenoid and anterior/inferior capsulolabral structures for any pathology.
- If a Bankart lesion is found, it is repaired using either bony drill holes or suture anchors. The sutures are left untied until completion of the reconstruction of the humeral head defect.
- The humeral head retractor is removed and the humerus is extended and brought into maximal external rotation to expose the Hill-Sachs lesion.
- A flat, narrow retractor is then placed in a position over the reflected undersurface of the subscapularis tendon and behind the neck of the humerus on the posterior cuff in order to lever out the humeral head and present the Hill-Sachs lesion for reconstruction.

Procedure

Step 1

- After adequate exposure of the Hill Sachs defect, a micro-sagittal saw is used to smooth and reshape the

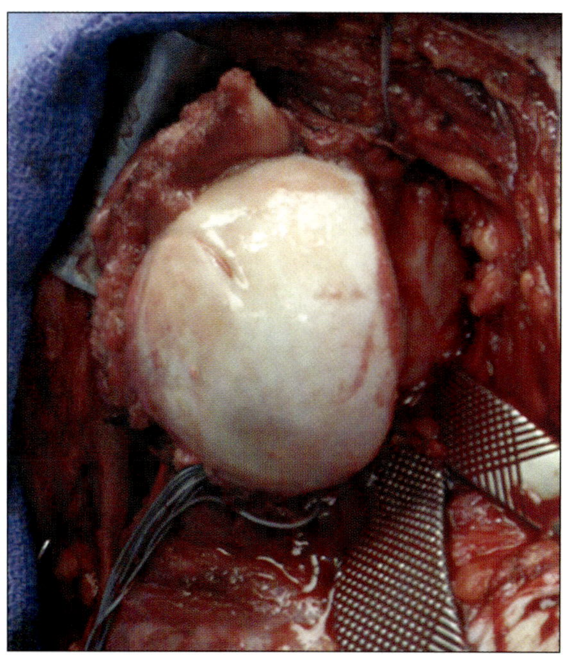

FIGURE 7

Pearls

- *In order to best restore the native anatomy and improve chances of appropriate healing, care should be given to creating precise, flat surfaces along the base and sides of the defect that will allow for the best fit for the donor allograft. This can be accomplished by further smoothing the defect edges with a hand rasp.*

defect into a chevron-type configuration and to provide a bed of bleeding subchondral bone onto which the allograft will be fixed (Fig. 7). The chevron-type defect should be constructed so as to correspond to a wedge-shaped piece of matching allograft humeral head that will be press-fitted into the defect (Fig. 8).

- Required measurements of the defect are then obtained. Figure 9 shows a schematic of the base (x), height (y), length (z), and outside partial circumference (c) of the defect; the graft is sculpted to match the defect to the nearest millimeter.

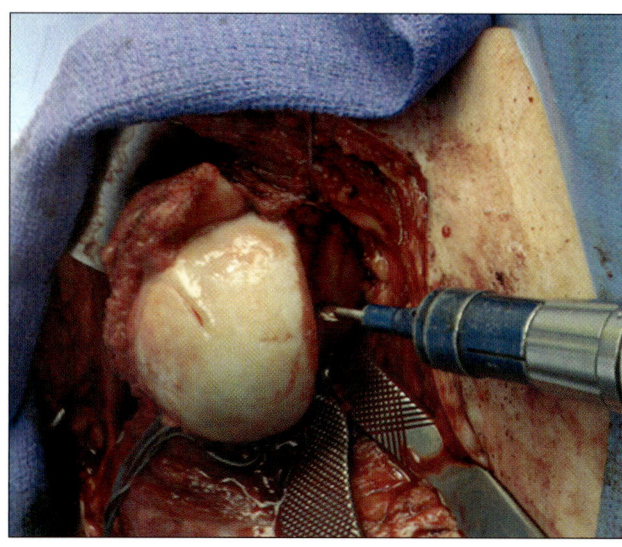

FIGURE 8

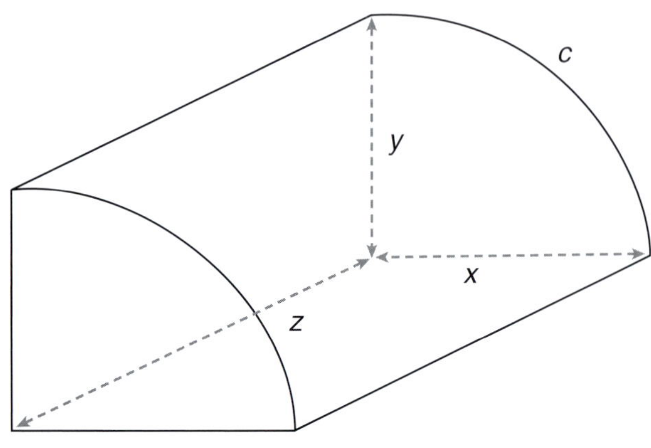

FIGURE 9

PEARLS

- *It is best to err on the side of creating a larger allograft plug that can be fine-tuned to fit the defect, as little can be done if the allograft piece is too small. If the donor piece has some irregular contours at the edges, bone graft can be used to fill in these small edges of incongruity to exact a better fit of the allograft (see Fig. 13).*

PITFALLS

- *Failure to recognize that adjustments in one plane will affect the final size of the allograft in the other two dimensions will result in a graft that is mismatched to the recipient defect.*

STEP 2

- The anatomic quadrant of the matched humeral head allograft that corresponds to the location of the defect on the humeral head is identified and marked (Fig. 10).
- A chevron-type defect is cut from the allograft humeral head. This wedge is approximately 2–3 mm larger in all dimensions than the measured defect (Fig. 11).
- The allograft segment is then provisionally placed into the Hill-Sachs defect and resized in all three planes. Excess length is then carefully trimmed with the micro-sagittal saw. It is also very important to reshape the graft in the other two planes to ensure appropriate size and match.

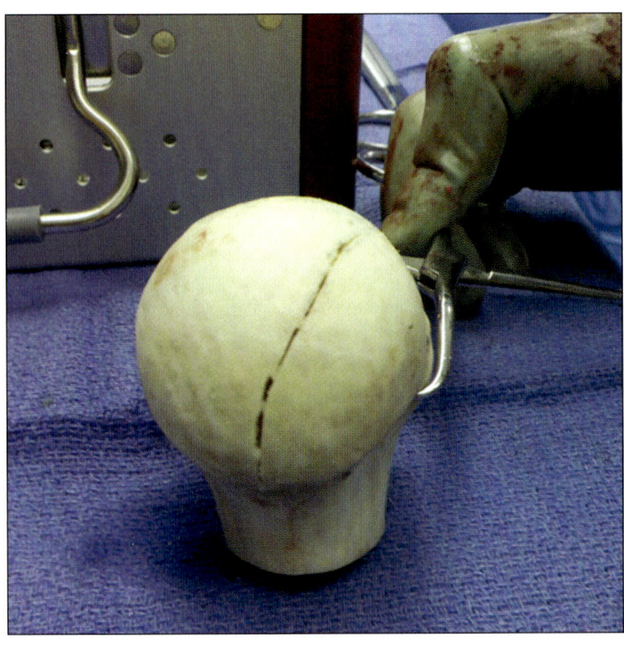

FIGURE 10

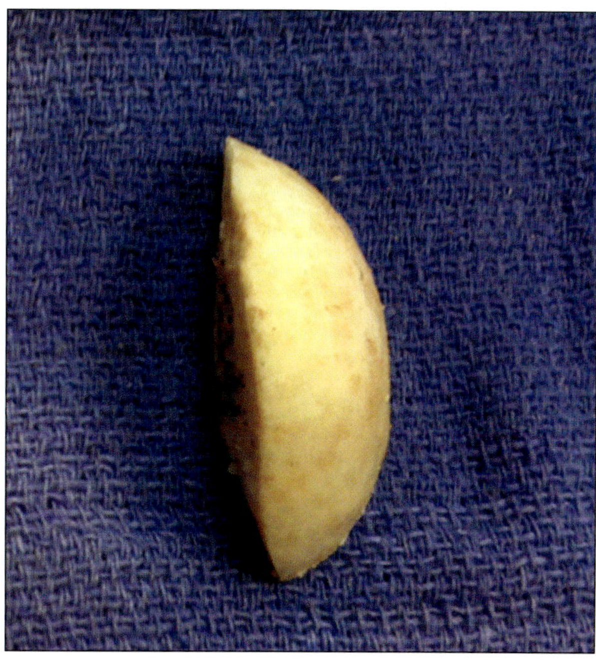

FIGURE 11

Controversies

- Headless, variable-pitch compression screws may also be used for allograft fixation. Nonetheless, it is absolutely imperative that the screw heads be countersunk below the articular cartilage. Moving the shoulder through a range of motion intraoperatively will help ensure this.

- Fine-tuning of graft size is then continued in one plane at a time until a perfect size match is achieved in all planes, including base, height, length, and outside partial circumference.

Step 3

- Once the appropriate size and configuration are obtained, the allograft is placed into the defect and aligned so as to achieve a congruent articular surface.
- The allograft is then provisionally secured in place with two or three smooth 0.045-inch Kirschner wires (Fig. 12).

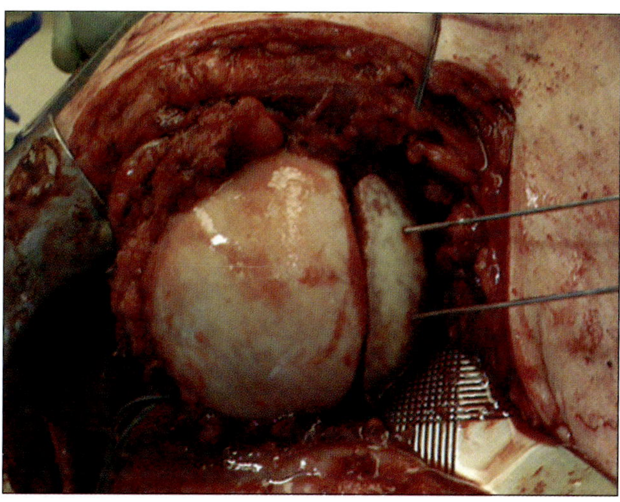

FIGURE 12

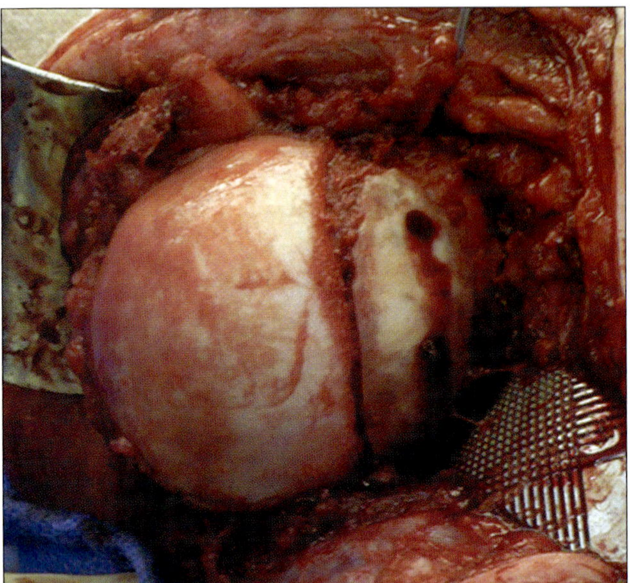

FIGURE 13

- The wires are then sequentially replaced with 3.5-mm fully threaded cortical screws placed in a lag fashion. The screw heads are countersunk so that they are below the level of the articular surface. Figure 13 presents an intraoperative view of the the final fixation of the allograft secured with two screws.

Step 4

- The joint is then copiously irrigated, and the shoulder is taken through a range of motion to ensure that the reconstructed humeral head provides a smooth, congruent articulating surface.
- Absorbable suture is used to close the capsulotomy, and any previously placed sutures that were used to repair the capsulolabral pathology (if present) are tied.
- The subscapularis tendon is then reapproximated to its stump anatomically with nonabsorbable suture, taking care not to shorten the tendon.
- The conjoined tendon, deltoid, and pectoralis major muscles are allowed to fall back into their normal anatomic positions, and the deltopectoral interval is not closed.
- The subcutaneous layer is closed with a 2-0 absorbable stitch, and a running 4-0 absorbable subcuticular suture is used to approximate the skin.

Postoperative Care and Expected Outcomes

- After surgery, the patient is placed immediately in a shoulder immobilizer and given a sling for comfort.
- Full passive range of motion as tolerated is allowed immediately.
- Due to the subscapularis detachment, the patient is protected against active and resisted internal rotation for a period of 6 weeks. After the initial 6-week period, patients are allowed terminal stretching and strengthening exercises.
- Shoulders are imaged with repeat radiographs at 6 weeks and 6 months. Postoperative radiographs showing anatomic allograft reconstruction of an engaging Hill-Sachs defect are shown in Figure 14A and 14B. A CT scan is obtained at 6 months as well to assess for consolidation and incorporation of the graft.
- The patient is generally not cleared for return to sport or strenuous overhead activity until at least 6 months after the date of surgery and with radiographic evidence of consolidation of the graft.
- Outcomes
    - Published reports of allograft reconstruction of humeral head defects are mostly limited to case reports or small case series, with follow-up data ranging from 2 to 5 years.
    - In the largest study of anatomic allograft reconstruction of humeral head defects in patients

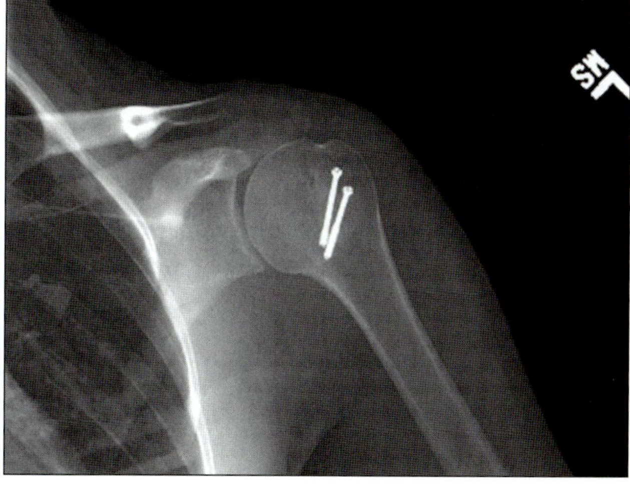

A

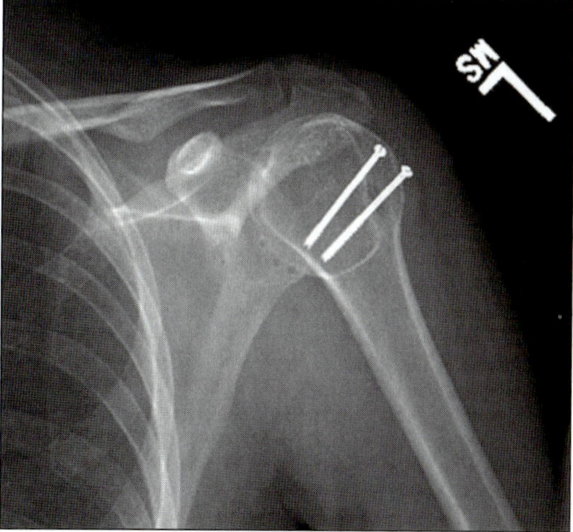

B

FIGURE 14

who failed previous attempts at surgical stabilization, this technique of allograft reconstruction has been shown to be effective (Miniaci and Gish, 2004). Patients demonstrated improvement in stability, loss of apprehension, and high subjective approval, allowing return to near-normal function with no further episodes of instability at average of 50 months' follow-up.

- More recent case series looking at the treatment of reverse Hill-Sachs lesions with matched allograft reconstruction following posterior locked shoulder dislocations have also shown good results, with improvements in patient satisfaction rates and functional assessment scores.

■ Complications

- Complications that have been reported after humeral osteoarticular allograft reconstruction of Hill-Sachs lesions include radiographic follow-up evidence of partial graft collapse, early evidence of osteoarthritis, continued sensation of catching and/or subluxation, and hardware complications in extreme external rotation (which was relieved after removal of the screws 2 years postoperatively).
- Although infrequently a cause for clinical concern, Hill-Sachs defects can be the source of significant disability and recurrent instability in a subset of patients. Anatomic allograft reconstruction of these defects is a viable treatment option resulting in favorable clinical outcomes.

Evidence

Currently in the literature, there are no prospective, randomized Level I trials that clinically or biomechanically compare the various treatment options for large defects of the humeral head. Most published reports examining osteoarticular allograft reconstruction for the treatment for Hill-Sachs defects are limited to case series with few patients and short-term follow-up.

Bock P, Kluger R, Hintermann B. Anatomical reconstruction for reverse Hill-Sachs lesions after posterior locked shoulder dislocation fracture: a case series of six patients. Arch Orthop Trauma Surg. 2007;127:543-8.

This case series presented the results of six patients with reverse Hill-Sachs lesions, sustained from traumatic dislocation, diagnosed between 5 and 180 days from time of injury. All patients were treated with elevation of the depressed articular surface, then filling of the defect with the graft and cartilage fixed on top of the graft via Mitek suture anchors introduced under the affected area. At a mean follow-up of 63 months, results were found to be excellent for two patients and good for the remaining four patients. At last follow-up, no redislocation or graft collapse was seen. (Level IV evidence)

Burkhart SS, De Beer JF. Traumatic glenohumeral bone defects and their relationship to failure of arthroscopic Bankart repairs: significance of the inverted-pear glenoid and the humeral engaging Hill-Sachs lesion. Arthroscopy. 2000;16:677-94.

This case series analyzed the results of 194 consecutive arthroscopic Bankart repairs by suture anchor technique (performed by two surgeons with an identical suture anchor technique) in order to identify specific factors related to recurrence of instability. The average follow-up was 27 months. There were 101 contact athletes, and the authors identified significant bone defects on either the humerus or the glenoid. The authors found 14 recurrent dislocations and 7 recurrent subluxations. Of those 21 shoulders with recurrent instability, 14 had significant bone defects. For the group of patients without significant bone defects (173 shoulders), there were 7 recurrences (4% recurrence rate). For the group with significant bone defects (21 patients), there were 14 recurrences (67% recurrence rate). For contact athletes without significant bone defects, there was a 6.5% recurrence rate, whereas for contact athletes with significant bone defects, there was an 89% recurrence rate. The authors concluded that arthroscopic Bankart repairs give results equal to open Bankart repairs if there are no significant structural bone deficits. Contact athletes without structural bone deficits may be treated by arthroscopic Bankart repair. However, contact athletes with bone deficiency require open surgery aimed at their specific anatomic deficiencies.

Gerber C, Lambert SM. Allograft reconstruction of segmental defects of the humeral head for the treatment of chronic locked posterior dislocation of the shoulder. J Bone Joint Surg [Am]. 1996;78:376-82.

The authors presented a case series of four consecutive patients who had a chronic locked posterior dislocation of the glenohumeral joint, associated with a defect of the humeral head that was at least 40% of the articular surface, who were managed with reconstruction of the shape of the humeral head with use of an allogenic segment of the femoral head. Stability was restored and maintained in each patient at an average of 68 months after the procedure. Three patients reported little or no pain and no or slight functional restrictions in the activities of daily living, and they considered the result to be satisfactory. The fourth patient had mild pain and moderate to severe dysfunction secondary to avascular necrosis of the remaining portion of the humeral head after a symptom-free period of 6 years. (Level IV evidence)

Kropf EJ, Sekiya JK. Osteoarticular allograft transplantation for large humeral head defects in glenohumeral instability. Arthroscopy. 2007;23:322.e1-5.

This case report described a new approach to treating highly functional patients with recurrent anterior instability and a large humeral head defect. In this patient with a traumatic anterior shoulder dislocation and continued symptoms of shoulder instability, the anterior capsulolabral pathology was addressed arthroscopically, and the Hill-Sachs lesion was then addressed via a limited posterior approach to the humeral head. Osteoarticular allograft transplantation was performed by use of a single plug to fill the defect.

Martinez AA, Calvo A, Domingo J, Cuenca J, Herrera A, Malillos M. Allograft reconstruction of segmental defects of the humeral head associated with posterior dislocations of the shoulder. Injury. 2008;39:319-22.

This case series looked at six patients who underwent operative management of large humeral head defects involving at least 40% of the articular surface following posterior humeral head dislocation. Time between dislocation and surgery ranged from 7 to 8 weeks. All defects were treated with humeral head allograft reconstruction and followed for mean of 63 months. Four patients had improved subjective scores. Two patients had a poor clinical result, and were found to have flattening and collapse of the graft at their last radiographic follow-up. (Level IV evidence)

Miniaci A, Gish MW. Management of anterior glenohumeral instability associated with large Hill-Sachs defects. Tech Shoulder Elbow Surg. 2004;5:170-5.

In this largest case series reviewing osteoarticular allograft reconstruction for large humeral head defects, the authors performed the above-described procedure on 18 patients with failed previous attempts at surgical stabilization and defects comprising greater than 25% of the humeral head. Patients were assessed pre- and postoperatively with history, physical examination, radiographs (including plain films), and axial CT and MRI, as well as validated clinical evaluation measures (Constant-Murley shoulder scale, Western Ontario Shoulder Instability Index, and Short Form-36). All patients demonstrated improvement in stability, loss of apprehension, and high subjective approval, allowing return to near-normal function with no further episodes of instability at average of 50 months' follow-up. (Level IV evidence)

Yagishita K, Thomas BJ. Use of allograft for large Hill-Sachs lesion associated with anterior glenohumeral dislocation: a case report. Injury. 2002;33:791-4.

This case report described an alternative treatment for large defect of the posterosuperior aspect of the humeral head using allograft in a patient with chronic anterior dislocation of the right glenohumeral joint and a large impaction fracture of the posterosuperior aspect of the humeral head. A preserved frozen allograft of the femoral head was configured to fit the defect. The graft was then impacted firmly down into the defect without adjuvant internal fixation. Two years after surgery, the patient was doing well according to the authors, without complaints. Radiographs revealed incorporation of the graft and no evidence of collapse.

SECTION I

SHOULDER

Clavicle

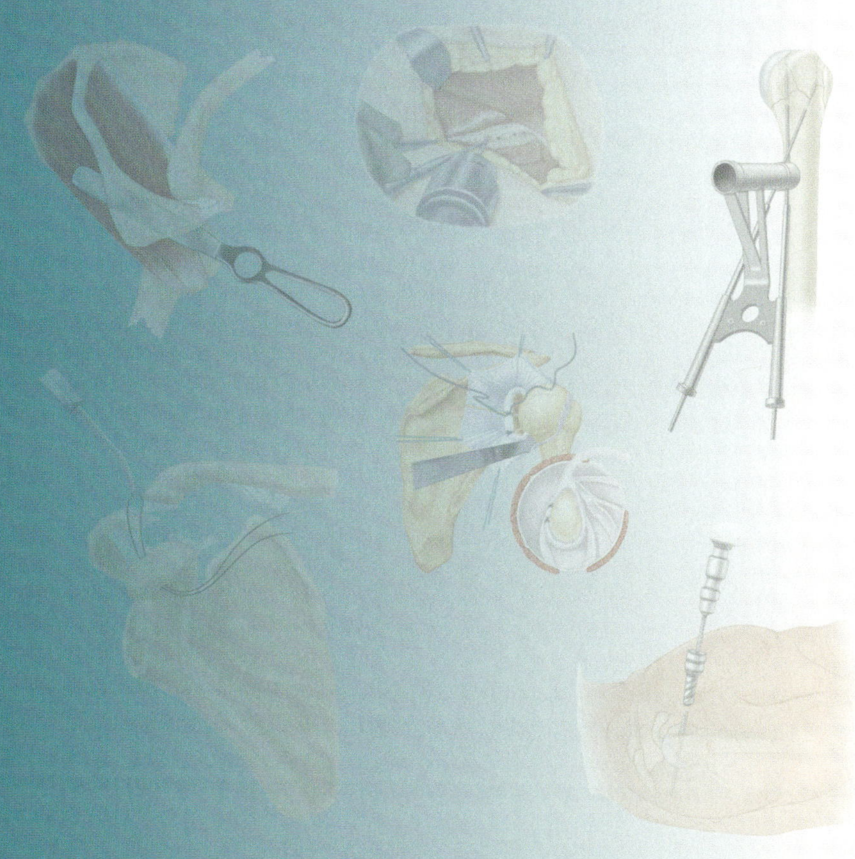

PROCEDURE 23

Open Distal Clavicle Excision

Bradley S. Raphael, Anne M. Kelly, Seth Sherman, and Edward V. Craig

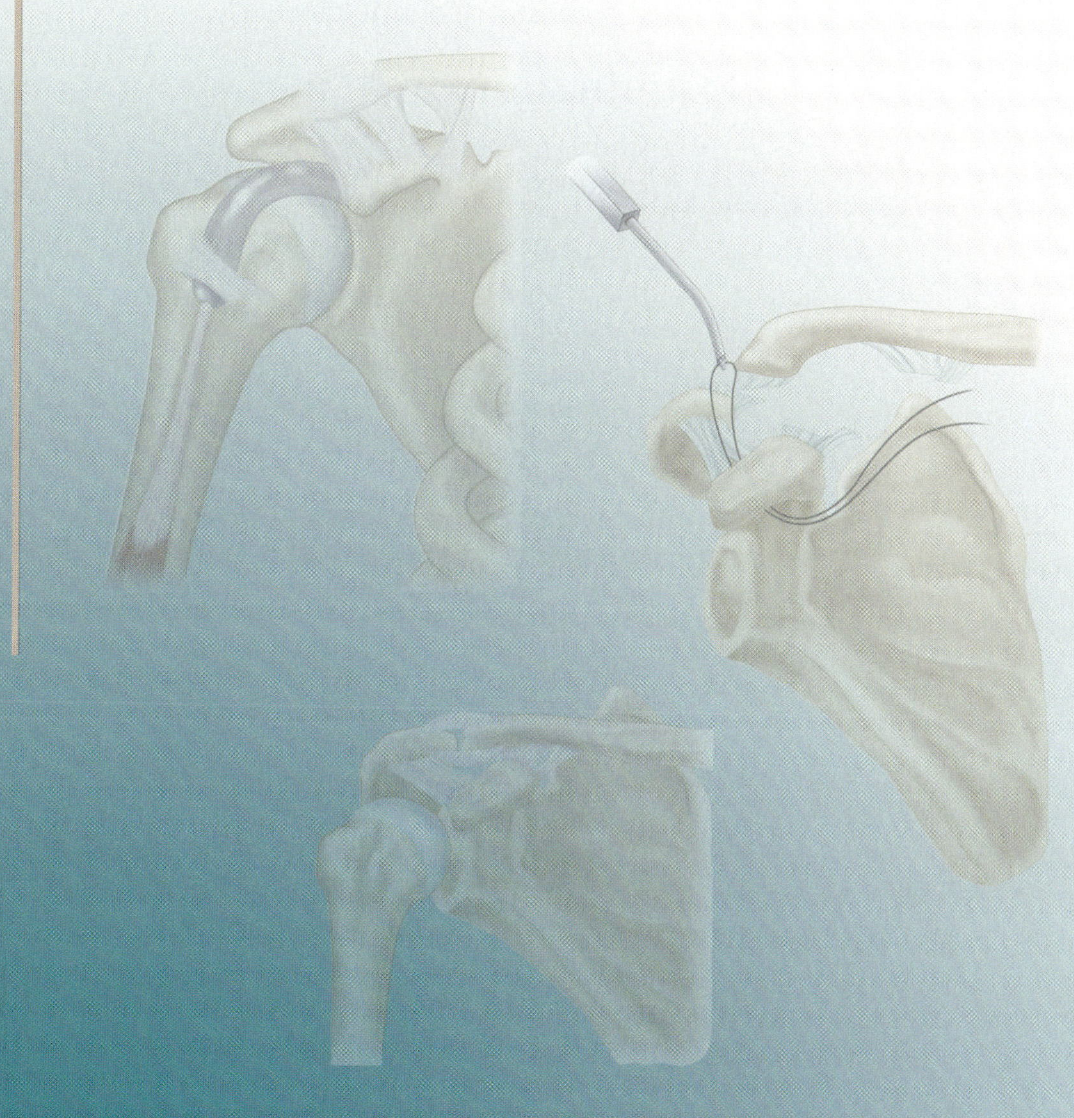

PITFALLS

- *Not indicated for grades III–V AC separation (Fig. 1; grade III), because the procedure can lead to increased symptoms in these patients. In these patients, open excision should be combined with a reconstructive procedure.*

Controversies

- Does not allow visualization of intra-articular pathology with overlapping symptoms (i.e., labral pathology).

Treatment Options

- Nonoperative treatment: Cortisone injections can provide relief, but are technician dependent. Due to the superficial location of the AC joint, steroid injections can cause skin discoloration or fat atrophy. Physical therapy, ice, anti-inflammatories, and activity modification can provide relief, but if the patient is still symptomatic after 6 months of conservative treatment, surgical intervention should be recommended.
- Arthroscopic distal clavicle excision offers the advantage of allowing a visual diagnostic examination of the glenohumeral joint before intervening and can be more cosmetic. This can identify concomitant pathologies (e.g., labrum, biceps, rotator cuff). Open excision usually takes less time with significantly less cost. However, both options demonstrate effective results.

Indications

- Distal clavicle fracture.
- Acromioclavicular (AC) arthritis.
- Hypertrophic osteoarthritis that, if treated arthroscopically, could take significantly more time, while causing more surrounding soft tissue damage.
- Distal clavicle osteolysis.
- Incomplete AC dislocation becoming symptomatic or causing early degenerative changes.
- If the symptoms are the result of AC joint instability, the coracoclavicular ligaments must be addressed and reconstructed simultaneously.

Examination/Imaging

- History
  - History of superior shoulder pain: This is generally present in a younger active athletic population following trauma or in a second group in the sixth and seventh decades with progression of degenerative disease.
  - History of trauma or injury to the affected joint: Even low-grade separation can lead to symptomatic degeneration in 42% of patients (Bergfeld et al., 1978).
  - Activities that reproduce AC joint compression or rotation can exacerbate symptoms (e.g. golf, weight lifting, overhead activity, sleeping).
- Physical examination
  - The patient is examined for AC joint tenderness. Provocative tests include the cross-body adduction stress test (Fig. 2), AC resisted extension, and active compression (Chronopoulous et al., 2004). It is useful to compare with the contralateral extremity.
  - Examination should be done for asymmetric bony anatomy, with prominence over the joint, as well as trapezial spasm.
  - Pain can mimic impingement or neurologic, labral, and rotator cuff pathology. However, AC joint pain is usually identified as tenderness localized to the superior aspect of the shoulder directly over the joint.
  - Lidocaine-steroid injections, if performed correctly, can be diagnostic as well as therapeutic. However, these can be very painful and difficult to perform given the small space and presence of osteophytes. It is important to distinguish between injecting lidocaine into the AC joint and the subacromial

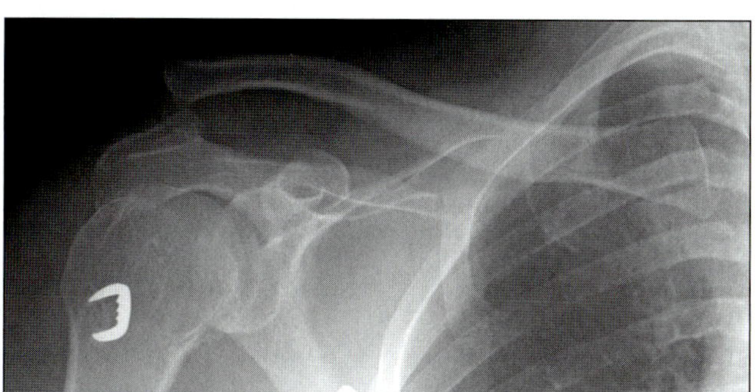

FIGURE 1

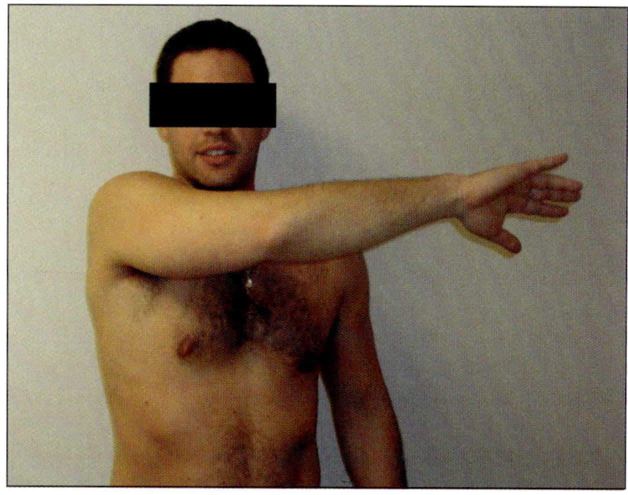

FIGURE 2

space for diagnostic purposes. Therefore, a small needle should be used for AC joint injections.

- Radiography
  - A Zanca view radiograph should be obtained (Fig. 3): this is an anteroposterior view with 10–15° of cephalic tilt, and the voltage decreased by 50% (Zanca, 1971).
  - Radiographic evidence of arthritis includes AC joint subluxation (Fig. 4), sclerosis, joint space narrowing, and osteophytes.
  - Radiographic evidence of degeneration does not correlate well with clinical findings.

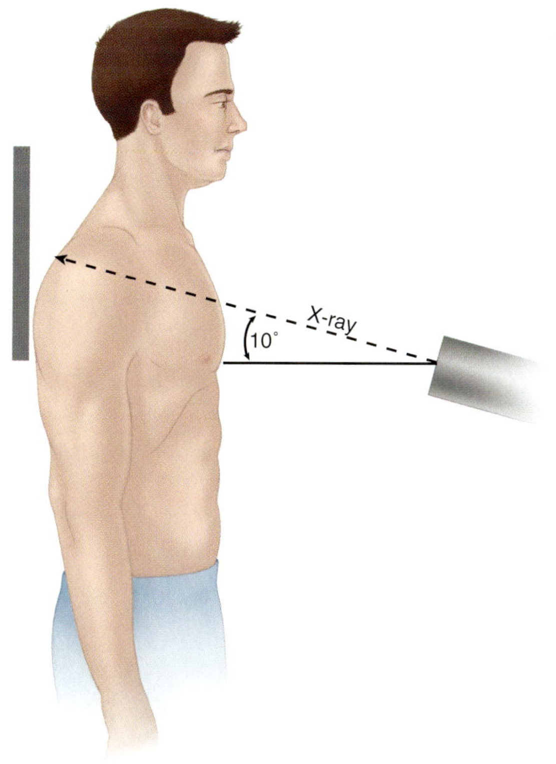

FIGURE 3

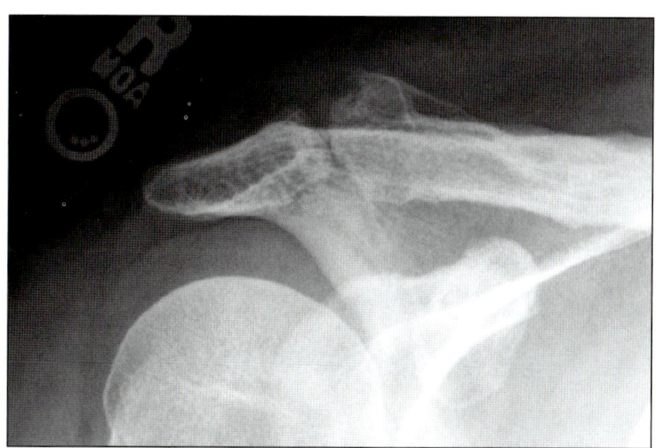

FIGURE 4

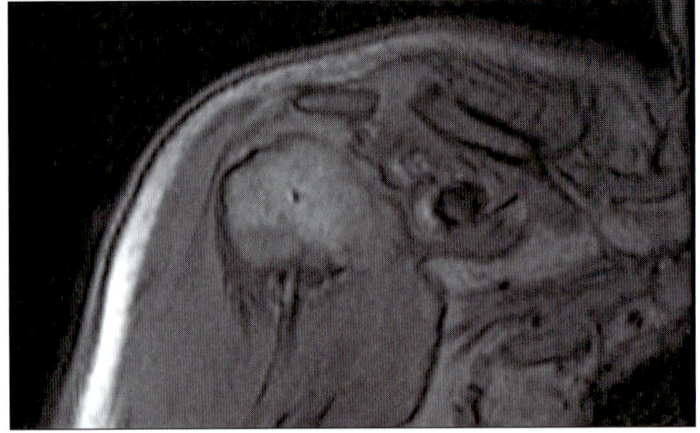
A

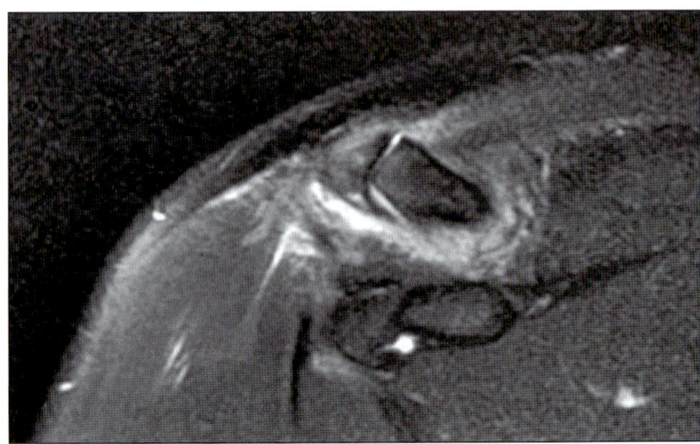
B

FIGURE 5

- Magnetic resonance imaging (MRI)
  - MRI is a sensitive study for AC arthritis, but not very specific.
    - In the MRI of symptomatic AC arthritis in Figure 5A, note the significant swelling within the AC joint capsule.
    - The MRI in Figure 5B shows edema in an asymptomatic arthritic AC joint.
  - A high rate of degenerative findings in asymptomatic patients (75%) has been reported (Needell et al., 1996).

Surgical Anatomy

- The primary components of the shoulder, as seen in the cadaver specimen in Figure 6, are the AC joint capsule (intact), the subscapularis muscle and tendon (intact), the biceps tendon, and the deltoid (reflected).

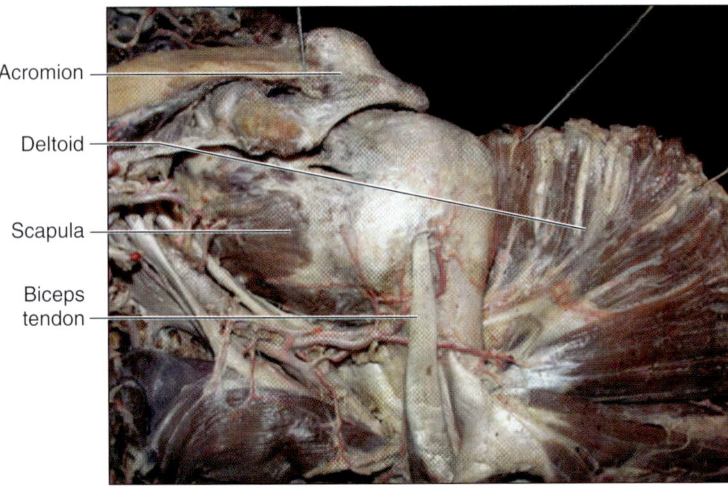

FIGURE 6

- The distal clavicle meets the acromion to form the diarthroidal AC joint and allow for three types of motion: rotation of the clavicle, tilting of the acromion, and anteroposterior gliding of the acromion.
- The joint surfaces are initially hyaline cartilage, but may transition to fibrocartilage with age.
- The average size of the adult AC joint is 9 × 19 mm (Bosworth, 1949).
- The AC joint has both dynamic (deltoid and trapezius) and static (AC and coracoclavicular ligaments) stabilizers (Fig. 7A).
  - The AC ligament controls horizontal stability and is the most important ligament stabilizer in daily activities.
  - The coracoclavicular (trapezoid and conoid) ligament is stronger, and controls vertical stability (Fig. 7B, *black arrow;* coracoacromial ligament, *white arrow*). The trapezoid ligament is medial to the distal clavicle excision border and should be preserved to prevent instability.

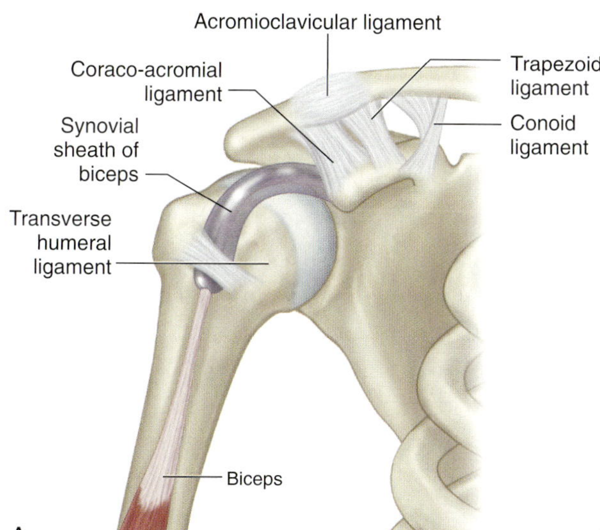

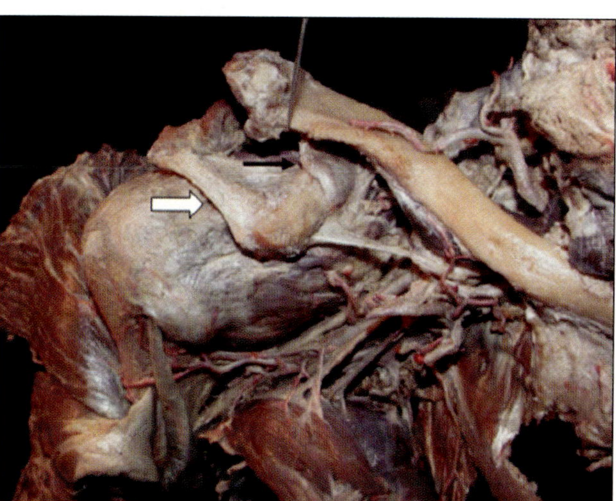

FIGURE 7

Pearls

- *Drape as medially as possible.*

Positioning

- Supine beach chair positioning is used, with the head at 20–30° of elevation.
- The head is stabilized with appropriate materials: either a foam donut or a helmet attached to the operating room table.
- Any hair in the operative field is shaved and removed.
- Preoperative antibiotics are administered.
- The entire upper extremity is prepped sterile.
  - The arm may be placed in an arm holder to stabilize the upper extremity after examination under anesthesia is performed.
  - The surgeon must have adequate clavicle exposure.
- The surface anatomy is marked to identify the location of the coracoid (Fig. 8, *black arrow*) and the AC joint (Fig. 8, *white arrow*).

Pitfalls

- *Avoid drifting too far anterior or posterior, where there is limited soft tissue for closure.*

Portals/Exposures

- After induction, an examination under anesthesia is performed to assess range of motion and any instability.
- A vertical saber incision is made over the AC joint measuring 3–4 cm in length (Fig. 9).
- The skin and subcutaneous tissues are retracted with small skin rakes.
- The soft tissue is elevated off the AC joint for exposure and palpation. Figure 10 shows an intraoperative subcutaneous dissection with skin retractors exposing the intact AC joint (*A*).
- Deep dissection is carried out subperiosteally along the clavicle by splitting the deltotrapezial fascia in line with the deltoid fibers.
- The perisoteum is incised over the clavicle with electrocautery, start 2 cm medial to the AC joint to create flaps for later closure.

Pitfalls

- *Limit resection to 10 mm of bone so as to not destabilize the joint. Poor results have been seen in patients with over 10 mm of resection.*
- *Destabilization of the AC joint should be avoided as this can lead to poor results.*

Procedure

Step 1

- Confirmation of AC joint location is made with a needle. Figure 11 shows a spinal needle in the AC joint, exposing the clavicle (C) and acromion (A).
- Thin Hohmann retractors are used anteriorly and posteriorly to protect soft tissue.

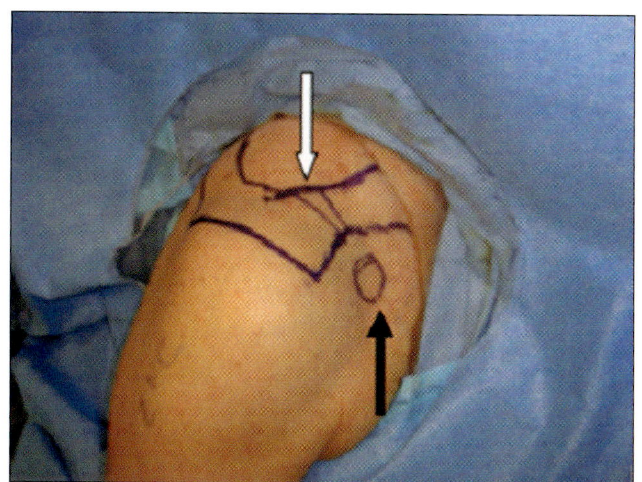

FIGURE 8

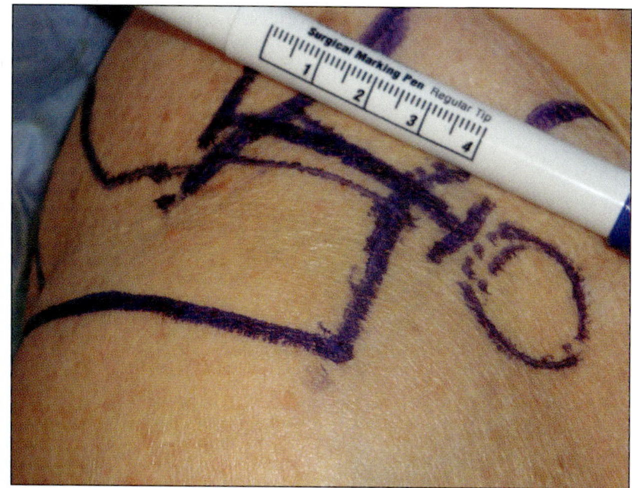

FIGURE 9

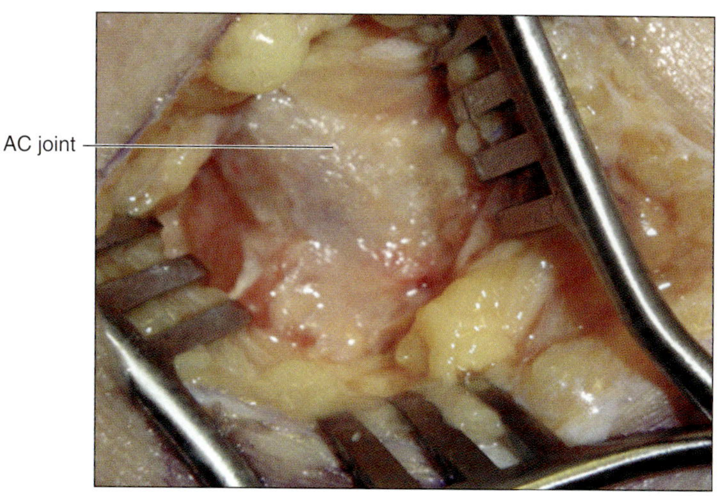

FIGURE 10

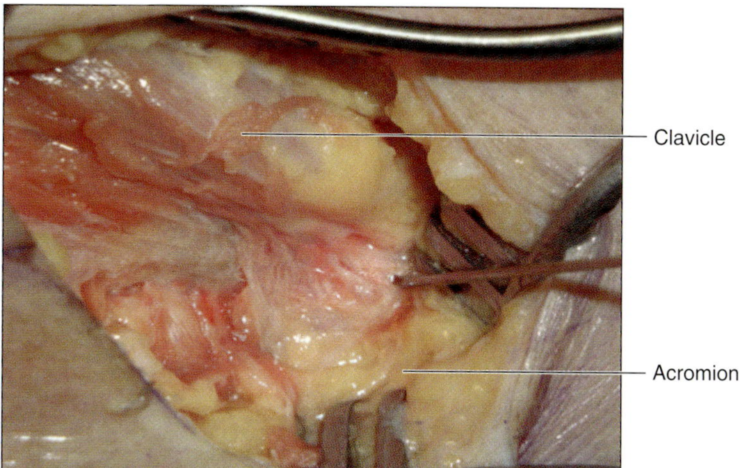

FIGURE 11

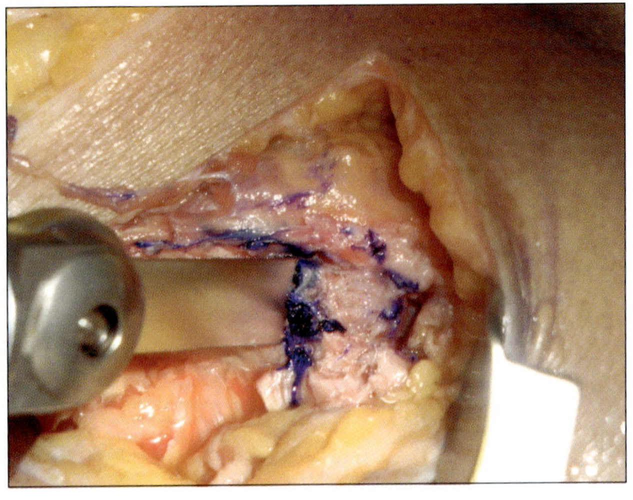
A

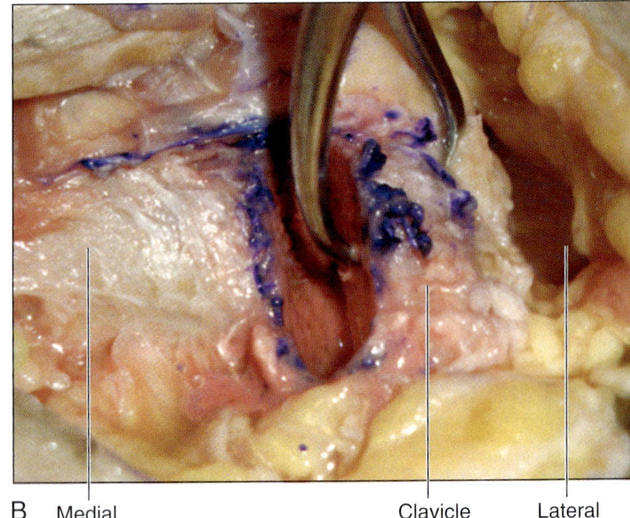

B

FIGURE 12

Controversies

- Poor results have been seen with distal clavicle resection used to treat fractures.
- Recent studies have looked at using 5 mm as the limit for distal clavicle excision to prevent AC joint destabilization (Branch et al., 1996).

Pearls

- *This technically straightforward, short procedure results in a small cosmetic incision.*
- *The surgeon should be able to place his or her index fingure in the resected space while taking the arm through cross-body adduction.*

- Using an oscillating saw, 10 mm of the distal clavicle is excised. In Figure 12A, the saw blade is at a blue line marking 10 mm of resection from the end of the clavicle. Note the slight lateral angle to the blade so as to resect a wedge of distal clavicle.
- A towel clamp is used to grasp the end of the resected section to aid in mobilization (Fig. 12B; C, distal clavicle).

Step 2

- Take the shoulder through the range of motion, including cross-body adduction, to digitally confirm the elimination of contact between the acromion and clavicle.
- Hemostasis can be achieved by utilizing bone wax on the exposed clavicle.
- Figure 13 is a bird's-eye view of a cadaveric specimen following 10-mm distal clavicle resection (C, clavicle; A, acromion; D, reflected deltoid). Note the intact trapezoid ligament (T).

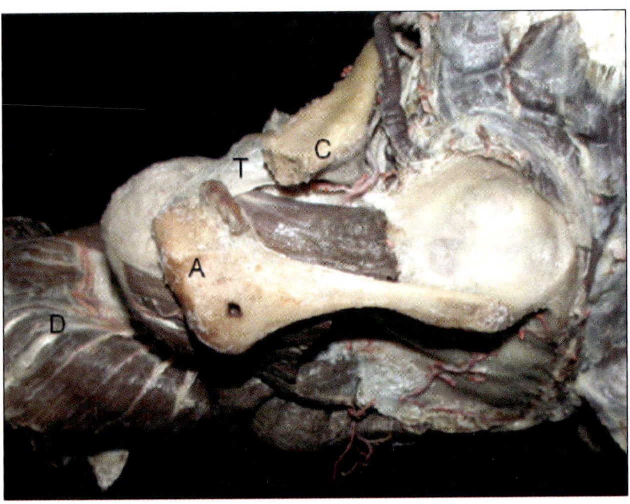

FIGURE 13

Postoperative Care and Expected Outcomes

- This is usually an outpatient procedure; the patient is usually discharged home in a sling with ice, anti-inflammatories, and a short course of narcotics.
- Elbow and wrist range of motion can begin immediately postoperatively while the patient remains in a sling.
- Active Codman and pendulum shoulder exercises can begin on postoperative day 7.
- After 2–3 weeks, the sling can be discontinued and the shoulder can be taken through a full range of motion.
- Rehabilitation consists of active and passive range-of-motion exercises as tolerated and should begin following suture removal on postoperative day 10–14. Goals of physical therapy should be active and passive range of motion while focusing on rotator cuff, trapezius (particularly if there were preoperative trapezius spasms), and deltoid strengthening. Patients can typically return to work after 5–7 days.
- Patients can typically return to athletic activity by 3 months.

Evidence

Alford W, Bach B. Open distal clavicle resection. Oper Techn Sports Med 2004;12:9-17.

The authors described an operative technique for open distal clavicle resection, as well as the history, presentation, imaging, and postoperative course.

Bergfeld JA, Andrish JT, Clancy WG. Evaluation of the acromioclavicular joint following first- and second-degree sprains. Am J Sports Med. 1978;6:153-9.

In this retrospective review, 133 patients with AC joint separation were followed for at least 6 months. They classified residual symptoms as either nuisance or significant.

Bosworth BM. Complete acromioclavicular dislocation. N Engl J Med. 1949;241:221-5.

In this early review article, the author examined the anatomy, etiology, pathology, and treatment for AC dislocation.

Branch TP, Burdette HL, Shahriari AS. The role fo the acromioclavicular ligaments and the effect of distal clavicle resection. Am J Sports Med. 1996;24:293-7.

This biomechanical cadaver study looked at the role of the AC ligaments in controlling scapular rotation. It examined each of the three orthogonal axes of rotation of the scapula with reference to the clavicle after sectioning the AC ligament before and after removing 5 mm of distal clavicle.

Chronopoulos E, Gill HS, Freehill MT, Petersen SA, McFarland EG. Complications after open distal clavicle excision. Clin Orthop Relat Res. 2008;(466):646-51.

This study was a retrospective review of complications in 42 patients who underwent distal clavicle excision. They report a substantially higher complication rate than previously reported. Complications included residual AC joint sensitivity, scar sensitivity, infections, and stiffness. (Level IV evidence)

Chronopoulos E, Kim TK, Park HB, Ashenbrenner D, McFarland EG. Diagnostic value of physical tests for isolated chronic acromioclavicular lesions. Am J Sports Med. 2004;32:655-61.

This retrospective case-control study examined provocative examination techniques in 35 patients who underwent distal clavicle excision. The goal of this study was to evaluate diagnostic values of physical tests, including cross-body adduction stress, resisted extension, and active compression.

Eskola A, Santavirta S, Viljakka HT, Wirta J, Partio TE, Hoikka V. The results of operative resection of the lateral end of the clavicle. J Bone Joint Surg [Am]. 1996;78:584-7.

This retrospective study examined the outcomes of 73 patients who underwent lateral clavicle resection. The average follow-up was 9 years; patients were split into three groups based on etiology (traumatic separation, fracture, osteoarthritis). The authors examined pain, strength, and range of motion, and also looked at the correlation of etiology with amount of resection and outcome. A poor result was more common in the patients who had a fracture.

Freedman BA, Javernick MA, O'Brien FP, Ross AE, Doukas WC. Arthroscopic versus open distal clavicle excision: comparative results at six months and one year from a randomized, prospective clinical trial. J Shoulder Elbow Surg. 2007;16:413-8.

This prospective randomized study compared outcomes after arthroscopic versus open distal clavicle excision in the treatment of refractory AC joint pain. Results were measured through the modified ASES form, visual analog pain scale, Short Form-36, and satisfaction questionnaire at 6 and 12 months postoperatively.

Horvath F, Kery L. Degenerative deformations of the acromioclavicular joint in the elderly. Arch Gerontol Geriatr. 1984;3:259-65.

The authors performed radiologic and locomotor examinations of the AC joint in relatively high numbers of elderly patients. They presented incidence, distribution by age, localization, and clinical symptoms of arthrosis.

Mumford EB. Acromioclavicular dislocation; a new operative treatment. J Bone Joint Surg. 1941;13:799-802.

This is an original article describing the operative technique of distal clavicle resection for AC joint pathology.

Needell SD, Zlatkin MB, Sher JS, Murphy BJ, Uribe JW. MR imaging of the rotator cuff: peritendinous and bone abnormalities in an asymptomatic population. AJR Am J Roentgenol. 1996;166:863-7.

This imaging study examined shoulder MRIs in 100 asymptomatic volunteers. The authors reported that changes characteristic of AC joint osteoarthrosis were present in three-fourths of the shoulders. However, its presence alone does not appear to be a reliable indicator of pain or tendon disease.

Rabalais RD, McCarty E. Surgical treatment of symptomatic acromioclavicular joint problems: a systematic review. Clin Orthop Relat Res 2007;(455):30-7.

The authors performed a literature review comparing open excision, direct (superior) arthroscopic excision, and indirect (bursal) arthroscopic excision.

Zanca P. Shoulder pain: involvement of the acromioclavicular joint. (Analysis of 1,000 cases). Am J Roentgenol Radium Ther Nucl Med. 1971;112:493-506.

This radiographic study described the "gold standard" method for plain film images of the AC joint.

PROCEDURE 24

Arthroscopic Distal Clavicle Resection

Jeffrey D. Watson and Anand M. Murthi

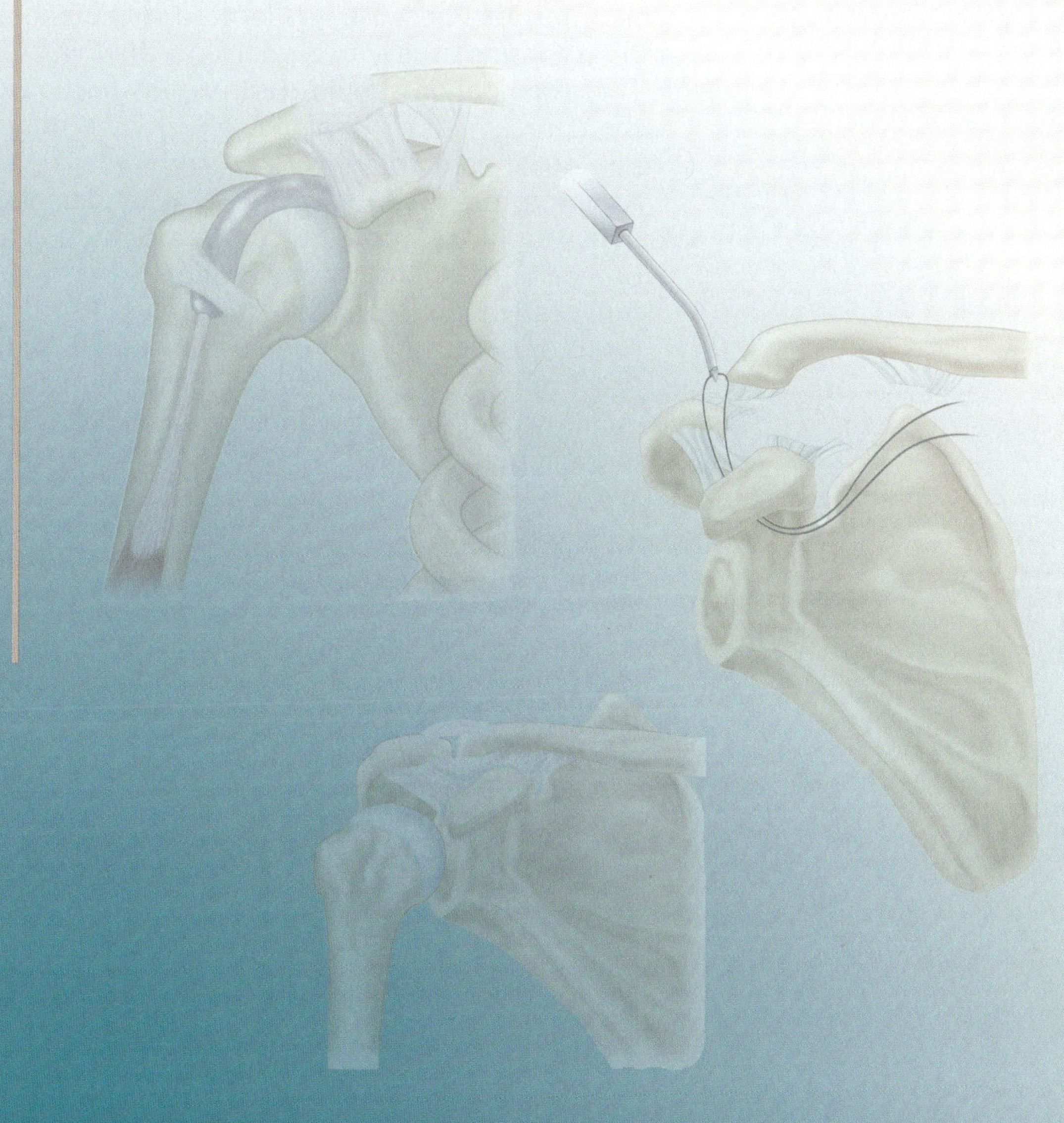

Treatment Options

- Nonoperative management with nonsteroidal anti-inflammatory medications, rest, activity modification, and physical therapy can be an effective treatment for AC joint pain.
- Open resection of the distal clavicle.
- Arthroscopic distal clavicle resection:
  - Indirect approach (Kay et al., 2003; Levine et al., 1998; Martin et al., 2001)
  - Direct approach (Flatow et al., 1995; Levine et al., 2006)

Indications

- Symptomatic acromioclavicular (AC) joint pain for which nonoperative management has failed.
- Pathologic conditions, including arthritis, posttraumatic arthritis, distal clavicle osteolysis, and AC joint synovitis (Flatow et al., 1995; Gartsman, 1993; Snyder et al., 1995; Zawadsky et al., 2000)

Examination/Imaging

- Examination of the AC joint is relatively straightforward because it is located subcutaneously and symptoms usually occur local to the joint.
  - The examination should start with inspection of the entire shoulder girdle. Swelling, deformity, and skin quality are noted.
  - A symptomatic AC joint typically is tender, and hypertrophic osteophytes can be palpated. Cross-body adduction at 90° of elevation is the classic provocative maneuver to test for pain. Pain and symptoms must be reproduced at the AC joint. Relief of pain after injection of local anesthetic confirms a pathologic condition of the AC joint.
- Plain radiographs
  - A standard shoulder series is obtained, including an anteroposterior (AP) view of the shoulder, a true AP view of the glenohumeral joint, and outlet and axillary views.
  - A Zanca view is optimal for visualization of the AC joint. This is a modified AP view obtained with the beam angulated 15° cephalad at 50% of the standard radiation dose (Fig. 1).

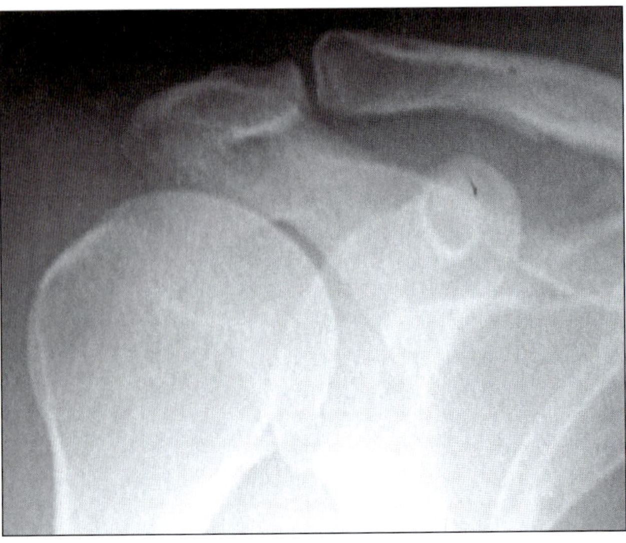

FIGURE 1

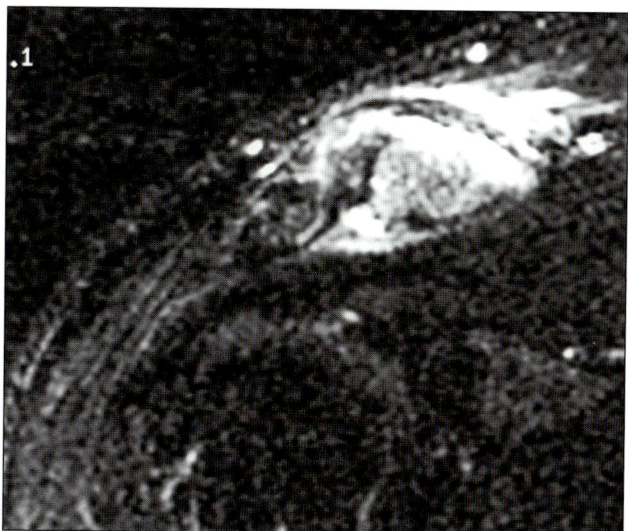

FIGURE 2

- Degenerative changes of the AC joint seen radiographically occur as part of the normal aging process, so radiographs *must* be correlated with physical examination findings.

- Magnetic resonance imaging (MRI)
  - Advanced imaging is not required to evaluate the AC joint. T_2-weighted MRI often shows edema within the clavicle and possibly the acromion (Fig. 2).
  - Like the findings of plain radiography, MRI findings might not correlate with physical examination findings.
  - The advantage of obtaining an MRI study is that it allows for thorough evaluation of the rotator cuff tendons and other shoulder pathologic conditions before operative treatment. MRI may also reveal inferior encroachment of clavicular osteophytes, which can be addressed during arthroscopic distal clavicle resection.

Surgical Anatomy

- The distal end of the clavicle and the medial facet of the acromion form the AC joint.
- The fibrocartilage disk resides within the AC joint between the hyaline cartilage–covered end of the distal clavicle and the medial facet of the acromion. Disk and cartilage degeneration is part of the pathoanatomy of a symptomatic AC joint.
- The capsular ligaments located anteriorly, posteriorly, superiorly, and inferiorly confer stability to the AC

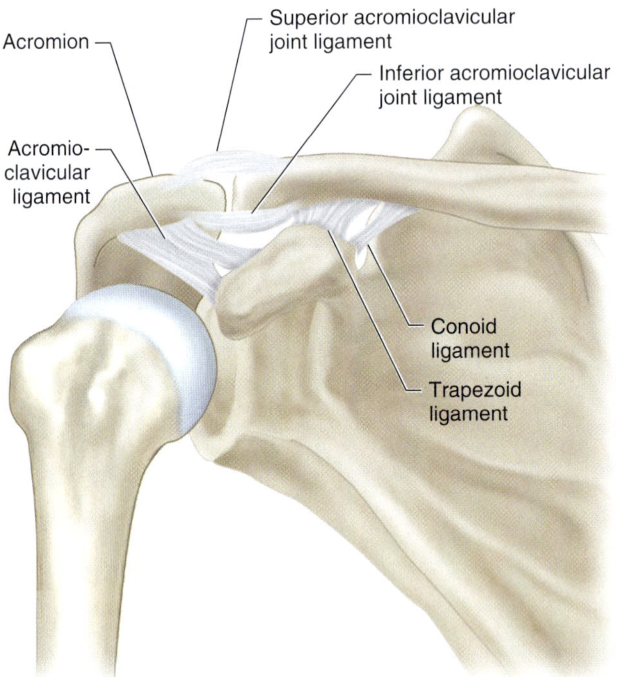

FIGURE 3

joint (Fig. 3). Iatrogenic resection of the superior, posterior and/or inferior (during direct distal clavicle resection) capsular ligaments during direct or indirect distal clavicle resection can result in horizontal AC joint instability.

Positioning

- The patient is placed in the beach chair (sitting) position with the operative shoulder and arm draped free (Fig. 4).

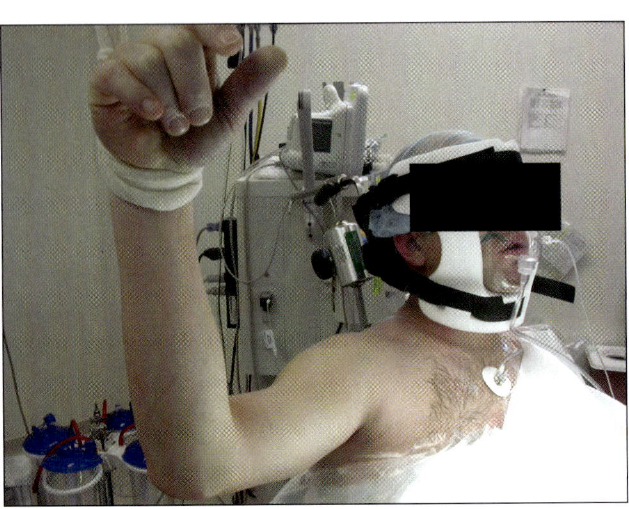

FIGURE 4

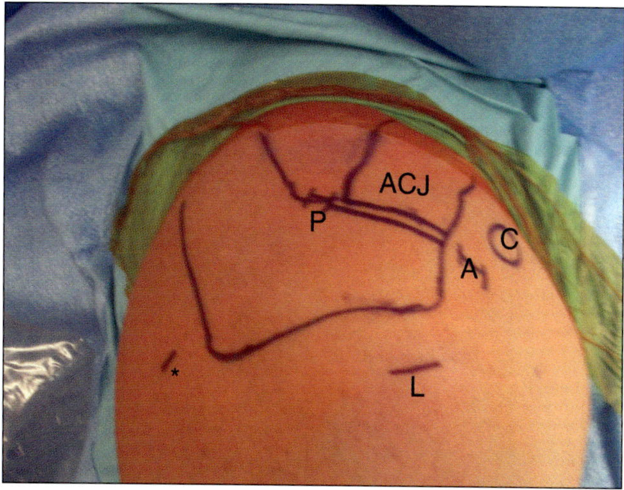

FIGURE 5

- The hand and forearm are placed in a stockinette.
- An armholder can be used to maintain the position of the extremity. The armholder is adjusted to place the extremity in the appropriate amount of flexion-extension, abduction-adduction, and internal-external rotation.

- The bony anatomy of the shoulder is outlined with a marking pen (Fig. 5). The anterior and posterior borders of the AC joint are identified for portal placement (in Fig. 5: A, anterior AC joint/glenohumeral portal; ACJ, AC joint; L, lateral subacromial portal; P, posterior AC joint portal; *, posterior glenohumeral/subacromial portal).
- This procedure may be performed in the lateral decubitus position as well.

Portals/Exposures

Direct Approach

- Anterior and posterior AC joint portals are created with a longitudinal incision through the skin in line with the joint.
- One or two 18-gauge spinal needles may assist in localizing a tight, arthritic AC joint.
- Once correct joint line position is confirmed, the anterior and posterior AC joint ligaments are opened with an obturator.

Indirect Approach

- A standard posterior portal is established for visualization of the glenohumeral joint and subacromial space.

Pearls

- *Correct joint line position for the direct approach can be confirmed by placing 18-gauge needles through the AC joint superiorly to align the AC joint externally.*

Pitfalls

- *In the direct approach, care should be taken to make the initial incision through only the skin to prevent iatrogenic injury to the superior or inferior AC joint ligaments.*

Pearls

- *For difficult exposures, begin with the smaller 2.7-mm scope and smaller burrs.*
- *Visualization of the AC joint can be facilitated by resection of a minimal amount of medial acromion.*

Pitfalls

- *Maintain the integrity of the superior and inferior AC ligaments to prevent horizontal instability of the clavicle.*

Instrumentation/ Implantation

- A standard 4.0-mm, 30° arthroscope generally is used, with a 2.7-mm scope on standby for difficult exposures. A cannula can be used (rarely) if space permits.
- An arthroscopic radiofrequency wand, 4.5-mm arthroscopic full radius, and/or aggressive shaver should be included to clear debris and clean bony surfaces. A 4.0- to 5.0-mm round or barrel burr is used to resect the distal clavicle, and an arthroscopic rasp can be used to smooth rough surfaces. A quality arthroscopic pump will allow hemostasis to be controlled and allow for proper irrigation of debris.

Pearls

- *The width of the barrel burr (usually 4 to 5 mm) can be used to gauge the amount of bony resection.*

- The anterior glenohumeral and AC joint portal is made inferior to and in line with the AC joint space.
- The lateral subacromial portal is made 1 cm posterior to the anterior edge of the acromion and under visualization from the posterior portal utilizing an outside-in technique, and confirmation of position is made with a spinal needle.

Procedure: Direct Approach

Step 1

- The arthroscope is first introduced into the posterior AC joint portal. From the posterior portal, the blunt metal obturator is visualized entering through the anterior portal.
- The obturator is used initially to sweep the AC joint clear of meniscus and debris. A radiofrequency wand can then be used to identify the distal clavicle and medial acromial surfaces. The surfaces are then cleaned subperiosteally while the integrity of the inferior and superior AC joint ligaments is carefully maintained.

Step 2

- A barrel burr is then introduced through the anterior AC joint portal. Usually 6–8 mm of distal clavicle is resected in male patients and 4–7 mm in female patients (see Video 1).
- With the arthroscope in the posterior AC joint portal, bony resection proceeds from anterior to posterior and inferior to superior directions (see Video 2).

Step 3

- Once the anterior distal clavicle resection is complete, switch the arthroscope to the anterior portal to allow for improved visualization during resection of the posterior clavicle. Because of the obliquity of the distal clavicle, more of the posterior clavicle will need to be resected.
- All edges are smoothed with an arthroscopic rasp (Fig. 6) (see Video 3).
- Resection amount may be measured with a clamp (see Video 4) or calibrated probe.
- Routine preoperative and postoperative Zanca views also may verify adequate resection of the distal clavicle (Fig. 7A and 7B).

Pearls

- *View from both portals to confirm resection, especially superiorly and posteriorly.*

Pitfalls

- *Avoid leaving a superior acromial ridge (overhang).*
- *Avoid underresection posteriorly as this may cause painful continued impingement.*

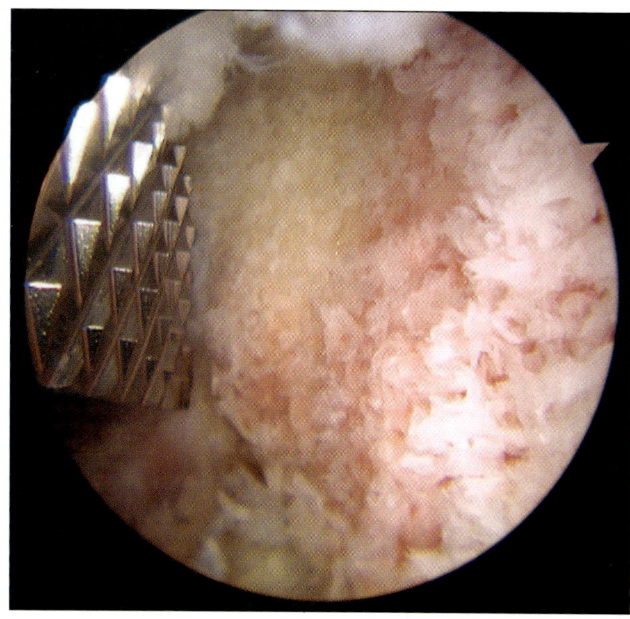

FIGURE 6

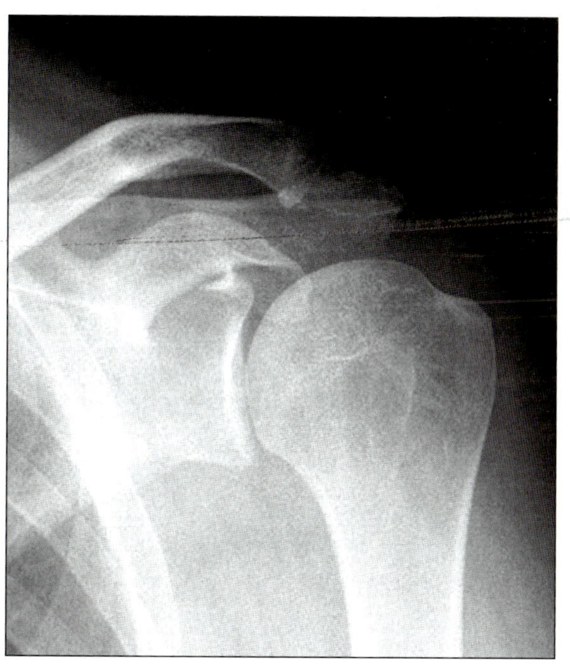

A

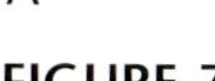

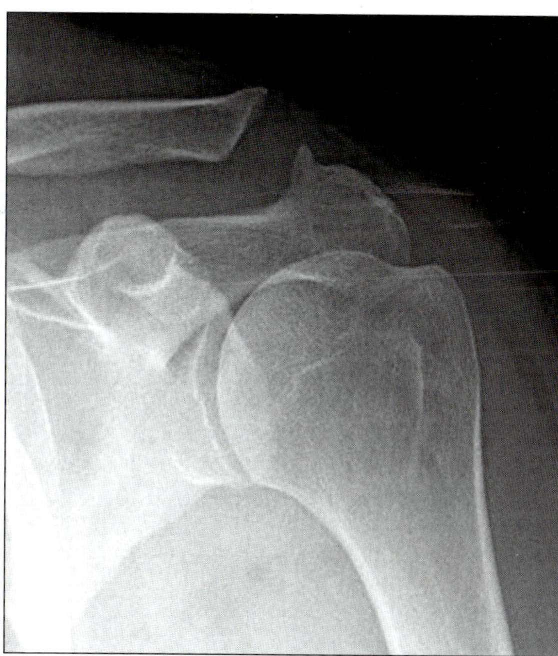

B

FIGURE 7

Procedure: Indirect Approach

STEP 1

- Diagnostic and therapeutic treatments of the glenohumeral joint are completed before attention is turned to the subacromial space.
- A subacromial bursectomy is performed with the use of the shaver and radiofrequency wand. Bursal tissue is cleared medially, sufficient to identify the AC joint.

PEARLS

- *Medial acromial facet decompression in addition to subacromial bursectomy often is necessary to adequately view the distal clavicle.*

STEP 2

- With the arthroscope in the posterior portal, the radiofrequency wand is introduced through the anterior AC joint portal to subperiosteally isolate the distal clavicle and medial acromion (viewed from posterior and inferior).
- Once the interval between the distal clavicle and acromion is identified, a barrel burr is placed in that space from the anterior portal. Again, 6–8 mm of distal clavicle usually is resected in male patients and 4–7 mm in female patients.
- Often upon reaching the midway point of distal clavicle resection, switching arthroscopic visualization to the lateral portal will facilitate resection of the posterior distal clavicle (see Video 4).

PEARLS

- *Complete release of the anterior AC ligament/capsule is necessary to introduce arthroscopic equipment, especially superiorly.*
- *Make sure to view from all portals (anterior, posterior, lateral) to confirm exposure, preparationl and resection.*

Instrumentation/ Implantation

- The equipment described for the direct approach can be used for the indirect approach to arthroscopic distal clavicle resection.

Postoperative Care and Expected Outcomes

- The arm is placed in a sling for comfort, and the patient is instructed to keep the incisions clean and dry.
- The patient is instructed to perform pendulum exercises and elbow, wrist, and hand range-of-motion exercises until the first postoperative visit.
- At 7–10 days after surgery, the sling is discontinued, and the patient's shoulder range of motion is advanced. Flexion with cross-body adduction is avoided for 6 weeks after surgery.
- Full range-of-motion and rotator cuff strengthening exercises are initiated at 6 weeks postoperatively.
- Patients can expect and should be educated on full return of function at 12 weeks.
- Several authors have reported outcomes of arthroscopic distal clavicle resection that compare favorably with open resection (Flatow et al., 1995; Levine et al., 1998).

- Complications of arthroscopic distal clavicle resection include inadequate resection, overzealous resection, iatrogenic instability, heterotopic bone formation, and infection.

Evidence

Flatow EL, Duralde XA, Nicholson GP, Pollock RG, Bigliani LU. Arthroscopic resection of the distal clavicle with a superior approach. J Shoulder Elbow Surg. 1995;4:41–50.

This study reviewed the results of 41 patients who underwent arthroscopic distal clavicle resection for AC joint disease. Follow-up duration averaged 31 months, and outcome was judged based on pain and function. (Level IV evidence [case series])

Gartsman GM. Arthroscopic resection of the acromioclavicular joint. Am J Sports Med. 1993;21:71–7.

This study was a retrospective review of 20 patients who underwent arthroscopy for distal clavicle resection. Follow-up was conducted at 2 years, and outcome was judged by pain, activities of daily living, work, and return to sports. (Level IV evidence [case series])

Kay SP, Dragoo JL, Lee R. Long-term results of arthroscopic resection of the distal clavicle with concomitant subacromial decompression. Arthroscopy. 2003;19:805–9.

This study was a retrospective review of 20 patients who underwent arthroscopic distal clavicle resection. Average follow-up duration was 6 years, and outcomes were judged by the UCLA and Constant scoring systems. (Level IV evidence [case series])

Levine WN, Barron OA, Yamaguchi K, Pollock RG, Flatow EL, Bigliani LU. Arthroscopic distal clavicle resection from a bursal approach. Arthroscopy. 1998;14:52–6.

This study was a retrospective review of 24 patients who underwent arthroscopic distal clavicle resection from a bursal approach. Average follow-up duration was 32.5 months, with pain scores being the primary outcome measure. This study also attempted to correlate technical factors that influenced outcome. (Level IV evidence [case series])

Levine WN, Soong M, Ahmad CS, Blaine TA, Bigliani LU. Arthroscopic distal clavicle resection: a comparison of bursal and direct approaches. Arthroscopy. 2006;22:516–20.

In this study, 24 patients who underwent arthroscopic distal clavicle resection from a bursal approach were retrospectively compared with 42 patients who underwent arthroscopic distal clavicle resection from a direct approach. Average follow-up duration was 6 years, and outcomes were judged by subjective pain score and the American Shoulder and Elbow Surgeons score. (Level IV evidence [case series])

Martin SD, Baumgarten TE, Andrews JR. Arthroscopic resection of the distal aspect of the clavicle with concomitant subacromial decompression. J Bone Joint Surg [Am]. 2001;83:328–35.

This study was a retrospective review of 31 patients (32 shoulders) who underwent arthroscopic resection of the distal clavicle with concomitant subacromial decompression. Average follow-up duration was 4 years 10 months, and outcomes were judged based on pain, clinical examination, and isokinetic testing. (Level IV evidence [case series])

Snyder SJ, Banas MP, Karzel RP. The arthroscopic Mumford procedure: an analysis of the results. Arthroscopy. 1995;11:157–64.

This study was a retrospective review of 50 patients who underwent arthroscopic distal clavicle resection. Average follow-up was at 2 years, with outcomes judged by physical examination and the UCLA shoulder score. (Level IV evidence [case series])

Zawadsky M, Marra G, Wiater JM, Levine WN, Pollock RG, Flatow EL, Bigliani LU. Osteolysis of the distal clavicle: long-term results of arthroscopic resection. Arthroscopy. 2000;16:600–5.

This study was a retrospective review of 37 patients (41 shoulders) who underwent arthroscopic distal clavicle resection for treatment of distal clavicle osteolysis. Average follow-up duration was 6.2 years, and outcomes were judged based on pain and functional scores. (Level IV evidence [case series])

PROCEDURE 25

Open Treatment of Acute and Chronic Acromioclavicular Dislocations

Andrew Green

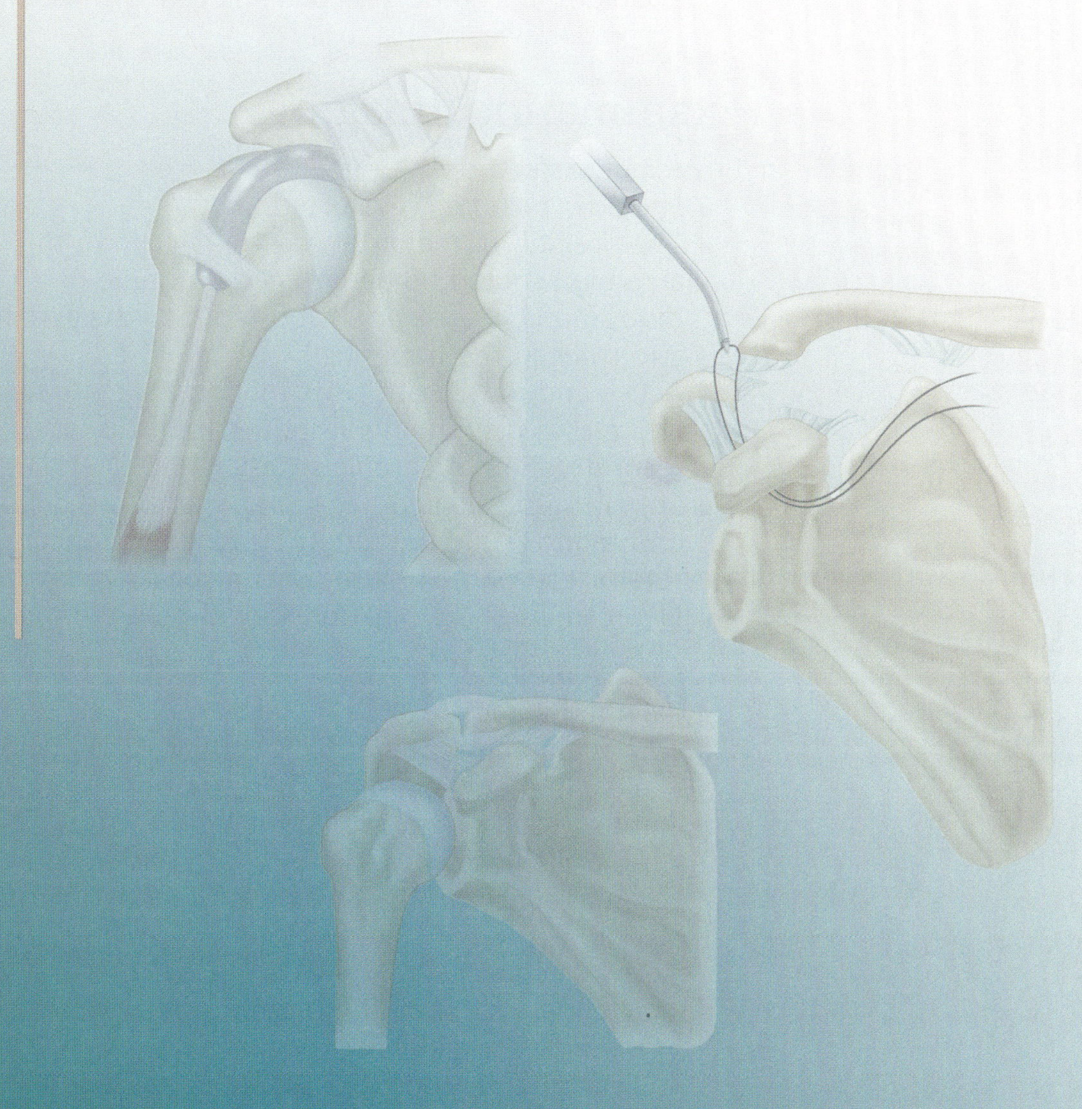

Pitfalls

- *Acute injury*
  - *Skin abrasion—wait until healed*
  - *Noncompliant patient*
- *Chronic injury*
  - *Noncompliant patient*

Controversies

- Acute repair of grade III injuries is controversial. There are advocates of both operative and nonoperative treatment. Operative treatment of acute injuries is the only treatment that will restore normal anatomy, but it is associated with greater risk of complications.

Indications

- Acute injury
  - Grade III in selected patients, including heavy laborers (lifting, carrying) and physically active athletic patients
  - Grades IV, V, and VI in most patients unless surgery is contraindicated due to medical or psychological factors
- Chronic injury
  - Grade II in patients with symptomatic anterior-posterior instability of the distal clavicle
  - Grades III, IV, and V in patients with symptomatic coracoclavicular instability

Examination/Imaging

Physical Examination

- Shoulder posture is evaluated.
- The position of the distal clavicle relative to the acromion should be determined. In grade IV dislocations, the clavicle is posterior to the acromion and stuck in the trapezius.
- Active and passive shoulder motion are evaluated, addressing glenohumeral stiffness prior to reconstruction of chronic separation.
- Strength is evaluated, including that of the deltoid and rotator cuff. The rare occurrence of concomitant rotator cuff pathology should be considered.
- Neurovascular examination should be performed.

Imaging Studies

- Plain radiographs
  - A true anteroposterior view is used to evaluate the glenohumeral joint and check for bony signs of rotator cuff pathology (Fig. 1A).
  - An axillary view will demonstrate posterior displacement of the clavicle in grade IV injuries (Fig 1B).
  - An outlet/scapular Y view is obtained to evaluate acromial anatomy; the presence of a spur might warrant acromioplasty.
  - Bilateral anteroposterior acromioclavicular views (Zanca view: 10–15° cephalad tilt of x-ray beam) should be obtained to evaluate the acromioclavicular joint position and arthritic changes, as well as the coracoclavicular relationship (Fig. 2).

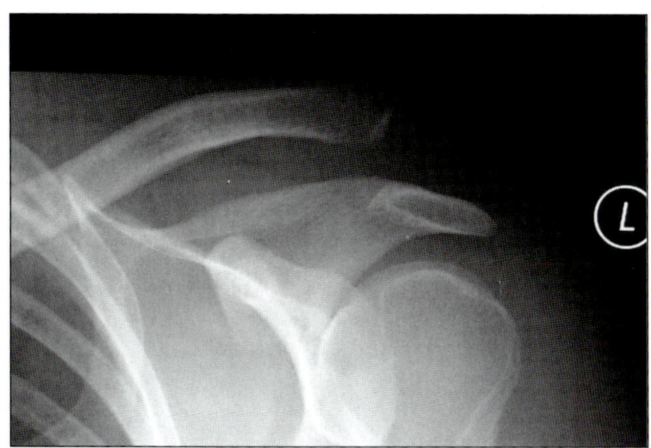

A

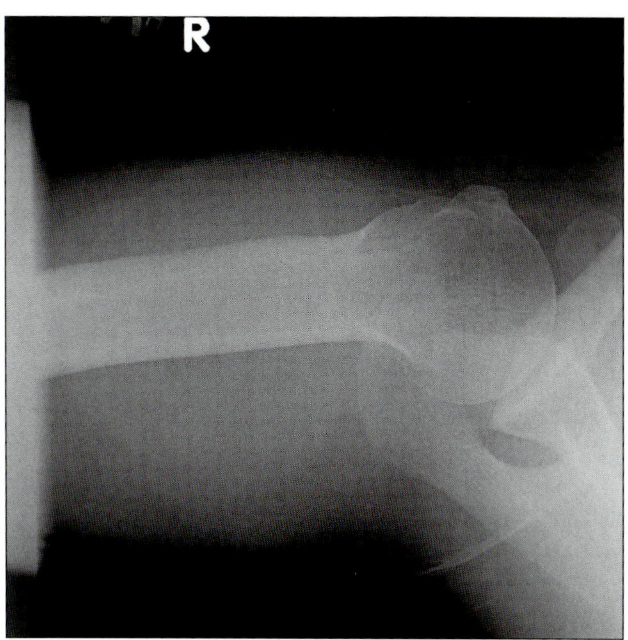

B

FIGURE 1

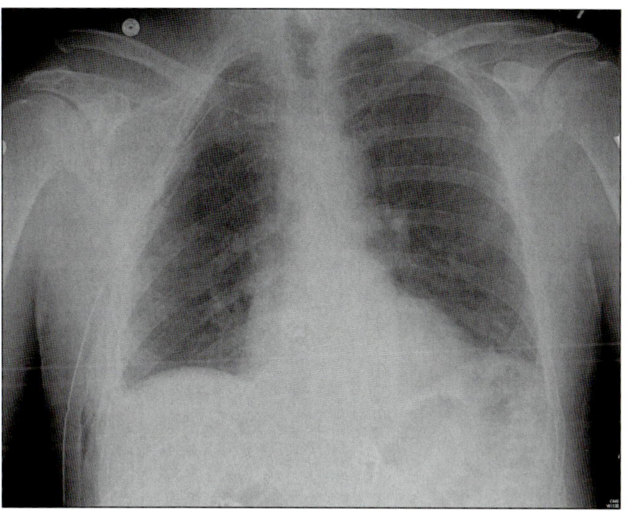

FIGURE 2

- Advanced imaging should be considered only if evaluation suggests rotator cuff or intra-articular glenohumeral pathology.
  - Magnetic resonance imaging may be indicated to evaluate the rotator cuff in chronic injury.

Surgical Anatomy

- Clavicle
  - The coracoclavicular ligaments attach to the undersurface of the distal clavicle lateral to the

Treatment Options

- Acute injury
  - Nonoperative treatment with physical therapy, including early shoulder range of motion and periscapular and rotator cuff strengthening. A short course (2–3 weeks) of sling support/immobilization for may be used for comfort, but immobilizers such as a Kenny-Howard brace should not be used.
  - Operative treatment with coracoclavicular suture, transarticular acromioclavicular pin fixation, coracoclavicular screw fixation, Weaver-Dunn acromioclavicular ligament transfer, and acromioclavicular hook plate.
- Chronic injury
  - Other surgical procedures, including coracoclavicular ligament reconstruction with tendon graft, conjoined tendon transfer, and Weaver-Dunn reconstruction—all augmented with coracoclavicular fixation.

juncture of the middle and lateral thirds of the clavicle.
  - The distal clavicle forms the medial articulation of the acromioclavicular joint.
- Acromion
  - The acromion forms the lateral aspect of the acromioclavicular joint with attachment of the acromioclavicular capsule and ligaments.
  - The anterior acromion is also the site of insertion of the coracoacromial ligament, which is used in the Weaver-Dunn repair.
- Acromioclavicular joint
  - The orientation of the joint varies from vertical to oblique from inferomedial to superolateral. The clavicle underlies the acromion in rare cases.
  - Acromioclavicular ligaments
    - The posterior acromioclavicular ligament is an important restraint to posterior translation of the acromioclavicular joint.
    - The superior acromioclavicular ligament contributes to a lesser extent to restraint of posterior translation of the acromioclavicular joint
    - The inferior acromioclavicular ligament contributes to restraint of anterior translation of the acromioclavicular joint.
  - The intra-articular meniscus is a fibrocartilaginous structure within the acromioclavicular joint. The true function is unknown, and the disk undergoes significant degeneration with aging.
- Coracoclavicular ligaments
  - The conoid and trapezoid are short, strong ligaments that connect the clavicle to the base of the coracoid.
  - The conoid ligament is a more medial structure that attaches on the conoid tubercle on the underside of the distal clavicle. The conoid tubercle is located at the juncture of the lateral and medial thirds of the clavicle.
  - The trapezoid ligament is more lateral and attaches on the trapezoid line of the inferior clavicle.
- Disruption of the acromioclavicular and coracoclavicular ligaments as occurs in grades III, IV, V, and VI injuries is shown in Figure 3.
- Muscular anatomy—The trapezius, pectoralis major, and anterior deltoid muscles attach to the distal clavicle and acromion, providing some dynamic stability to the acromioclavicular joint.

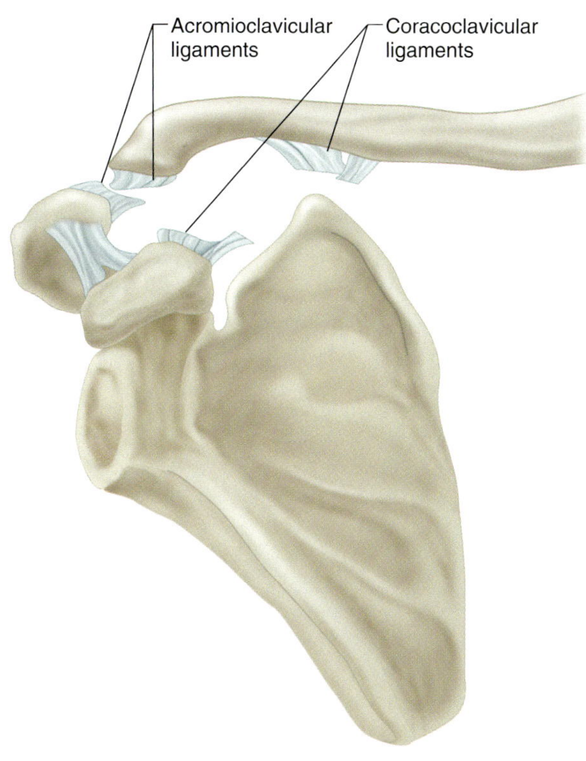

FIGURE 3

- Neurologic anatomy—The proximity of the brachial plexus, as well as the suprascapular and musculocutaneous nerves, is relevant to surgical reconstruction of the coracoclavicular ligaments.
- Vascular anatomy—Branches of the thoracoacromial artery that run in the vicinity of the distal clavicle can bleed during the dissection and exposure of the base of the coracoid.

Pearls

- *Drape high on the neck and inferior enough on the chest to have an adequate surgical field.*
- *Drape the operative arm free.*
- *Position the shoulder so that imaging can be used if needed.*

Pitfalls

- *Keep the neck aligned in neutral rotation and flexion/extension position to protect the cervical spine and prevent brachial plexus injury.*

Equipment

- Articulating sterile armholder
- Adjustable and articulating headrest
- Side pad

Positioning

- The patient is placed in the beach chair position, with the surgical field draped out, bony landmarks outlined, and the skin incision marked (Fig. 4).
- Neck alignment should be in neutral position with the head on an adjustable articulating headrest.
- An articulating armholder is used to support and position the arm during the procedure (see Fig. 4).
- A side pad is placed against the lateral chest to keep the patient from falling off the side of the table.

Portals/Exposures

- A superior surgical approach is used.
- An incision is made in Langer's lines over the distal end of the clavicle, beginning just posterior to the

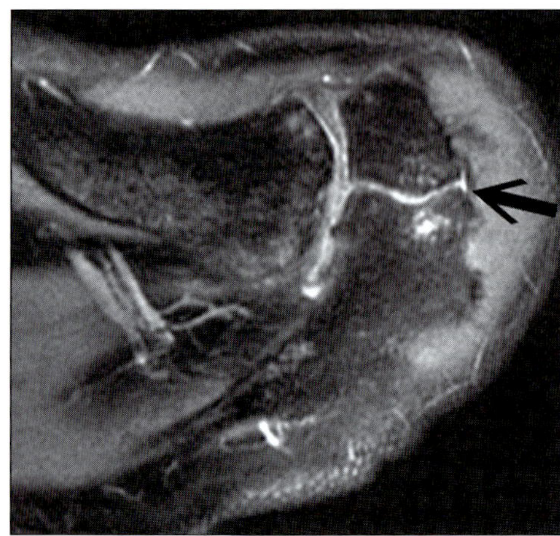

FIGURE 4

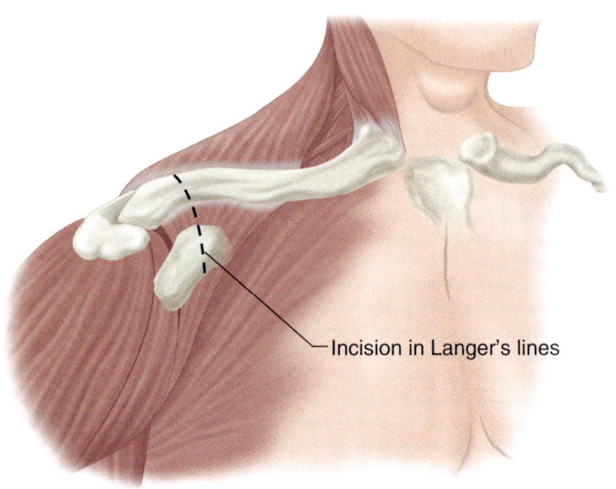

FIGURE 5

Pearls

- *An incision in Langer's lines will heal with a very cosmetic scar.*

Pitfalls

- *An incision that is too lateral limits exposure of the clavicle.*
- *An incision that is too medial limits access to the acromion.*
- *A longitudinal incision in line with the clavicle, across Langer's lines, may heal with a thick, uncosmetic scar.*

clavicle and extending toward the coracoid process (Fig. 5).

Procedure

Step 1: Skin Incision and Surgical Dissection

- Surgical dissection is performed following Langer's lines.
- Dissection extends through the subcutaneous tissue, using electrocautery for hemostasis.
- The skin and subcutaneous tissue are elevated to extend exposure medially and laterally to expose the distal 3–4 cm of the clavicle and the medial acromion.

Instrumentation/ Implantation

- Place a self-retaining retractor to hold the skin and subcutaneous tissue apart.

Pearls

- *Release enough capsule and soft tissue to facilitate anatomic reduction of the distal clavicle to the coracoid.*
- *Maintain anterior and posterior acromioclavicular ligament attachment to the acromion.*

Pitfalls

- *Excessive distal clavicle resection potentially destabilizes the acromioclavicular joint by releasing the acromioclavicular ligaments.*

Instrumentation/ Implantation

- Distal clavicle resection with power saw, osteotome, or chisel

Controversies

- Distal clavicle resection is controversial. Weaver-Dunn coracoacromial ligament transfer requires distal clavicle resection for ligament reattachment. Isolated coracoclavicular ligament reconstruction does not require distal clavicle resection. Preserving the distal clavicle may enable better acromioclavicular ligament repair and provide better acromioclavicular joint stability. Resection of the distal clavicle might facilitate reduction and prevent late acromioclavicular arthritis.

Step 2: Acromioclavicular Joint Exposure

- The acromioclavicular joint capsule and ligaments are elevated off the distal clavicle.
- The meniscus is débrided.
- An evaluation for arthritis is done. Distal clavicle resection should be considered in chronic cases (8–10 mm) with arthritis.

Step 3: Coracoclavicular Exposure

- Subperiosteal elevation of the anterior deltoid off the distal clavicle is performed.
- Subperiosteal elevation of the acromioclavicular capsule off the distal clavicle is done.
- The deltoid is retracted anteriorly.
- The surgeon must identify fatty tissue deep to the deltoid, and cauterize vessels.
- Blunt dissection is performed to the base of the coracoid.
- The posterior attachment of the acromial ligament to the coracoid is partially released.
- Blunt dissection continues medial to the coracoid, staying posterior to the pectoralis minor insertion and anterior to the suprascapular notch.

Step 4: Tendon Graft Preparation for Chronic Reconstruction

- A 6- to 7-mm diameter tendon graft is prepared using autologous or allograft semitendinosus tendon.
- The graft is pretensioned.
- Sutures are placed for passing the tendon graft around the coracoid and through drill holes in the clavicle.

Pearls

- *Identify the plane deep to the anterior deltoid to find the base of the coracoid*
- *Blunt dissection medial and lateral to the coracoid as well as underneath is done to develop a passage for sutures and any tendon graft.*

Pitfalls

- *Dissection around the base of the coracoid places nerves at risk. Avoid distal dissection posterior to the conjoined tendon as well as medial dissection into the suprascapular notch.*

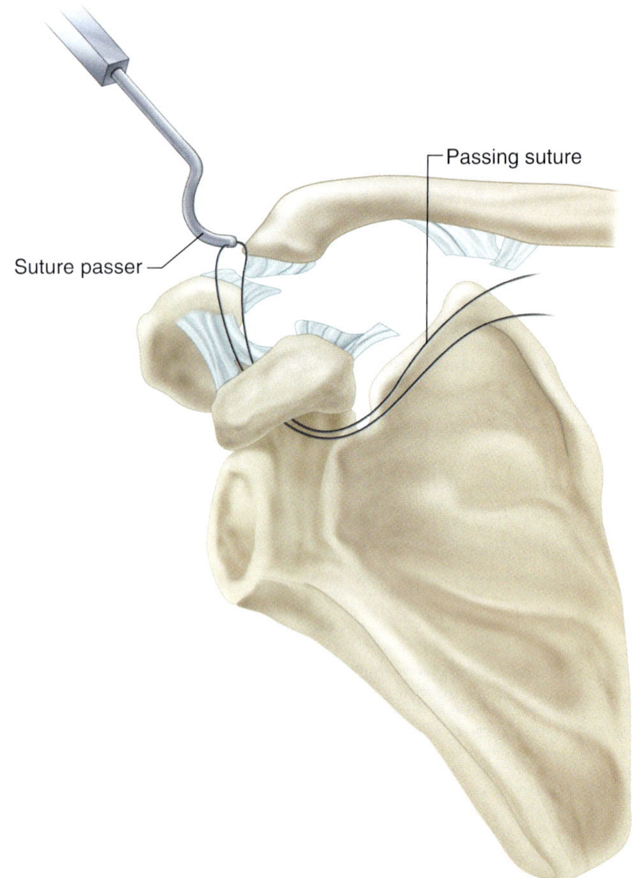

FIGURE 6

Instrumentation/ Implantation

- Right-angle retractors medial and anterior to coracoid: provide visualization medial to the base of the coracoid

Controversies

- Allograft versus autograft
- Allograft
  - No secondary graft site issues
  - Can pick the specific graft for size
  - Quicker procedure
- Autograft
  - No issues with disease transmission or weakening of tendon secondary to tissue processing

Pitfalls

- *Blunt spreading of tissue immediately under the coracoid will protect neurovascular structures.*

Instrumentation/ Implantation

- Curved suture passer—reusable crotchet hook versus disposable passer

Step 5: Passage of Fixation Sutures and Tendon Graft

- Acute repair
  - A curved suture-passing device is placed deep to the coracoid from lateral to medial, and a loop of #2 braided suture is passed to be used as a shuttle for the coracoclavicular fixation sutures (Fig. 6).
  - Fixation sutures are passed inferior to the coracoid.
- Chronic reconstruction
  - A curved suture-passing device is placed deep to the coracoid from lateral to medial, and a loop of #2 braided suture is passed to be used as a shuttle for the coracoclavicular fixation sutures as well as a tendon graft (see Fig. 6).
  - The tendon graft and fixation sutures are passed inferior to the coracoid.

Step 6: Clavicle Drilling

- Acute repair
  - The previously passed sutures are pulled around coracoid vertically and aligned with the clavicle to

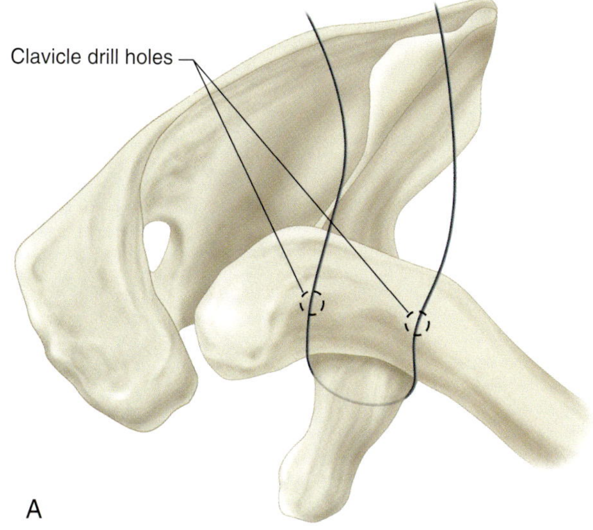

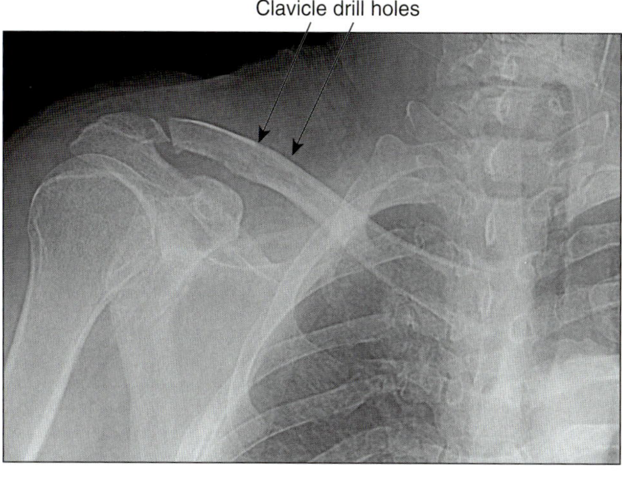

FIGURE 7

Controversies

- Tendon around/under the coracoid versus direct fixation to the coracoid with an interference screw
  - Direct fixation to the coracoid weakens the coracoid, which could lead to fracture.
  - Direct fixation may provide a more anatomic position of graft attachment to the coracoid.
  - Suture around the coracoid could potentially lead to cutting through and fracture.

Instrumentation/ Implantation

- Power drill or burr to make holes in the clavicle for suture and tendon passing

Instrumentation/ Implantation

- Curved suture-passing instrument to pass sutures and tendon graft under base of coracoid

mark placement of drill holes in the clavicle (Fig. 7A and 7B). The clavicle must be reduced to the acromion so that the holes are not placed too far laterally.
  - Holes are drilled with a 3.5-mm bit for isolated suture repair.
- Chronic reconstruction
  - The previously passed sutures are pulled around the coracoid vertically and align with the clavicle to mark placement of drill holes in the clavicle (see Fig. 7). Be sure that clavicle is reduced to the acromion so that the holes are not placed too far laterally.
  - Holes are drilled with a 6-mm drill bit for a 6- to 7-mm tendon graft.

Step 7: Coracoclavicular Fixation

- Acute repair
  - The coracoclavicular sutures (nonabsorbable no. 5 suture or 5-mm suture tape) are passed. Both ends of one suture are pulled up through both medial and lateral clavicle drill holes. The medial end of the other suture is passed up through the medial clavicle hole and the other end is passed anterior to the clavicle.
  - The clavicle is held reduced to the acromion with an awl pressing downward on the distal clavicle and with upward pressure on the arm through the elbow, and the sutures are tied (Fig. 8).
- Chronic reconstruction
  - Tendon ends are prepared with passing sutures.
  - Tendon ends are pulled up through the clavicle drill holes. The end pulled through medial hole

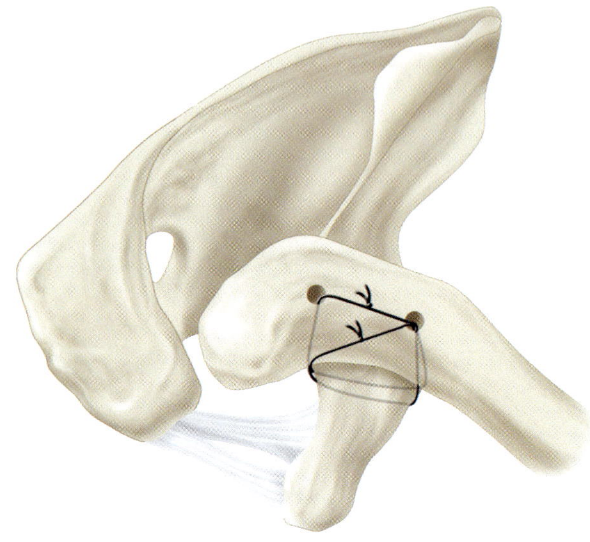

FIGURE 8

Controversies

- Coracoclavicular fixation can be achieved with heavy sutures, a coracoclavicular screw, a transarticular acromioclavicular screw or pins, or an acromioclavicular hook plate.

should be longer, and the end through the lateral hole long enough to overlap to the medial hole.

- Next the coracoclavicular sutures are passed. Both ends of one suture are pulled up through both medial and lateral clavicle drill holes. The medial end of the other suture is passed up through the medial clavicle hole and the other end is passed anterior to the clavicle.
- The clavicle is held reduced to the acromion with an awl pressing downward on the distal clavicle and with upward pressure on the arm through the elbow, and the sutures are tied (see Fig. 8). There should be little or no space between the underside of the clavicle and the base of the coracoid.
- The tendon graft is tied to itself between the clavicle drill holes and anchored with side-to-side sutures (Fig. 9).
- The long medial end of the tendon is brought across the acromioclavicular joint and passed through the acromioclavicular capsule tissue at the medial acromion to augment the acromioclavicular ligament repair (see Fig. 9).

Step 8: Deltotrapezial and Acromioclavicular Repair

- The deltotrapezial fascia is sutured over the clavicle with nonabsorbable suture.
- The acromioclavicular ligaments and capsule are repaired over acromioclavicular joint, incorporating the lateral extension of the tendon graft for a chronic reconstruction.

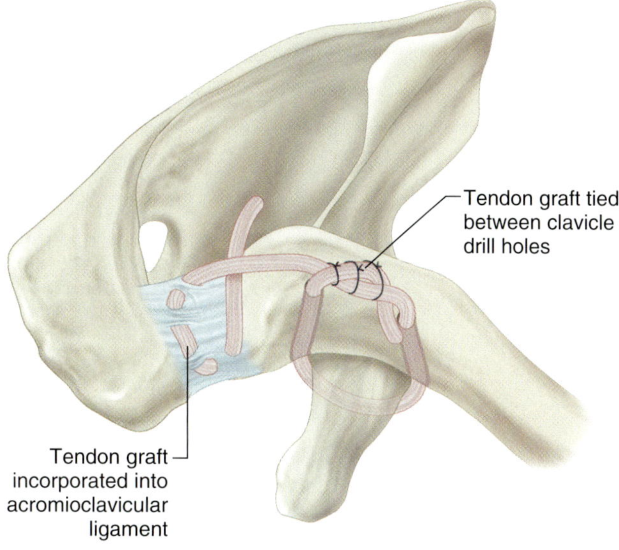

FIGURE 9

PEARLS

- *Avoid an unsupported position of the arm.*

PITFALLS

- *Overly aggressive early rehabilitation can lead to attenuation or failure of the repair or reconstruction.*

Postoperative Care and Expected Outcomes

- A sling and swathe or abduction brace (small cushion) immobilization is used to support the arm for 6 weeks. No shoulder motion is permitted for 2 weeks.
- After 2 weeks, supine passive self-assisted external rotation and scapular plane elevation to 90° are begun. All ranges of motion, passive and active-assisted, are begun after 6 weeks postoperative. Isometric deltoid exercises, and movement of the rotator cuff below chest level, are done for 6 weeks. Progressive resisted exercises are begun after 12 weeks postoperative.

Evidence

Ceccarelli E, Bondi R, Alviti R, et al. Treatment of acute grade III acromioclavicular dislocation: a lack of evidence. J Orthopaed Traumatol. 2008;9:105-8.

The authors reviewed published literature on the treatment of acute grade III acromioclavicular dislocations and found that there was insufficient literature to perform a meta-analysis. Nevertheless, they found that the reported clinical results of nonoperative and operative treatment are similar and that there are more complications with surgical treatment. Consequently, they concluded that nonoperative treatment is a valid method. (Level III evidence)

Deshmukh A, Wilson D, Zilberfarb J, Perlmutter G. Stability of acromioclavicular joint reconstruction. Am J Sports Med. 2004;32:1492.

The authors did biomechanical testing to compare acromioclavicular joint laxity of six different techniques of acromioclavicular reconstruction fixation. Testing was performed in intact cadaveric shoulders and after simulated type III acromioclavicular joint injury and reconstruction. The Weaver-Dunn reconstruction had the least stability with the greatest anterior-posterior and inferior-superior translation and had failed at the lowest load. None restored acromioclavicular stability to normal. Augmentation techniques were mostly similar but did not restore acromioclavicular stability to normal. They did not evaluate the effect of augmentation on Weaver-Dunn reconstruction.

Dimakopoulos P, Panagopoulos A, Syggelos S, et al. Double-loop suture repair for acute acromioclavicular joint disruption. Am J Sports Med. 2006;34:1112-9.

The authors reported the results of a double-loop suture technique for repair of acute grade III and V acromioclavicular dislocation. Of 38 patients, 34 were available for follow-up at a mean of 33.2 months (range, 18–59 months). The complications were minimal. There were two cases with slight loss of reduction (less than half of the width of the clavicle). The mean Constant-Murley score was 93.5 points (range, 73–100 points). (Level IV evidence)

LaPrade R, Wickum D, Griffith D, Ludewig P. Kinematic evaluation of the modified Weaver-Dunn acromioclavicular joint reconstruction. Am J Sports Med. 2008;36:2216-21.

In this study, the authors used electromagnetic tracking to determine acromioclavicular joint motion of intact cadaver specimens, after grade III acromioclavicular dislocations, and after a modified Weaver-Dunn reconstruction. The reconstruction restored near-normal values for acromioclavicular long-axis rotation and excursion of the acromioclavicular joint. Weaver-Dunn reconstruction resulted in slight anterior and inferior displacement of the clavicle.

Lee SJ, Keefer EP, McHugh HP, et al. Cyclical loading of coracoclavicular ligament reconstructions. Am J Sports Med. 2008;36:1990.

The authors used five cadaver specimens to compare acromioclavicular reconstruction with unaugmented Weaver-Dunn reconstructions, suture-augmented (one #5 Ethibond) Weaver-Dunn reconstructions, and semitendinosus graft augmentation. Cyclical loading was performed at low and high load. All of the unaugmented Weaver-Dunn reconstructions failed with low loading. None of the augmented Weaver-Dunn reconstructions failed at low load while all failed under high load. The semitendinosus graft reconstructions did not fail under the low- or high-load conditions.

Nicholas SJ, Lee SJ, Mullaney MJ, et al. Clinical outcomes of coracoclavicular ligament reconstructions using tendon grafts. Am J Sports Med. 2007;35:1912-7.

The authors reported the results of nine patients with grade V acromioclavicular dislocation who were treated with semitendinosus allograft reconstruction. There were no cases of loss of reduction. The tendon graft and a 5-mm Mersilene tape (Ethicon, Somerville, NJ) were passed under the coracoid and through a single drill hole in the clavicle. The tendon was tied into a double surgeon's knot that was augmented with side-to-side sutures. The outcomes were rated highly on the American Shoulder and Elbow Surgeons, Simple Shoulder Test, and Pennsylvania Shoulder scales, and there were no cases of loss of reduction. (Level IV evidence)

Tauber M, Gordon K, Koller H, et al. Semitendinosus tendon graft versus a modified Weaver-Dunn procedure for acromioclavicular joint reconstruction in chronic cases. Am J Sports Med. 2009;37:181-90.

In this study, the authors compared the outcomes of two consecutive cohorts of 12 patients who had surgical treatment of chronic grades III–V acromioclavicular dislocations with either an augmented Weaver-Dunn reconstruction or an augmented autogenous semitendinosus graft reconstruction. The outcomes as determined with American Shoulder and Elbow Surgeons and Constant scores were better for the semitendinosus reconstruction group. The authors found that there was a significant correlation between the clinical scores and the amount of the displacement under stress loading ($p < .05$). The coracoclavicular distance was significantly less in the semitendinosus group ($p = .027$). (Level III evidence)

PROCEDURE 26

Sternoclavicular Joint Reconstruction Using Semitendinosus Graft

Alfred A. Mansour III and John E. Kuhn

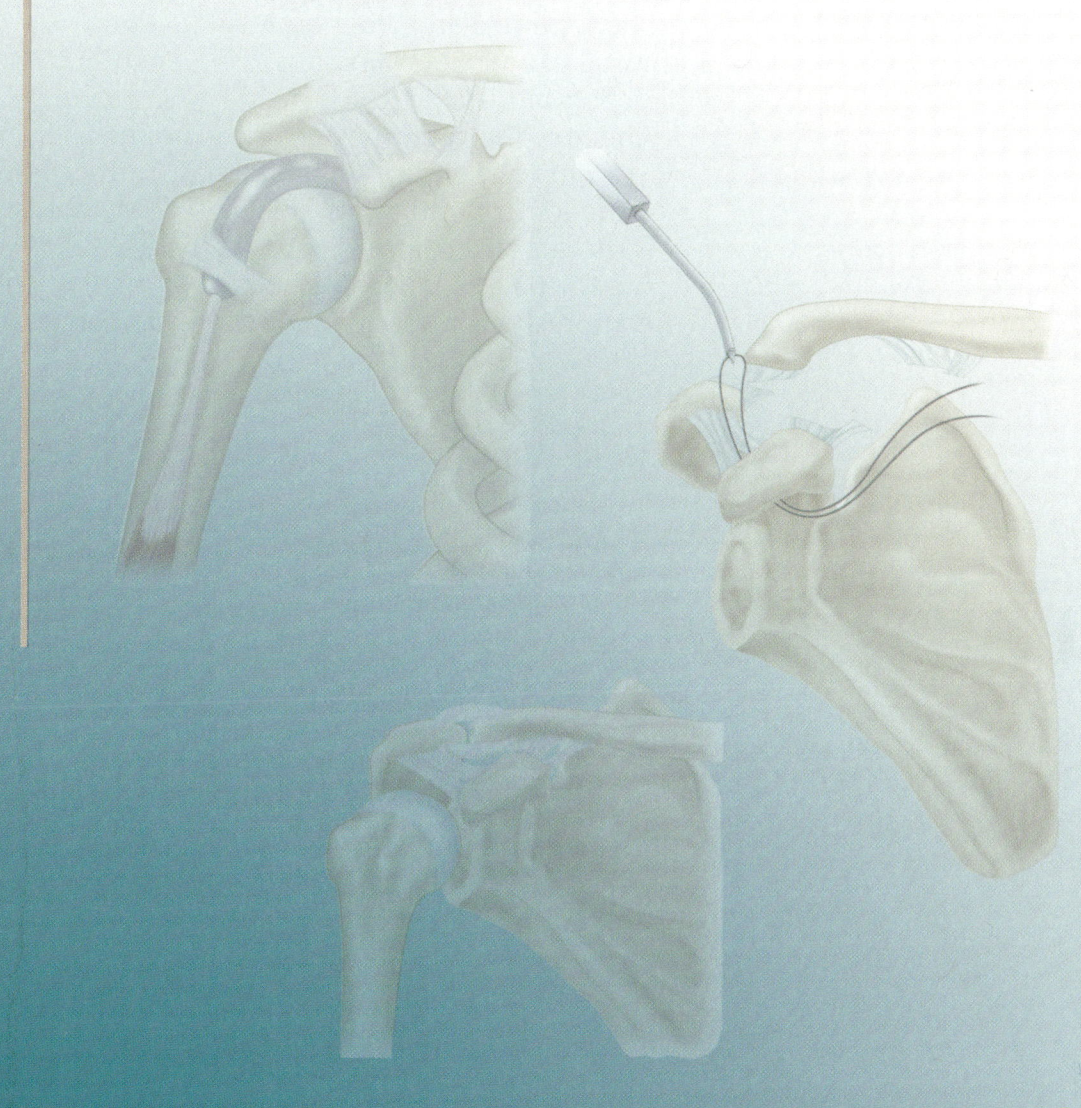

Pitfalls

- *Atraumatic voluntary sternoclavicular joint instability may be a contraindication for surgery.*
- *Patients with connective tissue disorders such as Ehlers-Danlos or Marfan syndrome may fail soft tissue reconstructions.*
- *Patients with fixed, displaced chronic anteriorly dislocated sternoclavicular joints may have minimal symptoms, and surgery is usually not necessary.*

Controversies

- Some patients with recurrent traumatic voluntary subluxations may benefit from surgery if nonoperative treatment fails and symptoms are disabling.

Indications

- Acute irreducible posterior dislocations
- Chronic posterior dislocations
- Symptomatic and functionally limiting irreducible anterior dislocations refractory to activity modification, physical therapy, and nonoperative treatment

Examination/Imaging

- Physical examination is characterized by pain over the sternoclavicular joint exacerbated with arm motion, particularly cross-body adduction.
- Physical examination findings also depend on the direction of instability.
  - Anterior dislocation/instability—The medial clavicle is prominent and palpable anterior to the sternum.
  - Posterior dislocation/instability—The sternal border is more easily palpable, and the typically present medial clavicle is recessed. Signs of mediastinal compression of vascular and/or respiratory

Treatment Options

- Acute Anterior Dislocations
  - Closed reduction under anesthesia can be performed, followed by sling immobilization for 6 weeks and then physical therapy, with return to activites after 12 weeks.
  - If closed reduction fails, leave the clavicle in a dislocated position and immobilize the arm in a sling for 6 weeks, follow with physical therapy and return to activities after 12 weeks.
  - Nonsurgical treatments include rest, a figure-of-8 brace or sling, and activity modification. Closed reduction is usually followed by bracing for 6 weeks.
- Acute Posterior Dislocations
  - Closed reduction under anesthesia can be performed with thoracic surgery available (the dislocated clavicle may be obscuring a mediastinal vessel injury). Successful reductions are held with a figure-of-8 brace for 6 weeks, followed by physical therapy for 6 weeks.
  - Failed closed reductions should undergo open reduction and either ligament repair or reconstruction.
- Chronic Posterior Dislocations
  - Open reduction and reconstruction is recommended as late complications may develop affecting mediastinal structures.
- Other techniques for sternoclavicular joint reconstruction have been described and include:
  - Burrows technique (subclavius tenodesis)
  - Rockwood technique (medial clavicle resection with costoclavicular ligament reconstruction)

structures may also be present, including venous congestion of the face or arm, trouble breathing, and dysphagia.

- Plain radiographs are of marginal value.
  - The "serendipity view" is a 40° cephalad tilt on an anteroposterior (AP) projection centered at the sternal notch. The clavicle will appear displaced superiorly to an imaginary horizontal line when compared with the normal clavicle for anterior dislocations and appear inferiorly to an imaginary horizontal plane when compared with the normal clavicle for posterior dislocations (Fig. 1).
- The most reliable imaging modality is computed tomography (CT). It has a higher sensitivity for detecting subtle subluxations of the sternoclavicular joint compared to plain radiographs (Fig. 2). CT is also useful for distinguishing medial clavicle fractures from joint injuries.

Surgical Anatomy

- Ligaments about the sternoclavicular joint (Fig. 3)
  - Costoclavicular ligament—originates on the anteromedial aspect of the first rib and inserts on the inferior surface of the medial clavicle, next to the articular margin of the clavicle head. It provides stability to the joint during elevation and rotation.
  - Interclavicular ligament—connects the superomedial region of the clavicle with the capsular ligaments and superior aspect of the

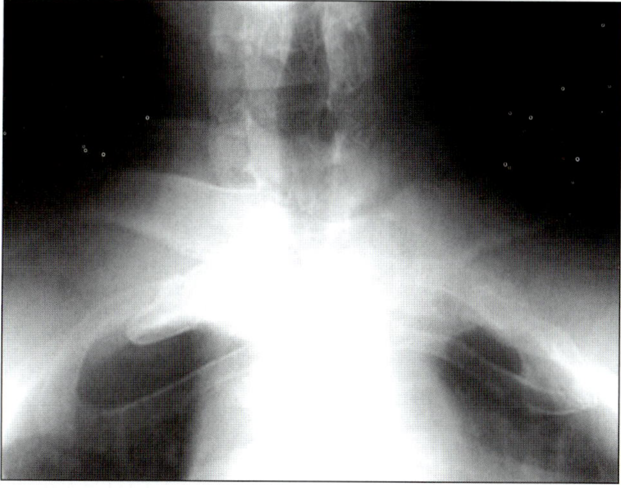

FIGURE 1

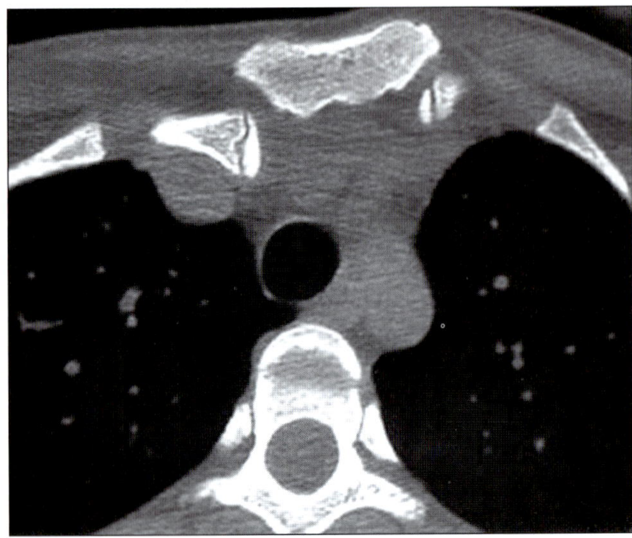

FIGURE 2

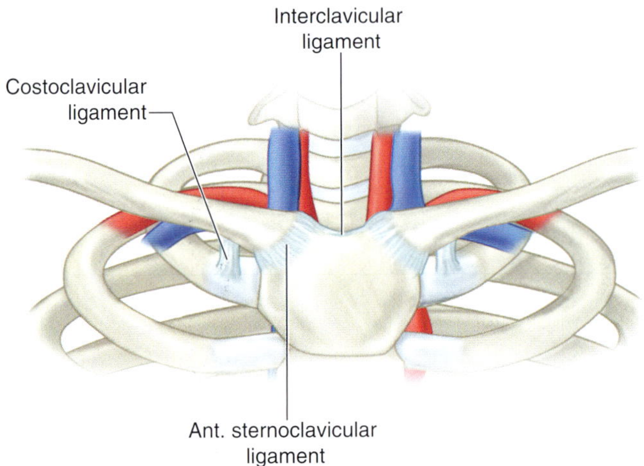

FIGURE 3

sternum. It functions in resisting inferior displacement of the medial clavicle.

- Capsular ligament—also referred to as the anterior and posterior sternoclavicular ligaments, which represent thickenings of the joint capsule. It functions in resisting upward rotation of the medial clavicle combined with downward rotation of the distal clavicle. The posterior capsule restrains anterior and posterior translation, and the anterior capsule restrains anterior translation.

- Retrosternal structures at risk include the great vessels, specifically the brachiocephalic artery and vein lying immediately posterior to the sternoclavicular joint (Fig. 4). These are at high risk for damage during reconstruction if care is not taken.

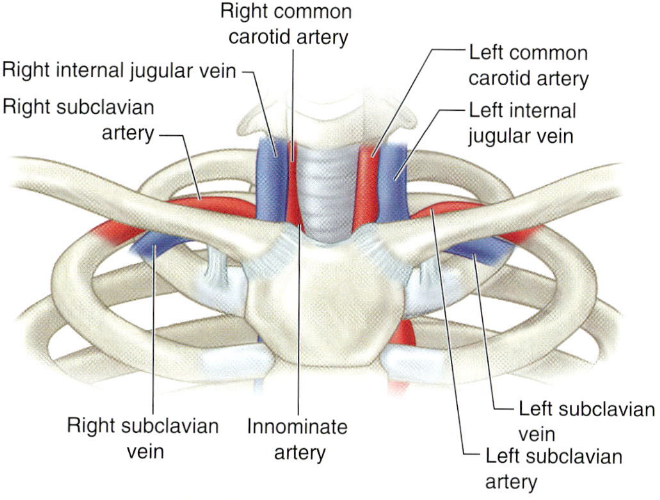

FIGURE 4

PEARLS

- *Wide exposure is necessary should bleeding of substernal structures occur and access to the neck or thoracic cavity is required.*
- *The arm and shoulder are prepped to allow for motion of the arm to help with reduction.*
- *For posterior instability, a small rolled towel may be applied behind the spine between the scapulae. This would not be used for anterior instability.*

Positioning

- The patient is positioned supine. The affected arm and the entire chest and neck are included in the prepped area (Fig. 5).
- The ipsilateral leg should also be prepped and draped for the semitendinosus harvest. A tourniquet is not used as this may hinder procurement of the graft.

Portals/Exposures

- A curvilinear incision is made following Langer's lines over the sternoclavicular joint to the midline.
- Skin and subcutaneous tissues are elevated as full-thickness skin flaps.

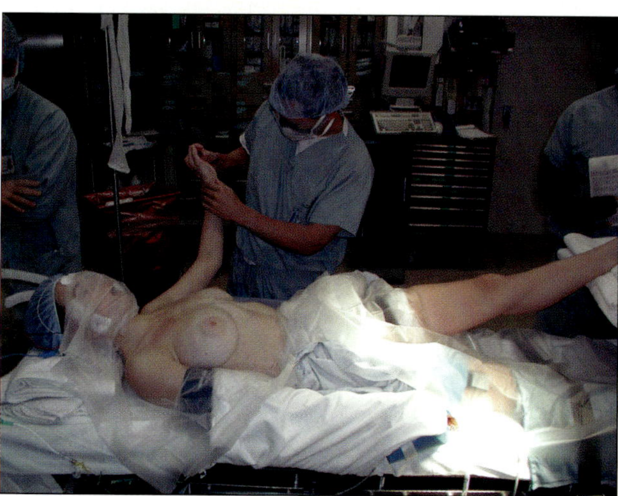

FIGURE 5

Pearls

- *Grasping the clavicle with a towel clip or bony tenaculum and pulling anteriorly while an assistant applies traction to the arm will assist in reducing posterior dislocations.*
- *The medial pectoralis may need to be stripped from the clavicle to allow mobility for reduction.*
- *The medial head of the clavicle is surprisingly deep in the AP plane.*
- *Rarely, the clavicle is not dislocated; rather, it is fractured. Look carefully at the CT scan to ascertain if the posterior cortex of the medial clavicle remains in an anatomic position.*

Pitfalls

- *The heads of the sternocleidomastoid muscle must not be detached from the clavicle or sternum, or, if they are disturbed, they must be repaired.*
- *Disruption of the posterior capsule when removing scar tissue from the joint may place the great vessels at risk of injury.*

Controversies

- Medial clavicle resection may be considered for difficult reductions; however, the loss of inherent bony stability will cause additional stress on the reconstruction and may lead to failure.

- The platysma is incised along the skin incision and dissected as separate cranial and caudal flaps.
- The heads of the sternocleidomastoid muscle and the sternal notch are identified.
- The joint capsule is incised parallel to the clavicle and carefully elevated from the manubrium and clavicle (Fig. 6A and 6B).

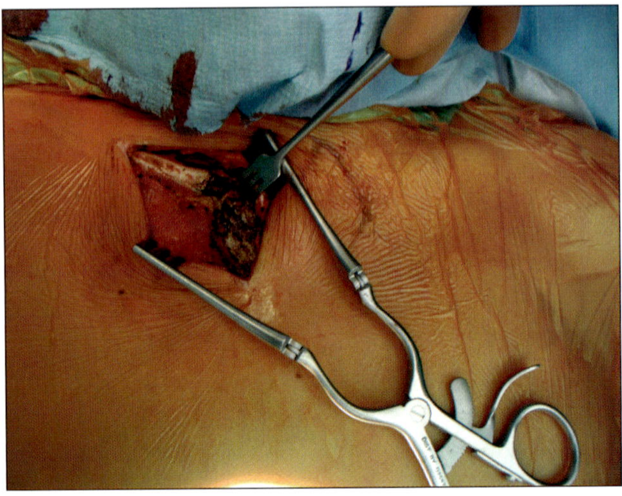

A

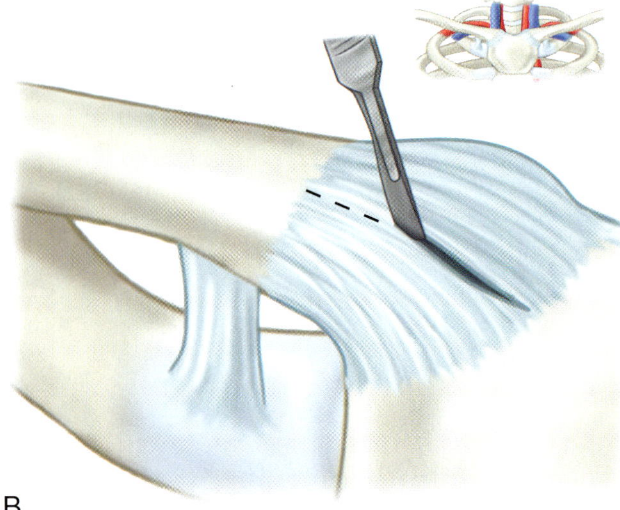

B

FIGURE 6

Pearls

- *When the tendon is identified and the adherent bands are removed, tugging on the graft should produce a springlike feel.*
- *Tensioning the graft with an ACL graft tensioning device will decrease stretching of the graft after implantation.*

Pitfalls

- *Not releasing the fascial slips adequately will hinder graft procurement and may lead to premature laceration of the graft, resulting in insufficient length.*

Instrumentation/Implantation

- Open-ended or closed tendon stripper of adequate diameter must be available to obtain the graft.

Controversies

- Allograft semitendinosus tendon graft may be used; however, no studies have directly compared allograft versus autograft.

- Scar tissue in the original joint space is removed carefully while protecting the capsule and ligaments.

Procedure

Step 1: Harvest of the Semitendinosus Autograft

- Semitendinosus graft harvesting may be performed at any time during the procedure, but harvesting at the beginning of the procedure allows tensioning of the graft to occur during the rest of the procedure and can be performed by an assistant simultaneously with the primary procedure.
- A 3- to 4-cm vertical incision is made approximately 5 cm distal to the medial knee joint line on the anteromedial crest overlying the pes anserinus. The sartorius fascia is exposed. The surgeon should palpate the gracilis tendon and split the sartorius fascia along the inferior border of the gracilis tendon in line with the tendon.
- The semitendinosus is located deep and inferior to the gracilis, and any fascial slips present are released. There may be numerous fascial slips to the medial gastrocnemius or sartorius fascia that, unless released, will make harvest difficult.
- The tendon is stripped using an open-ended tendon stripper, similar to that used for anterior cruciate ligament (ACL) reconstruction. The graft can then be released distally from the tibia for preparation.
- The muscle is removed from the proximal portion of the tendon with curved Mayo scissors or a periosteal elevator. Each end of the tendon graft is prepared by placing #2 nonabsorbable suture in a locking suture pattern with the suture ends left free (Fig. 7).

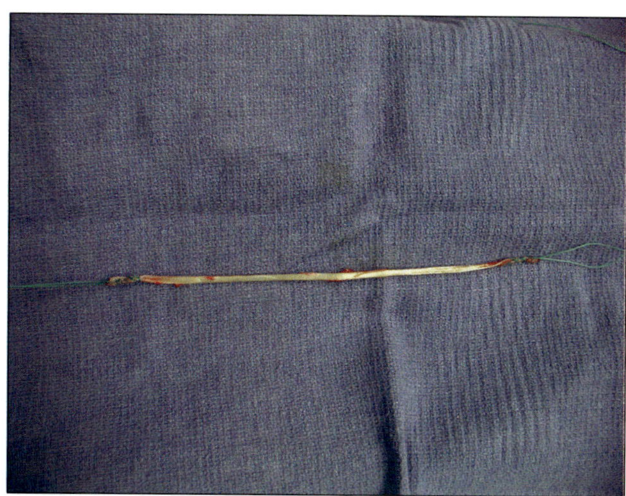

FIGURE 7

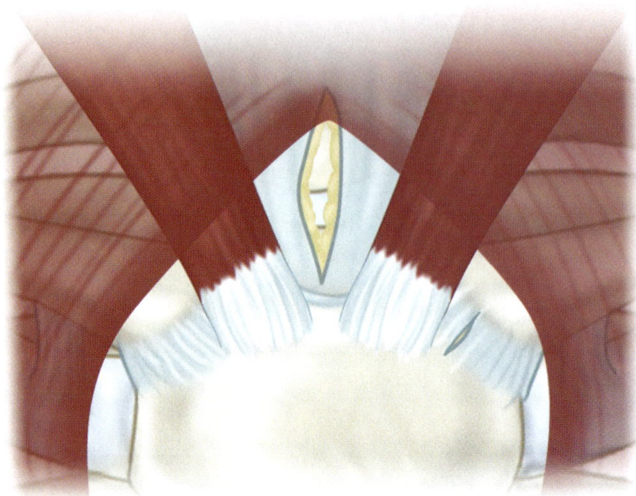

FIGURE 8

- The pes anserinus fascia is repaired and the wound closed in layers.

Step 2: Retrosternal Exposure with Protection of the Great Vessels

- This step is usually performed by a thoracic surgeon.
- A 3- to 4-cm vertical incision is made in the platysma above the sternal notch (Fig. 8). (This approach is often used for mediastinoscopy.)
- The retrosternal tissue is bluntly dissected from the undersurface of the sternum and medial clavicle, utilizing the finger in a sweeping motion, until the posterior surfaces are free of soft tissue.
- A malleable ribbon retractor is then placed behind the sternoclavicular joint, immediately behind the posterior manubrium, to protect the mediastinal structures and vessels during tunnel preparation (Fig. 9).

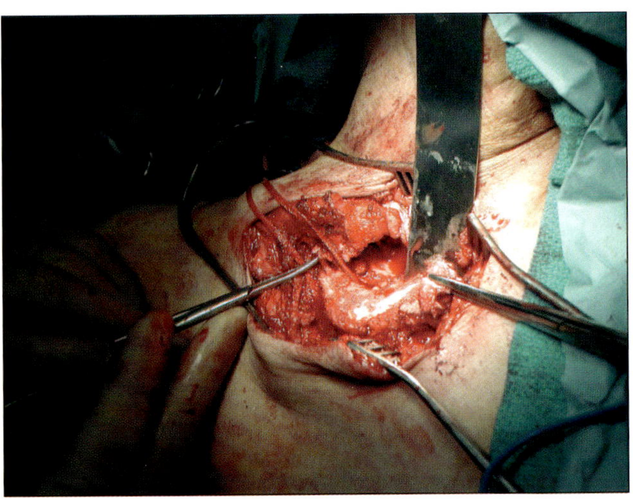

FIGURE 9

Pearls

- *Many orthopedic surgeons are unfamiliar with the substernal anatomy critical to this case. Having a thoracic surgeon immediately available and even assisting during the case is essential.*

Pitfalls

- *Sharp dissection deep to the sternum places the brachiocephalic vessels at great risk and should be avoided.*
- *Soft tissue from the back of the sternum and medial clavicle must be removed to allow tunnel creation.*

Instrumentation/ Implantation

- A malleable ribbon retractor or similar retractor should be used to protect the substernal structures.

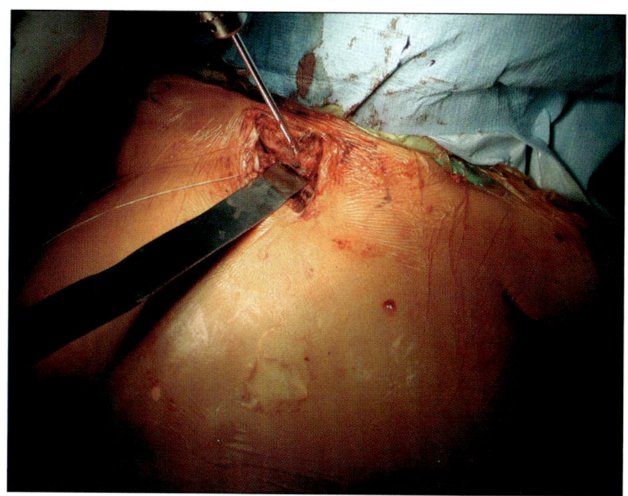

A

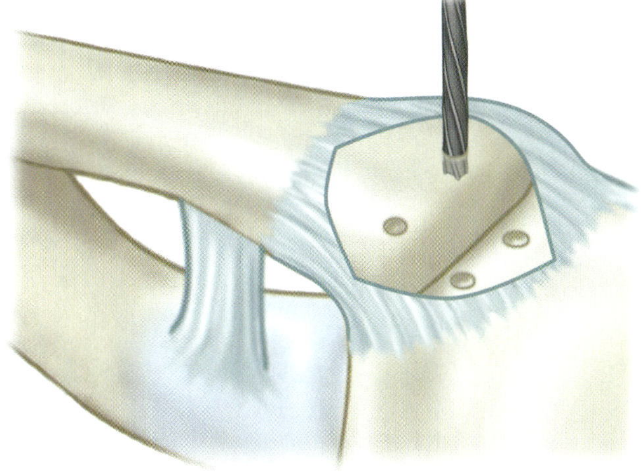

B

FIGURE 10

Step 3: Creation of Medial Clavicle and Sternal Tunnels

- A $^{1}/_{4}$-inch drill is used to create two parallel holes behind the subchondral plate of the articular surface of the clavicle (Fig. 10A).
- Two holes are also placed through the manubrium (Fig. 10B).
- Alternatively, the drill may be advanced partially through the posterior cortex and a curette can be inserted to gently complete the drill hole.

Instrumentation/ Implantation

- A $^{1}/_{4}$-inch drill bit and battery-powered drill are necessary for the creation of the tunnels.
- A small straight curette is also required for completion of or for enlarging the tunnels so the graft will be passed easily.

Pearls

- *Determining the position of the drill holes is done with the clavicle reduced. The drill holes should be placed as parallel as possible to prevent rotation of the clavicle when the graft is secured.*
- *When drilling through the back of the manubrium, a finger may be placed behind the sternum to prevent plunging. When it feels like the drill is close, the posterior hole may be finished with a curette.*
- *The ribbon retractor must be placed to prevent the drill from going deep into the mediastinum.*

Pitfalls

- *Advance the drill slowly to avoid plunging into the mediastinum.*
- *Protect the substernal vessels with a finger or ribbon retractor.*

Pearls

- *If the graft is large and difficult to pass through a tunnel, the tunnel may be widened using a curette.*
- *Repair the capule of the joint (poserior and/or anterior) before securing the graft to itself.*
- *Extra graft material can be brought back on itself and secured to other limbs of the graft.*

Pitfalls

- *Avoid overtightening the graft because it could lead to limited joint motion and clavicle malrotational, potentially leading to static scapular winging.*

Instrumentation/ Implantation

A Hewson-type suture passer will facilitate passing of the sutures used to pass the graft.

Step 4: Graft Passage

- Passing the graft
  - A Hewson-type suture passer or a handmade smooth wire loop is inserted from superficial to deep into one of the holes.
  - The end is identified deep to the sternoclavicular joint and pulled through the incision above the scapular notch.
  - A loop of #2 nonabsorbable suture is then passed through the hole in order to pass the tendon graft.
  - This step is repeated for the remaining three holes, creating a separate suture loop for each drill hole (Fig. 11A and 11B).
  - The end of the graft is passed through each drill hole by using the suture loops previously placed.
  - The free ends of the suture attached to the graft are captured by the suture loops and used to pass the graft through the tunnels (Fig. 12A and 12B).
- The graft is passed through the drill holes, forming parallel bands on one side and figure-of-8 crossed bands on the other side (Fig. 13). A more stable construct is expected if the graft is passed so that the parallel limbs are on the side of the instability.
- Graft passage for anterior instability
  - The first graft pass is from superficial to deep through the inferior hole in the manubrium.
  - The next pass is from deep to superficial through the superior clavicular hole.
  - The third pass is from superficial to deep through the superior hole in the manubrium.

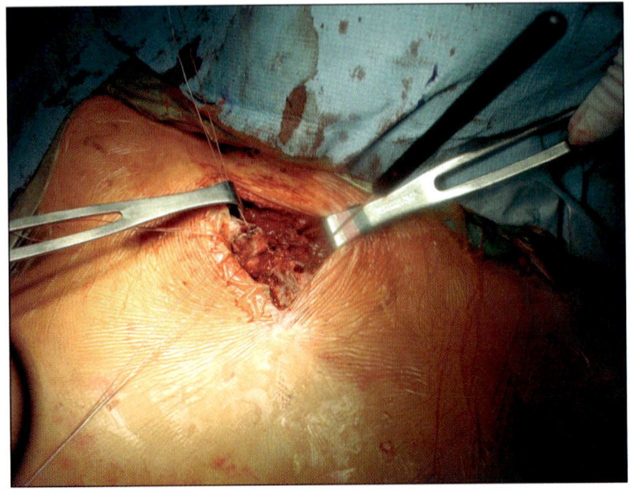

A

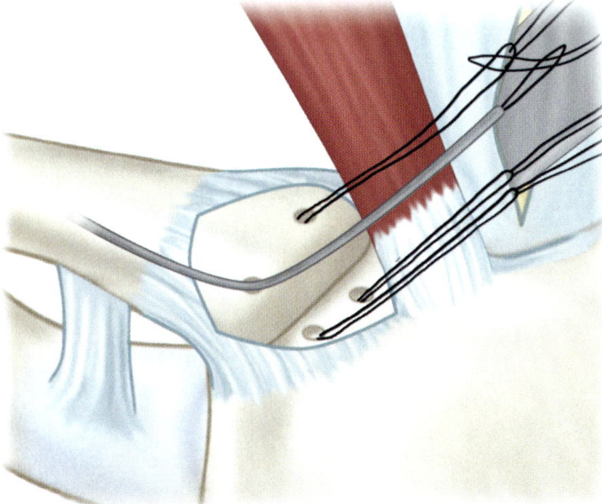

B

FIGURE 11

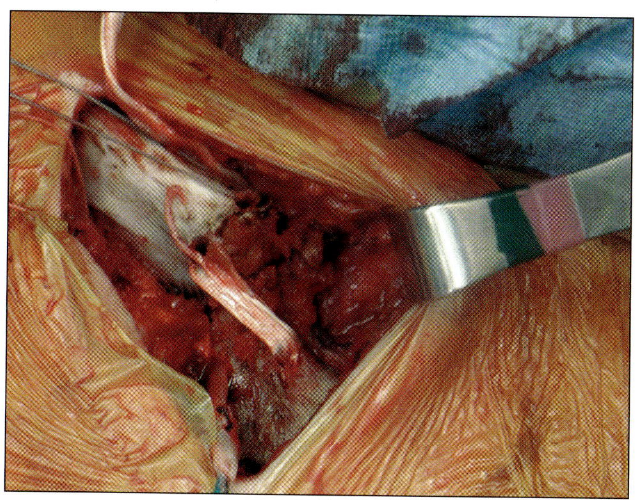

A

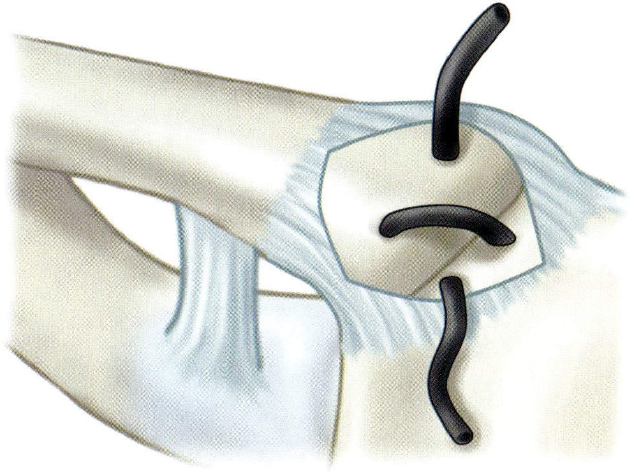

B

FIGURE 12

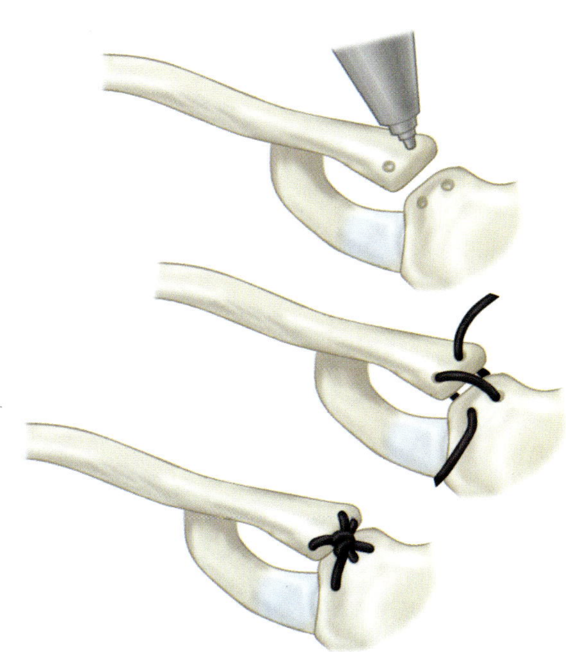

FIGURE 13

Controversies

- For severe instability, a second graft (e.g., palmaris longus) may be used as a loop around the first rib and clavicle. This dissection around the first rib is extremely risky as the internal mammary artery is at risk. A thoracic surgeon can assist in passing the graft around the first rib.

  - The final pass is from deep to superficial through the inferior clavicular hole.
  - The graft is tied to itself and sutured to itself with #2 nonabsorbable suture.
- Graft passage for posterior instability
  - The first graft pass is from superficial to deep through the inferior hole in the manubrium.
  - The next pass is from deep to superficial through the inferior clavicular hole.
  - The third pass is from superficial to deep through the superior hole in the manubrium.

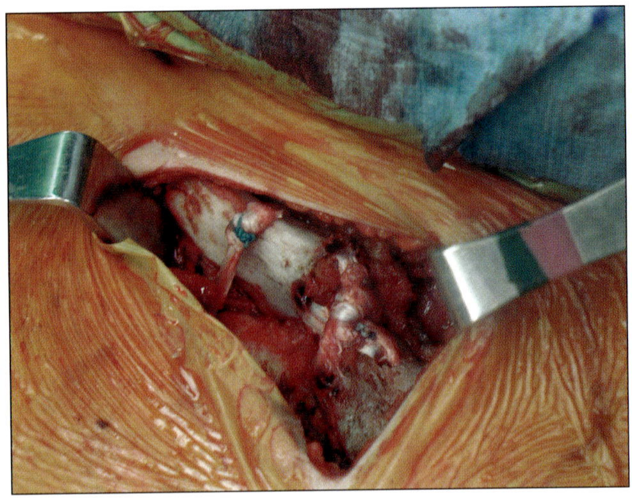

A

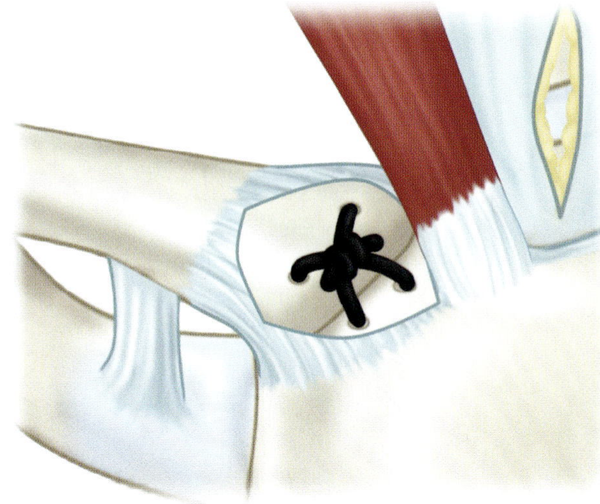

B

FIGURE 14

- The final pass is from deep to superficial through the superior clavicular hole.
- After the graft has been passed, the native anterior capsule (and if possible the posterior capsule) of the joint can be repaired with #2 nonabsorbable suture. Suture anchors will hold well in the medial clavicle adjacent to the edge of the cartilage surface. These can be used to augment the repaired capsule.
- The graft is tied and sutured to itself with #2 nonabsorbable suture (Fig. 14A and 14B).

Step 5: Wound Closure

- The wound is then copiously irrigated with normal saline.
- The sternal head of the sternocleidomastoid muscle must be anatomically repaired using suture anchors in the manubrium if it was detached during the exposure.
- The playsma is closed with 0 absorbable sutures over the reconstructed joint (Fig. 15A and 15B).
- The subcutaneous tissues and skin are then closed (Fig. 16).
- Posterior instability patients are placed in a figure-of-8 brace to keep the shoulders back. Anterior instability patients are placed in a standard arm sling.

Pearls

- *Meticulous closure of the capsule and reattachment of the sternocleidomastoid are the essential elements of closure.*

Instrumentation/ Implantation

- Small suture anchors will need to be available if repair of the sternocleidomastoid is to be performed.

Postoperative Care and Expected Outcomes

- The arm is immobilized (figure-of-8 brace for posterior instability and sling for anterior instability) for 4–6 weeks.

Pearls

- *Patients with generalized laxity may proceed more slowly in therapy.*

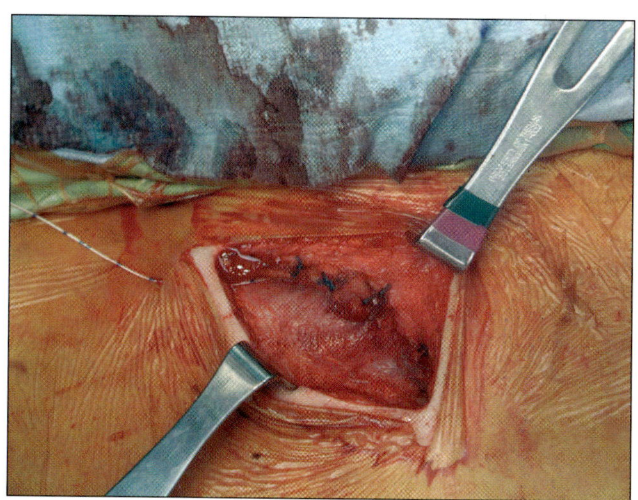
A

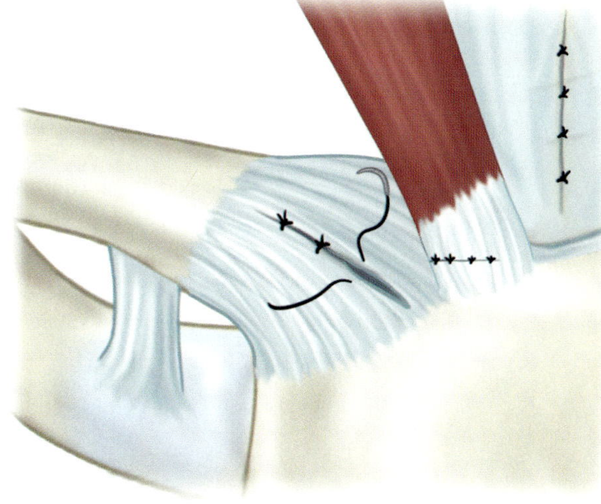
B

FIGURE 15

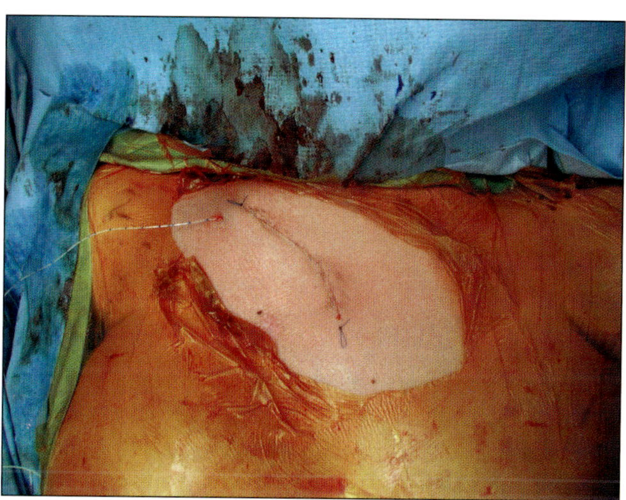

FIGURE 16

- At 6 weeks postoperatively, passive shoulder motion is initiated followed by active-assisted motion with the patient supine. Over the next 2–4 weeks, the patient's back is elevated for active assisted motion until 8–10 weeks after surgery, when exercises can be done upright.
- Active motion begins 8 weeks after surgery. Full motion is expected between 8 and 12 weeks.
- Strengthing of the shoulder should begin at week 12.
- Most patients have stable sternoclavicular joints and are satisfied with the outcome.
- Some patients exhibit complications, including infection, loss of reduction, and fracture through the drill holes.

Evidence

This is an uncommon injury. As such, we likely will never see randomized trials comparing different treatment strategies, and clinical decision making will be based on relatively low-level evidence.

Bae DS, Kocher MS, Waters PM, Micheli LM, Griffey M, Dichtel L. Chronic recurrent anterior sternoclavicular joint instability: results of surgical management. J Pediatr Orthop. 2006;26:71-4.

In this retrospective case series, patients with operatively treated chronic sternoclavicular joint instability treated with reconstruction were followed an average of 55 months. Functional outcome was assessed. (Level IV evidence)

Castropil W, Ramadan LB, Bitar AC, Schor B, de Oliveira D'Elia C. Sternoclavicular dislocation—reconstruction with semitendinosus tendon autograft: a case report. Knee Surg Sports Traumatol Arthrosc. 2008;16:865-8.

The authors presented a case report of semitendinosus autograft figure-of-8 reconstruction used for chronic traumatic sternoclavicular dislocation in a young athlete, with results of 1-year follow-up. (Level IV evidence)

Spencer EE, Kuhn JE. Biomechanical analysis of reconstructions for sternoclavicular joint instability. J Bone Joint Surg [Am]. 2004;86:98-108.

Biomechanical analysis using a cadaveric model compared three different sternoclavicular reconstruction techniques: intramedullary ligament reconstruction, subclavius tendon reconstruction, and semitendinosus figure-of-8 graft. Stiffness and peak load to failure were evaluated.

SECTION I

SHOULDER

Trauma

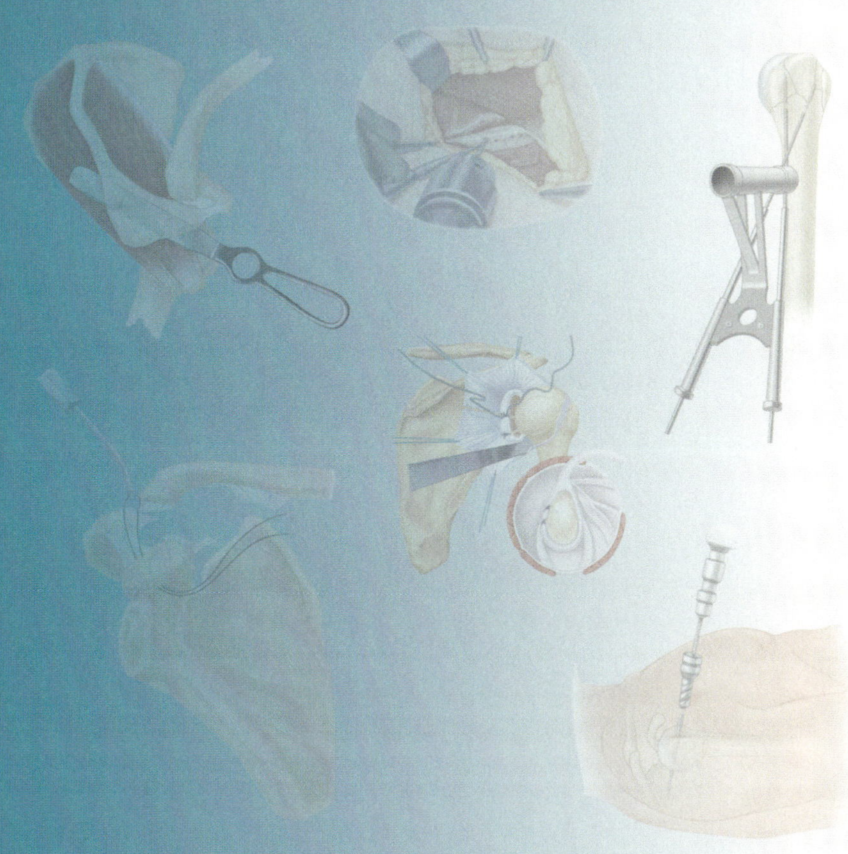

PROCEDURE 27

Open Reduction and Internal Fixation of Acute Midshaft Clavicular Fractures

Nata Parnes and Jesse B. Jupiter

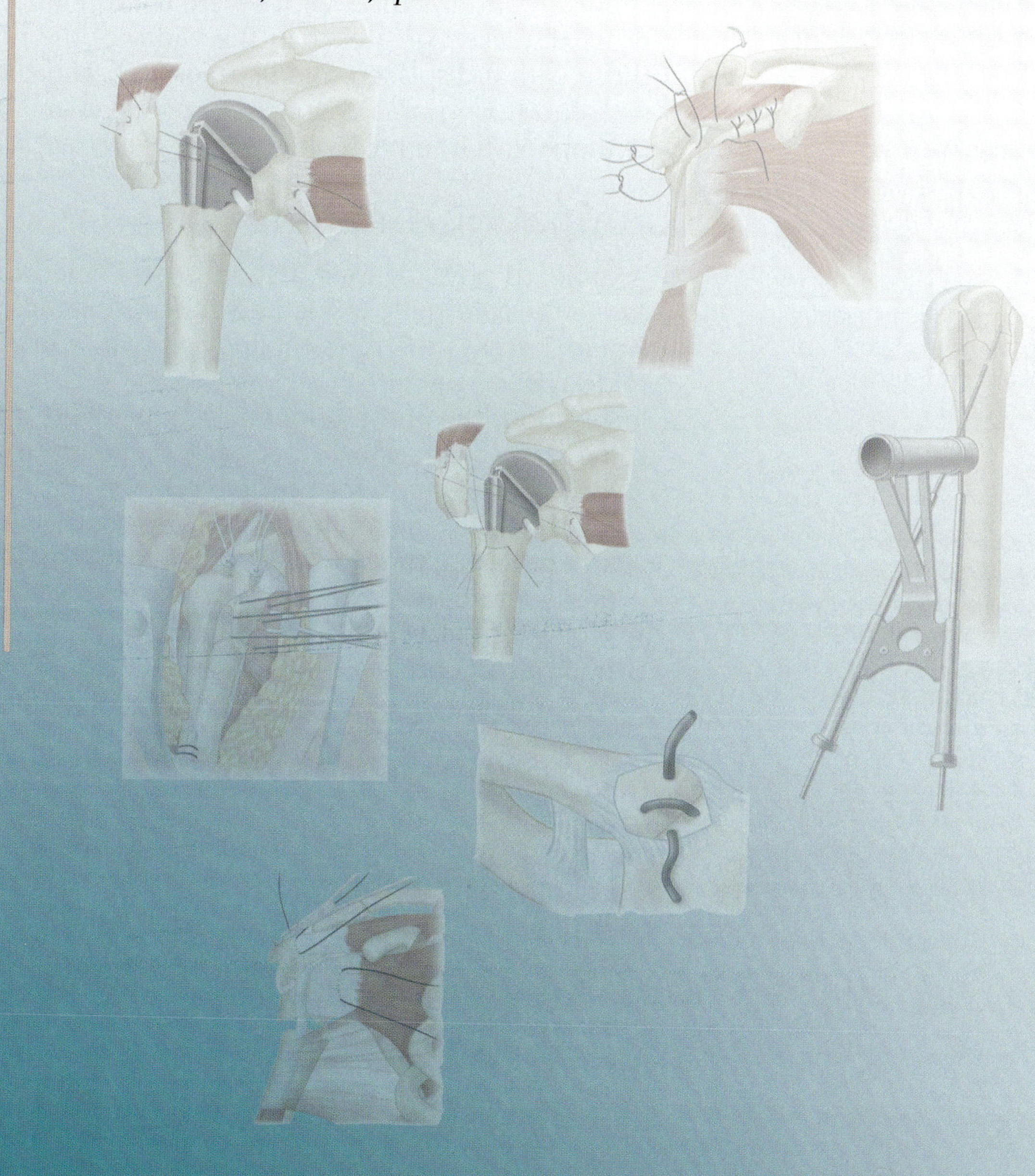

Pitfalls

- *Patients and surgeons should be aware of the following: In most patients who are treated nonoperatively, the fracture will heal and they will have good function (Nordqvist et al., 1998). Operative treatment carries some risks, and nonunion (Jupiter and Leffert, 1987) and malunion (Chan et al., 1999) can be salvaged with secondary procedures, if necessary.*

Controversies

- The need for operative treatment of floating shoulder injury has been questioned recently, but should be considered for patients who place substantial demands on the shoulders (van Noort et al., 2001).

Treatment Options

- Nonoperative treatment: Usually, a sling or figure-of-8 brace is applied in the acute setting. With either device, immobilization is, typically, for 2–6 weeks, based on the patient's level of comfort.
- Other techniques exist for fixation of clavicular fractures in addition to the plating procedure that is described here (intramedullary fixation).

Indications

- The primary goal is to restore shoulder function to the preinjury level.
- Indications for surgical treatment include open fractures, scapulothoracic dissociation, and fractures associated with skin compromise or with neurologic or vascular injury (Lange and Noel, 1993).
- Relative surgical indications include patients with multiple-system trauma in whom fixation of the clavicle will contribute to rehabilitation, a floating shoulder, and fractures with severe comminution, those displaced greater than the width of the bone, those with a displaced middle fragment, and those with shortening greater than 2 cm (Canadian Orthopaedic Trauma Society, 2007; Hill et al., 1997).

Examination/Imaging

- A standard physical examination is performed to assess for deformity, tenderness, and crepitation; Figure 1 shows the physical findings with a left midclavicular fracture.
- In addition, the entire upper extremity, chest, and spine are evaluated for concomitant injuries.
  - Include evaluation for possible rib fractures, pneumotorax, hemothorax, neurovascular injury, and other fractures or dislocation of the shoulder girdle and upper extremity.
  - When the fracture is accompanied by high-energy trauma, a complete body examination should be performed to avoid missing associated injuries.

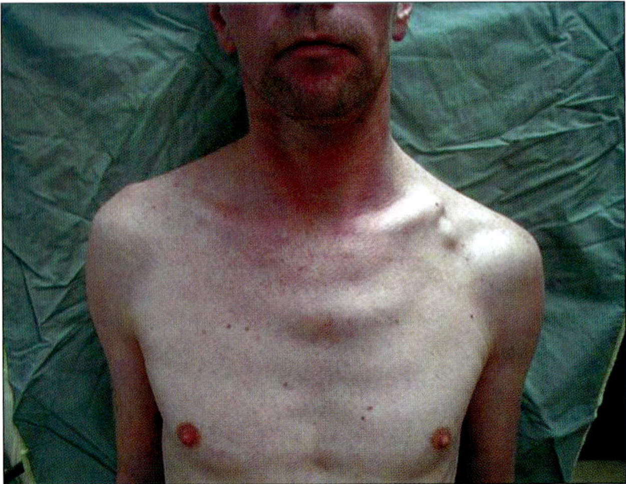

FIGURE 1

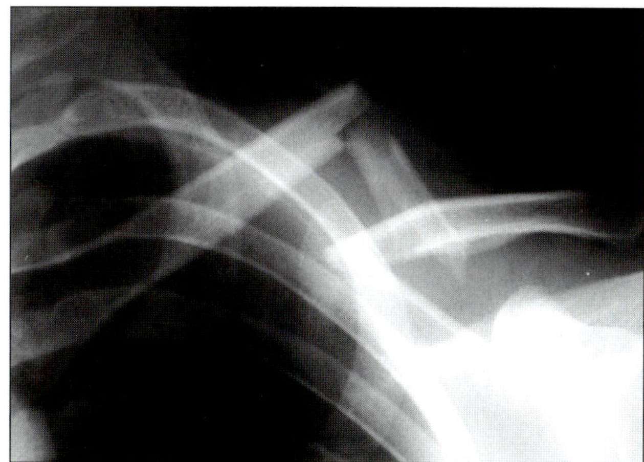

FIGURE 2

- Plain radiographs are obtained in anteroposterior and 45° cephalic tilt views.
  - Radiographic film should be large enough to evaluate the acromioclavicular and sternoclavicular joints and the remainder of the shoulder girdle and upper lung fields.
  - Radiographic evaluation assesses the fracture pattern, presence of comminution, displacement, and shortening or distraction of the fracture (Fig. 2). Overall displacement of fracture ends greater than 2 cm and displacement without bony contact, especially with a transversely displaced fragment, is strongly predictive of long-term sequelae (Hill et al., 1997).
  - An abduction lordotic view, in which the shoulder is abducted above 135° and the central ray angled 25° cephalad, is useful for clavicle evaluation after internal fixation.

PEARLS

- *The head and neck should be tilted away from the surgical site.*
- *A bump is placed behind the scapula to aid in the reduction.*

PITFALLS

- *Care must be taken during positioning and fracture manipulation to avoid stretching of the brachial plexus.*

Surgical Anatomy

- The clavicle is relatively subcutaneous, with only the supraclavicular nerves crossing the bone.
- The junction of the outer and middle thirds is the thinnest part of the bone (Fig. 3) and is the only area not protected by, or reinforced with, muscle and ligamentous attachments, thereby rendering it prone to fracture, particularly with axial loading (Huang et al., 2007).
- The muscles attachment to the clavicle creates the predictable deformity seen with fractures.
  - The proximal fragment is pulled superiorly and posteriorly by the sternocleidomastoid muscle.

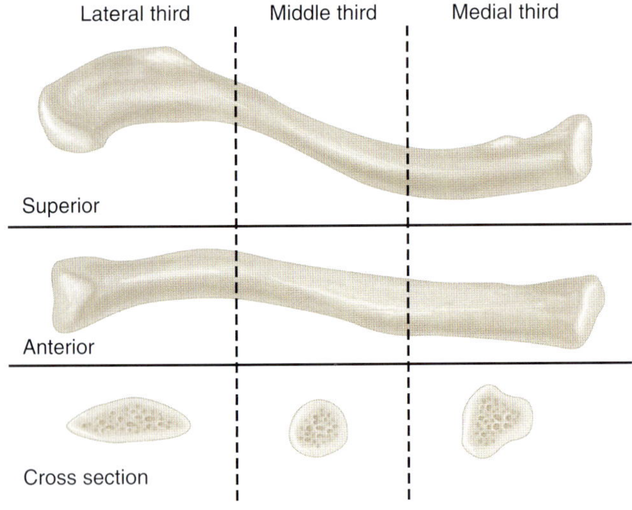

FIGURE 3

Equipment

- An arm-holding device, positioned on the ipsilateral side of the table, can help support the upper extremity and resist gravity during reduction and fixation of the fracture.

Pearls

- *Incision of the inferior skin after pulling it over the fracture site will prevent the wound from being in contact with the plate on the clavicle. This improves cosmesis and reduces wound complications.*

  - The distal segment sags forward and rotates inferiorly because of the weight of the upper extremity and the pull of the pectoralis muscle on the humerus.
- The clavicle is in intimate relation to the brachial plexus, subclavian artery and vein, and apex of the lung. These structures should be carefully protected during the surgical procedure.

Positioning

- The patient is placed in a supine, semi-sitting (beach chair) position. The arm should be prepped in the field to allow for traction and manipulation to assist in the reduction (Fig. 4).
- When there is a chance that bone graft will be needed, the iliac crest is prepped and draped.

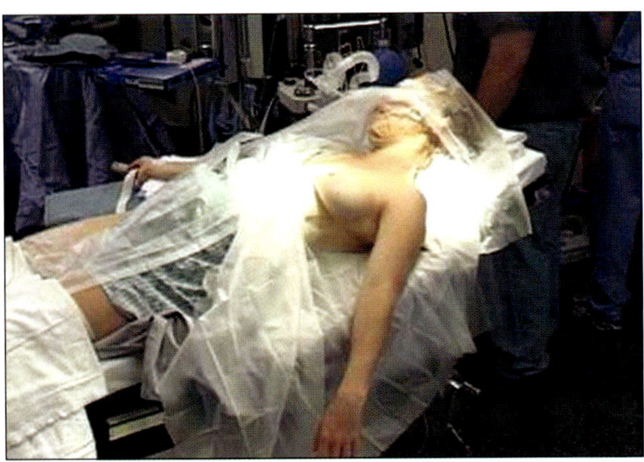

FIGURE 4

Controversies

- The skin incision can be made parallel or perpendicular to the clavicle's longitudinal axis. The perpendicular incision is claimed to produce a more aesthetic scar. The authors have used both perpendicular and parallel incisions and have found that the scars are not appreciably different in appearance.

Portals/Exposures

- A longitudinal incision is made in the skin, parallel and just inferior to the long axis of the clavicle (Fig. 5).
- The crossing supraclavicular nerves should be identified and protected (Fig. 6) to limit chest wall numbness and a potentially painful neuroma (Jupiter and Leibman, 2007).

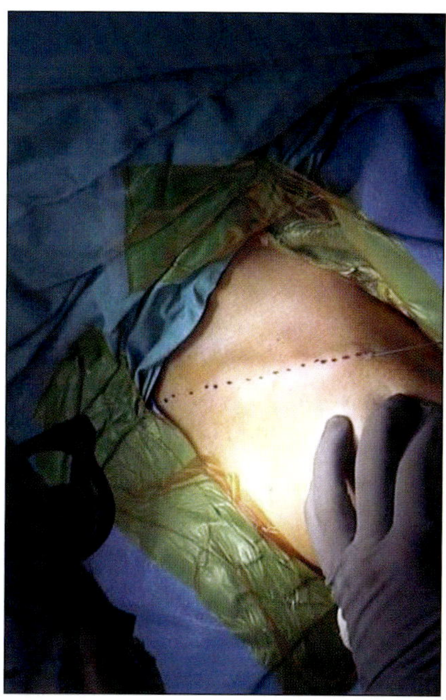

FIGURE 5

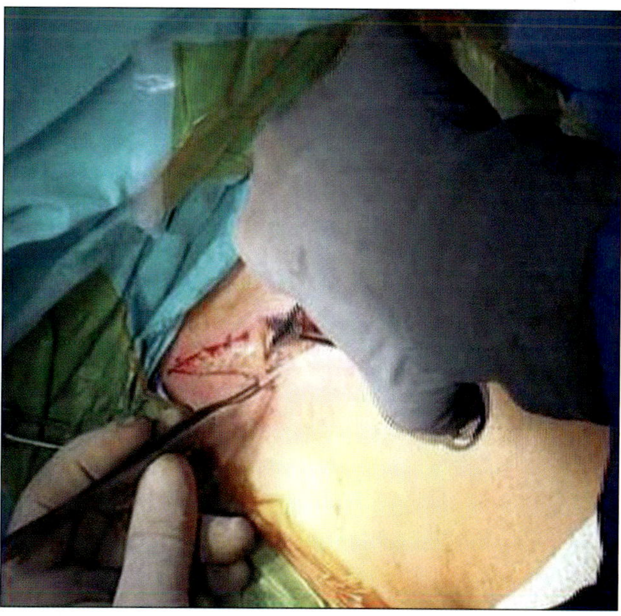

FIGURE 6

Pearls

- *The close proximity of the brachial plexus and the subclavian vessels make the use of oscillating drill bits recommendable.*
- *In complex multifragmentary fractures, the plate is best used as a bridge spanning the fragments, which is far more successful than dissecting each fragment.*
- *When the vascularity to the fragments has been preserved and there is no bone gap, no bone graft is needed.*

Pitfalls

- *Semitubular plates are not rigid enough and should not be used.*
- *Reconstruction plates are more easily contoured and have been used with success; however, they account for several failures to obtain union and would not be the authors' first choice.*
- *Locked plates are not necessary for the acute plating of nonosteoporotic clavicular fractures as there is no significant advantage in using them over conventional plating, and the cost is higher.*

Procedure

Step 1

- Minimal soft tissue dissection is recommended.
- The fracture site is exposed with minimal periostal and muscle attachment elevation to preserve the vascularity to the fragments (Fig. 7).

Step 2

- Reduction can be achieved by stripping the clavicle subperiosteally and manipulating the fragments with bone clamps. However, this compromises the vascularity of the clavicle.
- We prefer to use a temporary external fixator or small skeletal distractor to facilitate gradual restoration of alignment (Fig. 8).

Step 3

- For fixation, ideally, a 3.5-mm limited-contact dynamic compression plate (LCDC Plate, Synthes, Paoli, PA) or a plate of similar strength, with at least

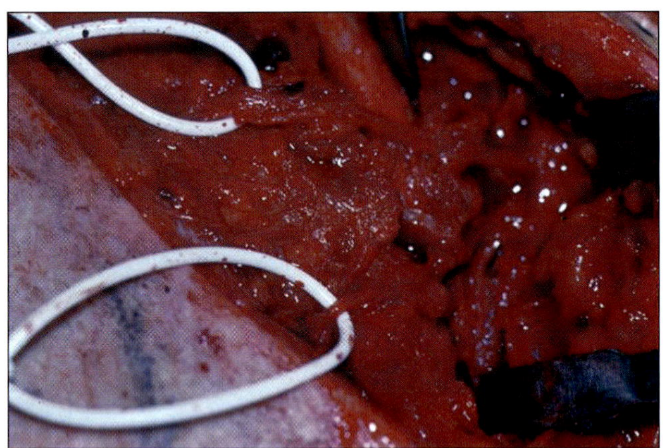

FIGURE 7

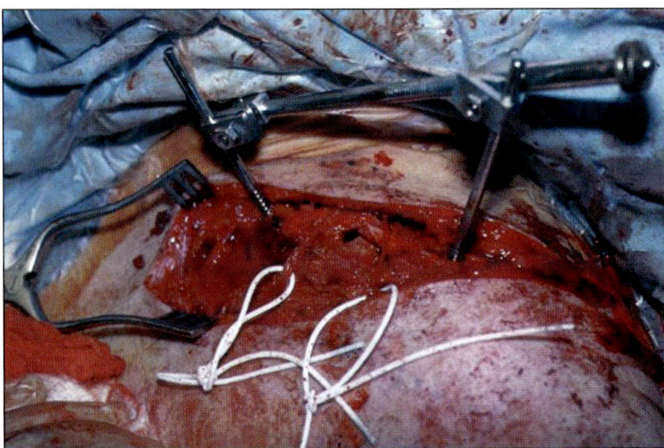

FIGURE 8

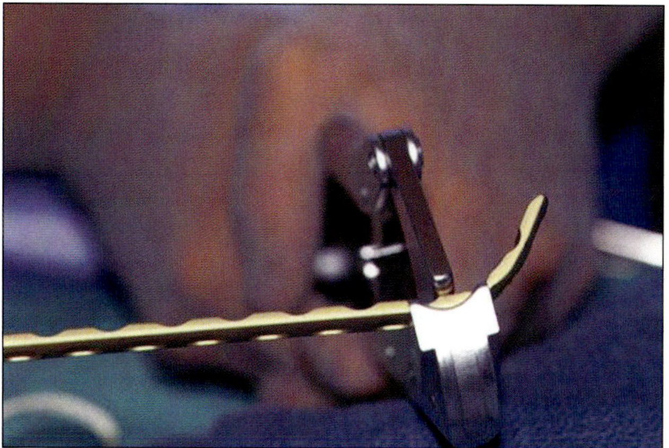

A

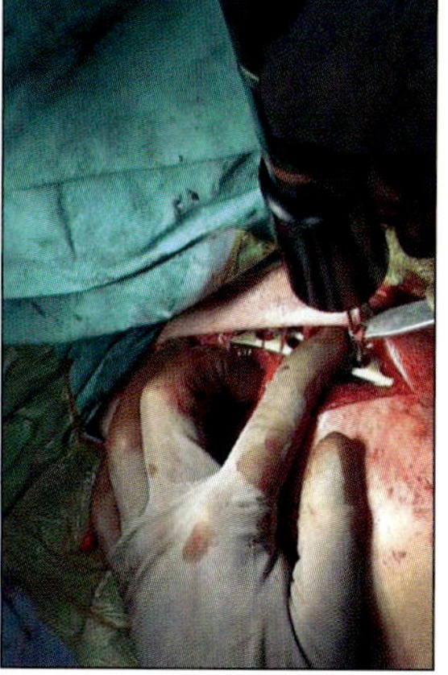

B

FIGURE 9

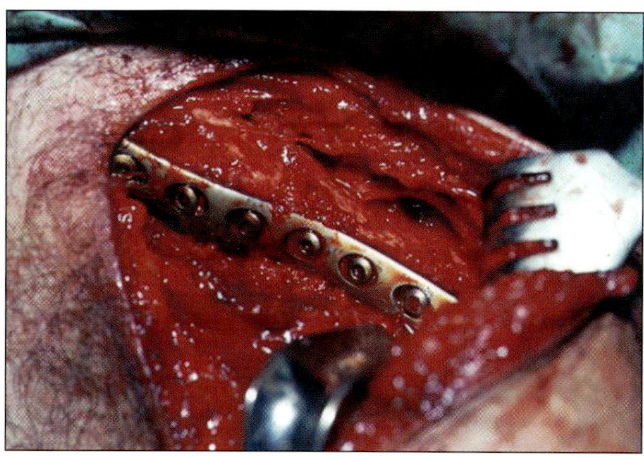

FIGURE 10

Controversies

- The plate can be placed on the anterosuperior or the anteroinferior side of the bone. An anteroinferior position, although less favorable biomechanically, allows for drilling in a direction that is away from the subclavian vessels and lung. It also keeps the plate from being placed under the incision. This position is, theoretically, less likely to cause irritation, thereby decreasing the need for plate removal. However, the anteroinferior position demands additional soft tissue stripping and a more difficult contouring of the plate compared to the anterosuperior position (Collinge et al., 2006).

six cortices on each side, should be used (Mullaji and Jupiter, 1994).

- The plate is contoured to match the clavicle anatomy (Fig. 9A).
- A minimum of three screws should be placed in each major fragment (Fig. 9B).
- Placement of interfragmentary screws (when the fracture pattern allows it) greatly enhances the stability of the construct.
- Figure 10 shows the final fixation of a clavicular fracture with an anteroinferior plate.

■ Anatomically shaped plates are recent developments and may prove useful. Flexible intramedullary nails are also effective for displaced transverse fractures.

Step 4

■ The wound is irrigated copiously and all bleeding should be controlled.

- The fascia is repaired over the plate, if possible, and the skin incision is closed. Suture closure is preferable to staples.

PEARLS

- *Clavicle rotation is relatively small until humeral elevation exceeds 90°; thus, early rehabilitation that avoids over-the-shoulder activity will significantly limit rotational forces at the site of a clavicular fracture.*

Postoperative Care and Expected Outcomes

- With a sufficiently stable construct, unrestricted shoulder motion is allowed, with the exception of overhead lifting during the first 6 weeks. Once healing is demonstrated, progressive strengthening exercises are permitted.
- A return to all occupational activities and recreational pursuits is usually possible by 4 months after operative treatment.
- In most cases plate removal is unnecessary. When the patient requests plate removal, we advise waiting at least 12 and preferably 18 months from the time of the injury and verifying reconstitution of the cortex under the plate.
- Most clavicular fractures heal without incident when length and alignment are maintained. Acceptable cosmetic and functional results should be expected. Satisfactory results occur less consistently when the fracture fails to heal or heals with a significant deformity.
- The complications that have been reported for this procedure are refracture, usually due to premature resumption of full activity or premature plate removal; nonunion; and malunion (Jupiter and Leffert, 1987; Chan et al., 1999).

Evidence

Canadian Orthopaedic Trauma Society. Nonoperative treatment compared with plate fixation of displaced midshaft clavicular fractures: a multicenter, randomized clinical trial. J Bone Joint Surg [Am]. 2007;89:1-10.

In this multicenter, prospective clinical trial, 132 patients with a displaced midshaft fracture of the clavicle were randomized to either operative treatment with plate fixation or nonoperative treatment with a sling. At follow-up of 1 year, better functional outcomes, lower rates of malunion and nonunion, and a shorter time to union were demonstrated in the operatively treated group. However, this group had higher complication and reoperation rates.

Chan KY, Jupiter JB, Leffert RD, Marti R. Clavicle malunion. J Shoulder Elbow Surg. 1999;8:287-90.

This study reported on four patients in whom a malunited fracture of the clavicle contributed to shoulder girdle dysfunction. In each patient, the functional status was improved after corrective osteotomy, realignment, and plate fixation.

Collinge C, Devinney S, Herscovici D, DiPasquale T, Sanders R. Anterior-inferior plate fixation of middle-third fractures and nonunions of the clavicle. J Orthop Trauma. 2006;20:680-6.

This consecutive clinical series studied 58 patients treated with an anterior-inferior 3.5-mm plate for middle-third clavicle fractures and nonunions. At a mean follow-up of 49 months (minimum follow-up was more than 24 months), a low complication rate was found.

Hill JM, McGuire MH, Crosby LA. Closed treatment of displaced middle third fractures of the clavicle gives poor results. J Bone Joint Surg Br. 1997;79:537-9.

This study evaluated 242 clavicular fractures in adults that had been treated conservatively. The study demonstrated that shortening at the fracture of greater than 20 mm has a highly significant association with nonunion and unsatisfactory result.

Huang JI, Toogood P, Chen MR, Wilber JH, Cooperman DR. Clavicular anatomy and the applicability of precontoured plates. J Bone Joint Surg [Am]. 2007;89:2260-5.

In this radiographic anatomic study, 100 pairs of clavicles were analyzed. The location and magnitude of the superior clavicular bow were determined with use of a digitizer and modeling software. With use of Adobe Photoshop technology, the precontoured Acumed Locking Clavicle Plate was freely translated and rotated along each clavicle to determine the quality of fit and the location of the "best fit."

Jupiter JB, Leffert RD. Non-union of the clavicle: associated complications and surgical management. J Bone Joint Surg [Am]. 1987;69:753-60.

This study described in detail the senior author's experience with clavicle nonunion treatment, and included results of surgical treatment in 23 patients with average follow-up of 2 years.

Jupiter JB, Leibman MI. Supraclavicular nerve entrapment due to clavicular fracture callus. J Shoulder Elbow Surg. 2007;16:e13-4.

This case report described the anatomy of the supraclavicular nerve and the reasons for its injury.

Lange RH, Noel SH. Traumatic lateral scapular displacement: an expanded spectrum of associated neurovascular injury. J Orthop Trauma. 1993;7:361-6.

This article described the management of four patients who satisfied the radiographic criteria for scapulothoracic dissociation and presented with a spectrum of neurovascular conditions.

Mullaji AB, Jupiter JB. Low-contact dynamic compression plating of the clavicle. Injury. 1994;25:41-5.

This article described the authors' experience of treating nine clavicle fractures with LCDC plate fixation. At an average follow-up of 17 months, union was secured in each case.

Nordqvist A, Petersson CJ, Redlund-Johnell I. Mid-clavicle fractures in adults: end result study after conservative treatment. J Orthop Trauma. 1998;12:572-6.

This retrospective study evaluated the clinical and radiographic outcomes of conservative treatment of 225 midclavicle fractures at an average of 17 years after injury.

Van Noort A, te Slaa RL, Marti RK, van der Werken C. The floating shoulder: a multicentre study. J Bone Joint Surg [Br]. 2001;83:795-8.

This retrospective study reviewed the outcome of 46 patients treated for floating shoulder by 79 surgeons in the Netherlands.

PROCEDURE 28

Intramedullary Fixation of Clavicle Fractures

Jason D. Doppelt and Robert J. Neviaser

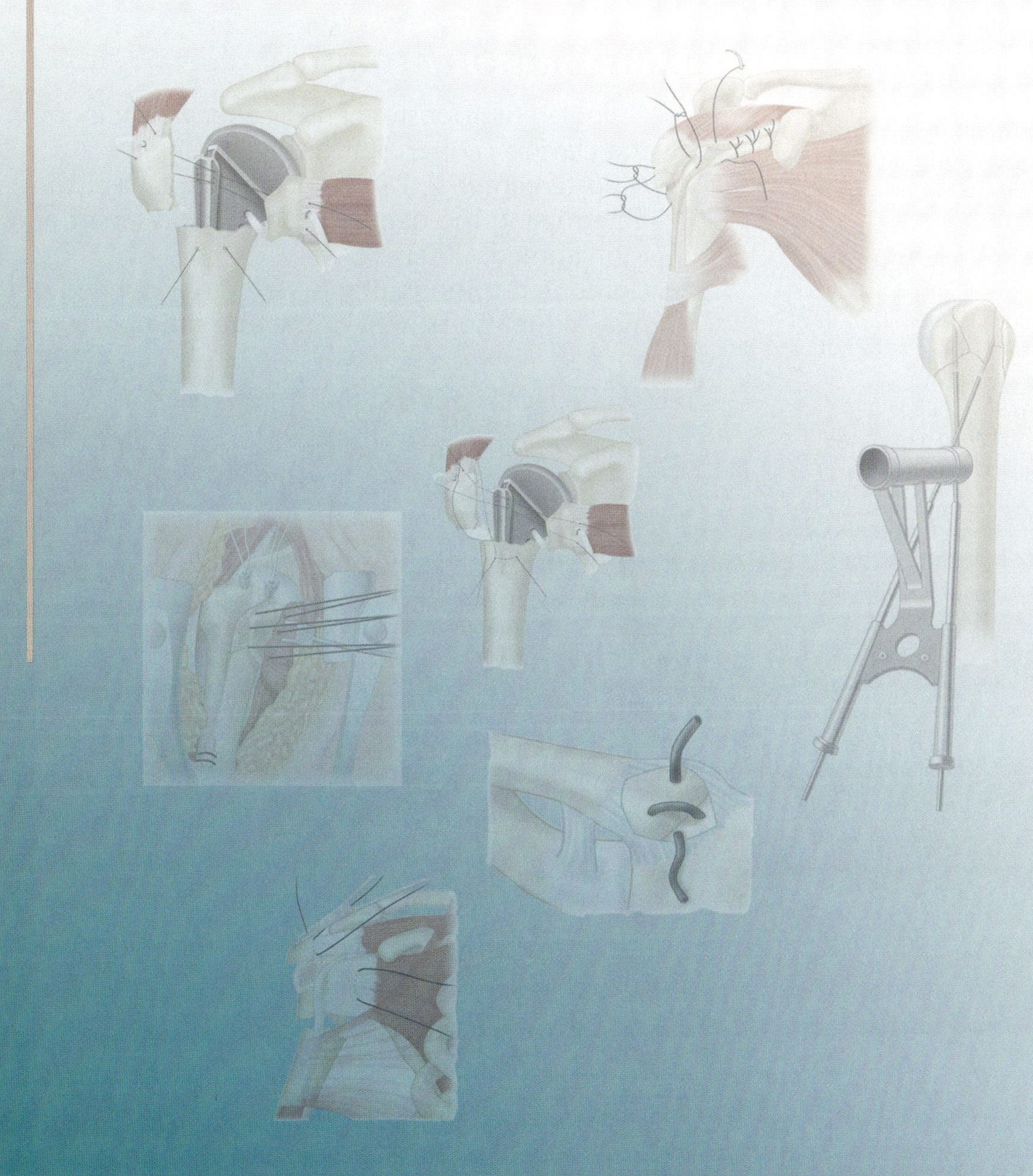

PITFALLS

- *Operative management of displaced fractures has been associated with superior results (Canadian Orthopaedic Trauma Society), but there is no consensus on the degree of unacceptable displacement.*

Controversies

- A satisfactory outcome is typical with operative intervention for malunions and nonunions, making early surgical intervention controversial.

Treatment Options

- Simple sling immobilization of the affected upper extremity
- Figure-of-8 bracing
- Percutaneous flexible intramedullary nailing (not commonly employed)
- Open reduction and internal fixation with an intramedullary device or plate and screws construct

PEARLS

- *Ensure that positioning of the image intensifier will allow unimpeded images without interfering with surgeon access.*

Equipment

- A pneumatic armholder can be employed if an assistant is not available.

Indications

- Open clavicle fractures or closed injuries with excessive skin tenting and possible conversion to an open fracture
- Management of a neurovascular injury
- Acute fractures with marked displacement or shortening more than 1.5 to 2 cm
- Certain polytrauma patients with bilateral upper extremity injuries, to facilitate rehabilitation
- Symptomatic nonunions

Examination/Imaging

- A single anteroposterior 15° cephalad radiograph of the clavicle is often sufficient (Fig. 1).
- A posteroanterior 15° caudal view may assist in determining the degree of shortening (Sharr and Mohammed, 2003).
- Computed tomography is very rarely needed but may aid in assessment of fracture union.

Surgical Anatomy

- The S shape of the clavicle requires careful attention when inserting an intramedullary device to avoid cortical penetration by the tip of the implant.
- The clavicle thins both medially and laterally, reducing the volume of the intramedullary canal.

Positioning

- The patient is placed in the sitting position with the upper extremity draped free to allow easy manipulation of the lateral fragment.

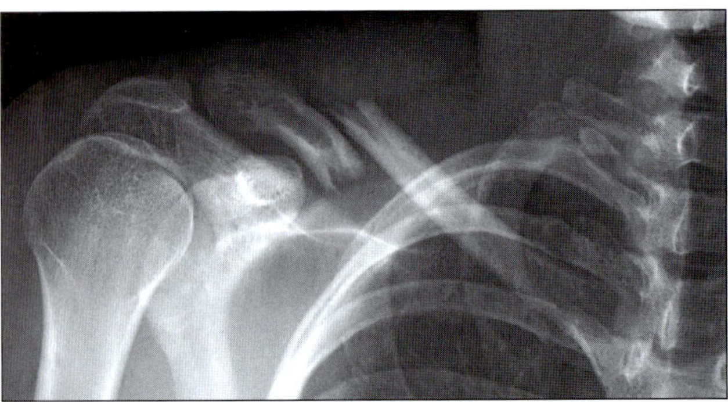

FIGURE 1

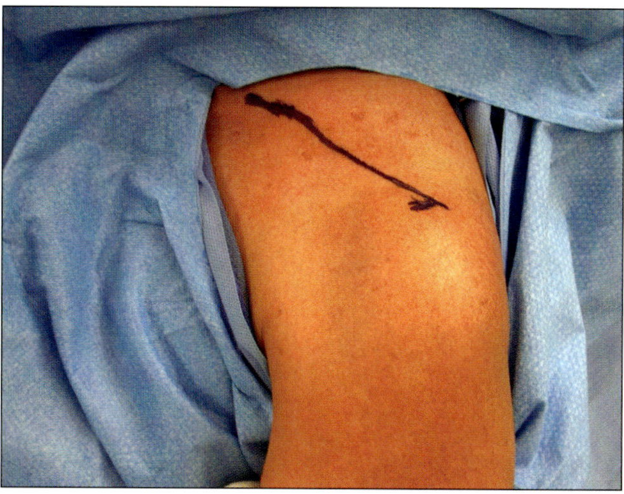

FIGURE 2

Pearls

- *The dissection should be done through a single plane to maintain fascial integrity for subsequent closure.*
- *The incision laterally should be centered over the posterior clavicle, as the start point for the implant is the posterior cortex.*

Pitfalls

- *The supraclavicular nerves will cross the plane of dissection and should be protected.*
- *Periosteal stripping should be avoided except at the very ends of the fracture.*

Portals/Exposures

- An anterior incision is made in line with the clavicle, centered over the fracture site (Fig. 2).
- Depending on the medial-to-lateral position of the fracture, the start point for the intramedullary device can be exposed by lateral extension of the same incision or by making a separate incision over the posterolateral prominence of the clavicle.

Controversies

- Some utilize a vertical incision over the fracture site, splitting the platysma to protect the supraclavicular nerves (Ring and Holovacs, 2005).
- A variety of intramedullary implants have been utilized, including Knowles pins, Hagie pins, Rockwood clavicle pins, and Kirschner wires. We prefer Knowles pins as they permit a compressive force across the fracture but have a low risk of medial migration due to the pin's hub. Additionally, they have relatively low prominence when the proper start point at the posterior cortex is utilized.

Procedure

Step 1

- After adequate exposure of the fracture site is obtained, a provisional reduction should be attempted.
- In acute fractures, cortical interdigitation will ensure restoration of the patient's anatomy.
- In highly comminuted fractures and nonunions, restoration of clavicular length is more challenging. In these situations, preoperative measurement of the contralateral clavicle may be helpful.

Pearls

- *Manipulation of the upper extremity will help align the lateral fragment with the medial fragment.*

Step 2

- The fracture is distracted to allow predrilling of the intramedullary canal with a 4.0-mm cannulated drill, both medially and laterally (Fig. 3A), to facilitate passing of the intramedullary device.
- The guidewire for this drill bit is passed first into the medullary canal, and the drill is passed into the canal over it for approximately a centimeter (Fig. 3B).

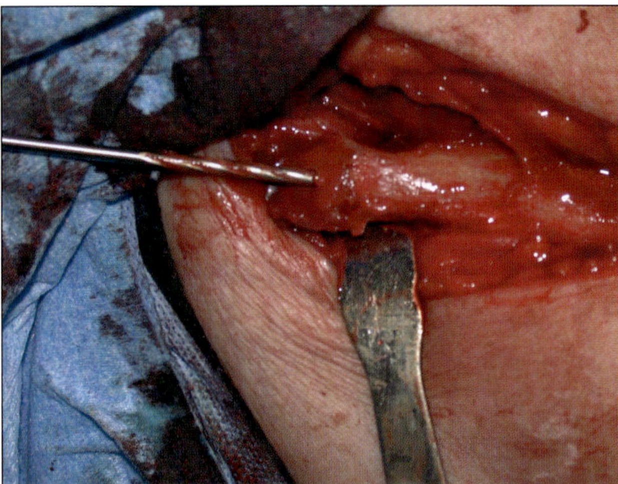
A

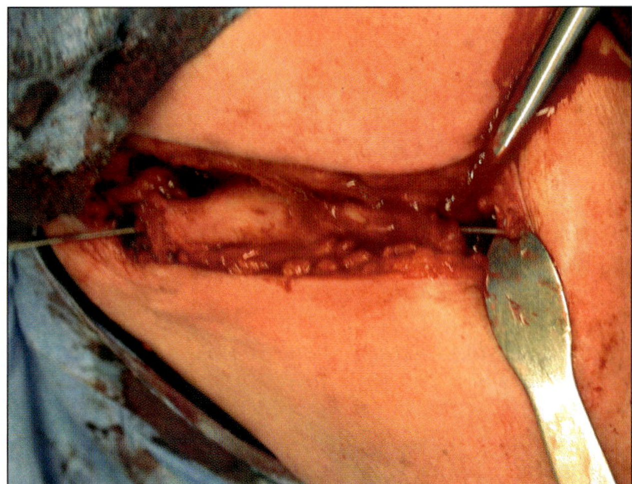
B

FIGURE 3

PITFALLS

- *Care must be taken when advancing the drill medially to avoid cortical penetration.*
- *Excessive forceful distraction at the fracture is thought to be a possible cause of postoperative brachial plexus palsy (Ring and Holovacs, 2005).*

Instrumentation/ Implantation

- Careful attention must be paid to the length of the implant.
  - Short pins are associated with insufficient fixation in the medial fragment as well as distraction at the fracture site if all of the threads are not advanced past the fracture.
  - An excessively long pin will penetrate the anteromedial cortex, which can cause symptomatic hardware prominence.

STEP 3

- The guidewire is passed from the fracture site retrograde to exit at the posterolateral aspect of the distal clavicle, slightly medial to the acromioclavicular joint (see Fig. 3B).
- A cannulated drill is then used over the wire to establish the lateral start point for the Knowles pin and continued for a centimeter or so down the shaft.
- A Knowles pin is introduced into the lateral starting point and advanced down the lateral fragment slowly until the tip appears at the fracture end of this fragment (Fig. 4).

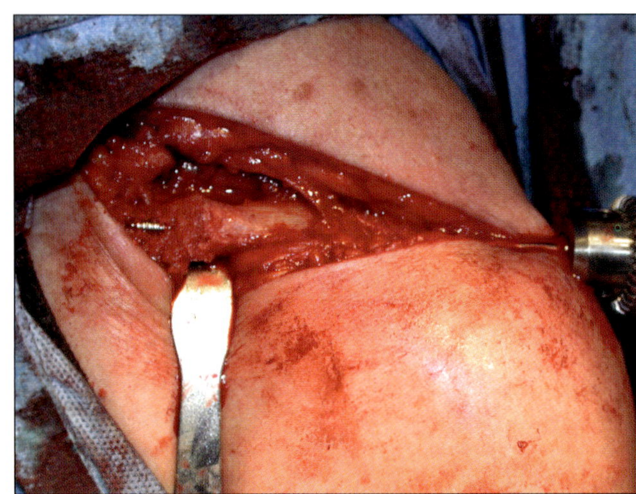

FIGURE 4

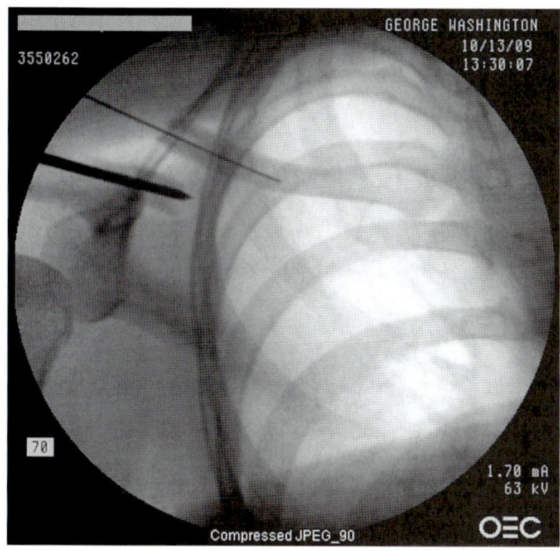

A

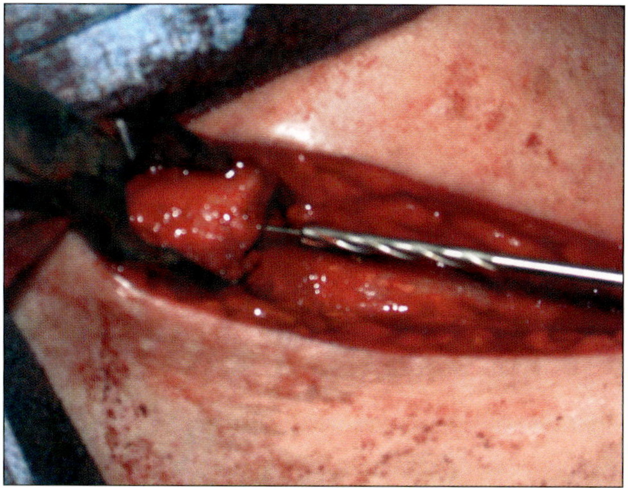

B

FIGURE 5

Step 4

- The medial fragment has been prepared with the guidewire (Fig. 5A) and the 4.0-mm cannulated drill (Fig. 5B) as described above (see Fig. 3).
- The tip of the Knowles pin is keyed into the drilled entrance point in the medial fragment and the fracture reduced (Fig. 6).
- The Knowles pin is then advanced into the medial fragment.
  - Initially, because the pin is terminally threaded, it appears to distact the fracture, but once the threads engage fully in the medial fragment, the fracture coapts nicely.
  - The pin is advanced until the hub seats behind the posterior cortex of the lateral fragment (Fig. 7A and 7B).

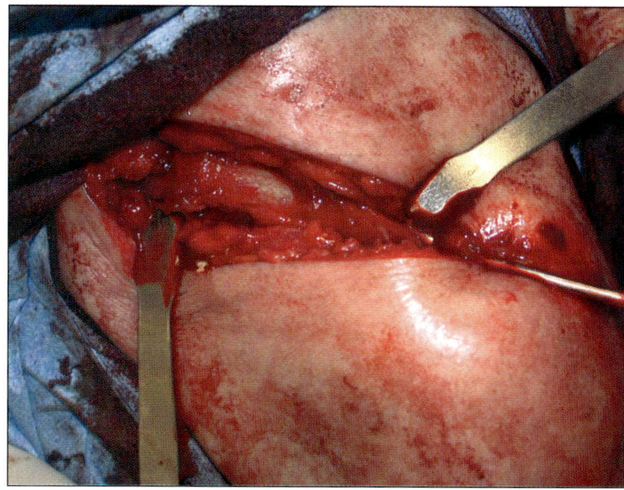

FIGURE 6

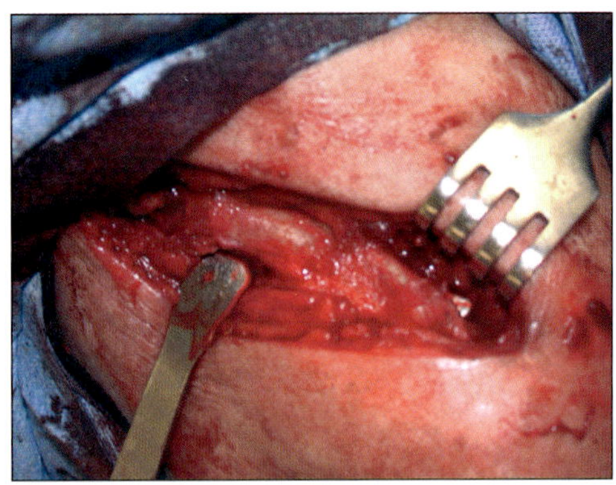

A

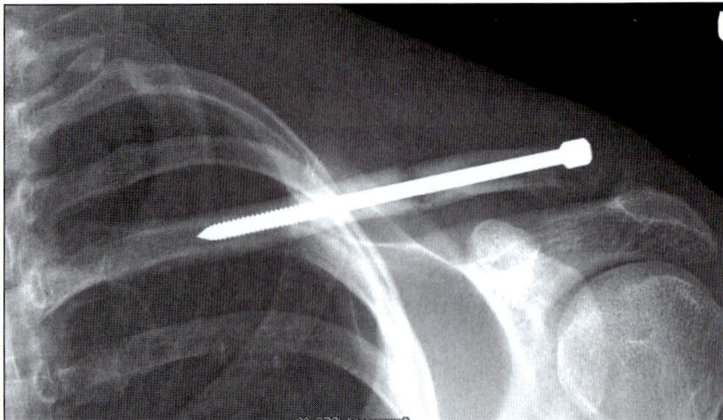

B

FIGURE 7

Pitfalls

- *Do not allow shoulder elevation above 40° for the first 6 weeks to prevent motion at the fracture site.*

Controversies

- Some authors advocate longer periods of immobilization; however, when stable fixation with a Knowles pin is achieved, the duration of immobilization can be reduced.
- Routine hardware removal is not necessary as implant prominence is not a common problem.

Postoperative Care and Expected Outcomes

- The involved upper extremity is immobilized in an immobilizer for a total of 6 weeks. The elbow, wrist, fingers, and thumb should be exercised frequently to prevent stiffness.
- After the first 2 weeks, the shoulder can be rotated with the elbow at the side and flexed forward, extended, and abducted between 30° and 40° at maximum to minimize stiffness but not more than the listed parameters to prevent toggling at the fracture site, which may impair union.

Evidence

Anderson K, Jensen PO, Lauritzen J. Treatment of clavicular fractures: figure of eight bandage versus a simple sling. Acta Orthop Scand. 1987;58:71-4.

This prospective randomized study evaluated 61 patients over a 3-month period. No functional or cosmetic difference was detected between the two forms of immobilization. A simple sling was associated with less discomfort. (Level II evidence)

Canadian Orthopaedic Trauma Society. Nonoperative treatment compared with plate fixation of displaced midshaft clavicular fractures. J Bone Joint Surg [Am]. 2007;89: 1-10.

This multicenter randomized trial followed 132 patients with displaced fractures. Open reduction and plate fixation was associated with improved Constant shoulder scores and DASH scores. The average time to union as well as the total number of nonunions was greater in the nonoperative group. The degree of displacement, however, was not clearly quantified by the authors. (Level I evidence)

Chu CM, Wang SJ, Lin LC. Fixation of mid-third clavicular fractures with Knowles pins. Acta Orthop Scand. 2002;73:134-9.

In this study, 78 patients were managed with 3.8-mm Knowles pin fixation and followed for 2–7 years. Only one patient went on to nonunion. In two cases the medial cortex was violated, causing hardware prominence requiring revision surgery. In one case the pin failed to provide sufficient fixation and was revised to a longer Knowles pin. There were no cases of pin migration or metal failure. (Level V evidence)

Keener JD, Dahners LE. Percutaneous pinning of displaced midshaft clavicle fractures. Tech Shoulder Elbow Surg. 2006;7:175-81.

A surgical technique for anterograde percutaneous pinning with an elastic titanium nail was presented. Adequate follow-up was available from 21 patients. An open reduction was required in 10 cases to allow passage of the implant across the fracture. There were three malunions, but only one required revision surgery. Six patients underwent pin removal due to skin irritation at the pin site. There were no cases of pin migration. (Level IV evidence)

Neviaser RJ, Neviaser JS, Neviaser TJ, Neviaser JS. A simple technique for internal fixation of the clavicle: a long term evaluation. Clin Orthop Relat Res. 1975;(109):103-7.

Eleven patients were followed from 1 to 20 years after Knowles pin fixation of middle-third clavicle fractures. All fractures healed uneventfully, and there were no intraoperative or postoperative complications. There were no cases of pin migration. No pins required removal. (Level IV evidence)

Ring D, Holovacs T. Brachial plexus palsy after intramedullary fixation of a clavicular fracture: a report of three cases. J Bone Joint Surg [Am]. 2005;87:1834-7.

In this study, 22 patients were managed with a Rockwood clavicle pin. Three patients were found to have a brachial plexus palsy on postoperative examination. Surgical exploration was not performed, and all three had complete or near-complete recovery. Excessive distraction at the fracture site during reaming of the intramedullary canal was thought to be the likely cause. (Level IV evidence)

Sharr JRP, Mohammed KD. Optimizing the radiographic technique in claviclar fractures. J Shoulder Elbow Surg. 2003;12:170-2.

Fifty patients with clavicle fractures were radiographically evaluated. The authors determined that a posteroanterior 15° caudad view more accurately detected shortening at the fracture site than the standard anterosuperior 15° cephalad view. (Level IV evidence)

Strauss EJ, Egol KA, France MA, Koval KJ. Complications of intramedullary Hagie pin fixation for acute midshaft clavicle fractures. J Shoulder Elbow Surg. 2007;16:280-4.

Intramedullary Hagie pin fixation in this series resulted in a 50% complication rate. There were three cases of skin breakdown, two cases of hardware breakage, and one case of persistent pain at the fracture site. The authors concluded that Hagie pins should not be used to manage clavicle fractures. (Level IV evidence)

PROCEDURE 29

Operative Treatment of Two-Part Proximal Humerus Fractures

Gerald R. Williams, Jr.

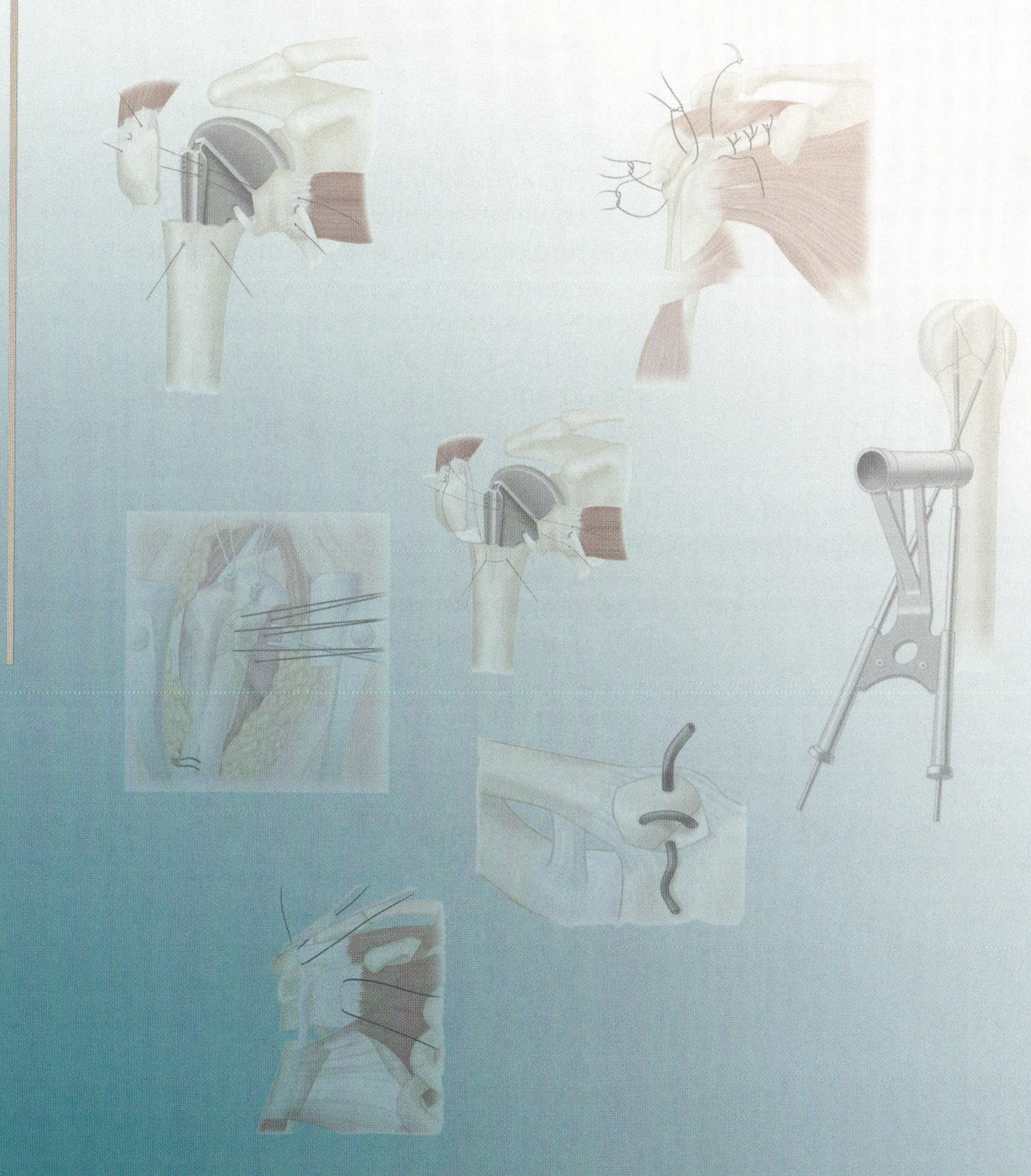

Figures 9-11 courtesy of Jorge Orbay, M.D.

Pitfalls

- *Superior greater tuberosity displacement (0.5 mm) is tolerated less well than posterior displacement (1.0 cm).*
- *Lesser tuberosity fragments that contain a substantial portion of the articular surface may block internal rotation with less than 1.0 cm of displacement.*

Controversies

- Displacement as a means of fracture classification has been shown to be unreliable in some studies, even with two-dimensional computed tomography (CT) scanning.
- Adequate radiographs and surgeon experience are important.
- Three-dimensional CT scanning may help.

Treatment Options

- Open reduction and internal fixation
- Closed reduction with percutaneous fixation
- Arthroscopically assisted reduction and internal fixation

Indications

- Surgical neck fracture with 1 cm of displacement or 45° of angulation
- Greater tuberosity or lesser tuberosity fracture with 1 cm of displacement
- Absence of medical contraindications to surgery

Examination/Imaging

- Physical examination should be focused on identifying concomitant injuries and verifying neurovascular integrity.
  - Concomitant injuries include
    - Ipsilateral upper extremity injuries/fractures
    - Rib fractures
    - Facial/head injuries
    - Lower extremity injuries
  - Neurological injuries are underappreciated and can occur in up to 82% of displaced fractures.
- Sensory examination is unreliable.
- Motor function should be confirmed and documented in each individual nerve (i.e., axillary, musculocutaneous, radial, median, and ulnar).
- Vascular injuries typically occur just proximal to the humeral circumflex vessels in the second part of the axillary artery.
  - Injuries are most often intimal tears with subsequent thrombosis
  - Extensive collateral flow exists between the third part of the subclavian artery and the third part of the axillary artery, making physical findings associated with even complete occlusion of the axillary artery potentially subtle (i.e., decreased radial pulse).
- Essential radiographs include an anteroposterior view in the scapular plane, a trans-scapular or Y view, and an axillary view: the trauma series.
  - Radiographs in at least two orthogonal planes are necessary when evaluating proximal humerus fractures. In Figure 1, the anteroposterior view (Fig. 1A) of this two-part proximal humerus fracture shows substantially less displacement than the axillary view (Fig. 1B).
  - Beware of a valgus-impacted head fragment in combination with or instead of greater tuberosity displacement.

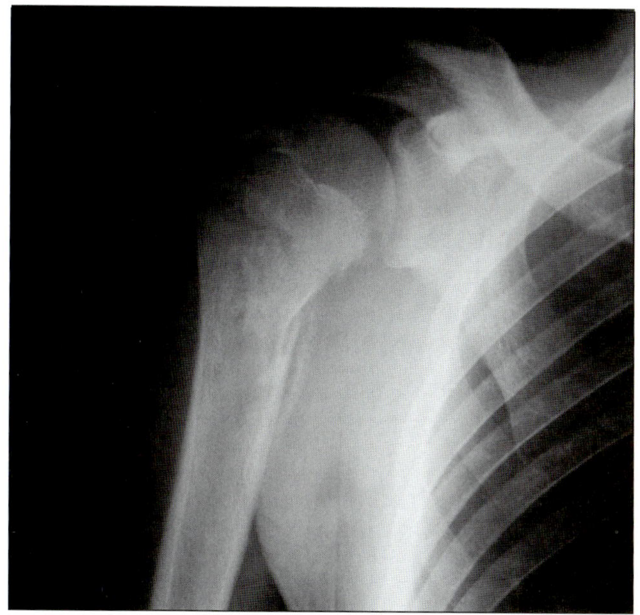
A

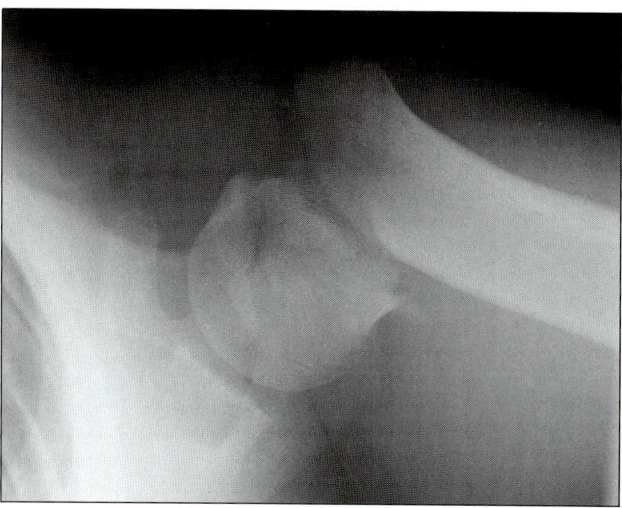
B

FIGURE 1

- CT scanning is indicated for quantifying tuberosity displacement or for excluding dislocation when an adequate axillary radiograph cannot be obtained.
- Arteriography may be indicated in displaced surgical neck fractures with only asymmetric pulses.
  - Axillary artery occlusion can be present in displaced surgical neck fractures even when the physical findings are subtle. The patient with the fracture seen in Figure 2A had an outwardly normal-appearing distal extremity with only a decrease in her radial pulse.
  - An arteriogram (Fig. 2B) revealed complete axillary artery occlusion.

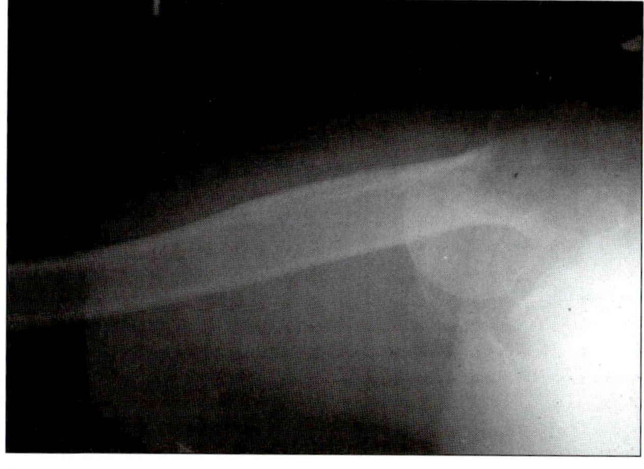
A

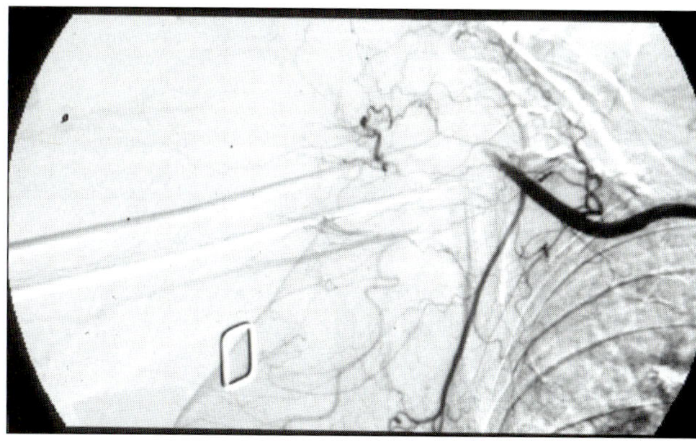
B

FIGURE 2

Surgical Anatomy

Osseous Structures

- The humeral neck-shaft angle averages 135° (range: 120-145°).
- Valgus impaction of the head can simulate or magnify greater tuberosity displacement.
- Fixation of the greater tuberosity without reduction of the head should be avoided.
- The tip of the greater tuberosity is, on average, 8 ± 3.2 mm inferior to the highest point of the humeral head. This relationship should be restored during reduction of greater tuberosity fractures.
- The greater tuberosity fracture line typically occurs approximately 5 mm posterior to the bicipital groove.

Soft Tissues: muscles, tendons, and ligaments

- The posterosuperior rotator cuff muscles (supraspinatus, infraspinatus, and teres minor) insert on the greater tuberosity through broad tendinous attachments (Fig. 3). The subscapularis inserts on the lesser tuberosity with a similar broad tendinous attachment.
  - These attachments lead to posterior and superior displacement following greater tuberosity fracture,

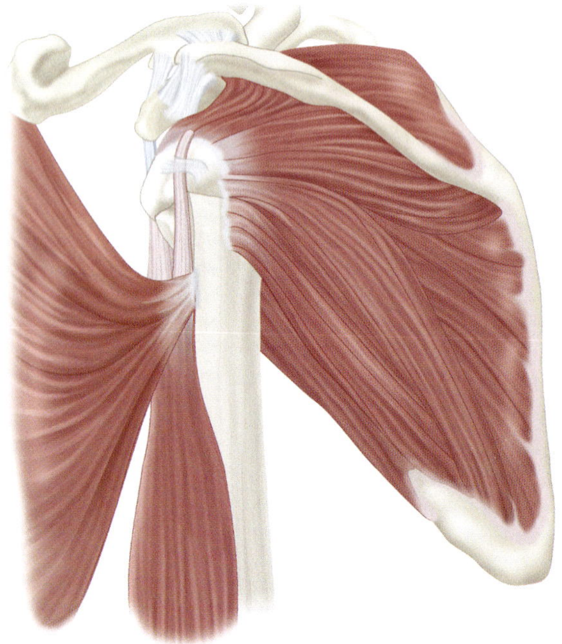

FIGURE 3

medial displacement following lesser tuberosity fracture, and abduction of the proximal fragment following surgical neck fracture.

- The rotator cuff tendons can be used to augment fixation using heavy, nonabsorbable sutures.
- The rotator interval lies between the subscapularis anteriorly and the supraspinatus posteriorly.
- Greater tuberosity fractures with severe posterior displacement may result in a longitudinal tear through the anterior third of the supraspinatus or the rotator interval.
- The long head of the biceps tendon lies deep to the tendon of the pectoralis major within the bicipital groove.
  - During open reduction and internal fixation (ORIF), identification of the long head of the biceps may assist in identifying greater or lesser tuberosity fracture lines.
  - During open surgical management of surgical neck fractures, the long head of the biceps may be damaged or entrapped in the fracture site.
- The tendon of the pectoralis major inserts on the lateral lip of the bicipital groove and causes an anterior and medial deforming force on the humeral shaft following surgical neck fracture (see Fig. 3).
  - When using a plate for fixation of a surgical neck fracture, it should lie approximately 5 mm posterior to the pectoralis major insertion on the lateral aspect of the proximal humeral shaft.
- The insertion of the deltoid muscle on the humeral shaft is extremely large. A small portion of the anterior insertion may be released to accommodate the distal portion of a fixation plate in surgical neck fractures.
- The conjoined tendon of the coracobrachialis and short head of the biceps arises from the tip of the coracoid and inserts on the medial aspect of the humeral shaft. Excessive medial retraction of this tendon should be avoided, especially in the presence of a concomitant brachial plexus injury or identified high penetration of the musculocutaneous nerve (see following section).

Soft Tissues: nerves and vessels

- The neurovascular structures adjacent to the proximal humerus include the brachial plexus and its peripheral branches (most notably the axillary nerve), the axillary artery, and the axillary vein (Fig. 4).

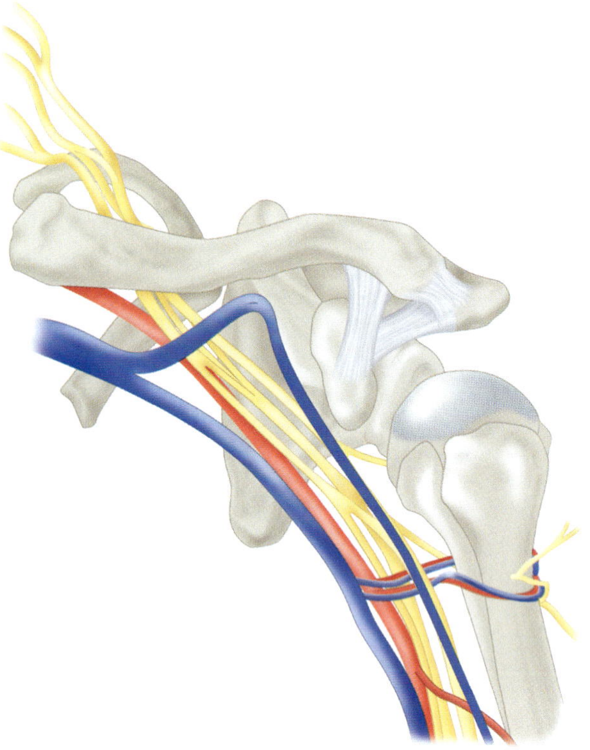

FIGURE 4

- Divisions from the trunks of the brachial plexus coalesce to form the medial, lateral, and posterior cords posterior to the pectoralis minor tendon. The cords are named according to their relation to the second part of the axillary artery.
- Distal to the pectoralis minor, the posterior cord gives rise to one of its terminal branches, the axillary nerve.
  - The axillary nerve traverses the anterior surface of the subscapularis to reach into the inferior aspect of the glenohumeral joint and enters the posterior aspect of the axilla through the quadrilateral space, where it divides into an anterior and a posterior division.
  - The posterior division of the axillary nerve innervates the teres minor muscle and a portion of the posterior deltoid muscle, and supplies sensation to the glenohumeral joint and a variable portion of the posterior skin.
  - The anterior division of the axillary nerve traverses the deep surface of the deltoid at the level of the surgical neck of the humerus approximately 4.5-5.0 cm distal to the lateral margin of the acromion. The anterior division of the axillary

nerve innervates a variable portion of the posterior deltoid, the middle deltoid, and the anterior deltoid. It also provides sensation to a variable portion of the skin over the deltoid.

- The musculocutaneous nerve is a terminal branch of the lateral cord of the brachial plexus that penetrates the conjoined tendon and innervates the brachialis and biceps muscles.
  - The musculocutaneous nerve penetrates the deep surface of the conjoined tendon approximately 5 cm, on average, distal to the tip of the coracoid. This site of penetration is extremely variable and can be as close as 1-2 cm from the tip of the coracoid.
- The axillary artery begins at the first rib and terminates at the teres major.
- The anterior and posterior humeral circumflex vessels are the first branches of the third portion of the axillary artery.
  - The posterior humeral circumflex artery traverses the quadrilateral space with the axillary nerve and supplies terminal vessels to the humeral head through the posteromedial calcar. Injury to these vessels may increase the likelihood of avascular necrosis.
  - The anterior humeral circumflex artery traverses the anterior surface of the inferior portion of the subscapularis, crosses the bicipital groove, and gives off the ascending branch. This branch travels superiorly, 2-3 mm posterior to the bicipital groove, and terminates in the arcuate branch that supplies a substantial portion of the humeral head. Injury to the arcuate branch or to the distal portion of the ascending branch increases the likelihood of avascular necrosis.

Positioning

- The semirecumbent or beach chair position, with the torso approximately 30-45° elevated, is used for the deltopectoral approach in ORIF of two-part surgical neck or lesser tuberosity fractures (Fig. 5). Note the mechanical arm holder (*arrow*), which can be helpful in maintaining arm position.
- The semi-sitting position, with the torso elevated approximately 70-80°, is used for the superior approach for two-part greater tuberosity fractures (Fig. 6). Note the C-arm entering the field from

Pearls

- *In either position, the hips and knees are flexed to relieve tension on the sciatic nerves.*
- *Mechanical compression boots may be used to prevent venous pooling.*
- *The entire shoulder girdle should be extended over the table to allow unfettered access for the C-arm.*

Pitfalls

- *Avoid traction on the neck and brachial plexus by stabilizing the head and neck in a neutral position.*
- *Avoid compression of lower extremity peripheral nerves and bony prominences.*
- *Check adequate radiographic visualization before preparation and draping.*

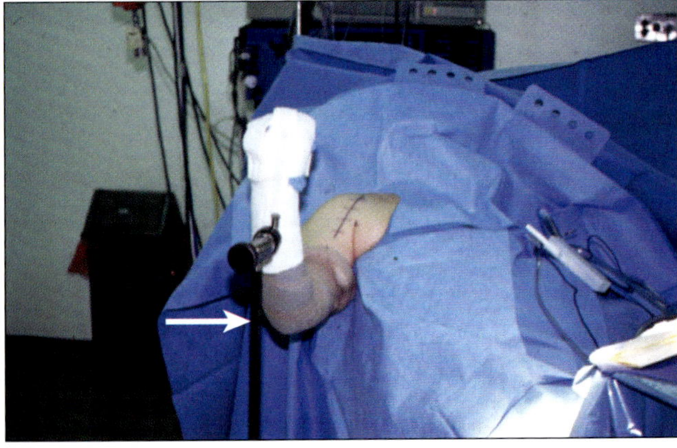

FIGURE 5

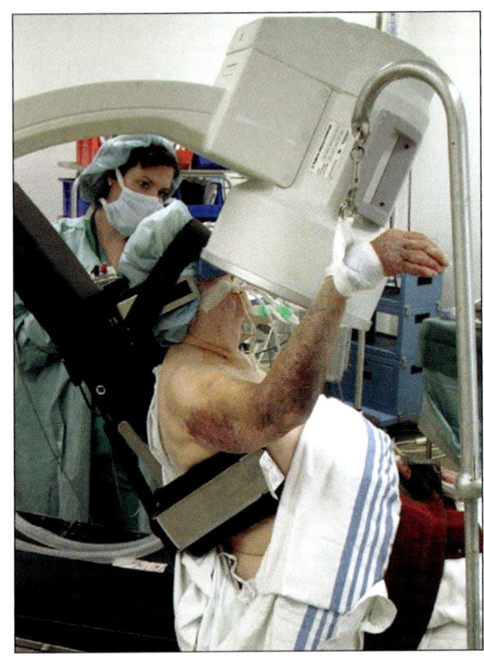

FIGURE 6

Equipment

- A specialized table with "fall-away" sections behind the shoulders is helpful.
- A C-arm and image intensifier should be used in every case.
- A mechanical arm holder or padded Mayo stand assists in maintaining reduction, especially in two-part surgical neck fractures.

Controversies

- The C-arm can be brought into the operative field from superiorly, parallel to the edge of the patient, or from the opposite side of the table. The opposite side of the table works well with the specialized, more narrow tables mentioned above.
- If the C-arm is to be brought in from superiorly, the anesthesia team needs to be moved accordingly.

superiorly. It can also be brought in from the opposite side of the table.

- Two-part surgical neck fractures
  - Semirecumbent (beach chair) position—deltopectoral approach, superolateral approach, or closed reduction with percutaneous pinning
- Two-part greater tuberosity fractures
  - Semi-sitting position—superior approach and closed or arthroscopically assisted approach
  - Semirecumbent (beach chair) position—deltopectoral approach
- Two-part lesser tuberosity fractures
  - Semi-sitting position—closed or arthroscopically assisted approach

- Semirecumbent (beach chair) position—deltopectoral approach

Portals/Exposures

- The deltopectoral approach (Fig. 7) is used for ORIF of two-part surgical neck fractures and lesser tuberosity fractures. Some surgeons also use it for ORIF of greater tuberosity fractures.
- The superior approach (Fig. 8) is most often used for open reduction and internal fixation of two-part greater tuberosity fractures.

Pitfalls

- *Two-part surgical neck fractures*
  - Closed reduction and percutaneous pinning should be reserved for patients with excellent bone quality and little or no medial comminution. The anterolateral (greater tuberosity–to–medial surgical neck) pin exits within 5 mm of the axillary nerve, and the pin interferes with the acromion.
  - In ORIF with the superolateral deltoid-splitting approach, which is not an extensile approach, fixation is potentially limited by the axillary nerve.
- *Two-part greater tuberosity fractures*
  - In ORIF with the superior approach, the potential exists for deltoid dehiscence. This approach is also limited distally because of the axillary nerve.

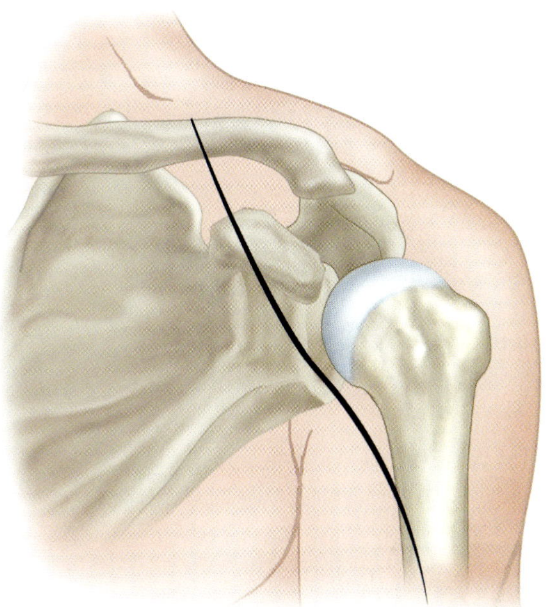

FIGURE 7

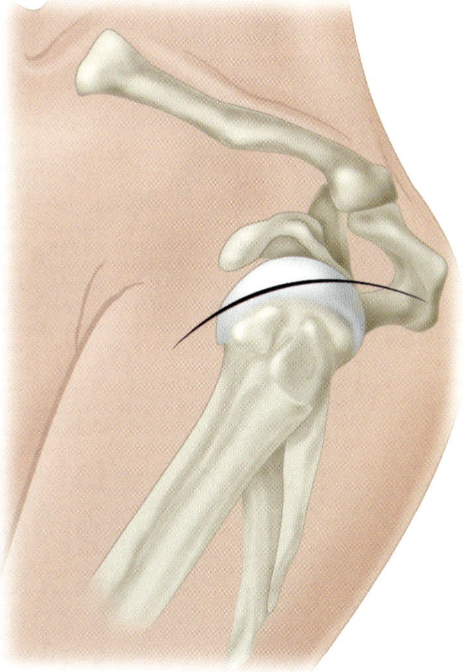

FIGURE 8

Instrumentation

- Closed reduction with percutaneous fixation
  - 2-mm, terminally threaded pins
  - Cannulated screw set (4.0-4.5 mm)
- Arthroscopically assisted treatment
  - Suture anchors
  - Cannulated screw set (4.0-4.5 mm)

Controversies

- Two-part surgical neck fracture
  - Superolateral deltoid-splitting approach versus deltopectoral approach
  - Intramedullary rods versus plates
- Two-part greater tuberosity fracture
  - Superior approach versus deltopectoral approach

Controversies

- The cephalic vein can also be retracted medially with the pectoralis major to decrease intraoperative trauma during retraction of the deltoid.
- Most of the branches draining into the cephalic vein enter from the deltoid and must be ligated if the vein is to be retracted medially.

- Two-part surgical neck fractures
  - Closed reduction with percutaneous pinning
    - Two anterolateral, retrograde, terminally threaded pins should suffice.
    - The surgeon may spread to bone or use an insertion sheath.
  - ORIF—deltopectoral approach (most common)
    - This is an extensile approach that does not cross the axillary nerve.
    - The arm is placed in a mechanical arm holder in 20-30° of flexion, neutral rotation, and 40-45° of abduction to relax the deltoid and pectoralis major.
  - ORIF—deltoid-splitting approach
- Two-part greater tuberosity fractures
  - Closed or arthroscopically assisted reduction and percutaneous fixation
    - Mild displacement
    - Good bone
    - Experienced surgeon
  - ORIF—superior approach (most common)
    - This approach is excellent for posterior visualization and reduction.
    - The surgeon may detach the anterior deltoid as in an open cuff repair.
  - ORIF—deltopectoral approach
    - A supraspinatus traction stitch should be used to control the fragment.
    - This is an extensile approach.
- Two-part lesser tuberosity fractures
  - Closed or arthroscopically assisted reduction and percutaneous fixation
    - Mild displacement
    - Good bone
    - Experienced surgeon
  - ORIF—deltopectoral approach (most common)
    - Extensile approach
    - Maintain anterior circumflex vessels
    - Biceps tenodesis

Procedure: ORIF of Surgical Neck Fracture with Locking Plate Through Deltopectoral Approach

Step 1: Superficial Dissection

- A 10- to 12-cm deltopectoral skin incision is made.
- The deltopectoral interval is developed.

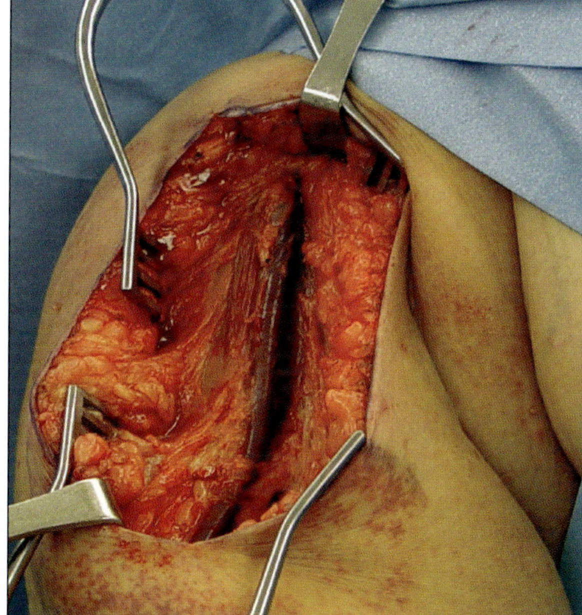

FIGURE 9

- The cephalic vein marks the deltopectoral interval and is most often kept with the deltoid and retracted laterally (Fig. 9).

Step 2: Deep Dissection

- The clavipectoral fascia is incised lateral to the conjoined tendon of the coracobrachialis and short head of the biceps.
- The axillary nerve is identified and the presence or absence of high penetration of the musculocutaneous nerve through the conjoined tendon is determined.
- The conjoined tendon is retracted medially and the deltoid laterally.
- The shaft is exposed distally between the deltoid and pectoralis insertion for placement of the plate.
- The long head of the biceps is identified and removed from the bicipital groove. Soft tissue tenodesis of the biceps to the pectoralis major is performed and the tendon is resected proximally to the tenodesis site.

Pearls

- *Normal anatomic planes and landmarks can be obscured because of the bleeding associated with acute fractures.*
  - Early identification of the long head of the biceps may facilitate identification of the fracture fragments as well as the lateral surface of the greater tuberosity and cuff insertion.
  - The biceps is easily identified by following the pectoralis major to its humeral attachment; the biceps is immediately deep to the pectoralis tendon insertion.
- *When exposing the humeral shaft distally, a small portion (0.5-1.0 cm) of the anterior portion of the deltoid insertion may be elevated to allow adequate room for the distal portion of the plate.*

Pitfalls

- *Avoid excessive dissection posterior to the superior aspect of the bicipital groove, as injury to the arcuate artery may occur.*
- *When a high penetration (within 2-2.5 cm) of the musculocutaneous nerve through the conjoined tendon is identified, limit retraction of the conjoined tendon, especially with self-retaining retractors.*

Controversies

- Potential difficulties with deltoid retraction is one of the arguments for using a superolateral, deltoid-splitting approach.
- Abduction of the arm not only aids in reduction of the fracture but also facilitates deltoid retraction.
- The deltopectoral approach is extensile and more versatile than the superolateral approach.

Pearls

- *The most important step is to provisionally fix the plate to the distal fragment in the middle of the shaft, between the deltoid and pectoralis major insertion, at the correct height. The correct height can be determined by passing the guide pin and verifying its position in the humeral head.*
- *If the fracture is particularly unstable, after provisionally fixing the plate to the shaft, the rotator cuff sutures that were used to control the proximal fragment can be passed through the plate and clamped to provide provisional fixation.*
  - The guide pin can then be passed through the proximal portion of the plate into the head.
  - The sutures are not tied until all proximal locking screws or pegs have been placed.

Pitfalls

- *It is important to verify adequacy of reduction when the plate is provisionally fixed to the distal fragment with one screw and the proximal fragment with the guide pin. Do not proceed with placing the proximal locking screws or pegs until the reduction is satisfactory in both planes.*
- *When placing the proximal locking screws or pegs, penetration of the head should be avoided if possible. Screw or peg length can be made 5 mm shorter than the subchondral surface to minimize intraoperative or postoperative penetration.*

Step 3: Provisional Reduction and Fixation

- The fracture is reduced by abducting the arm to bring the distal fragment to the proximal fragment.
  - Heavy nonabsorbable sutures are placed at the tendon-bone junction of the rotator cuff anteriorly, superiorly, and posteriorly to control the proximal fragment.
  - An elevator can be used to "guide" the reduction.
  - Position is maintained with a mechanical arm holder or padded Mayo stand.
- Reduction is confirmed with the C-arm in two planes.
- An appropriately sized plate is applied to the distal fragment in the center (anterior-posterior) of the shaft between the deltoid insertion and the pectoralis insertion.
  - The anterior edge of the plate should be 5 mm posterior to the lateral lip of the bicipital groove.
  - The appropriate height of the plate depends on the angles of the proximal locking screws and should be estimated using the C-arm.
  - The plate is provisionally fixed to the shaft manually or with a fracture clamp.
  - A guide pin is passed from the proximal portion of the plate into the head and its position confirmed in two planes with the C-arm.
  - One screw is placed in the distal portion of the plate, preferably in an oblong hole, to allow superoinferior adjustment if necessary.
  - Again reduction and hardware placement are confirmed in two planes with the C-arm. Figure 10

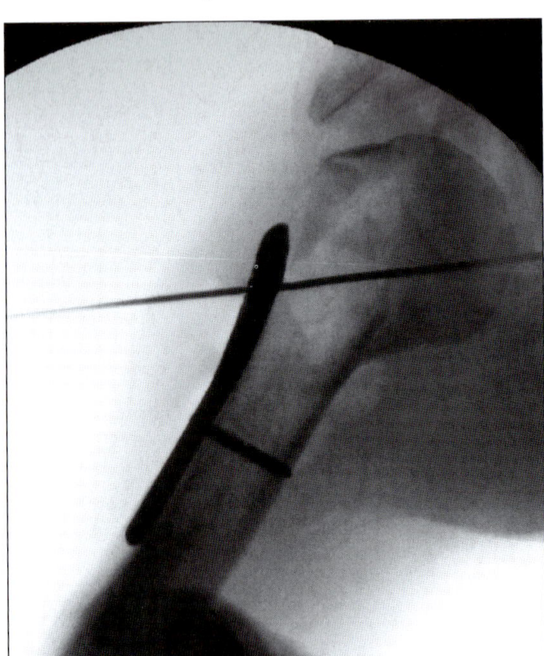

FIGURE 10

Instrumentation/ Implantation

- There are many proximal humeral locking plates on the market. Be familiar with the surgical details of whichever implant is being used.
- The implant used in this procedure (S3 plate; Depuy, Warsaw, IN) attempts to mimic the 135° neck-shaft angle of the humerus in its proximal locking screw or peg placement.
- The smooth profile and blunt tip of the pegs may decrease the likelihood of penetration.
- The screws in the distal portion of the plate can also be locked to the plate, but this is often not necessary.

Controversies

- There is controversy with regard to how long to make the proximal locking screws. It appears that intraoperative penetration may occur without recognition and that postoperative penetration may occur even if the screw was contained within bone intraoperatively. This has caused some surgeons to recommend very short screw placement. This has the potential disadvantage of not engaging the subchondral bone of the humeral head, which is often the only good bone in the proximal fragment.

shows a plate provisionally fixed to the shaft with one screw and to the head with a guide pin through the proximal portion of the plate.

- The reduction can be easily changed until multiple locking screws or pegs have been inserted into the head.
  - The most common errors are residual varus and/or apex anterior angulation.
  - If the reduction is not satisfactory in both the anteroposterior and lateral planes, the pin is removed, the fracture reduction is changed, and the pin is reinserted.
  - Loosening the screw in the distal portion of the plate slightly, especially if it was placed in an oblong hole, provides another degree of freedom when adjusting the reduction.

Step 4: Final Fixation

- The proximal locking pegs or screws are placed, confirming appropriate length with the C-arm.
- Remaining screws are placed in the distal portion of the plate.
- Previously placed sutures are passed through holes in the plate for additional fixation.
- Final confirmation is obtained with the C-arm. In Figure 11, the head is fixed to the plate with multiple divergent locking pegs and to the shaft with bicortical screws. Note the sutures from the rotator cuff to the plate.

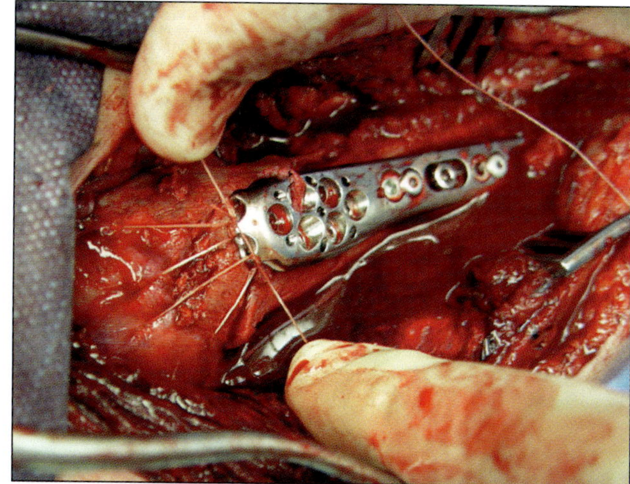

FIGURE 11

Procedure: ORIF of Greater Tuberosity Fracture Through Superior Approach

Step 1: Superficial Dissection

- A 6- to 8-cm skin incision is made paralleling the lateral border of the acromion in Langer's skin lines.
- Full-thickness skin flaps are developed medially to the acromioclavicular joint and laterally to expose the proximal deltoid.

Step 2: Deep Dissection

- The deltoid is split along the raphe between the anterior and middle deltoid starting at the lateral margin of the acromion and extending distally 3.5-4.0 cm.
  - The split should not go further than 4-5 cm to avoid injury to the axillary nerve, as seen in Figure 12.
  - The surgeon may release some of the anterior deltoid as in open cuff repair to improve exposure.
- The anterior deltoid is retracted anteriorly and the middle deltoid posteriorly.
- A partial bursectomy is performed to visualize the greater tuberosity fragment.

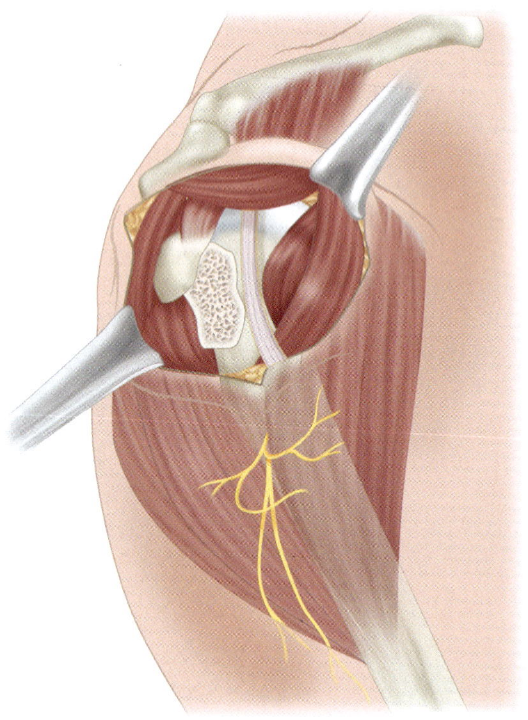

FIGURE 12

Pearls

- *A protective suture can be placed at the distal extent of the deltoid split to limit distal propagation and injury to the axillary nerve.*
- *In most cases, severe displacement of the greater tuberosity is prevented by an intact periosteal sleeve or supraspinatus tendon. Visualization of the entire fragment can be accomplished by internal and external rotation of the arm.*
- *With more severe displacement, visualization can be improved by releasing the anterior deltoid from the acromion.*

Pitfalls

- *The deltoid split must be limited to no more than 4.5 cm distal to the lateral margin of the acromion in order to avoid injury to the axillary nerve. This may limit exposure of the most distal extent of the fracture in some cases.*
- *If any portion of the anterior deltoid is to be released, a good cuff of tendinous tissue should be left of the deltoid muscle to ensure a robust repair to bone.*

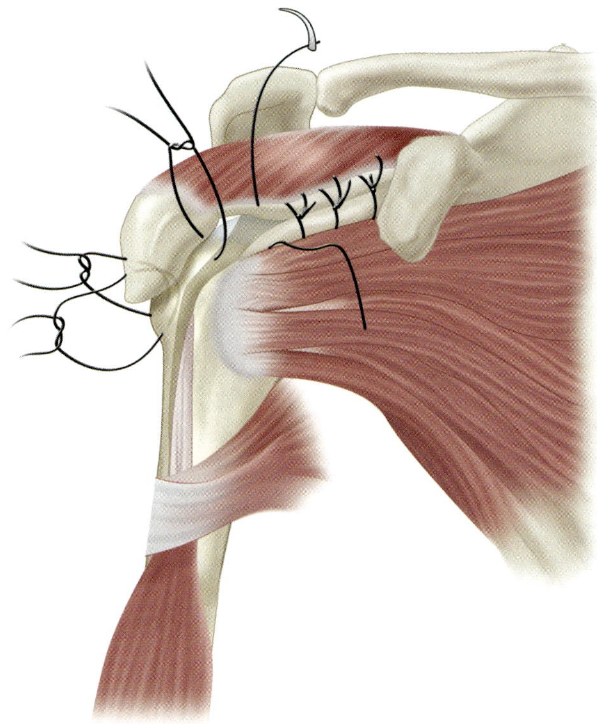

FIGURE 13

Pearls

- *If the fracture fragment is large and extends substantially distally, a second traction suture can be placed posterior and inferior to the first one. This allows better control of the proximal and distal portions of the fragment.*
- *The guide pins for the cannulated screws should be perpendicular to the lateral cortex and the fracture line so that placement of the screws results in orthogonal compression.*

Pitfalls

- *Placement of the guide pins too close to one another may result in fracture of the cortex between the two screws, interference or conflict between the washers on the two screws, and poor rotational stability of the fragment.*
- *Confirm placement of the pins in the subchondral bone of the humeral head without intra-articular penetration.*
- *Verify that the humeral head is anatomically positioned and not impacted into valgus.*

Step 3: Provisional Reduction and Fixation

- A heavy nonabsorbable suture is placed at the bone-tendon junction of the supraspinatus at the anterior leading edge of the fracture (Fig. 13).
- This suture, rotation of the arm, and an elevator are used to key the fracture into a reduced position.
- The fracture is provisionally fixed with a guide pin from a 4.0- or 4.5-mm cannulated screw set.
  - The pin should be placed approximately 1.0-1.5 cm posterior to the anterior edge of the fracture fragment, perpendicular to the lateral cortex, and approximately 1.0-1.5 cm distal to the bone-tendon junction.
  - The pin is advanced medially until it reaches the palpably hard subchondral bone of the humeral head.
  - Placement should be confirmed in two planes with the C-arm.
  - A second pin should be placed parallel and approximately 1.5-2.0 cm posterior and 1-1.5 cm distal to the first one.
  - Adequate reduction and pin placement should again be verified radiographically.

Instrumentation/ Implantation

- Multiple cannulated screw systems are available.
- The guide pins should be terminally threaded.
- Self-tapping screws are preferable.

Controversies

- Controversy exists with regard to whether fractures should be fixed with sutures rather than screws because of poor bone quality. In most cases, the subchondral bone of the humerus is adequate for screw fixation. The superior suture is combined with the screws improve fixation.

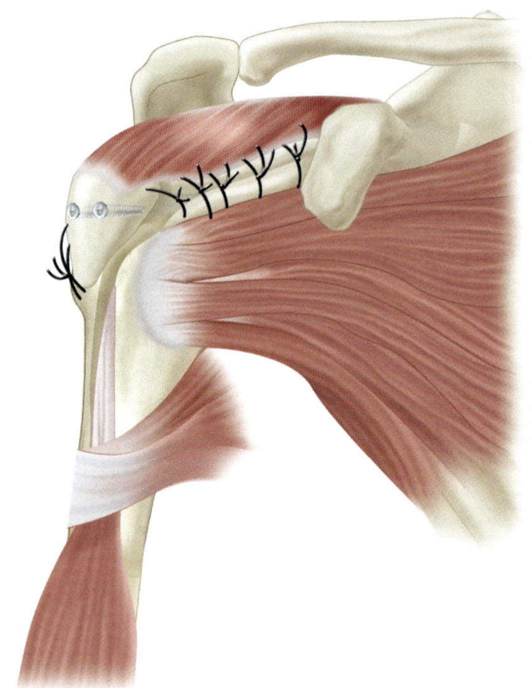

FIGURE 14

Pearls

- *A large cutting needle is usually sufficient to pass the deep limbs of the interfragmentary sutures through the fracture bed, deep to the bicipital groove, and out the lateral cortex of the humerus.*
    - If the bone of the lateral cortex is too hard to allow passage of the free needle, drill hole can be placed in the lateral cortex and a suture passer can be used to pass the suture.

Pitfalls

- *The anterior humeral circumflex vessels should be preserved.*
- *Avoid large suture anchors at the anatomic neck region as the cortical margin between the fracture bed and the anatomic neck is small (0.5-1.0 cm).*

Step 4: Final Fixation and Deltoid Closure

- Two appropriately sized cannulated screws with washers are placed over the guide pins (Fig. 14).
- One limb of the previously placed suture is passed through the bone-tendon junction of the greater tuberosity anterior to the fracture line.
- Final radiographic confirmation is obtained.
- The deltoid split is repaired and any portion of the anterior deltoid that was released to the bone of the acromion is reattached.

Procedure: ORIF of Lesser Tuberosity Fracture Through Deltopectoral Approach

Step 1: Superficial Dissection

- A 6- to 8-cm deltopectoral incision is made.
- The cephalic vein is retracted laterally with the deltoid and the pectoralis major is retracted medially.

Step 2: Deep Dissection

- The clavipectoral fascia is incised lateral to the conjoined tendon.

Controversies

- Screw fixation may also be used. If the screw is placed perpendicular to the fracture line, it may require bicortical fixation in relatively soft metaphyseal bone because it often exits lateral to the subchondral bone of the humeral head.

- The axillary nerve is identified and potential high penetration of the musculocutaneous nerve through the conjoined tendon is determined.
- The conjoined tendon is retracted medially and the deltoid laterally.
- The long head of the biceps tendon is identified superior to the pectoralis major insertion and the sheath and rotator interval are incised to the supraglenoid tubercle.
- A soft tissue biceps tenodesis to the upper border of the pectoralis major insertion is performed and the long head of the biceps is resected proximally.
- The lesser tuberosity fracture fragment is identified and the anterior humeral circumflex vessels are preserved.

Step 3: Provisional Reduction and Fixation

- Three heavy, nonabsorbable sutures are passed through the subscapularis bone-tendon junction from deep to superficial, starting superiorly and proceeding inferiorly (Fig. 15).
  - This will produce three sutures with one limb superficial and one limb deep to the lesser tuberosity.
- The lesser tuberosity is retracted medially to expose the anatomic neck of the humerus.
- Two suture anchors are placed at the level of the anatomic neck, one adjacent to the superior portion and one adjacent to the inferior portion of the lesser tuberosity fracture bed or footprint (Fig. 16).
  - The sutures are passed from the suture anchors in a mattress configuration from deep to superficial

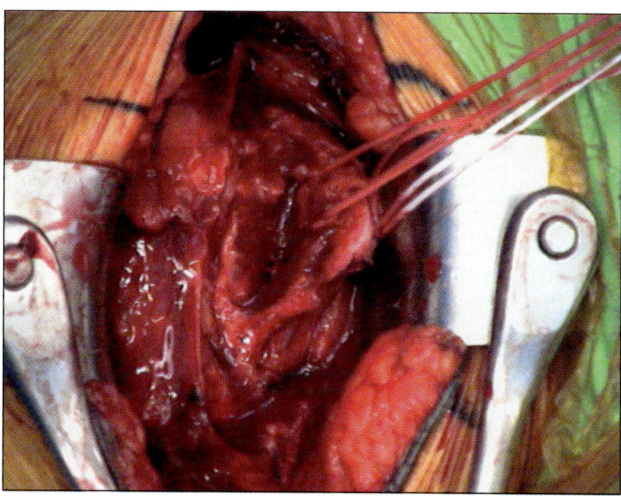

FIGURE 15

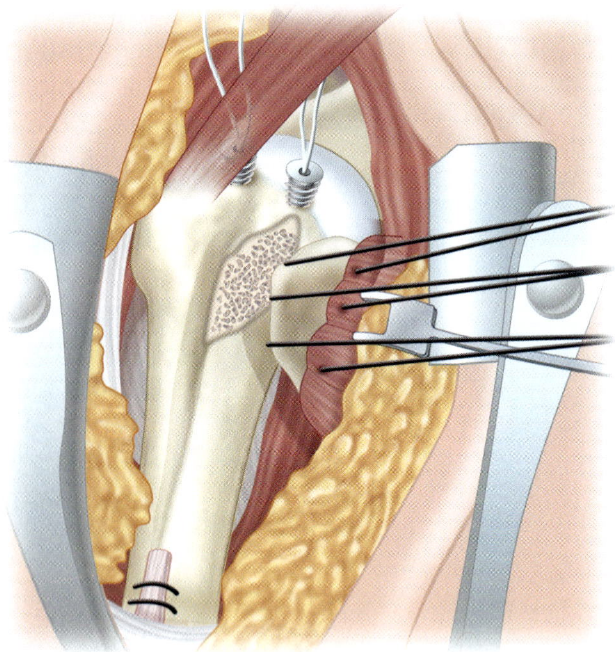

FIGURE 16

through the subscapularis bone-tendon junction, slightly medial to the previously placed nonabsorbable sutures.

- The deep limbs of the three initially placed sutures are passed through the lateral aspect of the fracture surface on the humeral metaphysis, deep to the bicipital groove, and out the lateral cortex, posterior to the bicipital groove. This can usually be done using large, cutting free needles.
- After passing the deep limbs of these three sutures, they are clamped to their partners.

Step 4: Final Fixation

- Three groups of sutures are used to fix the lesser tuberosity (Fig. 17).
  - The single soft tissue–to–soft tissue suture at the rotator interval (*dashed arrow*)
  - The three interfragmentary sutures passed around the lesser tuberosity and through the fracture bed and tied over the bicipital groove (*white arrows*)
  - The two medial sutures in the suture anchors at the anatomic neck (*black arrow*)
- While manually holding the lesser tuberosity in a reduced position, the rotator interval is closed laterally with a nonabsorbable suture. The rotator interval suture is tied first to hold the tuberosity in a reduced postion.

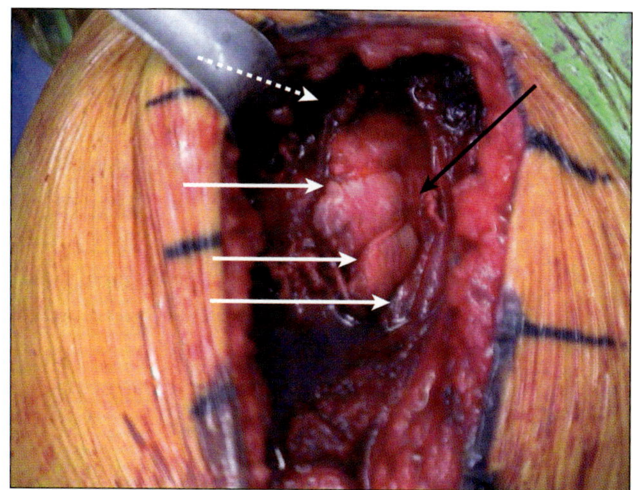

FIGURE 17

PEARLS

- *The rate at which rehabilitation progresses is, in part, a function of intraoperative fracture stability.*
  - The patient can be seen once between the first postoperative visit (7-10 days) and the 6-week postoperative mark to monitor the progress of the rehabilitation.
  - If the patient is compliant and the range of motion is returning as expected, passive exercises during the first 6 weeks can be performed at home.
- *Examine for neurologic injury closely during the first 6 weeks.*
- *Follow hardware position and fracture reduction closely.*

PITFALLS

- *Unrecognized neurologic injury.*
- *Unrecognized or underappreciated loss of reduction or hardware penetration.*
- *Overzealous rehabilitation, especially in the first 6 weeks.*

- The suture anchor sutures are tied second to prevent over-reduction when the last sutures are tied.
- The three interfragmentary sutures around the lesser tuberosity are tied last.
- Reduction is confirmed with the C-arm.

Postoperative Care and Expected Outcomes

- The postoperative care is similar for all procedures, assuming stable fixation was attained.
- The general philosophy regarding postoperative care is to allow a short period of healing, perform progressive passive range of motion for the first 6-8 weeks, and then add active range of motion, strengthening exercises, and a gradual return to activities.
- Complete recovery may take up to 1 year.
- Follow-up radiographs are taken at 7-10 days, 3 weeks, 6 weeks, 3 months, 6 months, and 1 year.
- Specific postoperative care:
  - 7-10 days: sling for comfort, pendulum exercises
  - 10 days–6 weeks: supine passive elevation, passive external rotation, pendulum exercises
  - 6-8 weeks: add passive end-range stretching and overhead pulley
  - 8-12 weeks: add active range of motion; rotator cuff, deltoid, and scapular muscle strengthening
  - 12-24 weeks: gradual return to activities
- Potential complications:
  - Loss of reduction
  - Hardware migration or intra-articular penetration

Controversies

- The frequency with which radiographs are taken is controversial. Radiographs at three time points within the first 6 weeks are justified because hardware problems and loss of reduction are most likely to occur and most easily addressed in this time frame.
- The timing, aggressiveness, and setting of postoperative rehabilitation is controversial.
  - There may not be one correct protocol for all patients, and rehabilitation must be individualized.
  - Weigh fracture stability, progression of range of motion on follow-up visits, and patient factors such as compliance, age, and bone quality to dictate rehabilitation decisions.

- Nonunion
- Malunion
- Avascular necrosis
- Posttraumatic arthritis
- Frozen shoulder
- Rotator cuff tear
- Nerve injury
- Complex regional pain syndrome (reflex sympathetic dystrophy)
- Vascular injury
- Infection

Evidence

Brunner F, Sommer C, et al. Open reduction and internal fixation of proximal humerus fractures using a proximal humeral locked plate: a prospective multicenter analysis. J Orthop Trauma. 2009;23:163-72.

In this study, 157 patients with 158 fractures treated with ORIF with a proximal humeral locking plate were followed for 1 year. Primary screw perforation was the most frequent problem (14%), followed by secondary screw perforation (8%) and avascular necrosis (8%). Mean Constant score was 72 points and mean Disabilities of the Arm, Shoulder, and Hand (DASH) score was 16 points. Good functional outcome can be expected. More accurate length measurement and shorter screw selection should prevent primary screw perforation. (Level IV evidence)

Egol KA, Ong CC, et al. Early complications in proximal humerus fractures (OTA Types 11) treated with locked plates. J Orthop Trauma. 2008;22:159-64.

Fifty-one consecutive patients treated with a proximal humerus locking plate for fracture or nonunion were analyzed for the development of an intraoperative, acute postoperative, or delayed postoperative complication. Radiographically, 92% of the cases united at 3 months after surgery, and two fractures had signs of osteonecrosis at latest follow-up. Sixteen complications were seen in 12 patients (24%). Eight shoulders in eight patients (16%) had screws that penetrated the humeral head. Two patients developed osteonecrosis at latest follow-up. The major complication reported in this study was screw penetration, suggesting that exceptional vigilance must be taken in estimating the appropriate number and length of screws used to prevent articular penetration. (Level III evidence)

Flatow EL, Cuomo F, et al. Open reduction and internal fixation of two-part displaced fractures of the greater tuberosity of the proximal part of the humerus. J Bone Joint Surg [Am]. 1991;73:1213-8.

Twelve patients, ranging in age from 34 to 72 years (average, 53 years), were evaluated at an average of 5 years (range, 2-8 years) after ORIF of a two-part displaced fracture of the greater tuberosity of the proximal part of the humerus. The anterosuperior deltoid-splitting approach, combined with rotation of the humerus, allowed adequate exposure of the retracted tuberosity. Internal fixation of the greater tuberosity with heavy, nonabsorbable sutures and careful repair of the rotator cuff permitted early passive motion. All fractures healed without postoperative displacement. Six patients had an excellent result and six had a good result; active elevation averaged 170°. There was one partial, transient palsy of the axillary nerve. (Level IV evidence)

Keener JD, Parsons BO, et al. Outcomes after percutaneous reduction and fixation of proximal humeral fractures. J Shoulder Elbow Surg. 2007;16:330-8.

This study included 35 patients from three institutions. Of these, 27 were followed up for a minimum of 1 year after surgery. The mean age at injury was 61 years. There were 7 two-part, 8 three-part, and 12 valgus-impacted four-part proximal humeral fractures. All fractures were reduced and stabilized with percutaneous techniques only. All fractures healed after the index procedure. The mean American Shoulder and Elbow Surgeons and Constant scores were 83.4 and 73.9, respectively. Four patients healed with malunion, and in four, glenohumeral joint osteoarthritis developed. (Level IV evidence)

Koike Y, Komatsuda T, et al. Internal fixation of proximal humeral fractures with a Polarus humeral nail. J Orthop Traumatol. 2008;9:135-9.

In this study, 54 shoulders of 54 patients (44 females, 10 males) underwent intramedullary fixation using the Polarus humeral nail. Fracture type by Neer classification was two-part in 29 shoulders, three-part in 22 shoulders, and four-part in 3 shoulders. All the shoulders after osteosynthesis obtained bone union. There was no osteonecrosis of the humeral head. Functional outcome measured by JOA score averaged 81 points; 43 patients (79%) had satisfactory to excellent results. Varus deformity was seen in four shoulders (8%) and deformity of the greater tuberosity in four (8%). (Level IV evidence)

Rowles DJ, McGrory JE. Percutaneous pinning of the proximal part of the humerus: an anatomic study. J Bone Joint Surg [Am]. 2001;83:1695-9.

In 10 fresh frozen cadaveric shoulders, the intact proximal part of the humerus was pinned under fluoroscopic guidance with use of an identical published technique. The proximal lateral pins were located at a mean distance of 3 mm from the anterior branch of the axillary nerve. Four of the 20 lateral pins were noted to penetrate the articular cartilage of the humeral head. The anterior pins were located at a mean distance of 2 mm from the tendon of the long head of the biceps (perforating the tendon in three specimens) and of 11 mm from the cephalic vein (perforating the vein in one specimen). The proximal tuberosity pins were located at a mean distance of 6 and 7 mm from the axillary nerve and the posterior humeral circumflex artery (tenting the structures in two specimens with internal rotation), respectively.

Sudkamp N, Bayer J, et al. Open reduction and internal fixation of proximal humeral fractures with use of the locking proximal humerus plate: results of a prospective, multicenter, observational study. J Bone Joint Surg [Am]. 2009;91:1320-8.

In this study, 187 patients (mean age, 62.9 ± 15.7 years) with an acute proximal humeral fracture were managed with open reduction and internal fixation with a locking proximal humeral plate. The Constant and DASH scores were determined for the injured and contralateral extremities at the time of the 1-year follow-up. The mean Constant score for the injured side was 70.6 ± 13.7 points, corresponding to 85.1% ± 14.0% of the score for the contralateral side. The mean DASH score was 15.2 ± 16.8 points. Sixty-two complications were encountered in 52 of 155 patients (34%) at the time of the 1-year follow-up. The most common complication, noted in 21 of 155 patients (14%), was intraoperative screw perforation of the humeral head. (Level IV evidence)

Visser CP, Coene LN, et al. Nerve lesions in proximal humeral fractures. J Shoulder Elbow Surg. 2001;10:421-7.

For this study, 143 consecutive proximal humeral fractures due to low-velocity trauma were included. According to the Neer classification, 93 were nondisplaced and 50 were displaced fractures. Denervation on the electromyogram was found in 96 patients (67%). The nerves most frequently involved were the axillary nerve (83 [58%]) and the suprascapular nerve (69 [48%]). Frequently a combination of nerve lesions was seen. Nerve lesions were much more frequent in displaced fractures (82% [41/50]) than in nondisplaced fractures (59% [55/93]). (Level III evidence)

PROCEDURE 30

Open Reduction and Internal Fixation of Three- and Four-Part Proximal Humerus Fractures

Julie Y. Bishop and Joseph Mileti

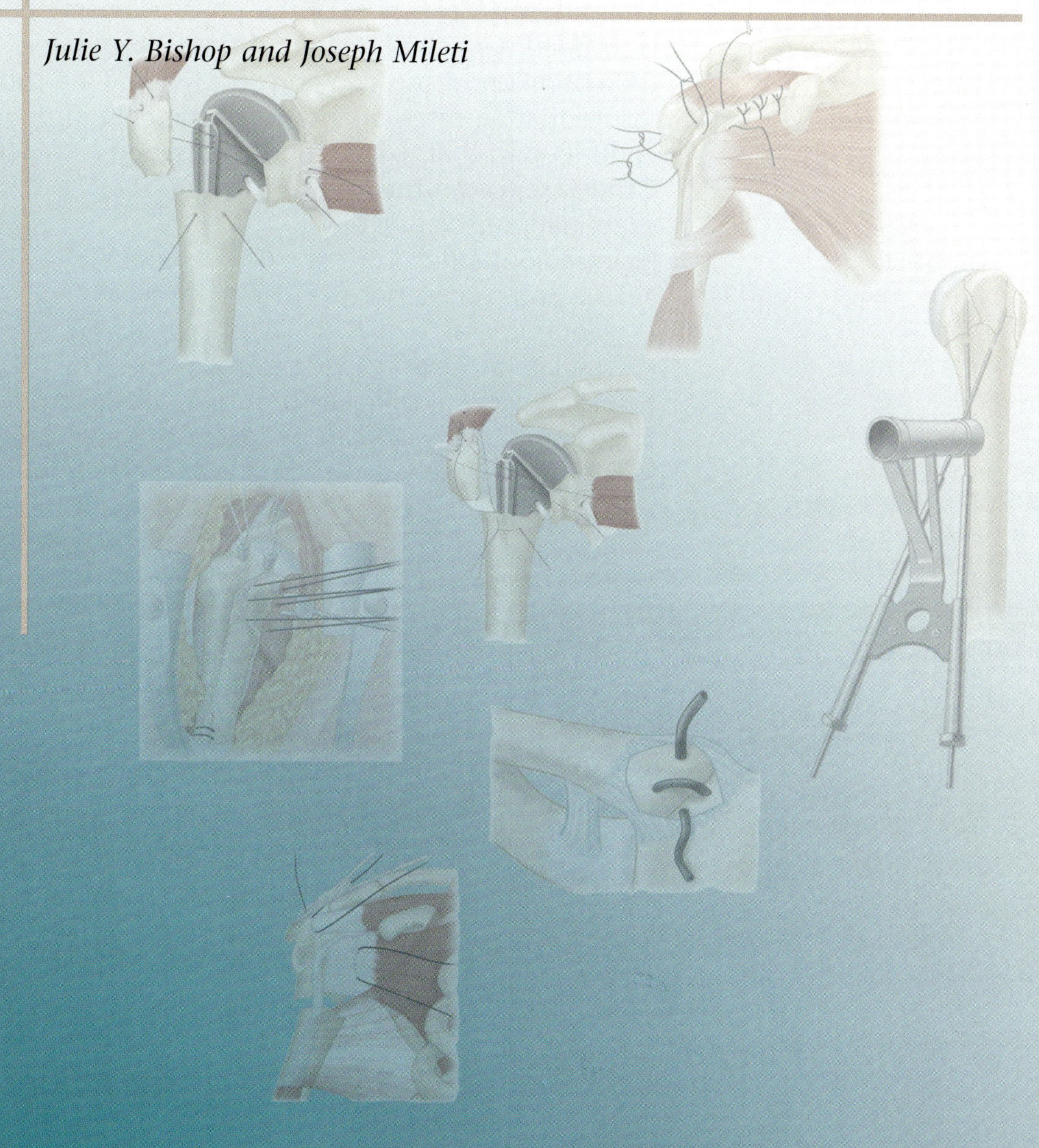

PITFALLS

- *Three-part fracture-dislocation of the proximal humerus*
- *Displaced four-part proximal humerus fractures, especially with the humeral head in varus alignment*
- *Very osteoporotic bone (may not be amenable to plate fixation)*
- *Substantial comminution of the medial calcar with loss of periosteal sleeve/hinge*

Controversies

- Substantial comminution of the GT
- The degree of osteoporotic bone that is acceptable for plate fixation

Indications

- Displaced/unstable three-part proximal humerus fractures that primarily involve displacement of the greater tuberosity (GT) and the shaft of the humerus.
- Four-part proximal humerus fractures are occasionally included if there is minimal displacement of one of the tuberosities, most often a nondisplaced crack in the lesser tuberosity (LT).

Examination/Imaging

- The most crucial aspect of the physical examination is to document the function of the axillary nerve and the condition of the skin and soft tissue. One should assure that all three quadrants of the deltoid do contract and that axillary nerve sensation is intact. Otherwise, given the known fracture, the examination is very limited.
- Plain radiographs
  - True anteroposterior (AP) view of the glenohumeral joint (Fig. 1A).
  - True lateral view in the scapular plane (Fig. 1B).
  - Axillary view: if difficult to obtain, a Velpeau axillary lateral view can be taken.
  - The true AP view is very important to determine accurately the degree of GT displacement. Often

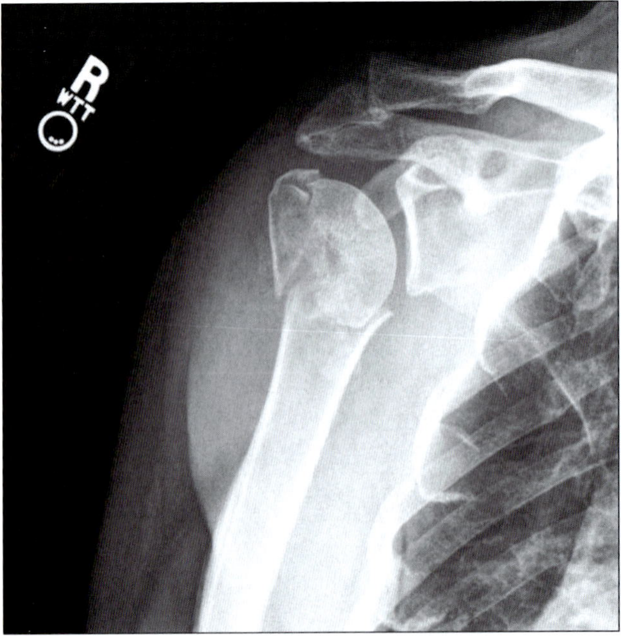

A

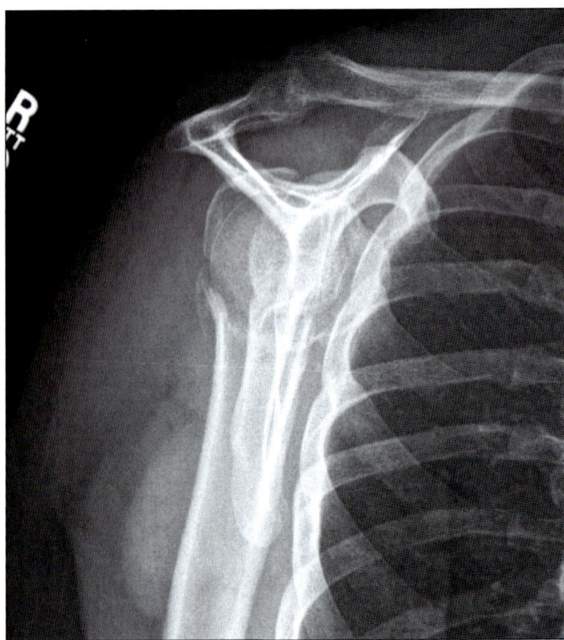

B

FIGURE 1

Treatment Options

- Nonoperative treatment is often acceptable in the older, sedentary patient provided enough overlap between shaft and humeral head exists for healing.
- Percutaneous pin fixation can be utilized for this fracture pattern.
- Heavy suture fixation alone is occasionally an option.

this view is taken with the arm in internal rotation and thus a profile view of the GT is not obtained (Fig. 2). In this circumstance, the treating physician may need to position the arm if the radiographic technician is not familiar with the correct technique to obtain this view. The arm is gently externally rotated about 20° and an AP of the scapula is taken (Fig. 3). The lateral view allows an

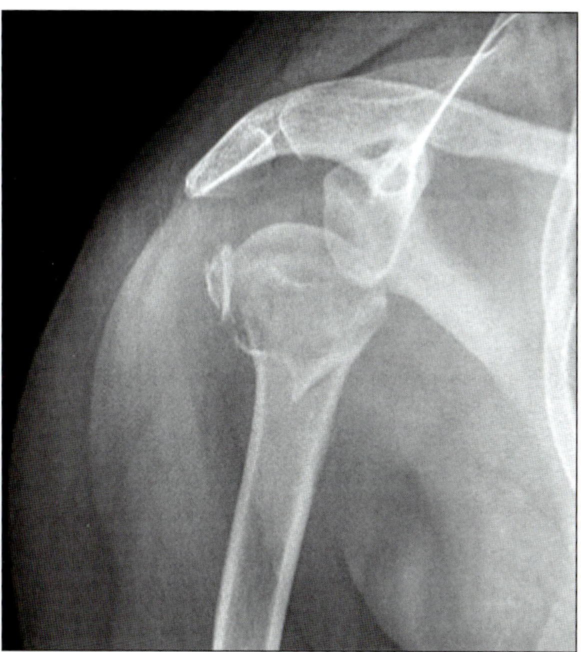

FIGURE 2

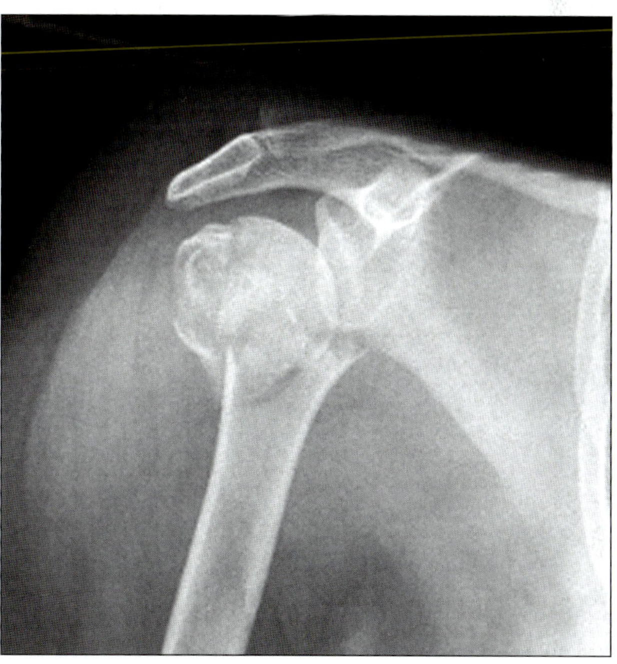

FIGURE 3

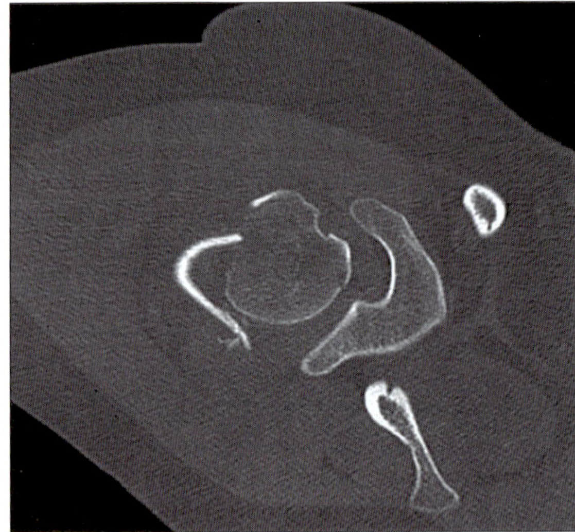

A

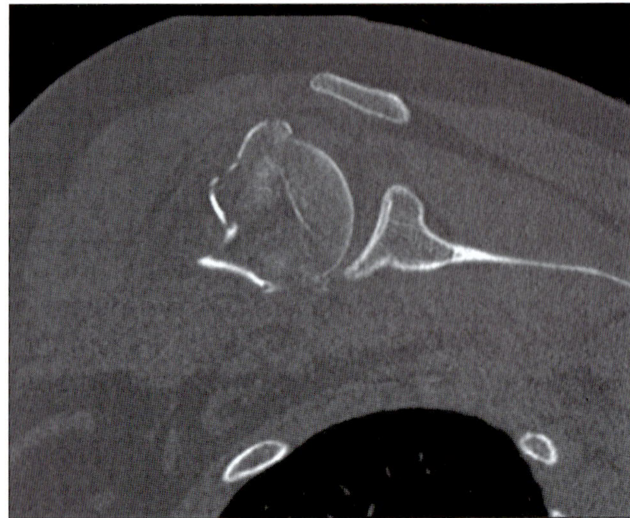

B

FIGURE 4

accurate determination regarding the angulation and degree of anterior displacement of the humeral shaft.

- Computed tomography (CT)
  - Although not always essential, CT scanning can allow more a detailed assessment of the degree of tuberosity involvement (especially any nondisplaced cracks into the LT) and any articular surface involvement.
  - Figure 4A shows a CT scan of the fracture in Figures 2 and 3, revealing a small crack in the LT, and the CT scan in Figure 4B shows the degree of displacement of the GT.

Surgical Anatomy

- The deltopectoral interval must be accurately identified, as inappropriate dissection planes can lead to severe denervation of the anterior quadrant of the deltoid.
- The coracoid and conjoined tendon must be identified because medial dissection to these structures may result in neurovascular damage (Fig. 5).
- The long head of the biceps (LHB) must be identified; it can be found just medial to the pectoralis major insertion (Fig. 6A; Freer elevator is on the LHB). This is an important anatomic landmark that can guide accurate fracture reduction, but also, this structure can be trapped in the fracture site, blocking reduction (Fig. 6B).

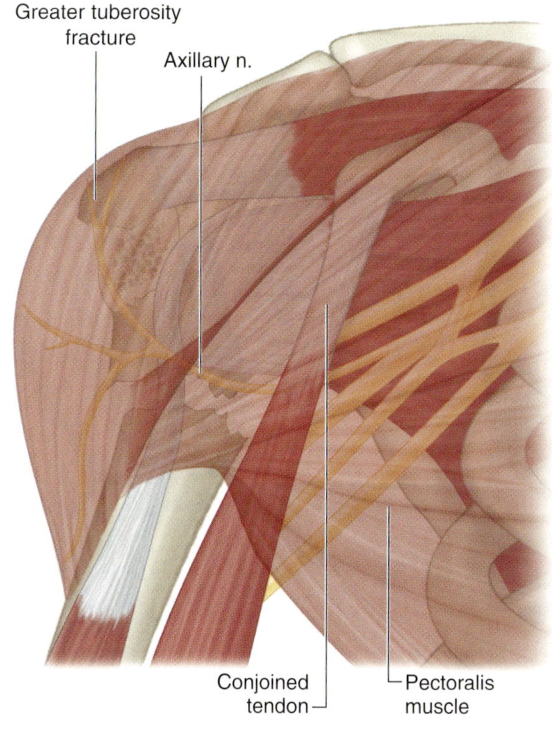

FIGURE 5

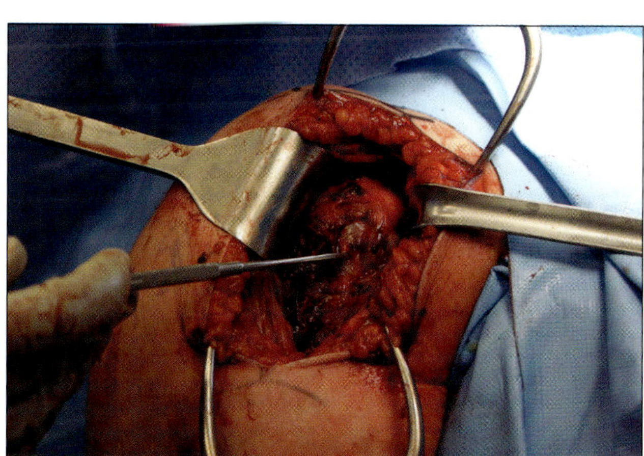

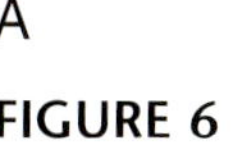

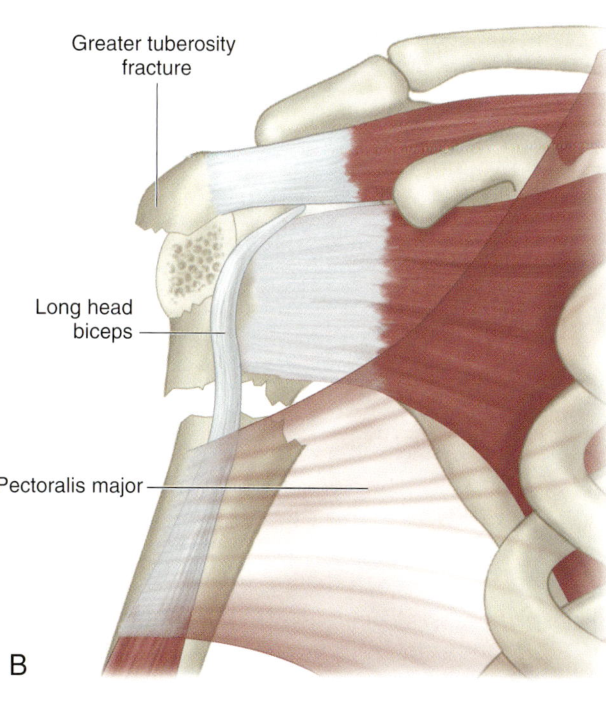

A B

FIGURE 6

- The axillary nerve must be identified in both locations:
  - Anteriorly in an inferior location to the subscapularis.
  - Posteriorly as it innervates the deltoid.
  - Care must be taken to avoid injury to the nerve when retracting the deltoid to gain exposure of a posteriorly displaced GT and when retracting anteriorly to expose and reduce the surgical neck.
- The subscapularis insertion onto the lesser tuberosity must be identified; it will most often be attached to the humeral head (HH) and not a displaced fragment.
- The GT fragment and the facets of the supraspinatus, infraspinatus, and teres minor and the corresponding rotator cuff attachments must be identified.
- The GT fracture line is almost always just posterior to the bicipital groove, another reason it is key to locate the LHB in the groove.

Equipment

- An appropriate shoulder/beach chair table that allows C-arm imaging
- Potentially an armholder/positioner that will not interfere with the image

Controversies

- Some debate exists as to whether the mini C-arm (Fig. 8A) or large C-arm (Fig. 8B) is more appropriate. The surgeon should try both and make the determination as to which one he or she is more comfortable using, as both can work well.

Positioning

- Beach chair positioning is commonly utilized for fracture fixation (Fig. 7).
- The beach chair positioner used must allow an unobstructed view of the proximal humerus for use of the C-arm for image intensification.
- An armholder may be used, but must not interfere with the C-arm.
- A padded Mayo stand can be used as well to support the arm; it can be easily adjusted for height and can move in and out.
- The patient's entire arm is prepped out for the surgery.

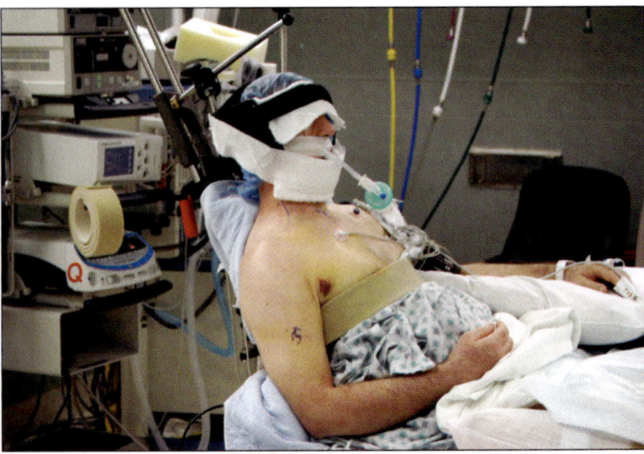

FIGURE 7

PEARLS

- *Bring the C-arm in first, prior to draping, to assure you are able to obtain appropriate intraoperative views—this key to a good outcome.*
- *The C-arm is often brought in from above the patient's head; assure there is enough space in the operating room for the machine.*
- *Make sure the C-arm screen is positioned so one can easily view the images.*
- *Assure that the patient's arm is draped out free from obstruction. If it is necessary to convert for any reason to a hemiarthroplasty, the surgeon must be able to extend, adduct, and externally rotate the arm to produce the shaft.*

PITFALLS

- *Care must be taken prior to draping the patient to absolutely assure one can obtain the images needed given the position the patient is in and the table the patient is on.*
- *Attention must be paid to the position of the patient's head, as the C-arm can push into the patient's head while rotating to obtain the correct image.*

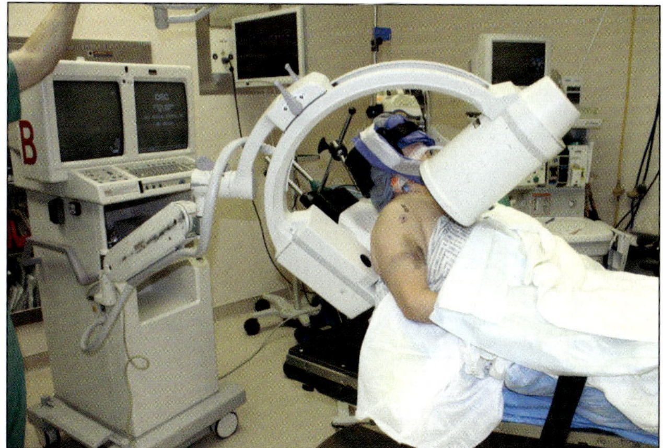

A

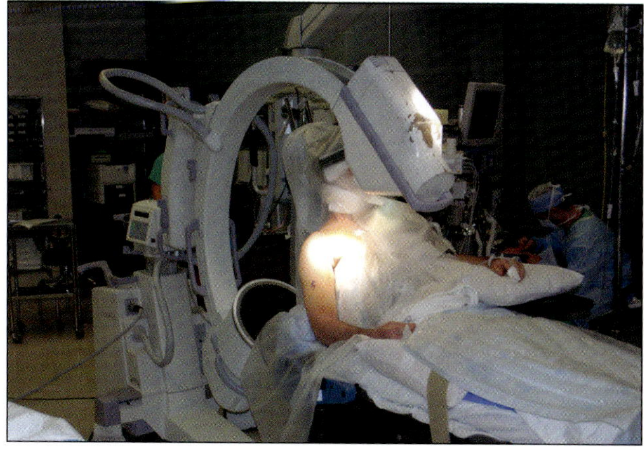

B

FIGURE 8

Pearls

- *The deltopectoral interval can be hard to find in the trauma situation; it is typically more medial than one expects.*
- *Rarely is the cephalic vein injured by the trauma; one should be able to find it.*
- *The LHB is a key structure: Always find it to assist with understanding the anatomy.*
- *Remember to minimize soft tissue stripping medially except as needed for reduction.*

Pitfalls

- *Frustration in finding the deltopectoral interval can cause one to erroneously create a new interval in the anterior quadrant of the deltoid.*
  - *This will limit exposure.*
  - *It also leads to deltoid atrophy/denervation.*
- *Failure to adequately clear fracture hematoma and early adhesion formation out from the SA space can interfere with accurate evaluation of the GT fragment.*

Portals/Exposures

- A deltopectoral approach is utilized (Fig. 9).
  - The incision is marked out ahead of time based on the location of the coracoid.
  - Swelling can affect the normal appearance of the shoulder and the expected position of the key landmarks.
- The deltopectoral interval and the cephalic vein are located (Fig. 10).
  - Swelling from the trauma can distort the anatomy.
  - The cephalic vein is located and taken either medial or lateral according to surgeon preference.

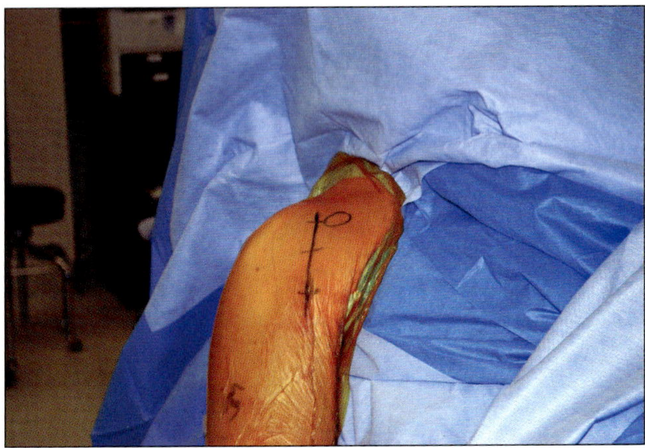

FIGURE 9

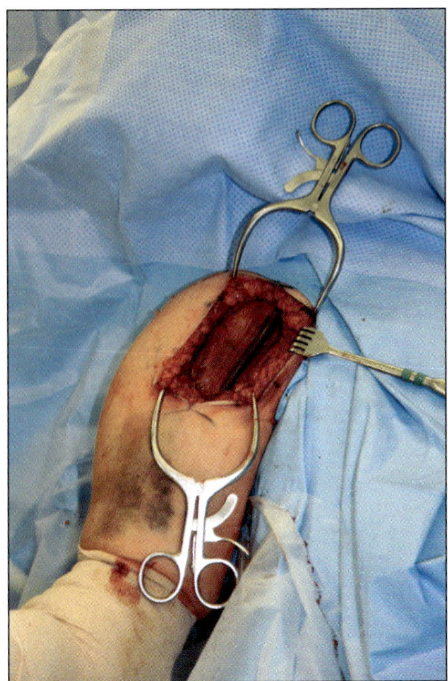

FIGURE 10

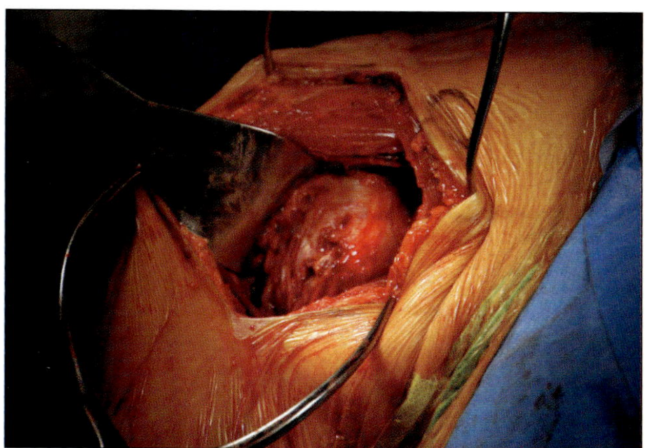
A

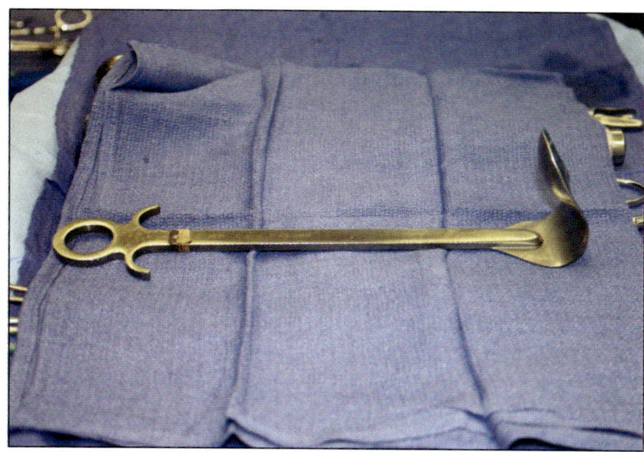
B

FIGURE 11

Instrumentation

- Specific instruments are available to retract the deltoid; they are very helpful with the exposure and will facilitate the procedure (Fig. 11B).

Pearls

- *The rotator cuff tendon is stronger than the tuberosities. The suture must be placed at the tendon-bone interface; do not attempt to place suture through the bone of the tuberosity.*

Pitfalls

- *The GT is often comminuted and/or osteoporotic; take care when handling it and try to only mobilize through sutures in the tendon.*

- The deltoid is retracted (Fig. 11A).
  - The area is irrigated to remove any hematoma.
  - Any subdeltoid adhesions are freed.
  - An appropriate retractor is placed.
- The coracoid and conjoined tendon are localized.
  - The conjoined tendon is gently freed off the underlying subscapularis. Often gentle finger dissection is best.
  - The conjoined tendon is retracted.
- The LT is identified.
  - The biceps tendon is localized and followed up in the bicipital groove (see Fig. 6A).
  - Its position is identified in relation to the shaft fracture and shaft displacement (rotation and angulation).
  - The LT is palpated—just medial is the subscapularis insertion.
- The GT is identified.
  - Any hematoma is cleared from the subacromial (SA) space.
  - The coracoacromial (CA) ligament is located.
  - The SA space is bluntly cleared by placing either one's finger or a blunt instrument such as a Cobb elevator under the CA ligament into the SA space.
  - Again, the LHB can be used to help identify the GT fracture as the fracture line is typically posterior to the groove.

Procedure

Step 1

- The tuberosities are mobilized.
- Lesser tuberosity

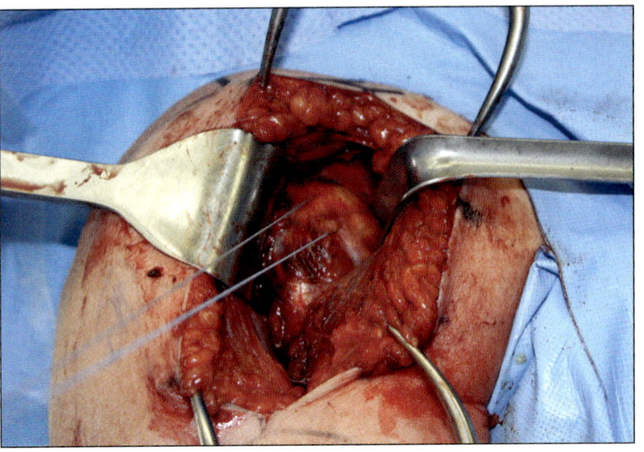

A

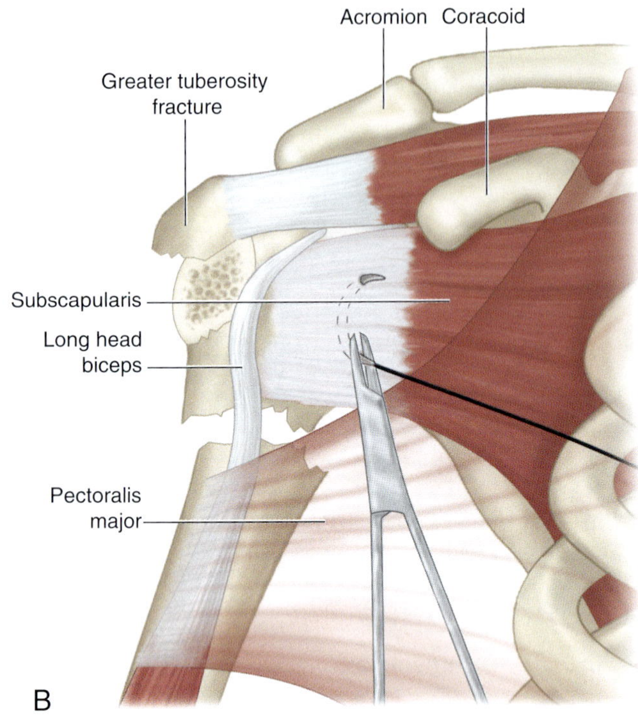

B

FIGURE 12

Instrumentation/ Implantation

- Use heavy suture to control the tuberosities.
- Use a large enough needle when placing the suture; otherwise, it will be difficult to pass the posterior suture in the infraspinatus (Fig. 14).

- The HH-LT complex is often internally rotated due to the unopposed pull of the subscapularis.
- Using heavy suture (#2 or #5 heavy suture), one or two vertical stitches are placed at the tendon-bone interface of the subscapularis (Fig. 12A and 12B).
- If the LT is not fractured or displaced, these stitches will provide traction to control rotation of the HH-LT complex.
- If the LT is cracked, it is typically nondisplaced and the soft tissue envelope is entirely intact.

- Greater tuberosity
  - The surgeon must assure that the fracture hematoma is cleared and a good view of the GT is possible. It is often posterior/superior and better seen if the arm is internally rotated and levered a bit against the deltoid retractor.
  - One heavy suture is placed at the tendon-bone interface of the supraspinatus facet. This will allow the surgeon to pull the GT more anterior, making the next pass into the infraspinatus a little easier.
  - A second suture is placed at the tendon-bone interface of the infraspinatus facet (Fig. 13A and 13B).

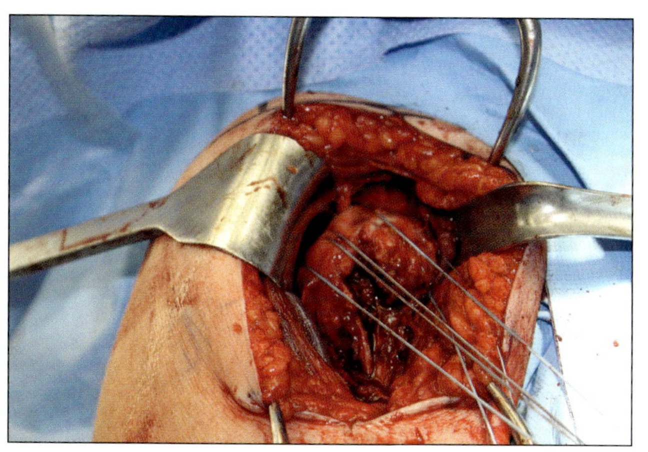
A

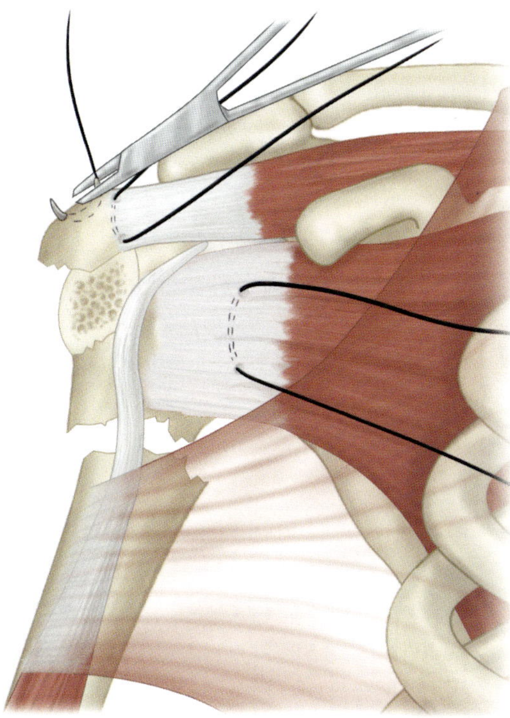
B

FIGURE 13

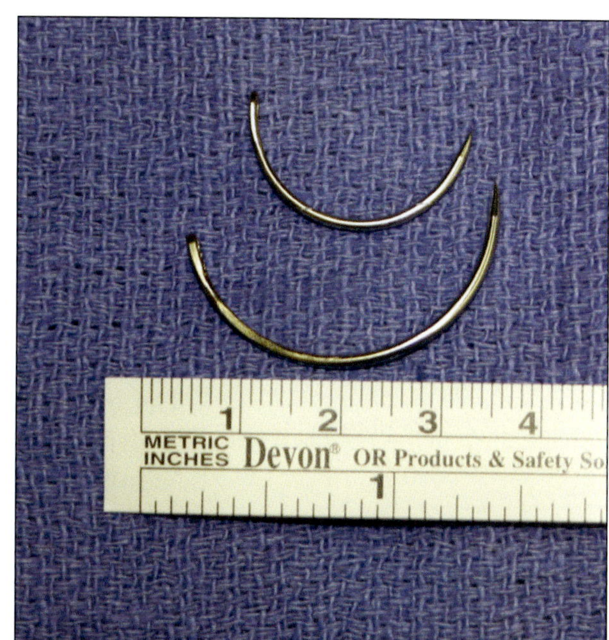

FIGURE 14

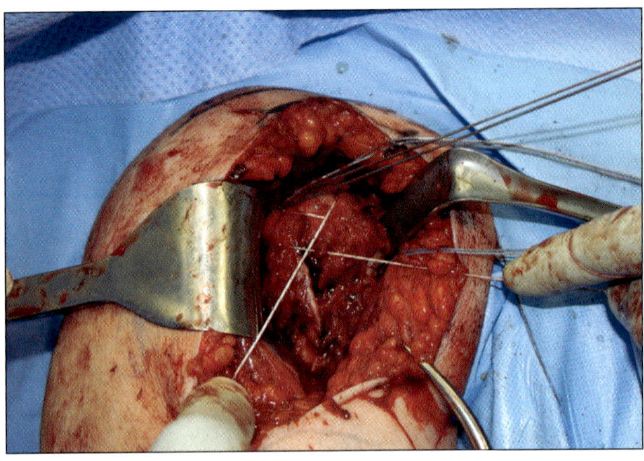

A

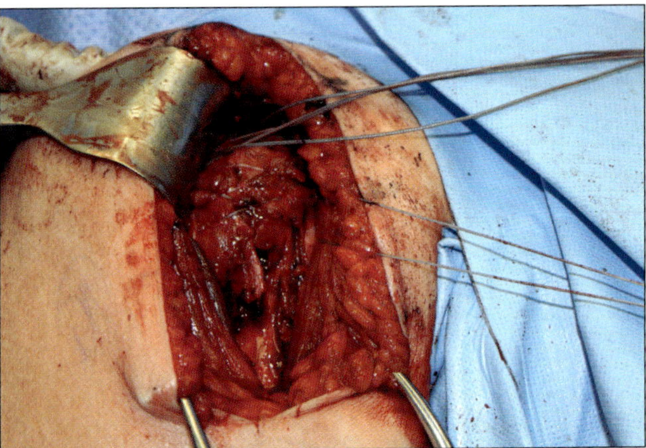

B

FIGURE 15

Pearls

- *Again, use the biceps as a landmark for tuberosity reduction. The bicipital groove is most often with the HH-LT complex.*
- *There is often a well-defined metaphyseal spike on the GT fragment that can be used to assist in keying the GT into place.*

Pitfalls

- *Take care not to over-reduce the GT, which can occur if one pulls too hard inferiorly on the traction sutures.*
- *Make sure that some traction sutures are available to reduce the HH to the shaft—do not use them all when reducing the tuberosities.*

Instrumentation/ Implantation

- If the HH is tipped into valgus, a Cobb elevator or similar instrument can be used to lever the head up.

Step 2

- The tuberosities are reduced (Fig. 15A and 15B).
  - Traction stitches at the tendon-bone interfaces of both tuberosities can be used to aid in reduction.
  - Pulling on the stitches in the subscapularis will externally rotate the HH out to the GT. Pulling anteriorly and inferiorly on the GT stitches will bring the GT around to reduce.
  - The biceps can be used as a landmark to line up the tuberosities.
  - If the rotator interval is open due to the degree of GT displacement, this can be used to evaluate GT reduction.
- The GT can then be repaired to the HH-LT complex with a heavy figure-of-8 suture at the tendon-bone interface of both tuberosities.
- The C-arm should be brought in to confirm the reduction prior to securing the suture fixation.
- Special care should be taken for the valgus-impacted HH.
  - It may be difficult to reduce the GT anatomically until the HH is out of valgus. A Cobb elevator or similar instrument can be used to lever the head up. Figure 16 shows a Cobb elevator through a GT fracture site pushing the HH out of valgus (Fig. 16A and 16B), and the head tipped out of valgus (Fig. 16C).
  - Bone graft can be considered to help support the reduced valgus HH in very osteopenic bone.
  - The medial periosteal sleeve is typically intact in this situation. It can be used as a hinge to reduce the valgus-impacted fracture.

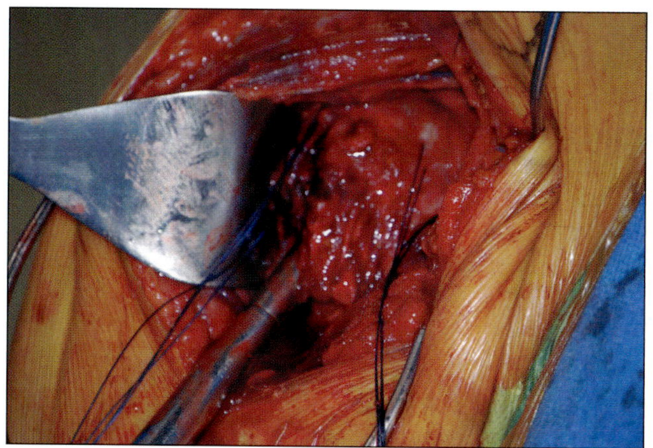

A

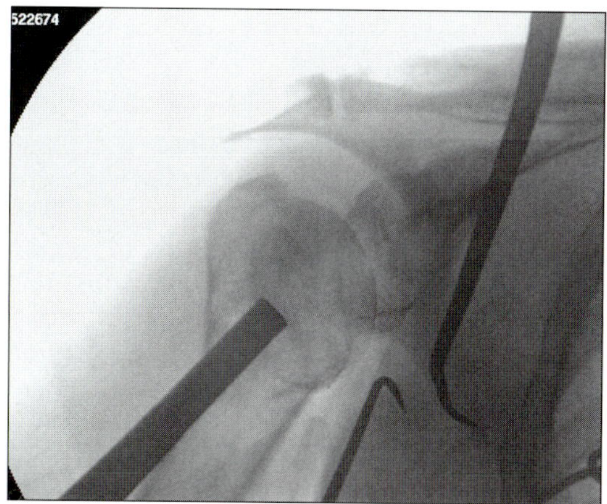

B

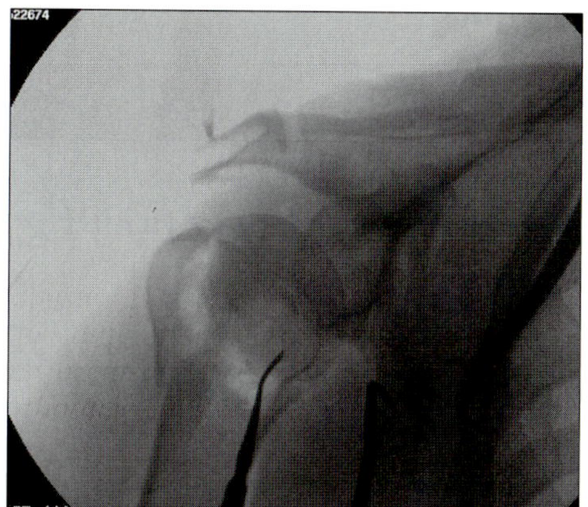

C

FIGURE 16

Step 3

- The HH-LT complex can now be reduced to the shaft, which is typically displaced medially and anteriorly, due to the pull of the pectoralis major. Again, the LHB can be used to assist with an anatomic reduction.
- The metaphyseal spike of the GT fragment will aid in keying the HH into the shaft anatomically (Fig. 17; Freer elevator is on the metaphyseal spike on the GT).
- If the HH construct is sitting in varus in relation to the shaft, the traction sutures still in the GT can be used to pull the head out of varus as reduction is obtained and the plate placed.
- The appropriate-size proximal humerus locking plate is selected: Typically fractures involving the surgical neck do not need a long locking plate and the standard size is adequate, with most allowing three bicortical screws in the shaft.

Pearls

- *Try to key the shaft just inside the HH to add to stability to the reduction.*
- *Over-reducing the GT on the shaft a few millimeters is acceptable.*
- *If the medial calcar is comminuted, impacting the shaft into the HH can add to stability.*

Pitfalls

- *If the lateral cortex of the shaft is reduced lateral to the HH-LT complex, there is a higher risk of the head falling into varus and the construct failing.*
- *Any soft tissue interposition can interfere with reduction.*
- *Remember to limit medial dissection and soft tissue stripping.*

Instrumentation/ Implantation

- Several proximal humerus locking plate systems exist and are acceptable for use.
- Make sure that you have a hemiarthroplasty system on backup in the event a HH resurfacing is needed.

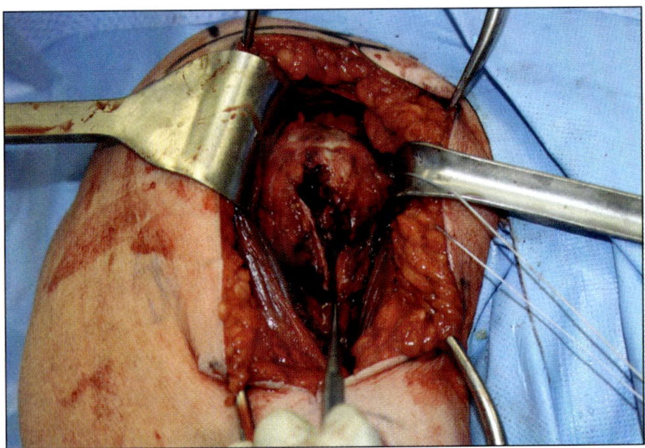

FIGURE 17

- Sutures can be placed through small Kirschner wire (K-wire)/suture holes on the plate prior to placing the plate on the humerus; they will be tied at the conclusion of fixation (Fig. 18).

Step 4

- The plate is provisionally fixed to the reduced construct with K-wires; or, some prefer to hold plate in place with the guide for the locking screws (Fig. 19A and 19B). Small holes for K-wires are available at the borders of the plating systems. The plate should be lateral to the bicipital groove and sit flush on the lateral cortex of the GT. The plate can be secured to the shaft with a K-wire as well. The C-arm is brought in to confirm that:
  - The plate is not too superior.
  - The plate is centered on the shaft distally.
  - The reduction is acceptable.

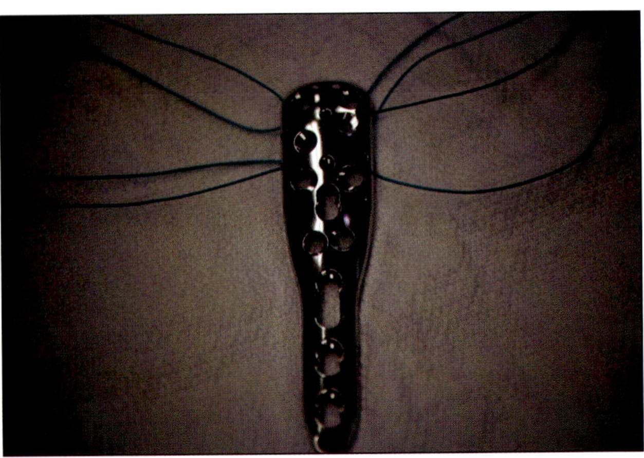

FIGURE 18

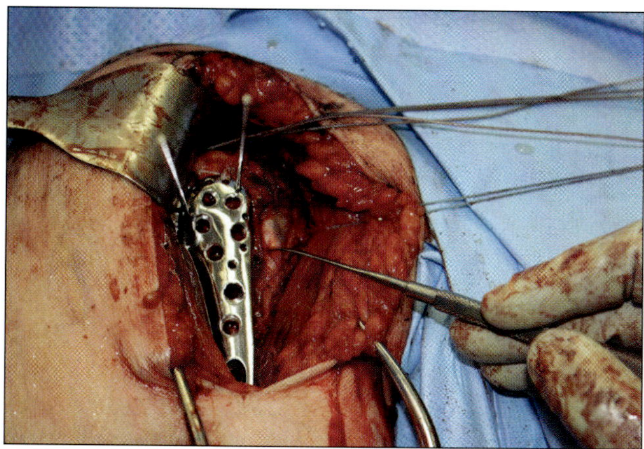

A

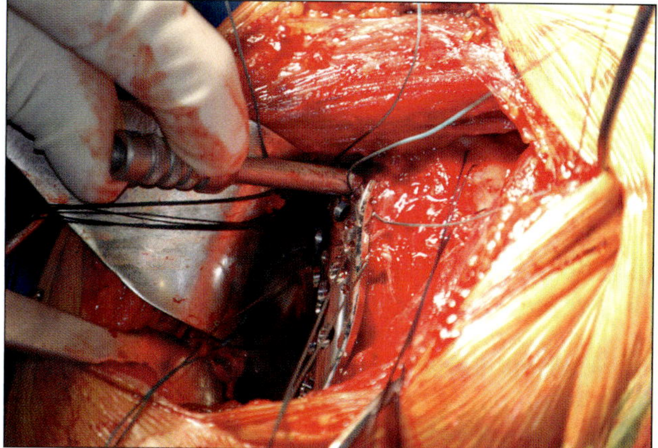

B

FIGURE 19

- Screw placement is done next.
  - A bicortical, nonlocking screw is placed in the shaft, preferably in the slotted hole on the chance that the plate height must be adjusted (Fig. 20). Often prior to placing this screw, the plate is not yet flush against the shaft. This screw will typically compress the plate nicely against the shaft and will lateralize the shaft relative to the HH.
  - The C-arm is brought in to confirm the height of the plate and adjust, if necessary, by loosening the bicortical screw in the slotted hole.
  - The plate is secured to the HH with two locking screws initially.
    - The bone can be very soft in the HH and one must drill very slowly, "tapping" the drill (or K-wire if cannulated screws are used) and stopping immediately upon hitting resistance against the subchondral bone. If the subchondral

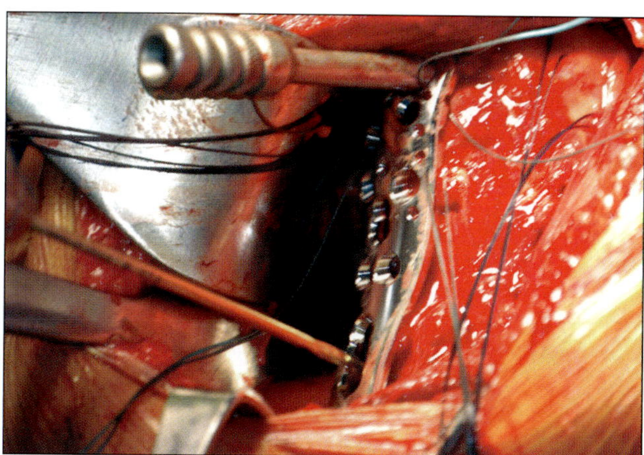

FIGURE 20

Pearls

- *If the subchondral bone is hard to identify, drill under live C-arm imaging. One should try to avoid perforation of the subchondral bone.*
- *The angled screws, in particular the posterior-directed screws, are especially susceptible to penetration through the HH.*

Pitfalls

- *The thickness of the rotator cuff at the supraspinatus facet can be deceiving and lead to placement of the plate too high, where it can impinge against the acromion (Fig. 22). The plate should not be above the actual bone of the GT, which is best identified with imaging. Intraoperatively it may look acceptable because it is still below or at the level of the rotator cuff, when actually it is above the facet.*

Controversies

- Not all proximal humerus locking plates utilize cannulated screws in the HH. If using a drill and a noncannulated screw, the surgeon must assure that he or she does not perforate the subchondral bone with the drill, which can lead to more damage than perforating with a K-wire. But, the drill may allow a better tactile sense of where the subchondral bone starts.

bone is perforated, it is very hard to accurately determine screw length.

- Very osteoporotic bone can be underdrilled well short of the subchondral bone. Osteoporotic bone will allow the depth gauge to penetrate deeper into the subchondral bone while minimizing the risk of HH penetration and still allowing the maximal screw length to be obtained.

- The order of initial reduction above can be reversed.
- Again the C-arm is used to confirm the accuracy of the construct, as the one shaft screw and two screws in the HH are sufficient to allow rotational control to thoroughly check plate position and fracture reduction.
- The remaining screws, which are typically all locking screws, are then placed in the HH. Then the final screws are placed in the shaft.
  - Close attention must be paid to the HH angled locking screw that starts on the shaft, as this screw is often long and can obtain good purchase in the head. The angled locking screw can be drilled into the head under live C-arm imaging to assure accuracy (Fig. 21).
  - Especially with medial comminution and calcar loss, this inferior, angled screw can provide solid support in the inferior HH.

- Final C-arm images are obtained from multiple angles and using live C-arm imaging; the surgeon must absolutely assure that no screws penetrate the articular surface of the HH.

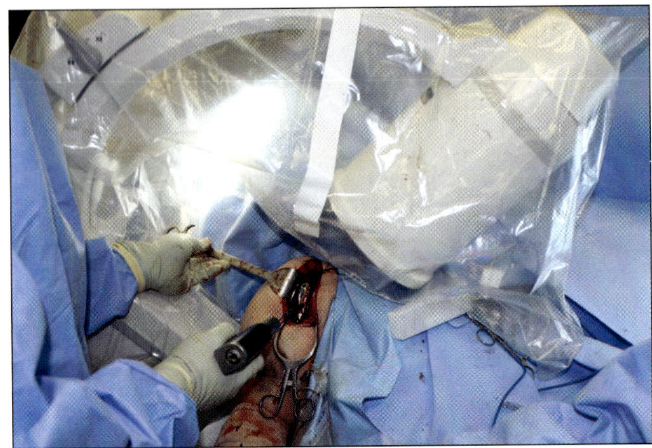

FIGURE 21

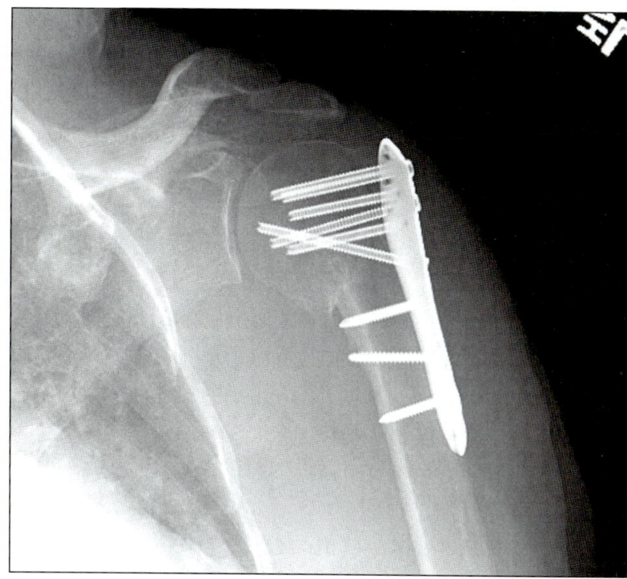

FIGURE 22

Step 5

- For added tuberosity fixation, GT traction stitches are secured through the K-wire holes or empty screw holes on the proximal locking plate.
- Alternatively, sutures that were put into holes on the plate prior to placing the plate can be used (Fig. 23).
- Sutures can be passed with a small free needle and are tied over the plate (Fig. 24).
- One or two lateral sutures are placed to close the rotator interval if opened.
- The final construct is confirmed visually and with C-arm imaging (Fig. 25).
- The wound is irrigated and closed in the standard fashion.

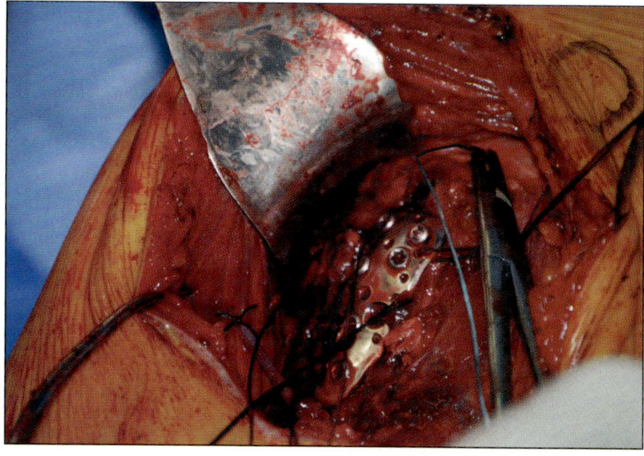

FIGURE 23

Pitfalls

- *The most common complications are*
  - *Unrecognized intraoperative errors, primarily malreduction and screw perforation of the HH, both of which can be avoided with accurate use of imaging intraoperatively.*
  - *Impingement due to high plate placement.*
  - *Hardware failure postoperatively, due to inadequate initial fixation or under-recognition of the degree of osteoporosis.*
  - *Fractures fixed in substantial varus are likely to fail, with the HH falling away from the plate into more varus. In Figure 27, the fracture is fixed in an acceptable amount of varus.*
  - *Avascular necrosis or hardware failure postoperatively due to lack of appreciation for the degree of initial displacement/four-part nature of the fracture.*
  - *Postoperative stiffness due either to plate impingement or generalized postoperative capsulitis.*

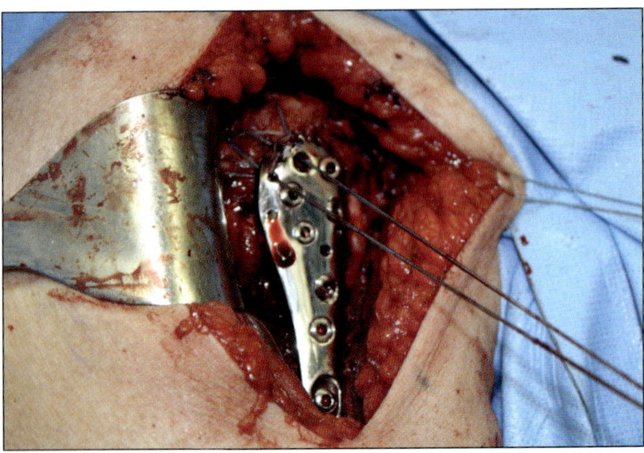

FIGURE 24

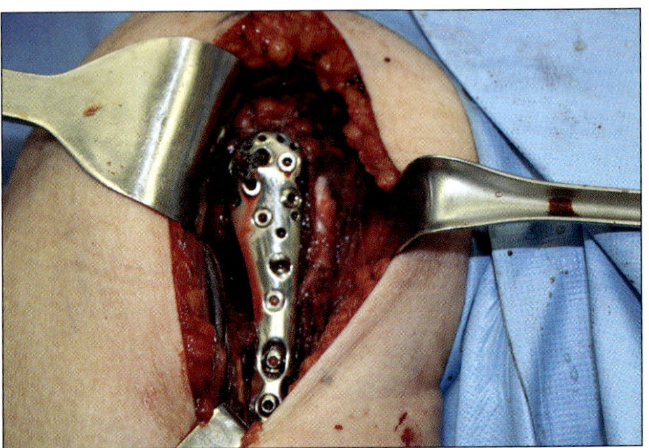

FIGURE 25

Postoperative Care and Expected Outcomes

- The patient is seen at 10 days, 6 weeks, 12 weeks, and 6 months. Radiographs are taken at each visit. Figure 26A and 26B show postoperative radiographs of the same fracture seen in Figures 2–4.
- A postoperative sling is utilized for 6 weeks.
- Ultimate decision making regarding postoperative range of motion (ROM) is based on multiple factors: bone quality, soft tissue quality, security of fixation, and overall patient condition.
- Pendulums and hand/wrist and elbow ROM start immediately.
- Passive ROM typically starts immediately relative to either patient tolerance or limits set within the operating room.

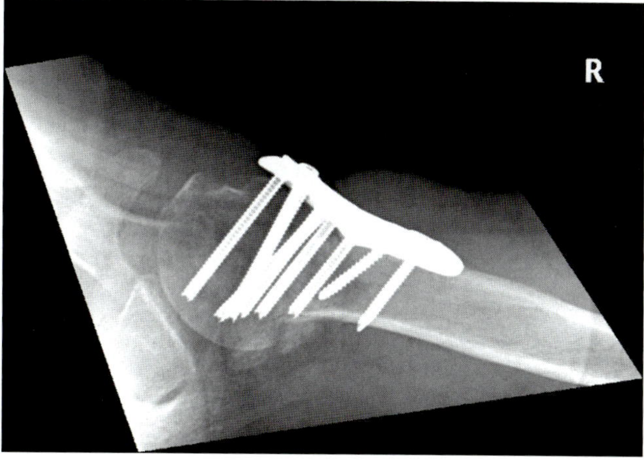

A

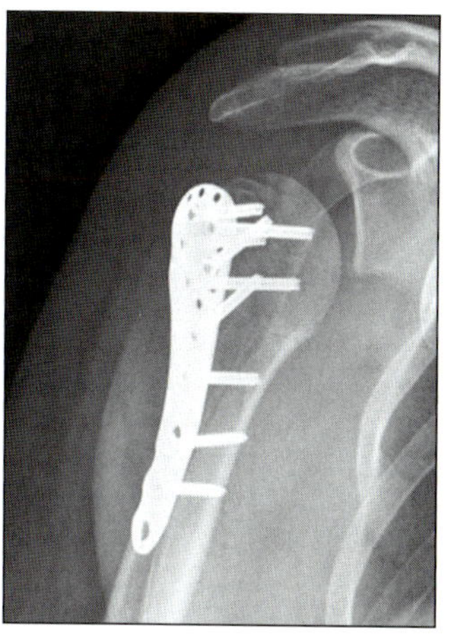

B

FIGURE 26

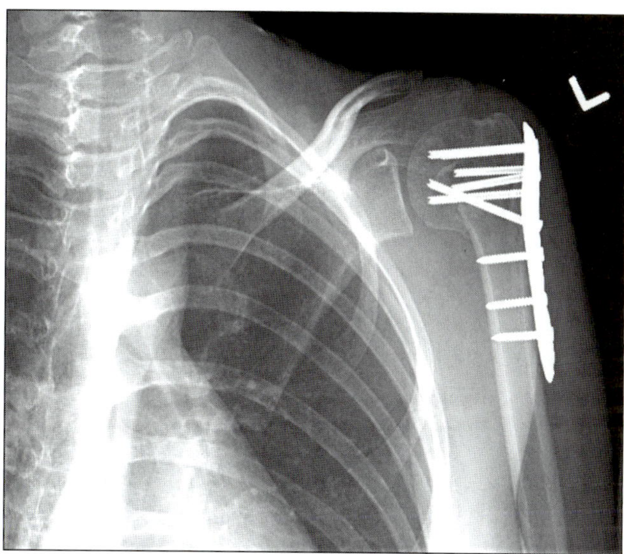

FIGURE 27

- Active-assisted ROM and progression to active ROM can start around week 6 or when evidence of tuberosity healing is seen.
- Terminal stretches and progressive strengthening with Therabands can start at week 12, at which time bone healing is expected. Progression is allowed within pain-free limits.

Evidence

Agudelo J, Schurmann M, Stahel P, et al. Analysis of efficacy and failure of proximal humerus fractures treated with locking plates. J Orthop Trauma. 2007;21:676-81.

This was a retrospective study of 153 patients treated with a proximal humerus locking plate for a displaced proximal humerus fracture. Loss of fixation primarily occurred in the presence of varus malreduction, and a neck-shaft angle of greater than 120° was recommended to maintain fixation and reduction. (Level IV evidence)

Bjorkenheim JM, Pajarinen J, Savolainen V. Internal fixation of proximal humerus fractures with a locking compression plate: a retrospective evaluation of 72 patients followed for a minimum of 1 year. Acta Orthop Scand. 2004;75:741-5.

This retrospective study looked at 72 patients treated with a proximal humerus locking plate for an osteoporotic frature, at 1 year from the procedure. Despite the osteoporotic bone, the functional outcomes were acceptable. Seven complications were reported.

Fankhauser F, Boldin C, Schippinger G, Haunschmid C, et al. A new locking plate for unstable fractures of the proximal humerus. Clin Orthop Relat Res. 2006;(430):176-81.

This prospective cohort study looked at 29 proximal humerus fractures treated with a locking proximal humerus plate. Most of the fractures were of a complex nature, and the Constant score at 1 year was 74.6. There were six complications and two cases of partial osteonecrosis. Overall, this was felt to be a reliable procedure in complex fractures. (Level II-1 evidence)

Gardner MJ, Weil Y, Barker JU, et al. The importance of medial support in locked plating of proximal humerus fractures. J Orthop Trauma. 2007;21:185-91.

Thirty-five patients who underwent locked plating for a proximal humerus fracture were followed until healing. In those cases that did not have adequate mechanical medial support, there was a higher rate of screw penetration and loss of humeral height. The authors concluded that a slightly impacted stable reduction and a well-placed superiorly directed oblique locked screw in the inferomedial region of the HH may allow more stable medial column support.

Owsley KC, Gorczyca JT. Fracture displacement and screw cutout after open reduction and locked plate fixation of proximal humeral fractures. J Bone Joint Surg [Am]. 2008;90:862.

This study looked at 53 patients treated by one surgeon with a locked proximal humerus plate for a proximal humerus fracture. The results showed an unexpectedly high rate of screw cutout and revision surgery, especially in patients older than 60 years with a three- or four-part fracture. The overall complication rate was 36%, but in patients older than 60, the rate was 57%.

Robinson CM, Page RS. Severely impacted valgus proximal humerus fractures: results of operative treatment. J Bone Joint Surg [Am]. 2003;85:1647-55.

In this study, 25 patients with a neck-shaft angle of greater than 160° and the GT displaced greater than 1 cm were followed for 1–2 years. Bone substitute was utilized to fill in the metaphyseal defect left once the HH was reduced out of valgus. All fractures went on to unite and, although there were six complications, none required reoperation. There were no cases of osteonecrosis at short-term follow-up. At 1 year, the mean Constant score was 80 points.

Solberg BD, Moon CN, Franco DP, et al. Surgical treatment of three and four-part proximal humeral fractures. J Bone Joint Surg [Am]. 2009;91:1689-97.

This retrospective study looked at 122 patients, age 55 or older, in whom a three- or four-part proximal humerus fracture was treated with locked plating (38 patients) versus hemiarthroplasty (48 patients). In this series, open repair with a locked humeral plate resulted in better outcome scores than did hemiarthroplasty in similar patients, especially those with a three-part fracture, despite a higher overall complication rate. However, the authors felt that open reduction and internal fixation of fractures with an initial varus pattern should be approached with caution and had a worse outcome than those with an initial valgus pattern. (Level IV evidence)

Sudkamp N, Bayer J, Hepp P, et al. Open reduction and internal fixation of proximal humeral fractures with use of the locking proximal humerus plate: Results of a prospective, multicenter, observational study. J Bone Joint Surg [Am]. 2009;91(6):1320-8.

This therapeutic study (a prospective case series) looked at functional outcomes and complication rates after open reduction and internal fixation with locking proximal humerus plates. One-year follow-up was obtained on 155 patients from nine different trauma centers. Sixty-two complications were noted in 52 of the 155 patients, and 34 of these were reported as directly related to the initial surgical procedure. (Level IV evidence)

PROCEDURE 31

Percutaneous Fixation of Proximal Humerus Fractures

Mark Tauber and Herbert Resch

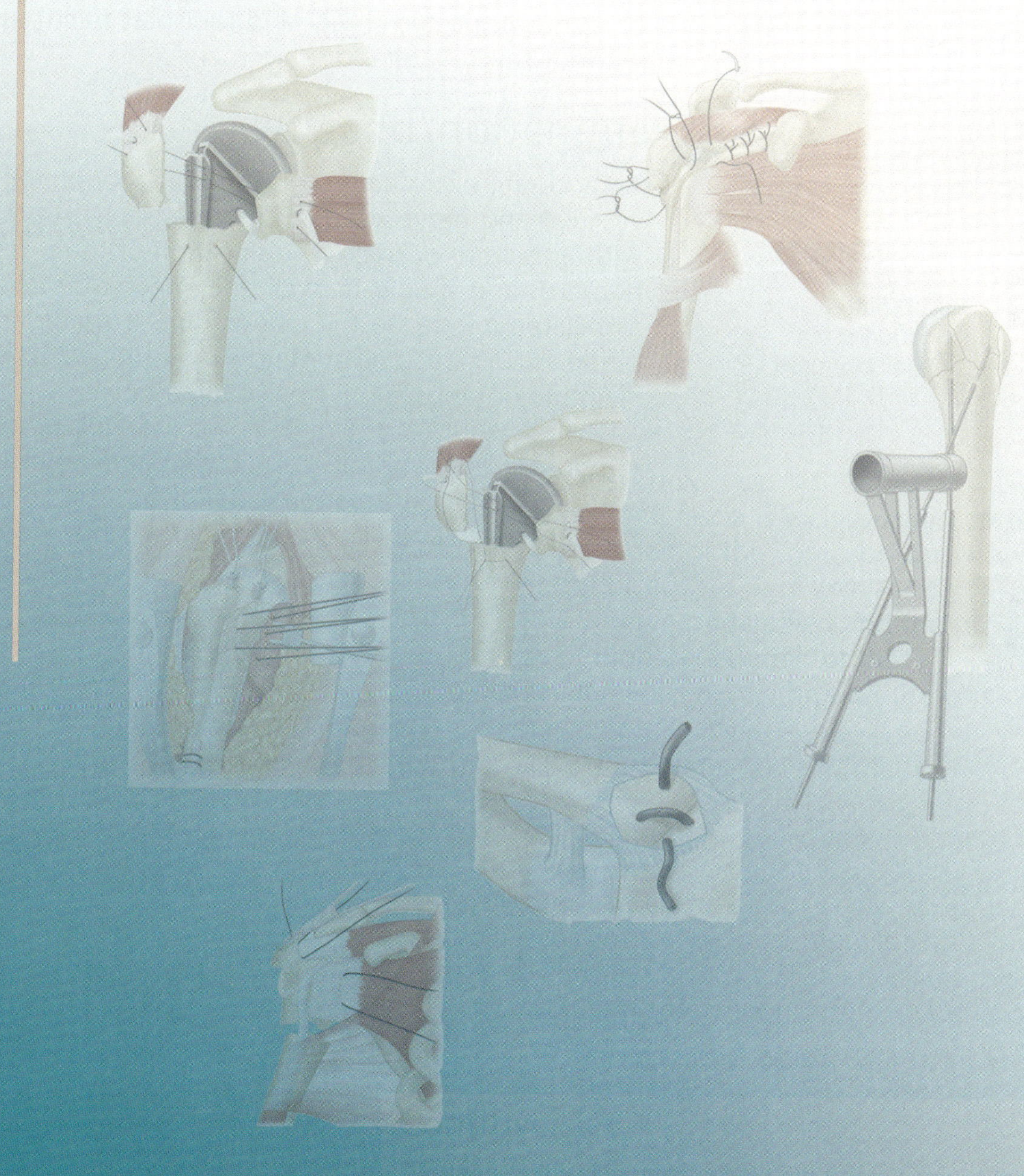

Pitfalls

- *Four-part fractures with severe lateral displacement of the articular segment ("true" four-part fractures according to Neer) and severely displaced fracture-dislocations (type VI according to Neer) represent less suitable indications for percutaneous fracture management and should remain in experienced hands.*

Controversies

- Unreducable fracture-dislocations necessitating open reduction and internal fixation and head-splitting fractures are considered as contraindications for percutaneous fixation, as are fractures with a comminuted metaphyseal zone or extension into the humeral shaft.

Indications

- Proximal humerus fractures fulfilling the criteria of displacement according to Neer, with displacement of the greater tuberosity of greater than 5 mm or an angle of ≥ 30° between the shaft and head fragment.
- Good indications are extra-articular fractures (e.g., fractures of the greater tuberosity or surgical neck fractures), and some intra-articular fractures (e.g., three-part fractures according to Neer involving the surgical neck with avulsion of the greater tuberosity or valgus-impacted three- and four-part fractures without severe lateral displacement).

Examination/Imaging

- An accurate examination of the intact peripheral vascular and nerve supply is indispensable in patients with a fracture or fracture-dislocation of the proximal humerus and should be well documented. Possible associated injuries to the elbow joint or shoulder girdle should be kept in mind.
- Plain radiographs should be obtained in anteroposterior (AP) (Fig. 1) and axillary views.
    - Two orthogonal radiographic views are crucial to study the fracture pattern, identifying the "fracture personality" and allowing for classification and

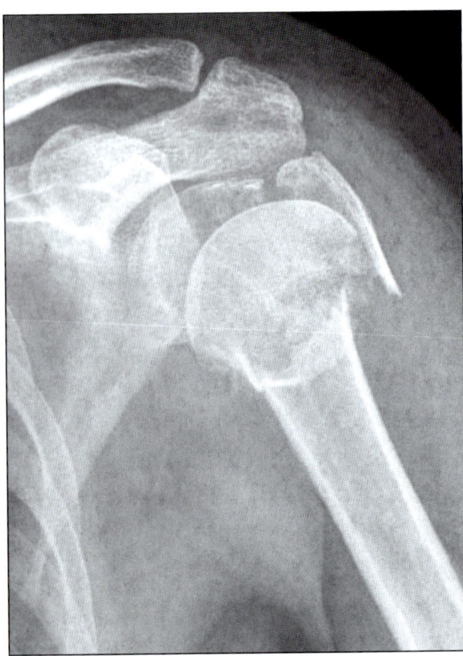

FIGURE 1

assessment of soft tissue structures as interfragmentary periosteal bridges. If an axillary view (which is preferred by the authors) is not possible to carry out, a trans-scapular view (Fig. 2) should be obtained.

- Performance of computed tomography with three-dimensional reconstruction in fractures of the proximal humerus involving three segments or more is recommended (Fig. 3). This imaging tool allows for three-dimensional viewing of the fracture, revealing interfragmentary relationships and details often misdiagnosed or undetected on plain radiographs.

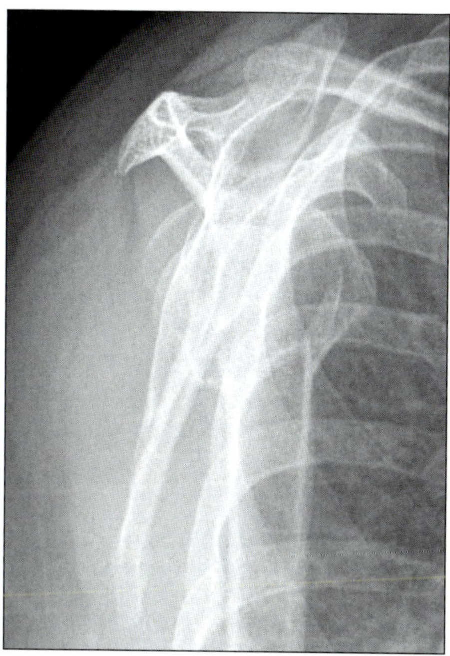

FIGURE 2

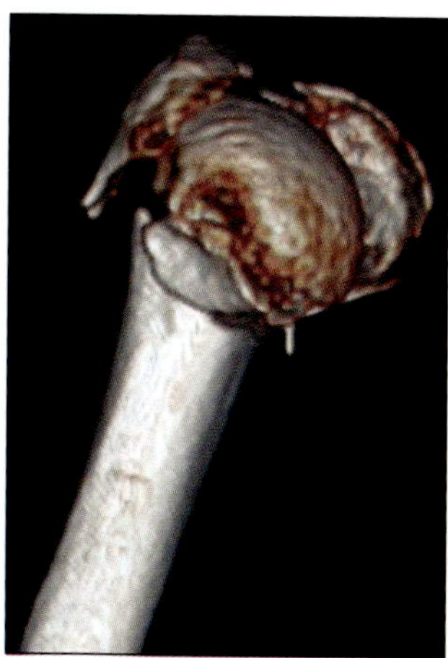

FIGURE 3

Treatment Options

- Alternative implants for osteosynthesis of proximal humerus fractures that are gaining more popularity are proximal intramedullary humerus nails and anatomically shaped proximal humerus plates with locking screws.
- Despite a reduced approach area, an obvious disadvantage of the nail is the fact that it is inserted through the rotator cuff. Furthermore, the range of screw insertion is limited, which may create difficulties in multifragmentary fracture patterns with dislocation of the tuberosities.
- The standard implant of open reduction and internal fixation is the angle-stable plate using locking screws. In spite of higher primary stability, the prevalence of complications such as screw cutout, screw malpositioning, nonunion, and avascular humeral head necrosis, most often in elderly patients with advanced osteoporosis, is reported to be higher than with percutaneous techniques.

Surgical Anatomy

- Detailed knowledge of shoulder biomechanics and fracture pathology is necessary. Interfragmentary relationships and periosteal junctions have to be known for successful closed reduction. The number of fragments (greater/lesser tuberosity, articular segment, humeral shaft) and acting muscle/tendon forces resulting in typical fragment dislocations must be identified and correctly interpreted.
- According to the injury mechanism, we distinguish two types of fractures:
    - Impaction fractures in falls on the extended arm with valgus impaction of the head fragment caused by the glenoid (Fig. 4). The medial "hinge-periosteum" usually is intact, as the lateral periosteal link is between the greater tuberosity and humeral shaft. These intact soft tissue junctions allow for closed reduction by simple raising of the articular head fragment using an elevator, making use of the "ligamentotaxis effect" (Fig. 5).

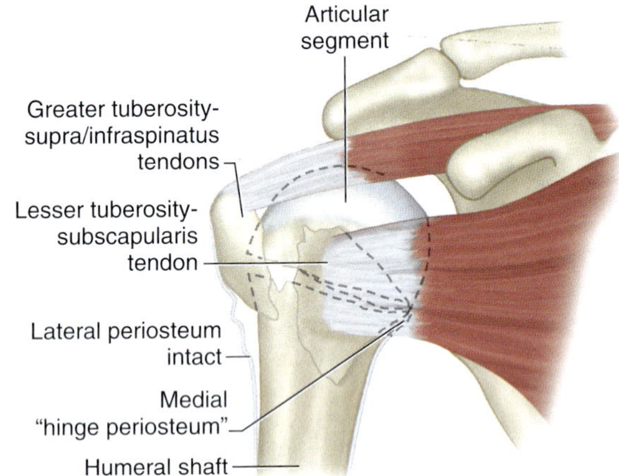

FIGURE 4

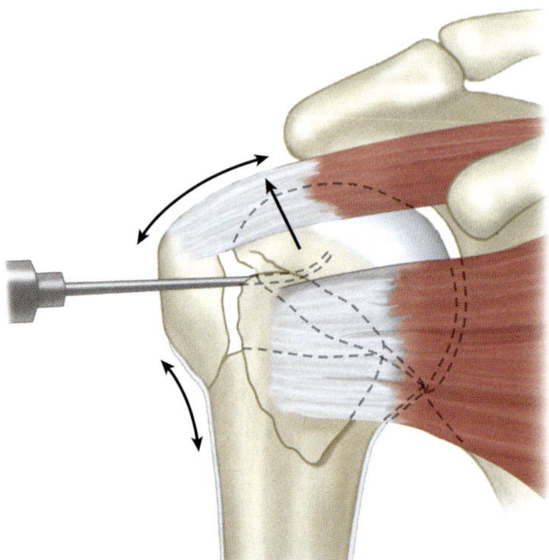

FIGURE 5

- Avulsion fractures caused by a combination of rotational, axial, and muscle forces. The interfragmentary periosteal links are commonly disrupted, rendering the maneuvers of closed reduction challenging. The greater tuberosity is displaced posterosuperiorly into the subacromial space following the tension force of the supra- and infraspinatus tendons. In three-part fractures with avulsion of the greater tuberosity, the articular head segment is internally rotated due to the tension force of the subscapularis tendon at its insertion on the lesser tuberosity (Fig. 6A). The humeral shaft is medialized and internally rotated secondary to the acting force of the pectoralis major tendon (Fig. 6B).

■ The axillary nerve and its branches are prone to damage at the lateral aspect of the shoulder. To avoid injury to this nerve, the Humerusblock implant must be set at least 5–6 cm distally to the surgical neck. Additional cannulated screws for tuberosity fixation should be inserted at the junction of the middle and posterior thirds of the humeral head through stab incisions using the trocar sheath with the blunt trocar to protect the nerve. In the area of the axillary nerve, no washers should be used to avoid entrapment of the nerve or its branches under a washer.

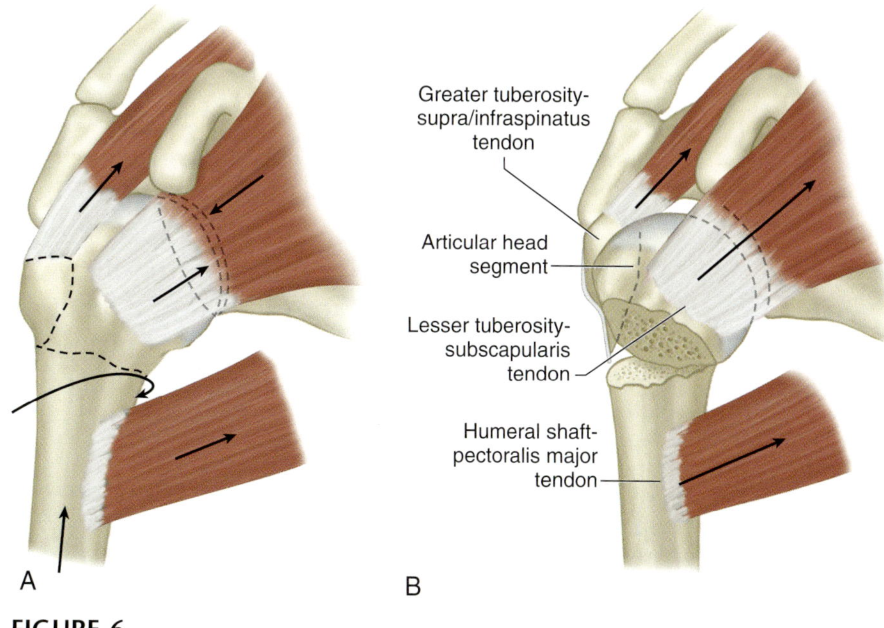

FIGURE 6

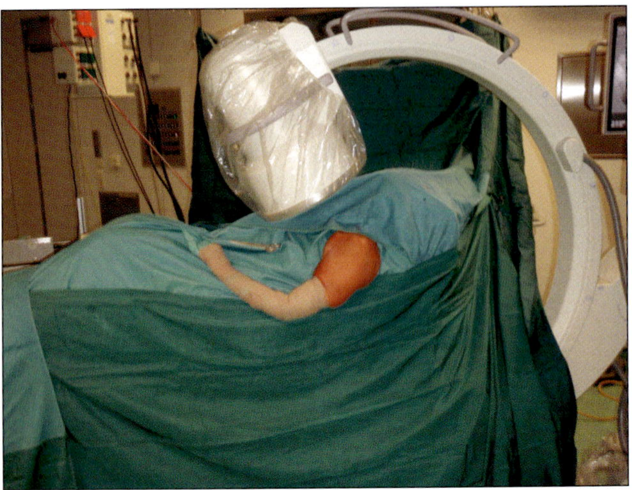

FIGURE 7

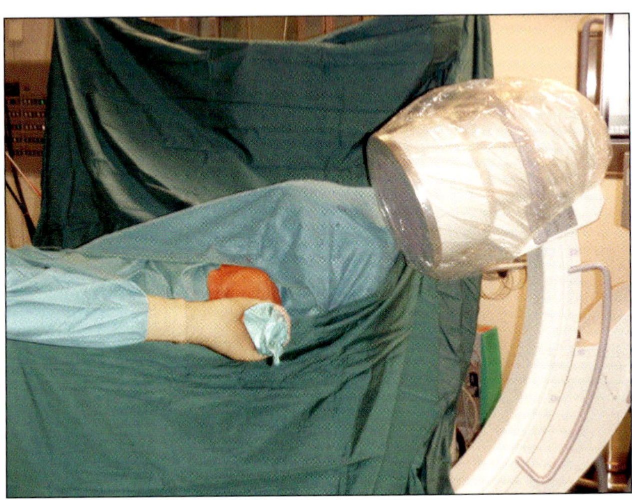

FIGURE 8

Pearls

- *The arm is held in neutral rotation by an assistant during implantation of the Humerusblock.*
- *The patient's head is held a little to the opposite side and stabilized in that position to permit adequate approach to the C-arm.*

Pitfalls

- *Care must be taken in fracture-dislocations in regard to the cervical spine. Because the patient's head is fixed during reduction maneuvers, the cervical spine and the brachial nerve plexus are at increased risk for traction injuries.*

Positioning

- The procedure is performed with the patient in the beach chair position.
- The arm is draped free to permit mobility.
- The image intensifier is positioned cranially, with the C-arm creating a right angle between the central beam and the humerus shaft (Fig. 7).
  - Rotation to 90° allows a direct axial view with the arm in 90° of abduction (Fig. 8).

Portals/Exposures

- A skin incision 3 cm in length is made on the lateral side of the upper arm, about 5–6 cm below the subcapital fracture line (Fig. 9).

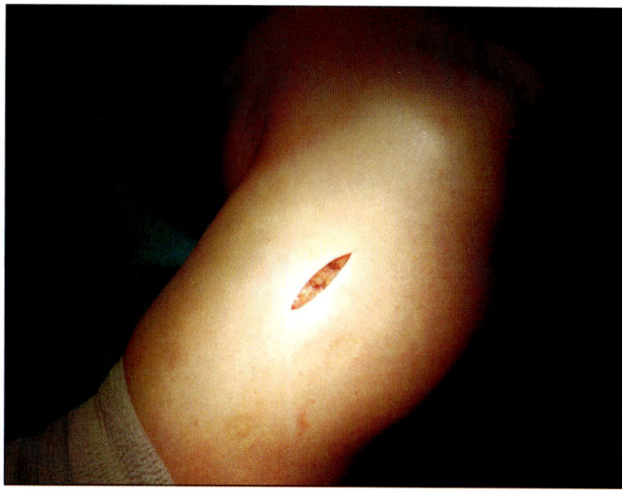
FIGURE 9

Pearls

- *To perform the skin incision at the correct height, we recommend radiologic control using the image intensifier (Fig. 13).*

- The deltoid muscle is split along its muscle fibers and the lateral humeral cortex is freed gently from soft tissues.
- The fracture gap between the greater tuberosity and the humeral head is always situated several millimeters lateral of the bicipital groove. It serves as the entry portal for the elevator to tunnel under and lift the humeral head.
  - The corresponding stab incision for elevator insertion is made at the junction of the anterior and middle thirds of the humeral head under image intensification control (Fig. 10).
  - Through this incision, a bone hook can also be inserted to reduce the displaced greater tuberosity.

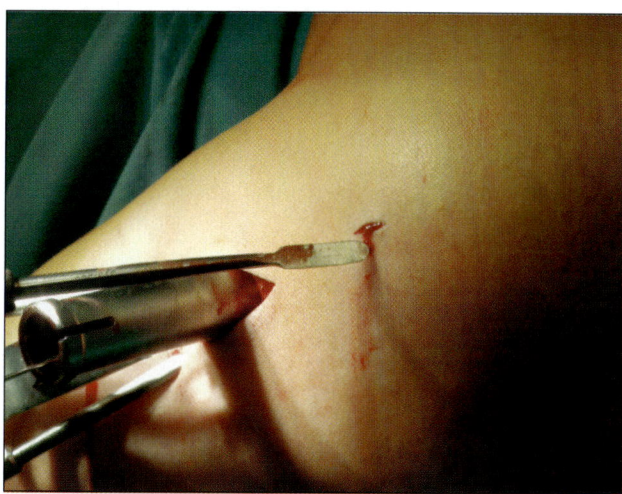
FIGURE 10

- To fix the reduced greater tuberosity, use of at least two cannulated screws is recommended to guarantee rotational stability. The stab incisions for insertion of these screws are placed at the junction of the middle and posterior thirds of the humeral head (Fig. 11).
- A displaced lesser tuberosity can be fixed through one to two additional stab incisions at the anterior aspect of the shoulder using two cannulated screws (Fig. 12A and 12B).

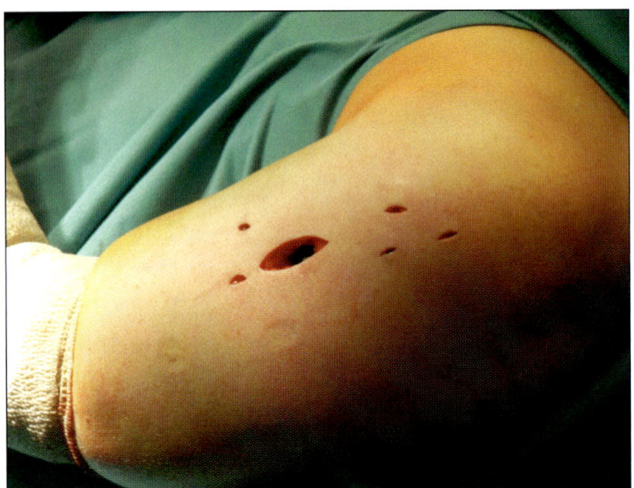

FIGURE 11

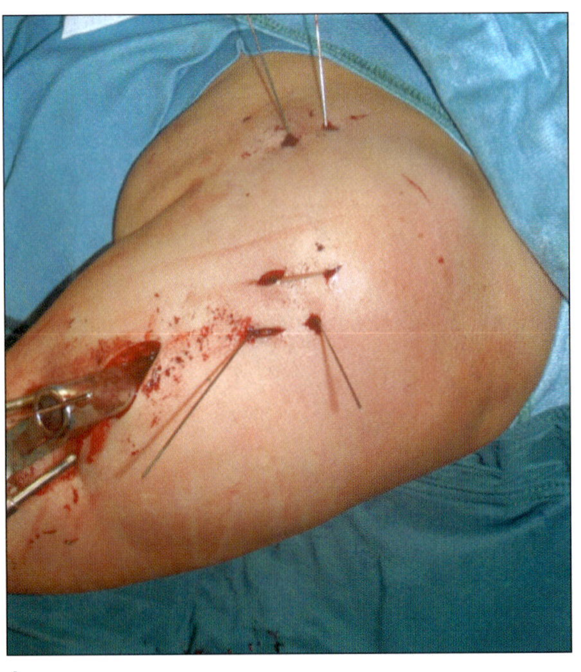

A

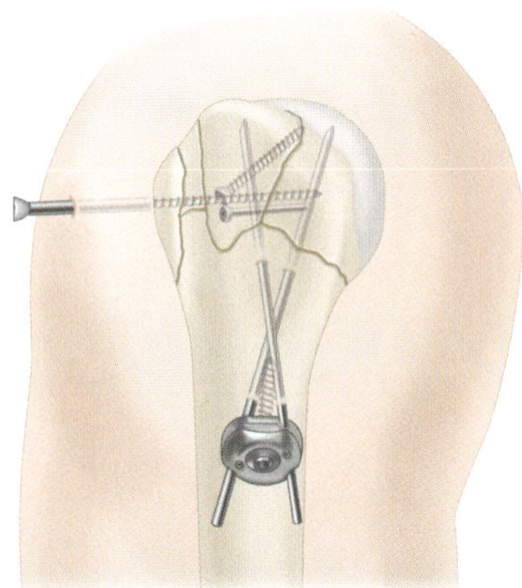

B

FIGURE 12

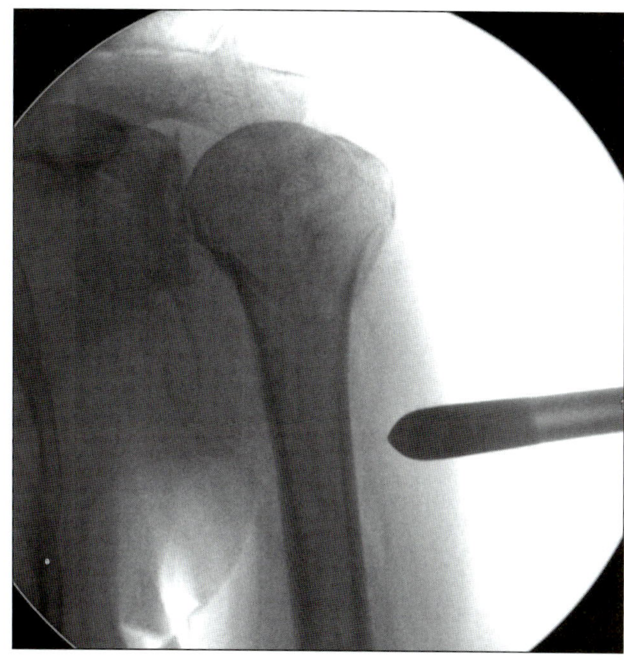

FIGURE 13

PEARLS

- *Exact positioning of the Humerusblock strictly at the lateral humeral cortex represents a key step for success of the procedure. If it is not centered in the middle of the shaft, direction of the K-wires to the humeral head center is not possible, resulting in eccentric rotational forces.*

PITFALLS

- *If image intensification shows the tip of the guidewire for the cannulated screw exactly at the outermost lateral border of the diaphysis, then the position will appear correctly in midshaft in the axial view (Fig. 18A). If the tip of the guidewire is protruding into the shaft, then the tip has been positioned too far anterior or too far posterior and needs to be corrected (Fig. 18B). During this step, the assistant must hold the arm strictly in neutral rotation.*

Procedure

Step 1

- Through the lateral skin incision and the split deltoid muscle, a Humerusblock is placed at the lateral humerus shaft cortex using the aiming device (Fig. 14).
  - The implant used is a metallic button with preformed gliding holes for two 2.2-mm Kirschner wires (K-wires) crossing inside at an angle of 30°.

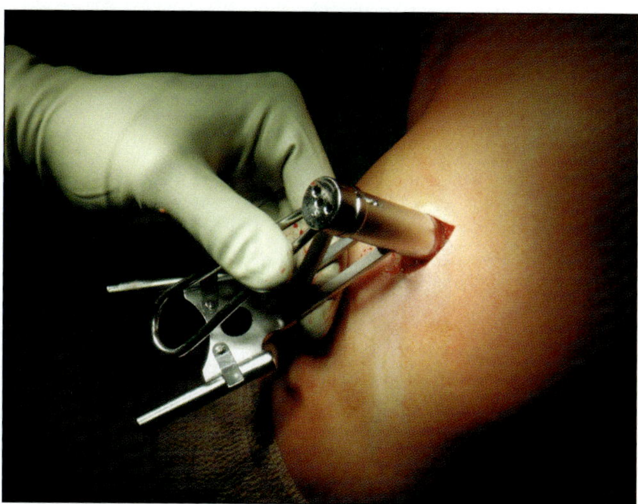

FIGURE 14

Instrumentation/ Implantation

- Humerusblock (Synthes, Oberdorf, Switzerland)

  - The holes can be locked by fixation screws inside the metallic cylinder (Fig. 15).
- The Humerusblock is fixed to the humeral shaft by a 4-mm self-tapping cannulated cortical screw (in most cases 40 mm in length), which initially is not completely tightened to allow varus or valgus adjustement of the block for directing the two K-wires.
- The centering sleeves for both K-wires are introduced into the aiming device and advanced through two small stab incisions to the Humerusblock. Laterally, the aiming device must be exactly aligned with the longitudinal axis of the shaft (the lateral humeral epicondyle can be used as reference point) so that the 2.2-mm K-wires can be correctly positioned in the humeral head (Fig. 16A and 16B).

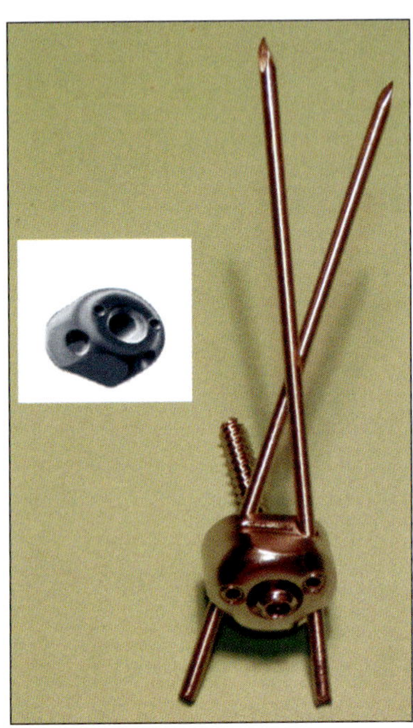

FIGURE 15

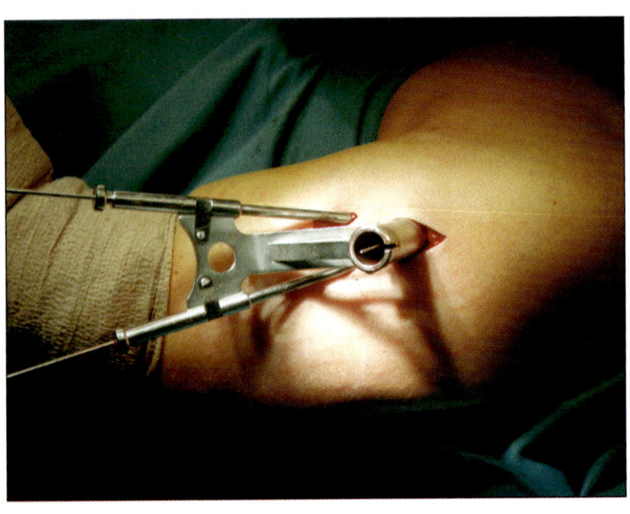

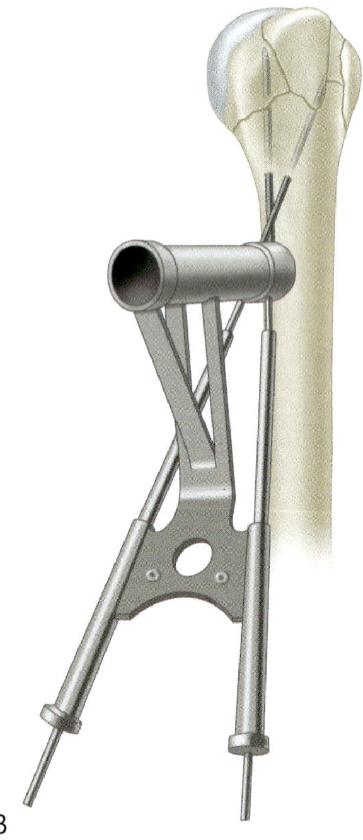

A B

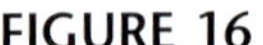

FIGURE 16

Pearls

- *The fracture gap between the greater tuberosity and the humeral head serves as the entry portal for the elevator. It is always situated several millimeters lateral of the bicipital groove (Fig. 21). Very often the avulsed greater tuberosity will be guided by the intact lateral periosteum and realigned when the rotator cuff is restored to normal tension.*

Pitfalls

- *Close attention is required while raising the articular head segment using the elevator. In elderly patients with advanced osteoporosis, the bone quality is poor, increasing the risk of perforation of the the subchondral cortical lamellae with the elevator.*
- *When drilling the two K-wires into the articular segment, perforation of the tips through the subchondral cortex, which would increase the risk for loss of reduction, must be avoided. Accurate imaging control in both planes (AP and axillary) is indispensable during the stepwise drill.*
- *The tips of the K-wires should be directed to the area between the superior glenoid pole and the top of the humeral head. Thus, in the case of secondary subsidence of the humeral head fragment ("guided sliding" of the head) resulting in perforation by the tips of the K-wires, damage to the glenoid cartilage can be avoided when shoulder motion is started.*

- The two K-wires are drilled through the lateral humeral cortex just below to the subcapital fracture level (Fig. 17).

Step 2

- Reduction of the humeral head must be controlled under image intensification in two planes. In subcapital fractures, the antecurvation pushing the humerus shaft posteriorly must be addressed.
- In valgus impacted three- or four-part fractures (see Figs. 1–3), the first step of reduction is raising the articular segment using an elevator (Fig. 19).

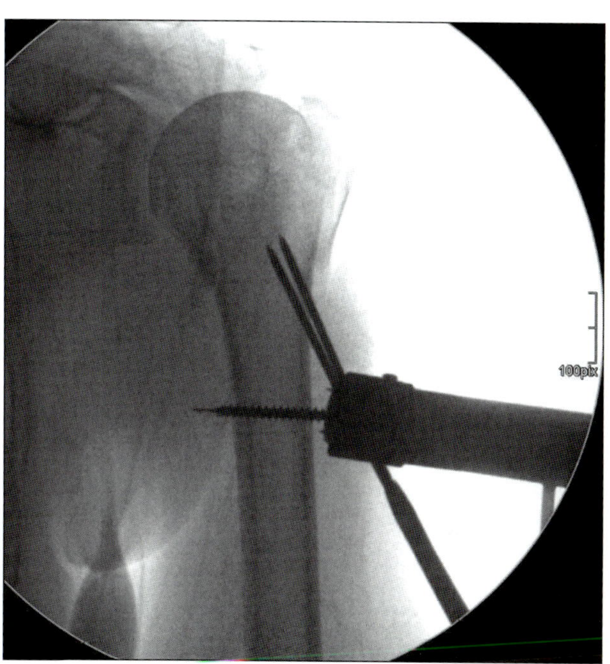

FIGURE 17

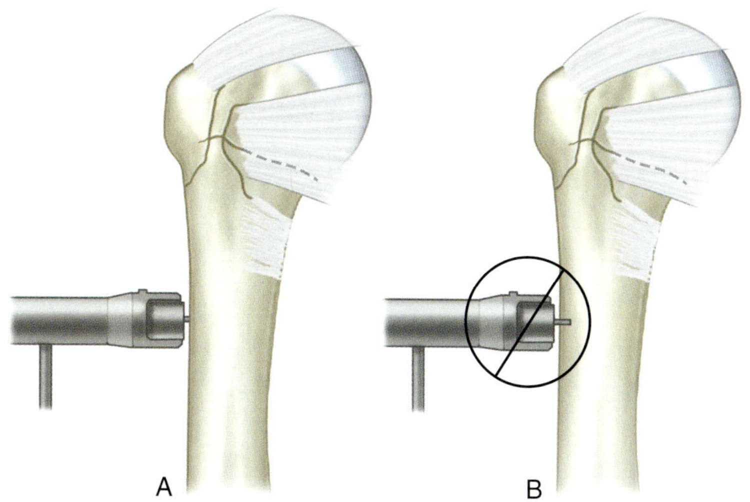

FIGURE 18

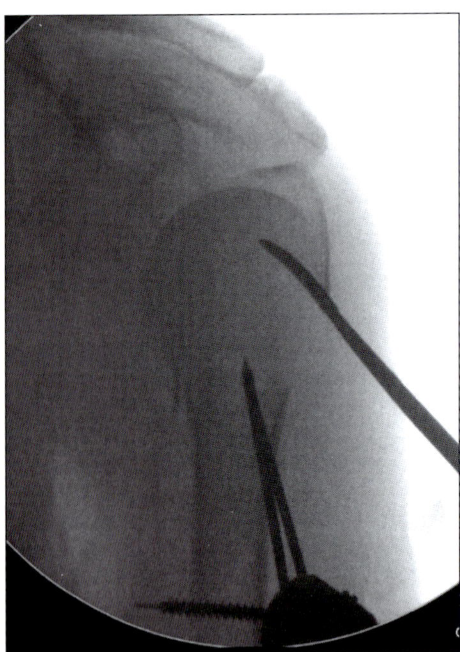

FIGURE 19

Pitfalls

- *If the articular head segment is not raised sufficiently with remaining minimal valgus impaction, anatomic reduction of both, the lesser and greater tuberosity, is not possible. In this case, the two K-wires must be drawn back at the subcapital fracture level and the head fragment raised up again using the elevator.*

- If the valgus impaction is offset with the articular segment in the anatomic position, the two K-wires are drilled forward into the subchondral bone (Fig. 20A and 20B) to secure the articular segment.

Step 3

- If in four-part fractures the lesser tuberosity shows displacement, a hook retractor or an elevator is used to reduce it. The reduction maneuver is easy to

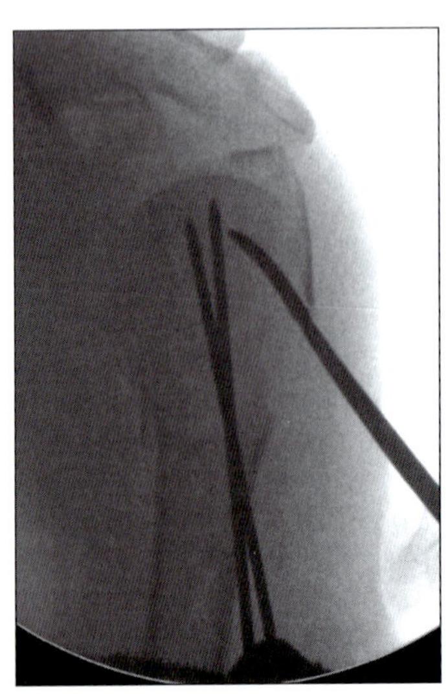

A

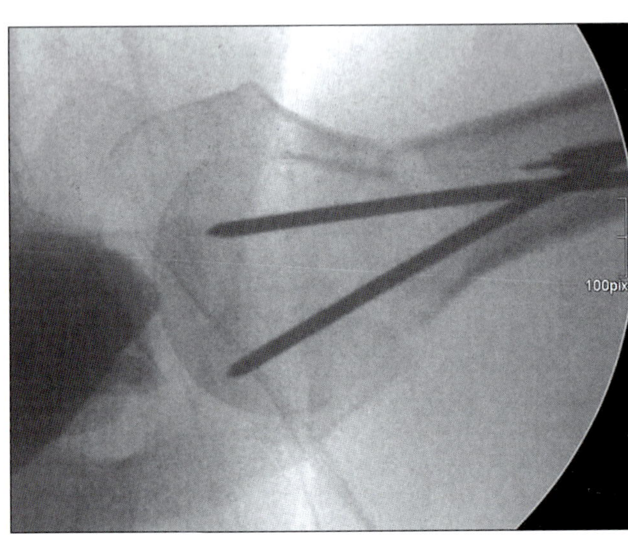

B

FIGURE 20

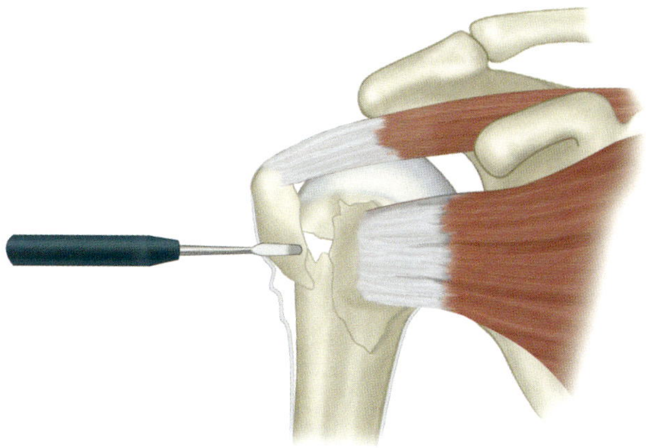

FIGURE 21

control in the axillary view. The hook is inserted directly at the tendon's insertion area on the lesser tuberosity (Fig. 22A) and pulled laterally (Fig. 22B).

- Temporary fixation is performed using a drill-guidewire combination set that allows direct setting of 2.7-mm cannulated titanium screws.
  - The set comprises cannulated, self-tapping screws with a diameter of 2.7 mm and 10–40 mm in length. The screws are inserted over a guidewire that is part of a drill-guidewire combination (diameter of 2.2 mm), allowing for temporary fixation of the tuberosities (Fig. 23A and 23B).
  - If image intensification shows correct reduction and position of the guidewire, the drill is removed while the guidewire remains in place. A titanium

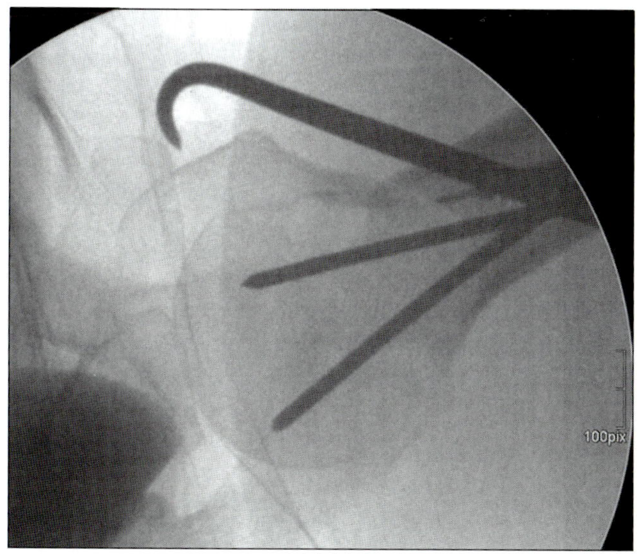

A

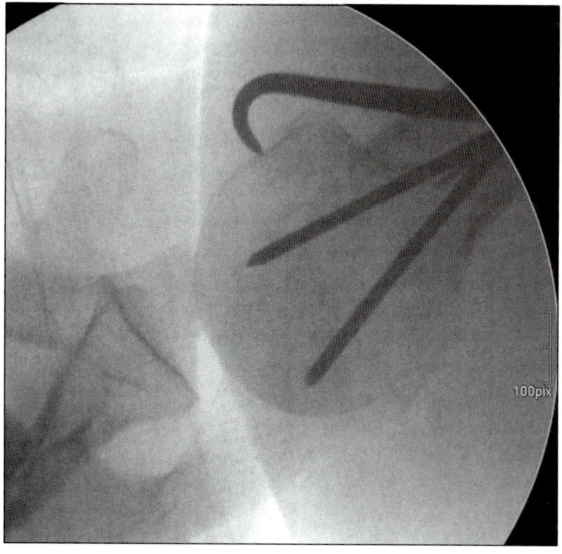

B

FIGURE 22

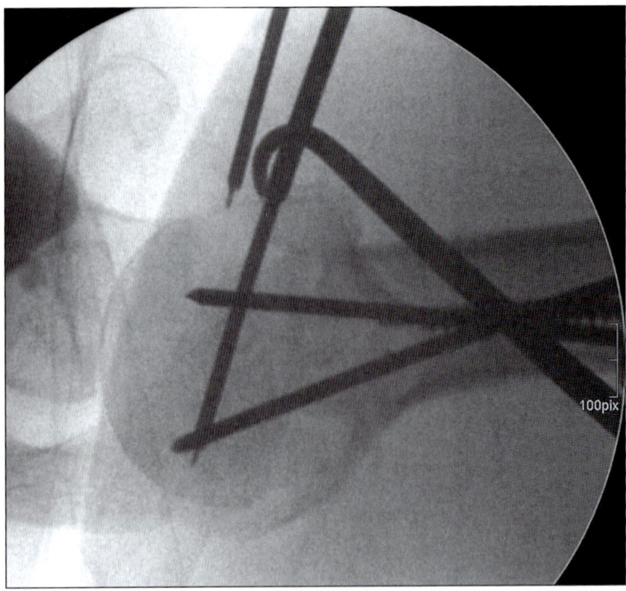

A

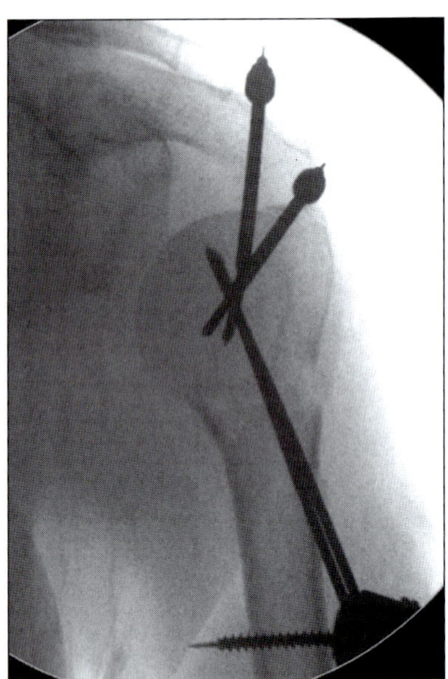

B

FIGURE 23

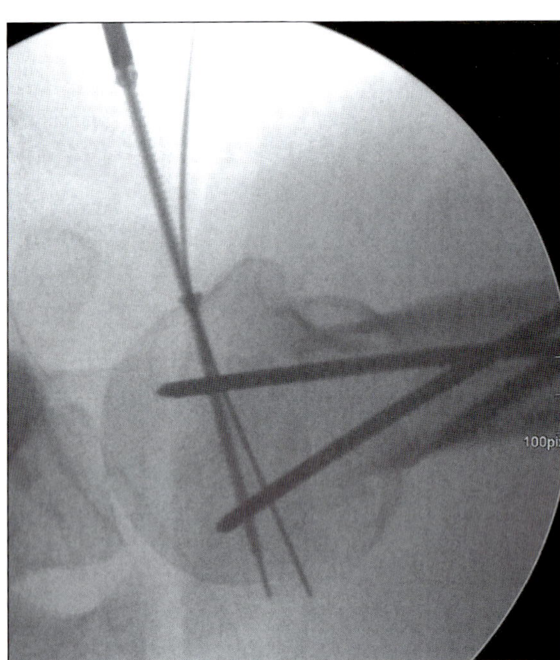

FIGURE 24

Instrumentation/ Implantation

- The hook retractor (Fig. 25) is inserted through the stab incision at the junction of the middle and anterior thirds of the humeral head.
- A special Arthroscopic and Percutaneous Screw Fixation System (Stryker Leibinger Micro Implants, Freiburg, Germany) is used.

screw, usually 40 mm long, is then inserted over the guidewire (Fig. 24).

- Fragment fixation is recommended to be performed using two cannulated screws, guaranteeing rotational stability.

Step 4

- The greater tuberosity also is reduced using a pointed hook retractor (Fig. 26).

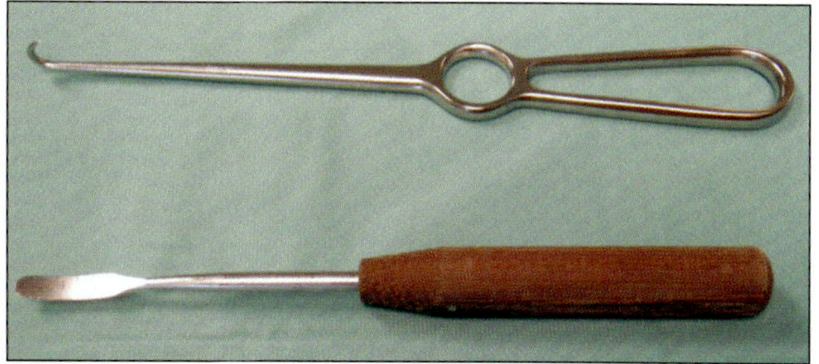

FIGURE 25

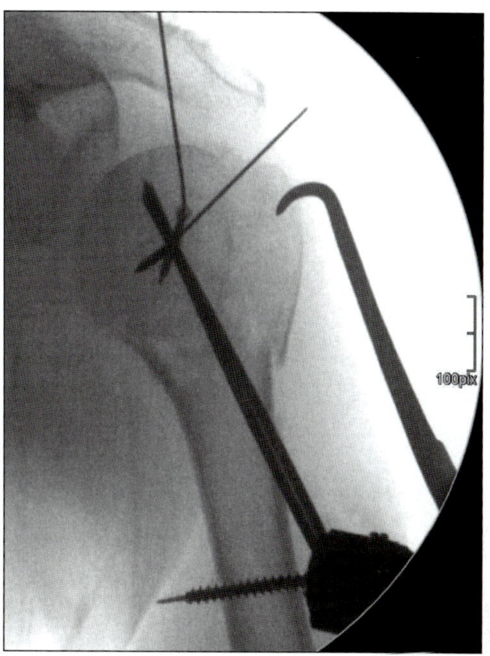

FIGURE 26

PEARLS

- *A greater tuberosity that appears to be well aligned in a.p.- view might be substantially displaced posteriorly. Residual displacement can be visualized by shifting the angle of the C-arm caudally.*

  - This instrument is inserted through a stab incision and engaged at the footprint of the supraspinatus tendon.
  - By pulling against the tension direction of the supra- and infraspinatus tendons anteroinferiorly, the greater tuberosity can be reduced anatomically (Fig. 27).
- The same principles for tuberosity fixation using cannulated screws as used for the lesser tuberosity are valid. After temporary fixation with the drill-guidewire combination (Fig. 28), the cannulated screws are inserted over the guidewires (Fig. 29).
- An axillary control view is mandatory (Fig. 30) to check exact reduction of the tuberosity and correct positioning of the screws.

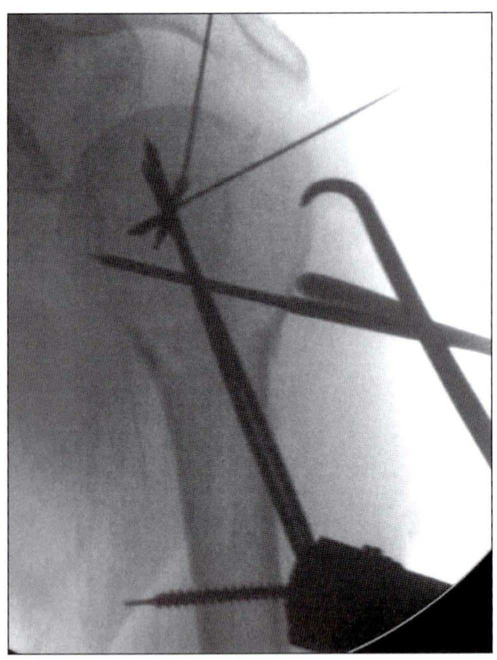

FIGURE 27

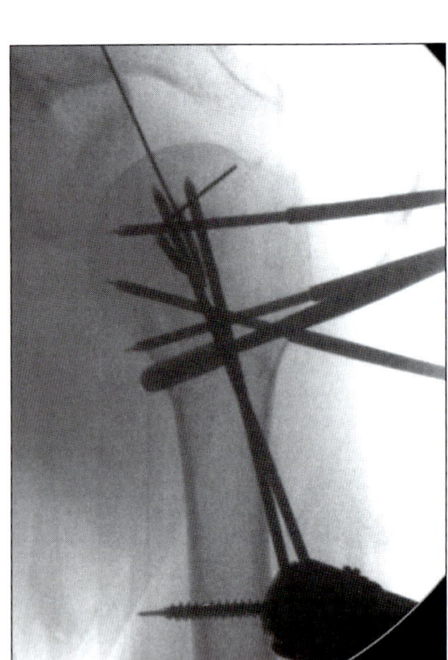

FIGURE 28

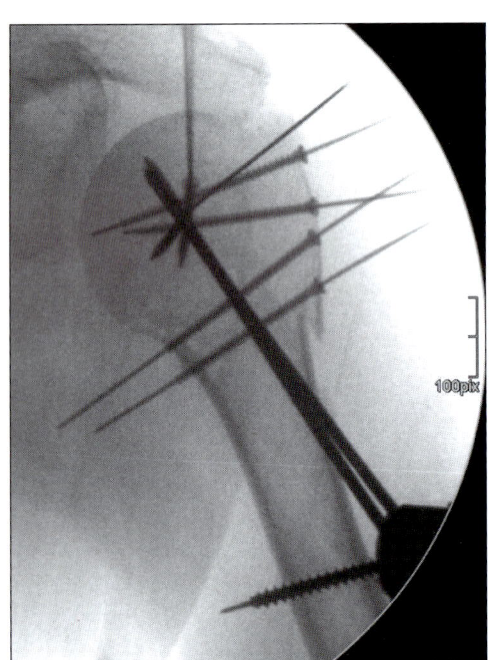

FIGURE 29

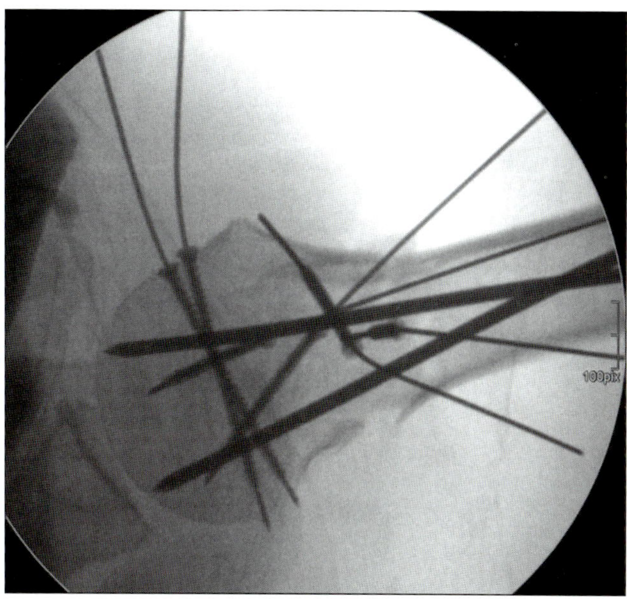

FIGURE 30

PEARLS

- *The guidewires of the cannulated titanium screws should not be removed until definitive fixation of all fragments is concluded. Without guidewires, screw removal can be challenging.*
- *Usually, the Humerusblock is not placed directly on the bone. Some tension can be exerted on the Humerusblock/K-wire system by slight tightening of the fixation screw.*

STEP 5

- The two K-wires are shortened at 5 mm from the Humerusblock after withdrawal of the centering sleeves and the aiming device.
- The guidewires of the cannulated screws are removed and a final radiologic image is taken to ensure correct reduction (Fig. 31).
- If necessary, suction drains are placed.
- The wound is closed in layers (Fig. 32).

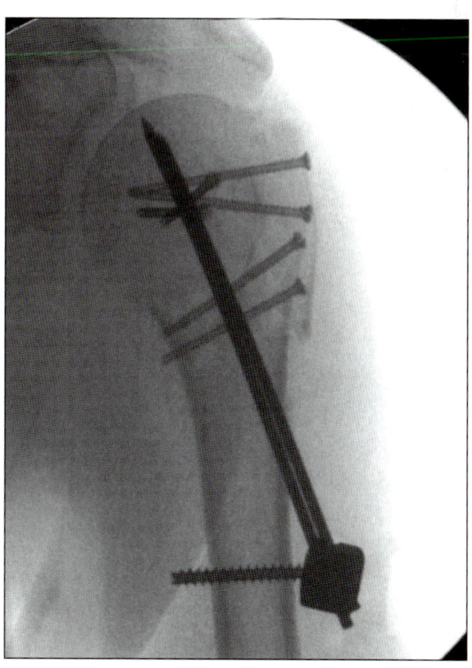

FIGURE 31

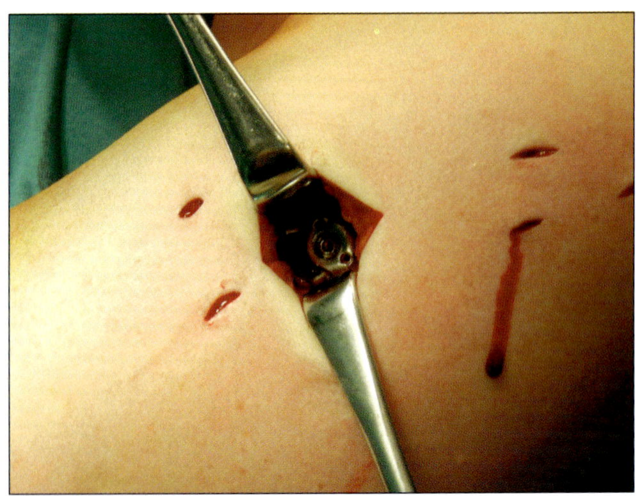

FIGURE 32

PEARLS

- *If K-wire perforation occurs, exercises of the shoulder must be stopped and the K-wires have to be withdrawn below the subchondral cortex to prevent cartilage damage of the glenoid.*
- *Before definitive removal of the Humerusblock after 6–8 weeks, the K-wires should be withdrawn intraoperatively to the subcapital fracture level, and shoulder motion in all planes with rotation must be reviewed under imaging intensification. If the head fragment shows stable fixation to the shaft, the Humerusblock can be removed.*

PITFALLS

- *We recommend not removing the cannulated screws for tuberosity fixation routinely. It can be difficult to detect the flat screw head in the cortical bone. If protruding the cortex, the screws can be removed.*

Postoperative Care and Expected Outcomes

- The shoulder is immobilized in a light bandage for 3–4 weeks depending on the degree of stability achieved, bone quality, and number of fragments.
- On the first postoperative day, passive exercises in the scapular plane, avoiding rotation of the arm, are started.
- Active movement and rotation exercises are allowed after removal of the bandage.
- Radiographs are obtained at intervals of 1 week to identify subsidence of the head fragment along the two K-wires ("guided" sliding of the head) in time to prevent perforation of the tips of the K-wires.
- The Humerusblock is removed after 6–8 weeks depending on the presence of radiologic signs of callus formation.

Evidence

Bogner R, Huebner C, Matis N, Auffarth A, Lederer S, Resch H. Minimally-invasive treatment of three- and four-part fractures of the proximal humerus in elderly patients. J Bone Joint Surg [Br]. 2008;90:1602-7.

The authors presented a retrospective radiologic and clinical follow-up of 50 patients older than 70 years of age after percutaneous fixation of three- and four-part fractures of the proximal humerus. The average Constant score was 61.2 points for three-part fractures and 49.5 points for four-part fractures. The rate of posttraumatic avascular necrosis (8%) was reduced as compared to open reduction and internal fixation. (Level III evidence)

Calvo E, de Miguel I, de la Cruz JJ, Lòpez-Martìn N. Percutaneous fixation of displaced proximal humeral fractures: indications based on the correlation between clinical and radiographic results. J Shoulder Elbow Surg. 2007;16:774-81.

The authors correlated the clinical outcome according the Constant score with the radiologic outcome regarding the quality of reduction in 74 patients (average age 70.9 years) with displaced proximal humeral fractures treated with closed reduction and percutaneous pinning. Reduction was good in 72%, with the worst radiographic results in four-part fractures. The average Constant score was 65.8 points. The clinical outcome correlated with the quality of reduction. The authors concluded that percutaneous pinning should be reserved for two-part fractures, with the exception of three-part fractures in elderly patients, who may better tolerate incomplete reduction. (Level III evidence)

Resch H, Huebner C, Schwaiger R. Minimally invasive reduction and osteosynthesis of articular fractures of the humeral head. Injury. 2001;32(Suppl 1):25-32.

Indications, surgical technique, and results of minimally invasive treatment of articular fractures of the humeral head were reported. Nine patients with B1 and B2 and 18 patients with C1 and C2 fractures were followed up. The age- and gender-related Constant score averaged 91% for B1 and B2 fractures, whereas it was 87% for C1 and C2 fractures. The posttraumatic avascular humeral head necrosis rate of the C1 and C2 fractures was 11%.

Resch H, Povacz P, Frohlich R, Wambacher M. Percutaneous fixation of three- and four-part fractures of the proximal humerus. J Bone Joint Surg [Br]. 1997;79:295-300.

The results after percutaneous fixation of three- and four-part fractures of the proximal humerus using pins and cannulated screws in patients with an average age of 54 years were reported. After an average follow-up period of 24 months, the nine patients with a three-part fracture showed a Constant score of 91% with no signs of avascular necrosis. The 18 patients with four-part fractures, of whom 13 had a valgus-type fracture, had an average Constant score of 87%. with avascular necrosis in 2 patients. (Level III evidence)

PROCEDURE 32

Hemiarthroplasty for Proximal Humerus Fracture

Steven M. Klein, Mark A. Mighell, and Mark A. Frankle

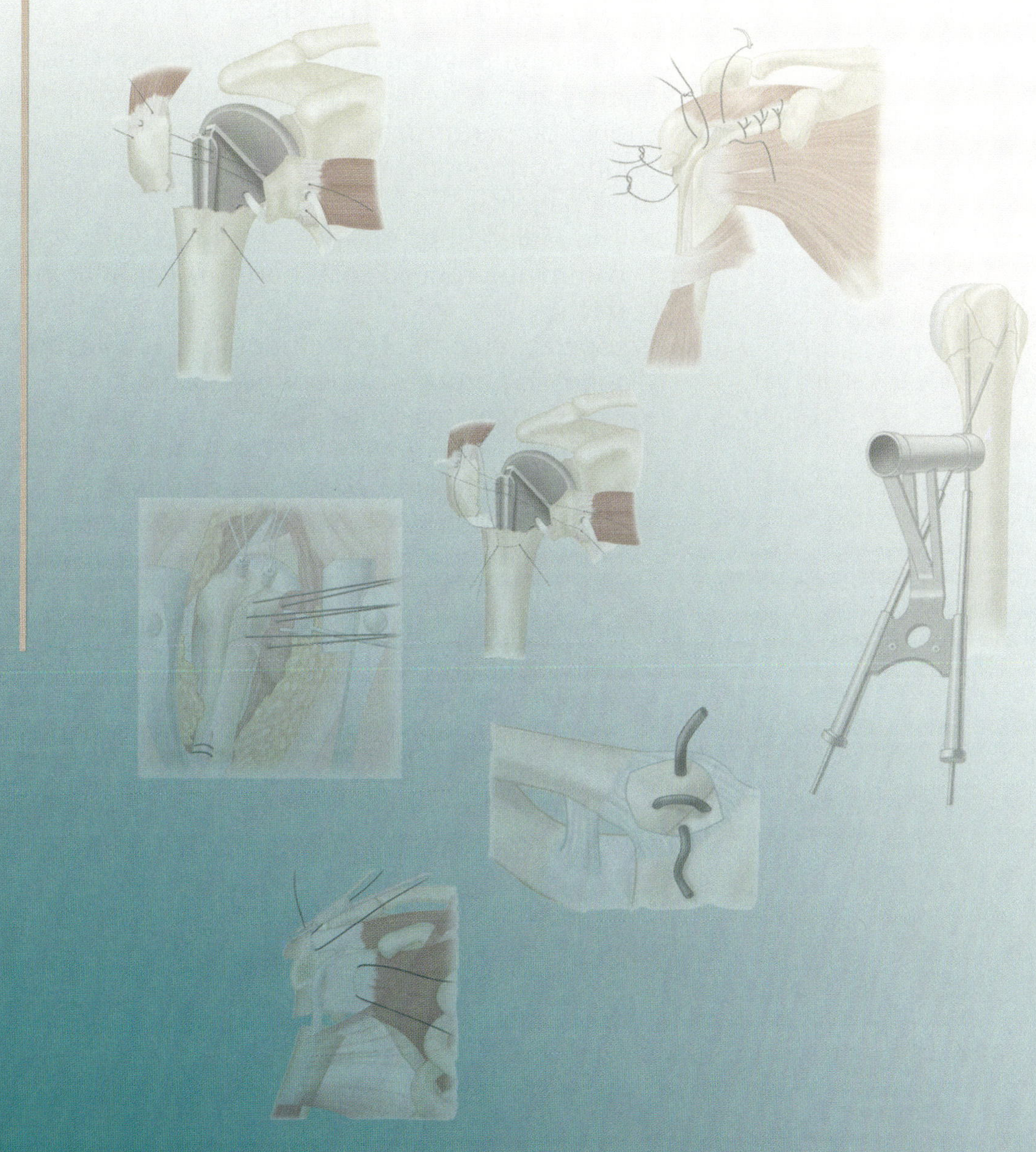

Figure 10 and Figure 12A from Mighell MA, Kolm GP, Collinge CA, Frankle MA. Outcomes of hemiarthroplasty for fractures of the proximal humerus. J Shoulder Elbow Surg. 2003;12:569-77.
Figure 12B and Figure 13 from Frankle MA, Mighell MA. Techniques and principles of tuberosity fixation for proximal humeral fractures treated with hemiarthroplasty. J Shoulder Elbow Surg. 2004;13:239-47.

Pitfalls

- *Patients with multiple comorbidities have diminished outcomes with hemiarthroplasty for fracture compared to healthier counterparts (Kabir et al., 2009).*
- *Patients with concurrent rotator cuff pathology are not ideal candidates for hemiarthroplasty.*

Controversies

- Indications for reverse shoulder arthroplasty include fractures in the setting of:
  - Glenohumeral arthritis.
  - Rotator cuff pathology.
  - Elderly patients where the likelihood of tuberosity healing is remote (Bufquin et al., 2007; Sirveaux et al., 2008).

Treatment Options

- Nonoperative management
- Open reduction and internal fixation
- Reverse shoulder arthroplasty

Indications

- Comminuted four-part fractures
- Three- and four-part fracture/dislocations
- Head-splitting fractures
- Impaction fractures of the humeral head with involvement of greater than 50% of the articular surface
- Anatomic neck fractures in patients greater than 40 years old

Examination/Imaging

- A thorough physical examination for associated injuries and a detailed neurovascular examination should be performed.
- Routine orthogonal radiographs should be obtained in all patients.
  - The radiographs in Figure 1A and 1B show a comminuted head-splitting proximal humerus fracture.
- Preoperative computed tomography (CT) is useful for diagnostic purposes and surgical planning.
  - The CT scan in Figure 1C shows a comminuted head-splitting proximal humerus fracture commonly treated with hemiarthroplasty.
  - Figure 2 illustrates a comminuted proximal humerus fracture that is not amenable to open reduction and internal fixation.
- Imaging of the contralateral arm should be obtained to determine the proper humeral length and head size.
- Intraoperative fluoroscopy is useful to assess height and tuberosity reduction.

Surgical Anatomy

- Deltoid
  - Fibers of the anterior deltoid run parallel as they extend from the clavicle to their broad area of insertion on the humerus. This orientation can act as a landmark in identifying the deltopectoral groove.
  - The pull of the deltoid may cause proximal migration of the distal segment.
- Pectoralis major
  - The fibers of the clavicular head of the pectoralis major take a more transverse course toward their insertion in the humerus when compared to the deltoid.

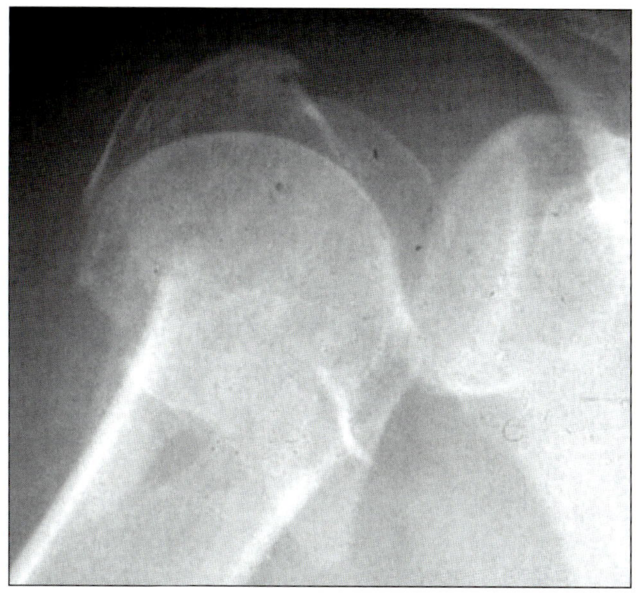

A

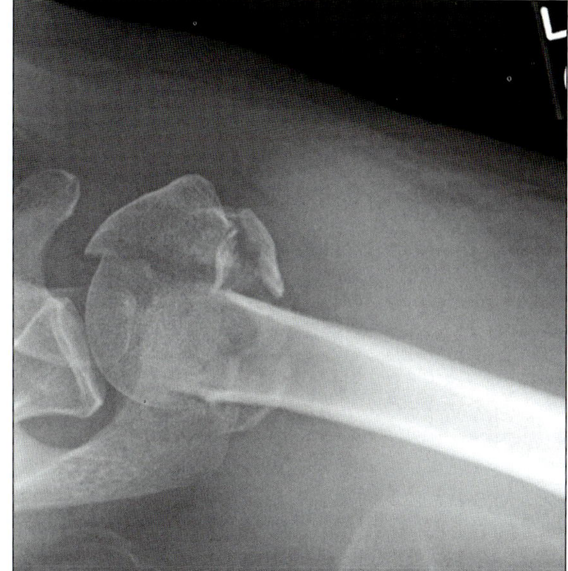

B

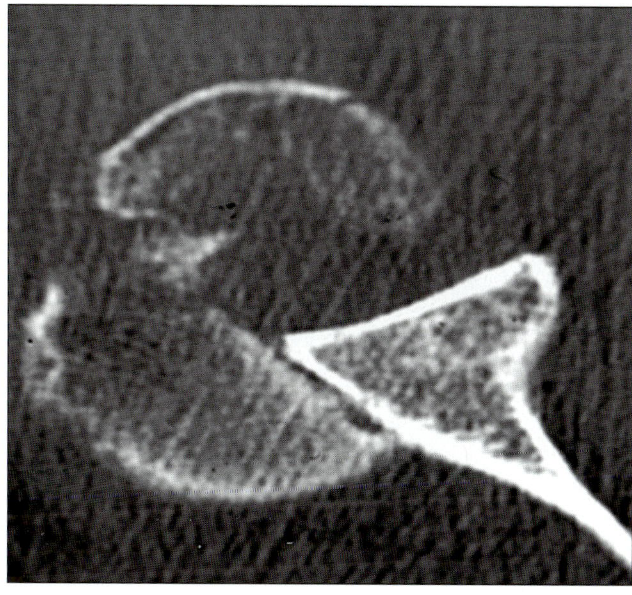

C

FIGURE 1

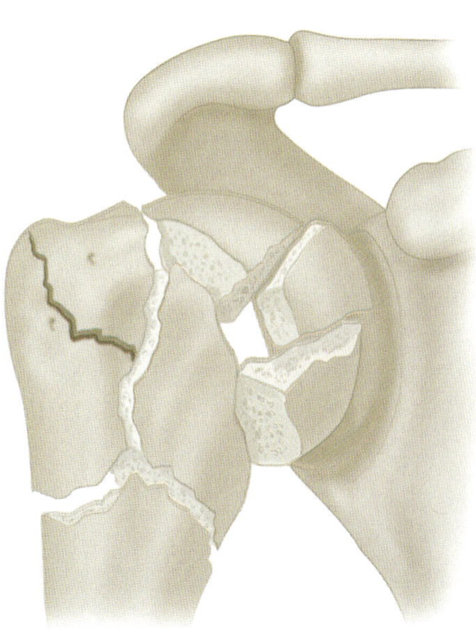

FIGURE 2

- Force exerted by the pectoralis major may cause the distal fragment to assume a valgus and internally rotated position.

- The long head of the biceps tendon is identified beneath the pectoralis major insertion and as it passes into the biceps groove (Fig. 3A).

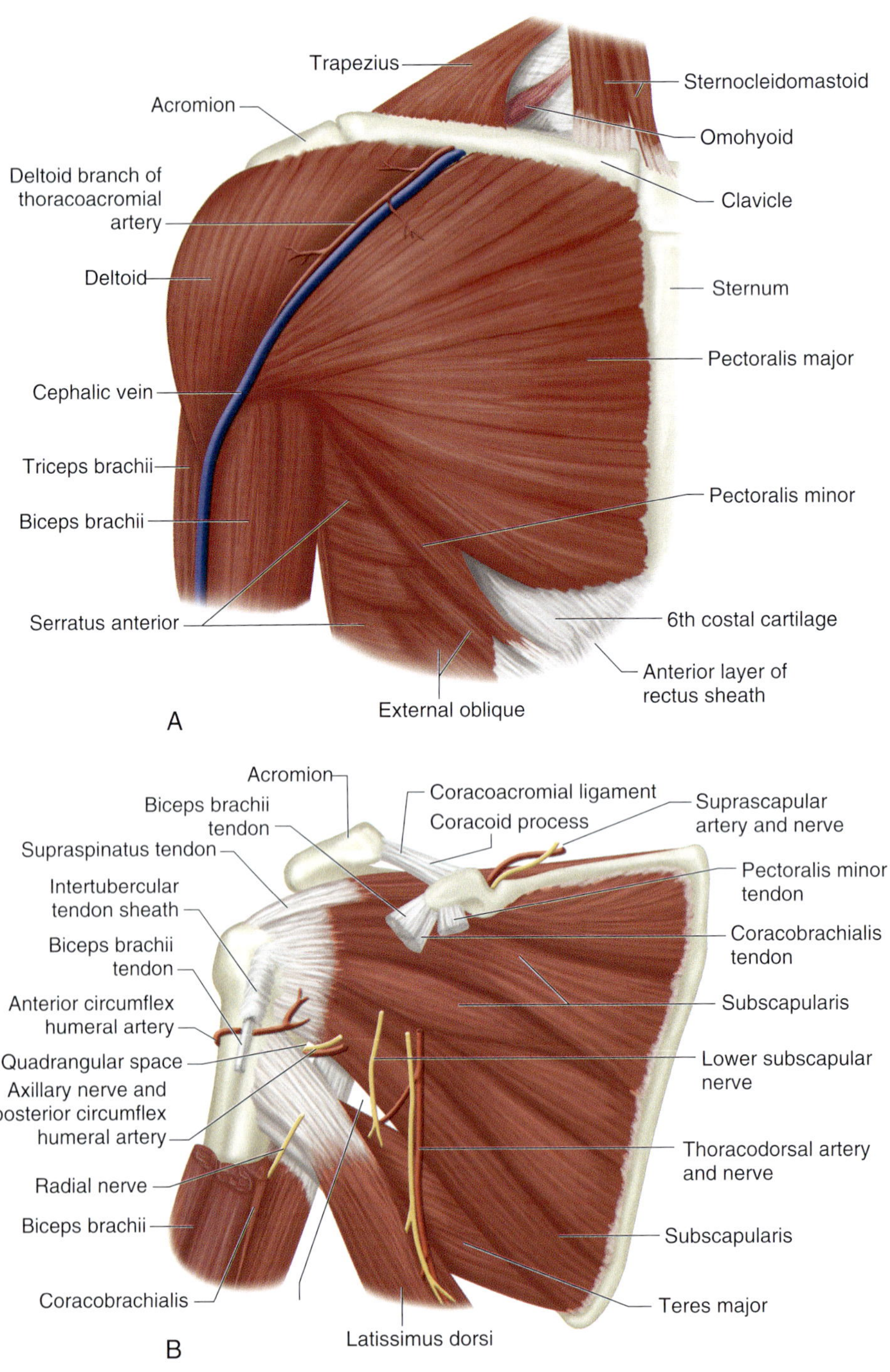

FIGURE 3

- The cephalic vein passes through the clavipectoral fascia to drain into the axillary vein. The vein presents a landmark for the deltopectoral interval and is almost always present.
- The axillary nerve may be identified within the subcoracoid space and along the inferior border of the subscapularis (Fig. 3B). External rotation of the humerus with the arm at the side brings the tendinous portion of the subscapularis away from the nerve. Abduction will draw the nerve closer to the surgical field.

Positioning

- Patients are placed in the modified beach chair position.
  - The foot of the bed is lowered and the bed is then re-flexed approximately 20°.
  - The back of the bed is raised to place the patient's torso 70–80° from the horizontal plane.
  - Once the patient is in position, the head is secured to a well-padded head holder.
  - Meticulous padding of bony prominences, with particular attention to the ulnar and peroneal nerves, is performed.
  - Positioning should ensure that the operative shoulder, including the scapula, is freely mobile (Fig. 4).
- The table is then turned approximately 90° relative to the anesthesiologist.

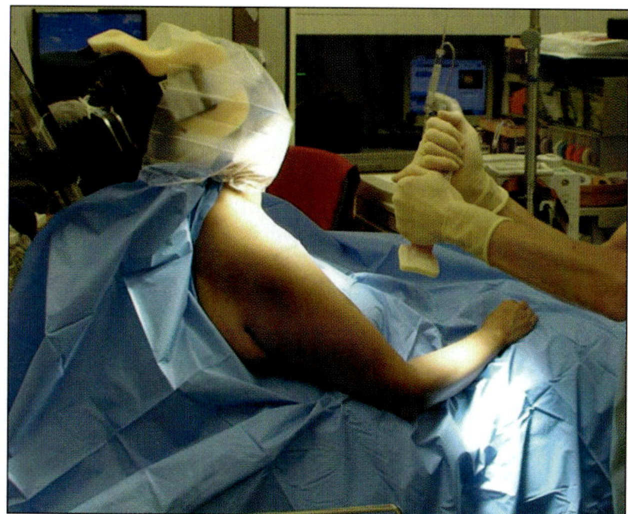

FIGURE 4

Pearls

- *An interscalene block minimizes postoperative pain.*
- *The endotracheal tube should be positioned on the opposite side of the surgical field to prevent inadvertent dislodgment.*
- *Patients at risk for cervical spine instability require preoperative evaluation.*

Pitfalls

- *Arm extension and adduction is necessary for adequate exposure and placement of the humeral component.*
- *Cervical spine hyperextension can cause serious neurologic injury.*
- *Slightly bending the knees avoids strain on the lumbosacral spine.*

Equipment

- Beach chair positioner
- Radiolucent fracture table

Controversies

- Patients can be placed in varying degrees of bed inclination (more horizontal vs. more upright) depending on surgeon preference.
- Alternatively, a radiolucent table can be useful in a polytrauma setting.

- Fluoroscopic imaging is obtained by positioning the C-arm parallel to the patient at the head of the bed (Fig. 5A and 5B). This allows for an unobstructed view of the shoulder and avoids interference with the anesthesiologist.
  - Fluoroscopy can also be done in the supine position (Fig. 6A and 6B).
- The C-arm is rotated over the top so that an anteroposterior view is obtained. Adequate imaging is confirmed prior to sterile prepping.
- The operative arm is draped free.

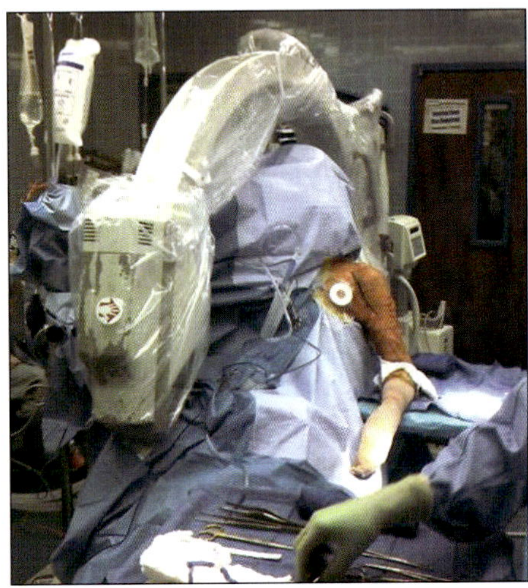

A

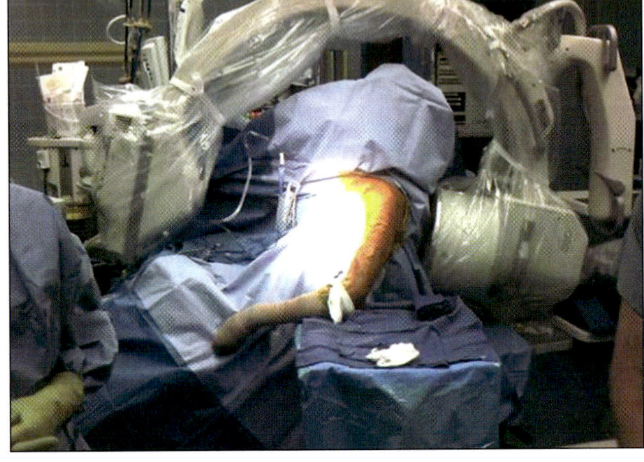

B

FIGURE 5

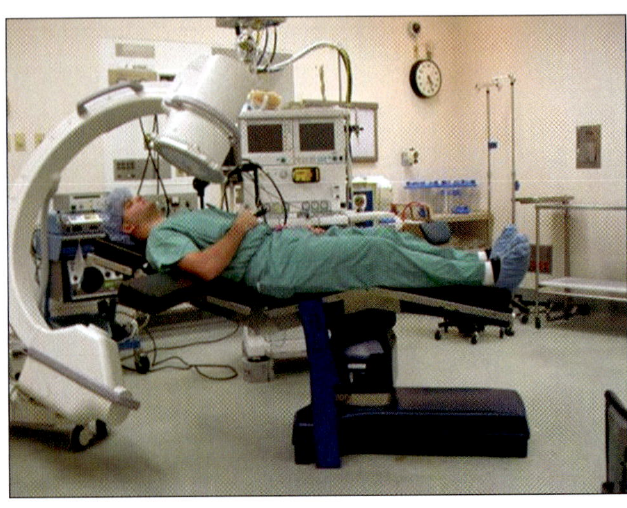

A

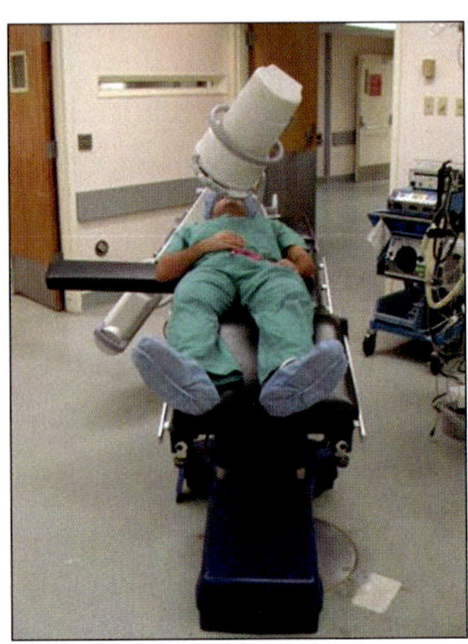

B

FIGURE 6

Pearls

- *The axillary nerve is not routinely dissected free during exposure.*

Pitfalls

- *Avoid excessive retraction of the anterior deltoid.*
- *Adequately release the subdeltoid bursa to prevent excessive tension on the deltoid insertion.*
- *Do not dissect medial to the coracoid.*

Instrumentation

- Well-padded Mayo stand to support the arm
- Browne deltoid retractor (Innomed Inc., Savannah, GA)

Portals/Exposures

- For the deltopectoral approach, the incision begins from approximately 5 cm medial to the acromioclavicular joint and extends in a line over the coracoid to end at the midhumerus near the proximal insertion of the pectoralis major. Identification of the deltopectoral interval is aided by locating the "fat stripe" at the most proximal portion (Fig. 7A).
- The cephalic vein is identified within the deltopectoral interval (Fig. 7B) and usually is taken medially to minimize trauma to it during lateral retraction of the deltoid.
- The subdeltoid, subacromial, and subcoracoid spaces should be developed. The axillary nerve may be palpated in the subcoracoid recess along the inferior border of the subscapularis. Any hemorrhagic bursa and hematoma are removed.

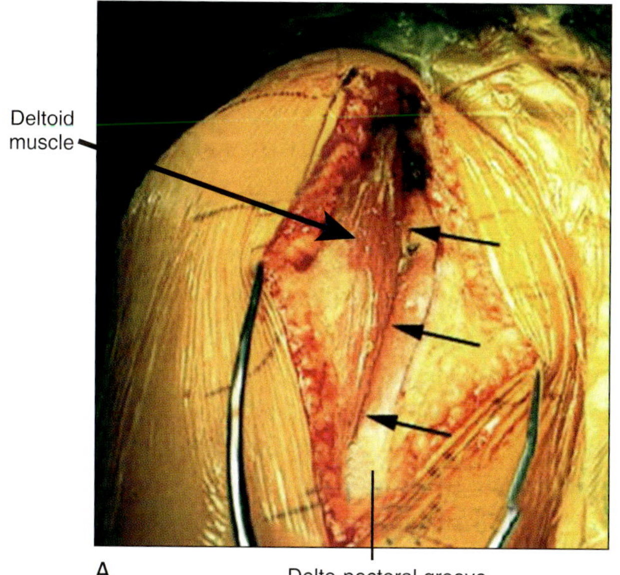

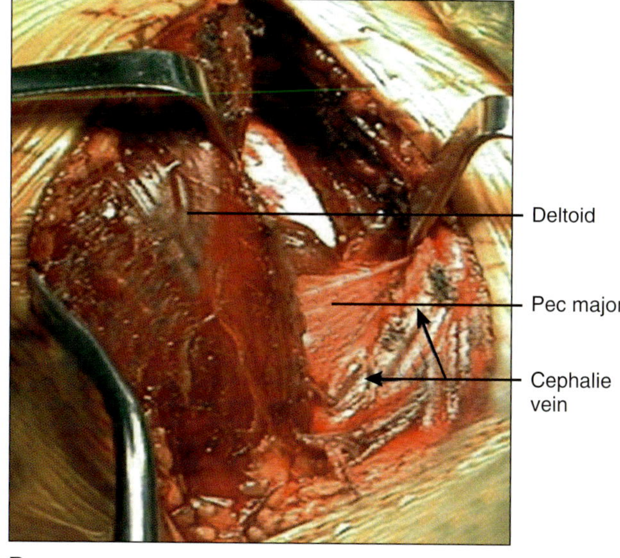

FIGURE 7

Pearls

- *A wide variety of fracture-specific systems is available, each with unique design features. We recommend using whichever implant the individual surgeon feels provides the best prospect of an anatomic reconstruction in his or her hands.*

Pitfalls

- *Understand how to utilize design-specific features to aid in the reconstruction prior to entering the operating room.*

Controversies

- It is unclear whether a specialized fracture prosthesis alters outcome (Loew et al., 2006).

Procedure

Step 1: Implant Selection

- Multiple fracture-specific implant systems are now available. Each offers features such as guides to help place the prosthetic device at the correct height and version as well as design alterations to enhance tuberosity reduction and fixation. Important implant characteristics to consider when choosing an implant include:
  - Modularity—A wide variety of head and stem sizes should be available to assist in obtaining an anatomic reconstruction.
  - Simple version guide—Multiple methods exist, including simple guide rods and extramedullary fracture jigs. In addition, fins on the proximal body may be positioned to assist in obtaining proper version and fragment reduction.
  - Centralizer—This feature may assist in preventing varus/valgus displacement.
  - Small proximal porous ingrowth body—This feature will allow for easier reconstruction of the tuberosities without the complication of overtensioning or the need to debulk the fragments. Various fracture stems utilize different methods to address this challenge. Examples of specific features include a small offset proximal segment and hollow sections within the body to allow for additional bone graft.
  - Available area for suture placement—A smooth medial surface allows for cerclage suture passage and minimizes the risk of suture breakage. Fins on the prosthesis may be fenestrated to allow for additional suture passage to secure tuberosity fragments.
  - Irregular proximal body geometry—An irregular shape improves the effects of cerclage compared with a smooth circular shape, which should help counteract the pull of the rotator cuff musculature (Frankle and Mighell, 2004; Frankle et al., 2001).
  - Secure distal fixation—Cement fixation or bony ingrowth technology can provide adequate distal fixation and prevent malrotation.
    - The prosthesis may be cemented in the shaft portion only and bone grafted proximally to facilitate tuberosity healing. Systems are available that provide the option to place the prosthesis without cement.

Step 2: Mobilization of the Tuberosities

- The major fracture line between the greater and lesser tuberosities is identified. This fracture is usually located just posterior to the bicipital groove. An osteotome may be used as an aid to "deconstruct" the fracture and separate the tuberosities (Fig. 8A and 8B).
- The supraspinatus may be split in line with its fibers extending from the fracture site to the level of the supraglenoid tubercle in order to enter the joint.
- The lesser tuberosity is identified and a traction stitch is placed at the tendon-bone interface. Mobilization of the tuberosity allows for access to the glenohumeral joint (Fig. 9A and 9B).

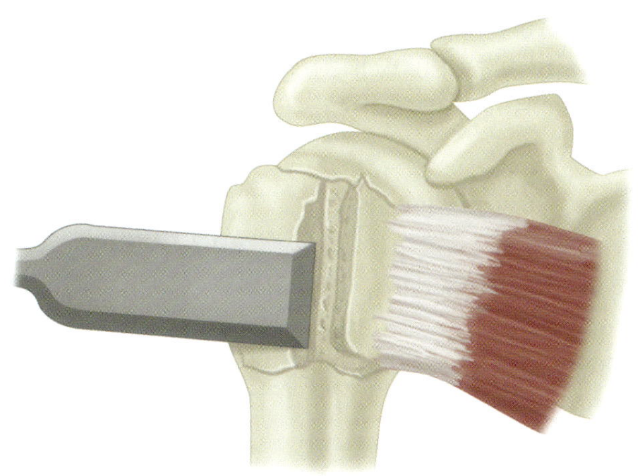

A

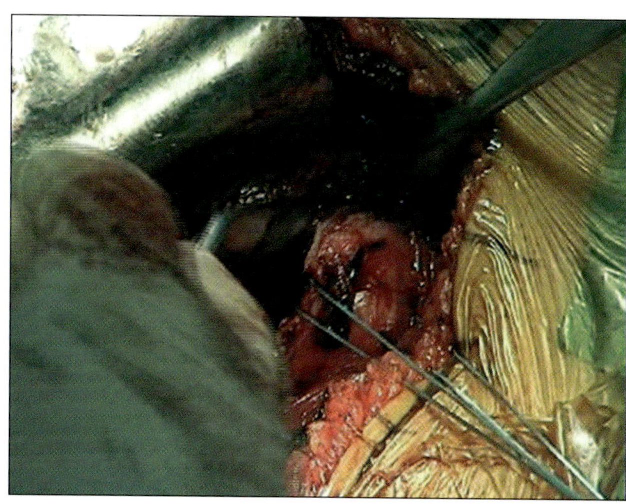

B

FIGURE 8

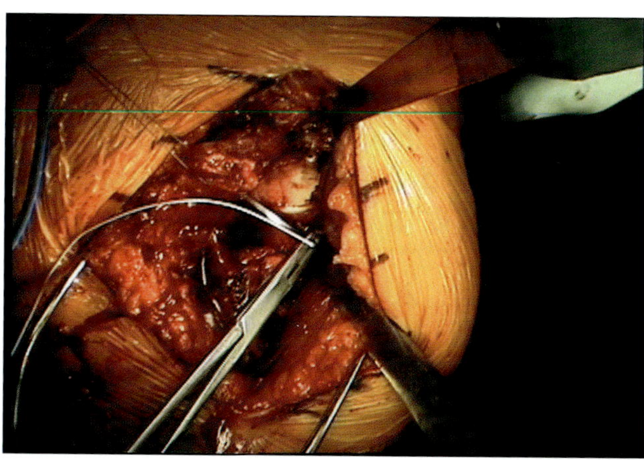

A

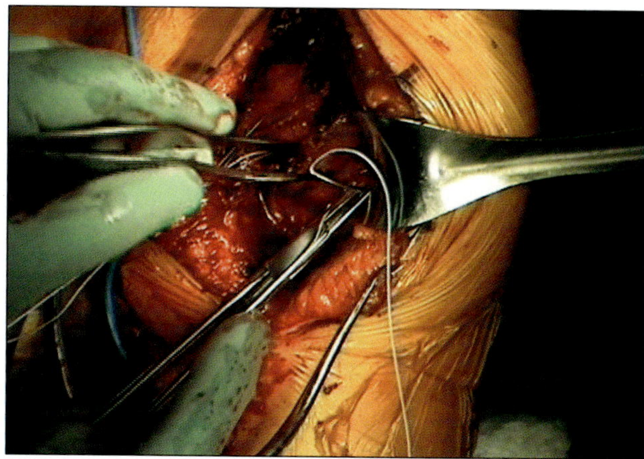

B

FIGURE 9

Pearls

- *Using small skin hooks can help pull the tuberosity fragment into the operative field with minimal damage to fragments.*
- *Minimize trauma to tuberosity fragments using a "no-touch" technique.*

Pitfalls

- *Excessive handling can lead to fragmentation of the osteoporotic greater tuberosity segment.*
- *Never debulk tuberosity fragments.*

- Head fragment(s) are identified and removed.
  - Cancellous bone from the humeral head is used for bone graft.
- The glenoid is evaluated for any trauma or degenerative arthritis.
- The greater tuberosity is often retracted posterior and superior. Abducting and internally rotating the arm can improve the exposure of these fragments.
- A traction stitch placed into the supraspinatus may be utilized to deliver the fragment into the wound. Once exposed, multiple heavy sutures are placed at the supraspinatus tendon–bone interface and used to manipulate the fragments.
- Banking larger diameter needles off the Browne deltoid retractor posteriorly may facilitate suture placement into the greater tuberosity fragment.
- Small greater tuberosity fragments may require additional suture from the humeral shaft to a Krakow stitch in the supraspinatus in order to prevent suture pullout and further fragmentation (Frankle and Mighell, 2004).

Pearls

- *Body size of the prosthesis should be minimized to allow for tension-free tuberosity reduction.*
- *The key to good function is anatomic tuberosity union.*
- *Voids are filled with bone graft and not cement.*

Pitfalls

- *Use of the distal biceps groove for alignment causes 10–20° of excessive retroversion (Boileau and Walch, 1997).*
- *Excessive retroversion limits internal rotation and increases traction forces on the repair (Frankle et al., 2001).*
- *Improper height, version, or head size compromises functional outcome (Frankle and Mighell, 2004).*

Step 3: Placement of Prosthesis

- The humeral canal is sequentially hand reamed to the appropriate size in preparation for cement fixation.
- Two drill holes are placed along the lateral humeral cortex approximately 1 cm distal to the surgical neck fracture, with one hole on each side of the bicipital groove. Two heavy sutures are placed through the drill holes for vertical fixation.
- The humeral component is trialed to assess for proper height. This determination is aided by:
  - Medial calcar—A portion is usually intact, and the medial collar of the prosthesis should be flush with remaining calcar. Figure 10A and 10B show assessment of height using a medial calcar reference and head-tuberosity distance (HTD).
  - Pectoralis major tendon—The average distance from the proximal edge of the tendon to the highest point of the humeral head is 5.6 ± 0.5 cm (Murachovsky et al., 2006).
  - Tuberosity position—With the trial head in place, the tuberosities should reduce to the shaft and remain beneath the humeral head without undue tension.
    - Head-to-tuberosity distance should be approximately 10 mm (Mighell et al., 2003).

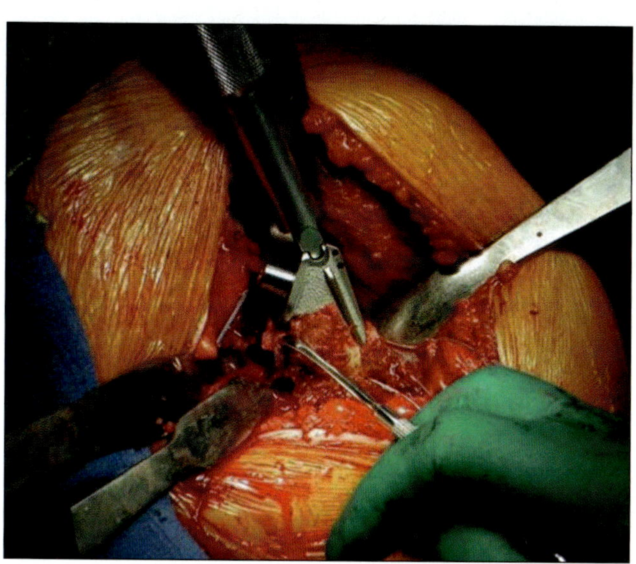
A

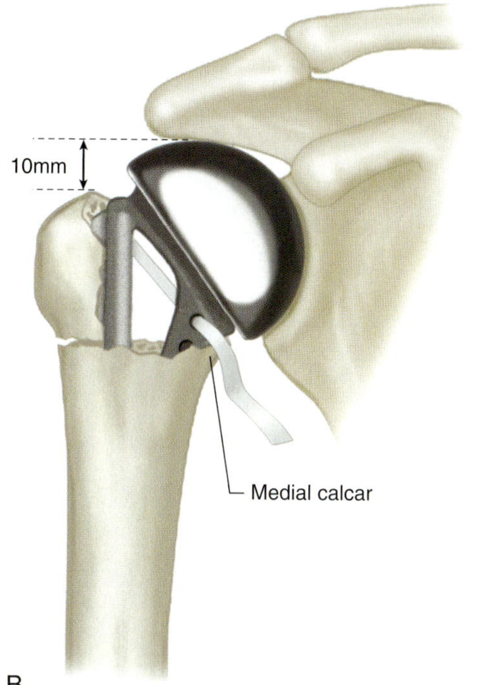

B

FIGURE 10

- Proper version is determined.
  - Forearm—An alignment guide can be used to place the prosthesis in 20–30° of retroversion with respect to the forearm.
  - Biceps groove—The proximal portion of the groove can be used as a landmark to align with the anterior fin of the prosthesis and recreate the appropriate amount of retroversion in most prosthetic designs with at least two fins.
  - In Figure 11, version is checked using a guide rod (Fig. 11A), bicipital groove alignment with an anterior fin (Fig. 11B), and the transepicondylar axis (Fig. 11C).
- Version is marked on the humeral shaft.
- Head size can be estimated using the removed head segment and the glenoid vault.
- A trial reduction of tuberosities around the stem and trial head is done to ensure proper fit.
  - The greater tuberosity should abut the anterior fin of the prosthesis in a three-fin design and should overhang the lateral fin.
- A cement restrictor is placed and cement is pressurized into the humeral canal.
- Two heavy sutures are placed around the neck of the prosthesis.

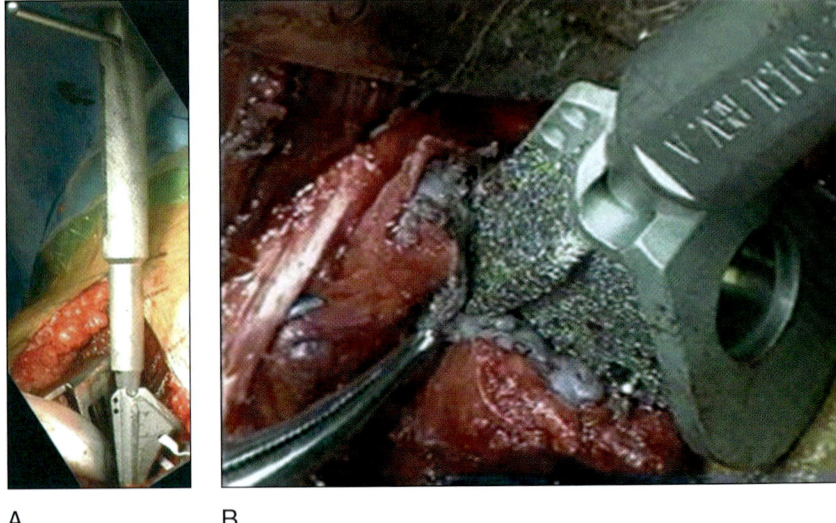

A B

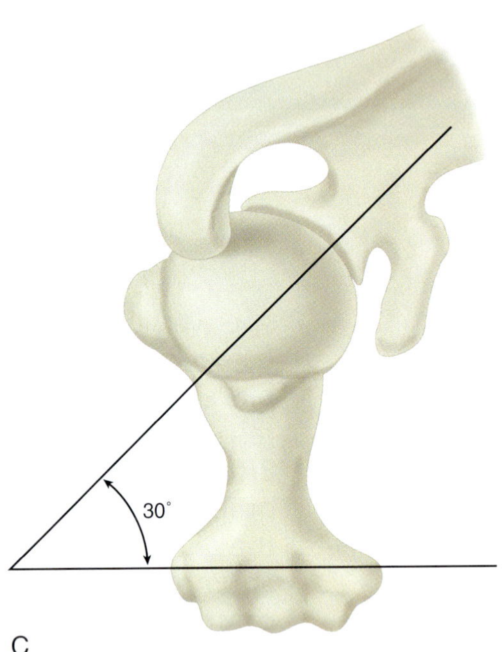

C

FIGURE 11

- Excess cement is removed as the prosthesis is placed.
- Bone graft from the humeral head is packed around the proximal portion of the neck of the prosthesis.
- Proper humeral head implant size may be judged by assessing the head fragments removed and/or by measuring the size of the patient's glenoid.
- The cement is allowed to cure and then the humeral head implant is impacted.

Pearls

- *Meticulous suture management allows for efficient tuberosity fixation.*
- *Flouroscopy intraoperatively can minimize the possibility of malreduction.*
- *Kirschner wires may help with provisional tuberosity placement.*

Pitfalls

- *Improper tuberosity placement (malreduction either vertically or horizontally) or inadequate tuberosity fixation will result in a poor outcome.*

Step 4: Reconstruction of Tuberosities

- Cerclage sutures
  - Heavy sutures are passed around the body of the prosthesis and then through the greater and lesser tuberosities at the bone-tendon junction (Fig. 12A).
  - Maximal tuberosity stability is provided by one or two heavy cerclage sutures around the tuberosities

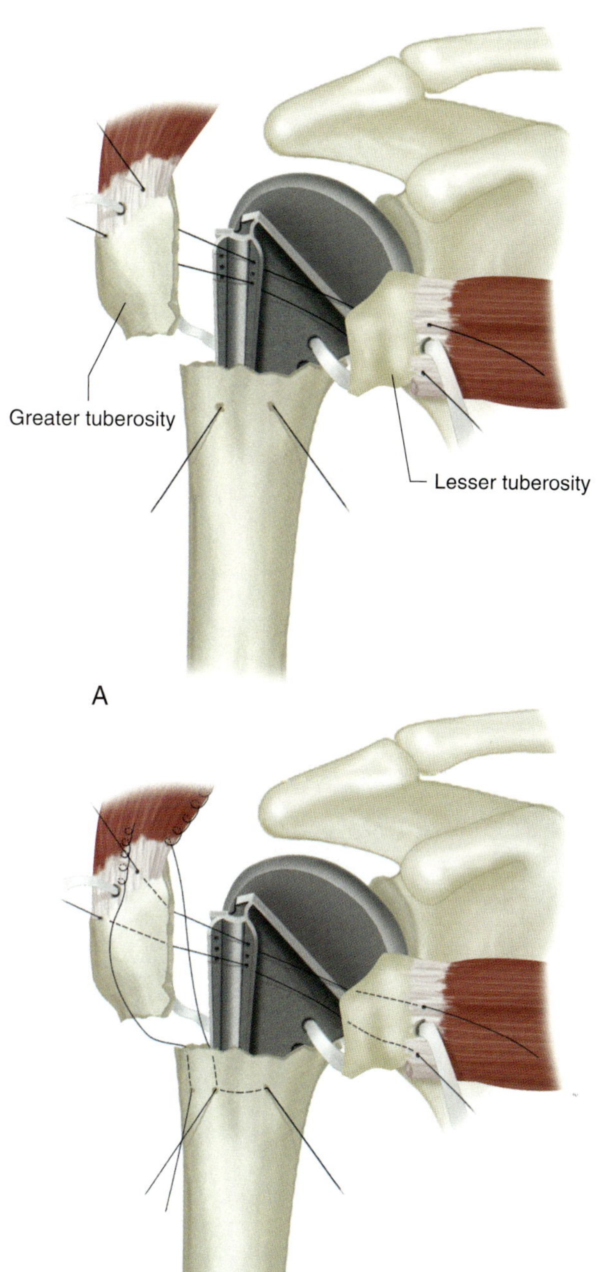

FIGURE 12

and prosthesis (Fig. 12B). A prosthesis with irregular geometry enhances the effectiveness of this construct (Frankle and Mighell, 2004; Frankle et al., 2001).

- Horizontal fixation—These sutures are passed from the greater to the lesser tuberosity at the bone-tendon junction laterally. Holes in the anterior fin of the prosthesis may be used to pass suture through.
- Tuberosity reduction—The C-arm can be used to check tuberosity position prior to final fixation.
  - The greater tuberosity should be approximately 10 mm from the top of the humeral head articular surface.
  - The greater tuberosity is then secured to the anterior fin in its reduced position.
- Cerclage sutures and horizontal fixation are secured after proper reduction is confirmed. Figure 13A and 13B show the suture fixation final construct.
- Vertical fixation—The tuberosities are secured to the shaft by passing one shaft suture through the construct anteriorly and one posteriorly in a figure-of-8 fashion.
- The arm is abducted approximately 20° prior to securing the vertical suture fixation to relieve tension on the construct.

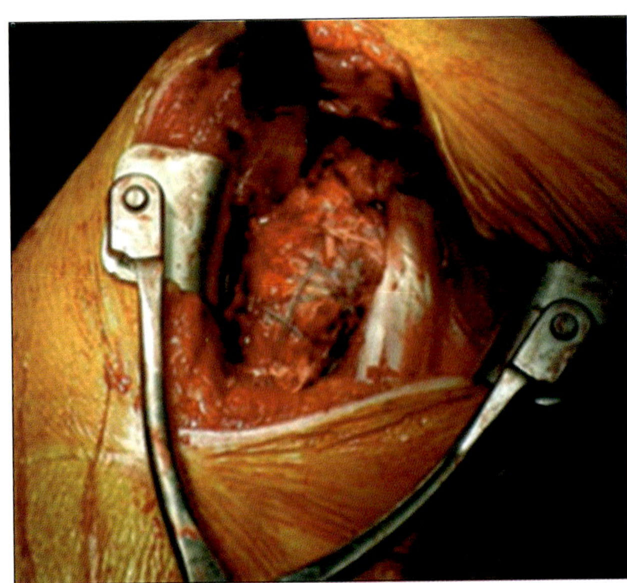

A

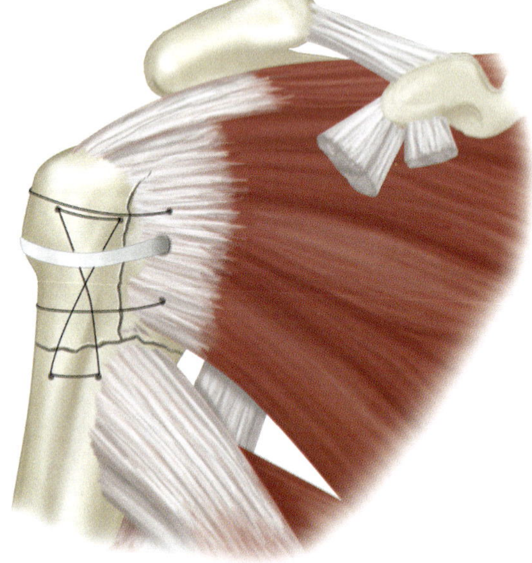

B

FIGURE 13

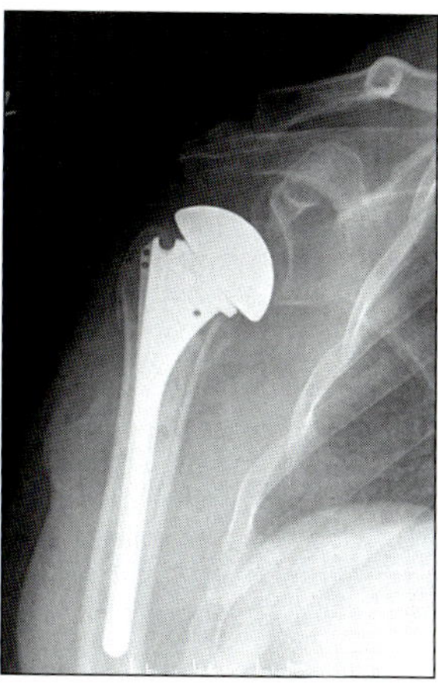
A

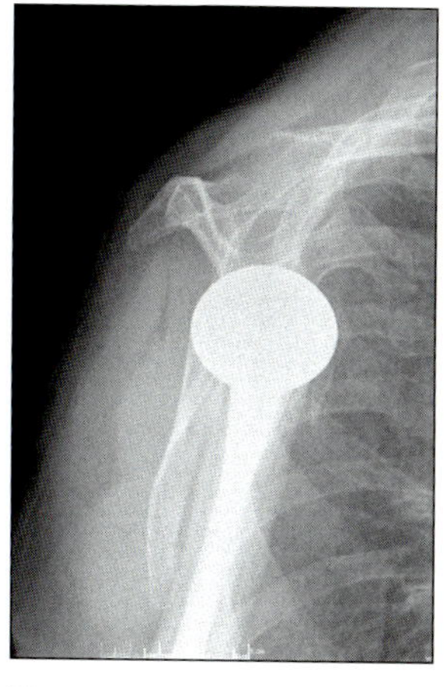
B

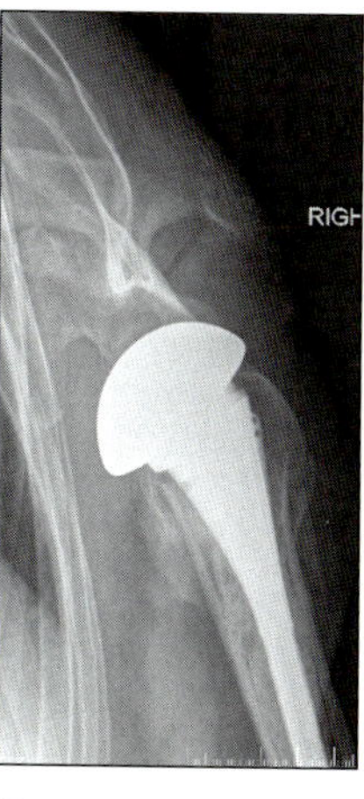

C

FIGURE 14

- Stability of the tuberosities is evaluated throughout the range of motion both visually and fluoroscopically. Figure 14A–C shows final radiographs of hemiarthroplasty for fracture.

STEP 5: CLOSURE

- The wound is copiously irrigated.
- A standard closure is performed in layers.
- The patient is placed into a shoulder immobilizer postoperatively.

PEARLS

- *Drains may be used if there is concern for hematoma.*

Postoperative Care and Expected Outcomes

- The shoulder immobilizer is used for 4–6 weeks or until evidence of tuberosity healing.
- The patient performs pendulum exercises only.
- After 6 weeks, the patient begins active-assisted range of motion and use of the arm for activities of daily living. Lifting restrictions of 5 pounds or less are imposed.
- The patient may begin to progress to activity as tolerated at 3 months. Heavy lifting and sport restrictions continue until 6 months.

PEARLS

- *The recovery period may last for greater than a year.*

PITFALLS

- *Early, aggressive therapy for range of motion puts the patient at risk for tuberosity failure.*

Evidence

Boileau P, Walch G. The three-dimensional geometry of the proximal humerus: implications for surgical technique and prosthetic design. J Bone Joint Surg [Br]. 1997;79:857-65.

The three-dimensional geometry of the proximal humerus was studied on human cadaver specimens. Findings demonstrated that the geometry of the proximal humerus is extremely variable. The authors evaluated the effectiveness of the bicipital groove as a means of determining retroversion of the prosthesis. If the biceps groove is used as a landmark at the level of the shaft, the fracture prosthesis was found to be retroverted an additional 10° with respect to the transepicondylar axis. Variations in the geometry of the humerus may not be accommodated by the designs of most contemporary human proximal humerus fracture systems.

Bufquin T, Hersan A, Hubert L, Massin P. Reverse shoulder arthroplasty for the treatment of three- and four-part fractures of the proximal humerus in the elderly: a prospective review of 43 cases with a short-term follow-up. J Bone Joint Surg [Br]. 2007;89:516-20.

The authors presented the results of 43 patients with three- and four-part proximal humerus fractures treated acutely with a reverse shoulder arthroplasty. The mean patient age was 78 years. At a mean follow-up of 22 months, the active forward elevation was 97°. The authors concluded that, compared with conventional hemiarthroplasty, satisfactory mobility was obtained despite frequent migration of the tuberosities. (Level IV evidence)

Frankle MA, Greenwald DP, Markee BA, Ondrovic LE, Lee WE. Biomechanical effects of malposition of tuberosity fragments on the humeral prosthetic reconstruction for four-part proximal humerus fractures. J Shoulder Elbow Surg. 2001;10:321-6.

In this study, nonanatomic tuberosity reconstruction led to significant impairment in external rotation kinematics and an eightfold increase in torque requirements ($p = .001$). In contrast, anatomic reconstruction produced results indistinguishable from normal shoulder controls. This study underscores the importance of rotational alignment of tuberosities during reconstruction. Failure to properly position tuberosity fragments in the horizontal plane may result in insurmountable postoperative motion restriction.

Frankle MA, Mighell MA. Techniques and principles of tuberosity fixation for proximal humeral fractures treated with hemiarthroplasty. J Shoulder Elbow Surg. 2004;13:239-47.

This paper presented a review of the literature on outcomes and complications of shoulder hemiarthroplasty. The authors also reviewed the pertinent anatomic landmarks that help achieve a proper reduction of the tuberosities and defined the biomechanical and clinical consequences of malunion and nonunion. The importance of achieving a stable, anatomic tuberosity fixation was underscored. This requires a reproducible technique, a reliable instrumentation system, and a fracture prosthesis that can optimize tuberosity reconstruction.

Frankle MA, Ondrovic LE, Markee BA, Harris ML, Lee WE. Stability of tuberosity reattachment in proximal humeral hemiarthroplasty. J Shoulder Elbow Surg. 2002;11:413-20.

This study compared different tuberosity reconstruction methods for four-part humeral fractures. The use of a circumferential medial cerclage during hemiarthroplasty for four-part humeral fractures decreased interfragmentary motion and strain, maximized fracture stability, and facilitated postoperative rehabilitation.

Kabir K, Burger C, Fischer P, Weber O, Florczyk A, Goost H, Rangger C. Health status as an important outcome factor after hemiarthroplasty. J Shoulder Elbow Surg. 2009;18:75-82.

A group of 28 patients over the age of 60 years was treated with hemiarthroplasty for proximal humerus fracture and divided according to their health status. The authors found that diminished functional outcomes were seen in patients with three or more medical comorbidities and taking a minimum of three medications. Additionally, the inability to comply with physiotherapy was associated with worse outcomes. (Level III evidence)

Loew M, Heitkemper S, Parsch D, Schneider S, Rickert. Influence of the design of the prosthesis on the outcome after hemiarthroplasty of the shoulder in displaced fractures of the head of the humerus. J Bone Joint Surg [Br]. 2006;88:345-50.

The authors reviewed the results of hemiarthroplasty for three- and four-part fractures in a group of 39 patients. During the first half of the study, a standard third-generation anatomic prosthesis was used; for the second half, a fracture-specific prosthetic design was utilized. Outcomes measured, including range of motion, rates of tuberosity healing, and Constant score, showed no statistically significant difference between the groups. Functional results were found to be significantly better with tuberosity healing. (Level II evidence)

Mighell MA, Kolm GP, Collinge CA, Frankle MA. Outcomes of hemiarthroplasty for fractures of the proximal humerus. J Shoulder Elbow Surg. 2003;12:569-77.

Outcomes of 80 shoulders treated with hemiarthroplasty were reviewed. At follow-up, 93% of patients were pain free and satisfied with their results. The mean American Shoulder and Elbow Surgeons score was 76.6, the mean Simple Shoulder Test score was 7.5, forward flexion was 128°, external rotation was 43°, and internal rotation was to L2. The authors recommended placement of the greater tuberosity 10 mm below the superior aspect of the prosthetic humeral head. (Level IV evidence)

Murachovsky J, Ikemoto RY, Nascimento LG, Fujiki EN, Milani C, Warner JJ. Pectoralis major tendon reference (PMT): a new method for accurate restoration of humeral length with hemiarthroplasty for fracture. J Shoulder Elbow Surg. 2006;15:675-8.

The authors dissected 20 cadavers (40 shoulders), and the distance between the upper border of the pectoralis major tendon insertion on the humerus and the top of the humeral head was measured (PMT). The PMT averaged 5.6 ± 0.5 cm. In only 4 of 40 shoulders did this distance exceed 6.0 cm, and there was no correlation between the size of the patient and this measurement. The PMT is a useful landmark that will aid in accurate restoration of humeral length when reconstructing complex proximal humeral fractures where landmarks are otherwise lost because of fracture comminution.

Sirveaux F, Navez GN, Roche O, Mole D, Williams MD. Reverse prosthesis for proximal humerus fracture, technique and results. Tech Shoulder Elbow Surg. 2008;9:15-22.

The authors discussed acute treatment of proximal humerus fractures with a reverse shoulder arthroplasty in cases with poor prognostic factors for treatment with hemiarthroplasty. Technical aspects of the procedure were reviewed. Data for 15 patients with a mean age of 78 who were treated acutely with a reverse shoulder arthroplasty for fracture were presented. At an average follow-up of 46 months, mean forward elevation was 107° and 14/15 patients had greater than 90°. The authors noted that external rotation recovery appeared dependent on tuberosity healing. (Level IV evidence)

PROCEDURE 33

Surgical Treatment of Scapular Fractures

Donald H. Lee

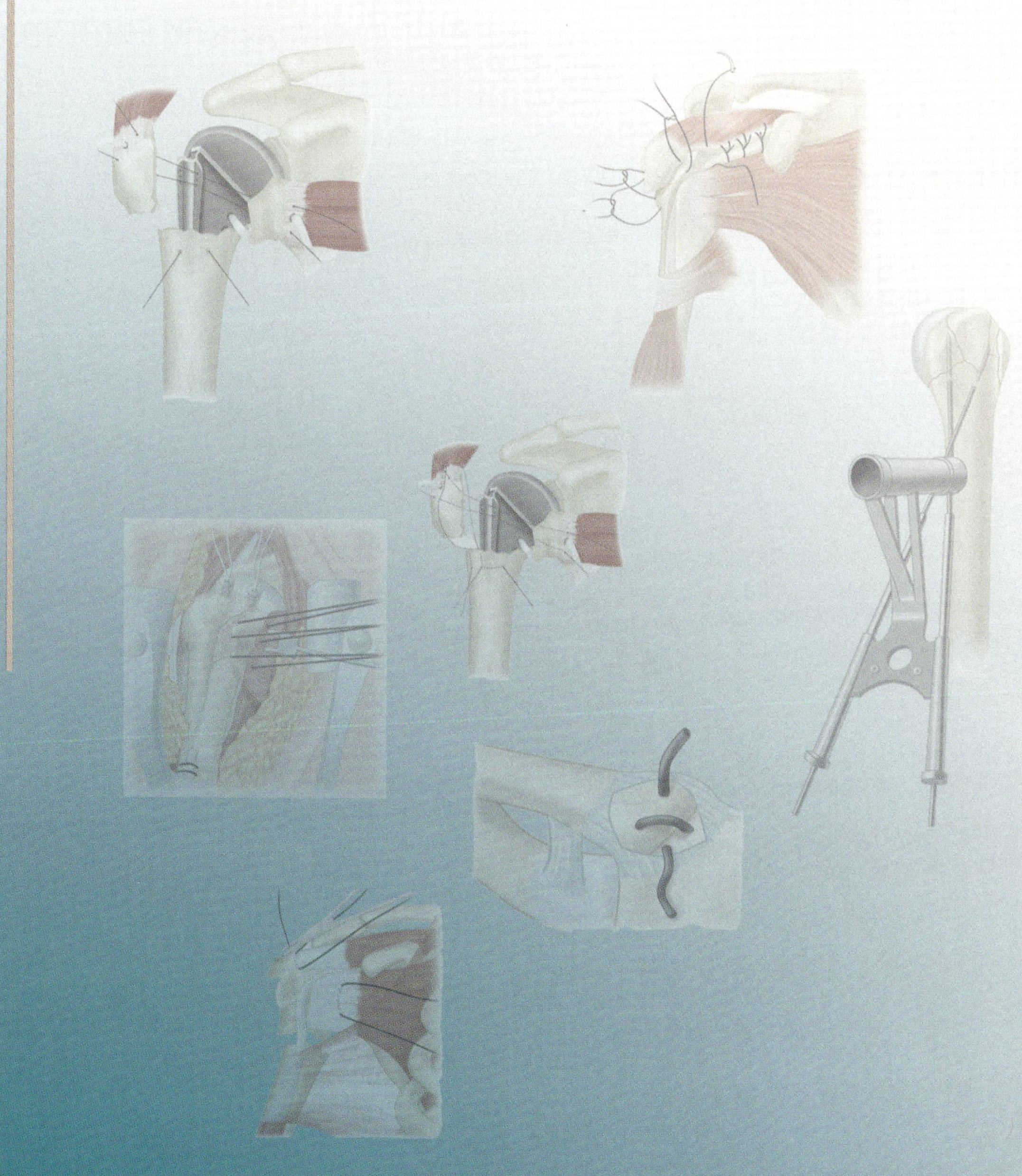

PITFALLS

- *With a high incidence of associated injuries, staging the operative procedures may be needed.*
- *Knowledge of the surgical anatomy and adequate surgical experience are needed.*
- *With combined approaches for complex fractures, surgery may take several hours to perform. The patient must be sufficiently medically stable to undergo a long surgical procedure.*

Indications

- Significantly displaced intra-articular glenoid cavity fractures (Fig. 1)
  - Glenoid rim fractures
    - With displacement ≥ 10 mm
    - Involvement of ≥ one quarter of the anterior glenoid rim
    - Involvement of ≥ one third of the posterior glenoid rim
  - Articular stepoff ≥ 5 mm
  - Failure of the humeral head to lie within the center of the glenoid cavity
  - Severe separation of glenoid fragments
- Glenoid neck extra-articular fracture (Fig. 2)
  - With more than 1 cm of translation *or*

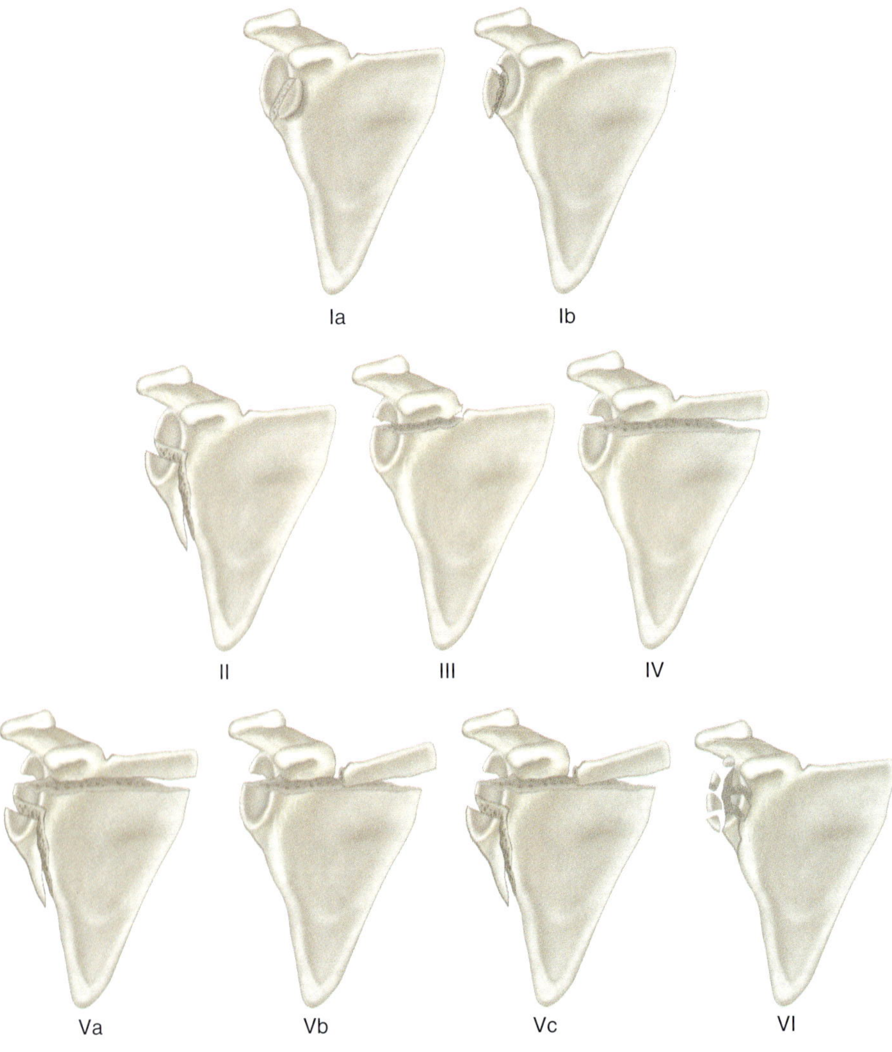

FIGURE 1

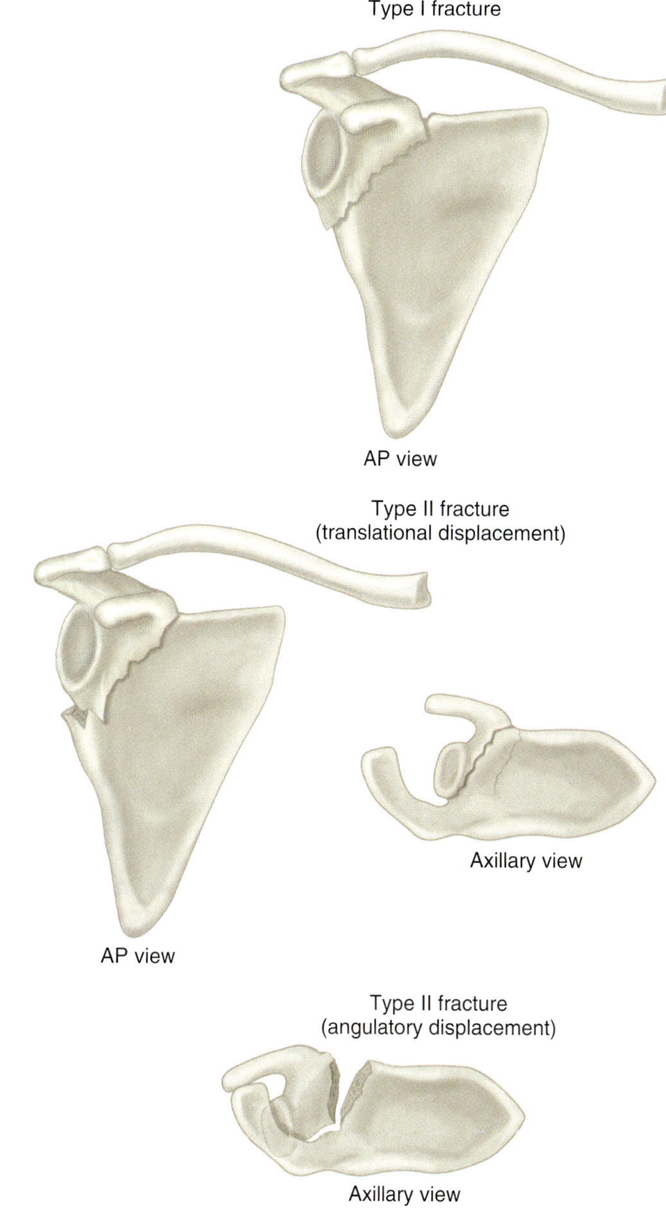

FIGURE 2

Controversies

- The majority of scapular fractures are treated nonoperatively.
- Surgical stabilization of complex scapular fractures requires extensive surgical dissection which may result in scarring and potential loss of motion and weakness.

  - With 40° of angulation in either the coronal or sagittal plane
- Glenoid neck fracture with associated clavicle fracture ("floating shoulder")
- Significantly displaced acromial fractures
- Significantly displaced coracoid fractures
- Disruptions of the superior shoulder suspensory complex
  - Coracoid fracture with grade III disruption of the acromioclavicular (AC) joint
  - Ipsilateral coracoid and acromial process fractures

- Fracture of the base of the coracoid process and glenoid neck fracture
- Coracoid process fracture and type I distal clavicle fracture
- Acromial fracture and grade III disruption of the AC joint
- Segmental acromial fracture
- Glenoid cavity fracture and disruption of the superior shoulder suspensory complex

- Rare indications for scapular body fractures
  - Lateral spike entering the glenohumeral joint
  - Intrathoracic penetration of fracture fragment
  - Removal of scapular malunion producing pain
  - Scapular nonunion

Examination/Imaging

- Evaluation for associated injuries
  - Skin, head, chest wall, pulmonary, abdominal, and pelvic injuries
  - Ipsilateral shoulder girdle and upper extremity injuries
- Neurologic examination
- Vascular examination
- Radiographs
  - Anteroposterior view of the scapula (Fig. 3A)
  - Trans-scapular Y view of the scapula (Fig. 3B)
  - Axillary view of the glenohumeral joint (Fig. 3C)
- Computed tomography scans (Fig. 4A–E)
  - Three-dimensional reconstructions (Fig. 5A–D)

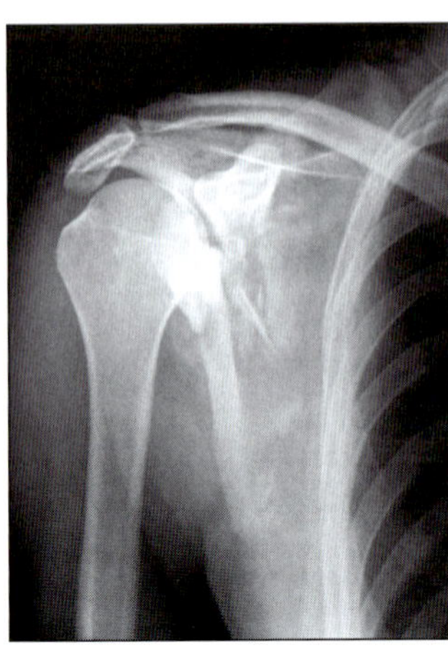
A

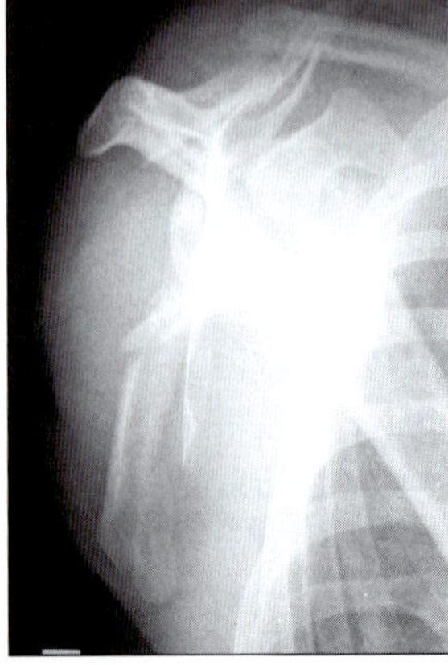
B

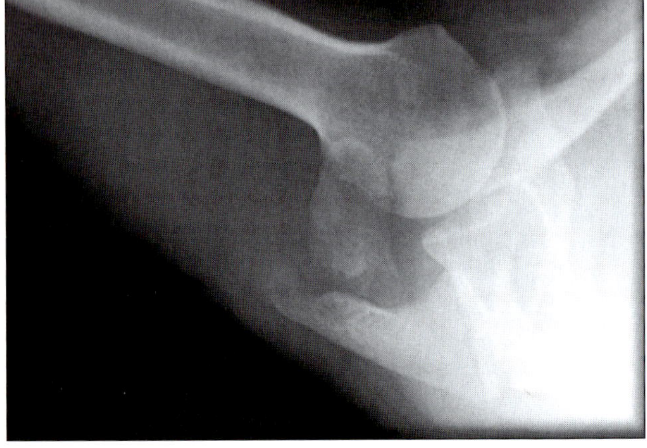
C

FIGURE 3

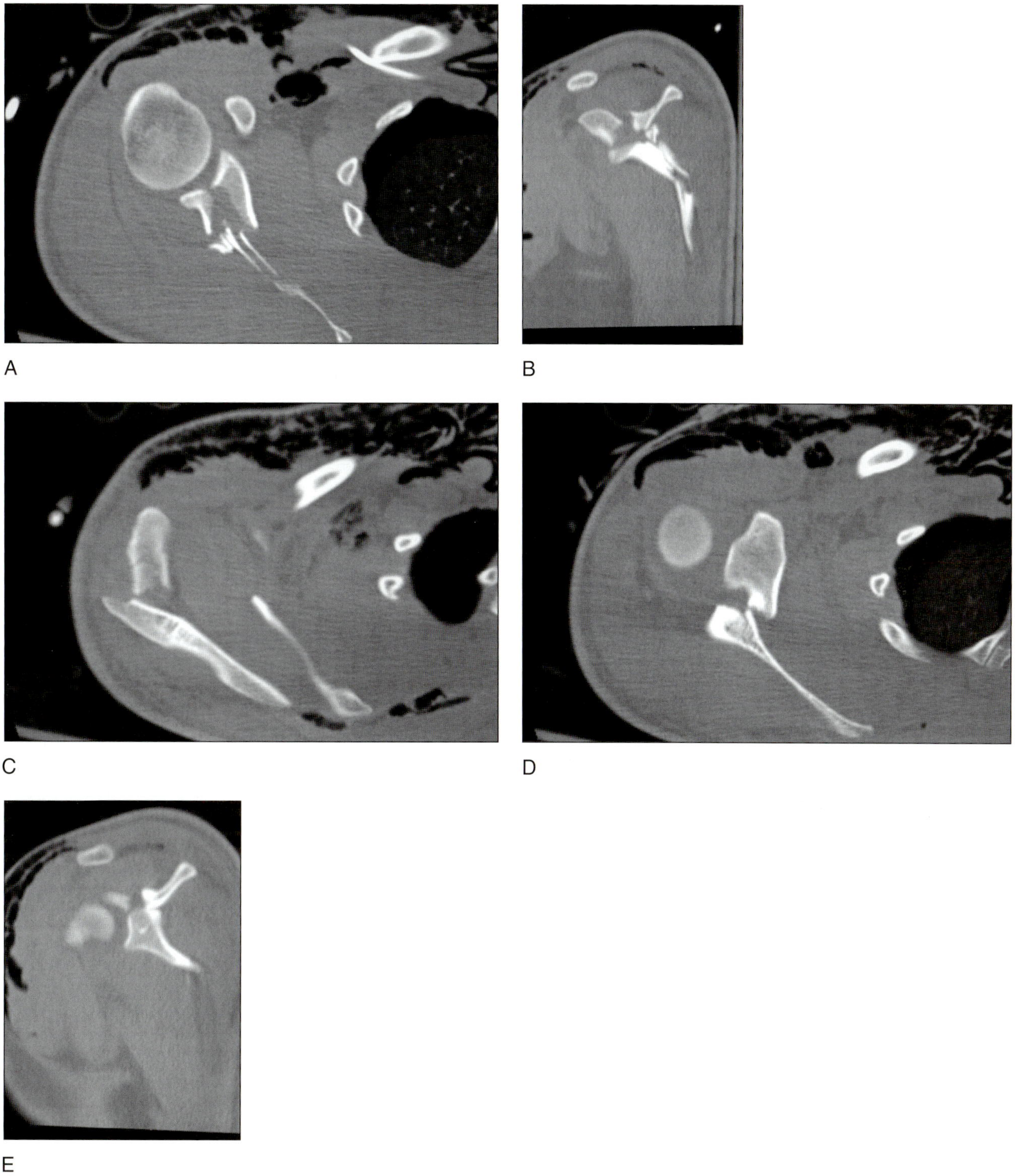

A

B

C

D

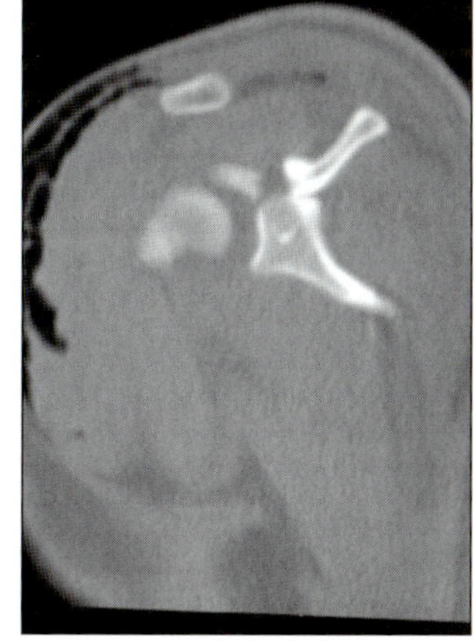

E

FIGURE 4

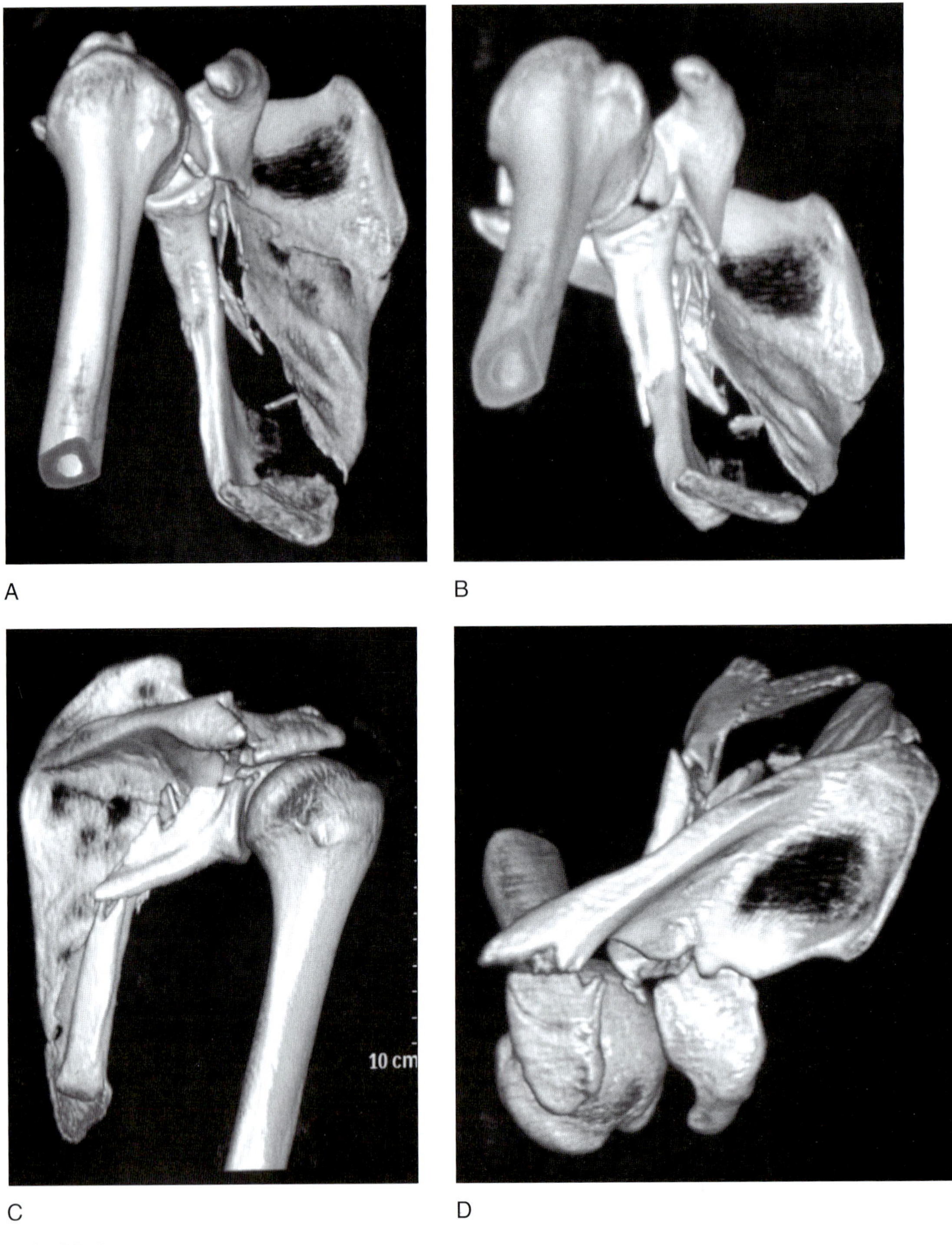

FIGURE 5

Surgical Anatomy

- Skeletal anatomy (Fig. 6A and 6B)
  - Four areas of the scapula have adequate bone stock for internal fixation:
    - Glenoid neck
    - Scapular spine

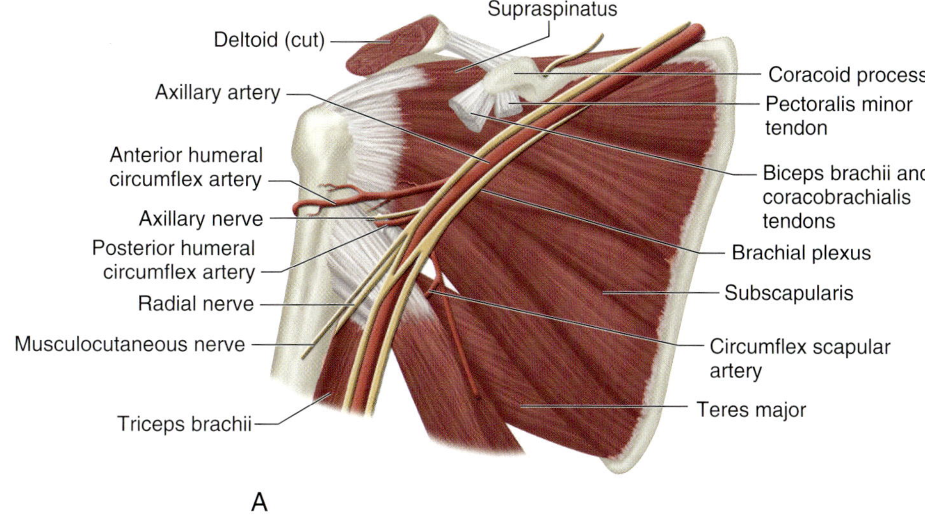

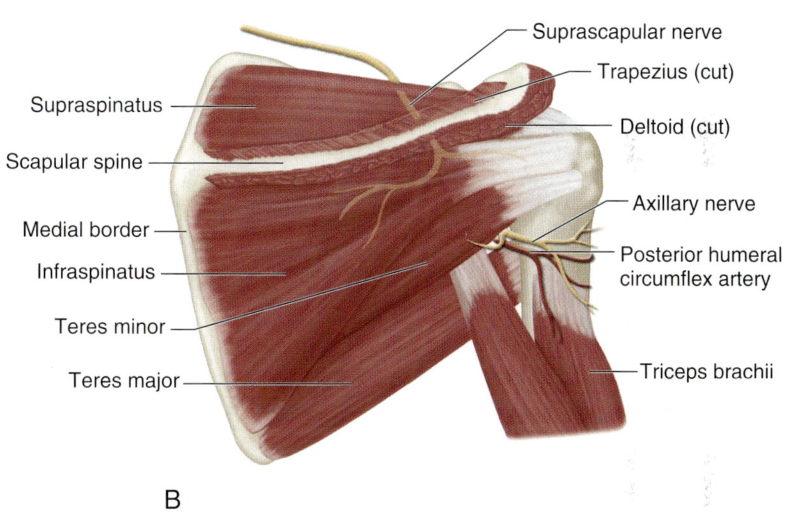

FIGURE 6

- ◆ Lateral border of the scapula
- ◆ Coracoid process

- ■ Soft tissue (muscular and tendon) attachments (see Figs. 6A and 6B)
- ■ Location of neurologic structures
  - Brachial plexus
  - Musculocutaneous nerve
  - Axillary nerve
  - Suprascapular nerve
  - Radial nerve
- ■ Location of vascular structures
  - Axillary artery
  - Anterior and posterior humeral circumflex arteries
  - Circumflex scapular artery

Positioning

- The lateral decubitus position is most commonly used for posterior approaches and for combined anterior, posterior, and/or superior approaches.
  - The affected arm is prepped and drape free (Fig. 7A and 7B).
  - An axillary roll is used.
  - The head, neck, chest, and pelvis are properly secured.
  - Care is taken to pad bony prominences and peripheral nerves (e.g., peroneal nerve).
  - The entire shoulder girdle is prepped, including the areas superiorly to the neck, anteriorly to the midline, distally to the midthorax level, and posteriorly to the spinous processes.
- The beach chair position is used for anterior and superior/anterior-superior approaches.
  - The affected arm is prepped and draped free.
  - The head and neck are properly secured.
  - The chest wall and pelvis are properly secured to the table.
  - A bump is placed along the medial border of the scapula to push the scapula forward.
  - Alternatively, a special beach chair positioner can be used to increase exposure to the posterior shoulder area.
- The prone position for posterior approaches is not commonly used.
  - The affected arm is draped free or placed at the patient's side.

Pearls

- *Preoperative placement of C-arm fluoroscopy will ensure that adequate fluoroscopy views are obtained during surgery.*
- *Care is taken during preparation and draping of the patient to ensure that there is adequate surgical exposure both anteriorly, posteriorly, and superiorly (see Fig. 7A and 7B).*
- *Endotracheal intubation is preferred so that the patient can be fully paralyzed (if needed) during surgery.*

Pitfalls

- *Failure to properly secure the head/neck and torso, especially during beach chair positioning, may result in loss of proper patient positioning during surgery.*

Equipment

- For lateral decubitus position
  - Beanbag
  - Peg board
- For beach chair position
  - Standard operating room bed versus specialized beach chair positioner

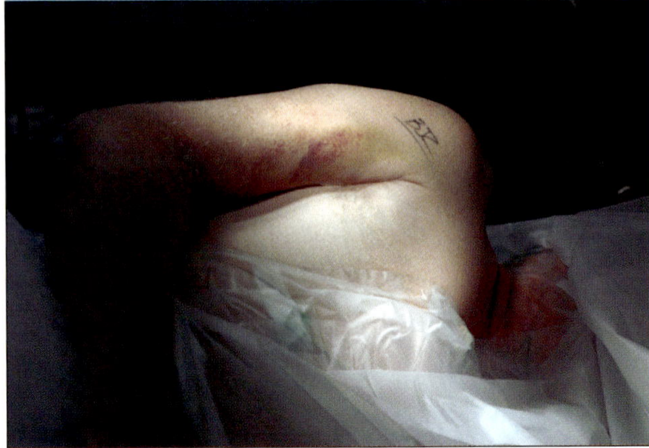
A

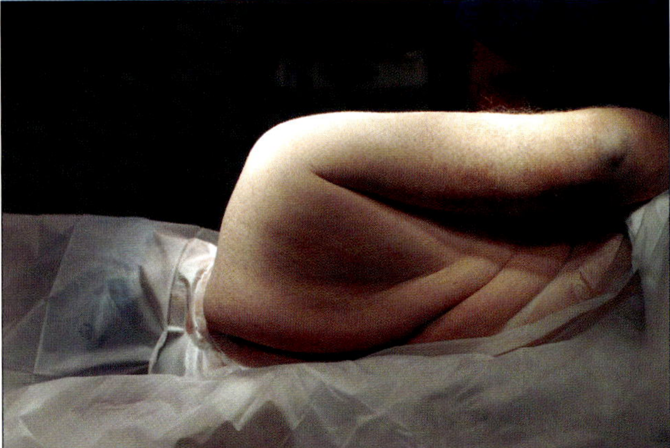
B

FIGURE 7

- The head and neck and endotracheal tube are properly secured.
- Care is taken to pad all bony prominences.

■ C-arm fluoroscopy is recommended.

- With lateral decubitus positioning, the C-arm is positioned over top of the patient (Fig. 8).
- With beach chair positioning, the C-arm is position at the head of the bed and brought in from a cephalad position (Fig. 9).

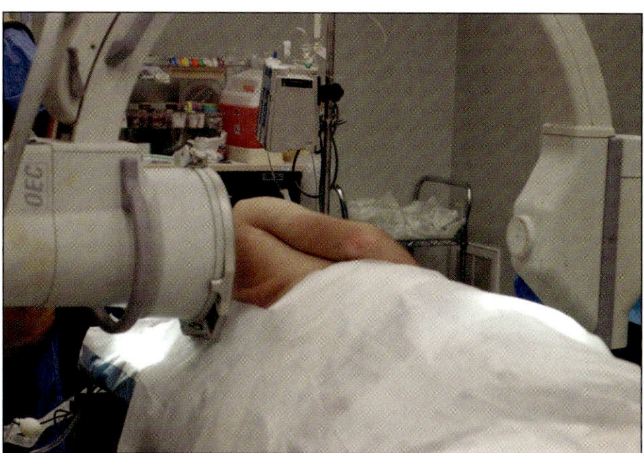

FIGURE 8

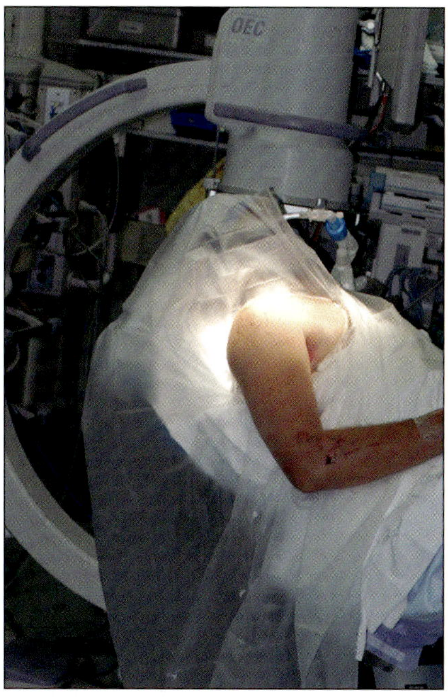

FIGURE 9

Portals/Exposures

Anterior Deltopectoral Approach

- The anterior deltopectoral approach is used for anterior glenoid rim fractures, intra-articular glenoid fossa fractures, and superior glenoid fossa fractures, including coracoid fractures.
- The skin incision starts superiorly near the coroacoid process, near the midclavicle, and extends distally and obliquely over the deltopectoral interval toward the deltoid insertion (Fig. 10) (see Anterior Shoulder Incision video).
- The deltopectoral interval is developed with the cephalic vein retracted laterally (preferred) or medially.
- The clavipectoral fascia is incised along the lateral edge of the conjoined tendon up to coracoacromial ligament but leaving the ligament intact (see Clavipectoral Fascia Dissection video).
- The coracoid (if needed) is exposed.
- The anterior inferior humeral circumflex artery is identified and cauterized or ligated.
- A subscapularis tenotomy or subscapularis release off the lesser tuberosity is performed with release of the underlying joint capsule (see Subscapularis Release videos 1 and 2).
- The anterior capsule, with a sleeve of periosteum, can be elevated along the anterior and medial humeral neck to increase exposure.
- The rotator interval is released.
- A humeral head retractor is used to expose the glenoid (see Glenoid Fracture Exposure video)

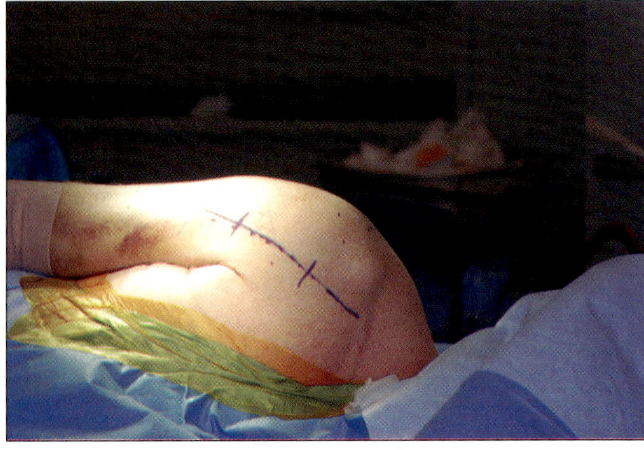

FIGURE 10

Posterior Approach

- The posterior approach is used for posterior glenoid rim fractures, intra-articular glenoid fossa fractures, glenoid neck fractures, scapular body (including scapular spine) fractures, and acromial fractures.
- The skin incision starts at the posterolateral corner of the acromion and horizontally parallels the scapular spine and then extends vertically along the medial border of the scapula (Fig. 11) (see Posterior Scapular Incision videos 1 and 2).
- The deltoid and trapezius (for later repair) with overlying fascia are elevated from the scapular spine (see Posterior Fascial Dissection videos 1 and 2 and Scapular Spine Dissection videos 1 and 2).
- For acromial fractures, the incision can be extended further anteriorly and laterally to expose the acromion subperiosteally (see Acromial Fracture Dissection videos 1–3).
- Along the medial border of the scapula, the fascia overlying the interval between the rhomboids and infraspinatus/teres minor is incised (see Scapular Medial Border Dissection videos 1 and 2).
- Inferior to the scapular spine, the interval between the deltoid and infraspinatus is developed.
- For the Judet approach, the infraspinatus and teres minor are elevated off of the infraspinatus fossa from a medial to lateral direction, allowing visualization of the scapular body and scapular neck (see Infraspinatus–Teres Minor Dissection video).
- For the modified Judet approach, the interval between the infraspinatus and teres minor is dissected, allowing for exposure of the glenoid neck.

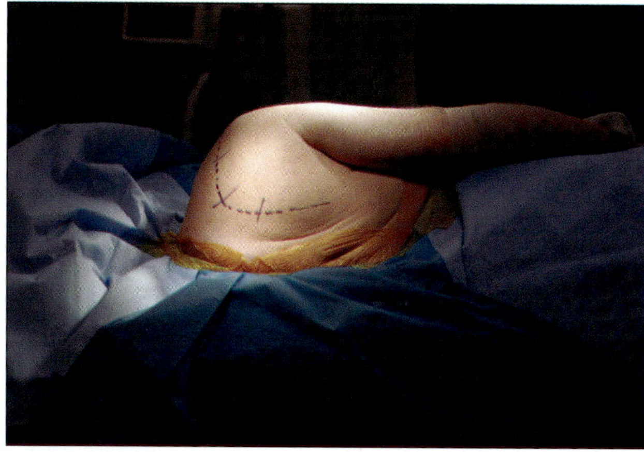

FIGURE 11

Pitfalls

- *Anterior approach*
  - *The incision should avoid the anterior axillary fold to prevent a scar contracture in this area.*
  - *Excessive traction on the conjoined tendon is avoided to prevent injury to the musculocutaneous nerve.*
  - *Care is taken to protect the axillary nerve inferiorly.*
- *Posterior approach*
  - *Limited interval approaches may give incomplete exposure of the scapular body and neck fractures.*
  - *Exposure to the posterior superior portion of glenoid neck is limited with the posterior approach, and may require elevation of the supraspinatus, endangering the suprascapular nerve.*
  - *Care is taken when dissecting the infraspinatus near the spinoglenoid notch to prevent undue traction on the suprascapular nerve.*
- *Superior and anterior superior approach*
  - *Care is taken to protect the supraclavicular nerves.*
  - *Provides only limited exposure of the glenoid fossa.*

Instrumentation

- Self-retaining retractors
- Glenoid retractors

- For exposure of glenoid intra-articular fractures, a tenotomy of the infraspinatus and teres minor (if needed) and posterior capsulotomy are performed (see Posterior Glenoid Fracture Exposure with Probe video).
- Alternatively, a modified posterior subdeltoid approach to the scapula is performed by using an extended posterior axillary fold incision.
  - The arm is abducted 90°, allowing deltoid relaxation and retraction of the deltoid superiorly.
  - A modified Judet interval approach can then be used (see above).

Superior or Anterior-Superior Approach

- The superior or anterior-superior approach is used for coracoid fractures, superior glenoid fossa fracture involving the coracoid process, acromial fractures, and clavicle fractures.
- The skin incision can include a saber-cut incision along Langer's skin lines or a transverse incision, slightly inferior and parallel to the clavicle (for clavicle fractures).
- The deltoid can be split between the anterior and middle thirds.
- A portion of the deltoid can be reflected off the anterior aspect of the acromion and clavicle for exposure.
- The rotator interval can be opened to expose the glenoid.
- For clavicle fractures, the platysma is incised and a subperiosteal dissection of the clavicle is performed.

Approach by Fracture Type

- Extra-articular glenoid neck fractures
  - For fractures involving the inferior glenoid fossa or lateral border of scapula, the interval approach between the infraspinatus and teres minor (modified Judet approach) is recommended.
  - For fractures requiring greater exposure of the glenoid neck and scapular body, elevation of the infraspinatus and teres minor from the infraspinatus fossa (Judet approach) is recommended.
- Intra-articular glenoid fossa fractures
  - For anterior glenoid fossa fractures, a deltopectoral approach with subscapularis tenotomy or subscapularis release from the lesser tuberosity and anterior capsulotomy is used.
  - For superior glenoid fossa/coracoid fractures
    - A superior deltoid splitting approach can be used.

Controversies

- Some types of intra-articular glenoid fractures may be treated with fluoroscopically assisted and/or arthroscopically assisted percutaneous internal fixation.

        - Alternatively, a deltopectoral approach with percutaneous placement of interfragmentary compression screws, and subscapularis tenotomy or subscapularis release from the lesser tuberosity, can be used.
    - For posterior glenoid fossa fractures, a posterior approach with infraspinatus and teres minor tenotomy and posterior capsulotomy is used.
- Acromial fractures
    - For fractures involving the acromion, the incision used for the posterior approach along the scapular spine is extended anteriorly along the acromion and a subperiosteal approach to the acromion is used.
- Clavicle fractures
    - An incision is placed parallel and slightly inferior to the clavicle.
    - Alternatively, a saber-cut type of incision along Langer's skin lines can be used.
- Coracoid fractures
    - A deltopectoral approach with percutaneous placement of cannulated screws can be used.
    - Alternatively, a superior approach can be used.

Pitfalls

- *Extremely comminuted fractures of the glenoid fossa and neck (type VI fractures) may be better treated nonoperatively.*

Procedure

Step 1: Fracture Exposure

- The fracture margins are visualized by removal of fracture hematoma, fibrous tissue, and/or callus using Cobb elevators and curettes (see Scapular Fracture Exposure videos 1 and 2).
    - Figure 12 shows an anterior glenoid exposure.
    - Figure 13 shows a Judet exposure of the scapular body.

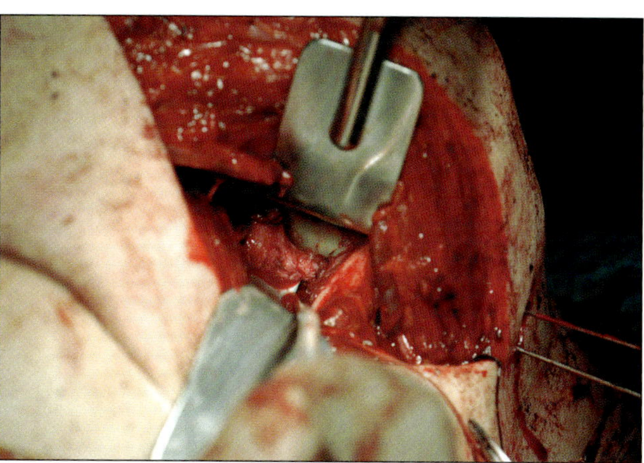

FIGURE 12

Instrumentation/ Implantation

- Threaded Schantz pins
- Curettes
- Cobb elevators
- Kirschner wires

- Threaded Shantz pins can be placed into fracture fragments (e.g., coracoid process, scapular spine, glenoid neck) to help mobilize fracture fragments.
- Kirschner wires can be used for provisional fracture fixation.

Step 2: Fracture Fixation

- Glenoid neck fractures
    - A 3.5-mm pelvic contoured reconstruction plate or precontoured scapular plate is placed along the posterior aspect of the glenoid fragment and along the lateral border of the scapula (Fig. 14A and 14B).
    - Alternatively, a contoured U-shaped 3.5-mm pelvic reconstruction plate is placed along the inferior aspect of the scapular spine and lateral border of the scapula, incorporating the scapular neck fracture (Fig. 15) (see Posterior Scapular Plate video).

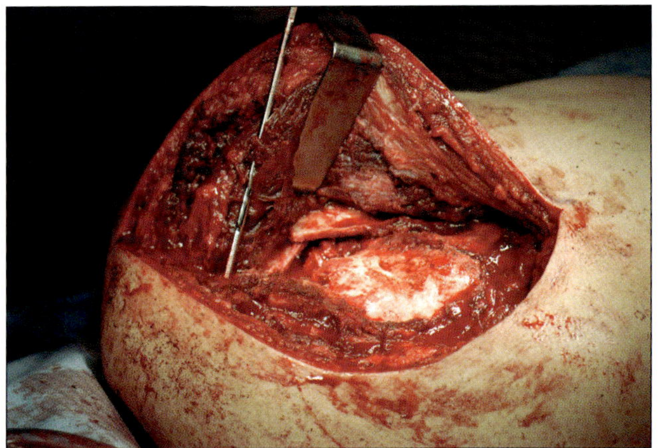

FIGURE 13

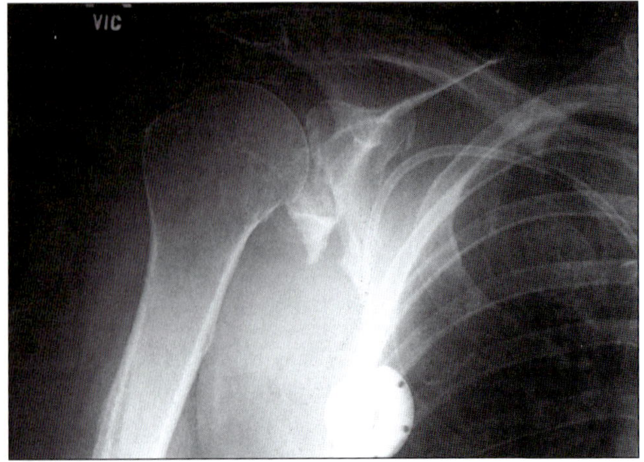

A

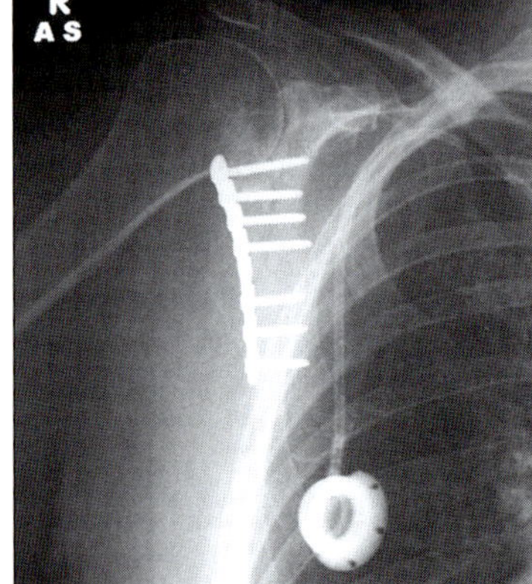

B

FIGURE 14

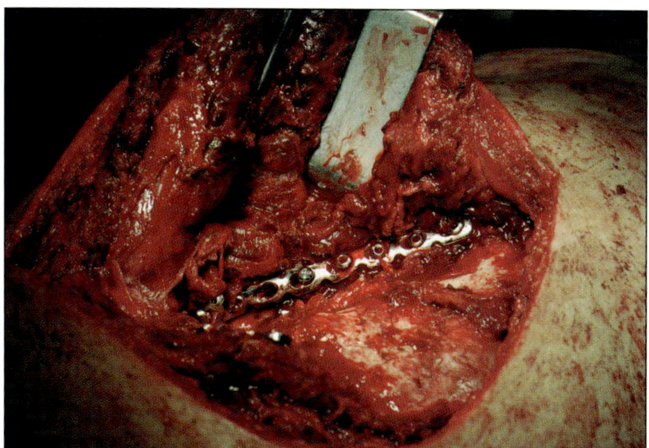

FIGURE 15

- Another alternative includes using two separate plates, one along the lateral border of the scapular body and posterior glenoid and the second along the scapular spine (Fig. 16A and 16B).
- Postoperative radiographs (of case shown in Figures 3, 4, and 5) show the final appearance in anteroposterior (Fig. 17A), axillary (Fig. 17B), and trans-scapular Y (Fig. 17C) views.

▪ Glenoid rim fractures (Fig. 18A–C)
  - For fixable fracture fragments, internal fixation is performed with interfragmentary compression screw fixation with cannulated screws (Fig. 19A and 19B).

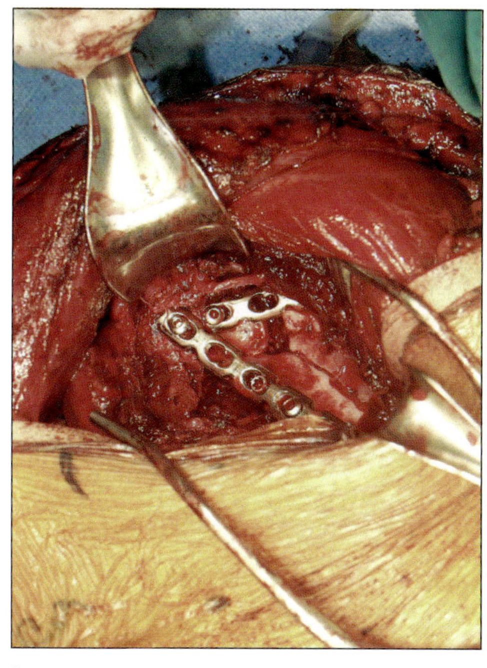

A

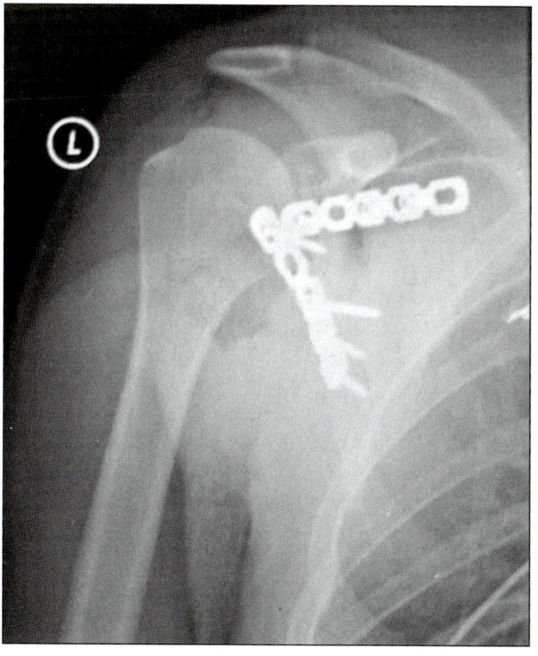

B

FIGURE 16

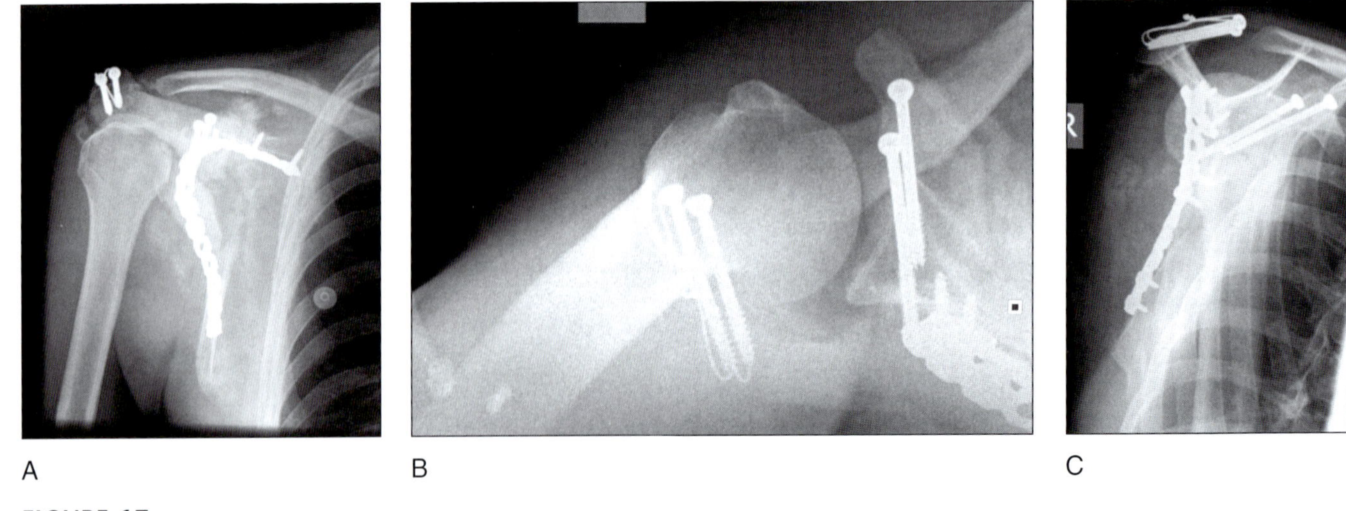

A B C

FIGURE 17

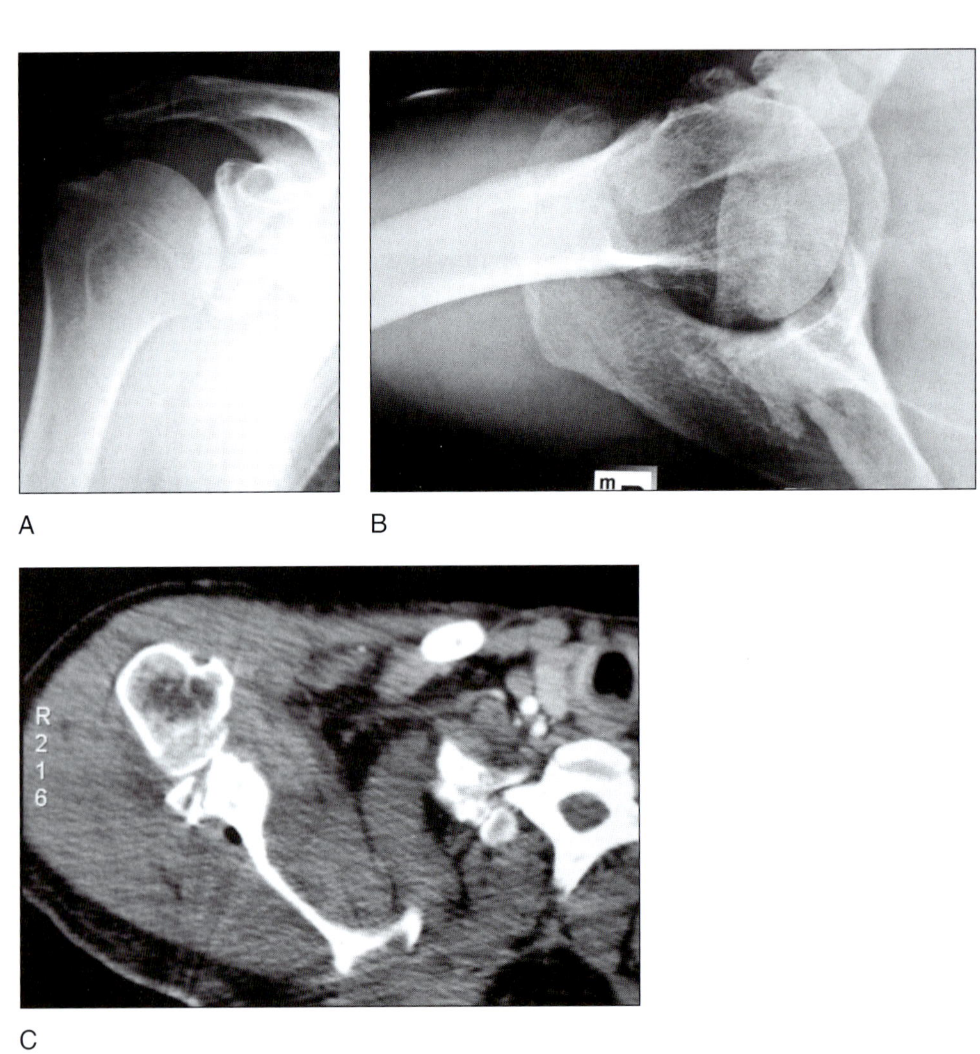

A B C

FIGURE 18

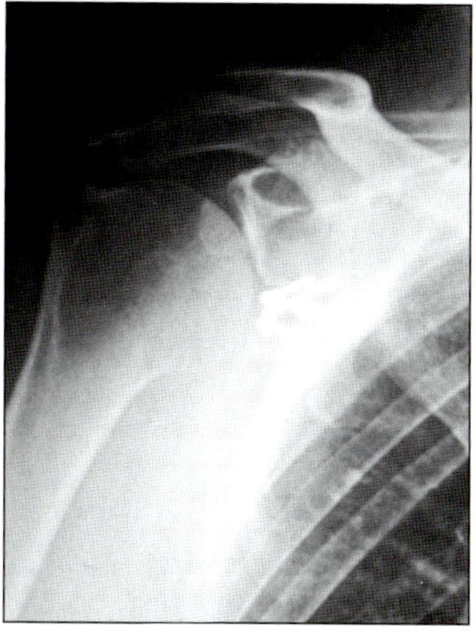

A

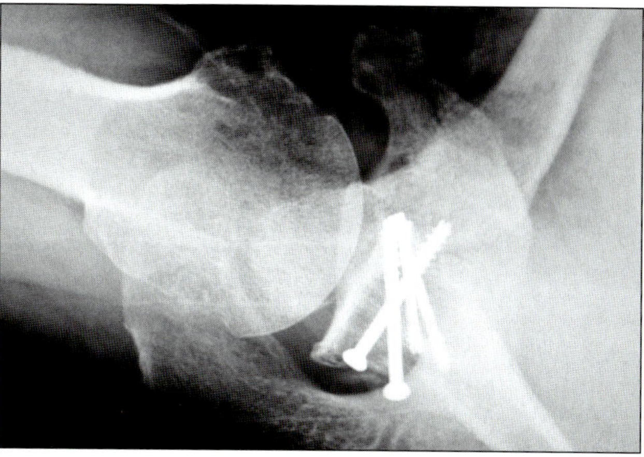

B

FIGURE 19

Pearls

- *For acromial fractures treated with cannulated screws and tension band wiring, the cannulated screws are kept short and buried within the bone, to allow for tensioning of the figure-of-8 wires.*

Pitfalls

- *Care must be taken to protect the:*
  - *Suprascapular nerve (with placement of hardware near the spinoglenoid notch and internal fixation of superior glenoid rim fractures)*
  - *Musculocutaneous nerve (with fractures involving the coracoid process)*
  - *Axillary nerve (with fractures involving the inferior glenoid rim)*

- For a comminuted fracture, fragment excision and bone grafting (e.g., tricortical iliac crest graft) is performed.
- For a small avulsion fracture (bony Bankart lesion), fragment excision and repair of periarticular soft tissue to the glenoid rim is performed.

- Glenoid fossa fractures
  - For a superior glenoid fracture fragment, interfragmentary compression screw fixation to the remaining glenoid is performed (see Superior Glenoid Screw videos 1–3) (see Fig. 17A–C).
    - Guidewires are placed percutaneously or through the anterior incision and under fluoroscopic guidance.
    - The wires are placed along the superior margin of the glenoid at the base of the coracoid process into the remaining glenoid. Care is taken to ensure that the wires remain extra-articular.
    - A cannulated drill bit is used over the guidewire and the appropriate screw length is measured.
    - The appropriate-length screw is placed over the guidewire.
  - For comminuted glenoid fossa fractures, the major fracture fragment is reduced and internally fixed using a contoured reconstruction plate or interfragmentary compression screw fixation, followed by fixation of the smaller fracture fragment (see Fig. 17A–C).
- For double disruptions of the superior shoulder suspensory complex (e.g., glenoid neck fracture and clavicle fracture)
  - Clavicle fractures are repaired with precontoured plate fixation.

Instrumentation/ Implantation

- Contoured 3.5-mm reconstruction plates (locking or nonlocking)
- Precontoured plates (clavicle, acromial, scapular plates)
- Cannulated interfragmentary compression screws
- Kirshner wires for provisional fracture fixation
- Schantz screws for manipulation of fracture fragments
- Malleable wire for tension band fixation (acromial fractures)

Controversies

- Glenoid neck fractures associated with concomitant clavicular fracture may be indirectly stabilized with clavicular fixation.
- Isolated, minimally displaced fractures of the coracoid and acromion can frequently be treated nonoperatively.

- Acromial fractures are repaired in one of two ways:
  - Tension band technique using cannulated screws (preferred) or tension band with Kirschner wires (see Fig. 17A–C) (see Acromial Fracture Dissection videos 1–3 and Acromial Fracture Fixation videos 1–4)
  - Precontoured plate fixation
- Coracoid fractures are repaired in one of two ways:
  - Interfragmentary screw fixation
  - Fragment excision (small tip fractures) with reattachment of the conjoined tendon to the remaining coracoid process with nonabsorbable sutures

Step 3: Wound Closure

- Anterior approach
  - The subscapularis is closed with #2 nonabsorbable sutures for tenotomy or transosseous sutures for subscapularis release from the lesser tuberosity (see Subscapularis Repair video).
  - The rotator interval is closed.
  - Wound closure in done in layers.
  - A suction drain is inserted as needed.
- Posterior approach
  - With the Judet approach: the infraspinatus and teres minor are replaced into the infraspinatus fossa, repairing the medial edge of the muscles to soft tissue along the medial border of the scapula with #2 nonabsorbable sutures (see Infraspinatus Repair videos 1–3).
  - The deltoid and trapezius and overlying fascia are repaired to one another or with transosseous sutures into the scapular spine with #2 nonabsorbable sutures (see Deltoid-Trapezius Repair videos 1 and 2).
  - The skin is closed in layers (see Final Wound Closure videos 1 and 2).
  - A suction drain is inserted as needed.

Postoperative Care and Expected Outcomes

- Sling and swathe immobilization are employed for approximately 6 weeks.
- Early passive range-of-motion exercises are permitted for 4–6 weeks.
- Active range of motion is begun at 6 weeks.
- Strengthening exercises are begun at 3 months.

- Functional outcome is dependent upon fracture type, adequacy of fracture reduction and fixation, and postoperative rehabilitation.

Evidence

Ada JR, Miller ME. Scapular fractures: analysis of 113 cases. Clin Orthop Relat Res. 1991;(269):174-80.

Aulicino PL, Reinert C, Kornberg M, et al. Displaced intraarticular glenoid fractures treated by open reduction and internal fixation. J Trauma. 1986;26:1137.

Bauer G, Fleischman W, DuBler E. Displaced scapular fractures: indication and long term results of open reduction and internal fixation. Arch Orthop Trauma Surg. 1994;114:215.

Brodsky JW, Tullos HS, Gartsman GM. Simplified posterior approach to the shoulder joint: a technical note. J Bone Joint Surg. 1987;69:773-4.

Goss TP. Fractures of the glenoid cavity. Current Concepts review. J Bone Joint Surg [Am]. 1992;74:299-305.

Goss TP. Fractures of the glenoid cavity (operative principles and techniques). Tech Orthop. 1994;8:199.

Goss TP. Fractures of the glenoid neck. J Shoulder Elbow Surg. 1994;3:42-52.

Goss TP. Fractures of the scapula. In Rockwood CA, Matsen FA III, Wirth MA, Lippitt SB (eds). The Shoulder, ed 3. Philadelphia: Elsevier, 2004:413-54.

Hardegger FH, Simpson LA, Weber BG. The operative management of scapular fractures. J Bone Joint Surg [Br]. 1984;66:725.

Ideberg R. Fractures of the scapula involving the glenoid fossa. In Bateman JE, Welsh RP (eds). Surgery of the Shoulder. Philadelphia: BC Decker, 1984:63-66.

Ideberg R, Grevsten S, Larsson S. Epidemiology of scapular fractures. Acta Orthop Scand. 1995;66:395.

Kavanagh BF, Bradway JK, Cofield RH. Open reduction of displaced intra-articular fractures of the glenoid fossa. J Bone Joint Surg [Am]. 1993;75:479.

Leung KS, Lam TB, Poon KM. Operative treatment of displaced intra-articular glenoid fractures. Injury. 1993;24:324.

Miller ME, Ada JR. Injuries to the shoulder girdle. In Browner BD, Jupiter JB, Levine AM, Trafton PY (eds). Skeletal Trauma, ed 2. Philadelphia: WB Saunders, 1992:1291.

Nordqvist A, Petersson C. Fracture of the body, neck or spine of the scapula. Clin Orthop Relat Res. 1992;(283):139-44.

Pace AM, Stuart R, Brownlow H. Outcome of glenoid neck fractures. J Shoulder Elbow Surg. 2005;14:585-90.

Schandelmaier P, Blauth M, Schneider C, Krethek C. Fractures of the glenoid treated by operation: a 5- to 23-year follow-up of 22 cases. J Bone Joint Surg [Br]. 2002;84:173-7.

Van Noort A, te Slaa RL, Marti RK, van der Werken C. The floating shoulder: a multicentre study. J Bone Joint Surg [Br]. 2001;83:795-8.

Zdravkovic D, Damholt VV. Comminuted and severely displaced fractures of the scapula. Acta Orthop Scand. 1974;45:60-5.

SECTION I

SHOULDER

Miscellaneous

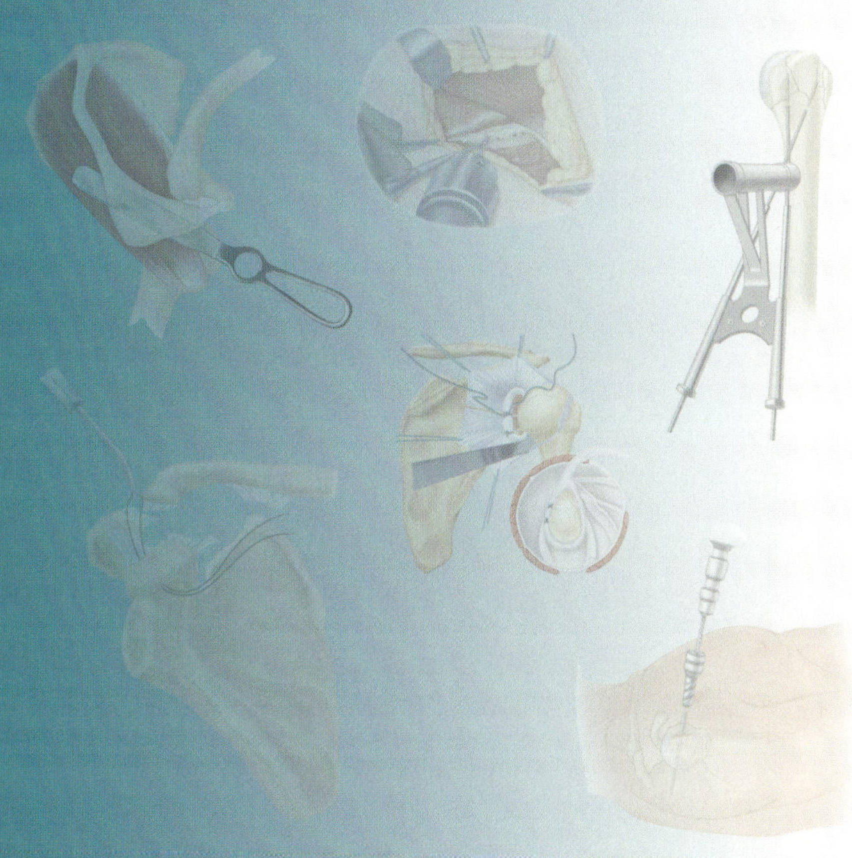

PROCEDURE 34

Arthrodesis of the Shoulder

Jason J. Scalise and Joseph P. Iannotti

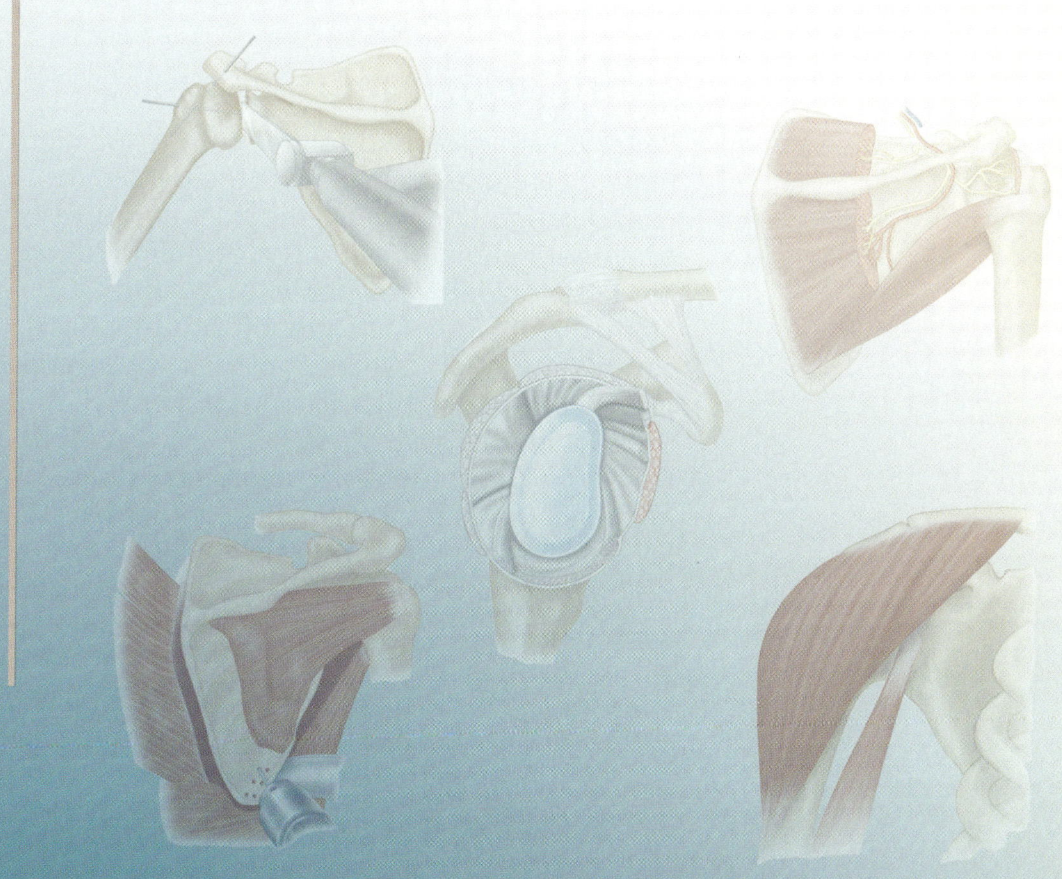

Figure 10 modfied from Scalise JJ, Iannotti JP. Glenohumeral arthrodesis after failed prosthetic shoulder arthroplasty. J Bone Joint Surg [Am]. 2008;90:70-7; reprinted with permission.

Controversies

- Older patients with low functional demands may benefit from resection arthroplasty in place of the more surgically complex arthrodesis (Braman et al., 2006).

Treatment Options

- Interfragmentary screw fixation without plate fixation has been utilized and requires less dissection. However, higher rates of nonunion have been reported when plate fixation is not incorporated (Ruhmann et al., 2005).

Indications

- Refractory shoulder pain and dysfunction resulting from brachial plexus injuries, failed shoulder arthroplasty, recalcitrant shoulder instability, or combined deltoid and rotator cuff dysfunction where other treatment options would not likely provide a durable solution.
- For younger individuals with the above conditions and with demands of considerable strength at low angles of the shoulder, arthrodesis has been advocated.

Examination/Imaging

- Patients with profound rotator cuff dysfunction require careful examination of the deltoid for consideration of a reverse shoulder arthroplasty. Poor or absent deltoid function is a contraindication to reverse shoulder arthroplasty.
- Normal scapulothoracic motion and muscular control, including trapezius and levator scapulae function, is required to allow postoperative motion of the shoulder girdle.
- Patients with a progressive neurologic disease involving the shoulder generally do not have favorable results with arthrodesis.
- Plain radiographs
  - Anteroposterior (AP), true AP, and axillary views of the glenohumeral joint should be obtained.
    - Figure 1 shows an AP view of a loose glenoid component with lack of tuberosities indicating a dysfunctional rotator cuff (*left*). An axillary view demonstrates greater tuberosity malunion to the glenoid (*right*).
    - Clinical examination demonstrated painful, chest level–only function and extreme deltoid atrophy and dysfunction.
  - Radiographs are evaluated for the extent of proximal humeral bone loss (e.g., in the setting of a failed humeral prosthesis) and the potential need for intercalary bone grafting.
  - Radiographs are also evaluated for extreme glenohumeral joint destruction as may be seen with Charcot's arthropathy. This finding should prompt evaluation of the cervical spinal cord for possible syrinx. Failure of arthrodesis in these patients is especially likely and should be avoided.

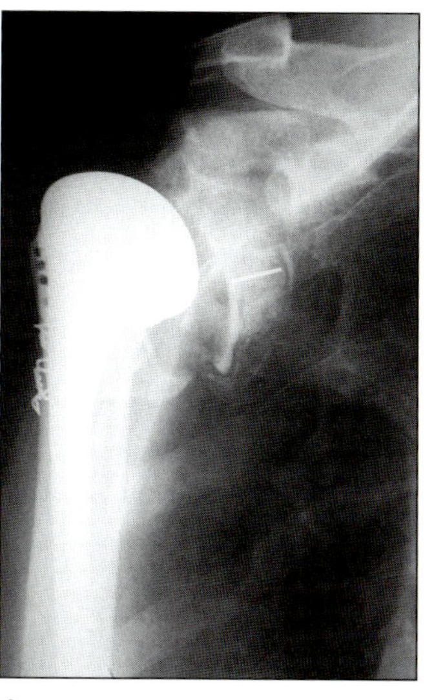
A

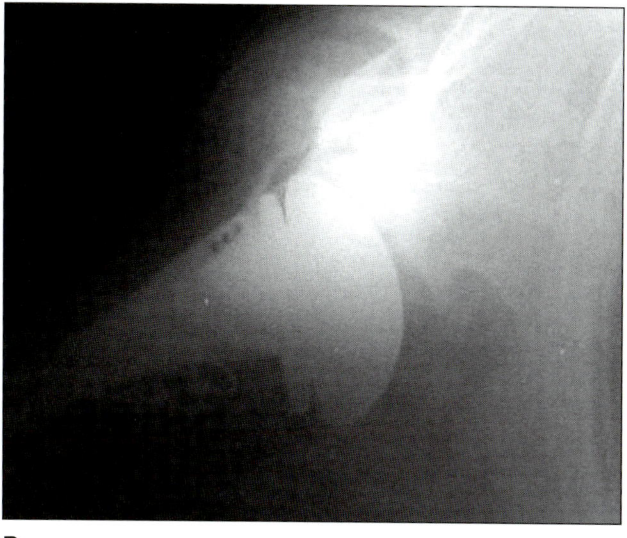
B

FIGURE 1

Surgical Anatomy

- The deltoid originates from the posterior, lateral, and anterior acromion as well as the distal clavicle (Fig. 2).
- Its insertion is at the deltoid tuberosity on the lateral humeral shaft.

PEARLS

- *The authors prefer to use an arthroscopy table for this procedure, which will allow complete exposure of the front and back of the shoulder. It will also allow for fluoroscopic or radiographic examination of the shoulder.*

Positioning

- The patient is placed in the modified beach chair position (Fig. 3).
- The operative extremity should have the ability to be fully adducted and extended. Full access to the posterior aspect of the shoulder is also required.
- General anesthesia combined with an interscalene block with an indwelling catheter will provide excellent pain relief for up to 2 weeks. In many cases, we discharge the patient with the catheter in place for the first postoperative week.

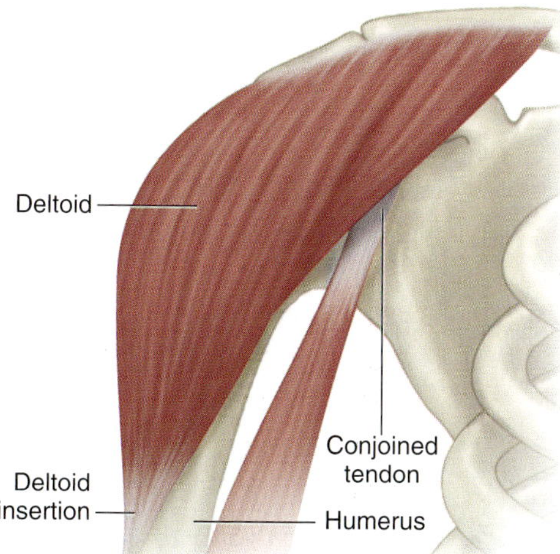

FIGURE 2

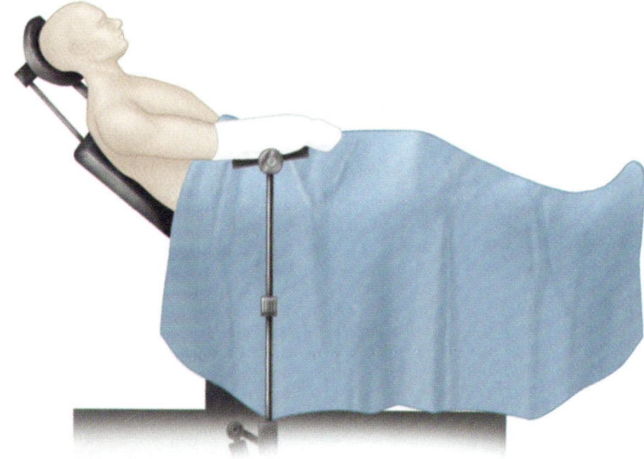
FIGURE 3

Equipment

- A sterile arm holder can be used and has the advantage of offering hands-free positioning of the humerus throughout the case (see Fig. 3).

Pearls

- *It is preferred to not denervate the deltoid to prevent loss of the soft tissues that cover the humerus and plate after fusion. It is for this reason that the deltoid origin is elevated to gain wide exposure rather than using a limited split in the deltoid, making the deep exposure more difficult.*

Portals/Exposures

- The incision is made over the spine of the scapula and curves anteriorly toward the midportion of the acromion lateral to the acromioclavicular joint and then distally between the anterior and middle deltoid for 6–7 cm (Fig. 4A and 4B).
- A large skin flap is made between the subcutaneous tissues and anterior deltoid to the deltopectoral interval and superiorly enough to expose the origin of the anterior deltoid on to the clavicle.
- The anterior and middle portions of the deltoid are elevated off the clavicle laterally and distally, exposing the entire rotator cuff and proximal humerus. In Figure 5, the atrophied deltoid has been elevated from its origin on the distal clavicle and acromion in a single full-thickness flap. If deltoid dysfunction is a component of the pathology, the deltoid may be atrophic or detached from its origin.

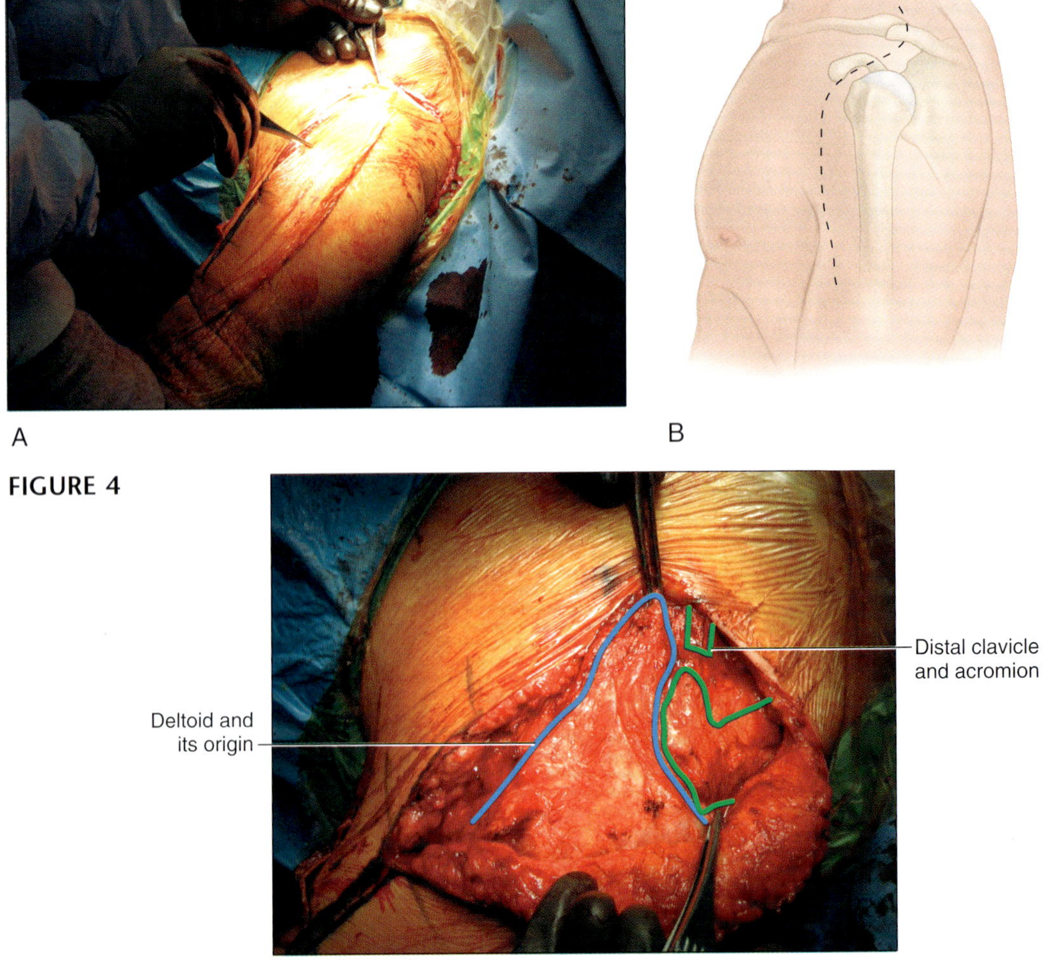

FIGURE 4

FIGURE 5

If so, this scar tissue is resected from the distal clavicle and anterior and lateral acromion, affording broad exposure.

- If the rotator cuff is intact, the subscapularis is elevated off the lesser tuberosity and retracted medially. The supraspinatus is resected from the greater tuberosity to the musculotendinous junction to allow the necessary exposure for the subsequent humeral head osteotomy and to allow for bone contact between the top of the humeral head osteotomy and the decorticated undersurface of the acromion.

Procedure

Step 1

- The glenoid surface is prepared by removing all of the articular cartilage and planing the surface flat with an oscillating saw or high-speed burr in the orientation of the joint line.
- The undersurface of the acromion is cut to a flat surface, removing as little bone as possible.
- The arm is then positioned with the forearm in 35–40 degrees of internal rotation and the humerus in about 20° of abduction and 20° of forward flexion in reference to the coronal plane of the body and the midsagittal line.
- The humeral head is then placed in contact with the prepared glenoid surface and shifted superiorly to contact the acromion with the humerus oriented in its preferred and final position (Fig. 6). When proper position of the humerus is determined, Steinmann pins are driven through acromion and glenoid to hold the position. This is temporarily held with two 4.5-mm Steinmann pins.

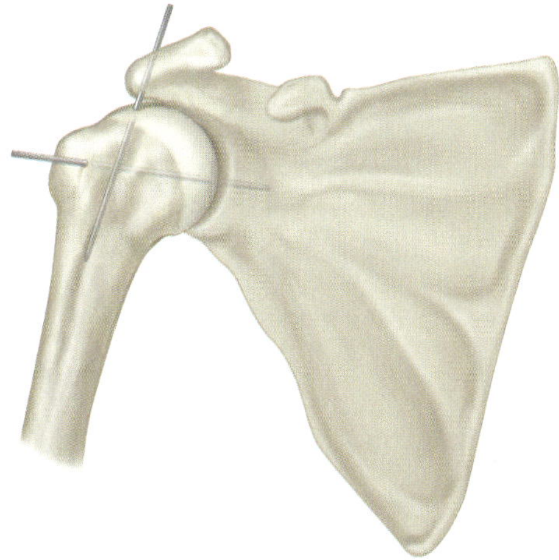

FIGURE 6

PEARLS

- *In patients with a large frame due to a barrel chest or high body mass index, greater degrees of abduction and forward positioning of the humerus can be achieved while still allowing for adduction to contact the side of the body or abdomen.*
- *Higher degrees of adduction or forward elevation will allow for a greater amount of active elevation after fusion.*
- *Removing and replacing the Steinmann pins allows adjustments to individualize the fusion position for the patient, allowing for a function arc of motion after fusion.*

- One pin enters the midacromion and then the humeral head to exit the anterior cortex of the humerus near its metaphyseal-diaphyseal region.
- A second 4.5-mm smooth pin enters the humeral head laterally below the greater tuberosity and enters the glenoid in a lateral-to-medial orientation.

STEP 2

- The arm is removed from the holder and gently taken through a range of motion to ensure that the arm can comfortable come to the side of the body and the forearm can contact or nearly contact the abdomen.
  - With forward flexion and abduction, the humerus can elevate to about 80° and the hand can touch the patient's forehead.
  - Internal rotation will result in the hand reaching posterior to the greater trochanter of the ipsilateral hip.
- Under all circumstances, it is very helpful to adjust the fusion position to allow for the above criteria for passive range of motion.
  - The position of fusion is a range of 10–20° of abduction, 10–20° of flexion, and 35–45° of internal rotation.
  - This position will generally allow the patient to reach his or her mouth, waist, buttock, and contralateral shoulder, facilitating activities of daily living.

STEP 3

- With the position finalized, the oscillating saw is used to cut the medial and superior portions of the humeral head parallel to the glenoid and undersurface of the acromion, respectively, in order to maximize bony contact (Fig. 7).

PEARLS

- *The initial cut is made medially, then superiorly.*
- *The Steinmann pins will need to be backed out of the bones and the humeral head then rotated to provide full exposure of the head; the osteotomy is completed keeping the plane established from the initial cut.*

PITFALLS

- *Ideally, the humeral head is cut so that most of the head remains to maximize bone volume for screw fixation.*

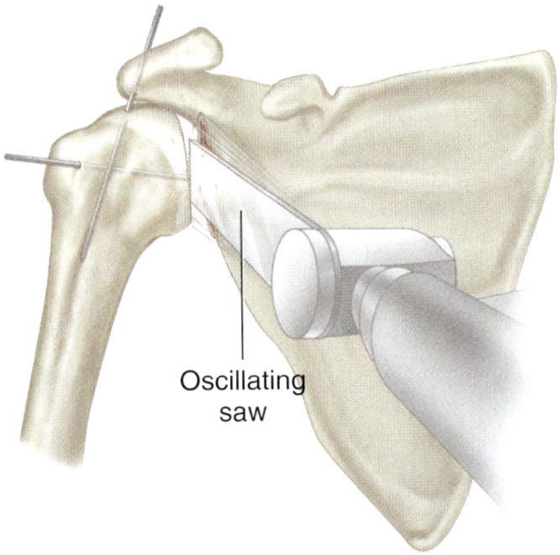

FIGURE 7

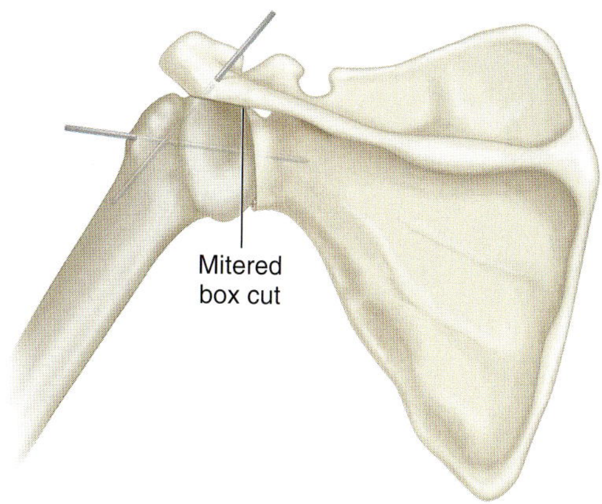

FIGURE 8

- After making both cuts, the head forms a "mitered box cut" that should fit within the cut surfaces of the glenoid and acromion (Fig. 8).
- While holding the surfaces in direct apposition, the position of the arm is checked. The osteotomy surfaces can still be adjusted to change arm position.

Step 4

- A 4.5-mm reconstruction plate or locking plate is contoured to the spine of scapula coming over the lateral acromion and lateral portion of the proximal humerus.
  - Ideally the plate is placed so to completely avoid the Steinmann pins, or those holes are incorporated into the plate holes.
  - A second 4.5-mm hole is placed into the lateral part of the humeral head and into the glenoid. This is tapped for a partially threaded 6.5-mm cancellous screw with a washer.
  - The Steinmann pins are then replaced with 6.5-mm partially threaded screws.
- The most important screws for holding the plate are those mentioned above as well as one additional screw that is placed just posterior to the acromion into the spine of the scapula and then into the neck of the glenoid to its inferior extent.
  - Additional cortical screws are placed in the distal part of the plate (three or four) and proximally in the spine of the scapula (two or three).
  - Fixation distally does not need to be significantly past the metaphyseal-diaphyseal region of the upper humerus.

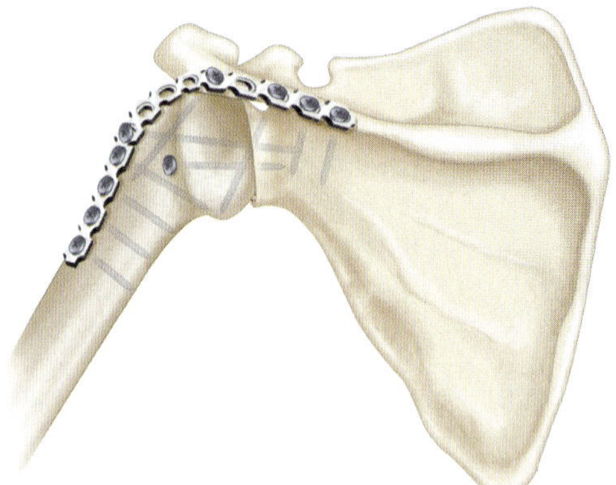

A

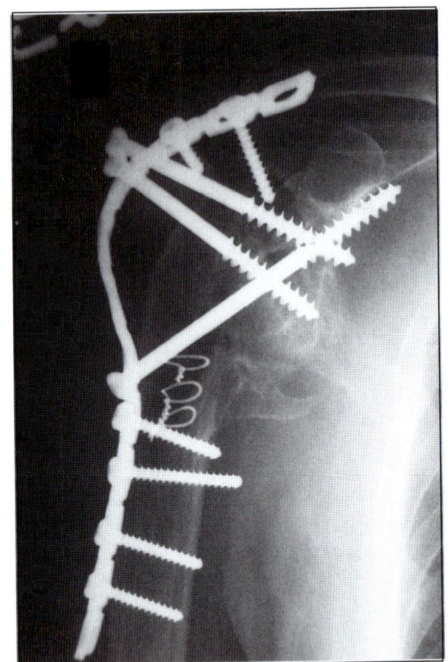

B

FIGURE 9

PEARLS

- *The plate can be inset into the lateral acromion by removal of a small part of the lateral acromion.*
- *It is important to be sure that the threads of the screw remain in the glenoid and do not distract the osteotomy surfaces.*
- *A fluoroscopic AP view or AP radiograph is helpful at this point to verify position of the osteotomy and screws.*

PITFALLS

- *If screws are placed through the plate, care must be taken such that the screw head is flush with the plate. A prominent screw in this area will almost always result in the need for removal after surgery.*
- *Minimize trauma to the deltoid or axillary nerve. Although the deltoid does not provide function to the shoulder after fusion, it provides important soft tissue coverage and a more cosmetic contour to the shoulder.*

  - Figure 9A shows the final fixation construct with contoured plate and interfragmentary screw fixation, also seen in the radiograph in Figure 9B.
- Additional bone grafting is not required for primary fusions if the bone is preserved by the methods outlined.
- The subscapularis is then repaired to the lesser tuberosity and the deltoid is reattached to the acromion and clavicle transosseously using nonabsorbable sutures.
- One or two limbs of a small drain are placed deep to the deltoid.
- A standard layered closure is then performed.

Step 5: For Situations with Proximal Humerus Bone Loss

- After wide exposure of the proximal humerus and glenoid as outlined above, wide resection of the soft tissue debris that is often surrounding the glenoid is performed.
- If tuberosities are present, preparation of the proximal humerus is much the same as described previously. The blood supply inherent to the tuberosities should be protected as it adds a greater potential for fusion to occur.
- A bulk femoral head allograft can be shaped and positioned between the plate and the proximal humerus to provide bone volume for supplemental fixation and osteogenic potential.

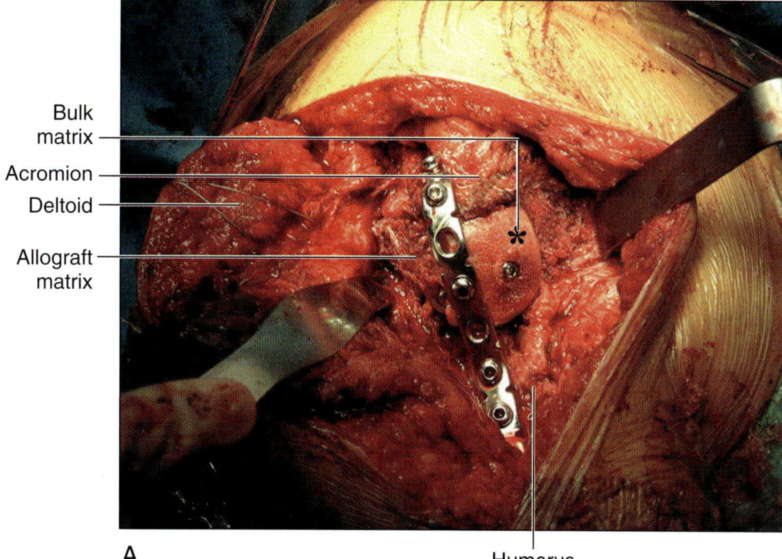

A

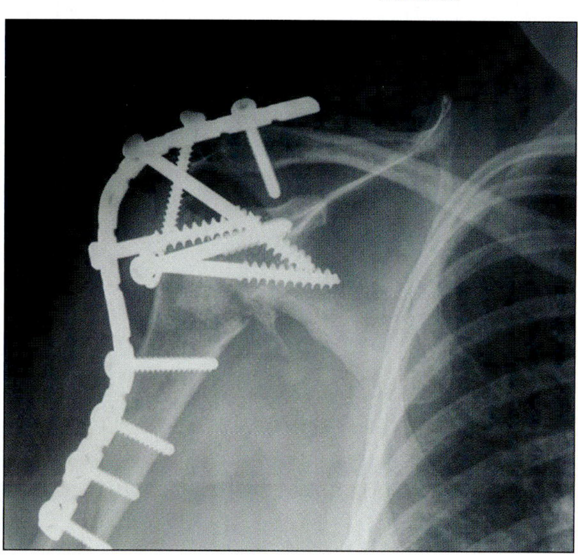
B

FIGURE 10

- Figure 10A shows a right shoulder after arthrodesis for treatment of a failed prosthetic arthroplasty.
  - The large-fragment reconstruction plate has been contoured over the spine of the scapula and acromion proximally and the humeral diaphysis distally.
  - The bulk allograft (*asterisk*), secured with interfragmentary fixation, is seen medial to the plate. A mixture of autologous bone marrow aspirate and allograft matrix (m) is seen packed around the fusion site anteriorly and posteriorly (ac, acromion; d, deltoid (retracted); h, humerus).
  - An AP radiograph of the same patient, made 2 years postoperatively, demonstrates a solid fusion (Fig. 10B).

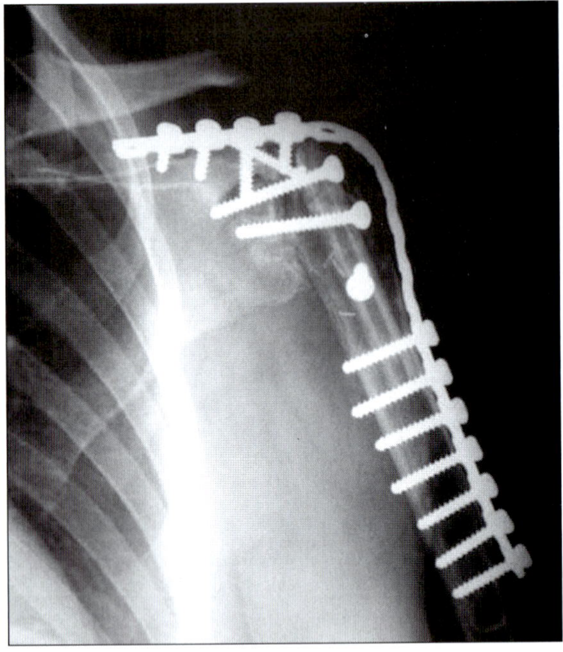

FIGURE 11

- For defects greater than 7 cm, a vascularized free fibula autograft can be considered and has the potential advantage of a bringing an increased healing potential with its blood supply and the needed volume of bone graft. Figure 11 shows a successful arthrodesis after failed hemiarthroplasty utilizing a fibular autograft to span the large proximal humeral defect left after prosthesis removal.
    - The bone gap is measured with traction on the arm to achieve normal or near-normal arm length, thus giving the fibula harvest team a target length of fibula to prepare.
    - The graft is harvested to provide at least 6 cm more bone length than the measured bone deficiency (top of the glenoid fossa to the proximal end of the humeral shaft).
    - The humeral shaft medullary canal is prepared so that the fibula autograft can be placed within the medullary canal, and at least two cortical (4.5-mm) screws are placed into the humeral shaft transfixing the autograft.
    - As before, fusion position for the arm is determined. The portion of the glenoid that comes into contact with the fibula autograft is contoured with a high-speed burr, creating a trough such that the dowel-like fibula autograft may rest within it.

PEARLS

- *If the greater tuberosity is intact or healed to the humeral shaft, its integrity should be preserved if possible given that it has an inherent blood supply that can be used to promote the fusion.*
- *A longitudinal osteotomy of the anterior humeral cortex can facilitate removal of a stubborn humeral prosthesis by allowing the bond between the humerus and prosthesis to be gently loosened.*
- *Two teams are preferred. In most cases, the existing prosthesis can be removed and the site prepared for the autograft during the time required to remove and prepare the vessels for revascularization.*

Pitfalls

- *Glenohumeral arthrodesis following failed shoulder arthroplasty should be considered a salvage procedure when other established revision options have failed or would not be likely to yield a favorable outcome.*
- *Arthrodesis is a much more difficult procedure but may be preferred for a younger patient who wishes to have better shoulder-level elevation.*

- Two 4.5-mm cortical screws are placed into the proximal fibula autograft and then into the glenoid vault.
- A large-fragment pelvic reconstruction plate or standard large-fragment plate is contoured as described above and fixed with cortical and cancellous screws.
- The fibula autograft is then vascularized by the microvascular team.
- After vascularization, cancellous bone graft (allograft or iliac crest autograft, or autologous bone marrow aspirate and allograft matrix) is used at both the proximal and distal osteosynthesis sites.

Postoperative Care and Expected Outcomes

- The arm is placed in a 20° abduction (pillow) sling for 10–12 weeks after surgery.
  - In cases of substantial humeral bone loss with extensive bone grafting, a shoulder spica cast may be preferred.
- The patient is allowed to remove the sling for waist-level activities to include dressing, bathing, and eating.
- Radiographs are taken at 2, 6, and 12 weeks postoperative.
  - Fusion is sufficient at 12 weeks in most patients to allow for scapula exercises and discontinuance of the abduction (pillow) sling.
  - In cases of substantial bone loss, the immobilization period may be 12–16 weeks or until radiographic evidence of the fusion is present.
- Radiographic evidence of only minimal healing at 6–8 weeks after surgery should prompt the surgeon to consider revision surgery in which the fusion site is bone grafted before hardware loosening or failure occurs.

Pearls

- *Particular attention should be given to the possibility of delayed union or nonunion in cases of arthrodesis in the presence of large bone defects.*

Pitfalls

- *Nonunion may occur in as many as half of the cases with substantial bone loss.*

Evidence

Clare DJ, Wirth MA, Groh GI, Rockwood CA Jr. Shoulder arthrodesis. J Bone Joint Surg [Am]. 2001;83:593-600.

The authors provided an excellent review of the techniques and outcomes of shoulder arthrodesis.

Scalise JJ, Iannotti JP. Glenohumeral arthrodesis after failed prosthetic shoulder arthroplasty. J Bone Joint Surg [Am]. 2008;90:70-7.

In this study, the most common complication was nonunion that required revision surgery. The authors stressed the complex nature of the surgery. Realistic expectations from surgeon and patient are indicated. (Level IV evidence [case series])

Richards RR, Beaton D, Hudson A. Shoulder arthrodesis with plate fixation: functional outcome analysis. J Shoulder Elbow Surg. 1993;2:225-39.

In this study, plate fixation technique provided robust fixation and high rates of union in cases of primary arthrodesis. (Level IV evidence [case series])

Ruhmann O, Schmolke S, Bohnsack M, Flamme C, Wirth CJ. Shoulder arthrodesis: indications, technique, results, and complications. J Shoulder Elbow Surg. 2005;14:38-50.

In this retrospective analysis of 43 patients with arthrodesis using screw fixation or plate and screw fixation, pseudarthrosis appeared to be less frequent in cases of plate arthrodesis compared with screw arthrodesis. Pseudarthrosis was observed in one of the patients in whom bone graft was not used. The use of bone graft in the setting of bone loss was suggested by the authors to help avoid nonunion. Use of plates resulted in better fusion rates but also correlated more often with infection, postoperative fractures of the humerus, and the necessity for hardware removal. (Level III evidence [case control])

Braman JP, Sprague M, Bishop J, Lo IK, Lee EW, Flatow EL. The outcome of resection shoulder arthroplasty for recalcitrant shoulder infections. J Shoulder Elbow Surg. 2006;15:549-53.

This case series demonstrated satisfactory outcomes for resection arthroplasty in low-demand, elderly patients. (Level IV evidence [case series])

PROCEDURE 35

Open and Arthroscopic Suprascapular Nerve Decompression

Jonathan E. Buzzell and Sumant G. Krishnan

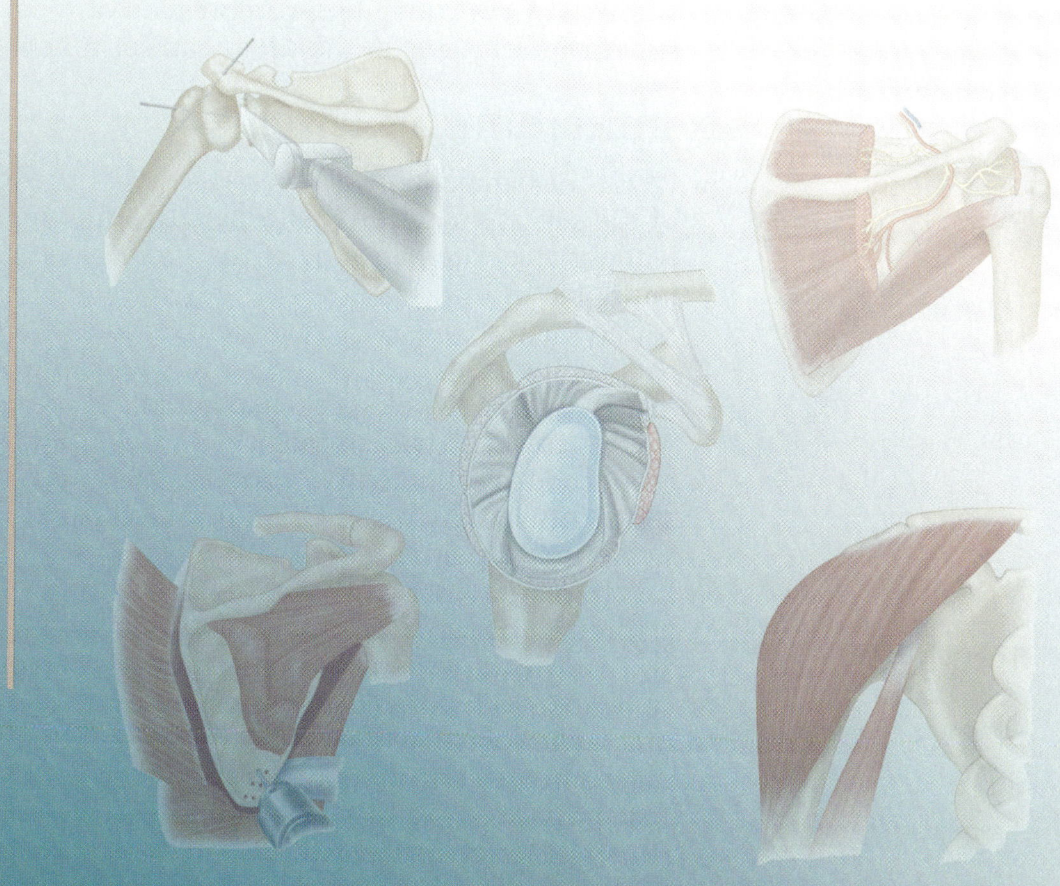

Pitfalls

- *Failure to identify/treat additional pathology*
- *Failure to consider suprascapular nerve compression, attributing symptoms to rotator cuff or other pathology*

Controversies

- Arthroscopic decompression utilizes the anteromedial portal medial to the coracoid. This portal is safe when the surgeon remains along the medial border of the coracoid.

Treatment Options

- Observation for clinical improvement over a period of 2–3 months

Indications

- Pain over the posterior and lateral aspects of the shoulder and/or weakness of the supraspinatus and infraspinatus muscles
- Greater amount of supraspinatus and infraspinatus atrophy and/or fatty infiltration than would be expected for a small cuff tear or normal cuff
- Massive, retracted cuff tear that causes traction injury to the suprascapular nerve
- Electromyography (EMG)/nerve conduction velocity study (NCV) documenting compression of the suprascapular nerve at the suprascapular notch

Examination/Imaging

- Physical examination will reveal decreased strength of the supraspinatus and infraspinatus with or without associated atrophy of the supraspinatus and infraspinatus musculature.
  - Cervical disk disease should be ruled out as a cause of symptoms.
  - A complete neurological examination of the affected side is performed.
- Diagnostic injection of 1% lidocaine over the suprascapular notch can be used to evaluate symptomatic pain relief.
- Plain radiographs are obtained to check for acromioclavicular and glenohumeral joint arthritis, and for greater tuberosity and acromion changes consistent with chronic cuff impingement.
- Magnetic resonance imaging is performed to identify perilabral ganglion cysts that could cause compression at the spinoglenoid notch.
- EMG/NCV is performed to evaluate for suprascapular nerve compression at the suprascapular notch and supraspinatus/infraspinatus muscle fibrillation potentials.

Surgical Anatomy

- The suprascapular nerve originates from the upper trunk and receives contributions from the C5 and C6 nerve roots.
  - The nerve follows the omohyoid muscle posteriorly and turns inferiorly at the suprascapular notch.
  - It is relatively fixed at the notch by the overlying transverse scapular ligament (Fig. 1).

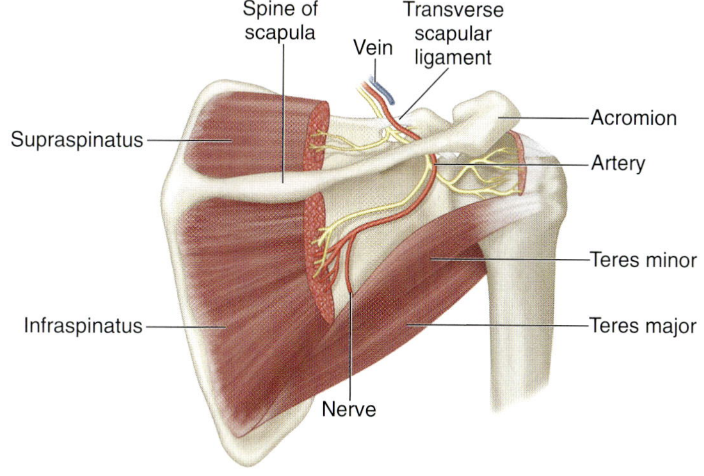

FIGURE 1

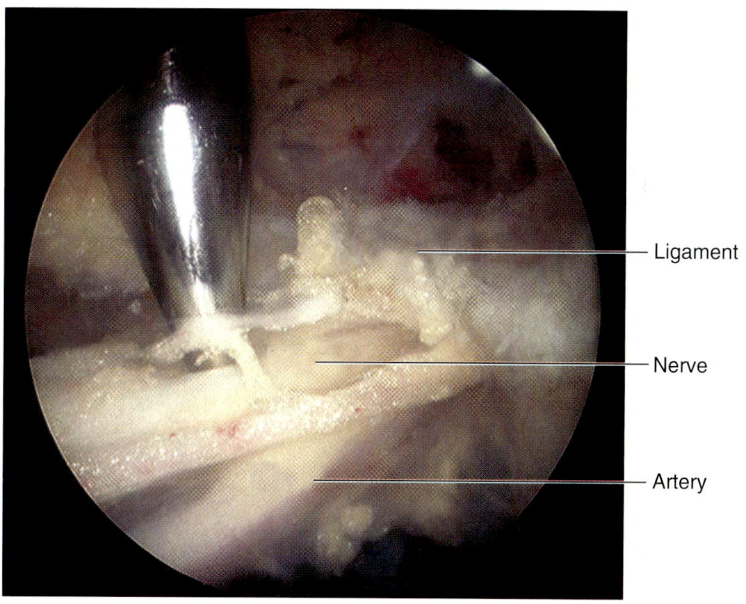

FIGURE 2

- After exiting the notch, the suprascapular nerve provides two branches to the supraspinatus muscle and several small sensory branches to the glenohumeral joint capsule. The nerve continues inferiorly to the spinoglenoid notch, at which point it arborizes into two to four motor branches to the infraspinatus.

- The suprascapular artery is a branch of the thyrocervical trunk and it typically runs on top of the transverse scapular ligament, lateral to the nerve. A subligamentous suprascapular artery variant has been described (Fig. 2).
- The suprascapular notch is at the junction of the base of the coracoid and the scapular body. It is

easily located arthroscopically by following the medial border of the coracoid process. Anatomic variations exist in the osseous and ligamentous structure comprising the notch (Rengachary, 1979).
  - The most common notch is U-shaped (48%), and the least common is a shallow V-shaped notch (3%).
  - Ligamentous variations include ossification, hypertrophy, bifid or trifid ligament, and other congenital malformations.
- The conoid and trapezoid ligaments attach to the dorsum of the coracoid and are safe during the approach along the medial border of the coracoid.

Pearls

- *Utilization of the McConnell head positioning device ensures that the neck and shoulder girdle are free of the operating table.*

Pitfalls

- *Inadequate positioning makes an open or arthroscopic approach to the nerve very difficult.*

Positioning

- The modified beach chair position (dinner chair position) is used. The patient is on a beanbag to help maintain stability on the table (Fig. 3). Two or three pillows are placed under the knees to maintain knee flexion, preventing tension on the sciatic nerve.
- During positioning, the beanbag is rolled and tucked under the distal tip and medial border of the scapula to maintain the scapula in a stable position throughout the procedure. The patient's back is nearly vertical.
- The nonoperative upper extremity rests on the patient's lap with the elbow, wrist, and hand well padded. A safety strap is used in all cases.

Equipment

- McConnell head and arm positioning devices (McConnell, Greenville, TX)
- Beanbag, size #30

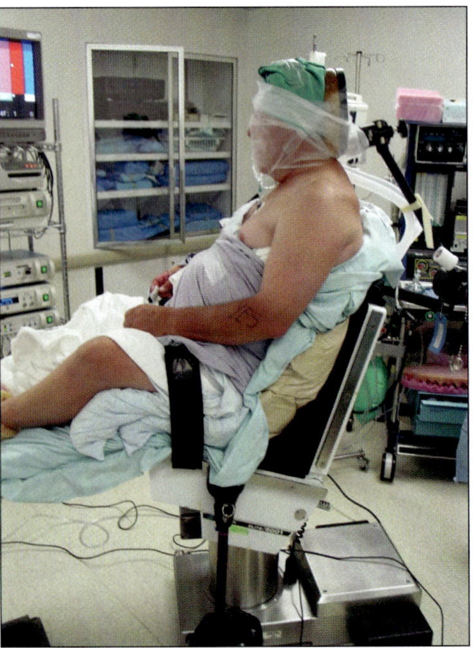

FIGURE 3

PEARLS

- *An anterolateral viewing portal should be used when dissecting to the coracoid.*
- *Shoulder flexion to 30° facilitates working under the deltoid.*
- *The coracoacromial ligament leads to the coracoid.*
- *A surgical assistant should place a hand over the supraspinatus to alert the surgeon of supraspinatus muscle twitches during dissection.*

PITFALLS

- *Improper head positioning and bulky surgical drapes will hinder the surgeon's ability to work through the open surgical wound or arthroscopically through the superior working portal.*

Portals/Exposures

- Open approach: A 2- to 3-cm incision is made along the posterior clavicular margin centered 2 cm medial to the posterior border of the acromioclavicular joint.
- Arthroscopic approach: Arthroscopic portals are placed as shown in Figure 4.
- Additional arthroscopic portals are required for suprascapular nerve decompression (Fig. 5). These include the anteromedial portal, placed medial to the coracoid, and an additional "notch" portal 2–3 cm medial to the posterior border of the acromioclavicular joint. This notch portal is made last, and proper placement is verified arthroscopically with a spinal needle.

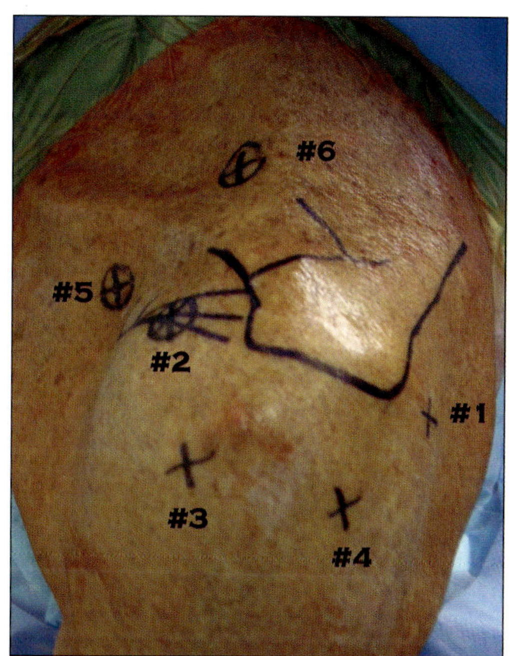

FIGURE 4

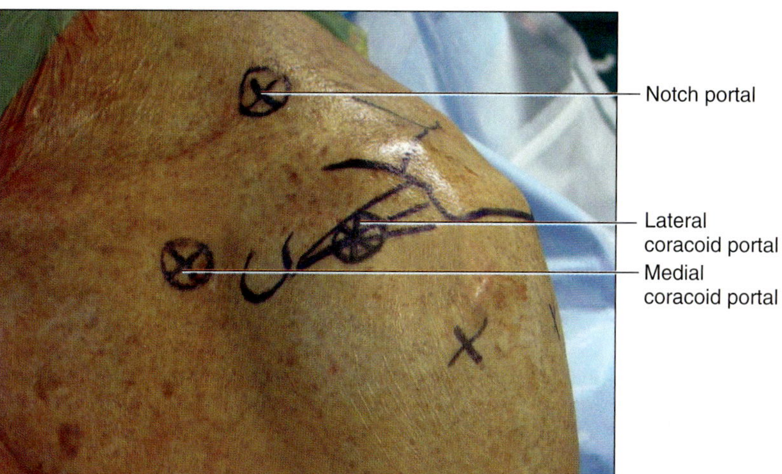

FIGURE 5

Instrumentation

- Three 4.5-mm Dyonics arthroscopic cannulas
- VAPR device (DePuy-Mitek, Raynham, MA)
- Basket forceps
- Shaver

Pearls

- *Placing the patient's arm in slight flexion to relax the anterior deltoid will facilitate work in the anterior shoulder girdle.*

Procedure: Arthroscopic Suprascapular Nerve Decompression

Step 1

- Diagnostic arthroscopy of the glenohumeral joint is performed, and any perilabral cyst identified preoperatively is decompressed.
- Subacromial decompression is performed.
- Biceps tenodesis is performed (if indicated).
- Rotator repair is performed (if indicated).
- Distal clavicle excision is performed (if indicated).
- The camera is placed in the anterolateral viewing portal (portal #3).
- Working through the anterior portal (portal #2), the coracoacromial ligament is followed to the coracoid process using the ablation wand (Fig. 6).

Step 2

- The anteromedial portal is established, first identifying proper placement with a spinal needle, such that the trajectory is straight down the medial border of the coracoid process.
- With a blunt trochar, the surgeon gently probes posteriorly along the medial border of the coracoid to identify the path of dissection. The stout coracoclavicular ligaments can be palpated to identify their location to prevent inadvertent injury to these important structures.

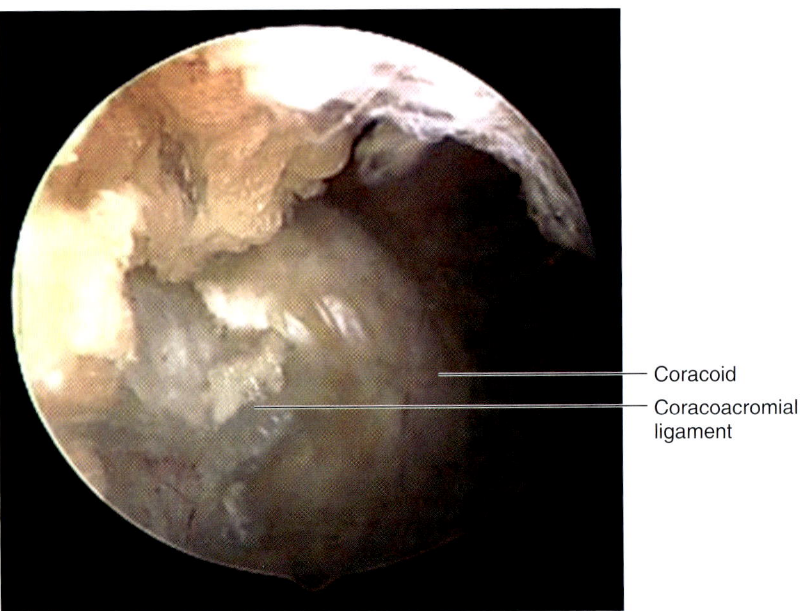

FIGURE 6

PEARLS

- *The surgical assistant is crucial to help identify when the surgeon is near the suprascapular nerve during dissection, and will notify the surgeon when the supraspinatus muscle twitches.*

PITFALLS

- *Working along the top of the coracoid process, rather than the medial border, can cause the surgeon to inadvertently transect the coracoclavicular ligaments and destabilize the acromioclavicular joint.*

- The surgical assistant places a hand on the patient's supraspinatus and informs the surgeon of any twitches in the muscle.
- Using the ablation wand, the surgeon carefully dissects along the medial border of the coracoid. Looking over the top of the anterior tip of the coracoid with the camera "eyes" down will ensure that he or she is working along the medial border (Fig. 7).
- When the supraspinatus twitches, the location of the suprascapular notch has been identified. Dissection is stopped and a blunt trochar is placed, under direct visualization, at the suprascapular notch through the anteromedial portal.

STEP 3

- Under direct visualization, a second viewing cannula is inserted through the anterior portal (portal #2) so that its tip is in contact with the previously placed trochar at the notch in the anteromedial portal (chopsticks maneuver) (Fig. 8).
- The camera is switched to the anterior portal. This will allow the surgeon to look down the medial border of the coracoid when dissecting to the suprascapular nerve and artery and the intervening transverse scapular ligament.
- Using the VAPR device, tissue is dissected off the medial border of the coracoid (Fig. 9A) and bluntly swept from lateral to medial (Fig. 9B). The ablation wand may be used to bluntly sweep tissue, but it is crucial that it is not activated during blunt dissection.

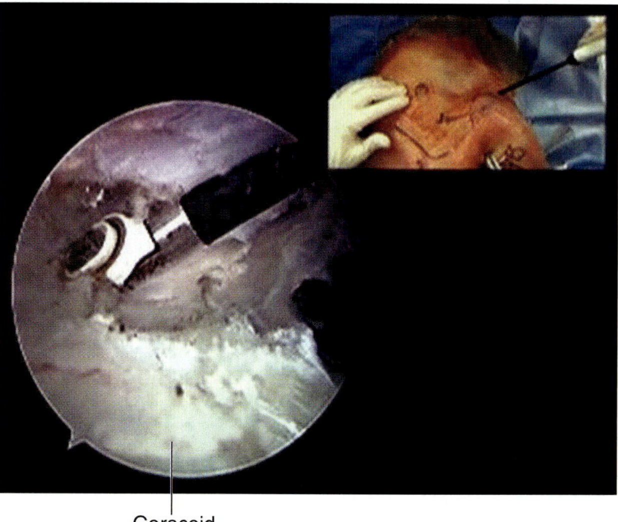

FIGURE 7

Pearls

- *Dissect tissue off the medial border of the coracoid.*
- *Bluntly sweep from lateral to medial to clear tissue from view.*
- *Work posteriorly toward the suprascapular notch.*
- *Be aware of anatomic variations.*

Pitfalls

- *Straying superiorly can cause injury to the coracoclavicular ligaments.*
- *Impatiently progressing toward the notch without adequately clearing tissue away from view will cause the surgeon to work without optimal visualization of the neurovascular structures.*

- The first assistant continues to maintain a position with one hand over the supraspinatus muscle belly to aid in safe dissection of the nerve.
- Using this technique, alternately dissecting and sweeping, the surgeon proceeds toward the suprascapular notch where the nerve, ligament, and artery are safely identified.
- Once the nerve, artery, and intervening ligament are identified, a viewing cannula is placed on top of the transverse scapular ligament through the anteromedial portal.

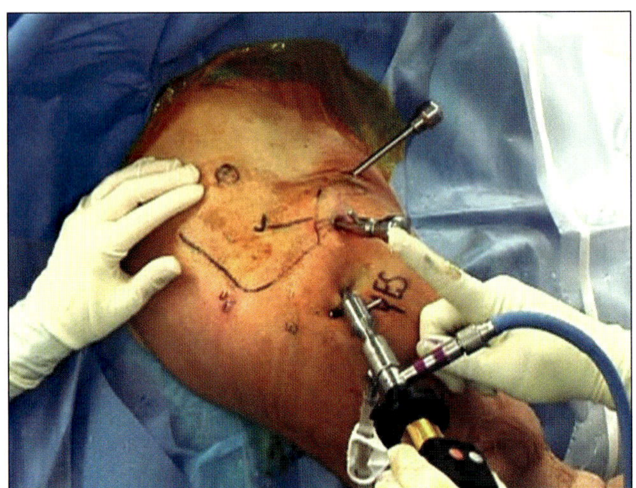

FIGURE 8

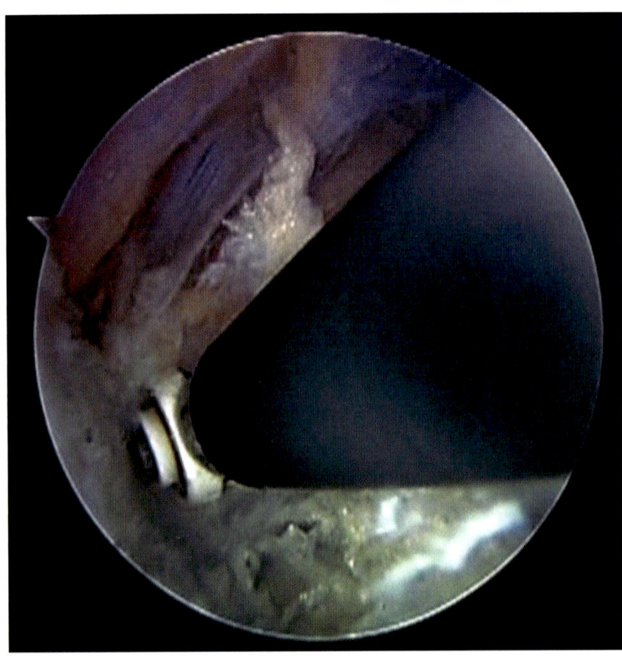

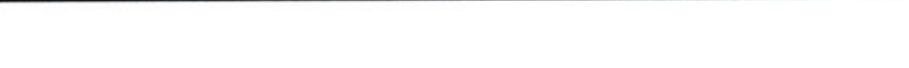

A

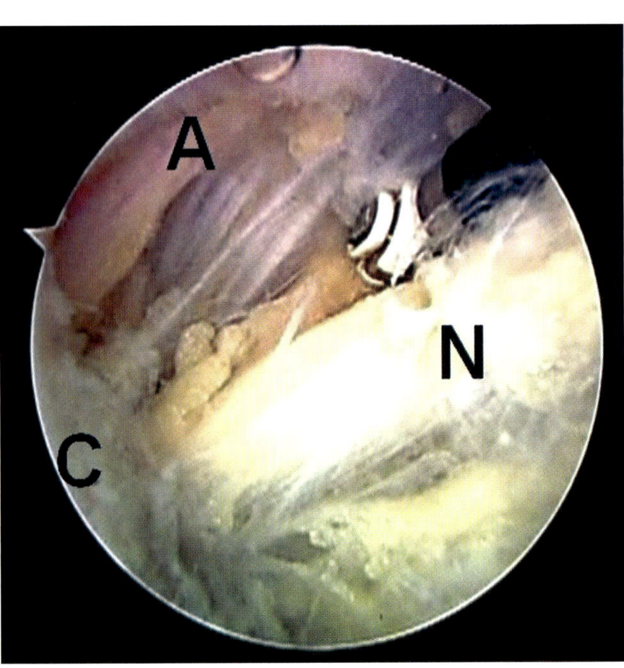

B

FIGURE 9

Instrumentation/ Implantation

- Three 4.5-mm Dyonics arthroscopic cannulas
- VAPR device

Controversies

- Contrary to traditional teaching, the anteromedial portal is safe if the surgeon adheres to the anatomy.

Step 4

- With the camera in the anteromedial viewing portal, the surgeon has a direct view of the suprascapular artery and nerve and the intervening transverse scapular ligament (Fig. 10).
- A spinal needle is inserted 2–3 cm medial to the posterior border of the acromioclavicular joint to verify proper position of the superior working portal (notch portal).
- The skin is incised and blunt dissection is performed through the trapezius muscle in line with its fibers to the working site.
- With a blunt trochar, the artery is gently swept away from the ligament to release any soft tissue connections that may impede transection of the transverse scapular ligament.
- A basket forceps is gently inserted through the superior working portal and used to remove the ligament from the coracoid (Fig. 11).
  - Under direct visualization, the ligament is excised from the medial border of the coracoid base. Between bites, tissue is bluntly swept from lateral to medial, continuing this process until all fibers of the ligament have been cut from the coracoid. Bluntly sweeping from posterior to anterior will

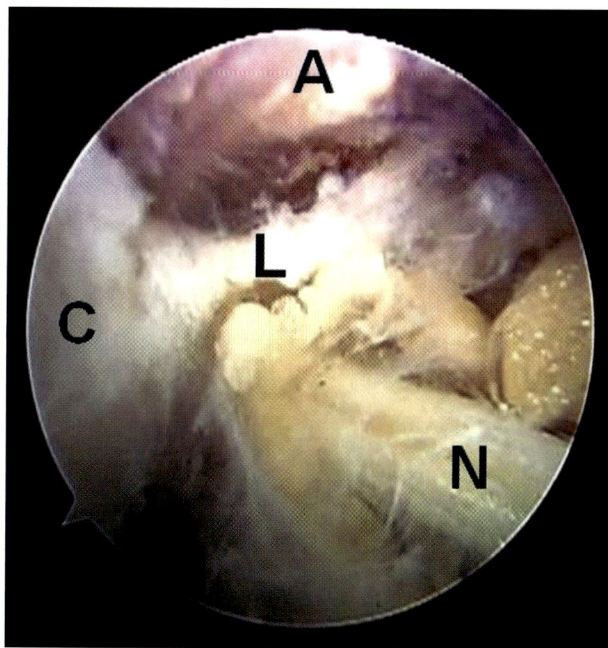

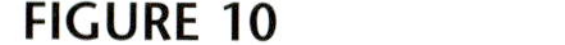

FIGURE 10

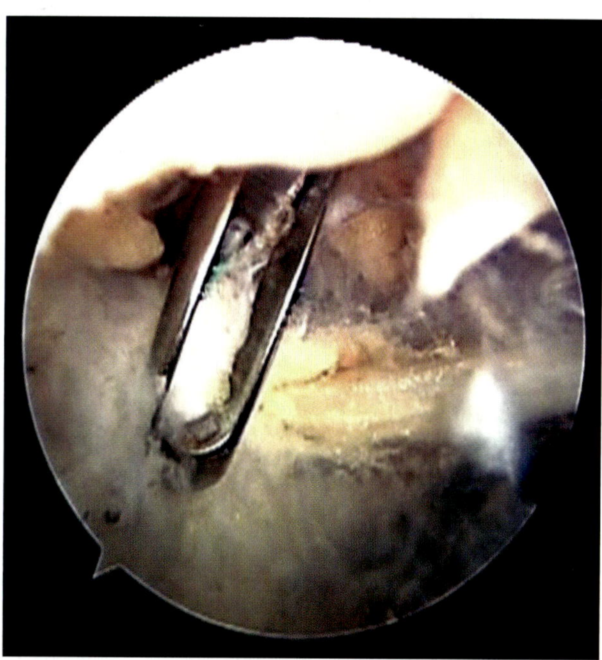

FIGURE 11

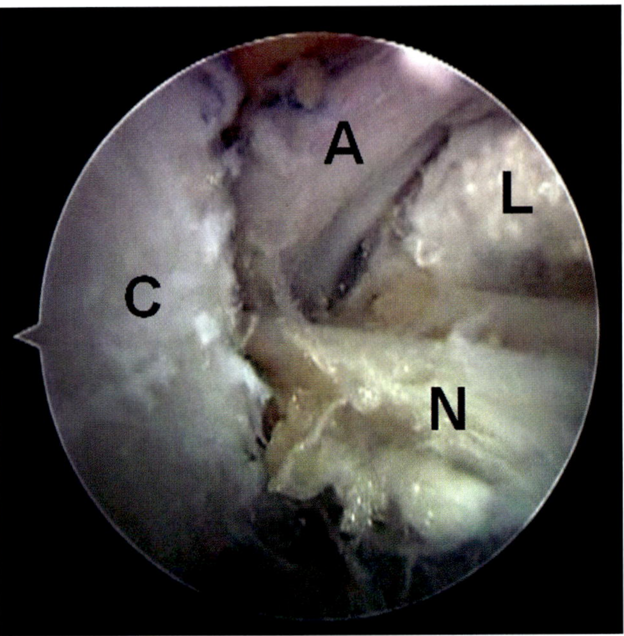

FIGURE 12

allow the surgeon to palpate any remaining fibers requiring removal.
- Figure 12 shows the suprascapular nerve, artery, and transected transverse scapular ligament.

- Once the ligament has been released, a shaver is inserted to débride the previous site of attachment along the medial coracoid base. The ligament is bluntly swept medially to create space between the coracoid and the ligament stump to prevent recurrent compression.
- With a blunt trochar, the nerve is palpated to ensure that it moves freely in the suprascapular notch, and the surgeon should verify with photos that it remains in continuity.
- Portals are closed with subcutaneous 3-0 absorbable suture and steri-strips.
- Sterile bandages are applied.
- Patient is placed in a sling for comfort. The duration of time in the sling is determined by concomitant pathology as determined by the treating surgeon.

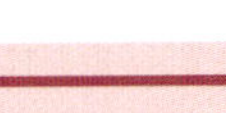

Pearls

- *Always keep the shaver opening toward the coracoid with gentle, if any, suction.*

Pitfalls

- *Impatiently dissecting along the medial border of the coracoid can injure the suprascapular artery and/or nerve.*
- *Injury to the suprascapular artery will cause bleeding that is difficult to control with electrocautery while simultaneously protecting the suprascapular nerve.*

Instrumentation/ Implantation

- Basket forceps
- Full-radius shaver

Procedure: Open Suprascapular Nerve Decompression

Step 1

- A 2- to 3-cm incision is centered 1–2 cm medial to the posterior border of the acromioclavicular joint, placed along the anterior border of the scapular spine (Fig. 13).

- The skin is incised.
- Electrocautery is used to incise through the trapezial fascia (Fig. 14A and 14B).
- Blunt dissection through the trapezius muscle may be performed by sequentially placing Army-Navy retractors in a stepwise fashion until the full depth of the muscle has been penetrated.
- The depth of the wound is now over the supraspinatus muscle fascia (Fig. 15).

Pearls

- *A head lamp and loupe magnification are useful.*
- *Retracting the supraspinatus muscle belly inferiorly/posteriorly will pull the suprascapular artery away from the ligament.*

Pitfalls

- *Working through a small incision can make visualization difficult. Make the incision large enough to see the vital structures.*

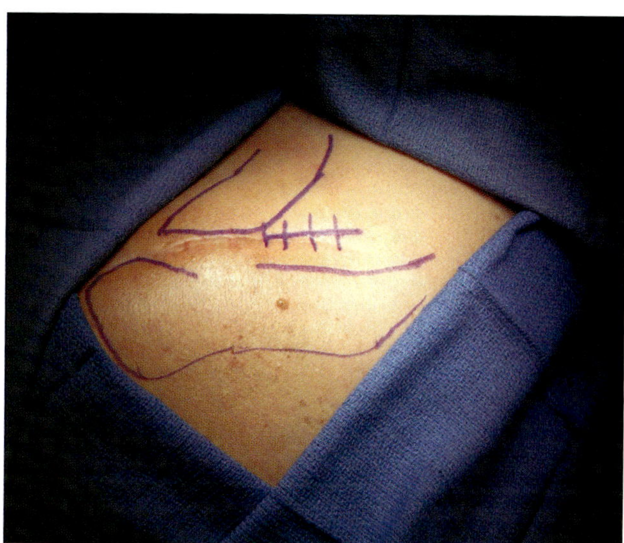

FIGURE 13

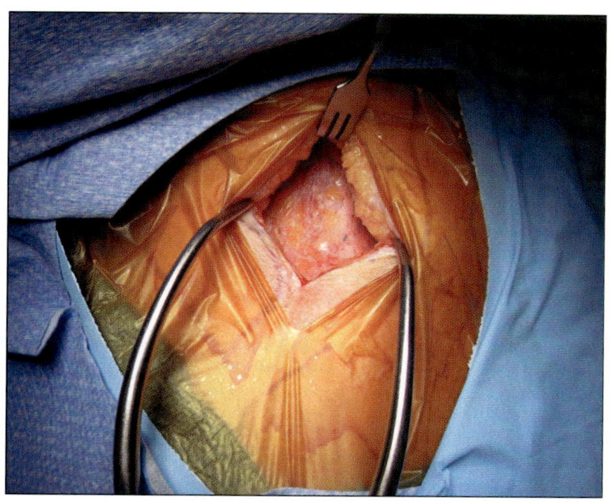

A

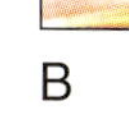

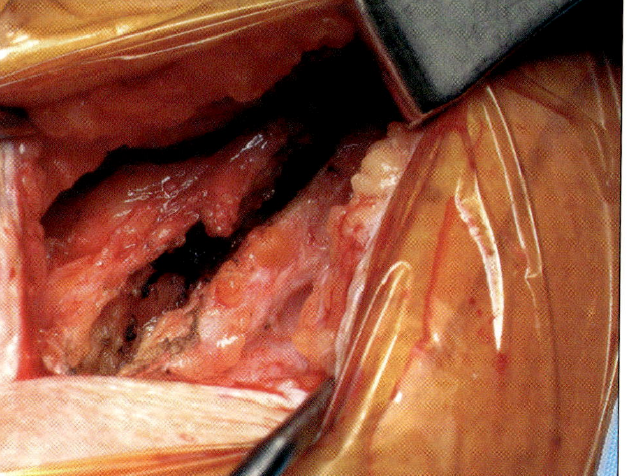

B

FIGURE 14

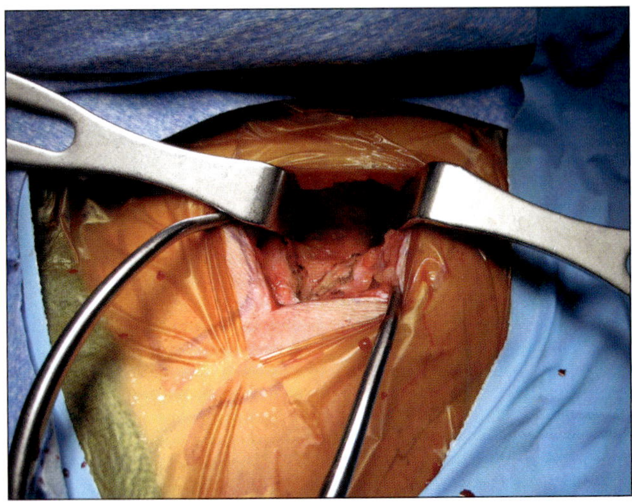

FIGURE 15

Instrumentation/ Implantation

- Head lamp (per preference)
- Loupes
- Soffield retractor set
- Kittner dissecting sponges
- Right-angle clamp
- No. 15 blade

Step 2

- The supraspinatus is gently retracted inferiorly (posteriorly). This will pull the artery free of the ligament.
- The transverse scapular ligament is identified with digital palpation (Fig. 16).
- Soft tissues are swept away from the ligament, artery, and nerve with a Kittner sponge.
- The ligament is sharply divided, taking care to identify and protect the artery and nerve (Fig. 17).

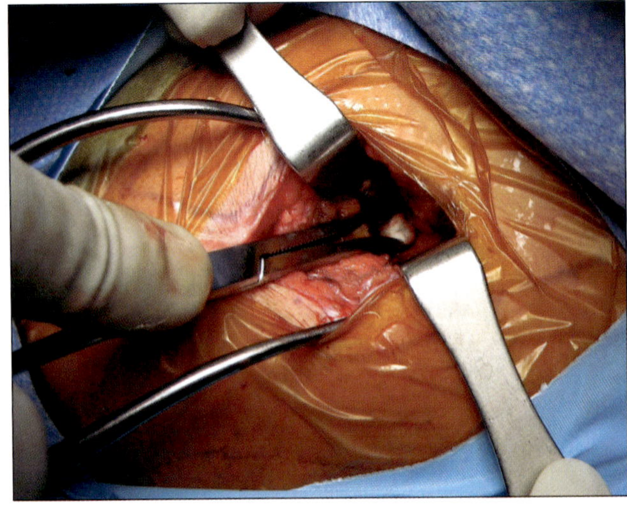

FIGURE 16

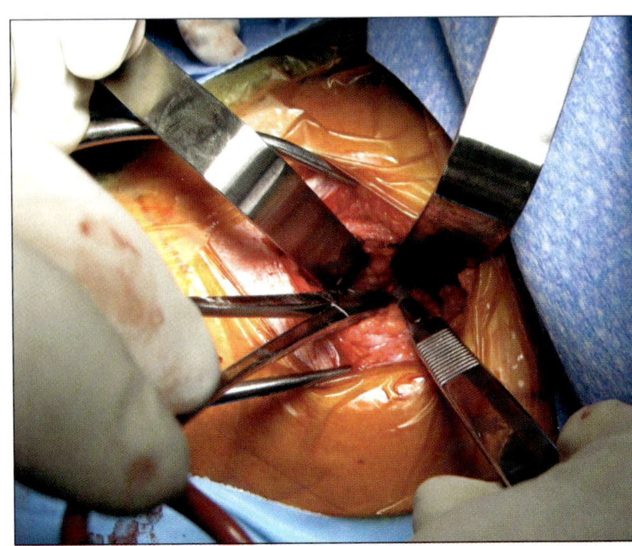

FIGURE 17

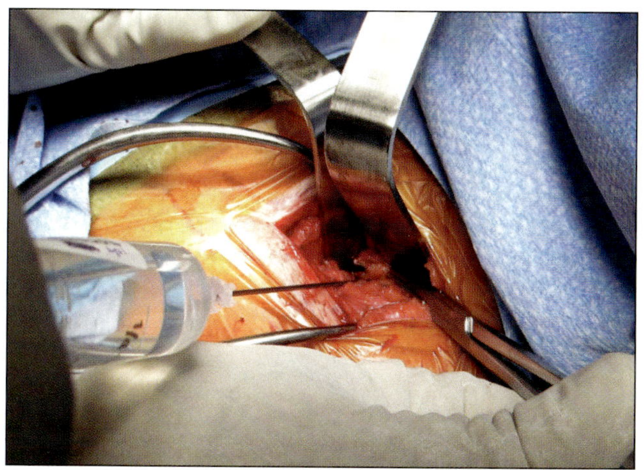
A

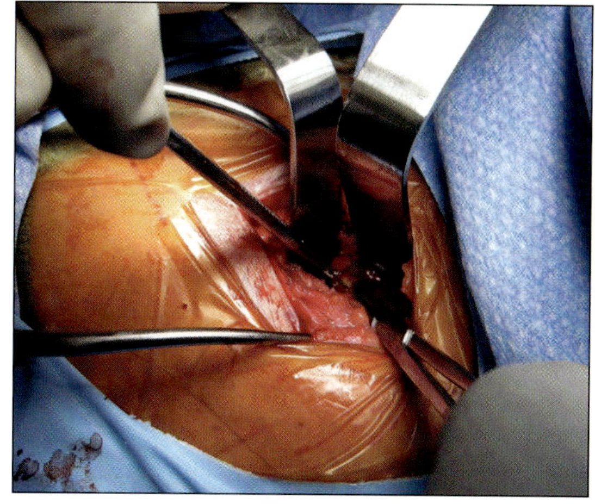
B

FIGURE 18

- For suprascapular neurectomy, the nerve is injected with 0.25% bupivacaine (Marcaine) (Fig. 18A) prior to dividing the nerve (Fig. 18B).
- The wound is irrigated, and the trapezial fascia, dermis, and skin are closed.

Postoperative Care and Expected Outcomes

- For isolated suprascapular nerve decompression, patients are placed in a sling for comfort.
- Full passive and active-assisted range of motion are allowed. Any further restrictions of motion postoperatively will be dictated by concomitant procedures (rotator cuff repair, distal clavicle resection, biceps tenodesis).

Evidence

Bhatia DN, de Beer JF, van Rooyen KS, du Toit DF. Arthroscopic suprascapular nerve decompression at the suprascapular notch. Arthroscopy 2006;Sep;22(9):1009-13.

The authors describe an alternative method of arthroscopic decompression of the suprascapular nerve. The technique described is a variation of the method described by Lafosse. No clinical followup is described.

Krishnan SG. Arthroscopic suprascapular nerve decompression using anterior portals: technique and results. Presented at the Annual American Academy of Orthopaedic Surgeons meeting, San Diego, 2007.

Lafosse L, Tomasi A, Corbett S, et al. Arthroscopic release of suprascapular nerve entrapment at the suprascapular notch: technique and preliminary results. Arthroscopy. 2007;Jan;23(1):34-42.

Ten patients with EMG/NCS evidence of SSN compression neuropathy underwent arthroscopic SSN decompression. Eight of 10 had postoperative EMG/NCS 6 months postoperatively demonstrating partial (1/8) or complete (7/8) normalization of motor latency and action potential. There were 9 of 10 excellent and 1 of 10 with satisfactory clinical outcomes. (Level IV evidence)

Rengachary SS, Burr D, Lucas S, et al. Suprascapular entrapment neuropathy: a clinical, anatomical and comparative study, Part 2: anatomical study. Neurosurgery 1979;5:447-51.

The dimensions of the suprascapular notch in two hundred eleven adult scapulae were examined. A classification system was developed based the dimensions of the suprascapular notch. Six types of suprascapular notch were observed ranging from notch absence (type I), a wide notch (types II-IV), to a narrow constricted with notch (type V) with a bony bridge (type VI). Transitions tended to occur between Types II, III, and IV. (Level IV evidence [anatomic study])

Ticker JB, Djurasovic M, Strauch RJ, et al. The incidence of ganglion cysts and other variations in anatomy along the course of the suprascapular nerve. J Shoulder Elbow Surg. 1998;Sep-Oct;7(5):472-8.

Seventy-nine adult human scapulae form 41 cadavers were dissected and evaluated. The suprascapular notch was U-shaped in 77% and V-shaped in 23%. Notch morphology was symmetric bilaterally in 89%. Variations in the transverse scapular ligament were observed in 23%. A ganglion cyst altering the course of the suprascapular nerve was present in 1%. (Level IV evidence [anatomic study])

PROCEDURE 36

Scapular Surgery I

W. Ben Kibler

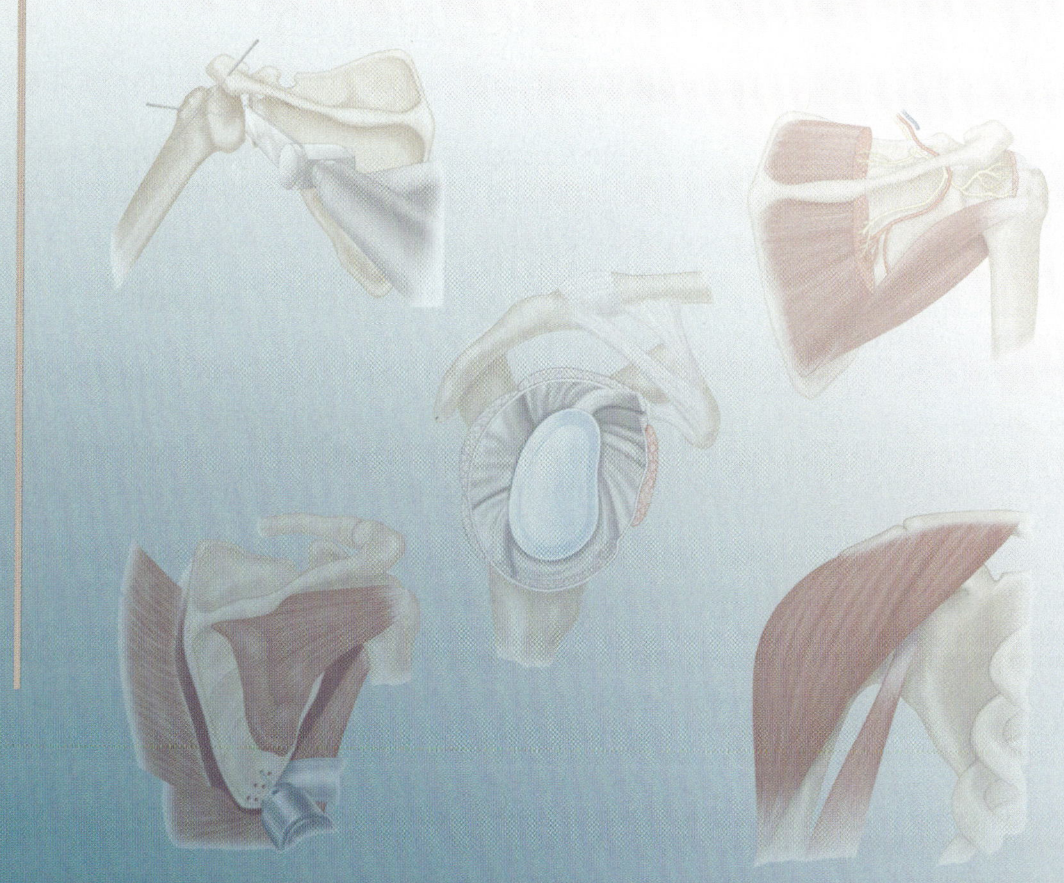

Figures 1, 5, and 7 modified from Kuhn J, Plancher K, Hawkins R. Scapular winging. J Am Acad Orthop Surg. 1995;3:319-25.

Eden-Lange Transfer for Trapezius Muscle Palsy

Indications

- Scapular dyskinesis and winging due to paralysis of the trapezius muscle resulting from injury to the accessory nerve (Acta Orthopaedica Scandinavica, 1973)

Examination/Imaging

- Atrophy of both upper trapezius and lower trapezius muscles.
- Characteristic scapular posture of posteroinferior tilt and drooping of entire shoulder due to trapezius palsy (Fig. 1).
- Inability to shrug shoulder.
- Difficulty in elevating the arm, especially in forward flexion or over 90°.
- Electromyography—denervation in muscle.
  - Beware of false-negative examination if needle is placed through the atrophic trapezius into the normal rhomboids.
- Imaging is of minimal efficacy.

Surgical Anatomy

- Palpable medial scapular border
- Scapular spine
- Rhomboid muscle attachments on medial scapular border (Fig. 2)
- Levator scapulae attachment along superior medial border superior to scapular spine
- Infraspinatus attachment along medial scapular border

Positioning

- Prone, chest rolls, padding under both shoulders (Fig. 3)
- Unaffected arm on armboard
- Affected arm tucked at side, padded
- Slight reverse Trendelenburg position, slight tilt to operative side
- Draped out with towels
- Entire scapula in field, medial border identified (Fig. 4)

Pitfalls

- *Distinguish from partial injury to the accessory nerve to the lower trapezius only*
- *Distinguish from dyskinesis and winging due to serratus anterior palsy (Kuhn et al., 1995)*
- *Distinguish from secondary dyskinesis and winging (Kuhn et al., 1995; Rubin and Kibler, 2002)*
  - *Glenohumeral joint injury with muscle inhibition and altered muscle activation*
  - *Scapular muscle detachment*
  - *Shoulder soft tissue contractures*
  - *Clavicle fractures with nonunion or shortened malunion*
  - *Acromioclavicular joint injury: high-grade separations or instability secondary to excessive distal clavicle resection*

Treatment Options

- Strengthening of surrounding muscles—usually of minimal benefit
- Neurolysis/repair of injured accessory nerve (Wright, 1975)

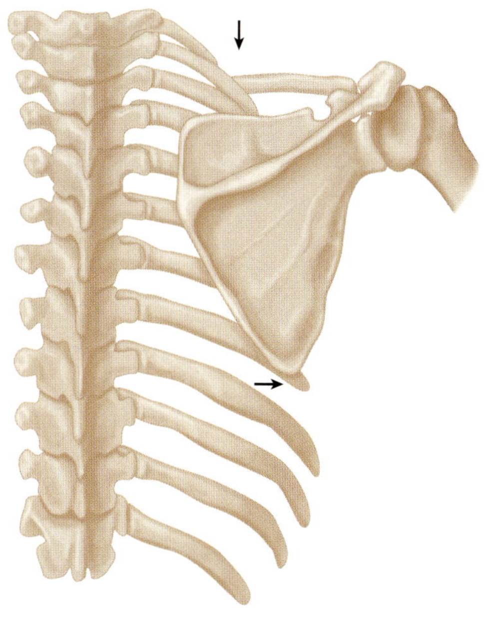
FIGURE 1

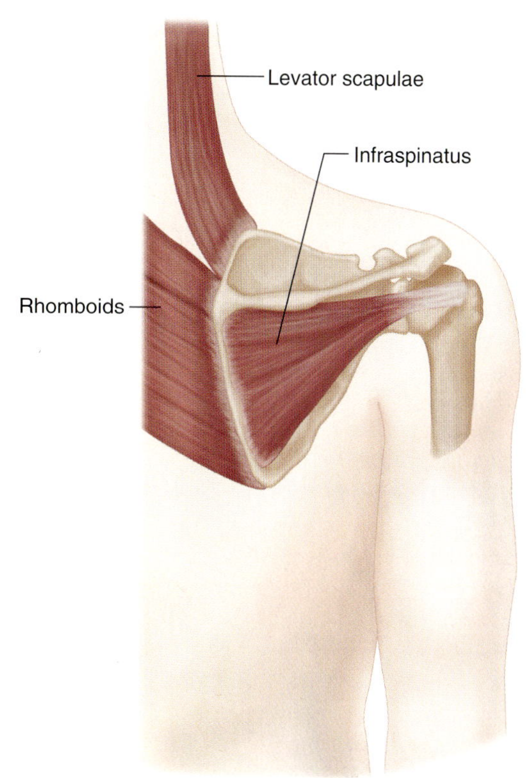

FIGURE 2

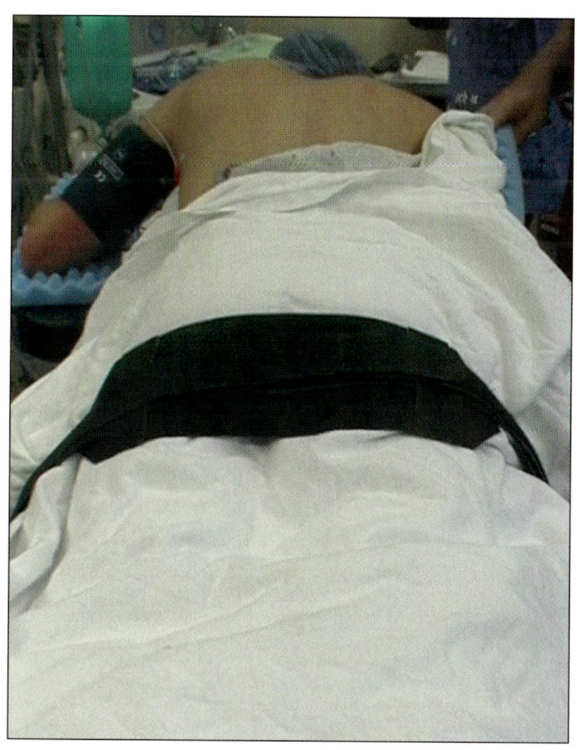
FIGURE 3

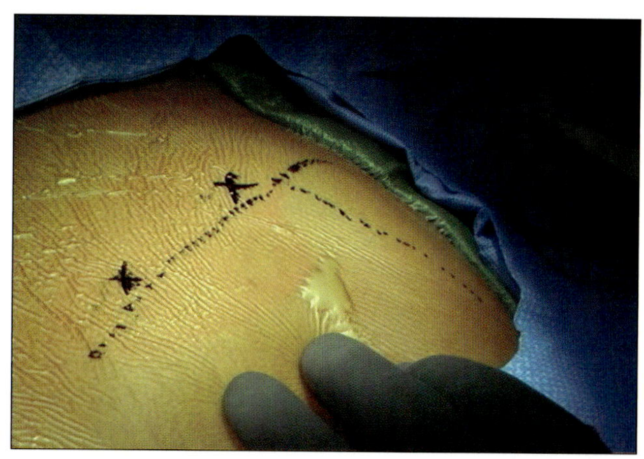
FIGURE 4

Portals/Exposures

- Longitudinal incision along entire medial scapular border, curving laterally over and superior to scapular spine (Bigliani et al., 1985)

Procedure

Step 1

- Develop the incision down to fascia.
- Identify the atrophic lower trapezius over the medial scapular spine.
- Identify the rhomboids along the entire medial border.
- Identify the levator scapulae under the atrophic upper trapezius (Kuhn et al., 1995).

Pearls

- *Dissect through the atrophic trapezius to identify the levator.*

Step 2

- Mobilize the rhomboids and levator off the medial border (Fig. 5).
- Mobilize the infraspinatus off the entire medial scapular border and spine and retract it 4–5 cm.

Pearls

- *Use electrocautery to remove the muscle attachment.*
- *Use a periosteal elevator to mobilize and bring tissues to the dorsal aspect.*

Step 3

- Place pairs of dorsal-to-ventral drill holes in the scapular body 4–5 cm lateral to the scapular border (Fig. 6A).
- Make the holes of each pair about 8–10 mm apart, and make each pair about 1.5–2 cm apart.

Pearls

- *Use a 2.0- to 2.4-mm drill bit.*
- *Use a wide-bladed periosteal elevator on the ventral side to protect the underlying structures.*

Step 4

- Place a pair of superior-to-inferior drill holes in the scapular spine at approximately the midpoint of the spine (Fig. 6B).

Pearls

- *Check the length of the mobilized levator and adjust the drill hole position on the spine so the transfer will be under a slight amount of tension.*

Step 5

- Use mattress sutures for the repair.
- Place the rhomboid stitches from dorsal to ventral through the muscle/tendon, dorsal to ventral through one of the bone holes, then ventral to dorsal through the other hole of the pair, then ventral to dorsal through the muscle/tendon.
- Place the levator sutures from superior to inferior in the muscle/tendon, superior to inferior through one of the holes, inferior to superior through the other hole of the repair, and inferior to superior through the muscle/tendon.
- Tie the sutures so there is slight tension on the repair. Tie the rhomboid from inferior to superior on the body, then tie the levator (Fig. 7).

Pearls

- *Manually position the scapula in a retracted posture before placing the sutures to maximize the effect of the transfer.*
- *Use #2 nonabsorbable suture material.*
- *Use a wide-bladed periosteal elevator to protect the underlying structures.*

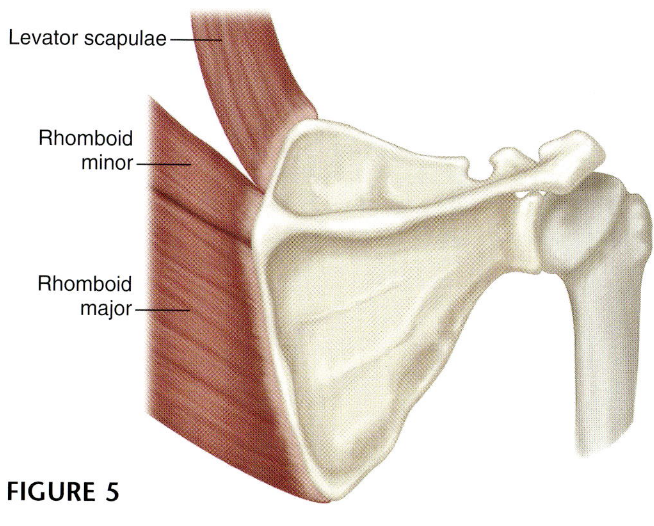

FIGURE 5

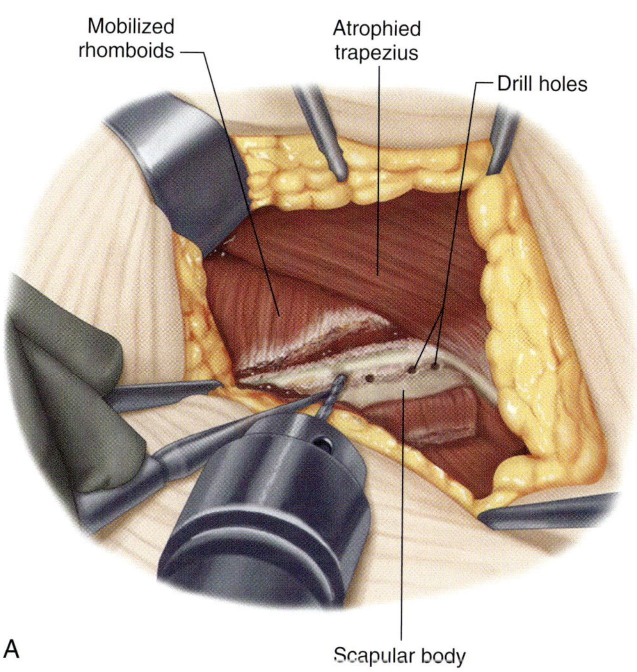

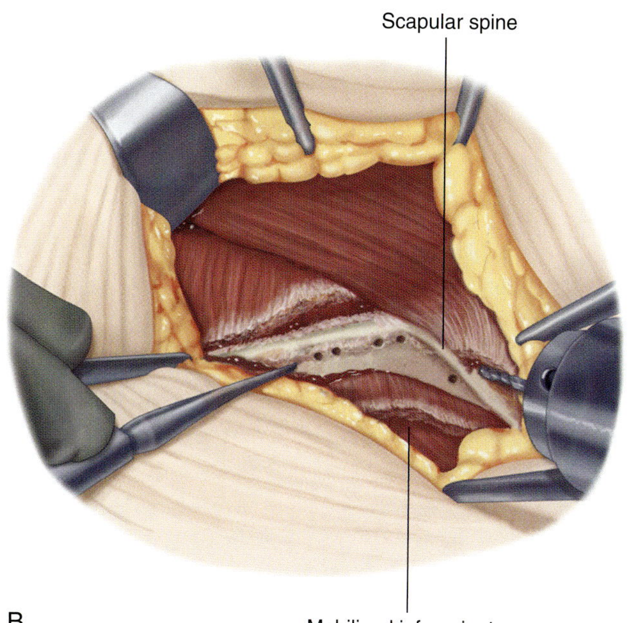

FIGURE 6

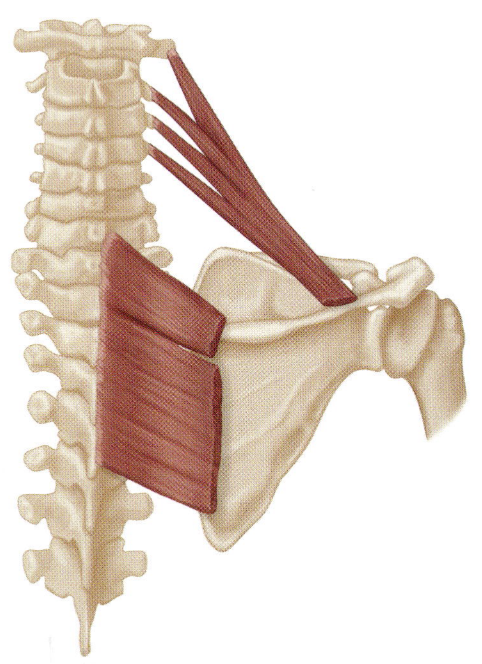

FIGURE 7

PEARLS

- *The muscle transfer sutures can be used to help secure the repair, but the infraspinatus should be reattached at its medial extent.*

PEARLS

- *Provide instructions for specific exercises on paper.*

PEARLS

- *Inform the patient that this is primarily a salvage procedure, that the transferred muscles will be weaker than normal, and that they are not ideally positioned to perform all the duties of the normal trapezius muscles. However, pain relief, better posture, and increased ability to accomplish activities up to 90° can be expected.*

STEP 6

- Reattach the infraspinatus at its normal length over the top of the muscle transfer.

STEP 7

- Close in layers: fascia, subcutaneous tissue, then skin.
- A pain pump may be placed in the subcutaneous tissue.

Postoperative Care and Expected Outcomes

POSTOPERATIVE CARE

- Postoperative sling with neutral wedge—no internal rotation or forward flexion for 3–4 weeks.
- May exercise within first 10 days—scapular pinches.
- At 4 weeks, may be out of sling, may start closed chain exercises in forward flexion and abduction up to 90°.
- At 6 weeks, may exercise above 90°—closed chain progressing to open chain. No eccentric loading with arm extended for 8 weeks.
- No heavy or repetitive lifting for 16 weeks.

EXPECTED OUTCOMES (KUHN ET AL., 1995)

- Variable relief of medial border pain
- Improved resting position of scapula in retraction and upward elevation—less drooping
- Improved muscle strength in forward arm activities, especially up to 90°
- Variable and unpredictable change in ability to accomplish overhead activities

Evidence

Bigliani LU, Perez-Sanz JR, Wolfe IN. Treatment of trapezius paralysis. J Bone Joint Surg [Am]. 1985;67:871-7.

This paper reviewed the presentation, treatment, and outcomes in a cohort of 18 patients with trapezius palsy. Patients treated nonoperatively did not do well, with continued symptoms. The operative approach of lateral transfer of the levator scapulae and rhomboids resulted in improved function and decreased deformity. The paper contains a detailed description of the surgical technique. (Level III evidence)

Kuhn J, Plancher K, Hawkins R. Scapular winging. J Am Acad Orthop Surg. 1995;3:319-25.

This review paper discussed scapular winging from all causes. It showed the different pathoanatomy responsible for each type of winging, discussed the clinical presentation of each type, and summarized treatment options. It also differentiated between primary and secondary winging. (Level III evidence [review])

Rubin B, Kibler WB. Fundamental principles of shoulder rehabilitation: conservative to postoperative management. Arthroscopy. 2002;18(Suppl):29-39.

This review paper discussed the spectrum of causation of scapular dyskinesis. It pointed out the causes of secondary winging, both proximal and distal to the scapula, that are not related to neurologic injury, and described methods of evaluation for these. These causes must be ruled out before doing muscle transfers for nerve injury. (Level IV evidence)

Treatment of paralysis of the trapezius muscle by the Eden-Lange operation. Acta Orthop Scand. 1973;44:383-88.

This paper reviews the surgical technique of muscle transfer to compensate for trapezius muscle deficiency due to paralysis.

Wright TA. Accessory spinal nerve injury. Clin Orthop Relat Res. 1975;(108):15-8.

This paper reviewed the pertinent anatomy of the accessory spinal nerve and demonstrated its vulnerability in posterior cervical neck dissection. It described the clinical presentation of trapezius palsy, including postural deformity, weakness, atrophy, and decreased ability to raise the arm. (Level IV evidence)

PROCEDURE 36

Scapular Surgery II

W. Ben Kibler

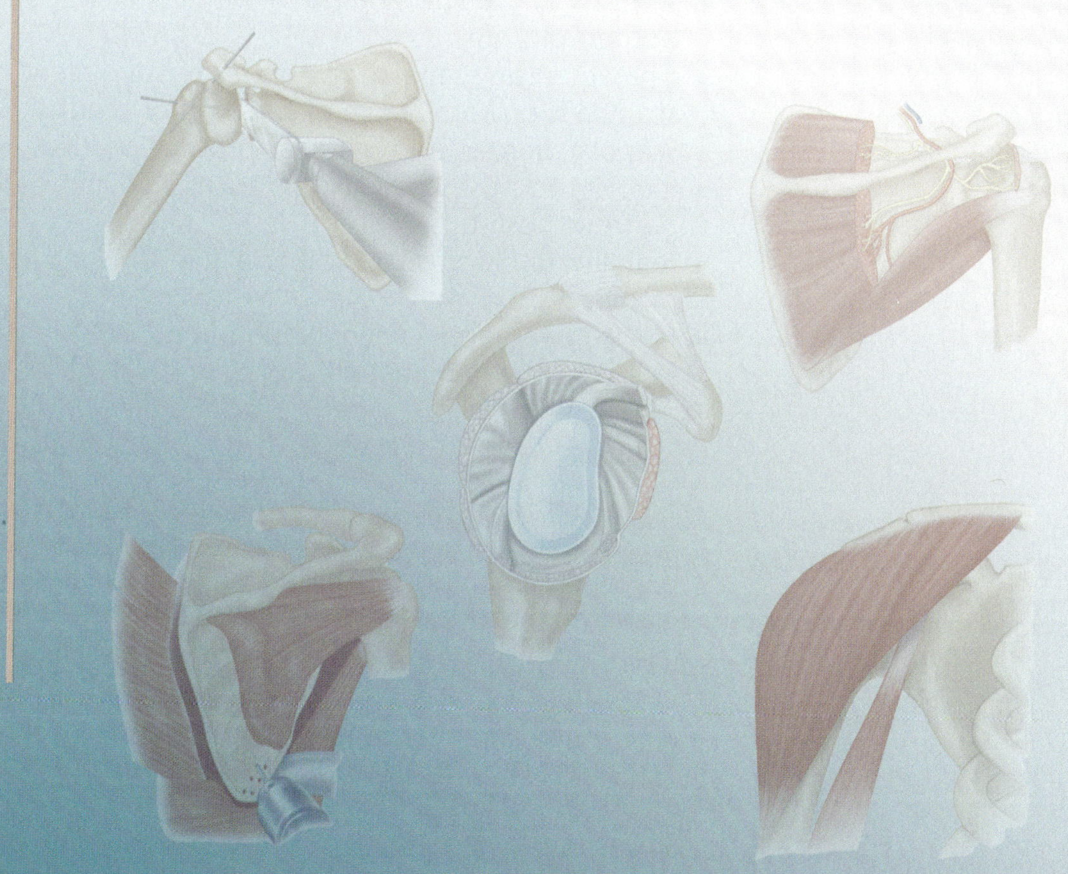

Figures 1, 3–5, 8, and 9 modified from Kuhn J, Plancher K, Hawkins R. Scapular winging. J Am Acad Orthop Surg. 1995;3:319-25.

Pectoralis Major Transfer for Serratus Anterior Palsy

Indications

- Serratus anterior muscle palsy due to long thoracic nerve injury (Post, 1995; Steinman and Wood, 2003)

Examination/Imaging

- Atrophy of serratus anterior along lateral scapular border and ribs.
- Characteristic scapular posture of posteroinferior scapula tilt, prominence of the inferior medial scapular border, and scapular protraction (Fig. 1).
- Inability to push against resistance, inability to perform push-ups.
- Inability to elevate arm, especially in forward flexion or over 90°.
- Electromyography—denervation in muscle.
- Imaging is of minimal efficacy.

Surgical Anatomy

- Pectoralis major attachment on anterior humerus (Fig. 2A)
  - Notice separate sternal and clavicular heads
  - Sternal head passes deep to the clavicular head and inserts more inferiorly on the humerus (Connor et al., 1997; Povacz and Resch, 2000)
- Latissimus dorsi muscle running along the lateral border of the scapula (Fig. 2B)
- Inferior medial scapular border, with serratus anterior attachment along inferior one fourth of ventral surface and infraspinatus attachment along dorsal surface
- Ipsilateral thigh, with fascia lata

Positioning

- Lateral decubitus
- Beanbag support
- Affected arm, anterior chest, and entire periscapular area prepped out
- Lateral thigh prepped and draped from greater trochanter to knee

Pitfalls

- *Absence of proven long thoracic nerve injury*
- *Distinguish from dyskinesis and winging due to trapezius palsy (Kuhn et al., 1995)*
- *Distinguish from secondary dyskinesis and winging (Rubin and Kibler, 2002)*
  - *Glenohumeral joint injury with muscle inhibition and altered muscle activation*
  - *Scapular muscle detachment*
  - *Shoulder soft tissue contractures*
  - *Clavicle fractures with nonunion or shortened malunion*
  - *Acromioclavicular joint injury: high-grade separations or instability secondary to excessive distal clavicle resection*

Treatment Options

- Strengthening of surrounding muscles—usually of minimal benefit; no muscles are capable of stabilizing the scapula as effectively
- Neurolysis/repair of injured long thoracic nerve

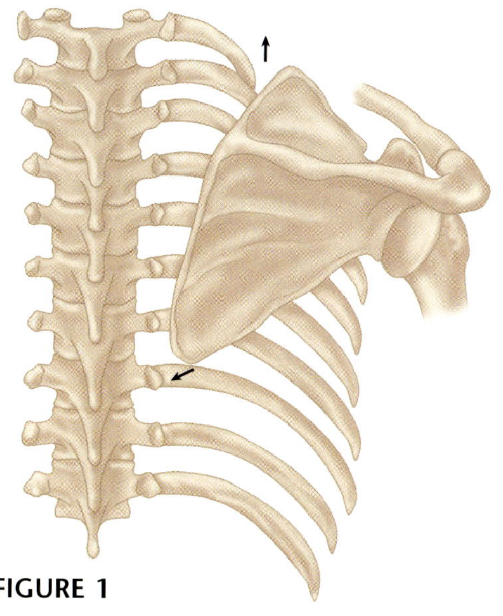

FIGURE 1

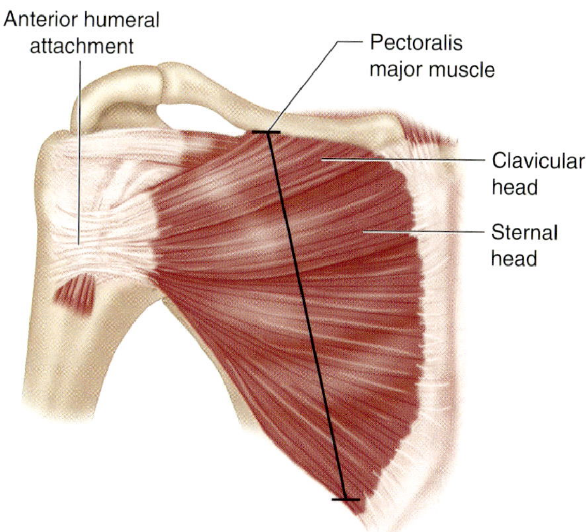

A

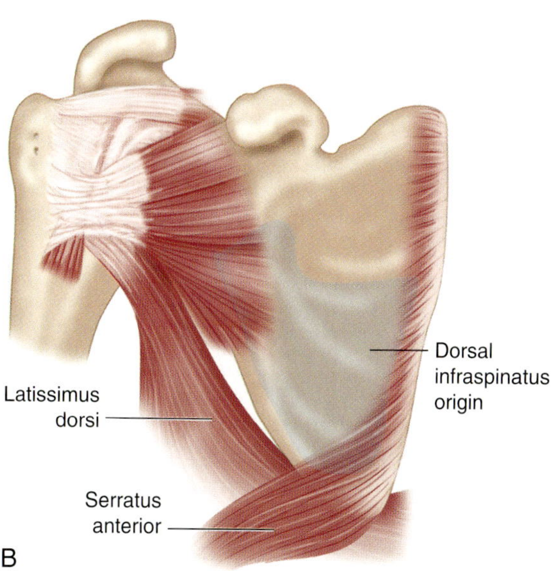

FIGURE 2 B

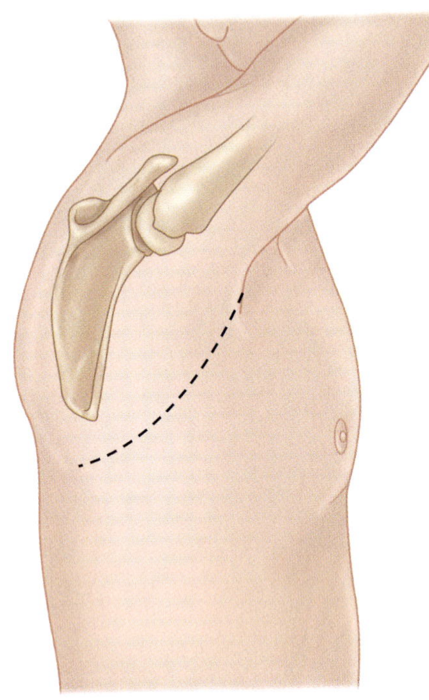

FIGURE 3

Portals/Exposures

- One long incision is made from the coracoid and pectoralis anteriorly, under the axilla, to the inferior scapular border (Fig. 3) (Post, 1995; Kuhn et al., 1995).
- Alternatively, two separate incisions are made, one anteriorly over the coracoid and pectoralis, the second posteriorly over the inferior scapular border (Povacz and Resch, 2000).
- A lateral longitudinal incision is made over the lateral thigh, if needed.

Procedure

Step 1

- Develop the incision through the superficial tissues.
- Anteriorly, identify the deltopectoral interval, trace the pectoralis to its humeral attachment, and detach the deeper inferiorly located sternal head of the pectoralis major (Fig. 4).

Step 2

- If needed, harvest a graft from the fascia lata, at least 12 cm in length and 4 cm in width.
- Suture it to the pectoralis tendon (Fig. 5).

Step 3

- Develop a tunnel under the latissimus dorsi to pass the graft (Fig. 6).

Pearls

- *Mobilize the tendon by dissection along the border between the two heads (Povacz and Resch, 2000).*

Pearls

- *Use multiple nonabsorbable sutures to create a secure graft-tendon interface.*
- *Occasionally in thin or small patients, the pectoralis will be long enough by itself. Check the length of the mobilized pectoralis tendon before taking the graft (Povacz and Resch, 2000).*

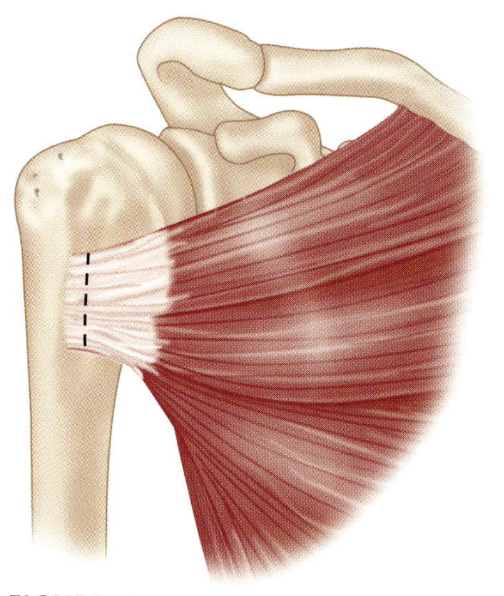

FIGURE 4

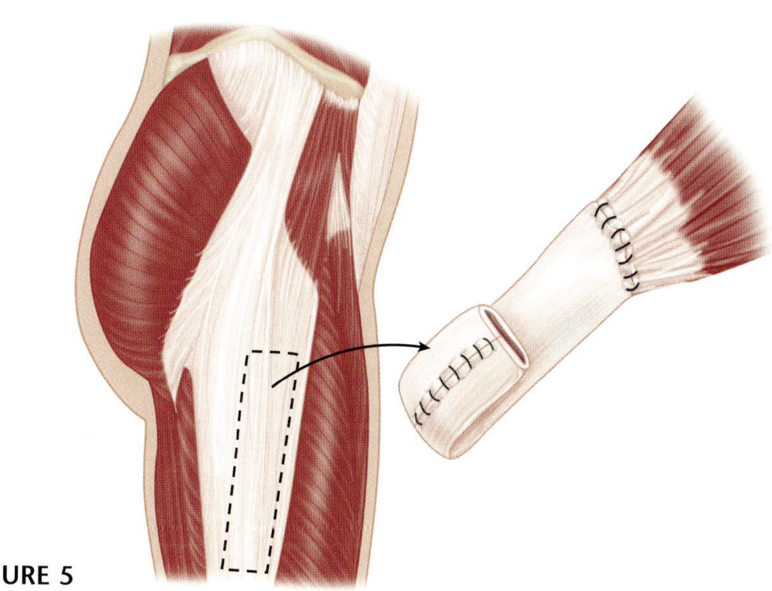

FIGURE 5

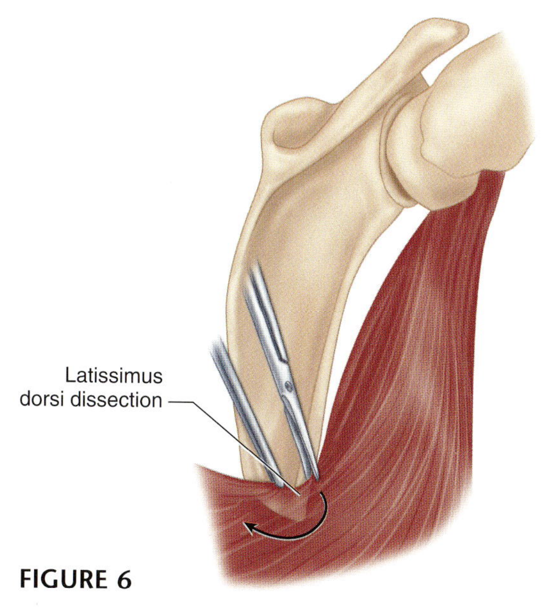

FIGURE 6

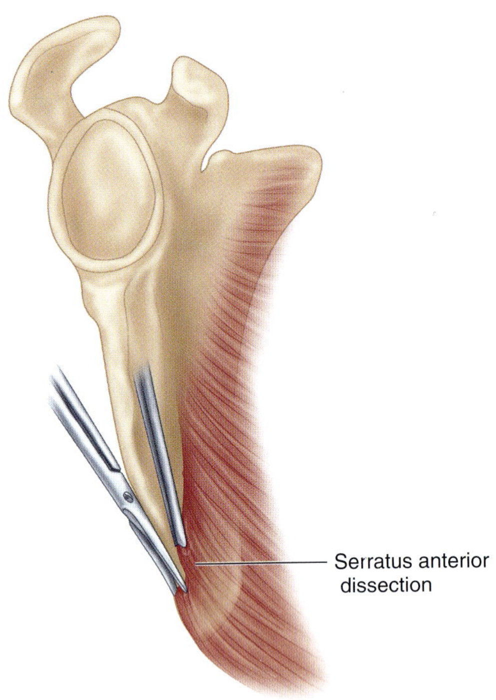

FIGURE 7

Step 4

- Posteriorly, develop a tunnel on the ventral surface of the scapula along the serratus anterior muscle (Fig. 7).

Step 5

- Dorsally, mobilize the infraspinatus off the inferior medial and lateral scapular borders for about 4–5 cm.
- Ventrally, mobilize the atrophic serratus anterior.

Step 6

- Create a hole in the scapular body to accept the graft (Fig. 8).
  - Orient the hole on a superior-to-inferior axis parallel to the medial border.
  - It is best to make the hole as close to the inferior tip as possible, but make sure that the thick medial and lateral scapular cortices are intact to allow secure fixation of the graft.

Step 7

- Pass the tendon/graft from the ventral surface to the dorsal surface, and loop it around the medial border.
- Place the scapula in a posture of retraction and posterior tilt before securing the distal end back on itself (Fig. 9).

Pearls

- *Bluntly dissect using scissors and forceps. It is easier to dissect from anterior to posterior around the chest wall.*
- *Always be aware of the contents of the axilla, which will be adjacent and superolateral to the dissection.*

Pearls

- *Use a micro-saw to create the hole.*
- *Make the hole wide and long enough to pass the tendon/graft.*

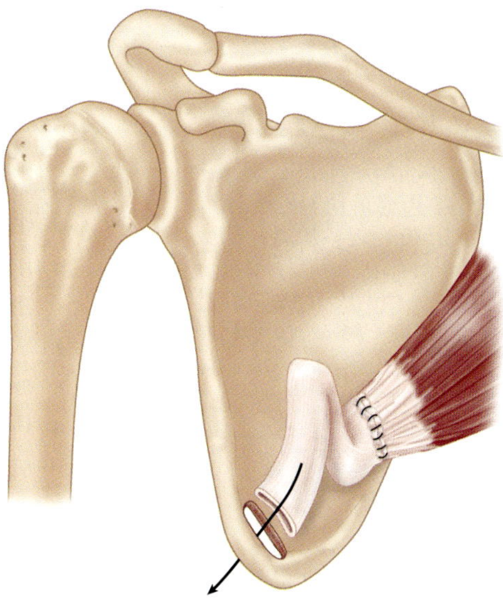
FIGURE 8

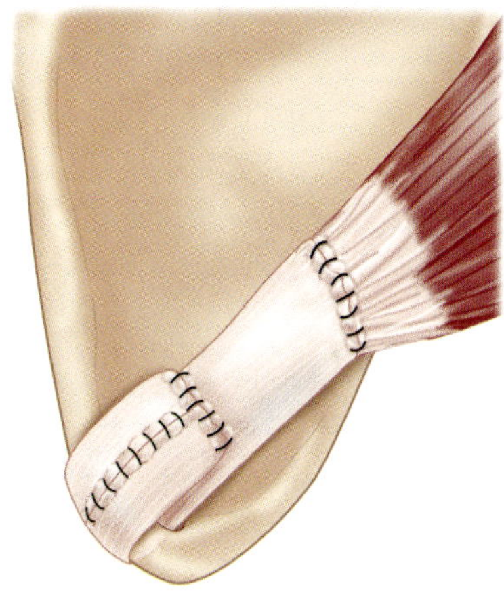
FIGURE 9

Step 8

- Close in layers: fascia, subcutaneous tissue, then skin.
- Place drains as needed.
- May use pain pump in subcutaneous tissue if no drains are used.

> **Pearls**
>
> - *Pass the graft and then secure it with multiple sutures of nonabsorbable material on the ventral scapular surface (Povacz and Resch, 2000).*

Postoperative Care and Expected Outcomes

Postoperative Care

- Postoperative sling with neutral wedge—no internal rotation or forward flexion for 3–4 weeks.
- May do trunk extension and core stability exercises at 7–10 days.
- At 4 weeks, may be out of sling, may start passive arm motions and closed chain exercises in forward flexion and abduction up to 90°.
- At 8 weeks, may exercise above 90°—closed chain progressing to open chain. No eccentric loading with arm extended for 12 weeks.

> **Pearls**
>
> - *Provide instructions for specific exercises on paper.*

PEARLS

- *Inform the patient that this is primarily a salvage procedure. The transferred muscle will be weaker and is not in phase to provide a high level of stability in scapular retraction. However, pain relief, better posture, and increased ability to accomplish activities up to 90° and pushing can be expected.*

- May progress to active open chain exercises at 12 weeks.
- No heavy or repetitive lifting for 16 weeks.

Expected Outcomes

- Good relief of posterior scapular pain
- Improved scapular posture
- Improved arm strength, especially up to 90° abduction and forward flexion
- Variable ability to accomplish repetitive vigorous overhead activities
- Possibly some decrease in active internal rotation strength

Evidence

Connor PM, Yamaguchi K, Manifold SG, et al. Split pectoralis transfer for serratus anterior palsy. Clin Orthop Relat Res. 1997;(341):134-42.

This clinical review described the technique of transforming a portion of the pectoralis major, often with a graft. (Level IV evidence)

Kuhn J, Plancher K, Hawkins R. Scapular winging. J Am Acad Orthop Surg. 1995;3:319-25.

This review paper discussed scapular winging from all causes. It showed the different pathoanatomy responsible for each type of winging, discussed the clinical presentation of each type, and summarized treatment options. It also differentiated between primary and secondary winging. (Level III evidence [review])

Povacz P, Resch H. Dynamic stabilization of winging scapula by direct split pectoralis transfer. J Shoulder Elbow Surg. 2000;9:76-8.

This paper described a technique of split pectoralis transfer through two incisions that results in a direct attachment of the transferred tendon to the scapula. The authors reported good results, but showed that maximum recovery may take 6 months. (Level IV evidence)

Rubin B, Kibler WB. Fundamental principles of shoulder rehabilitation: conservative to postoperative management. Arthroscopy. 2002;18(Suppl):29-39.

This review paper discussed the spectrum of causation of scapular dyskinesis. It pointed out the causes of secondary winging, both proximal and distal to the scapula, that are not related to neurologic injury, and described methods of evaluation for these. These causes must be ruled out before doing muscle transfers for nerve injury. (Level IV evidence)

Steinman S, Wood M. Pectoralis major transfer for serratus anterior paralysis. J Shoulder Elbow Surg. 2003;12:555-60.

This paper reported the results of pectoralis transfer with a graft in a cohort of patients with serratus anterior palsy. The results showed some improvement in position, but limitations in external rotation strength; 6 of 9 patients achieved good or excellent results. (Level III evidence)

PROCEDURE 36

Scapular Surgery III

W. Ben Kibler

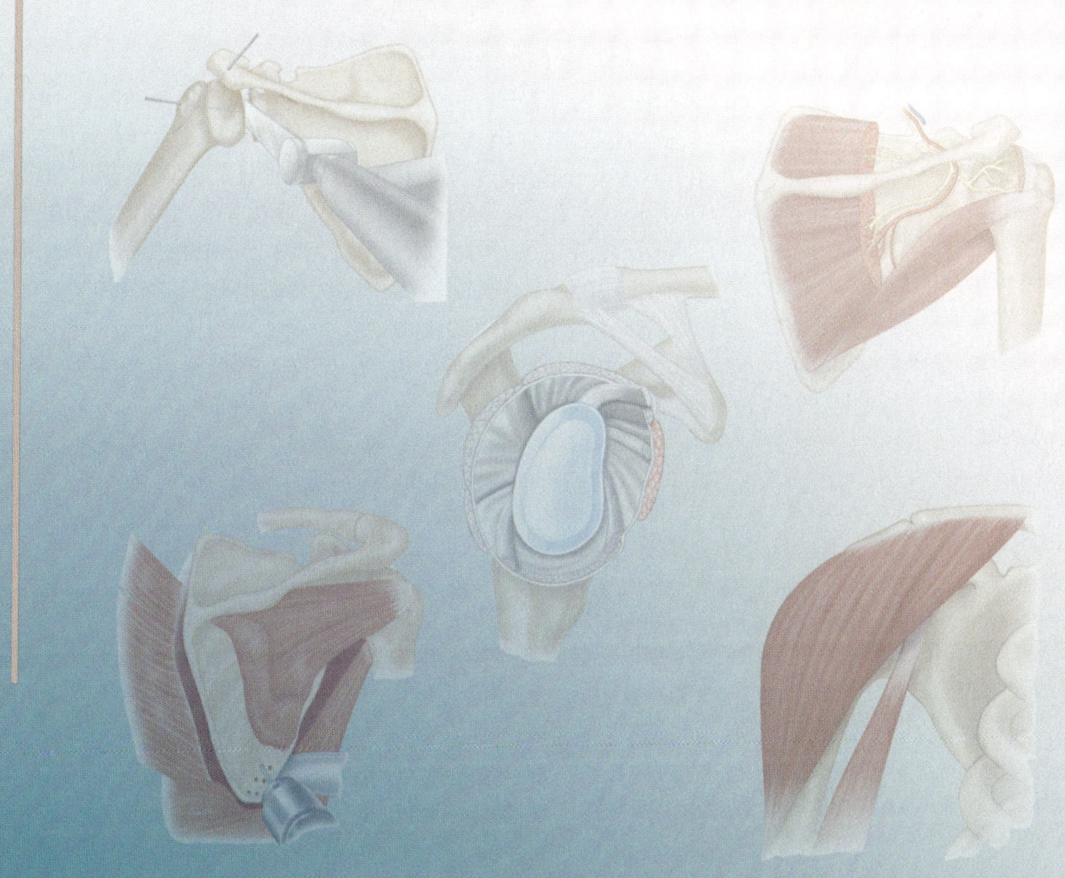

Figure 1 modified from Kuhn J, Plancher K, Hawkins R. Scapular winging. J Am Acad Orthop Surg. 1995;3:319-25.

Rhomboid/Latissimus Dorsi Transfer for Serratus Anterior Palsy

Indications

- Serratus anterior muscle palsy due to long thoracic nerve injury
- Failed pectoralis major transfer

Examination/Imaging

- Atrophy of serratus anterior along lateral scapular border and ribs.
- Characteristic scapular posture of posteroinferior scapula tilt, prominence of the inferior medial scapular border, and scapular protraction (Fig. 1).
- Inability to push against resistance, inability to perform push-ups.
- Inability to elevate arm, especially in forward flexion or over 90°.
- Electromyography—denervation in muscle.
- Imaging is of minimal efficacy.

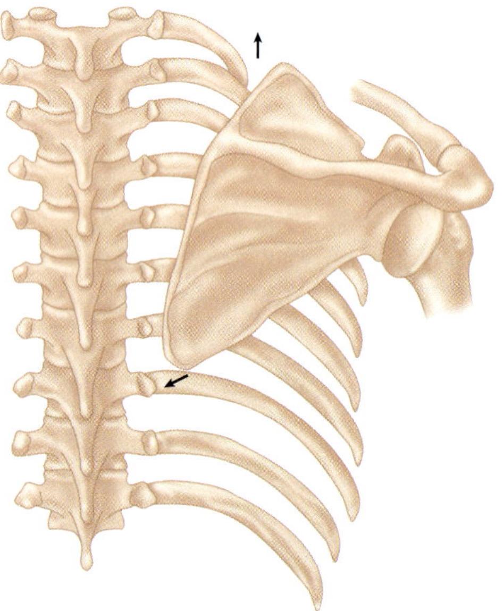

FIGURE 1

Pitfalls

- *Absence of proven long thoracic nerve injury*
- *Distinguish from dyskinesis and winging due to trapezius palsy (Kuhn et al., 1995)*
- *Distinguish from secondary dyskinesis and winging (Rubin and Kibler, 2002)*
  - *Glenohumeral joint injury with muscle inhibition and altered muscle activation*
  - *Scapular muscle detachment*
  - *Shoulder soft tissue contractures*
  - *Clavicle fractures with nonunion or shortened malunion*
  - *Acromioclavicular joint injury: high-grade separations or instability secondary to excessive distal clavicle resection*
- *Establish failure of the pectoralis transfer rather than muscle weakness.*

Treatment Options

- Strengthening of surrounding muscles—usually of minimal benefit; no muscles are capable of stabilizing the scapula as effectively
- Neurolysis/repair of injured long thoracic nerve

Surgical Anatomy

- Palpable scapular medial border
- Rhomboid muscle attachment on medial scapular border (Fig. 2A)
- Infraspinatus muscle attachment along medial scapular border
- Inferior scapular tip with latissimus dorsi attachment (Fig. 2B)

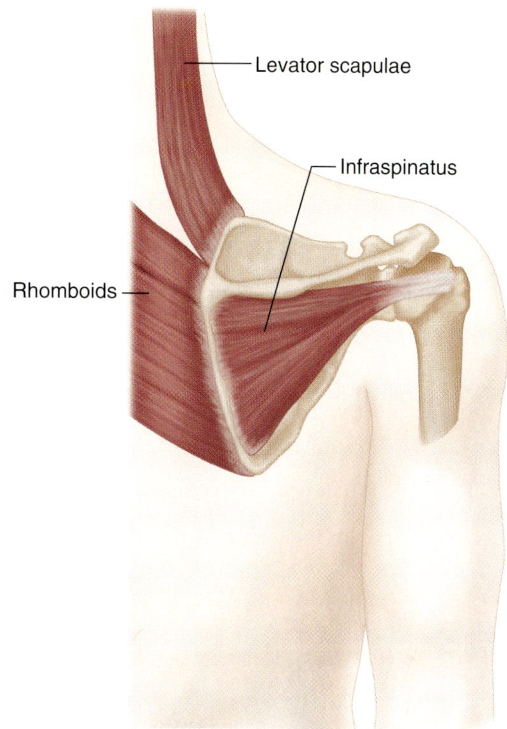

A

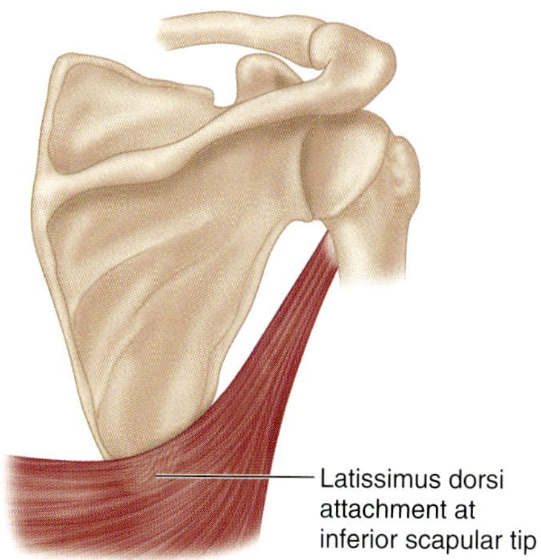

B

FIGURE 2

Positioning

- Prone, chest rolls, padding under both shoulders (Fig. 3)
- Unaffected arm on armboard
- Affected arm tucked at side, padded
- Slight reverse Trendelenburg position, slight tilt to operative side
- Draped out with towels
- Entire scapula in field, medial border identified (Fig. 4)

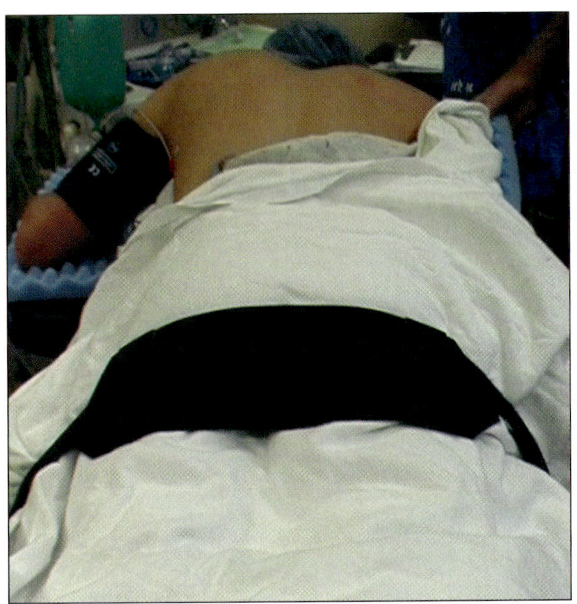

FIGURE 3

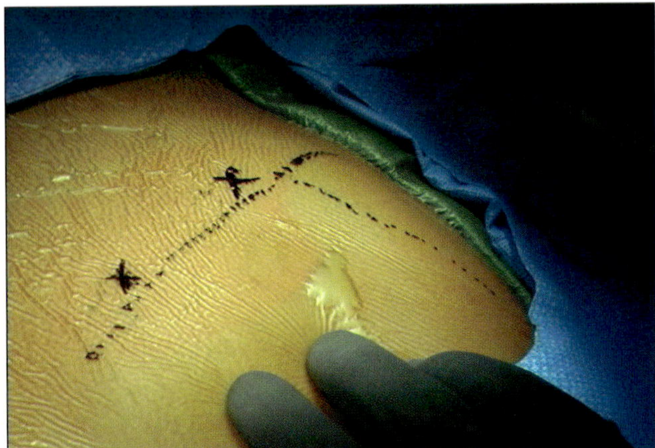

FIGURE 4

Portals/Exposures

- Longitudinal incision along entire medial scapular border down to inferior tip

Procedure

Step 1

- Develop the incision down to fascia.
- Identify the rhomboids along the entire medial border.
- Identify muscle attachments of the latissimus dorsi along the inferior lateral scapular border.

Step 2

- Mobilize the rhomboids off the medial border and the latissimus off the lateral border and bring them onto the dorsal aspect of the scapula (Fig. 5) (Herzmark, 1951).

Step 3

- Mobilize the infraspinatus off the entire medial scapular border and the inferior tip and retract it 2–3 cm.

Step 4

- Place pairs of dorsal-to-ventral drill holes in the scapular body 2–3 cm from the scapular border (Fig. 6). Place one set of holes along the lateral border.
- Make the holes of each pair about 8–10 mm apart, and make each pair about 1.5–2 cm apart.

Pearls

- *Use electrocautery to remove the muscle attachment.*
- *Use a periosteal elevator to mobilize and bring tissues to the dorsal aspect. This will create a V-shaped pouch at the inferior tip*

Pearls

- *Use a 2.0- to 2.4-mm drill bit.*
- *Use a wide-bladed periosteal elevator on the ventral side to protect the underlying structures.*

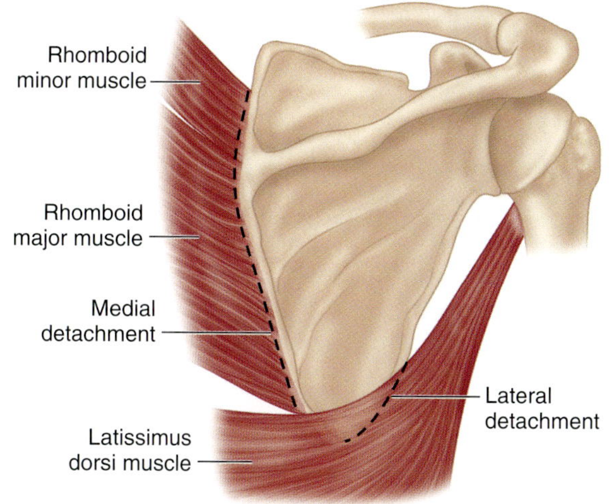

FIGURE 5

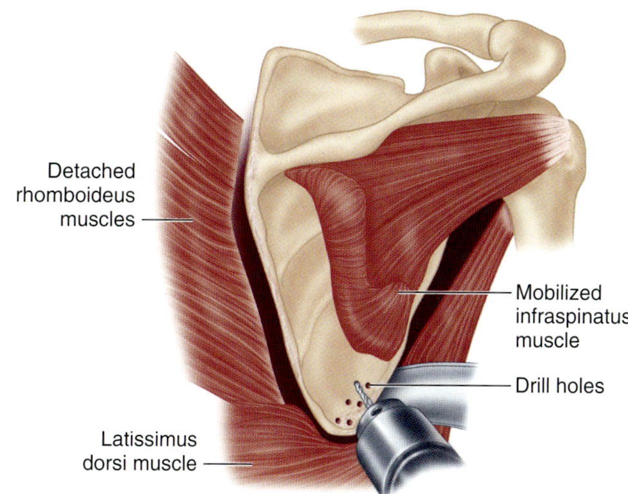

FIGURE 6

Step 5

- Use mattress sutures for the muscle transfer.
- Place the rhomboid stitches from dorsal to ventral through the muscle/tendon, dorsal to ventral through one of the bone holes, then ventral to dorsal through the other hole of the pair, then ventral to dorsal through the muscle/tendon (Fig. 7).
- Tie the sutures so there is slight tension on the repair. Tie from superior to inferior along the medial border.
    - Before tying the most inferior medial stitch, tie the inferior lateral sutures. Then tie the inferior medial suture over the inferior lateral suture, closing the V-shaped pouch over the inferior tip. This creates a dynamic vector for control of the inferior tip.

Pearls

- *Manually position the scapula in a retracted posture before placing the sutures to maximize the effect of the transfer.*
- *Use #2 nonabsorbable suture material.*
- *Use a wide-bladed periosteal elevator to protect the underlying structures.*

Step 6

- Reattach the infraspinatus at its normal length over the top of the muscle transfer (Fig. 8).

Pearls

- *The muscle transfer sutures can be used to help secure the repair, but the infraspinatus should be reattached at its medial and inferior extent.*

Step 7

- Close in layers: fascia, subcutaneous tissue, then skin.
- A pain pump may be placed in the subcutaneous tissue.

Pearls

- *Provide instructions for specific exercises on paper.*

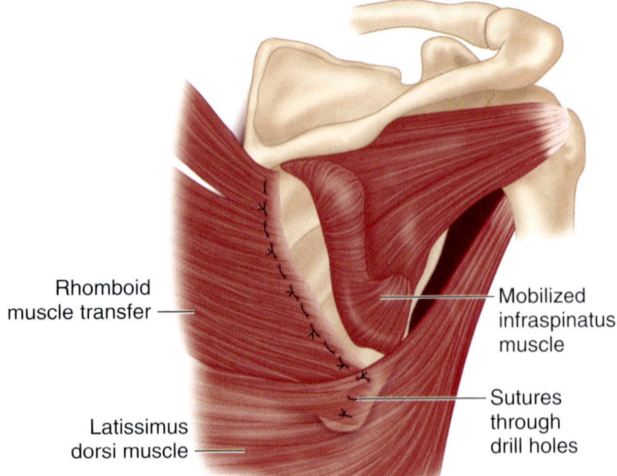

FIGURE 7

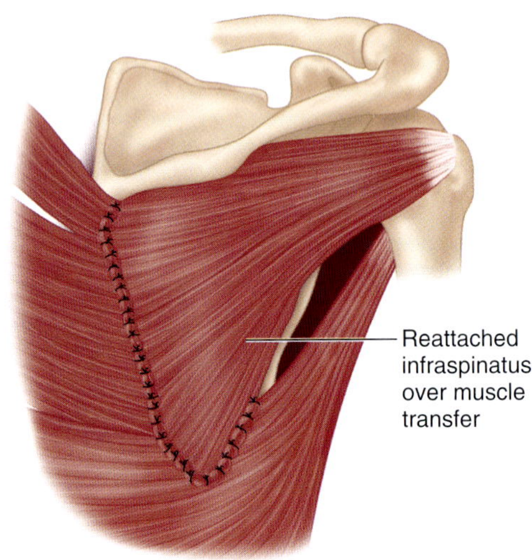

FIGURE 8

Pearls

- *Inform the patient that this is primarily a salvage procedure. The transferred muscles will be weaker. A consistent maintenance program for strengthening of the rhomboids, lower trapezius, and latissimus dorsi is necessary to maintain the dynamic force couples for scapular stability. However, pain relief, better posture, and increased ability to accomplish activities up to 90° and pushing can be expected.*

Postoperative Care and Expected Outcomes

Postoperative Care

- Postoperative sling with neutral wedge—no internal rotation or forward flexion for 3–4 weeks.
- May exercise within first 10 days—scapular pinches.
- At 4 weeks, may be out of sling, may start closed chain exercises in forward flexion and abduction up to 90°.
- At 6 weeks, may exercise above 90°—closed chain progressing to open chain. No eccentric loading with arm extended for 8–10 weeks.
- At 10 weeks, may start open chain loading.
- No heavy or repetitive lifting for 16 weeks.

Expected Outcomes

- Improved scapular posture
- Improved arm strength, especially up to 90° abduction and forward flexion
- Variable ability to accomplish repetitive vigorous overhead activities

Evidence

Herzmark MH. Traumatic paralysis of the serratus anterior relieved by transplantation of the rhomboidei. J Bone Joint Surg [Am]. 1951;33:235-8.

This paper described the technique of rhomboid muscle transfer for serratus anterior palsy. It described good functional results, but showed that maximum strength is maintained by continued exercises. (Level IV evidence)

Kuhn J, Plancher K, Hawkins R. Scapular winging. J Am Acad Orthop Surg. 1995;3:319-25.

This review paper discussed scapular winging from all causes. It showed the different pathoanatomy responsible for each type of winging, discussed the clinical presentation of each type, and summarized treatment options. It also differentiated between primary and secondary winging. (Level III evidence [review])

Rubin B, Kibler WB. Fundamental principles of shoulder rehabilitation: conservative to postoperative management. Arthroscopy. 2002;18(Suppl):29-39.

This review paper discussed the spectrum of causation of scapular dyskinesis. It pointed out the causes of secondary winging, both proximal and distal to the scapula, that are not related to neurologic injury, and described methods of evaluation for these. These causes must be ruled out before doing muscle transfers for nerve injury. (Level IV evidence)

PROCEDURE 37

Adhesive Capsulitis

Patrick J. McMahon

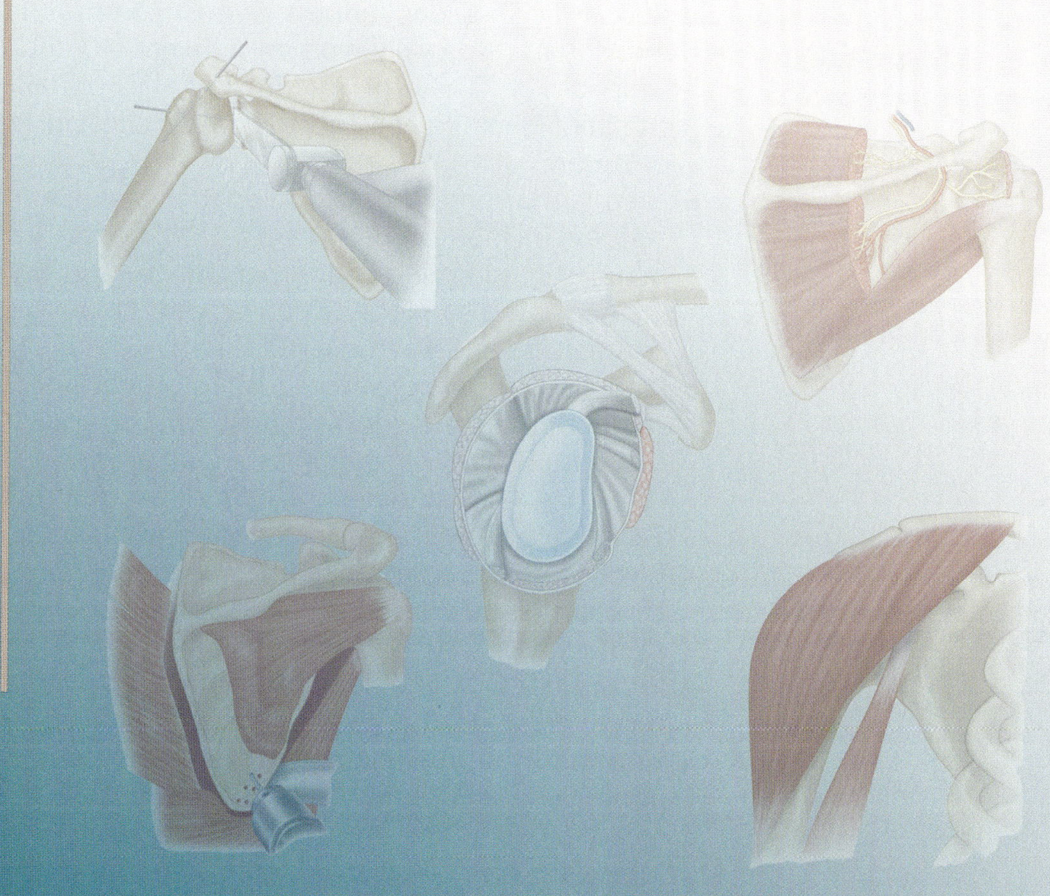

PITFALLS

- *It is vital to differentiate idiopathic adhesive capsulitis from posttraumatic etiologies. Many patients with idiopathic shoulder stiffness can recall some sort of antecedent trauma, but it is usually minimal. Those with distinct trauma, such as a prior fracture, rotator cuff tear, or surgical procedure, have a posttraumatic etiology, which often necessitates different treatments. All clinicians should be aware that traumatic injuries and the procedures to repair them may result in restricted shoulder motion.*
- *Examination under anesthesia is an essential first step in operative treatment of idiopathic adhesive capsulitis. Malingering and those patients with very low tolerance to pain can be identified by normal range of motion or restoration of normal range of motion with minimal manipulation.*

Controversies

- Some surgeons think operative treatments need not be avoided during the freezing phase.

Indications

- Failure to progress with nonoperative treatments is the primary indication for surgery.
  - Nonoperative treatments are successful for most cases of idiopathic adhesive capsulitis. The specific treatments vary, but include progressive range-of-motion exercises both actively and passively (i.e., stretching).
  - Posttraumatic adhesive capsulitis may be recalcitrant to rehabilitation alone.
- Idiopathic shoulder stiffness is most common in older individuals, especially women between 40 and 60 years of age. The articular surfaces are normal and the joint is stable, yet there is a restriction in range of motion.
- Factors that predispose to idiopathic shoulder stiffness include cervical, cardiac, pulmonary, neoplastic, neurologic, and personality disorders. The incidence is also higher in those with Dupuytren's contracture and Peyronie's disease.
- Patients with diabetes mellitus are also at a high risk of developing shoulder stiffness, with 10–35% of diabetics having restriction of shoulder motion. Diabetics who have been insulin dependent for many years have the greatest incidence and bilateral involvement. Because of this close association, clinicians should ask their patients with shoulder stiffness about symptoms of diabetes; 70% of individuals with shoulder stiffness may have diabetes or a prediabetes condition (Tighe and Oakley, 2008).
- Common to most etiologies of posttraumatic adhesive capsulitis is scarring between the tissue layers. While some stiffness after shoulder surgery is typical and usually resolves with time and appropriate rehabilitation, the shoulder should not be neglected after any surgery about the shoulder girdle. This includes axillary or cervical lymph node dissections, especially when combined with radiation therapy, cardiac catheterization in the axilla, and coronary artery bypass grafting with sternotomy and thoracotomy.

Examination/Imaging

Idiopathic Adhesive Capsulitis

- Often called adhesive capsulitis or frozen shoulder, idiopathic shoulder stiffness is a painful condition characterized by significant restriction in both active and passive range of motion.
- The restrictions of shoulder motion are global. That is, none of the shoulder planes of motion is spared.
  - Often the first motion the patients notices to be affected is internal rotation, demonstrated by an inability to bring the arm up the back to the same level as the normal shoulder.
  - Figure 1 demonstrates restriction in range of motion in external rotation of the left shoulder compared to the right. While restriction of range of motion is global and affects all planes, external rotation is easiest to quantify since it is less painful than other motions.
- The clinical presentation of idiopathic shoulder stiffness is classically described as having three phases: an initial, painful, "freezing" phase followed by a middle "stabilizing" phase and lastly a resolution, or "thawing," phase. Most likely there are only two phases and the course is U-shaped (Fig. 2) and occurs over a long period of time, making it seem as though there is a middle stabilizing phase with little progression.
  - Idiopathic adhesive capsulitis starts with pain, typically achy in nature with sudden jolts as attempts at rapid motion exacerbate the chronic

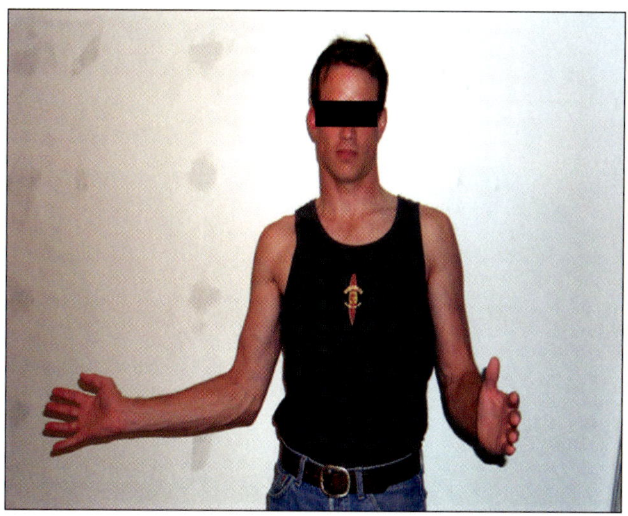

FIGURE 1

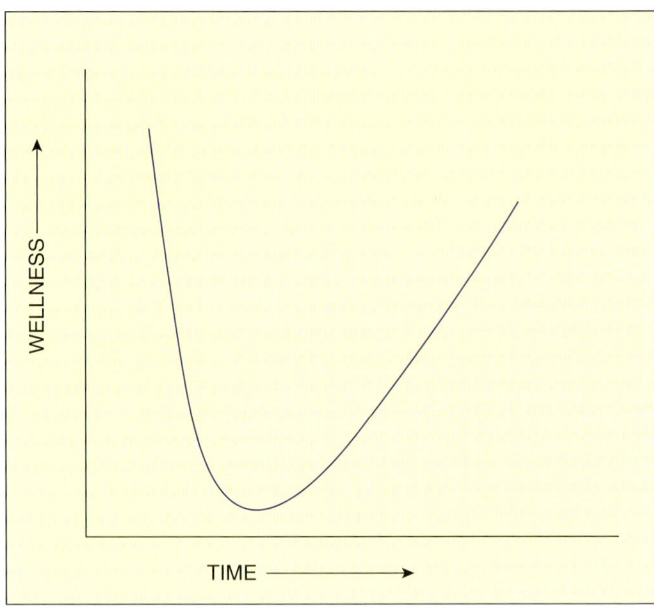

FIGURE 2

discomfort. There is pain at night, and shoulder motion becomes progressively limited.

- Patients often hold their arm at their side and in internal rotation with the forearm across the belly. Some who seek medical advice end up being treated for nonspecific shoulder pain with a sling in this position. This inflammatory phase often lasts between 2 and 9 months and is accompanied by progressive stiffness, with shoulder motion being restricted in all planes.
- Fortunately, pain then progressively decreases. With time, patients are able to use the shoulder with little or no pain, within the restricted range of motion, but attempts to exceed this range are accompanied by pain.
- The patient's symptoms seem to plateau, sometimes for extended periods.
- In the resolution or thawing phase, the shoulder slowly and progressively becomes more supple. This phase can be as short as a few months, but more commonly lasts nearly a year and can last for a few years.

- Radiographs reveal the absence of arthritis, which has a similar clinical presentation, the only difference being the presence of crepitus in patients with arthritis.
- Magnetic resonance imaging (MRI) reveals decreased rotator interval size, and arthography demonstrates marked reduction in joint capacity; often the affected

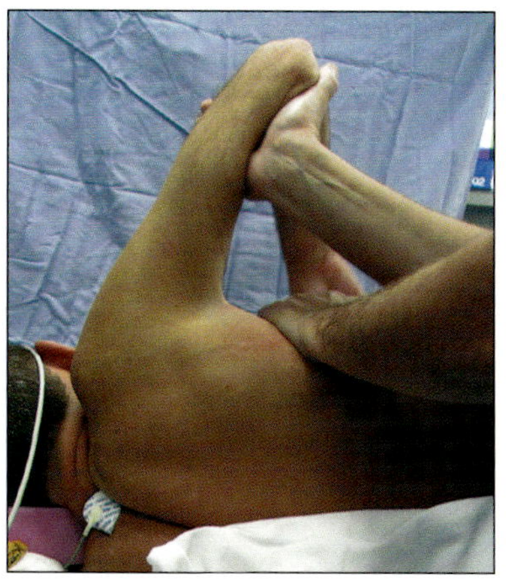
A

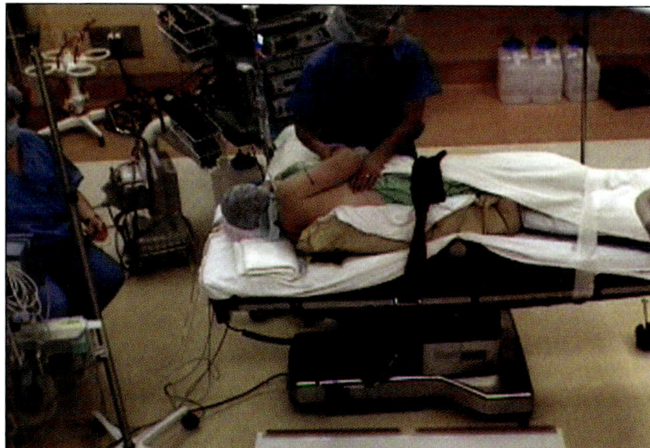
B

FIGURE 3

shoulder will not take more than a few milliliters of dye, whereas the normal capacity is 20–30 ml.

Posttraumatic Adhesive Capsulitis

- The assessment of posttraumatic adhesive capsulitis differs from that of idiopathic adhesive capsulitis. Prior to treatment, the cause of the stiffness should be determined. A prior fracture may have resulted in malposition of the bones, or a head injury may have resulted in heterotopic ossification.
- The location of the scarring must be found. Physical examination is helpful, but imaging is also helpful and in addition to radiographs may include computed tomography and/or MRI.

Treatment Options

- Traditionally, surgeons have avoided operative treatments during the freezing phase for fear of aggravating the condition.
- When operative treatments are chosen, manipulation under anesthesia and capsular distention, long the mainstays of intervention, are now being replaced by selective, arthroscopic capsular release.
  - Figure 3A demonstrates the proper way to perform a manipulation under anesthesia. The examiner's hands are place on the scapula and the humerus, rather than more distally on the upper extremity. This stabilizes the bones and minimizes applying too much force that can result in fracture.
  - Figure 3B shows a manipulation under anesthesia in the lateral decubitus position (see video). Manipulation under anesthesia can also be performed similarly in the supine position.

Surgical Anatomy

- While the pathophysiology of idiopathic adhesive capsulitis is uncertain, the pathoanatomy is limited to contracture of the glenohumeral capsule. Most prominently involved is the anterosuperior capsule, the rotator interval, and specifically the region of the coracohumeral ligament.
- The thin redundant joint capsule has almost twice the surface area of the humeral head to allow a large range of joint motion. Different regions of the joint capsule provide stability at different joint positions. With the arm at the side, the superior portion of the capsule is taut and the inferior portion is lax. With overhead elevation, this relationship reverses.
- There are folds or thickenings that are most easily visible on the inside of the capsule, which have been termed *glenohumeral ligaments*. Traditionally the

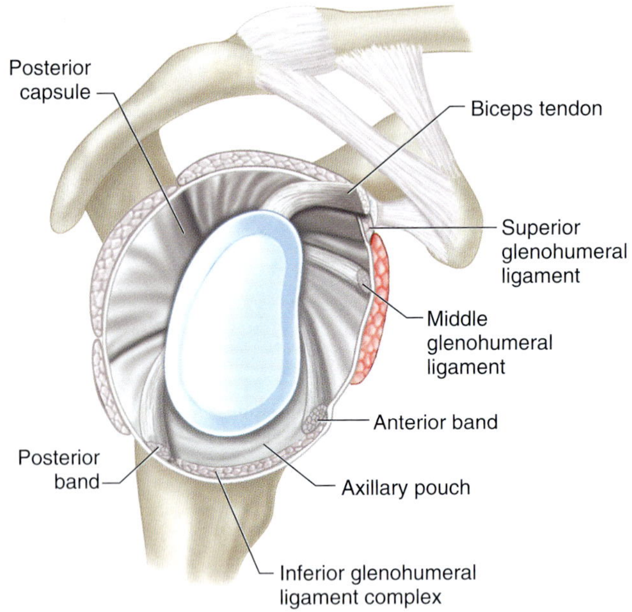

FIGURE 4

anterior capsule has been described as being composed of the superior, middle, and inferior glenohumeral ligaments (Fig. 4). While use of the term *ligament* is generally accepted, it needs some clarification.

- Ligaments are soft tissue structures that connect bones. They are most commonly bandlike, with parallel collagen fibers running between their insertion sites, and have clearly defined edges, such as the medial collateral ligament of the knee.
- The glenohumeral capsule as a whole may be considered a sheetlike ligament connecting the humerus and the scapula. The collagen fibers are not organized in a parallel fashion, the margins of the folds are indistinct, and functional study does not indicate it to have bandlike properties. This may be the reason that the "ligaments" of the anterior capsule have been described with variable prevalence; different authors have had varying success in identifying them. Also, with the shoulder in abduction and external rotation, even the most consistently reported fold in the anteroinferior capsule, the anterior band of the inferior glenohumeral ligament, is often indistinct.
- While terminology may be currently causing confusion in anatomic, biomechanical, and clinical studies, there is little doubt that different regions of the capsule have differing roles in joint function.

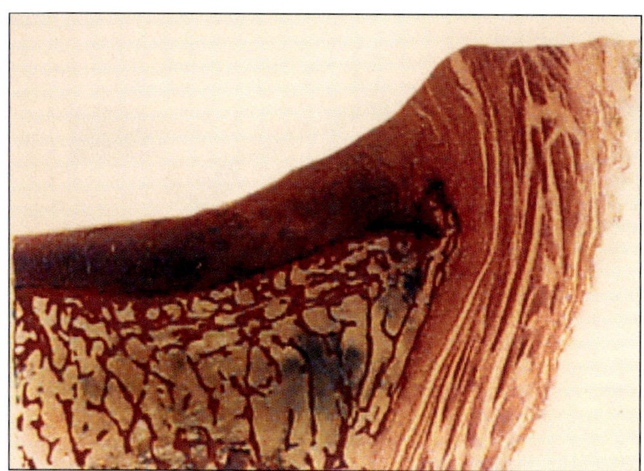

FIGURE 5

- The capsule inserts into the glenoid labrum and onto the glenoid bone. The glenoid labrum acts not only as an attachment site for the capsuloligamentous structures but also as an extension of the articular cavity. Its presence deepens the glenoid socket by nearly 50%, and the triangular cross section of the labrum acts as a chock to help prevent subluxation (Fig. 5). It must be preserved.
- The axillary nerve and the posterior humeral circumflex artery pass inferior to the subscapularis muscle, then the inferior glenohumeral joint capsule, and then inferior to the teres minor muscle through the quadrilateral space, also bordered by the teres major, the triceps, and the humerus.
  - More specifically with regard to the capsule, the axillary nerve passes caudal to the capsule, and its position relative to the capsule varies with shoulder position; its distance from the capsule diminishes with abduction of the shoulder. With the arm at the side, it courses 1–1.5 cm lateral to the anteroinferior glenoid rim at the 5 o'clock position (right shoulder). As the nerve courses posterior, it is located increasing more lateral to the glenoid rim. It is 2–2.5 cm from the posteroinferior glenoid rim at the 7 o'clock position (right shoulder) (Esmail et al., 2005).
  - It can be injured, especially during arthroscopic capsular release procedures, and is most prone to be injured with release of the anteroinferior capsule. Loss of axillary nerve function results in denervation of the deltoid and teres minor muscles and loss of sensation over the proximal lateral aspect of the arm.

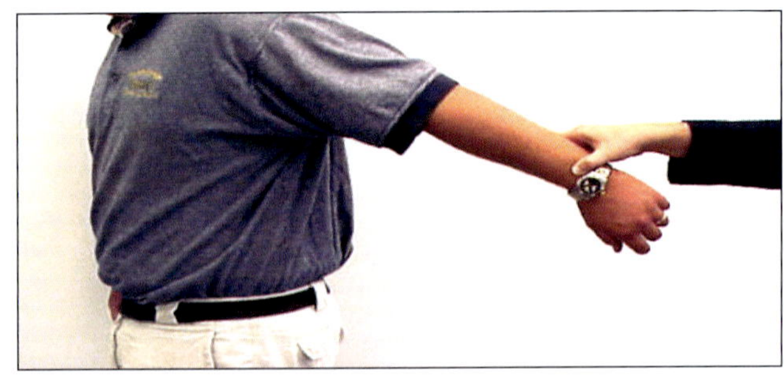

A

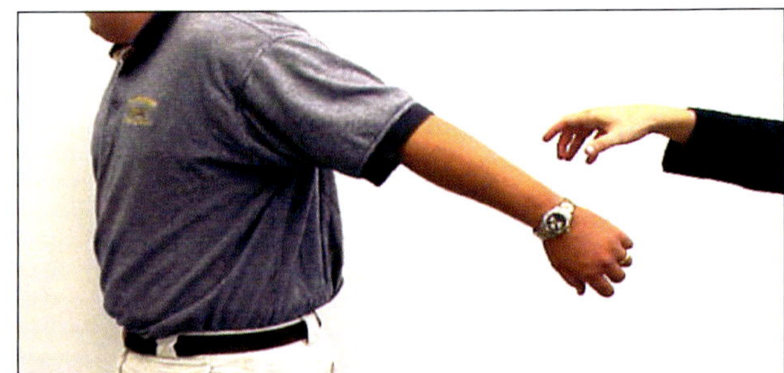

B

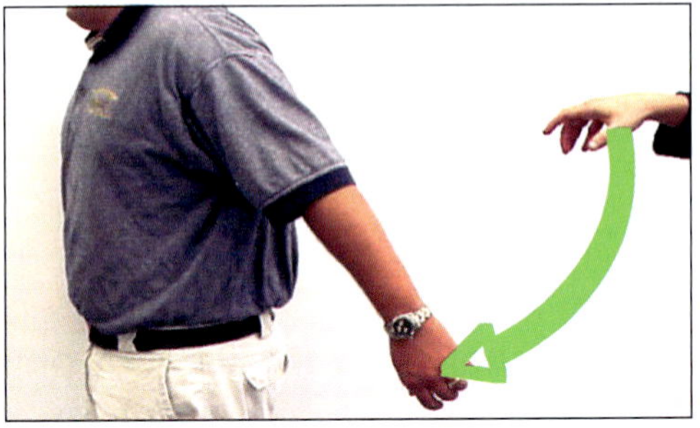

C

FIGURE 6

- The deltoid extension lag sign is indicative of axillary nerve injury. To perform this test, the examiner elevates the arm into a position of near-full extension (Fig. 6A). The patient is then asked to hold the arm in this position while the examiner releases the arm (Fig. 6B). If there is complete deltoid paralysis, the arm will drop (Fig. 6C). For partial nerve injuries, the magnitude of the angular drop, or lag, is an indicator of deltoid strength.

Positioning

- Shoulder arthroscopy can be done in either a beach chair or lateral decubitus position.
- Figure 7 shows a view from the bottom of the bed of shoulder arthroscopy being done in the lateral decubitus position.

Pitfalls

- *All bony prominences should be well padded.*
- *In the lateral decubitus position, there should be special attention to the "down" leg so as to protect the peroneal nerve.*

Portals/Exposures

- Visualization of the joint can be the most difficult part of arthroscopic capsular release. A standard posterior portal is used.
  - A standard anterior portal, between the long head of the biceps and the subscapulairs tendon, is also used.

Pearls

- *Addition of epinephrine to the arthroscopic fluid helps with visualization.*

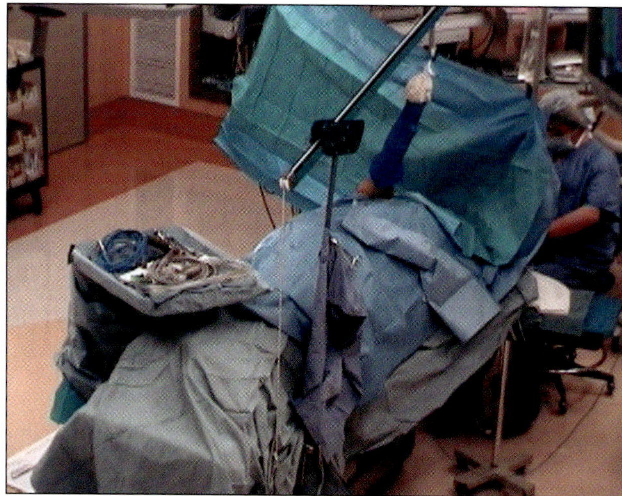

FIGURE 7

- Rarely, a second anterior, 5 o'clock portal is needed for release of the anteroinferior capsule.
- Also rarely, a second posterior, 7 o'clock portal is needed for release of the posteroinferior capsule.

- When the restriction in range of motion is severe, the intracapsular space is also markedly diminished, and this may make it very difficult to introduce the arthroscope. If the joint can be manipulated in abduction, tearing of the inferior capsule usually results in enough increase in intracapsular space for the arthroscope to be introduced. If not, and attempts are unsuccessful, a small posterior incision can be made and the arthroscope can then be introduced with direct visualization.
- Sometimes the anterior capsule cannot be seen after the arthroscope has been placed into the joint. Then, the anterior cannula can be placed with an inside-out technique.
  - Care must be taken to place this cannula in its correct position, lateral to the coracoid, but sometimes this is not possible for fear of injuring the articular surfaces. In this situation, a second posterior portal off the posterolateral corner of the acromion, similar to the portal of Wilmington, is helpful.
  - The superior joint capsule can be incised first, in a posterior-to-anterior position direction, and often "springs apart" when cut (Fig. 8A and 8B). Continuing the release to the superior part of the rotator interval results in sudden and, happily, increased intracapsular space.

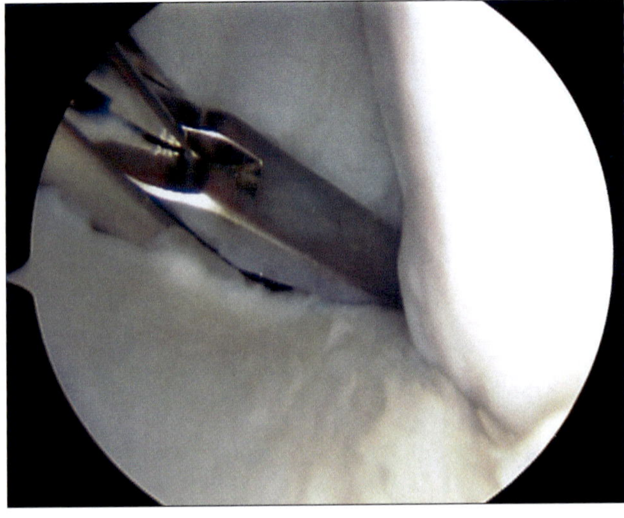
A

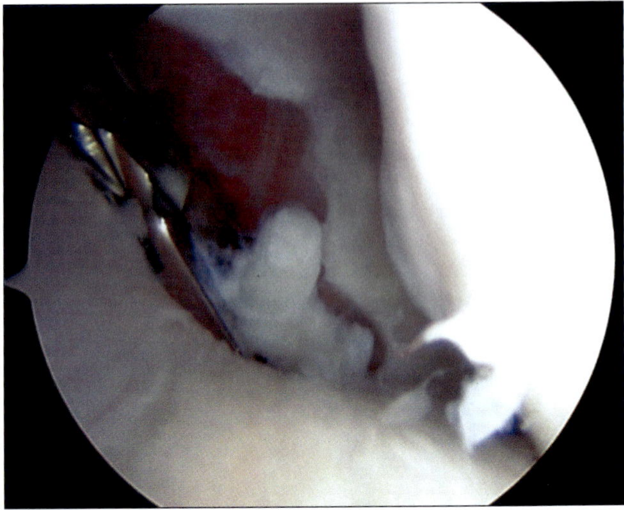
B

FIGURE 8

Pearls

- *Release of the rotator interval capsule results in increased external rotation with the arm at the side.*
- *Release of the anteroinferior capsule results in increased external rotation with the arm abducted.*
- *The superior border of the subscapularis must be indentified to minimize its injury.*

Pitfalls

- *The anteroinferior capsule should be released adjacent to the labrum to minimize risk of injury to the axillary nerve.*

Procedure: Idiopathic Adhesive Capsulitis

Step 1

- The procedure is begun with use of a mechanical up-biter, although electrocautery can also be used. The anterior cannula is pulled just outside the capsule and the up-biter turned down for release of the rotator interval that is below the portal (Fig. 9).

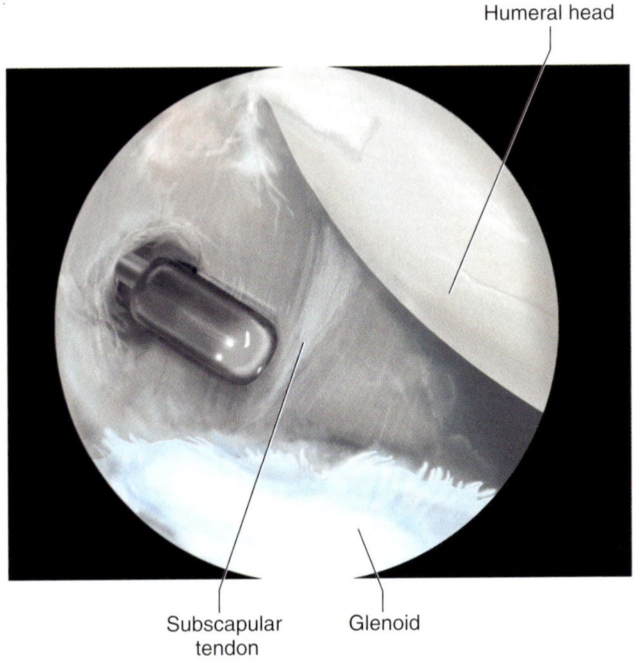

FIGURE 9

This often exposes the posterior surface of the coracoid.

- The tip of the up-biter is first used as an elevator to separate the capsule from the underlying tissue (Fig. 10A), and then the capsule is incised (Fig. 10B).
- Release of the remainder of the anterior capsule from superior to inferior ensues, exposing the posterior surface of the subscapularis.

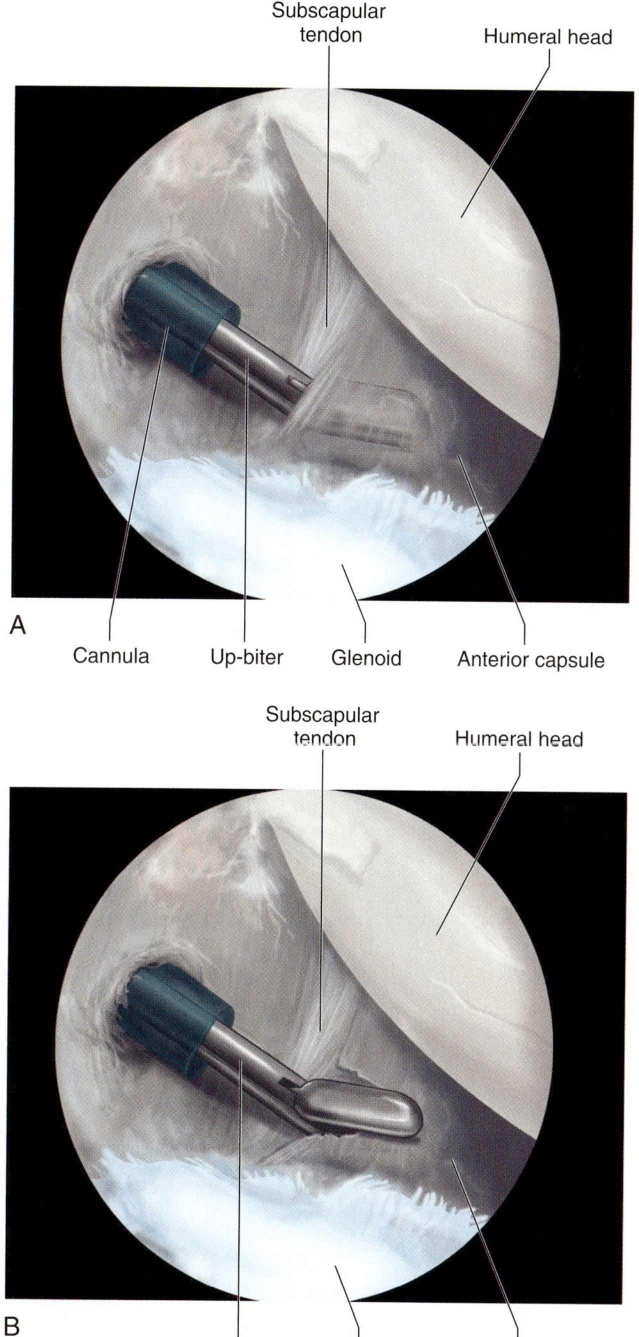

FIGURE 10

- The anteroinferior capsule is then released.
- Not only should the capsule be divided, but a portion should be removed to minimize the chances of recurrence.
- I use a shaver to remove the capsule once it is cut (Fig. 11).

PEARLS

- *Release of the rotator interval above the anterior portal is sometimes difficult because it is obscured by the long head of the biceps tendon. A "switching stick" can be placed through the same portal as a retractor for the tendon.*

STEP 2

- The up-biter is then turned up for release of the rotator interval that is above the portal.
- Electrocautery can also be used to incise and remove the capsule (Fig. 12). A release of the medial-most portion of the superior capsule first makes the release easier as there is often supraspinatus muscle under the capsule at this location rather than tendon.

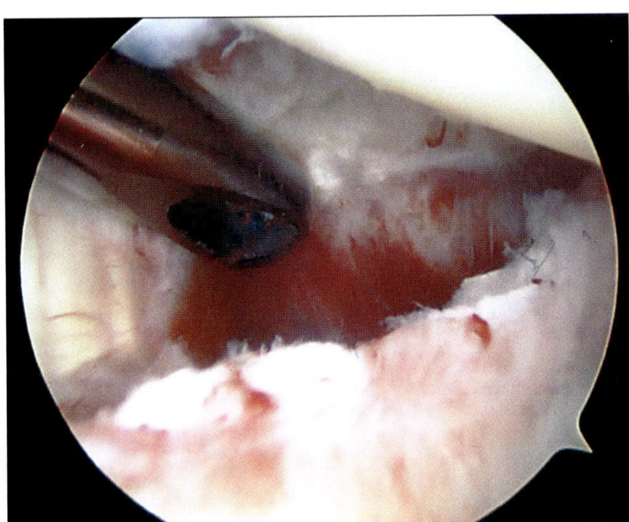

FIGURE 11

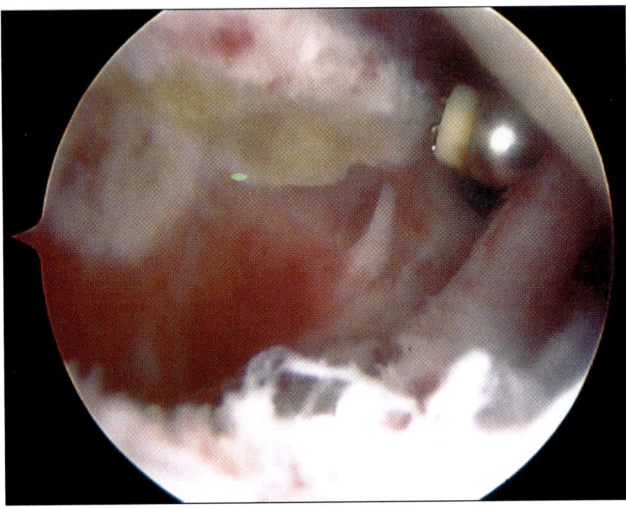

FIGURE 12

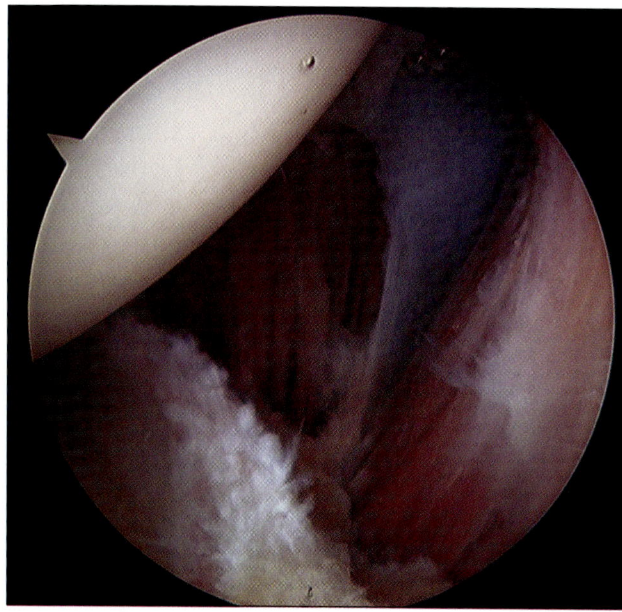

FIGURE 13

Pearls

- *Release of the posterior capsule results in increased internal rotation.*
- *Some surgeons prefer not to release the inferior capsule to minimize risk of injury to the axillary nerve and instead tear it with gentle manipulation, now possible after the remainder of the capsule has been resected.*

Pitfalls

- *Do not use undue force in manipulation of the joint. Instead, put the arthroscope back into the joint and assess the capsule for insufficient release.*

Step 3

- The arthroscope is then switched to the anterior portal and the posterior capsule (Fig. 13) and lastly the posteroinferior capsule are resected to complete the release of the inferior capsule.
- The arthroscopic instruments are now removed, and range of motion is assessed.
- Gentle manipulation is performed as decribed earlier, the only difference being that the force of two fingers is usually all that is needed to achieve the desired range of motion.

Procedure: Posttraumatic Adhesive Capsulitis

Step 1

- Surgical intervention for posttraumatic adhesive capsulitis may require both arthroscopic and open releases. Athroscopic release is performed when the capsule and the subacromial space are involved. Scarring in other locations outside the joint is best repaired with an open technique. The most common location of these releases is related to open anterior surgery done with a deltopectoral approach.
- Release should include the intervals between the clavipectoral fascia and the deltoid and pectoralis muscles, between the conjoined tendon and deltoid muscles, and between the coracoid and the rotator

interval. Scarring between the coracoid and the subscapularis should also be released.

- Then, the area over the superior margin of the subscapularis can be accessed to release scarring between the subscapularis and the glenoid as well.
  - A finger or an osteotome can be placed between the posterior surface of the subscapularis and the anterior glenoid neck. However, this may risk injury to the axillary nerve, so tenotomy of the subscapularis tendon is best in all patients but those in whom the scarring is least severe. The scarring can then be released, and the capsule can also be excised if the scarring is severe.
  - The subscapularis tendon can also be lengthened. The downside is that the repair must be protected from excessive stretching during the aggressive postoperative rehabilitation.

Step 2

- For contracture of the supbscapularis muscle, lengthening of the subscapularis or arthroscopic tenotomy may be required. One centimeter of lengthening of the subscapularis will result in 15–20° of external rotation.

Step 3

- Adhesions of the long head of the biceps can be treated with tenotomy, and this may be done with an arthroscopic technique. But as other releases with an open technique are common with posttraumatic adhesive capsulitis, it is often done with an open technique as well.
- Tenodesis is not indicated as it is not compatible with the aggressive postoperative rehabilitation necessary after the releases.

Postoperative Care and Expected Outcomes

- A physical therapy program is begun immediately.
- The sling is removed and strengthening ensues as pain permits.
- Commonly, 2–3 months of physical therapy are needed, as well as a home exercise program that continues for another few months, for patients to achieve satisfactory outcomes.
- A return of 80% shoulder range of motion, on average, is usual.

Pearls

- *Some surgeons insist that rehabilitation begin immediately, on the day of surgery. I prefer to begin physical therapy, with emphasis on progressive range-of-motion exercises both actively and passively (i.e., stretching), within a few days of surgery.*

Evidence

Bal A, Eksioglu E, Gulec B, Aydog E, Gurcay E, Cakci A. Effectiveness of corticosteroid injection in adhesive capsulitis. Clin Rehabil. 2008;22:503-12.

Eighty patients with adhesive capsulitis were randomly assigned to two groups both of which underwent a 12-week comprehensive home exercise program. Group 1 patients were given an intra-articular corticosteroid and group 2 patients were given intra-articular serum physiologic. Mean actual changes in abduction range of motion, Shoulder Pain and Disability Index total score, and Shoulder Pain and Disability Index pain score were statistically different between the two groups at the second week, with the better scores determined in group 1. However, there were no significant differences between the groups at the 12th week. Medians of University of California–Los Angeles scores in the second week were significantly different between the two groups ($p = .02$), with better scores in group 1; however, the difference in 12th week scores was insignificant. The authors noted that Intra-articular corticosteroids have the additive effect of providing rapid pain relief, mainly in the first weeks of the exercise treatment period.

Esmail AN, Getz CL, Schwartz DM, Wierzbowski L, Ramsey ML, Williams GR Jr. Axillary nerve monitoring during arthroscopic shoulder stabilization. Arthroscopy. 2005;21:665-71.

Twenty consecutive patients with glenohumeral instability were monitored prospectively during arthroscopic shoulder surgery, and axillary nerve mapping was recorded before the stabilization portion of the procedure.

Hand C, Clipsham K, Rees JL, Carr AJ. Long-term outcome of frozen shoulder. J Shoulder Elbow Surg. 2008;17:231-6.

In this study, outcomes for 269 shoulders in 223 patients with a diagnosis of primary frozen shoulder were evaluated primarily using the Oxford shoulder score. The mean follow-up from symptom onset was 4.4 years (range, 2–20 years). The mean age at symptom onset was 53.4 years; with women affected more commonly than men (1.6:1.0). Twenty percent of patients reported bilateral symptoms, but there were no recurrent cases. In the long term, 59% of patients had normal or near-normal shoulders and 41% reported some ongoing symptoms. The majority of these persistent symptoms were mild (94%), with pain being the most common complaint. Only 6% had severe symptoms with pain and functional loss. Those with the most severe symptoms at condition onset had the worst long-term prognosis ($p < .001$).

Hand GC, Athanasou NA, Matthews T, Carr AJ. The pathology of frozen shoulder. J Bone Joint Surg [Br]. 2007;89:928-32.

The authors treated 22 patients with a diagnosis of primary frozen shoulder resistant to conservative treatment by manipulation under anesthesia and arthroscopic release of the rotator interval, at a mean time from onset of 15 months (range, 3–36 months). Biopsies were taken from the site, and histologic and immunocytochemical analysis was performed to identify the types of cell present. The tissue was characterized by the presence of fibroblasts, proliferating fibroblasts, and chronic inflammatory cells with an infiltrate predominantly made up of mast cells, with T cells, B cells, and macrophages also present. The pathology of frozen shoulder thus includes a chronic inflammatory response with fibroblastic proliferation that may be immunomodulated.

Kim KC, Rhee KJ, Shin HD. Adhesive capsulitis of the shoulder: dimensions of the rotator interval measured with magnetic resonance arthrography. J Shoulder Elbow Surg. 2009;18:437-42.

This study was performed to define the dimensions of the rotator interval (RI) in adhesive capsulitis using magnetic resonance arthrography preoperatively to clarify and evaluate pathology. In a retrospective review, 26 shoulders with adhesive capsulitis were compared to 47 shoulders without adhesive capsulitis. Those with adhesive capsulitis were significantly different in height, base, RI area, RI index, and RI ratio.

Levine WN, Kashyap CP, Bak SF, Ahmad CS, Blaine TA, Bigliani LU. Nonoperative management of idiopathic adhesive capsulitis. J Shoulder Elbow Surg. 2007;16:569-73.

Charts of 234 patients treated for adhesive capsulitis were reviewed retrospectively, with study endpoints defined as resolution of symptoms with nonoperative treatment or operative treatment. A total of 105 shoulders in 98 patients were identified with follow-up to endpoint. Of these, 89.5% resolved with nonoperative treatment, including 17 (89.5%) of 19 diabetic shoulders. No significant difference was found for success of nonoperative treatment versus operative treatment or patient gender. Duration of treatment in successfully nonoperatively treated patients averaged 3.8 ± 3.6 months. Patients who required surgery were treated with an average of 12.4 ± 12.1 months of nonoperative treatment. Initial forward elevation averaged 118° ± 22°, with average forward elevation at resolution of 164° ± 17°. External rotation improved from an average of 26° ± 16° pretreatment to 59° ± 18° posttreatment. The authors concluded that, with supervised treatment, most patients with adhesive capsulitis will experience resolution with nonoperative measures in a relatively short period. Only a small percentage of patients will eventually require operative treatment.

Milgrom C, Novack V, Weil Y, Jaber S, Radeva-Petrova DR, Finestone A. Risk factors for idiopathic frozen shoulder. Isr Med Assoc J. 2008;10:361-4.

In this study, 126 new consecutive frozen shoulder patients from a shoulder clinic were compared to an age-matched control group of 98 consecutive patients from an orthopedic foot and ankle clinic and to the regional population disease prevalence registry. Among the frozen shoulder patients, 29.4% had diabetes and 13.5% had thyroid disorders. The risk ratio for diabetes in the frozen shoulder group was 5.9 for males and 5.0 for females. The risk ratio for thyroid disorders among females with frozen shoulder was 7.3. No significant difference was found in the prevalence of thyroid disorders between patients with frozen shoulder and the control group, but there was a significantly higher prevalence of diabetes in males and a trend for higher prevalence in females in the frozen shoulder group.

Thomas SJ, McDougall C, Brown ID, Jaberoo MC, Stearns A, Ashraf R, Fisher M, Kelly IG. Prevalence of symptoms and signs of shoulder problems in people with diabetes mellitus. J Shoulder Elbow Surg. 2007;16:748-51.

In this study of diabetes mellitus as a risk factor for frozen shoulder, the prevalence of frozen shoulder was found to be less than previously reported but still greater in diabetic patients. Frozen shoulder was defined as pain for more than 3 months and external rotation of less than 50% of the unaffected shoulder. Bilateral frozen shoulder was defined as external rotation of less than 30° in both shoulders. Shoulder pain was present in 25.7% of diabetic patients compared with 5.0% of general medical patients. The criteria for frozen shoulder were fulfilled in 4.3% of diabetic patients and in 0.5% of the general medical patients. Only duration of diabetes had a positive association.

Tighe CB, Oakley WS Jr. The prevalence of a diabetic condition and adhesive capsulitis of the shoulder. South Med J. 2008;101:591-5.

The authors studied the risk of diabetes and prediabetes in patients presenting with adhesive capsulitis of the shoulder. Consenting patients reporting no history of diabetes mellitus had blood testing for diabetes and prediabetes. The prevalence of diabetes in patients with adhesive capsulitis was 38.6% (34 of 88). The prevalence of prediabetes was 32.95% (29 of 88). The total prevalence of a diabetic condition in patients with adhesive capsulitis was 71.5% (63 of 88). Previous literature fails to reveal the incidence of newly diagnosed diabetes (2 of 88; 2%) and prediabetes (25 of 88; 28.4%) in patients presenting with adhesive capsulitis.

Wolf JM, Green A. Influence of comorbidity on self-assessment instrument scores of patients with idiopathic adhesive capsulitis. J Bone Joint Surg [Am]. 2002;84:1167.

The authors hypothesized that an increased number of comorbidities would be correlated with greater pain and worse function in patients with idiopathic adhesive capsulitis of the shoulder as measured by general and shoulder-specific self-assessment outcome tools. In 100 consecutive patients (71 women and 29 men, with a mean age of 52 years), comorbidities included medical factors and social factors. Patients with more comorbidities had significantly lower scores on the Disabilities of the Arm, Shoulder and Hand Questionnaire ($p = .0005$*) and the Short Form-36 subscale of physical function (*$p = .0009$*) as well as poorer scores on the Simple Shoulder Test and the Short Form-36 subscales of physical role, social function, emotional role, and mental health. There was no correlation between increased comorbidity and pain as measured on a visual analog scale, but the comfort/pain subscale of the Short Form-36 showed a significant correlation with increased comorbidity (*$p = .004$*).*

PROCEDURE 38

Arthroscopic Treatment of Calcific Tendinitis in the Shoulder

Kyle A. Caswell, Felix H. Savoie III, and Michael J. O'Brien

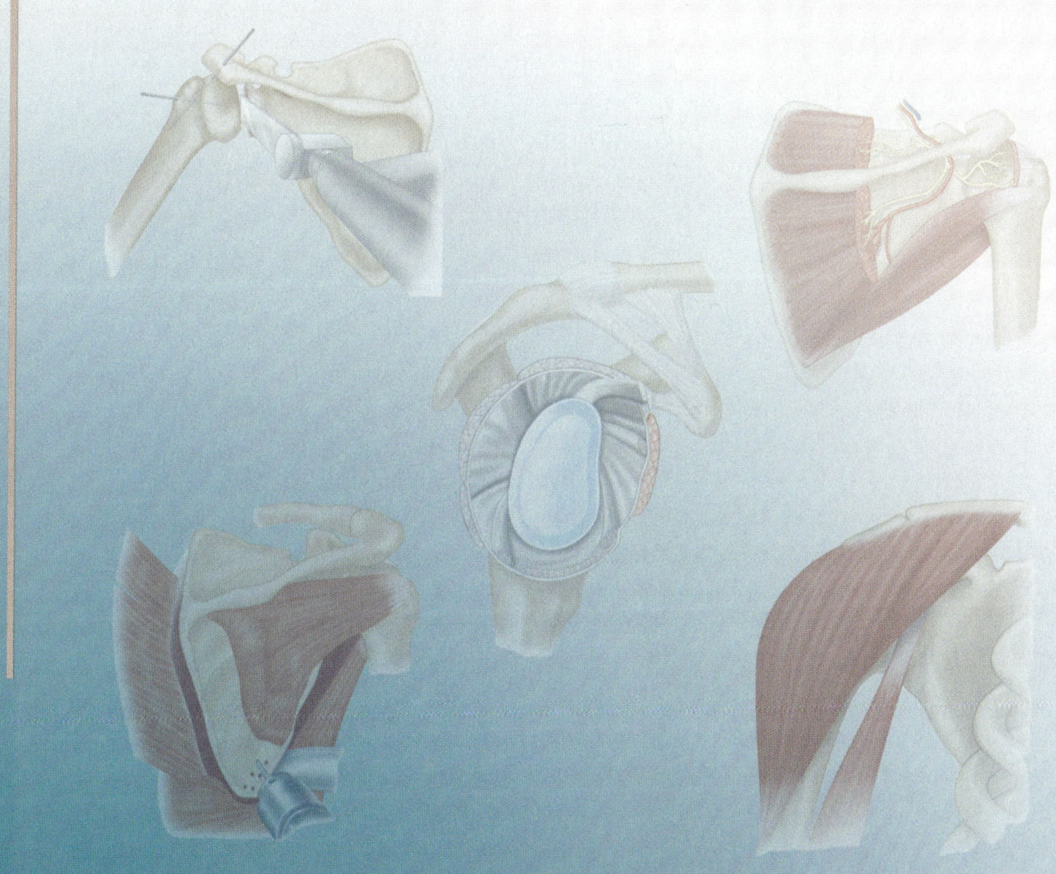

Figure 2 from Curtis A, Burbank K, Tierney J, Scheller A, Curran A. The insertional footprint of the rotator cuff: an anatomic study. Arthroscopy. 2006;22:603-9.
Figures 3 and 4 from Peruto CM, Ciccotti MG, Cohen SB. Shoulder arthroscopy positioning: lateral decubitus versus beach chair. Arthroscopy. 2009;25:891-6.
Figure 5 redrawn from Lo IKY, Lind CC, Burkhardt SS. Glenohumeral arthroscopy portals established using an outside-in technique: Neurovascular anatomy at risk. Arthroscopy. 2004;20:596-602.

PITFALLS

- *Failure to evaluate additional coexisting pathology: most commonly adhesive capsulitis*
- *Level of symptoms do not warrant surgical treatment*

Controversies

- Treatment and disease stage (Uhthoff and Loehr, 1997)
  - Nonoperative treatment: acute resorptive phase
  - Operative treatment: chronic formative phase when nonoperative measures have failed

Treatment Options

- Conservative
  - Steroid injections
  - Ultrasound-guided percutaneous needle aspiration
  - Extracorporeal shock-wave therapy
  - Disodium EDTA (chelating agent)
- Operative
  - Open surgery: not recommended
  - Arthroscopic removal: advantages include that it is an outpatient procedure, allows almost immediate rehabilitation, and reduces risk of postoperative stiffness (Ark et al., 1992)

Indications

- Pain and functional impairment of activities of daily living
- Progressive symptoms despite adequate nonoperative management, including injections, medications, and physical therapy
- Recurrence of symptoms after resolution with nonoperative treatment

Examination/Imaging

- Detailed history
  - Symptoms
  - Onset
  - Pain-relieving measures attempted
  - Nonoperative measures used before surgical evaluation
  - Activities of daily living affected
  - Impaired work performance
  - Impaired sports-related activities or hobbies
- Clinical examination
  - Position of scapula (protraction-balanced?)
  - Palpation of the rotator cuff
  - Active and passive range of motion in internal rotation, external rotation, abduction, horizontal adduction, and forward flexion
  - Whipple test with and without scapular retraction
  - Inferior glide test to rule out coexisting adhesive capsultis
- Initial radiographs should include three-view shoulder films: anteroposterior, scapular Y, and axillary.
  - Anteroposterior shoulder views (Fig. 1A)
    - Neutral rotation
    - Internal rotation: reveals infraspinatus or teres minor tendon deposits
    - External rotation: isolates supraspinatus tendon deposits
  - Scapular Y view: helps determine if calcific tendinitis is causing impingement (Fig. 1B).
  - Axillary view: isolates subscapularis tendon deposits (Fig. 1C).
  - An additional supraspinatus outlet view helps determine if impingement is present.
  - Three views of the shoulder allow mapping of the exact location of the calcific tendinitis in three planes as a part of preoperative planning (*arrows* in Fig. 1A–C point to calcific tendinitis).

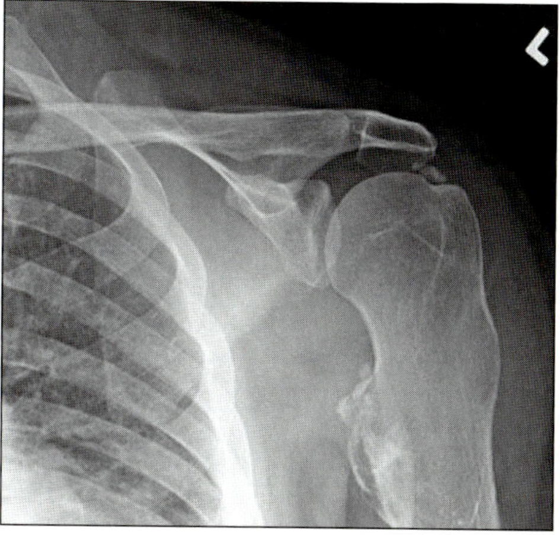

A

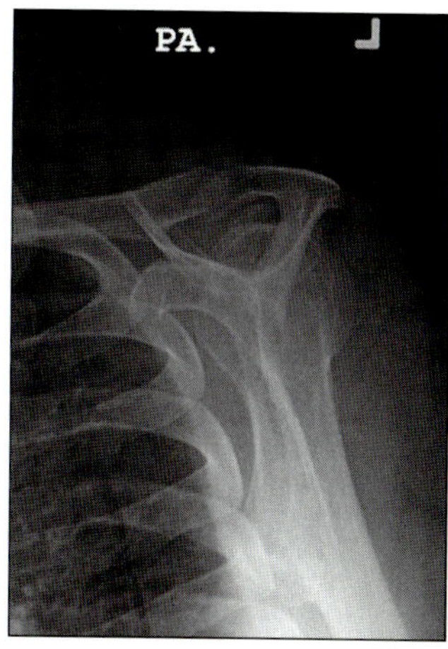

B

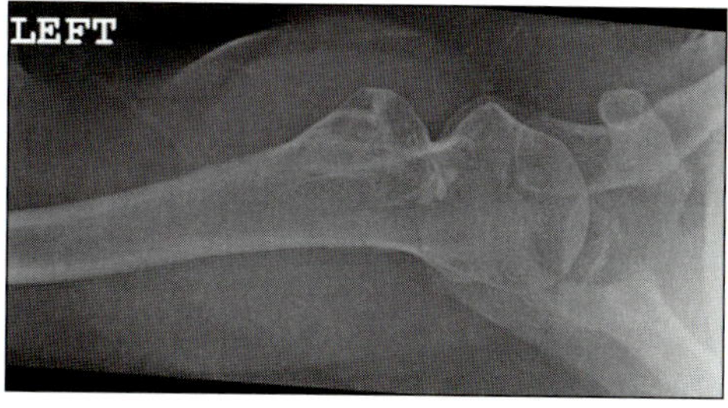

C

FIGURE 1

PEARLS

- *The patient should be positioned 20–30° posteriorly to place the glenoid surface parallel to the floor in the lateral decubitus position.*
- *The table should be rotated so the anesthesiologist moves toward the anterior waist of the patient to allow C-arm access to the shoulder.*

PITFALLS

- *Failure to place an axillary roll places neurovascular structures at risk in the lateral decubitus position.*
- *Failure to support the head and neck in a secure position causes traction to neurovascular structures in either position.*

- Computed tomography scanning can help isolate deposits not well localized on plain radiographs.
- Magnetic resonance imaging (MRI)
  - T_1 weighted: calcium deposits appear as areas of decreased signal intensity.
  - T_2 weighted: frequently reveals a perifocal band of increased signal intensity consistent with edema.

Surgical Anatomy

- Rotator cuff: supraspinatus, infraspinatus, subscapularis, and biceps tendons
  - Calcium deposits are usually not in contact with the bone insertion; they are at least 1.5–2.0 cm away from it (Uhthoff and Loehr, 1997).
    - Figure 2 shows lateral (Fig. 2A) and anterior (Fig. 2B) views of the rotator cuff and possible areas of calcific tendinitis.
  - Calcium deposit distribution: supraspinatus (most common) > infraspinatus > subscapularis (Gosens et al., 2009; Jerosch et al., 1998)
    - Supraspinatus with 51–90% of deposits (Gosens et al., 2009)

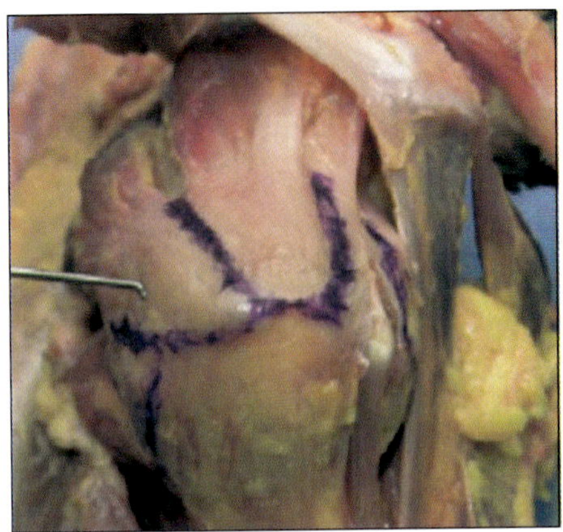
A

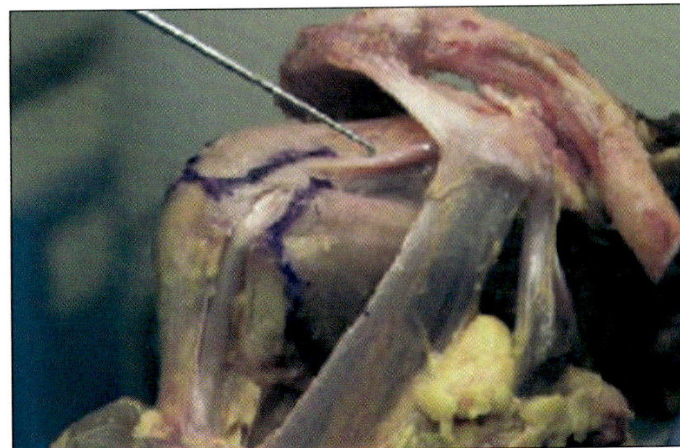
B

FIGURE 2

Equipment

- Lateral decubitus
  - Foam positioner: head support and airway protection
  - Reversed beanbag: positioning support and axillary roll
  - Boom with 10 lbs for traction
- Beach chair position
  - Table-specific head and neck support
- Pads for bony prominences

Controversies

- Either position is adequate.
- Beach chair position
  - Advantages: faster setup, reduced neurapraxia risk, improved arm mobility, and easier conversion to open procedure
  - Disadvantage: associated with hypotension and bradycardia leading to cerebral or spinal cord hypoperfusion

    - Infraspinatus with approximately 6% of deposits (Jacobs and Debeer, 2006)
    - Subscapularis with 3% of deposits (Gosens et al., 2009)
  - Coracoacromial and coracoclavicular ligaments
  - Deltoid attachment to the acromion

Positioning

- The patient can be placed in the lateral decubitus position on a beanbag with the affected arm exposed and a sterile hand holder placed to allow arm rotation (Fig. 3).
- Alternatively, the beach chair position can be used with an articulated armholder and protective head and neck support (Fig. 4).

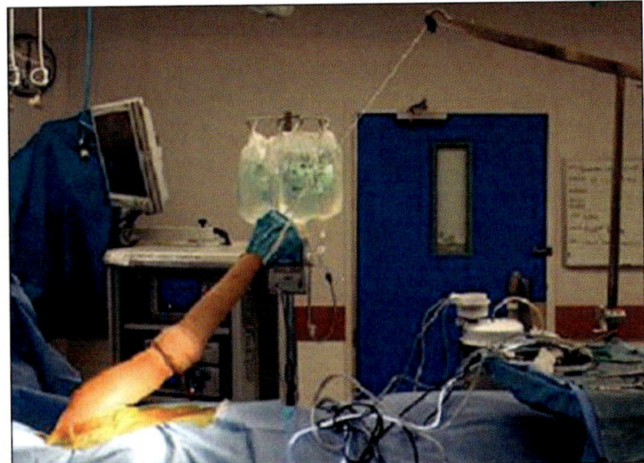

FIGURE 3

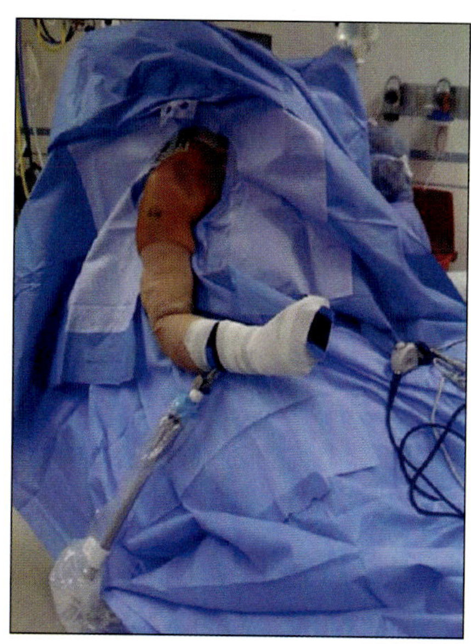

FIGURE 4

PEARLS

- *A spinal needle is placed to attain the appropriate position of the anterior portal while viewing from the posterior portal.*

PITFALLS

- *Posterior portal*
  - *If placed too far superiorly, then the infraspinatus tendon is at risk.*
  - *If placed too inferiorly, then the axillary nerve is at risk.*

Instrumentation

- 18-gauge needle
- #11 blade
- Cannula and blunt trocar
- 30° arthroscope
- Inflow system
- Motorized shaver
- Hand instruments to include punches, curettes, and awls
- Suction system controlled by hand control
- Video tower unit

Portals/Exposures

- Posterior portal (Fig. 5, *A*)
  - This portal is used for glenohumeral arthroscopy and subacromial bursoscopy.
  - It is located 2 cm inferior and 1 cm medial to the posteriolateral corner of the acromion.
  - The posterior portal passes through the posterior "soft spot" between the muscular bundles of the infraspinatus and enters parallel to the glenoid.

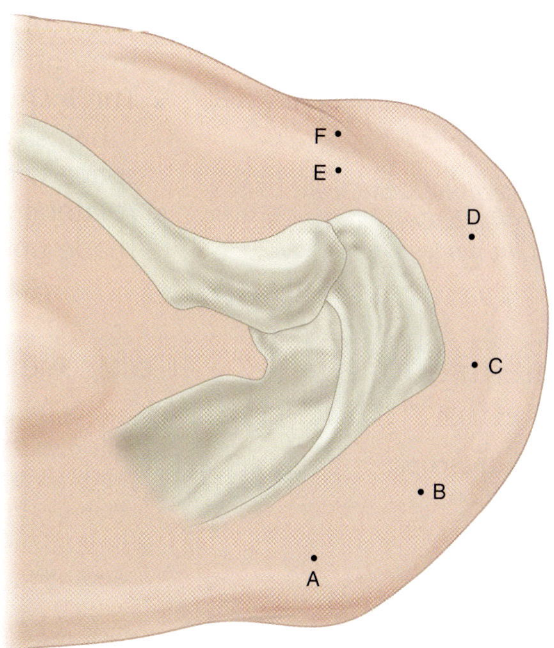

FIGURE 5

Pearls

- *Occasionally, intra-articular blebs are present. Bleb rupture may increase the adhesive capsulitis risk (Harvard Ellman, personal communication, 1988).*

Pitfalls

- *Iatrogenic damage to the articular cartilage*

Instrumentation/ Implantation

- Standard arthroscopic equipment

Controversies

- Glenohumeral exploration may increase pain length and delay return to work postoperatively (Sirveaux et al., 2005).
- We believe that the surgeon must perform a glenohumeral exploration.

Pitfalls

- *Production of bleeding by sweeping the subacromial bursa with instrumentation*
- *Failure to keep the arthroscope anterior to the bursal veil, which results in an inadequate picture*

Instrumentation/ Implantation

- Standard arthoscopic instrumentation

- Anterior portal (Fig. 5, *E*)
  - This portal is placed midway between the anteriolateral acromion and the coracoids.
  - It is located within the intra-articular triangle of the biceps superiorly, the superior portion of the subscapularis tendon inferiorly, and the anterior edge of the glenoid at the base.
- Lateral portal (Fig. 5, *C*)
  - This portal is located 3 cm lateral to the anterior lateral corner of the acromion and passes through the deltoid muscle.
- Superior portal
  - This portal is located off the anterolateral corner of the acromion.
  - It passes between the attachments of the lateral and anterior muscle groups of the deltoid.

Procedure

Step 1

- Diagnostic glenohumeral arthroscopy is performed to examine:
  - Glenoid and humeral head
  - Biceps tendon
  - Labrum in all aspects
  - Intra-articular rotator cuff

Step 2

- Subacromial exploration and lateral bursectomy are performed.
- The scope is placed in the subacromial space through the posterior portal.
- The instrument is gently swept over the greater tuberosity and down the humerus to create viewing space without producing increased bleeding.
- A lateral and, if necessary, an anterior portal are made under direct visualization.

Controversies

- Performing subacromial decompression
  - Reviewed literature shows no clinical difference in patients with or without a decompression (Ark et al., 1992; Jacobs and Debeer, 2006; Porcellini et al., 2004; Seil et al., 2006).
  - Indications are based on physical examination, radiographs, and MRI and confirmed by arthroscopic evidence.

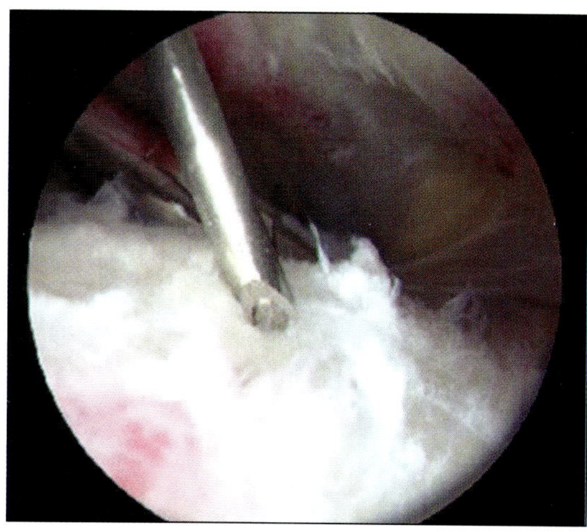

FIGURE 6

PEARLS

- *Fluoroscopy may be used to assist needle placement if localization difficulty occurs.*

PITFALLS

- *Inability to localize the calcium: it must be found before any débridement can be initiated.*

Instrumentation/ Implantation

- 18-gauge needle

PEARLS

- *Switch viewpoints and shaver between the lateral and posterior portals (see Fig. 8A and 8B).*
- *An accessory posterolateral portal improves the view (see Fig. 5, B).*
- *Calcium embedded in humeral bone is excised/microfractured to prevent recurrence and speed healing (see Fig. 9).*

STEP 3

- The spinal needle is used to localize the site of the calcific tendinitis (Fig. 6).
- Initial preoperative evaluation and three-view shoulder films (see Fig. 1A–C) should define the exact location of calcium in all three planes.

STEP 4

- The tendon is incised using the spinal needle or an arthroscopic knife to expose calcium deposits within the tendon (Fig. 7).
- Resection of the calcific tendinitis is performed.
  - A shaver is inserted into the incision and calcium evacuated from tendon and bone (Fig. 8A and 8B).
  - Figure 8C shows the extrusion of calcium deposit into the subacromial space.

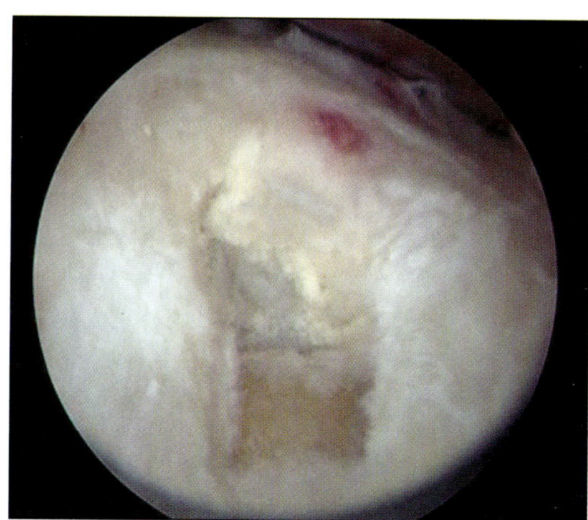

FIGURE 7

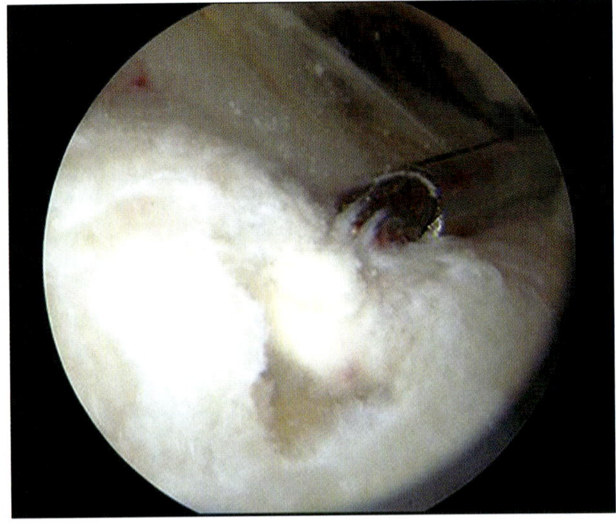

A

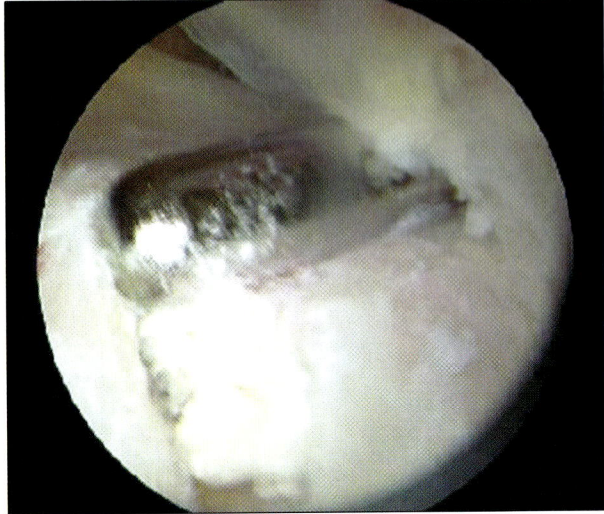

B

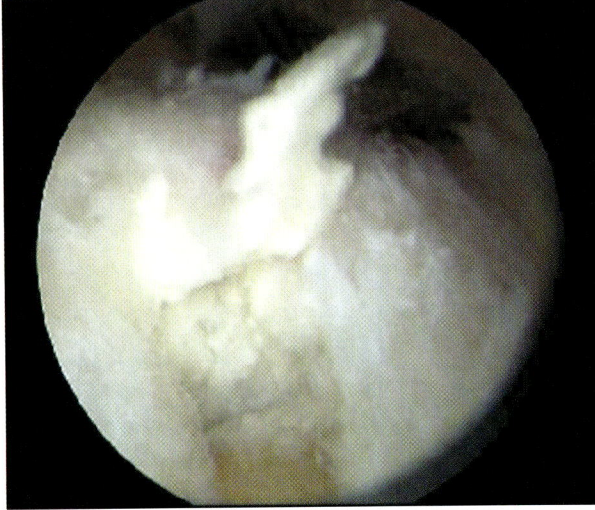

C

FIGURE 8

Instrumentation/ Implantation

- Standard arthroscopic instruments
- Banana blade
- Ring curette
- Microfracture awls

- The humerus is carefully examined for calcium deposits that may be present; once the calcium is removed, the humerus is microfractured (Fig. 9).
- When all apparent calcium deposits have been removed, the shoulder is checked via fluoroscopy or anteroposterior (Fig. 10A) and lateral (Fig. 10B) radiographs to ensure complete removal.

Postoperative Care and Expected Outcomes

- The patient is placed in an abduction sling postoperatively.
- Passive range-of-motion exercises are begun immediately to prevent shoulder stiffness.

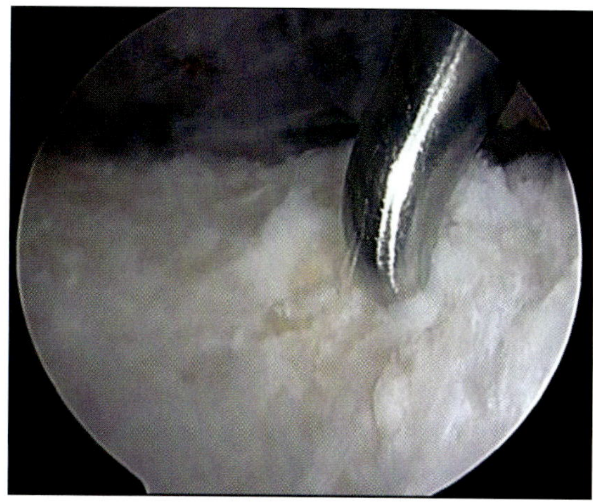

FIGURE 9

Controversies

- Partial versus complete excision of calcium: Jerosch et al. (1998) and Porcellini et al. (2004) recommend complete excision.
- Repairing rotator cuff after débridement
  - Removing cover: body resorbs deposit (Seil et al., 2006)
  - Studies suggest repair is unnecessary, but some advocate tendon repair with side-to-side sutures (Snyder, personal communication, 2005)

- Sling removal is allowed during the day, but the patient should continue to use the sling at night for 3–4 weeks following surgery.
- Pain-free waist-level cuff strengthening exercises are initiated after the first week.
- Physical therapy is begun in the second week to work on flexibility of the capsule.
- Exercise of the involved tendon may be delayed for 3–4 weeks to allow it to heal the defect.
- An integrative activity/work/sports-specific muscle strengthening program is begun at 6 weeks.

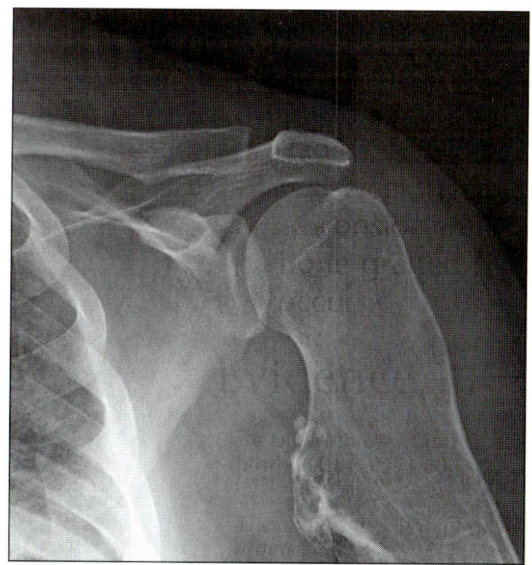

A

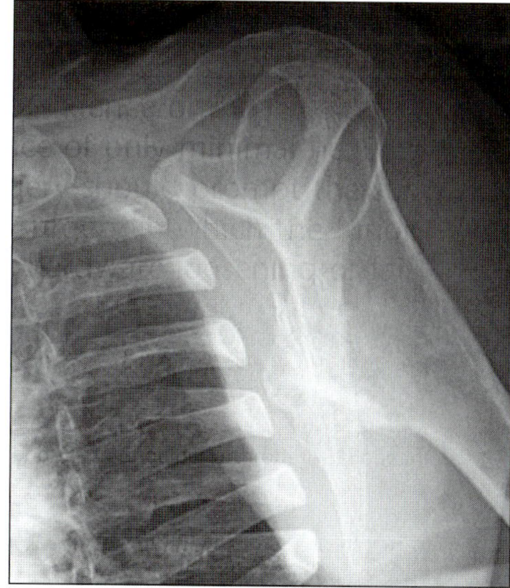

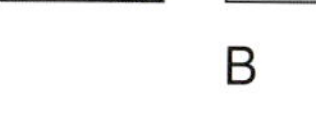

B

FIGURE 10

Pearls

- *Cryotherapy may be useful.*
- *Physical therapy: Capsular stretching/joint mobilization should be started on postoperative day 1 (if possible).*
- *Treat capsulitis with a low-dose oral steroid; supplement this with intra-articular/subacromial injections to decrease severity.*
- *Once the portals heal, aquatherapy helps the patient regain motion/function with little pain.*

Pitfalls

- *Failure to recognize the early onset of adhesive capsulitis*

- Potential complications
  - Adhesive capsulitis: This is the most common problem after resection of calcium deposits. It may be due to irritation of the lining of the shoulder from the calcium particles. Early recognition and treatment with oral and/or intra-articular/ subacromial corticosteroids may be helpful.
  - Failure to remove all of the calcium: Checking the resection during surgery with fluoroscopy will minimize this risk, but even so one should stress in the preoperative counseling sessions that the idea is not to remove all the calcium but to fragment it and allow the body to reabsorb the material.
  - Reoccurrence: This is rarely seen after resection.
  - Continued pain and stiffness: These are usually associated with adhesive capsulitis, and most cases resolve with medication and therapy.

Evidence

The following references are level IV to V evidence. No level I–III evidence was found.

Ark JW, Flock TJ, Flatow EL, Bigliani LU. Arthroscopic treatment of calcific tendinitis of the shoulder. Arthroscopy. 1992;8:183-8.

This was a retrospective study of 22 shoulders with an average of 23 months of follow-up. The study concluded that shoulder arthroscopy is an effective treatment to relieve pain in patients with refractory calcific tendinitis. (Level IV evidence [case series])

Codman EA. The Shoulder: Rupture of the Supraspinatus Tendon and Other Lesions in or About the Subacromial Bursa. Boston: Thomas Todd; 1934; 178-215.

Codman provides a detailed description of the pathology of the rupture, calcification and degeneration of the short rotator cuff. He presents the signs and symptoms of the pathology clearly and offers conclusions to management available at the time of publication. (Level V evidence [expert opinion])

Gosens T, Hofstee DJ. Calcifying tendinitis of the shoulder: advances in imaging and management. Current Rheumatology Reports. 2009;11(2):129-34.

This paper is a summary of current concepts related to calcific tendinitis of the rotator cuff. It discusses the past, present, and future research on this topic. It also provides a brief overview of non-operative and operative treatments and their controversies. (Level V evidence [expert opinion])

Jacobs R, Debeer P. Calcifying tendinitis of the rotator cuff: functional outcome after arthroscopic treatment. Acta Orthop Belg. 2006;72:276-81.

In this retrospective study of 61 patients with a mean follow-up of 15 months, the authors concluded that arthroscopic shaving and excision is a safe and reliable procedure for calcifying rotator cuff tendinitis. Also, neither acrominoplasty nor presence of residual calcifications after arthroscopic needling influenced the final outcome. Constant and DASH scores were used pre- and postoperatively for comparison. (Level IV evidence [case series])

Jerosch J, Strauss M, Schmiel S. Arthroscopic treatment of calcific tendinitis of the shoulder. J Shoulder Elbow Surg. 1998;7:30-7.

In this retrospective study of 48 patients with an average follow-up of 23 months, the authors stated that removal of as much calcific deposit as possible should be performed. Also, acromioplasty did not seem to make a difference. Their results were based on preoperative and postoperative assessment in parameters of pain, sports, sleep, work, activities of daily living, range of motion, and power. (Level IV evidence [case series])

Porcellini G, Paladini P, Campi F, Paganelli M. Arthroscopic treatment of calcifying tendinitis of the shoulder: clinical and ultrasonographic follow up findings at two to five years. J Shoulder Elbow Surg. 2004;13:503-8.

This was a retrospective study of 63 patients with a mean follow-up of 36 months. In a statistical analysis, higher Constant scores correlated with greater calcium deposit removal. Also, the authors stated that acromioplasty did not affect the clinical outcome. They recommended the complete removal of calcium deposits. (Level IV evidence [case series])

Seil R, Litzenburger H, Kohn D, Rupp S. Arthroscopic treatment of chronically painful calcifying tendinitis of the supraspinatus tendon. Arthroscopy. 2006;22:521-7.

In this retrospective review of 54 patients' results over 24 months, the authors concluded that arthroscopic treatment of chronically painful calcific tendinitis of the rotator cuff promises to be successful in more than 90% of the patients. (Level IV evidence [case series])

Sirveaux F, Gosselin O, Roche O, Turell P, Mole D. Postoperative results after arthroscopic treatment of rotator cuff calcifying tendonitis, with or without associated glenohumeral exploration. Rev Chir Orthop. 2005;91:295-9.

This was a retrospective review of 64 patients (32 with a glenohumeral exploration and 32 with a bursectomy alone) with a follow-up of 6 months. Postoperative pain was significantly higher and lasted longer (11 weeks versus 5 weeks), and return to work was delayed (12 weeks versus 5 weeks), in the glenohumeral group versus the bursal resection group, respectively. (Level IV evidence [case series])

Uhthoff H, Loehr J. Calcific tendinopathy of the rotator cuff: pathogenesis, diagnosis, and management. J Am Assoc Orthop Surg. 1997;5:183-91.

The pathology and pathoanatomy of calcific tendinopathy is reviewed in this paper. Optimal treatment results are discussed based on staging of the calcific tendinopathy. Acute and chronic calcific tendinitis are two phases of the same disease. If conservative management fails, surgery may become necessary, preferably in the formative phase of the disease. (Level V evidence [expert opinion])

SECTION II

ELBOW
Introduction

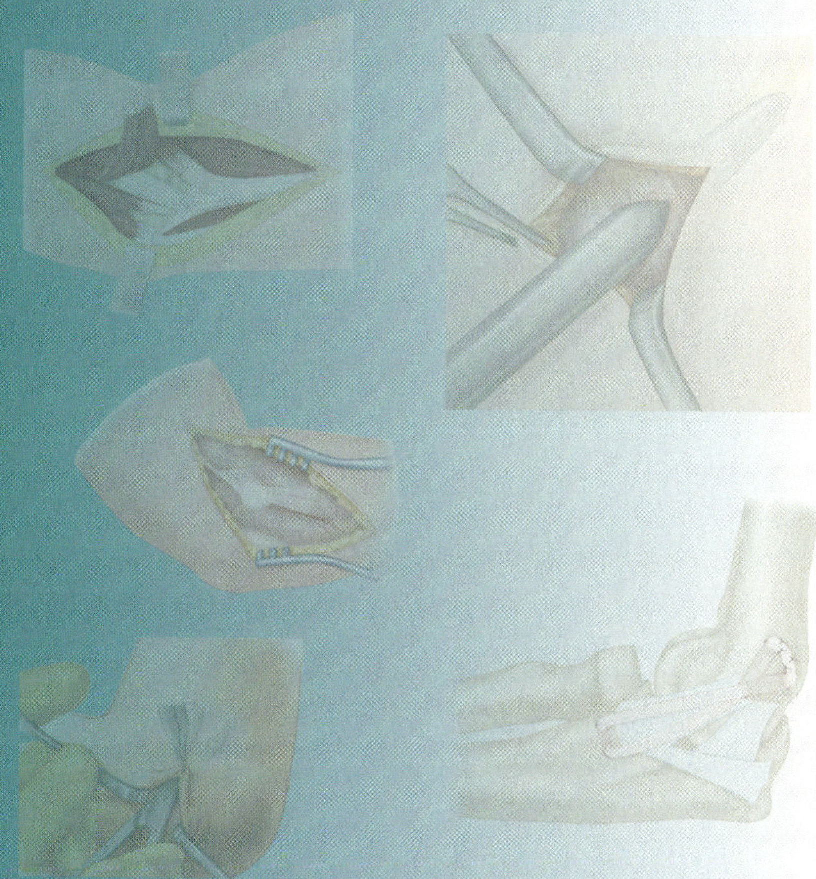

PROCEDURE 39

Surgical Approaches for Open Treatment of the Elbow I: Posterior Approach

Neil J. White and Robert J. Strauch

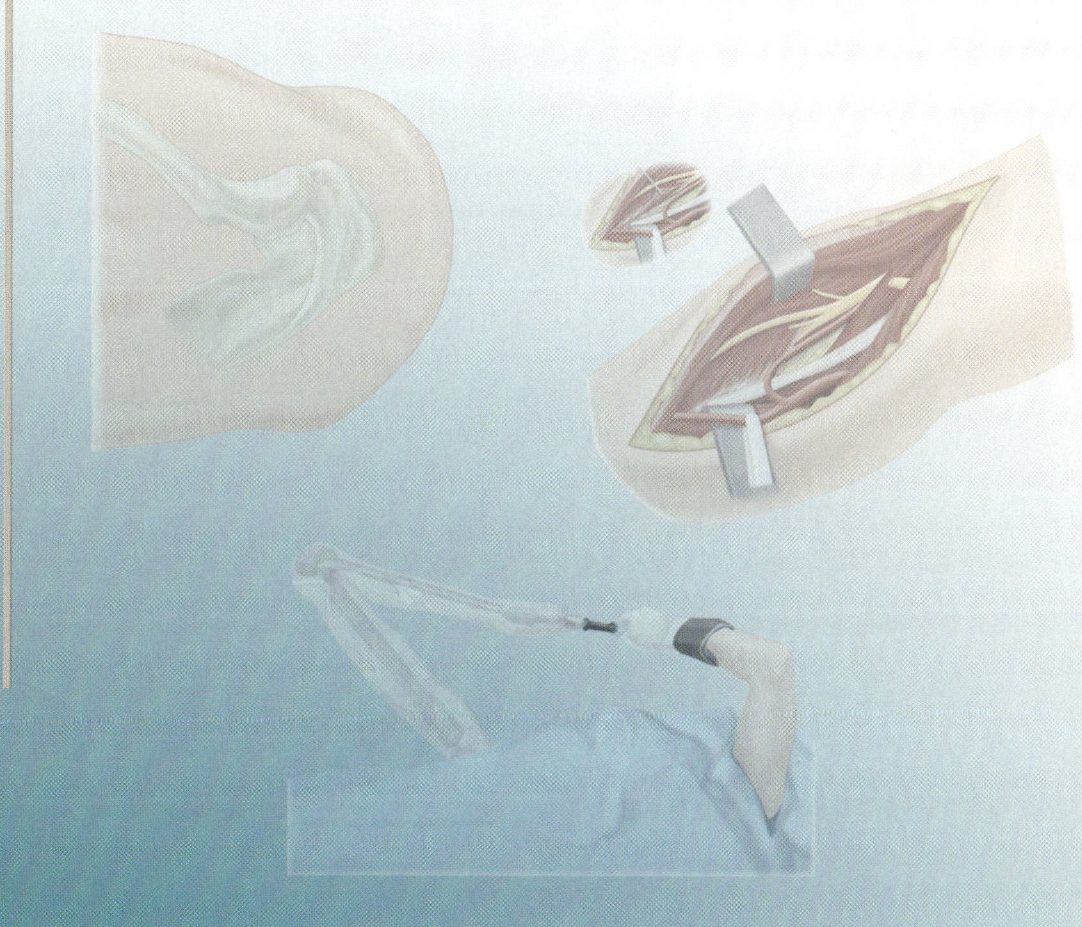

Surgical Approaches to the Elbow

- In recent years, there has been a growing interest and understanding concerning complex injuries about the elbow. Surgical approaches have been described that exploit virtually all muscle intervals circumferentially around the elbow, and many muscle-splitting approaches have also been described. This chapter is not an exhaustive list of surgical approaches. It is a guide to common and useful approaches that provide access to all areas of the elbow. Many alternates and modifications have been described, and ultimately, if the basic principles are followed any of these can be used. The elbow has a propensity for stiffness, and as such, early motion must be encouraged when possible regardless of approach.
- Most areas of the elbow can be accessed through a posterior or "global" skin incision, but this may require large skin flaps and increases the chance of developing a hematoma or seroma. Alternatively, separate medial and lateral skin incisions can be performed in isolation or combination to reduce this risk.
- There are usually several options for surgical exposure for a particular indication, with the ultimate decision being the surgeon's choice. For example, the coronoid can be accessed from the back, the front, and the medial side of the elbow. It can also be accessed from the lateral side if the radial head is absent. The surgeon needs to take into account the specific pattern of injury, the condition of soft tissues, and the need for potential future surgeries prior to making a surgical plan. The authors feel that, as long as several simple principles are followed, the surgeon can expect a good outcome related to the exposure:
  - Plan carefully to ensure that the approach selected will get you everywhere that you need to be (or has the ability to be extended).
  - Protect and preserve sensory nerves and crossing neurovascular structures by either keeping dissection within safe planes or identifying and protecting these structures. Minimize retraction and avoid self-retaining retractors.
  - Protect the collateral ligaments by understanding their anatomy and minimizing dissection and retraction. When ligaments must be taken down

for exposure, they also must be meticulously repaired.

- Respect the triceps mechanism. Surgical approaches that detach the triceps must be repaired securely. An olecranon osteotomy must be fixed with sound technique such that early motion can be encouraged. Similarly, splitting and reflecting of the triceps must be repaired soundly using bone tunnels as required.
- Encourage early motion when possible.

Posterior Approaches: Introduction

- The posterior approach is a versatile approach that can be used for virtually all fractures and reconstructive surgery about the elbow. Full-thickness skin flaps allow the surgeon to exploit a variety of inter- and intramuscular intervals to reach the humerus, elbow joint, and proximal forearm.
- Circumferential exposure of the joint can be achieved through this single incision. This has the additional benefit of avoiding skin bridges that may interfere with future surgery.
- This approach can be extended proximally.

Indications

- Triceps tendon repair
- Fixation of intra-articular and extra-articular fractures of the distal humerus
- Olecranon fracture fixation
- Complex fracture-dislocations of the elbow
- Reconstructive procedures such as total elbow arthroplasty

Examination/Imaging

- It is important to evaluate the skin for previous scars and incorporate these when possible.
- In the setting of revision procedures, the ulnar nerve may be embedded in scar tissue and easily injured. It is vital to have a complete understanding of previous procedures whenever possible.
- A detailed neurologic examination should be well documented before (and after) embarking on any elbow surgery.

Surgical Anatomy

- During the exposure, the ulnar nerve is identified and protected. A thorough understanding of its course is essential. In trauma or revision surgery, the ulnar nerve may not be in its normal position in the cubital tunnel; it is best identified outside of the zone of injury.
  - The ulnar nerve pierces the intermuscular septum, passing from anterior to posterior approximately 10 cm above the medial epicondyle (Shin and Ring, 2007).
  - The nerve follows the medial border of the triceps and passes across the elbow posteriorly under (posterior to) the medial epicondyle in the cubital tunnel.
  - It enters the forearm between the heads of the flexor carpi ulnaris (FCU).
    - It frequently gives a small branch to the medial aspect of the elbow joint before giving motor branches to the FCU muscle.
- The triceps comprises the entire musculature of the posterior arm. The long and lateral heads are superficial and blend to form a common tendon that inserts on the olecranon. The deep (medial) head inserts onto the deep surface of this tendon as well as the posterior olecranon.
  - The way in which the surgeon deals with the triceps dictates the deep dissection. Careful restoration of this mechanism (and early rehabilitation) is paramount to successful recovery, regardless of specific approach.

Positioning

- Depending on the indication, presence of skilled assistants, and surgeon comfort, this approach can be done in the supine, lateral, or prone position.
  - In the supine position, a large gown pack or bolster can be used to place the forearm across the patient's chest with the arm in a flexed adducted position (such that the humerus is vertical). An armboard is not used. This position requires a dedicated assistant to maintain arm position during the entire surgery. Alternatively, a pneumatic arm positioner is very useful. Such a positioner allows the limb to be held rigidly in space as per the surgeon's preference. It can be

Pearls

- *Ensure that adequate image intensification views are attainable prior to prepping and draping the patient. This is especially important if the surgeon is using new equipment or in a new hospital environment. The lateral view is best obtained by externally rotating the arm rather than moving the C-arm. In the situation of a stiff shoulder, internal rotation can be attempted. Alternatively, the C-arm can be rotated to a lateral position.*
- *Patients with previous anterior shoulder instability on the ipsilateral side are at risk of dislocation while under anesthetic. History of prior shoulder problems should be elicited, and care should be taken with external rotation of the arm in all patients.*

Pitfalls

- *A tourniquet can be used, but the surgeon must ensure that adequate proximal exposure is available. A sterile tourniquet may be preferred.*

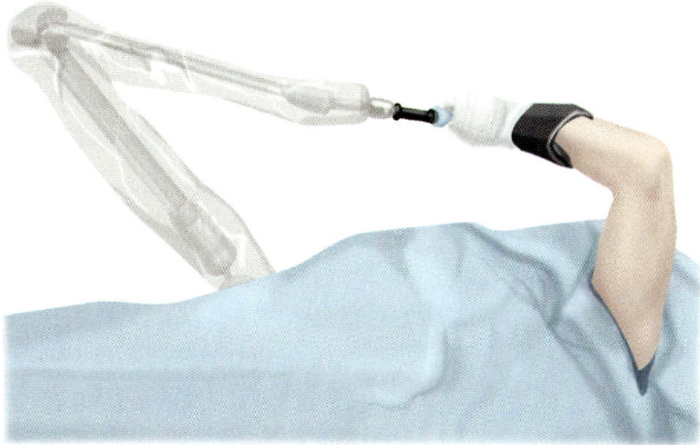

FIGURE 1

Equipment

- A pneumatic limb positioner (Tenet Spider) is very valuable when working in the supine position. The arm can be positioned anywhere in space and becomes rigid once the arm is locked (see Fig. 1).

easily repositioned with a surgeon-controlled foot pedal (Fig. 1).

- In the lateral position, the patient is angled slightly forward and the elbow hangs over a bolster (such that the humerus is horizontal). If image intensification is required, it is essential to ensure that adequate images are attainable prior to draping the patient.
- In the prone position, the arm simply hangs off a short armboard at the elbow. This probably gives the best visualization, but the surgeon incurs all of the potential complications of the prone position.

- We prefer the supine position with the arm flexed and adducted such that the humerus is vertical. We use a nonsterile bolster made of pillows under the drapes that is secured to the patient's chest with tape. This is often augmented with a small sterile gown pack.

Portals/Exposures

- Prior to starting, the patient should be prepped and draped using a free limb technique. The procedure can be completed with or without the use of tourniquet. If a tourniquet is not used, it is advisable to place an uninflated tourniquet or have a sterile tourniquet in the room.
- It is useful to mark the olecranon and the medial and lateral epicondyles with a sterile pen prior to planning the skin incision.
- The incision should start in the midline proximal to the olecranon and curve laterally or medially around the tip of the olecranon before returning to midline (Fig. 2). Crossing the tip of the olecranon should be avoided. This will prevent scarring and potential skin

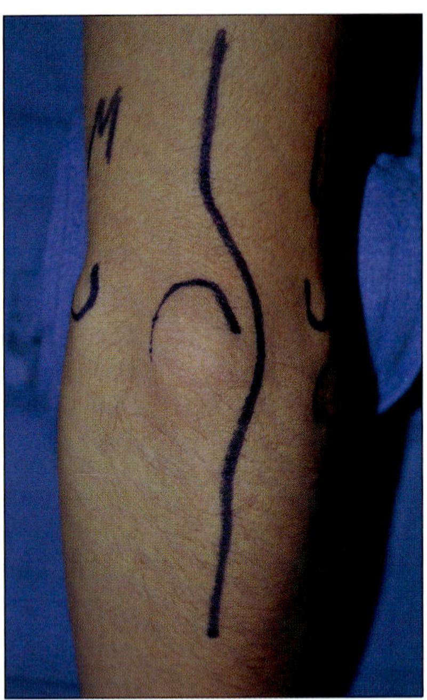

FIGURE 2

breakdown over the weight-bearing tip of the olecranon. The incision can easily be extended proximally or distally.

Procedure

Step 1

- A scalpel is used to develop skin and subcutaneous layers to the level of the triceps fascia. Electrocautery is used for hemostasis.
- The lateral flap is raised full thickness using scalpel dissection. It should be taken to the lateral border of the triceps proximally, and followed distally to the ulna.
- The medial flap needs to be developed with more trepidation. The ulnar nerve must be identified. In the context or trauma, the anatomy is often obscured within the zone of injury, and therefore the nerve is best identified outside of the zone of injury. This can be accomplished by palpating and carefully dissecting it free proximally along the medial border of the triceps.
- The nerve should be identified with a Penrose drain or vessel loops.
  - Do not place a clamp on the Penrose, as this can be prone to getting snagged and causing traction to the nerve. It is better to simply tie a knot in the drain or use skin staples or hemoclips.

Pearls

- *The length of the incision varies depending on the access required. The incision can be easily extended proximally or distally, as required during the procedure.*

Pitfalls

- *As this dissection extends proximal on the lateral side, it is not uncommon to encounter the radial nerve as it pierces the intermuscular septum from posterior to anterior. It is rarely seen closer than 7.5 cm from the distal articular surface of the elbow (Uhl et al., 1996; Zlotlow et al., 2006).*

- Once tagged, the ulnar nerve is dissected free to the insertion into the FCU muscle. A small branch to the joint capsule is consistently seen with careful dissection. Often this can be spared, but it may need to be cut sharply in order to transpose the nerve.
- It is essential to protect the nerve for the remainder of the case (this is easier said than done as the surgeon tackles complex intra-articular fractures).

Step 2

- Many options exist when navigating the triceps muscle. This depends heavily on the operative plan, visualization required, and surgeon preference/comfort. The chevron intra-articular osteotomy provides the best visualization of the joint, but carries a small risk of nonunion.
- Options for deep exposures include:
  - Triceps-sparing approach (work on either side of triceps)
  - Triceps-splitting approach
  - Intra-articular osteotomy
  - Extra-articular osteotomy
  - Triceps-reflecting (Bryan and Morrey) approach (Bryan and Morrey, 1982)
  - Triceps-reflecting anconeus pedicle (TRAP) approach (O'Driscoll, 2002)
- For distal humerus fractures, the medial and lateral border of the triceps can be exposed, allowing access to the medial and lateral columns. If the fracture is a simple intra-articular pattern or an extra-articular pattern, this may be enough exposure.
- A triceps-splitting approach can greatly enhance joint visualization, but the olecranon will continue to block direct joint visualization. If the split is developed medially and laterally over the olecranon such that the triceps tendon is disinserted, then repair of the tendon to bone must be performed at the conclusion of the procedure (Fig. 3A–D).
  - Many surgeons prefer a triceps split to visualize complex intra-articular fractures. One advantage is that it maintains the olecranon contour in which to rebuild the distal humerus. A towel clip on the olecranon with some traction opens the joint up to 5 mm in full flexion.
  - If the distal humerus is being removed for arthroplasty, it is possible to obtain excellent visualization of the joint without disturbing the triceps insertion.

Pearls

- *Note that the elbow joint cannot be as well visualized unless an osteotomy is performed. The contour of the olecranon hides the joint. Even with the osteotomy, the anterior joint is not seen.*
- *When performing a chevron osteotomy, the target should be the bare area of the olecranon articular cartilage.*

Pitfalls

- *It is common for the surgeon to attempt to spare the triceps and treat intra-articular distal humerus fracture by working on either side of the triceps. If the fracture needs an osteotomy, then this should be done early. It is reasonable to spend a few minutes assessing the need for an osteotomy, but the worst-case scenario is spending an hour or more trying to reduce the fracture and either settling for nonanatomic reduction or doing the osteotomy at that time. This makes for a long and frustrating procedure and often puts unnecessary traction on the ulnar nerve during the struggle. If the fracture is complex and intra-articular, it is best to do the osteotomy early.*
- *When performing osteotomy, rigorous technique is required to prevent associated complications, which can be as high as 36%.*
  - *It is tempting to use screw fixation alone (especially at the end of a long case). A tension band technique should always be used. The osteotomy is no different from an olecranon fracture. It requires adequate neutralization of the powerful triceps mechanism.*

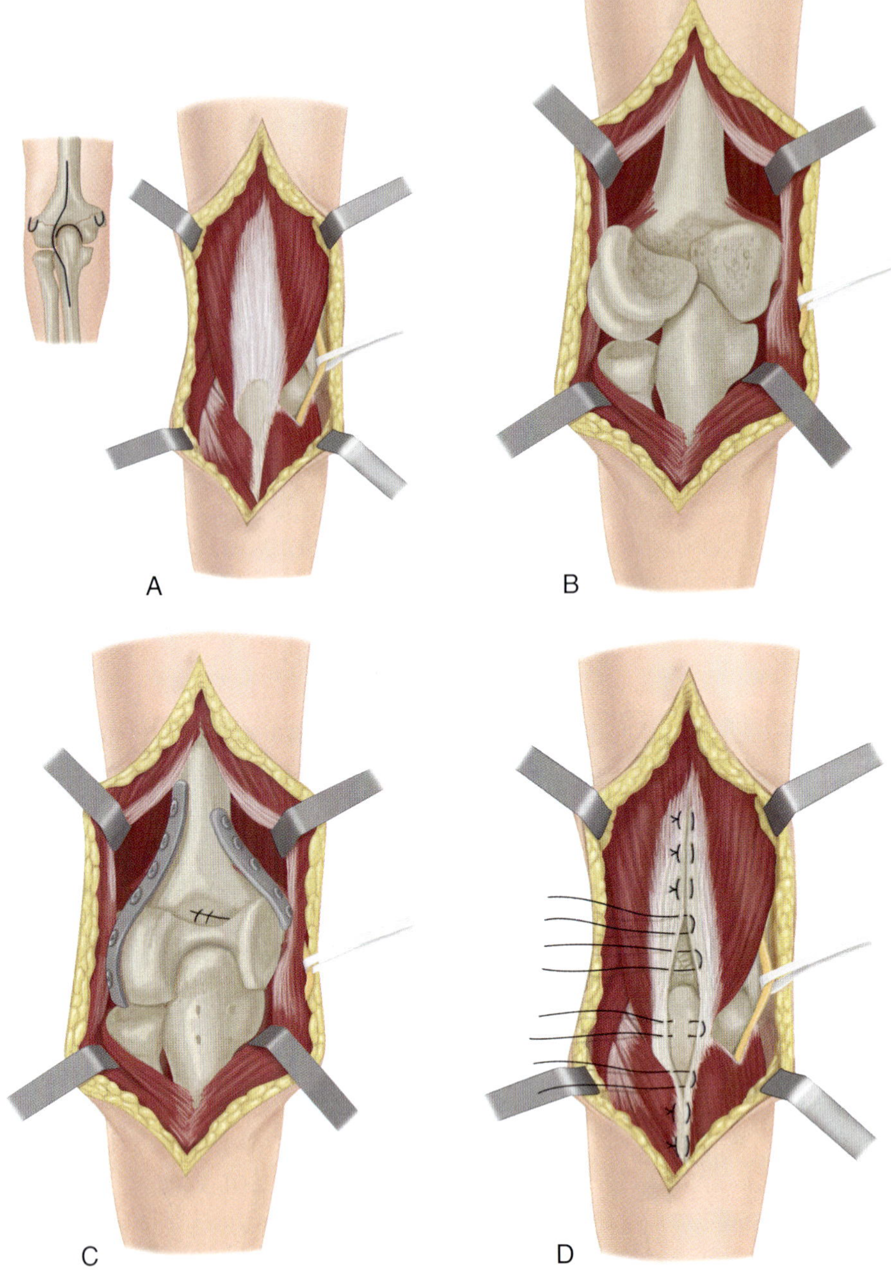

FIGURE 3

- If maximum articular exposure is desired, a classic chevron osteotomy can be performed. The principles include predrilling and tapping for later repair, marking the chevron with the apex distal, and using a sagittal saw to start the cuts. A narrow osteotome should be used to gently finish the osteotomy so as to prevent thermal necrosis of the articular cartilage. This maneuver also provides a jagged surface that

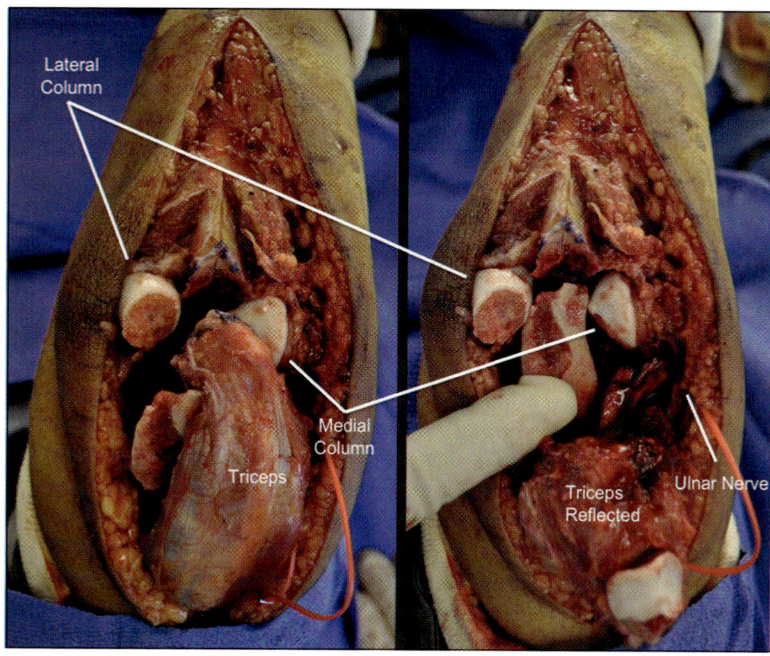

FIGURE 4

can be put back together in puzzle-piece fashion on repair, providing an easy anatomic reduction.

- Olecranon osteotomy is the most destructive approach, but it is safe, and it gives excellent visualization of the distal humerus. Note the difference in exposure from before (Fig. 4A) and after (Fig. 4B) the triceps muscle is reflected. Chevron osteotomy should be targeted at the anatomic bare area of the olecranon with the apex directed distally.
- Once the osteotomy is complete, exposure is wide. The olecranon and triceps should be kept moist throughout the procedure. Care must be taken not to place excessive traction on the radial nerve.

Step 3

- At completion of the operation, repair of this osteotomy can be accomplished using a large cancellous screw to fill the canal. This should be neutralized with a tension-band wire construct. Alternatively, Kirschner wires and a tension band or a plate can be used.
  - Twisting of a figure-of-8 wire should be done on the lateral side as to avoid ulnar nerve irritation.
- Fluoroscopic views should be taken in the lateral and anteroposterior planes to confirm anatomic reduction of the osteotomy and to ensure adequate hardware placement.

Pitfalls

- *The surgeon must be certain that the ulnar nerve is free and uncompressed after closure.*

Controversies

- Ulnar nerve transposition in trauma is controversial. Current data are not conclusive. It is important to clearly document the postoperative course of the nerve in case of any future surgery (Shin et al, 2007).

- The ulnar nerve is inspected, and can be transposed at this time. We routinely transpose the nerve when it is resting on hardware on the medial side. There is no evidence to support this part of the procedure.
  - A subcutaneous pocket is created anteriorly. A blunt elevator gently retracts the nerve as two or three sutures are passed from deep fascia to the subcutaneous layer at the level of the medial epicondyle. It is paramount to ensure the nerve has ample room in this pocket.
    - The course should be followed proximally and distally to ensure the nerve is free through its entire course.
- Subcutaneous tissue and skin are closed according to surgeon preference.
- A splint can be used for comfort through the first 1–2 weeks. Early motion is emphasized.

Postoperative Care and Expected Outcomes

- Early postoperative motion is paramount to a good result. This, of course, must be balanced with the risk of hardware failure or joint subluxation.
- Sutures are generally removed in the 10- to 14-day window.
- Therapy is initiated depending on procedures performed and patient motion.
- Injury to the ulnar nerve is reported to be as high as 13% (Shin and Ring, 2007). Patients have symptoms ranging from subjective numbness to significant motor weakness. This must be followed closely, and generally recovers with time.

Evidence

Bryan RS, Morrey BF. Extensive posterior exposure of the elbow: a triceps sparing approach. Clin Orthop Relat Res. 1982;116:188-92.

This paper described a medial-to-lateral triceps-reflecting approach to the distal humerus. This approach has been advocated to spare the triceps and allow for early rehabilitation.

O'Driscoll SW. Triceps-anconeus pedicle approach for distal humerus fractures and nonunions. Techn Shoulder Elbow Surg. 2002;3:33-8.

The author described a triceps-anconeus pedicle approach to the distal humerus. Through a posterior skin incision, a combination of medial and lateral approaches were used to reflect the entire triceps mechanism, with the anconeus gaining excellent exposure to the distal humerus.

Shin R, Ring D. The ulnar nerve in elbow trauma. J Bone Joint Surg [Am]. 2007;89:1108-16.

In this current concepts review of the ulnar nerve in elbow trauma, a summary of the literature suggested transposition, although recommendation is based on expert opinion alone.

Uhl RL, Larosa JM, Sibeni T, Martin LJ. Posterior approaches to the humerus: when should you worry about the radial nerve? J Orthop Trauma. 1996;10:338-40.

The authors performed an olecranon osteotomy approach on 75 cadavers, measuring the course of the radial nerve as it pierces the intermuscular septum. It was noted to be at risk an average of 9–10 cm from the distal articular surface, but as close as 7.5 cm on some specimens.

Zlotolow DA, Catalano LW 3rd, Barron OA, Glickel SZ. Surgical exposures of the humerus. J Am Acad Orthop Surg. 2006;14:754-65.

This paper provided an elegant evidenced-based review of surgical anatomy and exposures of the humerus, including a summary of the course of peripheral nerves from shoulder to elbow.

PROCEDURE 39

Surgical Approaches for Open Treatment of the Elbow II: Posterolateral (Kocher) and Kaplan Approaches to the Radial Head

Neil J. White and Robert J. Strauch

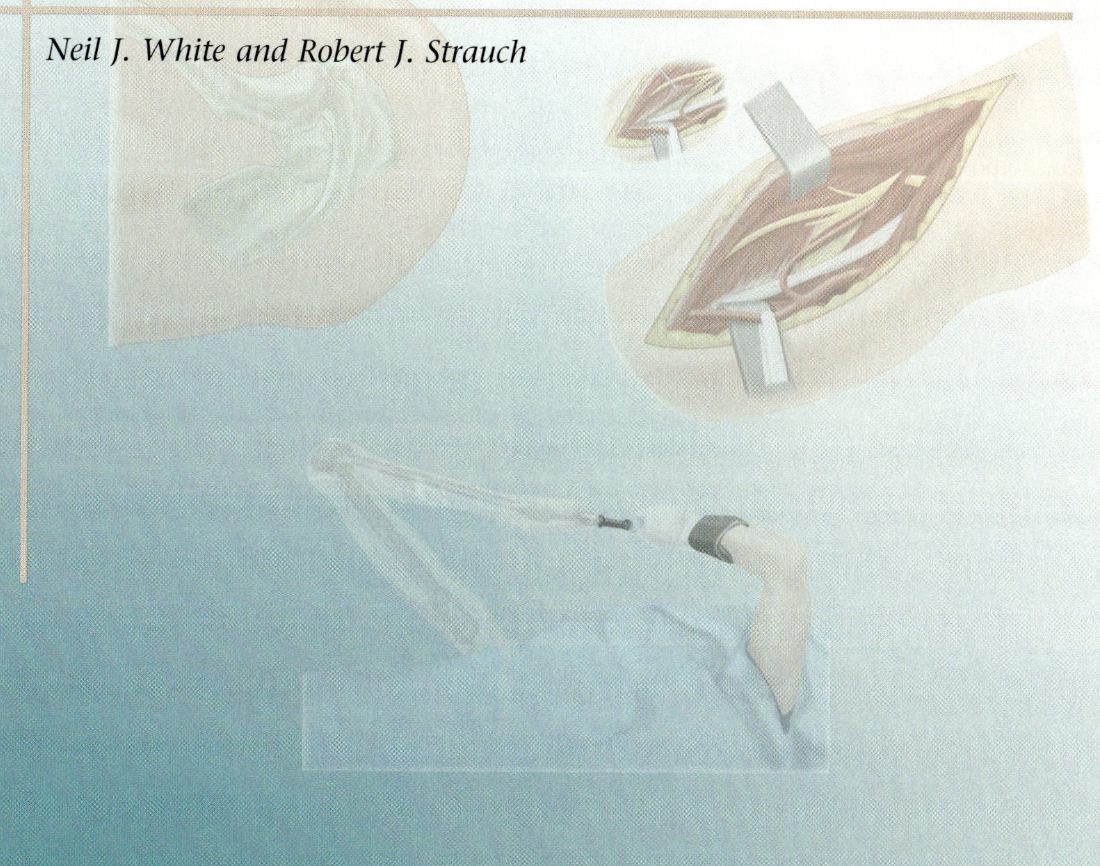

Pitfalls

- *Proximal extension (extended Kocher approach) requires takedown of the lateral ligaments to the elbow and subsequently mandates anatomic repair. This will allow excellent access to the elbow joint for contracture release, fracture fixation (especially lateral column or distal humeral articular shear fractures), or total elbow arthroplasty.*
- *Distal extension with the Kocher approach is limited as the approach technically ends on the ulna.*
- *The Kaplan approach lies in close proximity to the posterior interosseus nerve, although it is not visualized (it can be if desired). Caution should be exercised and the arm should be maintained in pronation during dissection.*

Treatment Options

- The Kaplan approach offers better exposure of the anterior elbow joint.
- Both the Kocher and Kaplan approaches can be utilized (column approach) in the same patient to visualize the anterior and posterior lateral elbow while preserving the lateral collateral ligament complex.

Indications

- Any surgery to the radial head
  - Fracture fixation
  - Radial head excision
  - Radial head replacement
- Posterolateral (Kocher) approach
  - Access to the radiocapitellar joint for infection or loose body removal
  - Access to the capitellum for fixation of fractures with proximal extension (Husband and Hastings, 1990)
- The Kaplan approach may prove a useful alternative when fracture fragments are anterior.

Examination/Imaging

- It is important to evaluate the skin for previous scars and incorporate these when possible.
- In the setting of revision procedures, the ulnar nerve may be embedded in scar tissue and easily injured if significant elbow flexion is gained. It is vital to have a complete understanding of previous procedures whenever possible.
- A detailed neurologic examination should be well documented before (and after) embarking on any elbow surgery.

Surgical Anatomy

- As in virtually all elbow surgery, one must understand the course of the posterior interosseus nerve (PIN) (although it is rarely seen through a Kocher interval). The PIN is at risk during lateral approaches to the elbow (Fig. 1). Its course and variations must be well understood.
  - The PIN takeoff is within 1–2 mm of the radiocapitellar joint (either slightly proximal or slightly distal to the joint) (Strauch et al., 1996).
  - It diverges posterolaterally to enter the supinator muscle between its deep and superficial bellies. In most specimens, the nerve remains intramuscular until the distal edge of the supinator, although anatomic variants have been identified where it runs directly on the proximal radius (Tornetta et al., 1997).
  - It is important to recognize that the nerve moves several centimeters with supination and pronation of the arm (Fig. 2A and 2B). Thus, pronation will

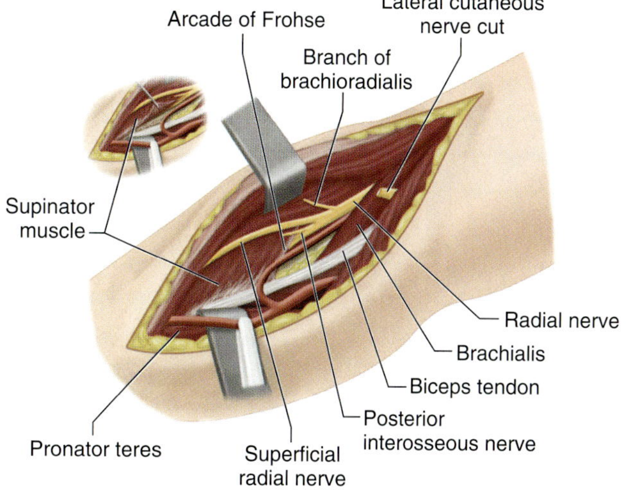

FIGURE 1

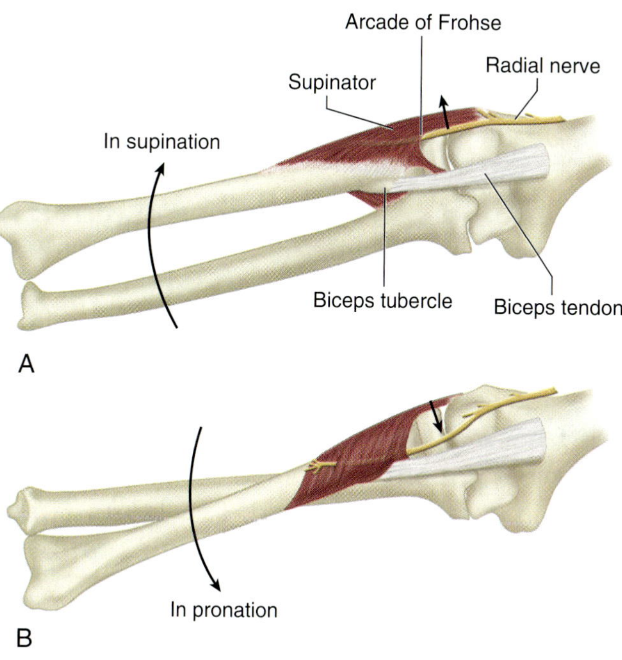

FIGURE 2

protect this structure during lateral approaches while supination will protect it for anterior exposures.

- Pronation moves the nerve anterior such that it crosses the radius more distally, thus protecting it during the posterolateral approach of Kocher.
- It has been shown in anatomic studies that blind subperiosteal dissection with the arm in pronation is safe for plate placement (Tornetta et al., 1997). We have no experience with blind dissection distal to the annular ligament and do not recommend it.

- A thorough understanding of the lateral ligaments of the elbow is also essential.
  - The lateral collateral ligament complex is made up of three distinct ligaments: the lateral ulnar collateral, the radial collateral, and the annular ligaments.
    - The radial collateral arises from the lateral epicondyle and merges indistinguishably with the annular ligament. The annular ligament encircles the radius, originating and inserting onto the ulna. Functionally this is a sling to suspend the radial head and maintain reduction of the proximal radioulnar joint and the radiocapitellar joint.
    - The lateral ulnar collateral ligament is a primary lateral stabilizer of the elbow. It originates at the isometric center of the capitellum and inserts onto the supinator crest of the ulna. Surgically these fibers appear confluent with the annular ligament distally.

PEARLS

- *If approaching an isolated radial head fracture, we prefer to have the patient supine with the arm abducted and internally rotated on an armboard. Using this technique allows for the shoulder to be moved to optimize visualization while working. It is easy to get excellent fluoroscopic views in this position.*
- *If working alone, the lateral position can be used. This allows the arm to rest over a bolster in an ideal position without the use of assistants.*
  - *Be certain that intraoperative images are easily attainable by testing standard views prior to prepping and draping the arm.*
- *A sterile tourniquet can be used if the surgeon may require more proximal exposure.*

Positioning

- For the Kocher approach, the patient can be positioned supine, lateral, or posterior depending on surgeon preference and the extent of the surgery performed.
- For the Kaplan approach, the patient is positioned in the supine position with the limb on a radiolucent hand table. This approach can also be done in the lateral position.

Portals/Exposures

- A sterile marking pen is used to draw the pertinent anatomy, including the lateral epicondyle and radial head. Even in the most swollen (or obese) of patients, the radial head is easily palpated while pronating and supinating the arm.
  - The Kaplan interval is anterior to the axis of rotation while the Kocher inteval is just posterior to this axis (Fig. 3A). The narrow sleeve of tissue between these intervals contains fibers of the lateral collateral ligament complex.
  - Generally, the skin incision for the Kaplan interval is slightly anterior to that of the Kocher; however, either interval can be accessed through either skin incision. The Kocher or Kaplan approach can be

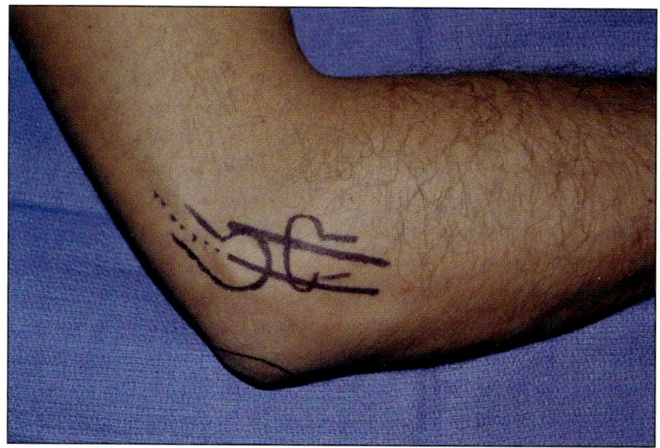

A

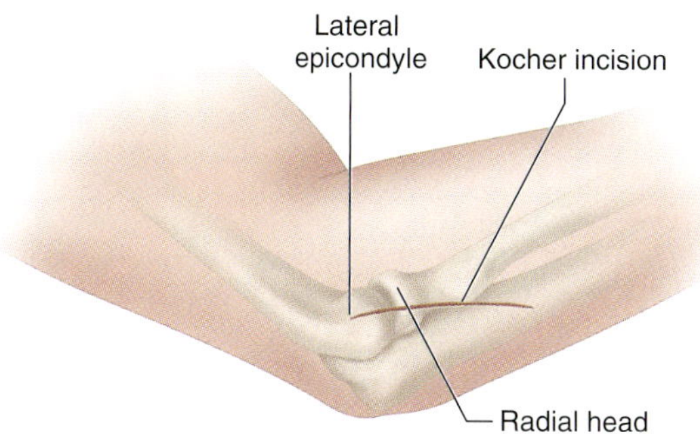

B

FIGURE 3

extended up the lateral column of the humerus (*dotted line* in Fig. 3A).

- With the Kocher approach, there are two options for skin incision.
  - The classic description is of an oblique skin incision starting at or slightly proximal to the lateral epicondyle and crossing the middle of the radial head directed toward the subcutaneous border of the ulna (Fig. 3B).
  - Alternatively, a posterior (global) skin incision can be used and a flap raised laterally to identify the deep interval. The advantage of this incision is its versatility in getting to all areas of the elbow and the ease with which it can be reused for any future surgery.
  - Regardless of incision, the fascial layer should be well exposed with generous flaps to ensure that the deep dissection is in the correct plane.
- With the Kaplan approach, after marking the key landmarks with a sterile marking pen, an incision is planned from 1 cm proximal to the lateral epicondyle and directed toward Lister's tubercle with the arm in neutral rotation (see Fig. 3B).

Procedure

Step 1

- Kocher approach
  - The dissection is carried out in the internervous and intermuscular plane between the anconeus (radial nerve) and the extensor carpi ulnaris (PIN). The raphe between these muscles can be identified by "falling" into the interval by finger palpation,

running the gloved finger perpendicular to the muscle fibers. It may help to sweep the muscle with a moist sponge. The anconeus muscle has a characteristic fan shape with the fibers directed more longitudinally in the proximal part of the muscle and more vertical in the distal part (Witt and Kamineni, 1998).

- Once through the skin and fascia, the Kocher interval can be identified.
  - The Kocher interval between the anconeus and extensor carpi ulnaris (ECU) is a challenge to identify (Fig. 4). Sweeping a sponge across the muscle layer may help to identify a subtle different orientation in muscle fibers. Once initially identified, the interval becomes obvious.
  - Once clearly identified, this interval can be developed sharply, exposing the capsule in the proximal wound and the supinator distally.
- The Pankovich approach is a modification of the Kocher exposure wherein the anconeus is widely elevated from distal to proximal off the olecranon and proximal ulna.

■ Kaplan approach
- Subcutaneous tissue is taken in line with skin to the extensor fascia. Beneath the subcutaneous tissue, the common extensor tendon is easily identifiable. Just anterior to this firm structure, the more muscular-appearing extensor carpi radialis longus (ECRL) is found, originating from the distal

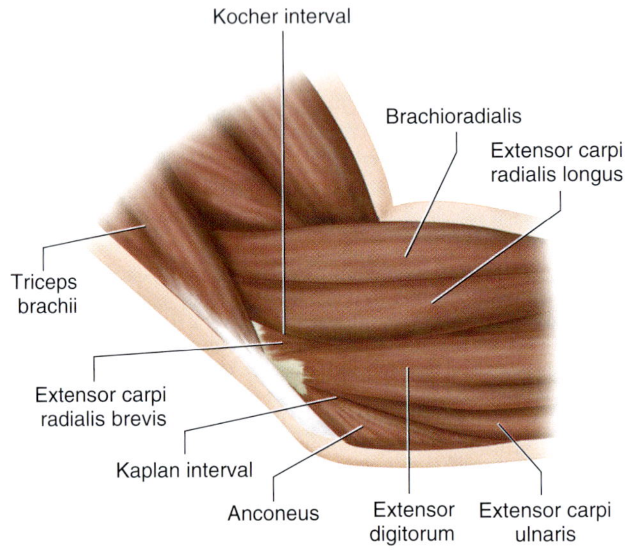

FIGURE 4

humerus. This is the superficial interval of the Kaplan approach.

- Once through this plane, the extensor carpi radialis brevis (ECRB) tendon, which is fibrous appearing and at a near right angle to the ECRL fibers, is seen. The interval between the ECRL/B and common extensor tendon is the Kaplan interval. The Kaplan interval can be identified between the common extensor tendon and the more muscular ECRL origin superficially (see Fig. 4). The deep dissection is carried out between the ECRB/L and the common extensor tendon.
- For better proximal visualization, the plane can be extended proximally along the lateral supracondylar ridge between the triceps and brachioradialis. This is rarely necessary for access to the radial head.

PEARLS

- *Once inside the joint, it is key to maintain forearm pronation while carefully gaining exposure in a subperiostal fashion along the radius. It is recommended to avoid crossing the annular ligament or passing the tuberosity of the radius. If the annular ligament is incised, it must be repaired.*

STEP 2

- Kocher approach
  - The capsule can be taken in line with the fascial dissection, exposing the radiocapitellar joint. Distally, with the arm fully pronated, the supinator can be teased off the radial neck in a subperiosteal fashion (Fig. 5). The dissection can be taken beyond the annular ligament if plate application is required. Although some anatomic papers quote as much as 6 cm from the joint line, we prefer to limit dissection to the level of the annular ligament.

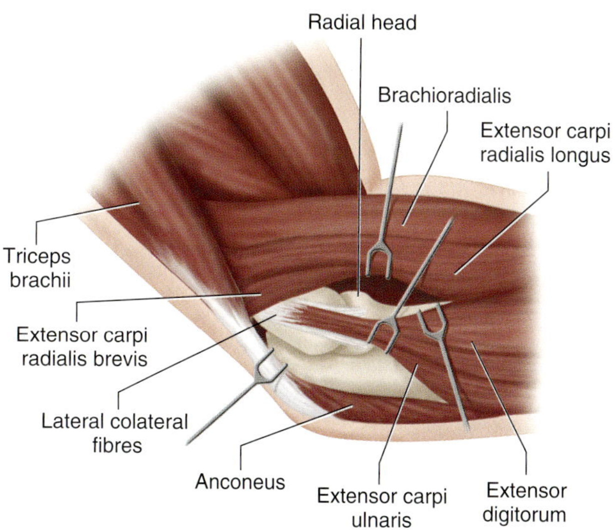

FIGURE 5

- The common extensor origin and the lateral ligament complex block proximal visualization. If more proximal exposure is required, the common extensor origin with its ligamentous complex can be reflected anteriorly while the triceps and anconeus are reflected posteriorly.
  - Feathering off a few millimeters of origin greatly increases exposure. It may also render the elbow unstable in varus, which allows the surgeon to open the joint substantially to access the coronoid (through a comminuted radial head), or to insert a radial head implant.
  - The ligamentous origin must be repaired in the precise isometric position in order to confer a stable elbow through the arc of motion. Failure to do so may result in iatrogenic posterolateral rotatory instability.

- Kaplan approach
  - Through this interval, the joint capsule can be seen proximally and the supinator muscle distally. With the arm maintained in full pronation, joint capsule is incised in line with the incision. Distally, the supinator can be carefully taken down at its origin (see Fig. 5). Distal extension requires entering the proximal aspect of the supinator muscle, and care must be taken to identify the PIN should further exposure of the radial neck be desired.
  - The Kaplan interval provides increase exposure to the anterior radial head, which is often helpful in trauma as it is this supinated anterior fragment that requires fixation. Both intervals can be developed as described in Procedure 39, Part III.

Step 3

- Kocher approach
  - On completing the operation, the lateral ligaments must be securely repaired back to the humerus using suture anchor(s) at the true center of rotation of the capitellum.
    - This is more anterior than expected on the lateral epicondyle. If doubt exists, a Kirschner wire can be placed in the lateral epicondyle at the suspected axis of rotation and a lateral image can confirm position prior to placement of a suture anchor.
  - The annular ligament, if taken down, must be securely repaired.
  - It is not always possible to close the capsule, but it will usually take a few sutures to approximate the borders.

Pearls

- *When repairing the lateral ligaments, a single stitch tied with a slipknot can be used to approximate the correct position. The elbow can then be taken through a range of motion to ensure that ligament tension is isometric, and then stressed in varus to ensure that the amount of tension is correct. This step can be repeated as needed until the tissue is appropriately tensioned.*

- The anconeus-ECU fascial split should be approximated and the skin closed according to surgeon preference.
- When there has been any suspicion of elbow instability, we obtain final images to confirm adequate joint reduction.

- Kaplan approach
  - Once the operative procedure is complete, it is usually possible to put a few stitches in the capsule. Subcutaneous tissue and skin are closed according to surgeon preference.

Postoperative Care and Expected Outcomes

- Postoperative care for these exposures is limited by the procedure performed, not the approach.
- As for all elbow surgery, early range of motion is encouraged where possible.

Evidence

Husband JB, Hastings H. The lateral approach for operative release of post-traumatic contracture of the elbow. J Bone Joint Surg [Am]. 1990;72:1353-8.

This paper described an extended posterolateral approach to the elbow for posttraumatic contracture release.

Kaplan EB. Surgical Approaches to the Neck, Cervical Spine and Upper Extremity. Philadelphia: WB Saunders, 1966.

This text presented Kaplan's original description of this approach. He highlighted the utility of exposure to the anterior aspect of the radial head in trauma. This interval remains unmodified since this publication.

Strauch RJ, Rosenwasser MP, Glazer PA. Surgical exposure of the dorsal proximal third of the radius: how vulnerable is the posterior interosseous nerve? J Shoulder Elbow Surg. 1996;5:342-6.

This elegant cadaver study evaluated the distance between the bicipital tuberosity and the PIN across the elbow. The nerve was seen an average of 2.3 cm from the most prominent point of the tuberosity (range, 1.8–3.2 cm).

Tornetta P 3rd, Hochwald N, Bono C, Grossman M. Anatomy of the posterior interosseous nerve in relation to fixation of the radial head. Clin Orthop Relat Res. 1997;(345):215-8.

This cadaver study examined the proximity of the PIN to a 4-cm mini-fragment radial head plate. The nerve was 5 ± 1.2 mm from the distal edge of the plate, with no nerve injuries noted in the 50 specimens. One of the cadavers displayed a known variant wherein the PIN lies directly on the radius.

Witt JD, Kamineni S. The posterior interosseous nerve and the posterolateral approach to the proximal radius. J Bone Joint Surg [Br]. 1998;80:240-2.

This cadaver study noted the PIN to be 6.0 ± 1.0 cm from the radial head, suggesting that, with the arm in full pronation, it is safe to dissect beyond the annular ligament.

PROCEDURE 39

Surgical Approaches for Open Treatment of the Elbow III: Anterior Approaches

Neil J. White and Robert J. Strauch

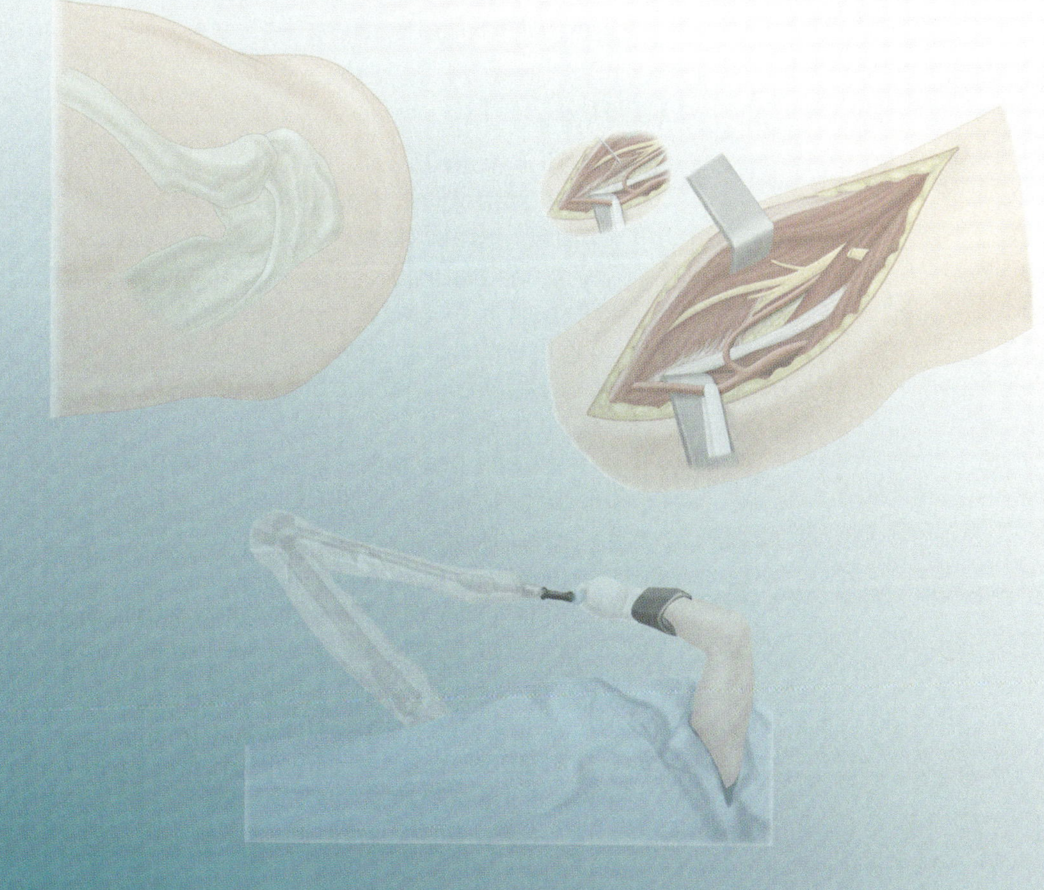

Anterior Approaches: Introduction

- In general, the anterior elbow approach is rarely used. Due to the presence of the brachial artery, numerous deep and superficial veins, and the median, radial, and lateral antebrachial cutaneous nerves, alternate approaches are generally favored. However, certain situations such as vascular compromise and nerve injury mandate use of anterior approaches.
- The anterior and anterolateral approaches are discussed together.

Indications

- Anterior approach
  - Exploration of the neurovascular structures of the antecubital fossa
    - After trauma or for entrapment syndromes
  - The distal half to two thirds is utilized for distal biceps tendon repair
    - The proximal extent of the exposure is dependent on the location of the retracted biceps tendon. The dissection must be taken proximal enough to allow for safe retrieval of this structure.
  - Tumor or infection
  - Exploration of neurovascular structures in supracondylar humerus fractures in children with associated vascular injury
- Anterolateral approach
  - Fractures of the capitellum
  - Anterior capsular release for elbow contractures
  - Tumor or infection

Examination/Imaging

- It is important to evaluate the skin for previous scars and incorporate these when possible.
- In the setting of revision procedures, the ulnar nerve may be embedded in scar tissue and easily injured. It is vital to have a complete understanding of previous procedures whenever possible.
- A detailed neurologic examination should be well documented before (and after) embarking on any elbow surgery.

Surgical Anatomy

- The key to this approach is an intimate understanding of the anterior neurovascular structures as they cross the elbow.
- The median nerve lies medial to the brachial artery at the level of the elbow joint. A helpful mnemonic is that the median nerve is "medial" (Fig. 1). The basilic vein is superficial and medial to these structures. The brachial artery runs with brachial veins on either side.
  - These structures travel distal together before crossing under the bicipital aponeurosis (see Fig. 1), where the median nerve dives between the two heads of pronator, and the brachial artery divides into the radial and ulnar arteries.
  - The radial artery travels under the medial edge of brachioradialis until it is palpable in the wrist. The ulnar artery lies on the brachialis and then the flexor digitorum profundus while being covered by the flexor-pronator mass.
- The radial nerve lies between the brachialis and brachioradialis, giving motor branches to each muscle (lateral brachialis only).
  - It crosses the joint in the radial tunnel, which spans from the radiocapitellar joint to the proximal aspect of the superficial head of the supinator (approximately 5 cm).

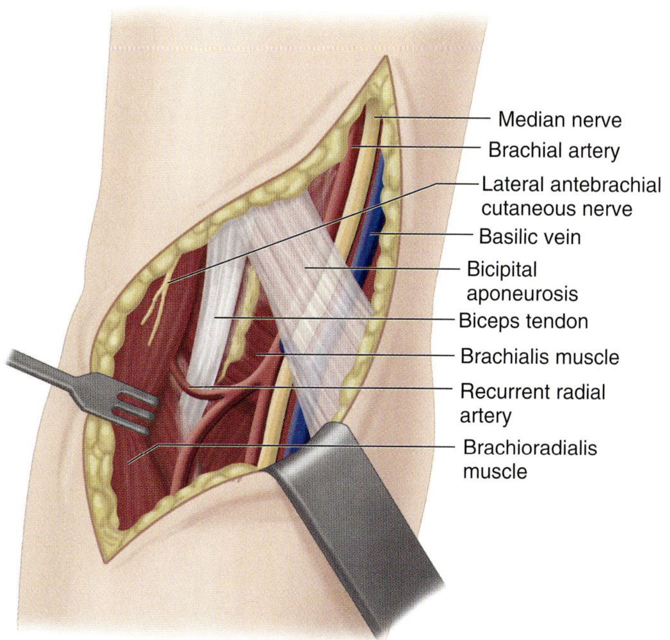

FIGURE 1

- The lateral antebrachial cutaneous nerve (LACN) is the most commonly injured structure when approaching the elbow anteriorly.
  - This terminal sensory branch of the musculocutaneous nerve pierces the brachial fascia approximately 3 cm proximal to the lateral epicondyle. It is most easily identified between the biceps tendon and the brachioradialis muscle in the distal aspect of the incision. In the proximal part of the incision, it can be seen between the brachialis and biceps.
  - We routinely identify and protect this vulnerable nerve with vessel loops.

PEARLS

- *If planning a distal biceps tendon repair, note that the tourniquet can entrap the retracted biceps muscle, making reattachment difficult. It should be released for the repair if the biceps is tight.*

PITFALLS

- *If not using a tourniquet, be sure to have a sterile one in the room.*

Positioning

- The anterior approach is done in the supine position with the arm on a radiolucent hand table.
- A sterile tourniquet is used.

Portals/Exposures

- A sterile marking pen is used to mark a curvilinear incision across the elbow crease (Fig. 2). It is important not to cross the crease at right angles. The distal limb of the incision is based on the medial border of brachioradialis and the proximal limb on the medial border of the biceps.

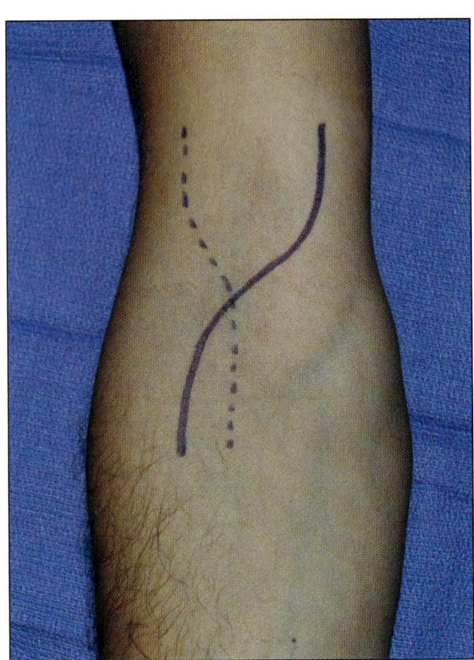

FIGURE 2

- The proximal skin incision can be placed over the lateral edge of the biceps if the pathology being addressed is on the anterolateral aspect of the elbow, such as a capitellar fracture (see Fig. 2).
- The anterior approach provides exposure of the neurovascular structures (*solid line* in Fig. 2), while an anterolateral skin incision (*dotted line*) better visualizes the radial nerve, joint capsule, or capitellum.

Procedure: Anterior Approach

Step 1: Superficial Dissection

- After sharp dissection is used to take skin, careful dissection should be used to raise generous skin flaps.
- Large veins will be encountered, and most of these can be retracted with the flaps. Occasionally crossing branches need to be ligated. We routinely use vascular clips.

Step 2: Protection of the LACN

- The LACN will often be identified as it emerges from fascia about 3 cm proximal to the lateral epicondyle. It is easiest to identify between the brachialis and biceps proximally or between the biceps tendon and brachioradialis distally.
- This nerve can also be found by identification of the cephalic vein. The nerve runs on the deep border of the vein.

Pearls

- *Injury to the LACN is the most common complication of this approach. Identify and protect the nerve with a vessel loop. Although less common, the posterior interosseous nerve is also at risk and a much more significant problem. Beware of rigorous retraction.*

Step 3: Deep Dissection

- The deep dissection is entirely dependent on the structure or structures that need be visualized
- Neurovascular Exposure
  - If visualization of the major neurovascular structures is required, then the bicipital aponeurosis should be identified and incised along the medial edge of the biceps tendon. We do not repair the bicipital aponeurosis. Note that the artery is just under this structure. A deep cut will injure the vessel. We prefer to protect the underlying vessels with a clamp when incising the aponeurosis.
    - Taking this layer provides instant exposure to the brachial artery and median nerve. These structures should be protected with vessel loops.

Pearls

- *For biceps tendon repair, the biceps tendon should be passed anatomically to its native insertion on the radius. Care must be taken not to "loop" any vessels or cutaneous nerves in doing so.*

Pitfalls

- *In the setting of distal biceps tendon repair, it is often tempting to retrieve the retracted tendon blindly. This may be problematic due to the multiple neurovascular structures in the area. This step should be completed under direct visualization.*

    - After these vital structures are protected, the surgeon will have an excellent view of the distal humerus.
    - The radial nerve is easily identified in the proximal wound between the brachialis and brachioradialis, if required.
- Biceps Tendon Repair
  - For biceps tendon repair, identification of the neurovascular structures is not necessary. Blunt dissection can be used along the medial border of brachioradialis to identify the radial tuberosity by palpation. The forearm must be placed in full supination to "deliver" the tuberosity to the incision.
    - Note that, although the bicipital aponeurosis is frequently injured with tendon rupture, it is occasionally intact. If it is intact, it generally prevents excessive retraction of the tendon.
    - Excessive deep retraction must be avoided in order to protect the posterior interosseous nerve (PIN). Particularly, Hohmann retractors around the lateral radial neck should be avoided.

Step 4: Closure

- Regardless of approach or procedure, we do not close any fascial layers.
- We deflate the tourniquet and gain hemostasis prior to closure, and then approximate the subcutaneous layer and skin only.

Procedure: Anterolateral Exposure

- The anterolateral approach provides access to the radial nerve, anterior capsule, and radiocapitellar joint (Fig. 3). To do this safely, the radial nerve must

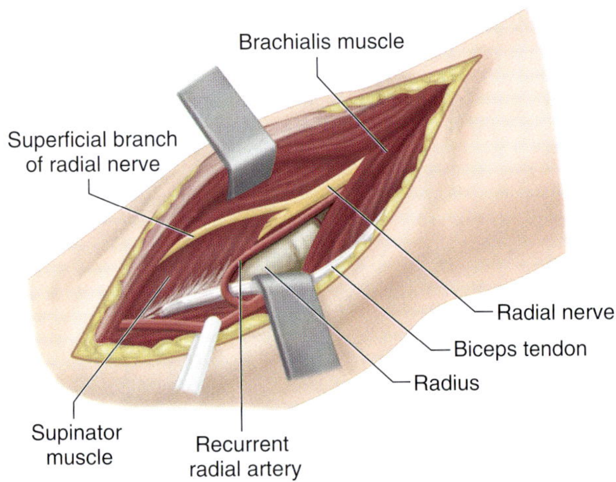

FIGURE 3

be identified and protected, and recurrent radial vessels may need to be cauterized.

STEP 1

- If the surgeon requires access to the radial nerve, anterior joint capsule, or capitellum, then, after using an anterolateral-based skin incision, the interval between the brachialis and brachioradialis is identified. Finger or blunt dissection is used to identify the radial nerve in this interval. The nerve is followed distally to its bifurcation, and fascia is taken down on the lateral aspect of biceps tendon.
- Recurrent branches of the radial artery will be identified, and must be ligated. If these branches are injured, they will retract, making bleeding difficult to control. It is not advisable to blindly cauterize in this wound.
- At this time, the elbow can be flexed and the forearm maximally supinated. The radial artery will be retracted medially with the pronator teres. Excessive retraction must be avoided. The joint capsule can now be incised to expose the capitellum.

STEP 2

- If exposure to the proximal radius is desired, two options are available.
    - The radial nerve can be traced from proximal to distal with identification of the two terminal branches: the superficial sensory and the PIN. (In some patients, a third discrete branch to the extensor carpi radialis brevis exists.) The PIN is most at risk. It can be followed into the supinator and freed, identified, and protected through the length of the wound. Note that there are several anatomic variants to the radial nerve anatomy at the elbow.
    - Alternatively, with the arm in full supination, the supinator muscle can be dissected sharply from its origin on the radius (be sure that you are at the true origin). This allows the deep muscle belly to protect the PIN from the surgeon. It is imperative to not vigorously retract this muscle. Take this dissection as far distally as required. It can be extended by a standard Henry's approach all the way to the wrist.
- The arm is pronated to bring the radius into view.
- The visible portion of the radial nerve should be completely free of tension at all times.

Step 3

- Regardless of approach or procedure, we do not close any fascial layers.
- We deflate the tourniquet and gain hemostasis prior to closure, and then approximate the subcutaneous layer and skin only.

Postoperative Care and Expected Outcomes

- Careful evaluation by pre- and postoperative neurovascular examination is mandatory with any approach about the elbow. Specifically, a detailed evaluation of the radial nerve and PIN as well as the anterior interosseous and median nerves is mandatory.
- Rehabilitation will be guided by the specific procedure performed. There are no limitations based on the approach. Early motion is encouraged when possible.

Evidence

Strauch RJ. Biceps and triceps injuries of the elbow. Orthop Clin North Am. 1999;Jan;30(1):95-107.

Urbaniak JR, Hansen PE, Beissinger SF, Aitken MS. Correction of post-traumatic flexion contracture of the elbow by anterior capsulotomy. J Bone Joint Surg Am. 1985;Oct;67(8):1160-4.

(Level IV evidence)

PROCEDURE 39

Surgical Approaches for Open Treatment of the Elbow IV: Anteromedial (Hotchkiss) Approach

Neil J. White and Robert J. Strauch

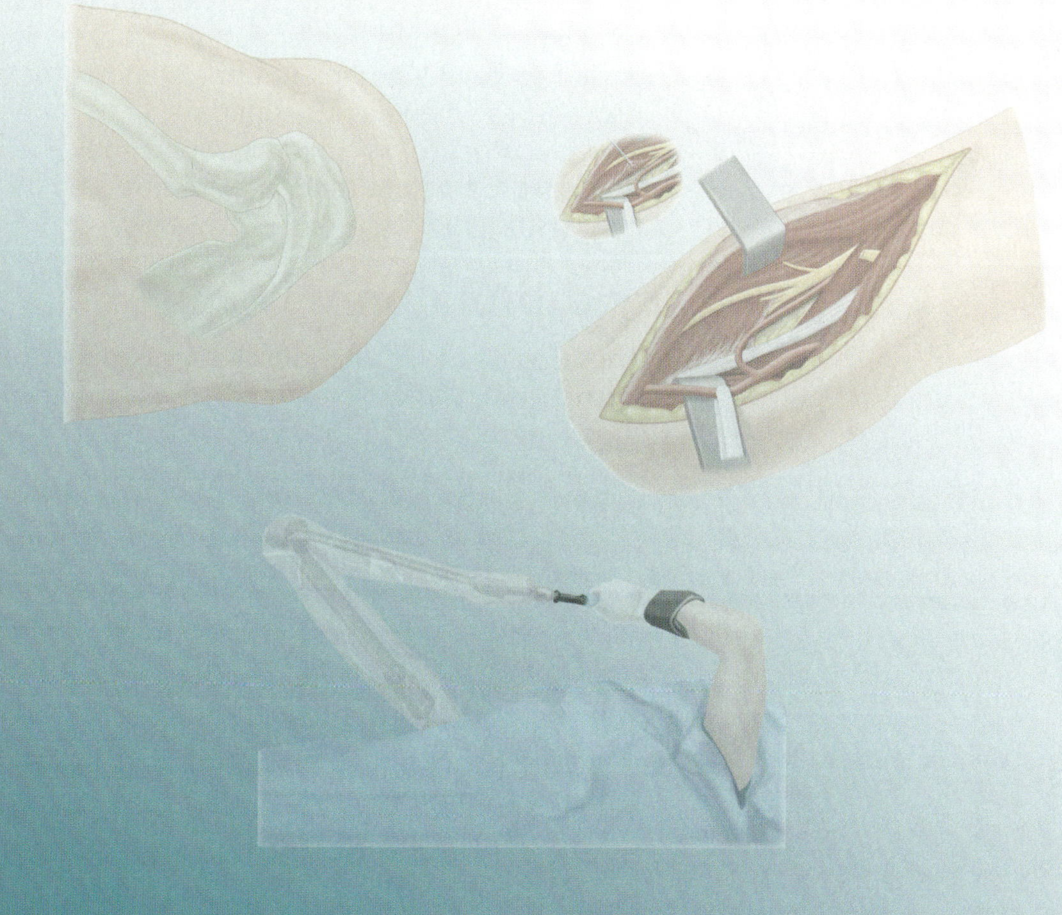

Indications

- Coronoid fractures
- Capsular release for stiff elbow
- Reconstruction of deficient medial collateral ligament (MCL)
- Access to joint for removal of heterotopic ossification

Treatment Options

- Coronoid fractures can often be accessed through the floor of the ulnar nerve. Exposure is limited to the base and midportion of the coronoid. The ulnar nerve is dissected free and the two heads of flexor carpi ulnaris are split. The anterior bundle of the MCL is usually attached to the coronoid fragment, and care must be taken to preserve it.

Examination/Imaging

- It is important to evaluate the skin for previous scars and incorporate these when possible.
- In the setting of revision procedures, the ulnar nerve may be embedded in scar tissue and easily injured. It is vital to have a complete understanding of previous procedures whenever possible.
- A detailed neurologic examination should be well documented before (and after) embarking on any elbow surgery.

Surgical Anatomy

- The medial side of the joint presents direct risk to the ulnar nerve. It must be identified and protected for most approaches to the medial elbow.
    - A notable exception to this rule is in the context of MCL reconstruction. A muscle-splitting "safe zone" has been described by Smith and colleagues (1996). This allows visualization of the coronoid insertion of the MCL without identifying or interfering with the ulnar nerve.
- There is no easy way into the elbow on the medial side. The large flexor-pronator muscle mass origin off the medial epicondyle is difficult to work above or below, and therefore it has been common to take it down subperiosteally, or perform a medial epicondyle osteotomy. More recently, Hotchkiss and others have described approaches that split the flexor-pronator mass (Hotchkiss, 1998).
    - The flexor-pronator mass consists of the pronator teres (PT), flexor carpi radialis (FCR), palmaris longus (PL), flexor digitorum superficialis and profundus, and flexor carpi ulnaris (FCU). All of the muscles except the FCU are median nerve innervated. The FCU has ulnar nerve innervation.
- At the capsular level, the MCL is at risk. It is paramount to preserve this structure. Aggressive traction on an intact MCL can cause ligament attenuation and chronic instability.

- The medial ligaments of the elbow are composed of three bundles. The anterior bundle is isometric and the most important structure for elbow stability against valgus load (Williams et al., 2004).

Pearls

- *If approaching the medial and lateral side of the elbow, we prefer to work in the supine position with the arm on an arm table. The shoulder can be externally and internally rotated to aid in visualization of the medial and lateral sides, respectively.*

Positioning

- The supine or lateral positions can be used for this approach, as previously described for the posterior approach (Procedure 40, Part I).
- If a medial skin incision is planned, the surgery can be done with the patient supine and the arm supinated on a hand table with the shoulder externally rotated. It is important that the patient has adequate shoulder motion for this position.

Pearls

- *In choosing an incision, surgeon preference plays the largest role. If access to the medial and lateral sides of the joint is necessary, separate medial and lateral incisions can be used. Alternatively, a midline posterior incision with generous full-thickness flaps gives access to any muscle interval.*

Portals/Exposures

- A direct medial or posterior skin incision can be used (Fig. 1).
  - If the medial skin incision is chosen, care must be taken to protect superficial sensory branches of the medial cutaneous nerve of the forearm.
  - If a posterior skin incision is used, a full-thickness flap is carefully developed at the level of the triceps fascia. The medial epicondyle and olecranon are used as landmarks. Usually, the ulnar nerve can be palpated proximal to the cubital tunnel.

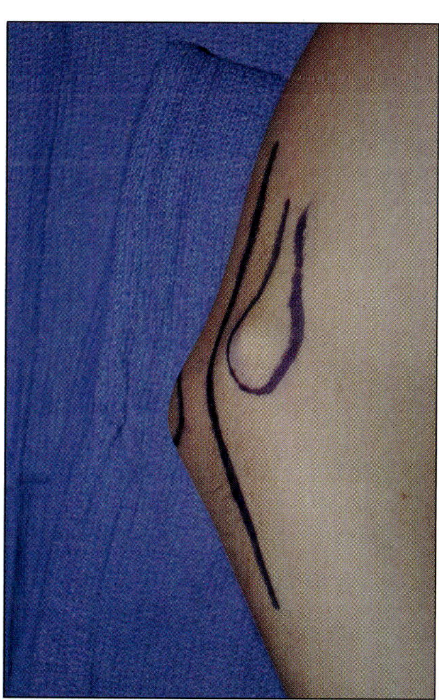

FIGURE 1

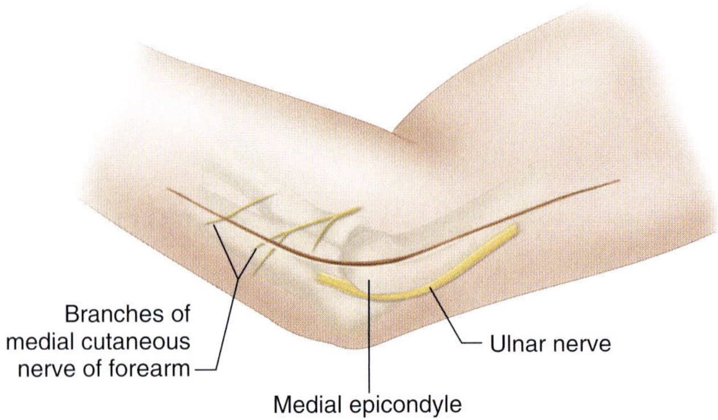

FIGURE 2

- A long skin incision is based on the course of the nerve crossing the elbow just posterior to the medial epicondyle (Fig. 2).
- The ulnar nerve is identified, and protected with a vessel loop or Penrose drain for the duration of the surgery.

Pearls

- *The proximal dissection of the brachialis must remain subperiosteal to protect the overlying median nerve and brachial artery.*
- *The morbidity from dividing the anterior half of the flexor-pronator mass is minimal if a secure soft tissue repair is performed. Core sutures can be utilized, and the tissue is generally substantial. If concerns exist, then drill holes or suture anchors can be used to augment the repair.*

Pitfalls

- *Excessive traction on the divided distal anterior half of the flexor-pronator mass can cause median nerve injury. If more distal exposure is required, an alternate approach is necessary.*

Procedure

Step 1

- The internervous plane between the FCU and FCR is identified and developed. If the PL exists (80–90%), then the plane is between the FCU and PL.
  - This interval can be recognized by perforating vessels that enter the fascia between these two muscles.
- Proximally, the supracondylar ridge is identified and the brachialis is dissected subperiosteally from its medial border off of the anterior humerus and joint capsule.
- The distal interval between FCU and FCR (or PL) is further developed to the level of the joint capsule.
  - The PL, FCR, and PT are identified and and elevated off the supracondylar ridge, leaving a cuff of tissue for later reattachment. The distal end is tagged with a suture for later identification and repair (Fig. 3). Keeping this dissection anterior to the FCU tendon ensures preservation of the MCL.
  - Deep dissection shows an excellent view of the coronoid process. The anterior bundle of the MCL is protected under the FCU tendon. The flexor-pronator mass must be securely repaired with suture anchors or drill holes at the end of the procedure.

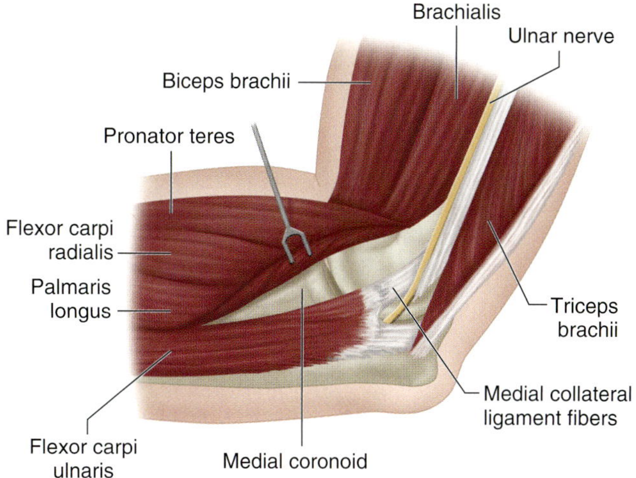

FIGURE 3

Controversies

- Many alternate deep dissections have been described, including complete flexor-pronator takedown, medial epicondyle osteotomy, and takedown of the posterior half of the flexor-pronator mass (FCU and flexor digitorum profundus). Regardless of the chosen method of deep dissection, the principles are unchanged: Protect and preserve the MCL and perform a secure repair of divided structures.

Step 2

- An anteromedial capsulotomy or capsulectomy is performed. Care is taken to remain anterior, ensuring preservation of the MCL.
- Access to the joint, trochlea, and coronoid is now obtained.
  - If planning an open reduction and internal fixation of the coronoid, care is taken to preserve the MCL, which is usually intact and inserting on the fracture fragment. After reduction, a medial plate can be applied or, alternatively, a back-to-front screw can be used to secure the coronoid. We use an anterior cruciate ligament guide and cannulated screw system if the fragment is large enough.
  - If planning MCL reconstruction, the dissection is taken posteriorly superficial to the capsule, exposing the origin and insertion of the anterior bundle of the MCL.

Step 3

- Closure involves secure repair of the anterior portion of the flexor-pronator mass (PL, FCU, and PT) using core sutures.
- The ulnar nerve is inspected for any evidence of injury. The decision to transpose the ulnar nerve is made according to surgeon preference.
  - We see no reason to transpose the nerve in a patient who has no nerve symptoms. (If medial or posteromedial hardware is used on the humerus, then we do routinely transpose the nerve.)
  - We routinely transpose the ulnar nerve when performing contracture release, and attempting to gain elbow flexion.

- Subcutaneous tissue and skin are closed according to surgeon preference.

Postoperative Care and Expected Outcomes

- Postoperative care is directed by the surgery performed and not the approach. Medial repair should be secure enough that it does not limit early range of motion.
- As for all elbow surgery, stiffness is common and early range of motion should be encouraged when possible.

Evidence

Hotchkiss R. Compass Universal Hinge: Surgical Technique. Memphis, TN: Smith and Nephew, 1998.

This text presented Hotchkiss' original description of the over-the-top approach to the medial elbow.

Smith GR, Altchek DW, Pagnani MJ, Keeley JR. A muscle-splitting approach to the ulnar collateral ligament of the elbow: neuroanatomy and operative technique. Am J Sports Med. 1996;24:575-80.

This anatomic and clinical study described and tested the muscle-splitting "safe zone" of the ulnar collateral ligament of the elbow. This has allowed for anatomic reconstruction with minimal dissection.

Williams RJ 3rd, Urquhart ER, Altchek DW. Medial collateral ligament tears in the throwing athlete. Instr Course Lect. 2004;53:579-86.

The authors presented an extensive review of the medial elbow in the throwing athlete, including ligamentous anatomy and biomechanics of the medial collateral ligament of the elbow.

PROCEDURE 40

Arthroscopy of the Elbow: Setup and Portals

Julie E. Adams and Scott P. Steinmann

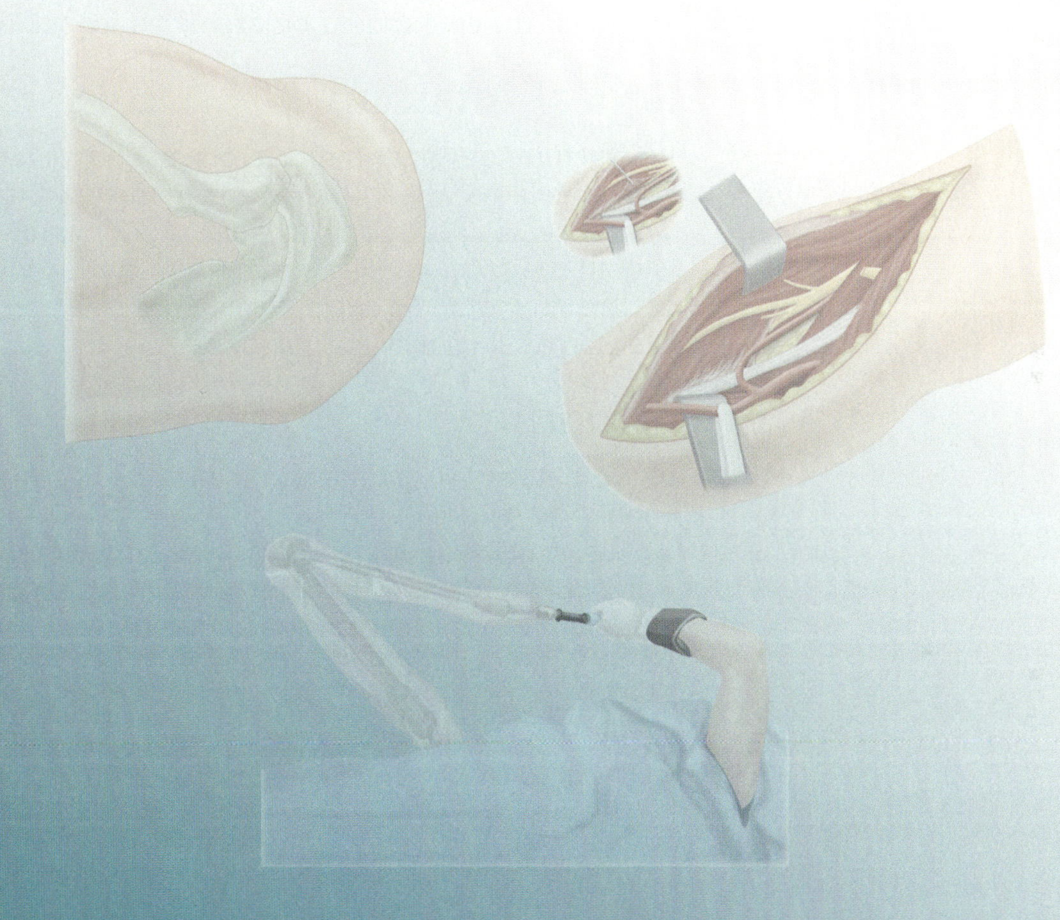

Pitfalls

- *Prior ulnar nerve transposition is not necessarily a contraindication to elbow arthroscopy, but requires caution and exact identification of the ulnar nerve, usually with a small incision.*
- *Ultrasound can also be used to localize and mark the course of the ulnar nerve prior to surgery; this should be done in the operating room with the elbow in flexion and extension. As typical in ultrasound, accuracy is dependent upon the skill and experience of the ultrasonographer.*

Controversies

- Arthroscopy of the elbow is a challenging procedure with a risk of injury to several neurovascular structures about the elbow.
- Injury to each of the susceptible nerves about the elbow has been described in the literature.

Pitfalls

- *Free access to the elbow is essential. Draping and positioning must allow 360° access to the joint, providing room for the surgeon's hands and the arthroscope.*

Indications

- Elbow arthroscopy can be indicated for treatment of elbow arthritis, stiffness, instability, osteochondral defects, fractures, and tendonitis and for débridement of a septic joint.

Examination/Imaging

- A careful physical examination and history should be taken to document previous elbow trauma or surgery, which may have distorted the anatomy.
- The ulnar nerve should be examined for subluxation.

Surgical Anatomy

- Structures at risk at the anterolateral portal include the radial nerve and the posterior antebrachial nerve.
- The median nerve is an average of 22 mm away from the anteromedial portal (Lindenfeld, 1990).
- Care should be taken to identify the ulnar nerve and ensure that it does not subluxate.

Positioning

- The patient is positioned in the lateral decubitus position (Fig. 1A).
- The arm is secured in a dedicated armholder.
- It is useful to "airplane" the bed slightly toward the surgeon.
- The elbow should be positioned just slightly higher than the shoulder.
- The arm should hang free, allowing access free access to the elbow (Fig. 1B).

Portals/Exposures

- Anterior portals (Fig. 2)
  - The anterolateral portal is just anterior to the sulcus between the capitellum and the radial head.
  - The anteromedial portal is established using an inside-out technique as described in Step 2. This portal usually lies approximately 1 cm distal and 1 cm anterior to the medial epicondyle.
  - A proximal anterolateral retraction portal may be established about 2 cm proximal to the lateral epicondyle.

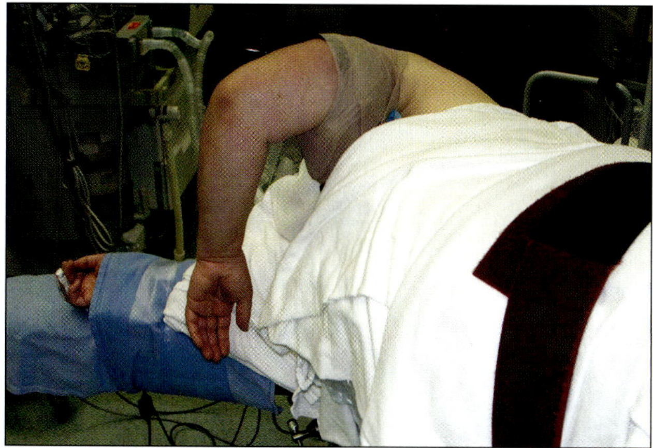

A

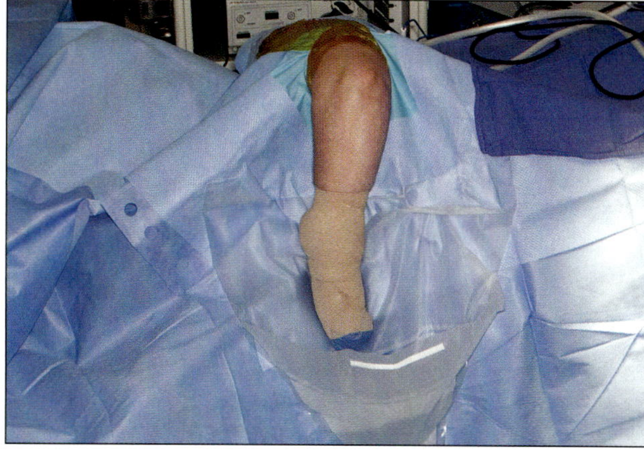

B

FIGURE 1

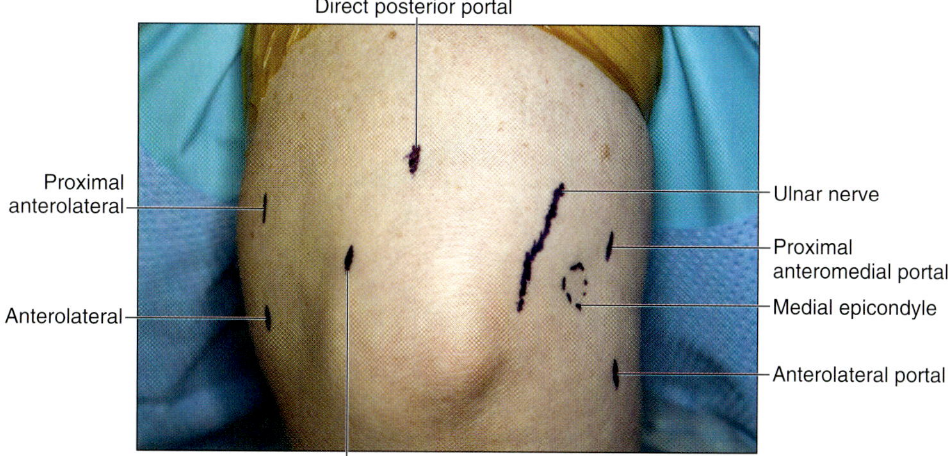

FIGURE 2

Equipment

- A conforming inflatable beanbag is useful under the patient to facilitate stable positioning.
- A dedicated armholder is used. This should support the arm proximal to the cubital fossa rather than putting pressure on this area, which can push soft tissue structures, such as neurovascular structures, into the joint.

Controversies

- Some authors prefer a supine or prone position.

- Posterior portals (see Fig. 2)
  - The posterolateral portal is used for visualization. It is at the lateral joint line level with the tip of the olecranon.
  - The direct posterior portal is a working portal made through the triceps 2–3 cm proximal to the tip of the olecranon. For this portal, the incision must be made down to bone through the thick triceps.
  - Retraction portals, if needed, may be placed 2 cm proximal to the direct posterior portal, situated either slightly medially or laterally.

Procedure

Step 1: Joint Distention

- The joint is distended with 20–30 ml of saline.
  - The fluid is introduced via an 18-gauge needle through the "soft spot": the center of a triangle

formed by the olecranon process, the lateral epicondyle, and the radial head.
- Fluid distention makes entry into the joint easier to achieve, and capsular distention pushes neurovascular structures away from the joint.

- Portal sites are established according to the order preferred by the surgeon; the procedure described below is the author's preference.

Step 2: Anterior Joint Arthroscopy

- The anterolateral portal is established first, just anterior to the sulcus between the capitellum and the radial head.
- Next, the anteromedial portal is established utilizing an inside-out technique with direct visualization.
  - The arthroscope is removed and the blunt trocar is replaced through the sheath.
  - The trocar is pushed directly across the joint until it tents the skin overlying the medial side of the elbow. The skin is then incised over this region and the trocar pushed through the remaining soft tissue.
  - A cannula may be placed over the trocar on the medial side, and the trocar is pulled back into the joint and out the lateral side.
- Retraction portals are established as needed.
- Arthroscopy proceeds with visualization with the arthroscope in the lateral side and the medial portal as the working portal; the working and viewing portals are swapped midway through the procedure.

Step 3: Posterior Joint Arthroscopy

- After the anterior joint arthroscopy is completed, attention is turned to the posterior portion of the elbow.

Pearls

- *Palpable landmarks and the intended portal sites must be marked out prior to insufflation of the joint, which may obscure landmarks (see Fig. 2).*
- *Portals should be established with the incision through the skin only, followed by blunt dissection to the capsule to avoid injury to neurovascular structures.*

Pitfalls

- *Suction tubing should be placed to gravity only, in order to prevent accidently shaving objects that may be sucked into the shaver.*

Controversies

- Some arthroscopists make the anterolateral portal first; others prefer to start with the anteromedial portal. Order of establishing portals is best determined by individual surgeon experience and preference and the pathology to be addressed.

Pearls

- *Portal sites are made by incising the skin only with a blade. Blunt dissection to the capsule is performed to avoid nerve injury. The blunt trocar and sleeve are then placed into the joint, and exchanged for the arthroscope.*

Instrumentation

- Arthroscopy is best performed with a standard 4-mm 30° arthroscope. A 2.7-mm arthroscope can be used, but in most cases the joint can accommodate a 4-mm arthroscope.
- Retractors such as a Howarth elevator or a large blunt Steinmann pin make the procedure easier and safer by enhancing visualization and retracting structures out of harm's way.
- Standard arthroscopic shavers and burrs are used; arthroscopic instruments may be procedure-specific devices (Fig. 3).
- Either a pump system or gravity may be used for inflow of saline; gravity systems are useful to limit pressure, which may cause fluid extravasation.

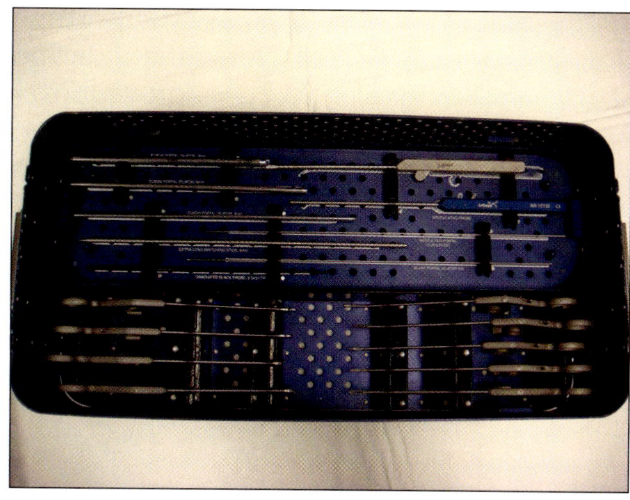

FIGURE 3

> **PITFALLS**
>
> - *As with any procedure about the elbow, risk of neurovascular injury is a real concern. In one series from the Mayo Clinic, 50 complications were seen following 473 elbow arthroscopies performed for various indications (Kelly et al., 2001). The most common complication was prolonged wound drainage; however, other complications included infection, nerve injury, and contractures. Although no permanent nerve injuries were seen in this series, injuries of each of the susceptible nerves about the elbow joint have been described. Careful examination preoperatively and attention to anatomy intraoperatively, in conjuction with appropriate portal placement, can help prevent injury.*

- Again, it is crucial to verify the position of the ulnar nerve. If necessary, a small incision may be made to confirm the location and to retract the nerve as needed.
- The posterolateral portal is the initial viewing portal. It is made with the elbow at 90° of flexion
- The direct posterior portal is initally the working portal.
- The posterior fossa is filled with fat and fibrous tissue, which must be débrided to gain a view. The shaver can be placed down to the bone and turned on to clear debris so that a view may be gained.
- After adequate visualization is achieved, pathology may be addressed as indicated; it is critical to respect the position of the ulnar nerve along the posteromedial capsule.

Step 4: Closure

- After the procedure is completed, range of motion is assessed and the portals are closed in the standard fashion with 3-0 nylon or Prolene sutures.
- A sterile compressive dressing is applied.
- A long-arm splint is placed posteriorly to immobilize the arm in full extension.

Postoperative Care and Expected Outcomes

- The arm is elevated overnight in the "Statue of Liberty" position.
- On postoperative day 1, the splint is removed and the neurovascular status is evaluated, with particular attention to the radial, median, and ulnar nerves.

- The postoperative protocol varies depending upon the indications. Unless structural reconstructive procedures were performed, in general, full active range of motion is initiated with no limitations on use of the arm.

Evidence

Adams JE, Steinmann SP. Nerve injuries about the elbow. J Hand Surg [Am]. 2006;31:303-13.

This review article detailed the anatomy and nerves around the elbow and how to avoid the nerves. (Level IV evidence)

Kelly EW, Morrey BF, O'Driscoll SW. Complications of elbow arthroscopy. J Bone Joint Surg [Am]. 2001;83:25-34.

This retrospective series documented complications in elbow arthroscopy among 473 patients treated for a variety of conditions. (Level III evidence)

Lindenfeld TN. Medial approach in elbow arthroscopy. Am J Sports Med. 1990;18(4):413-17.

This cadaveric study of 6 elbows investigated the proximity of neurovascular structures to portal sites and suggests a large margin of safety for the anteromedial portal site. (Level III evidence)

Savoie FH III. Guidelines for becoming an expert elbow arthroscopist. Arthroscopy. 2007;23:1237-40.

This expert opinion article presented indications, contraindications, and techniques of elbow arthroscopy. (Level IV evidence)

Schubert T, Dubuc JE, Barbier O. A review of 24 cases of elbow arthroscopy using the DASH questionnaire. Acta Orthop Belg. 2007;73:700-3.

These authors reviewed the results of elbow arthroscopy used to treat a variety of conditions. Patient outcomes and DASH scores were examined, as were complications. Conclusions were that arthroscopy is a safe and effective treatment option. (Level III evidence)

Steinmann SP. Elbow arthroscopy: where are we now? Arthroscopy. 2007;23:1231-36.

This expert opinion article presented past, present, and future considerations in elbow arthroscopy, and tips and techniques. (Level IV evidence)

SECTION II

Elbow

Elbow Arthroscopy

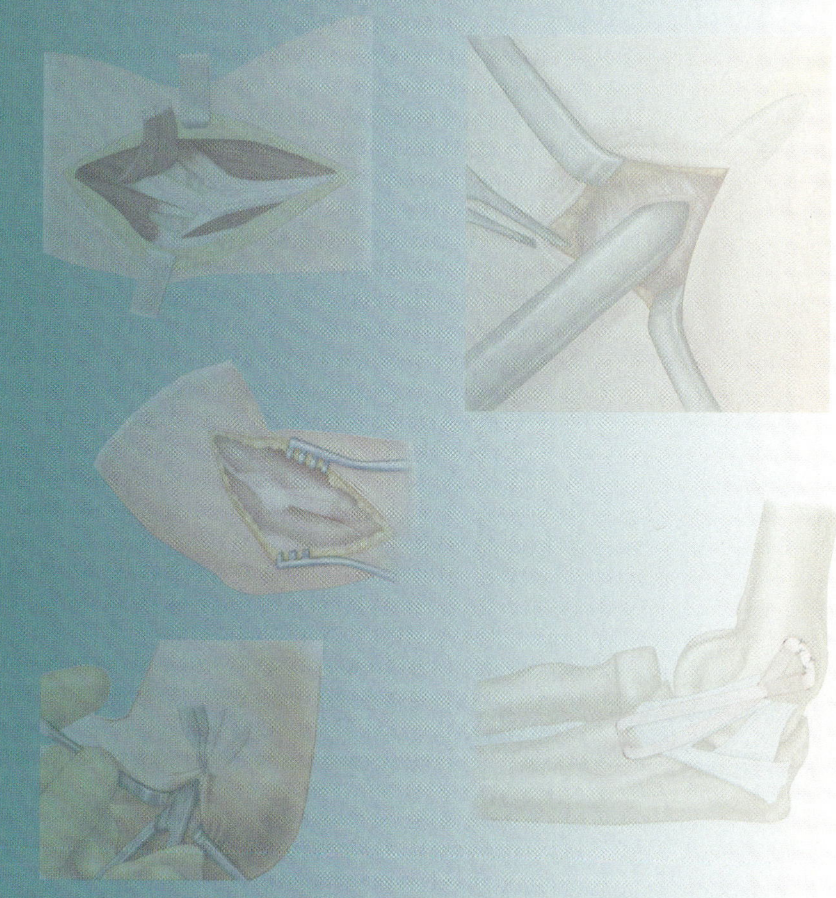

PROCEDURE 41

Elbow Arthritis and Stiffness: Open Treatment

Julie E. Adams and Scott P. Steinmann

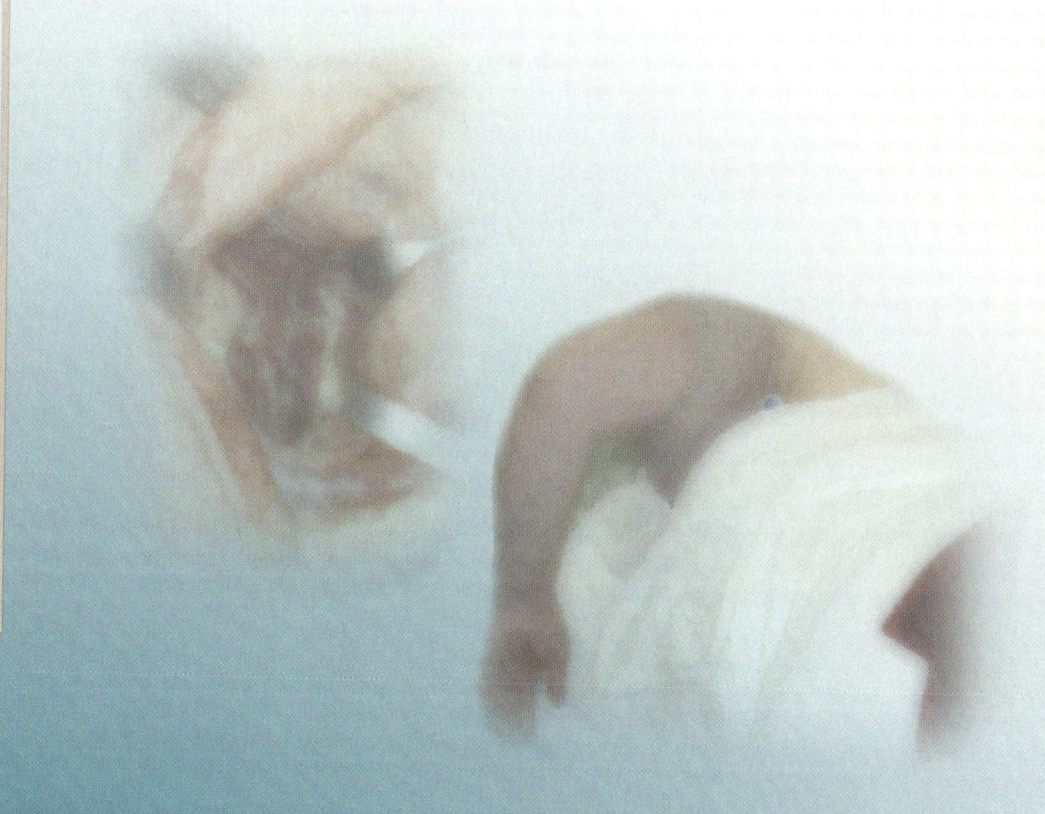

Pitfalls

- *In older or low-demand patients with severe symptoms and arthritis, total elbow arthroplasty may be an option.*
- *Depending upon the surgeon's skills and experience, arthroscopic treatment may be considered.*

Controversies

- Decision to perform open versus arthroscopic treatment is based upon the experience and discretion of the surgeon.
- In general, the authors use open débridements in the settings of prior fractures in which the hardware is to be removed, or other prior operative procedures in which the neuroanatomy is altered, or the patient is at higher risk of injury with an arthroscopic procedure.
  - If a prior surgical procedure was performed on the lateral side of the elbow, the radial nerve might be adherent and scarring of the lateral joint capsule may be present, making arthroscopic débridement risky.
  - Additionally, if prior surgery involved exposure of the ulnar nerve with possible scarring or heterotopic bone formation, then if motion is restored to the elbow, full release of the ulnar nerve is best done through an open approach.
- Nevertheless, open and arthroscopic procedures have similar clinical results that seem durable, and the existing literature does not provide support for choosing one procedure over the other; surgeon training and experience are important considerations in addition to the needs of the particular patient's situation.

Indications

- Symptomatic posttraumatic arthritis, osteoarthritis, or inflammatory arthritis of the elbow
- Symptomatic elbow stiffness

Examination/Imaging

- Routine plain film radiographs are usually all that is needed. However, computed tomography scanning with three-dimensional reconstructions is very helpful to define osteophytes and loose bodies.
- Range of motion is documented prior to the procedure. Figure 1 shows the preoperative extension (Fig. 1A) and flexion (Fig. 1B) in a 44-year-old male with significant elbow stiffness after radial head replacement for terrible triad injury.
- The status of the ulnar nerve, as well as the other important major peripheral nerves that cross the elbow, is documented prior to the procedure.
- Stability of the elbow is confirmed.

Surgical Anatomy

- Given the complex neuroanatomy about the elbow, a number of nerves are at risk.

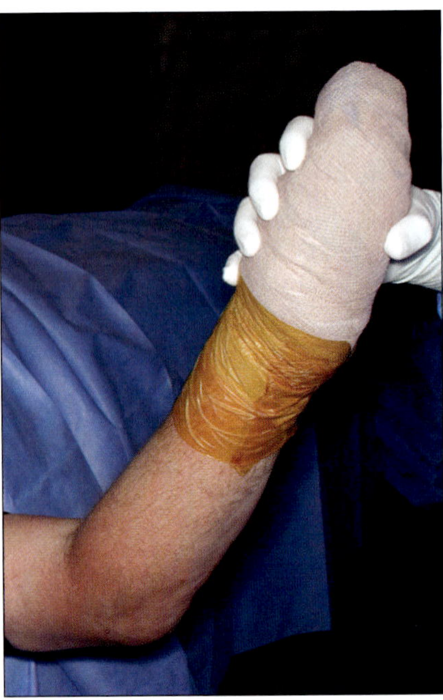

A

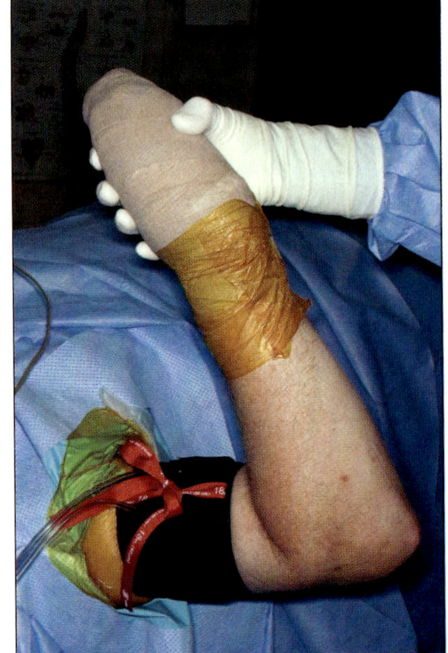

B

FIGURE 1

Treatment Options

- Consideration of splinting programs to increase motion, particularly in the posttraumatic setting, may be considered.
- Arthroscopic débridement or capsular release is an alternative.

- Laceration of a cutaneous nerve may lead to a troublesome numb patch or a painfull neuroma; injury to a major peripheral nerve can be devasting. Elevation of full-thickness flaps can help prevent this injury to cutaneous nerves.
  - The lateral antebrachial cutaneous nerve exits the brachial fascia approximately 3 cm proximal to the lateral epicondyle and then passes between the brachialis and biceps muscle, giving off anterior and posterior branches.
  - The medial antebrachial cutaneous nerve pierces the deep fascia of the mid or distal arm to become subcutaneous, and gives off anterior and posterior branches proximal to the medial epicondyle. The posterior branch of the medial antebrachial cutaneous nerve crosses over the ulnar nerve at a highly variable point above or below the medial epicondyle.
- The ulnar nerve travels subcutaneously along the medial aspect of the arm between the coracobrachialis laterally and the long and medial heads of the triceps posteriorly. The nerve then travels along the medial head of the triceps toward the medial epicondyle. It passes posterior to the epicondyle through the cubital tunnel; the posterior branch of the medial antebrachial cutaneous nerve crosses over the ulnar nerve between 6 cm proximal and 4 cm distal to the medial epicondyle.
- The median nerve travels lateral to the brachial artery and, at the elbow joint, it crosses anterior to the brachial artery to lie medial in the cubial fossa, where it is covered by the lacertus fibrosis. It then dips beneath the two heads of the pronator teres and travels through the forearm upon the dorsal surface of the flexor digitorum superficialis, which it supplies.
- The radial nerve travels along the posterior aspect of the humerus from about a quarter to halfway down the humerus. It emerges from the spiral groove 10 cm proximal to the lateral epicondyle and lies in close proximity to the humeral shaft. It traverses the lateral intermuscular septum to travel anterior to the lateral column of the humerus. The inferior lateral brachial cutaneous and posterior antebrachial cutaneous nerves arise from the radial nerve before it passes through the lateral intermuscular septum.
  - After passing through the lateral intermuscular septum, the radial nerve travels over the lateral edge of the brachialis muscle, providing muscular

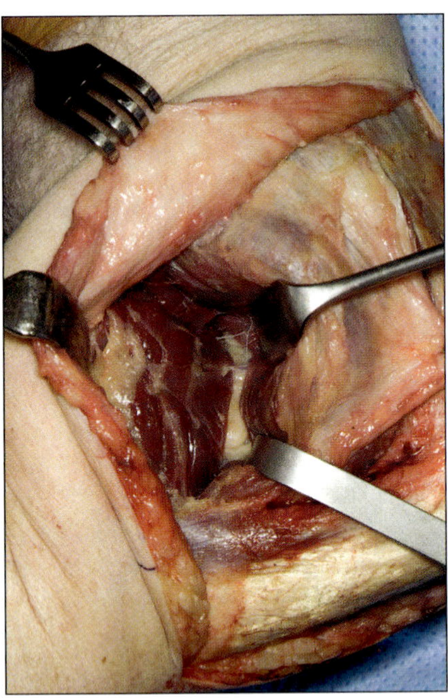

FIGURE 2

branches to the brachialis and extensor carpi radialis longus (ECRL) proximal to the elbow joint. The radial nerve then lies deep to the brachioradialis, extensor carpi radialis brevis (ECRB), and ECRL muscles and passes directly over the annular ligament (Fig. 2).

- At the level of the radial head, fibrous bands tether the radial nerve in close proximity to the radial head. The radial nerve bifurcates at this level, and gives off a deep branch that becomes the posterior interosseous nerve, and the superficial branch continues as the superficial radial nerve. Innervation to the ECRB arises at the level of the bifurcation of the nerve and is variable. The superficial branch of the radial nerve initially lies deep to the brachioradialis and superficial to the ECRL until it emerges from the lateral edge of the brachioradialis to travel subcutaneously to supply cutaneous sensation to the dorsoradial aspect of the hand.

Controversies

- The decision regarding position is based upon the experience and preference of the surgeon. We prefer a supine position, which is described in this section. Others prefer lateral or prone postioning, or supine with an armboard.

Positioning

- The patient is positioned in the supine position on the operating room table.
- Usually an arm table or hand table is not necessary; the arm may be placed across the chest over a bump.

- The arm should be prepped and draped to the axilla, with use of a sterile tourniquet.

Portals/Exposures

- Exposure for open débridement depends in large part upon the experience of the surgeon, the location of pathology, and the need for addional procedures such as ulnar nerve decompression at the elbow.
- A posterior utilitarian approach can allow access to both the medial and lateral aspects of the elbow if the surgeon raises full-thickness skin flaps.
- Alternatively, separate medial and/or lateral incisions may be made.

Pearls

- *To minimize risk of cutaneous nerve injury, a direct posterior incision over the olecranon and ulna with careful elevation of full-thickness flaps is recommended for open procedures.*
- *Use of full-thickness flaps helps prevent soft tissue healing complications and injury to cutaneous nerves.*

Pitfalls

- *If full-thickness skin flaps are not raised, difficulty with healing of the skin may be experienced.*

Procedure

Step 1

- Medially, the ulnar nerve is decompressed. The intermuscular septum is excised. The medial side of the triceps is elevated and the posterior capsular and joint are addressed.
- Osteophytes along the tip of the olecranon and olecranon fossa are excised. The olecranon fossa may be débrided with a burr or a trephine.
- Through the defect in the olecranon fossa, the tip of coronoid may be excised and the capsule released. The thickened and fibrotic capsule seen in osteoarthritis or posttraumatic arthritis is excised anteriorly and posteriorly.

Pitfalls

- *With either the posterior or the medial/lateral approach, it is important preserve the collateral ligaments.*

Step 2

- Using the "medial column approach," dissection proceeds along the supracondylar ridge, with elevation of the anterior muscles subperiosteally.
- Distally, the flexor-pronator muscles are divided in line with the fibers, preserving a cuff of tissue on the supracondylar ridge and a 1.5-cm portion of the FCU tendon to facilitate later repair.
- The dissection proceeds down to the capsule, which can be excised from proximal to distal and osteophytes removed.

Step 3

- A lateral approach can be used with elevation of the full-thickness flap from posteriorly, or a separate lateral incision may be made.
- The dissection proceeds along the supracondylar ridge of the humerus.

Pitfalls

- *The radial nerve is protected during the procedure (see Fig. 2).*

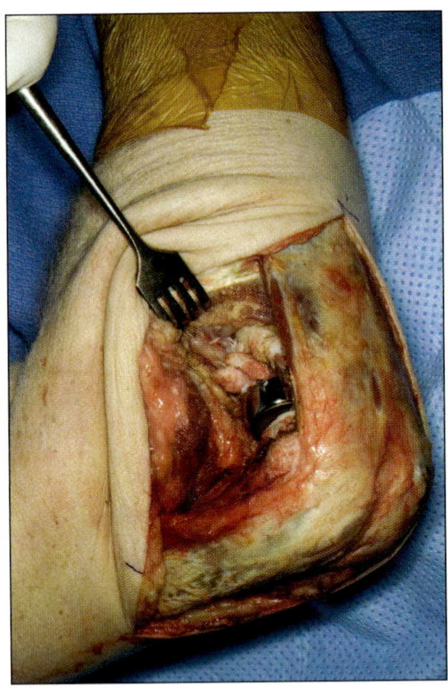

FIGURE 3

- Proximally, the origins of the brachioradialis and ECRL are elevated off the humerus, exposing the anterior elbow joint and giving access to the anterior capsule, which is excised (Fig. 3).
- Distally, the dissection can be continued in a muscle-splitting fashion between the ECRB and ECRL.
- Loose bodies and osteophytes are removed.
- Posteriorly, the triceps is elevated and the posterior capsule released and osteophytes removed.

Step 4

- After the procedure is completed, motion is assessed prior to leaving the operating room.
- It is sometimes useful to photograph the range of motion in flexion (Fig. 4A) and extension (Fig. 4B) so that the patient can visualize the range of motion achieved intraoperatively and hold this as a goal.
- Wounds should be closed in layers; staples may be used for the skin.
- A sterile compressive dressing is applied.
- A long-arm splint in full extension is applied. The plaster should be placed posteriorly.

Postoperative Care and Expected Outcomes

- The arm is elevated in the "Statue of Liberty" position overnight.

Controversies

- Heterotopic ossification prophylaxis, consisting of indomethacin 75 mg three times daily for 6 weeks, is initiated for patients with osteoarthritis or posttraumatic arthritis.
- If the patient has had prior heterotopic ossification, for which this procedure is being done, some use external beam irradiation with 700 cGy of radiation in a single dose up to 24 hours prior to the procedure or within 72 hours postprocedure.
- Splinting protocols, such as splints that may be adjusted from full extension to full flexion, are useful in most cases. The patient usually alternates hourly between the extremes of motion achieved at the time of surgery.
- Continuous passive motion (CPM) may be initiated using a CPM device with or without a nerve block; however, in the authors' experience, it is not usually necessary. In patients who are unable to practice motion on their own or in those with severe contractures, it may be of benefit, although a consensus regarding the indications and need for CPM is lacking.

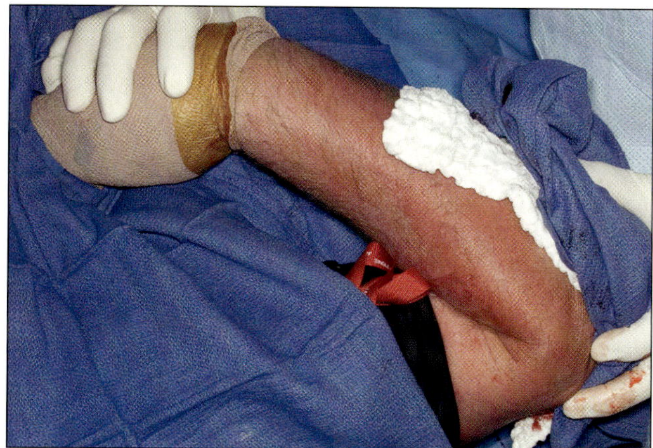

A

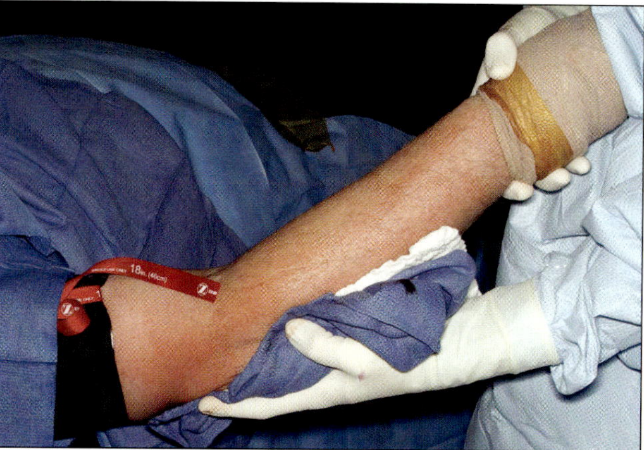

B

FIGURE 4

- On postoperative day 1, the splint is removed and the neurovascular status is evaluated, with particular attention to the radial, median, and ulnar nerves. Full active range of motion is then initiated.
- No limitations are placed on use of the arm.

Evidence

Antuña SA, Morrey BF, Adams RA, O'Driscoll SW. Ulnohumeral arthroplasty for primary degenerative arthritis of the elbow: long-term outcome and complications. J Bone Joint Surg [Am]. 2002;84:2168-73.

The authors evaluated long-term results and complications following ulnohumeral arthroplasty for primary osteoarthritis of the elbow. Forty-five patients underwent the procedure and were evaluated at average of 80 months postoperatively. Mean flexion-extension improved an average of 22°, and the Mayo Clinic Elbow Performance (MEP) score was excellent in 26 elbows. Because of several cases of ulnar nerve symptoms requiring subsequent operative procedures, the authors recommended care in evaluating the ulnar nerve preoperatively, with a low threshold to consider prophylactic decompression in those with severe motion loss, those with any preoperative symptoms, and those likely to require manipulation under anesthesia. (Grade A recommendation)

Cohen AP, Redden JF, Stanley D. Treatment of osteoarthritis of the elbow: a comparison of open and arthroscopic debridement. Arthroscopy. 2000;16:701-6.

In this series, the authors compared outcomes following arthroscopic débridement versus open débridement of the elbow for osteoarthritis, using the Outerbridge-Kashiwagi procedure and the arthroscopic modification. Both groups demonstrated improved range of elbow flexion, decrease in pain, and a high level of patient satisfaction. Increases in elbow extension, although improved in both groups, were more modest. Neither procedure included a capsular release. Comparison between the open and arthroscopic procedures demonstrated that the open procedure might be more effective in improving flexion, while the arthroscopic procedure seemed to provide more pain relief. No differences between overall effectiveness of the two procedures were noted. (Grade A recommendation)

Forster MC, Clark DI, Lunn PG. Elbow osteoarthritis: prognostic indicators in ulnohumeral debridement—the Outerbridge-Kashiwagi procedure. J Shoulder Elbow Surg. 2001;10:557-6.

The authors investigated 44 elbows that underwent ulnohumeral débridement. At mean follow-up of 39 months, 81% of patients were satisfied. Those with preoperative locking had poorer results, while those with ulnar nerve symptoms, severe symptoms, or duration of symptoms less than 2 years tended to do better postoperatively. Average arc of motion increased by 25° postoperatively. (Grade A recommendation)

Oka Y. Debridement arthroplasty for osteoarthrosis of the elbow: 50 patients followed mean 5 years. Acta Orthop Scand. 2000;71:185-90.

The author described outcomes in 50 elbows following débridement for osteoarthritis in athletes and laborers. At average follow-up of 59.5 months, pain relief and range of motion improvement were durable. Recurrence of osteophytes was noted; however, the symptoms were minimal. (Grade A recommendation)

Phillips NJ, Ali A, Stanley D. Treatment of primary degenerative arthritis of the elbow by ulnohumeral arthroplasty: a long-term follow-up. J Bone Joint Surg [Br]. 2003;85:347-50.

The authors reported on 20 ulnohumeral arthroplasties for osteoarthritis at mean follow-up of 75 months. Good or excellent results were obtained in 85% according to the DASH score and 65% according to the MEP score. Range of motion improved by 20°, and in 80% the results were durable over the follow-up time period. (Grade A recommendation)

Sarris I, Riano FA, Goebel F, Goitz RJ, Sotereanos DG. Ulnohumeral arthroplasty: results in primary degenerative arthritis of the elbow. Clin Orthop Relat Res. 2004;(420):190-3.

The authors presented results following ulnohumeral arthroplasty in 17 patients with osteoarthritis at an average follow-up of 36 months. Of these patients, 15 noted complete pain relief. Mean range of motion was 14–188°, with no major complications noted. (Grade A recommendation)

Tashjian RZ, Wolf JM, Ritter M, Weiss AP, Green A. Functional outcomes and general health status after ulnohumeral arthroplasty for primary degenerative arthritis of the elbow. J Shoulder Elbow Surg. 2006;15:357-66.

This paper presented the authors' patient-derived functional outcome measures following ulnohumeral arthroplasty for degenerative arthritis via an open posterior approach at mean follow-up of 85 months. Range of motion improved an average of 16° in the flexion-extension arc and 35° in pronation-supination. DASH scores were on average 9.75, MEP scores averaged 83, and Hospital for Special Surgery scores averaged 70. Patients described 11 elbows as painless, 4 as painful with use, and 3 as painful at rest. (Grade A recommendation)

Wada T, Isogai S, Ishii S, Yamashita T. Débridement arthroplasty for primary osteoarthritis of the elbow. J Bone Joint Surg [Am]. 2004;86:233-41.

The authors described outcomes after open débridement for osteoarthritis performed via a posteromedial approach and augmented by a second lateral approach in nine cases. At mean follow-up of 121 months, mean arc of motion was improved by 24°. Eighty-five percent of patients were satisfied with their elbow, and 76% returned to heavy labor occupations. (Grade A recommendation)

PROCEDURE 42

Elbow Arthritis and Stiffness: Arthroscopic Treatment

Julie E. Adams and Scott P. Steinmann

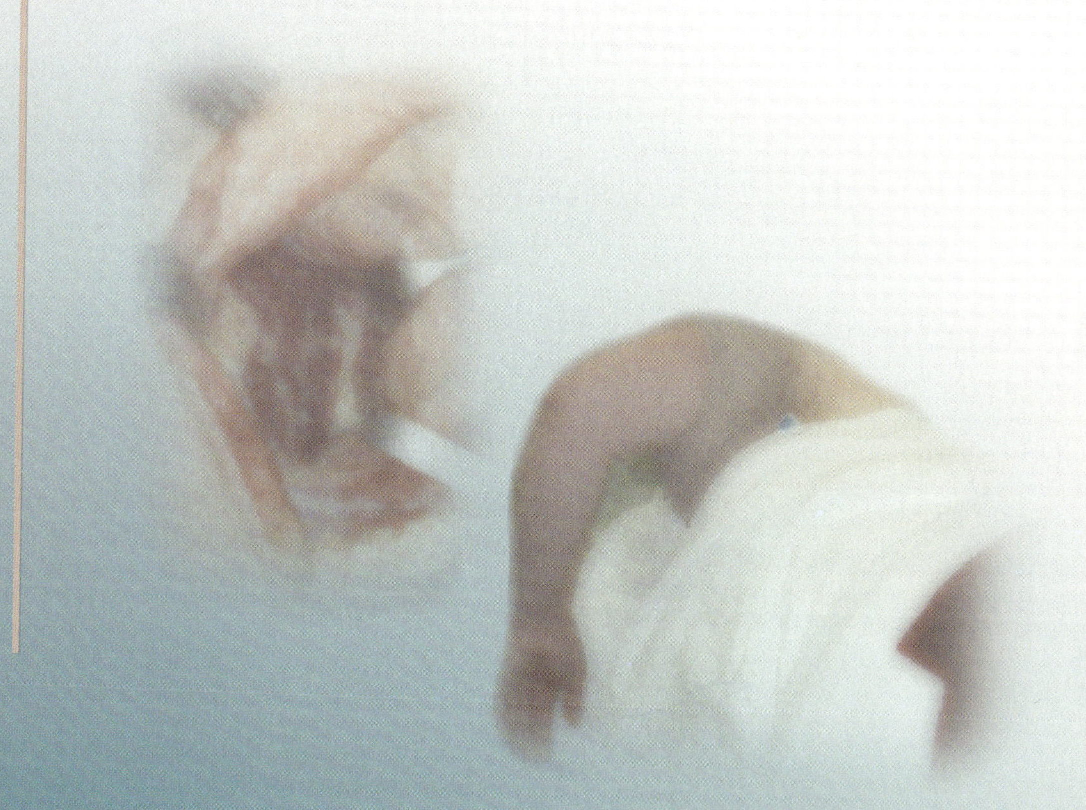

PITFALLS

- *Pain in the midarc of motion that is not associated with mechanical symptoms is suggestive of severe articular changes that may not respond to arthroscopic débridement.*
- *Patients with severe articular changes and/or instability may not respond to arthroscopic débridement.*

Controversies

- Decision to perform open versus arthroscopic treatment is based upon the experience and discretion of the surgeon.

Treatment Options

- Open contracture release or débridement can be considered.
- In older or low-demand patients with severe symptoms and joint destruction, total elbow arthroplasty may be an option.

Indications

- Symptomatic posttraumatic arthritis, osteoarthritis, or inflammatory arthritis of the elbow
- Functionally limiting contracture of the elbow

Examination/Imaging

- Routine plain film radiographs are usually all that is needed. However, magnetic resonance imaging or computed tomography scanning may be useful to define osteophytes and loose bodies.
- Range of motion is documented prior to the procedure.
- The status of the ulnar nerve, as well as the other important major peripheral nerves that cross the elbow, is investigated prior to the procedure. The position of the ulnar nerve and the presence of a subluxating ulnar nerve should be documented preoperatively.
- Stability of the elbow is confirmed.

Surgical Anatomy

- Anatomy for this procedure is discussed in Procedure 42.
- A number of major neurovascular structures and cutaneous nerves are at risk about the elbow. Injury to each of these susceptible structures has been described in the literature.

Positioning

- The patient is positioned on the operating room table in the lateral decubitus position.
- It is helpful to place an inflatable beanbag on the table, so that when the patient is placed on his side, the beanbag can be conformed to the patient and inflated, providing secure positioning. Likewise, safety straps are useful to secure the patient.
- The down arm is either tucked or preferentially secured to an armboard, which is placed in a position of forward elevation away from the body and oriented toward the head and the anesthetist.
- The operative arm is placed in a dedicated armholder that allows free access to the elbow.
- The arm may be prepped and draped to the axilla with use of a sterile tourniquet, or a nonsterile

PEARLS

- *It is critical to ensure that the antecubital fossa remains uncompressed and that the arm rests in the holder proximal to the antecubital region.*
- *The arm should be positioned such that the elbow is higher than the shoulder and the hand and forearm are free.*

PITFALLS

- *Placing the arm so that the armholder puts pressure upon the antecubital fossa will limit access to the elbow and will prevent full joint distention. Joint insufflation increases the space available in the joint and expands the fluid inside the capsule, pushing extracapsular neurovascular structures further away from potential harm.*

Equipment

- Inflatable beanbag
- Dedicated armholder

Controversies

- The decision regarding position is based upon the experience and preference of the surgeon. We prefer the lateral decubitus postion, which is described in this section. Supine or prone positioning has also been described.

tourniquet may be applied and the arm secured to the armholder with Coban.

- It is also useful to slightly "airplane" the table away from the surgeon to better position the elbow for optimal access.

Portals/Exposures

- The arm is set up (Fig. 1) and the portal sites and landmarks are marked as noted in Procedure 41.
- Portals for arthroscopic débridement are described in Procedure 41.

Procedure

STEP 1: PREPARATION

- The ulnar nerve should be examined and its location marked; the surgeon should be aware of a subluxating ulnar nerve. If prior surgery has been performed or there is any question of the nerve's location, a small incision may be made to identify and retract the nerve to protect it against inadvertent injury.
- The joint is distended with 20–30 ml of saline introduced via an 18-gauge needle through the "soft spot" (the center of a triangle formed by the olecranon process, the lateral epicondyle, and the radial head) or an intended portal site. Fluid distention makes entry into the joint easier to achieve and pushes the neurovascular structures away from the joint.
- Portal sites and order are established according to the preference and experience of the surgeon and

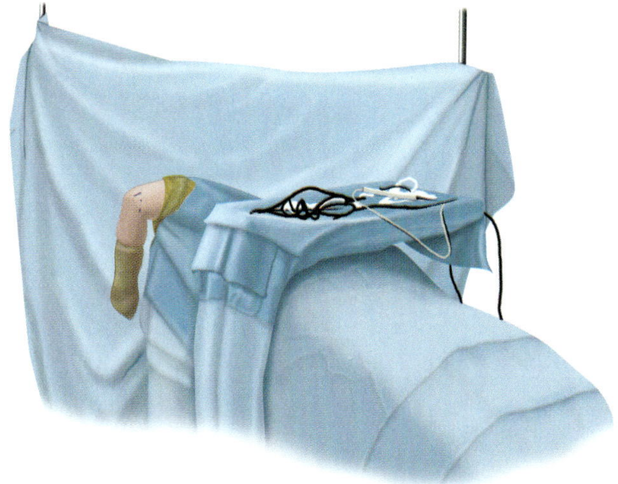

FIGURE 1

Pitfalls

- *Suction should be placed to gravity only, to prevent accidently shaving objects which may be sucked into the shaver.*

Controversies

- As noted previously.

Pearls

- *Depending upon the indications, the technique will vary. For stiffness, patients who lack flexion require addressing the posterior joint; those with lack of extension will require release and débridement anteriorly. Either compartment may be addressed first, depending on the pathology present. It is usually safest to release the posterior joint first, if this will be required, before swelling and fluid extravasation makes this difficult.*
- *Most patients with primary osteoarthritis or posttraumatic arthritis have some degree of joint contracture in addition to osteophyte formation and possibly loose bodies.*

the pathology to be addressed. For example, if the patient lacks flexion preoperatively, posterior work for capsular release is required. Conversely, if extension is a problem, anterior release may be needed. Retraction portals are placed to enhance visualization and to protect structures as needed.

Step 2: Anterior Capsulectomy and Débridement

- If anterior joint work is needed, visualization proceeds by initiating an anterolateral viewing portal.
- A 4.8-mm arthroscopic shaver is introduced through the anteromedial portal with retraction via a proximal anterolateral portal. The shaver is used to débride tissue and improve visualization.
- Loose bodies are removed throughout the procedure as they are visualized (Fig. 2). Arthroscopic graspers are useful for smaller loose bodies, but large loose bodies may be extracted through an enlarged portal using an Alyce clamp or needle driver rather than standard arthroscopic instrumentation. Alternatively, large loose bodies may be burred to an appropriate size for removal through standard portals.
- Bony work should be completed prior to capsulotomy or capsulectomy, as fluid extravasation after the capsule is removed will limit the time that arthroscopy can safely be continued.

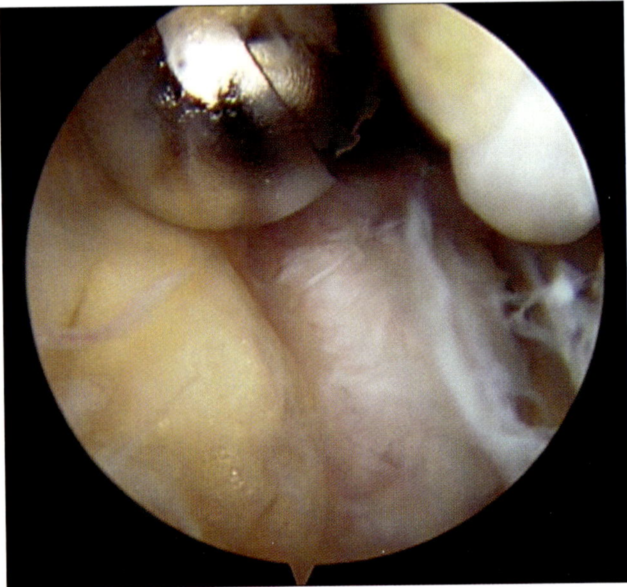

FIGURE 2

Instrumentation/ Implantation

- The standard arthroscopic equipment includes a 4-mm 30° arthroscope. Although a 2.7-mm arthroscope may be used, in most cases, it is not necessary. The standard arthroscopic 3.5- or 4.8-mm shaver and burr are used.
- Retractors such as a Howarth elevator or a large blunt Steinmann pin make the procedure easier and enhance visualization. Commercially available retractors are now available.
- Radiofrequency ablation is useful to control bleeding.
- Arthroscopic grabbers are often needed to retrieve loose bodies.
- Arthroscopic biters are useful to perform a capsulotomy; the capsulectomy may be completed by the shaver once a free edge is obtained.

- Osteophytes are removed with the shaver and burr from the coronoid and radial head fossae (Fig. 3).
- Following completion of the bony débridement (Fig. 4), if capsular release or capsulectomy is required, the anterior capsule is completely resected under direct visualization with the arthroscope in the lateral portal site.
- The anteromedial capsule is stripped off the humerus to expand space in the contracted joint. A variety of Howarth elevators or Steinmann pins may be used for retraction.

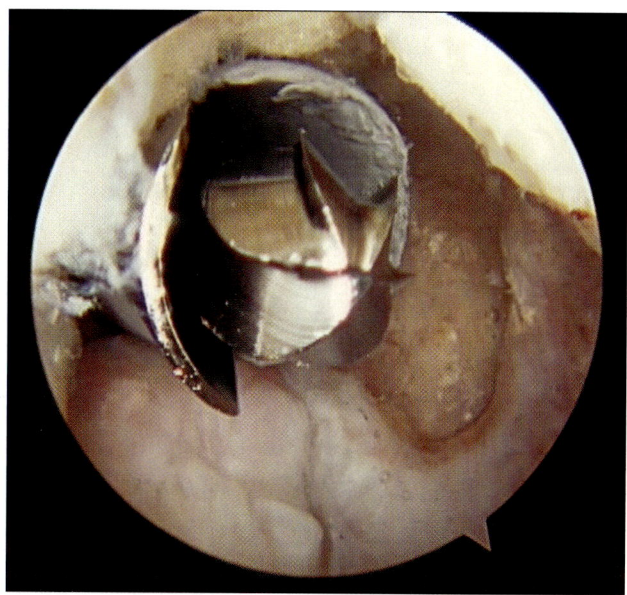

FIGURE 3

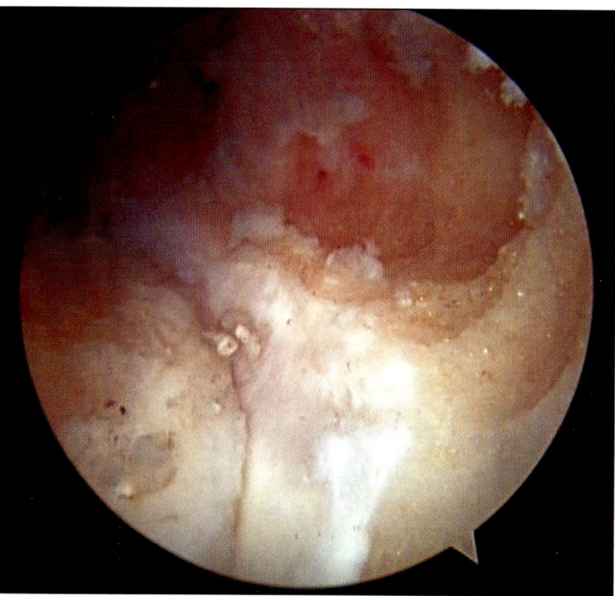

FIGURE 4

- The biter is used to gain a free edge of the anterior capsule, proceeding from medial to lateral and halting when the fat pad anterior to the radial head is encountered.
- The shaver is then used to completely resect the anterior capsule. The arthroscope is then placed in the medial portal and capsulectomy is completed.

PEARLS

- *When addressing the posteromedial capsule, care should be exercised to identify and protect the ulnar nerve (Fig. 5).*

Controversies

- The role of and need for ulnar nerve decompression remains a subject of discussion. Some authors perform ulnar nerve decompression in nearly every case, others peform this only when the patient has preoperative symptoms.

STEP 3: POSTERIOR JOINT DÉBRIDEMENT AND/OR CAPSULOTOMY

- Attention is turned to the posterior aspect of the joint.
- After a posterolateral viewing portal and a direct posterior working portal are created, the shaver is placed in the direct posterior portal and osteophytes are removed from the tip and sides of the olecranon and the rim of the olecranon fossa.
- Patients who lack flexion preoperatively will also require posterolateral and posteromedial capsular releases.
- In general, if a large restoration of motion is anticipated postprocedure, if preoperative ulnar nerve symptoms exist, or if preoperative flexion measures less than 90°, consideration should be given to ulnar nerve decompression or tranposition. This may be achieved via arthroscopic decompression if the surgeon possesses the requisite skill, or an open decompression and/or transposition.

STEP 4: CLOSURE

- After the procedure is completed, motion is assessed prior to leaving the operating room.

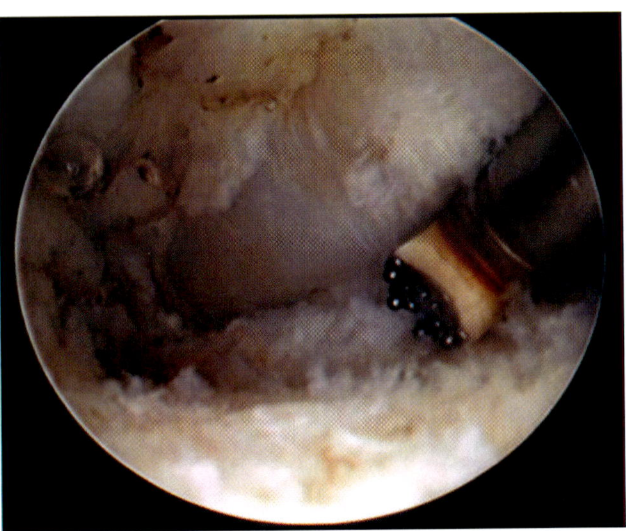

FIGURE 5

- Portals are closed with 3-0 nylon, and a sterile compressive dressing is applied.
- A long-arm splint in full extension is applied with the plaster placed on the posterior surface of the arm.

Controversies

- The role of and type of heterotopic ossification prophylaxis remain subjects of investigation. Certainly heterotopic ossification has been reported after arthroscopy, and seems to be related to intrinsic patient factors that remain poorly understood. We recommend heterotopic ossification prophylaxis, consisting of sustained-release indomethacin 75 mg once daily for 6 weeks, particularly for for patients with osteoarthritis or posttraumatic arthritis.
- Splinting protocols, such as splints that may be adjusted from full extension to full flexion, are useful in most cases. The patient usually alternates hourly between the extremes of motion achieved at time of surgery.
- The need for and role of continuous passive motion (CPM) remains a subject of discussion. It may be initiated using a CPM device with or without a nerve block; however, in the authors' experience, it is not usually necessary. In patients who are unable to practice motion on their own or in those with severe contractures, it may be of benefit, although a consensus regarding the indications and need for CPM is lacking.

Postoperative Care and Expected Outcomes

- At the first postoperative check, the neurovascular status is assessed. If the patient is intact, a regional block for pain control may be considered as needed.
- The arm is elevated in the "Statue of Liberty" position overnight.
- If the patient is admitted, it is helpful to "tie up" the arm to an orthopedic bed railing.
- On postoperative day 1, the splint is removed and the neurovascular status is evaluated, with particular attention to the radial, median, and ulnar nerves, if this has not already been performed. Full active range of motion is then initiated. No limitations are placed on use of the arm.
- Postoperative protocols such as a supervised physiotherapy program, use of splinting protocols to improve motion, or continuous passive motion devices may be considered.

Evidence

Adams JE, Wolff LH III, Merten SM, Steinmann SP. Osteoarthritis of the elbow: results of arthroscopic osteophyte resection and capsulectomy. J Shoulder Elbow Surg. 2008;17:126-31.

This retrospective review evaluated 41 patients (42 elbows) with primary osteoarthritis of the elbow who underwent arthroscopic osteophyte resection and capsulectomy with greater than 2 years of follow-up. Preoperative motion, pain, and Mayo Clinic Elbow Performance (MEP) scores were compared to those at final follow-up. At an average follow-up of 176.3 weeks, significant improvements were noted in mean flexion (from 117.3° preoperatively to 131.6° postoperatively, $p < .0001$*), extension (from 21.4° to 8.4°,* $p < .0001$*), supination (from 70.7° to 78.6°,* $p = .0056$*), and MEP scores (*$p < .0001$*), with 81% good to excellent results. Pain decreased significantly (*$p < .0001$*). Complications were rare (*$n = 2$*; heterotopic ossification and ulnar dysesthesias). (Level III evidence)*

Cohen AP, Redden JF, Stanley D. Treatment of osteoarthritis of the elbow: a comparison of open and arthroscopic debridement. Arthroscopy. 2000;16:701-6.

In this series, the authors compared outcomes following arthroscopic débridement versus open débridement of the elbow for osteoarthritis, using the Outerbridge-Kashiwagi procedure and the arthroscopic modification. Both groups demonstrated improved range of elbow flexion, decrease in pain, and a high level of patient satisfaction. Increases in elbow extension, although improved in both groups, were more modest. Neither procedure included a capsular release. Comparison between the open and arthroscopic procedures demonstrated that the open procedure might be more effective in improving flexion, while the arthroscopic procedure seemed to provide more pain relief. No differences between overall effectiveness of the two procedures were noted. (Grade A recommendation) (Level III evidence)

Kelly EW, Bryce R, Coghlan J, Bell S. Arthroscopic debridement without radial head excision of the osteoarthritic elbow. Arthroscopy. 2007;23:151-6.

This retrospective series evaluated the outcomes of 24 patients (25 elbows) with osteoarthritis of the elbow treated with arthroscopic débridement at average follow-up of 67 months. Twenty-four of 25 elbows were "better" or "much better" after surgery; 21 patients reported minimal or no pain. Range of motion in the flexion-extension arc improved an average of 21°. No complications were seen in this series. (Level III evidence)

Nguyen D, Proper SI, MacDermid JC, King GJ, Faber KJ. Functional outcomes of arthroscopic capsular release of the elbow. Arthroscopy. 2006;22:842-9.

This retrospective series described 22 patients who underwent arthroscopic contracture release with mean follow-up of 25 months. Twenty patients had capsulectomy while 2 underwent capsulotomy. Postoperatively, there were significant improvements in flexion, extension, and outcome scores. No complications were noted in this series. (Level III evidence)

Thoreux P, Blondeau C, Durand S, Masquelet AC. Anatomical basis of arthroscopic capsulotomy for elbow stiffness. Surg Radiol Anat. 2006;28:409-15.

In this cadaveric study, 10 elbows were dissected to examine the relationship of the neurovascular structures to the capule and the influence of varied elbow flexion upon these relationships. Ninety degrees of elbow flexion allowed the best capsular distention and moved the neurovascular structures further away. The radial nerve was consistently the closest structure; however, it was always separated from the capsule by the brachialis muscle. Based upon this anatomic dissection, the authors suggested technical parameters to conduct safer arthroscopic capsulotomy. (Level III evidence)

SECTION II

ELBOW
Arthroscopy

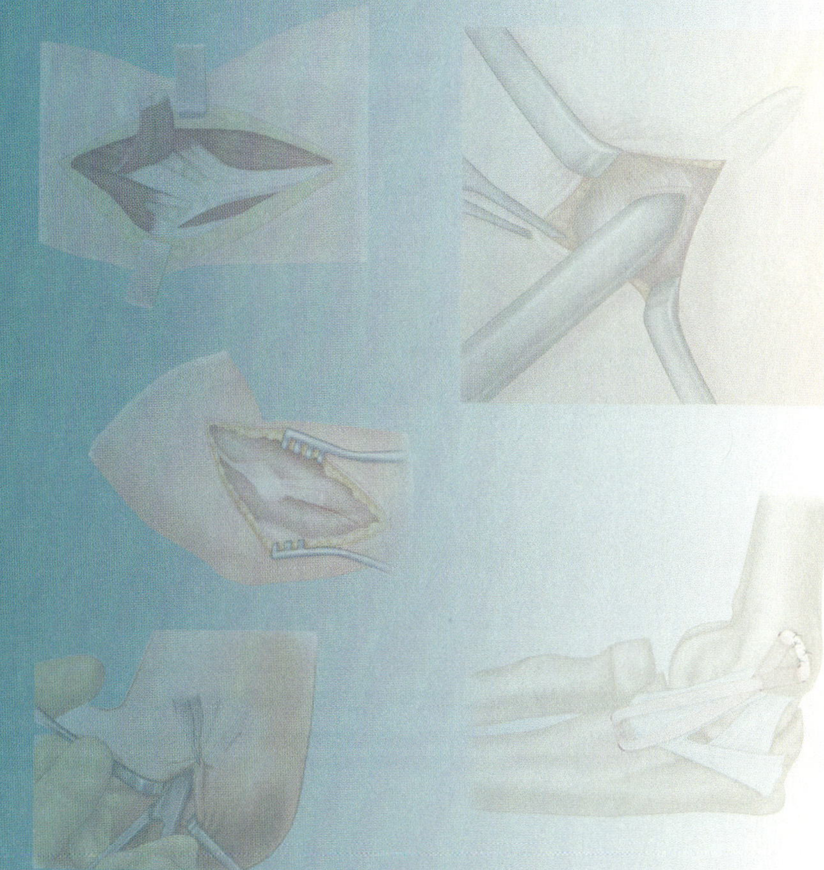

PROCEDURE 43

Radial Head Fractures: Radial Head Replacement

Donald H. Lee and John M. Erickson

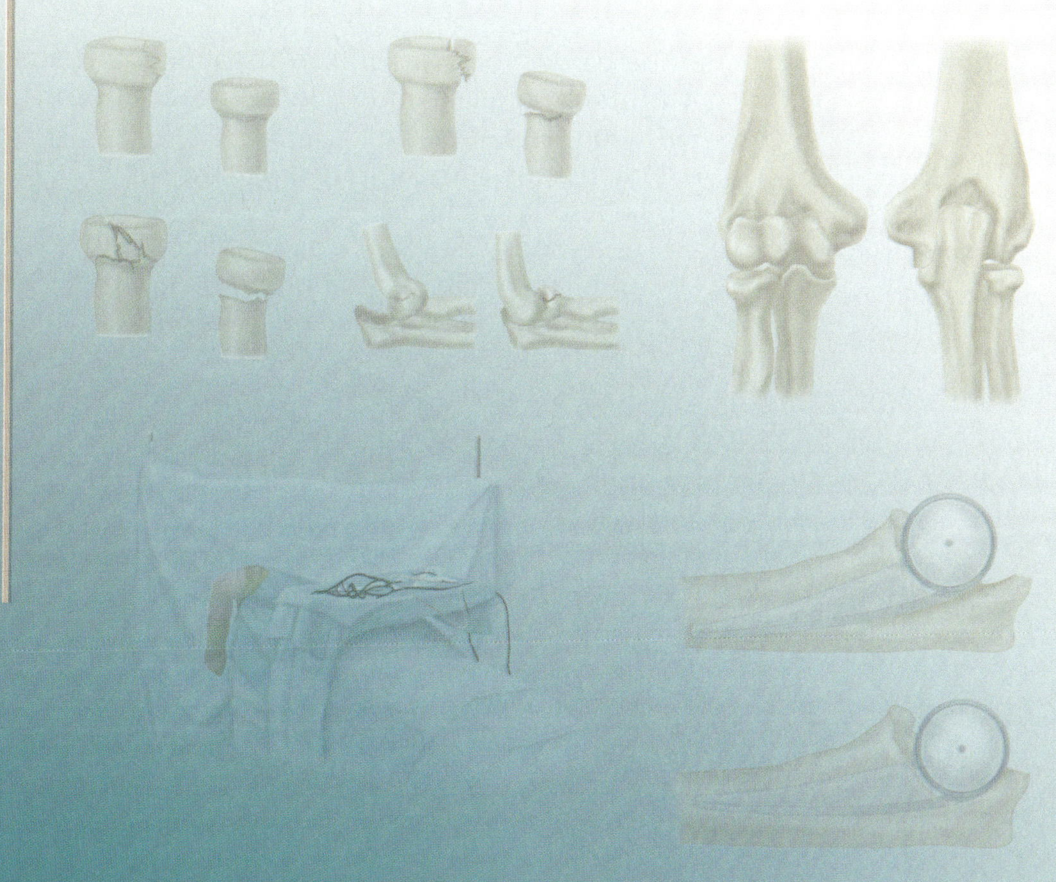

Pitfalls

- *Internal fixation of radial head fractures is generally indicated in fractures with three or fewer fragments.*
- *Radial head fractures with more than three fracture fragments, especially associated with a radial neck fracture, will be difficult to internally fix, and radial head arthroplasty is usually indicated.*

Controversies

- In the setting of a comminuted radial head fracture, patients should be assumed to have a complex injury pattern in which elbow instability is common.

Treatment Options

- Open reduction and internal fixation
- Metallic radial head replacement
- Radial head resection (rarely indicated in the acute setting)

Indications

- Comminuted, irreparable radial head fractures
- Radial head fractures with associated radial neck fracture
- Mason type III radial head fracture
- Mason type IV radial head fracture associated with elbow dislocation
- Complex or complicated radial head fracture associated with concomitant injury, including fracture of the coronoid and/or olecranon or associated ligamentous injuries (Fig. 1)

Examination/Imaging

- The elbow, forearm, and wrist should be examined for swelling, ecchymosis, tenderness, range of motion, and stability.
- Radiographs and computed tomography (CT) scans: (See also Procedure 57)
  - Anteroposterior (AP) elbow radiograph (Fig. 2A)
  - True lateral elbow radiograph (Fig. 2B)
  - Modified lateral radial head view (45° oblique elbow radiograph)
  - Posteroanterior and lateral wrist radiographs
  - CT scan with three-dimensional reconstructions

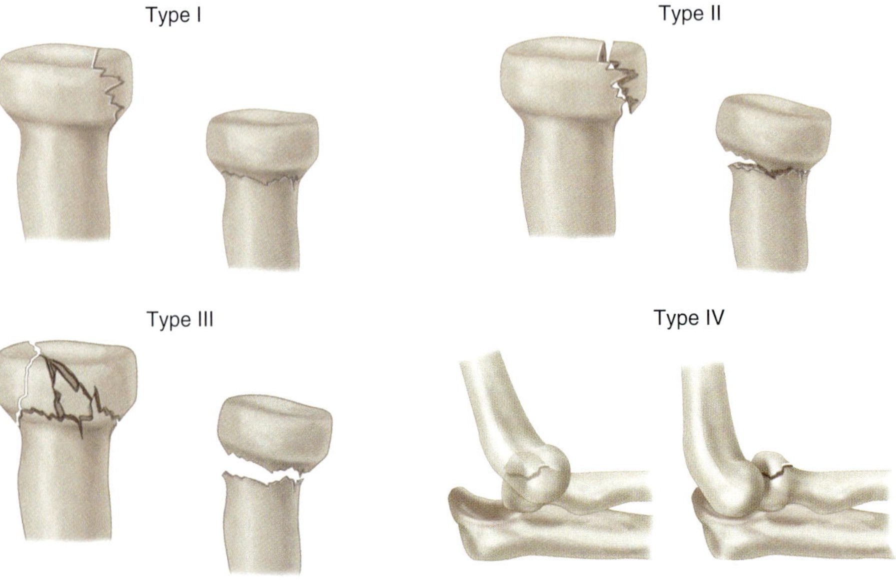

FIGURE 1

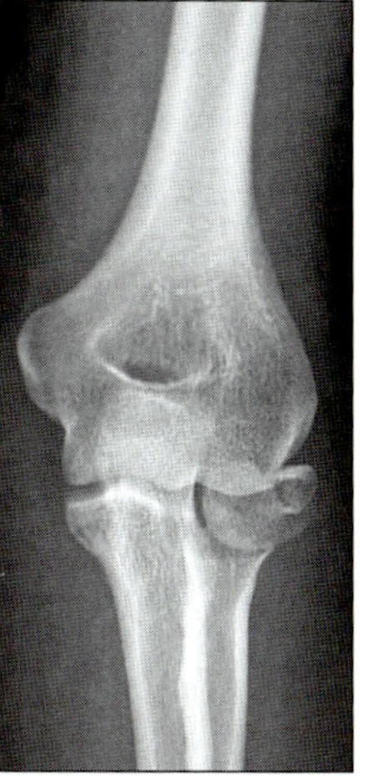
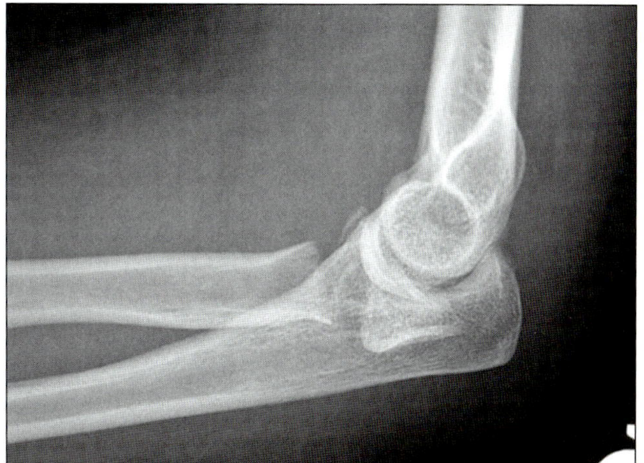

A B

FIGURE 2

Surgical Anatomy

- The proximal radius is important for valgus and posterolateral rotatory stability of the elbow and longitudinal stability of the forearm. The radiocapitellar joint transmits approximately 50–60% of the load across the elbow.
- Every attempt should be made to repair or replace the radial head, particularly in cases of elbow or longitudinal forearm instability.
- The posterior interosseus nerve (PIN) is intimately associated with the proximal radius as it passes through the supinator in its course from the anterior to the posterior aspect of the forearm (Fig. 3). Pronation of the forearm delivers the PIN medially and further from the surgical field. Placement of retractors around the radial neck should be minimized or such retractors used judiciously to avoid injury to the PIN.
- The lateral ulnar collateral ligament (LUCL) complex is at risk with lateral approaches to the elbow and is critical for elbow stability.
- It is important to remain anterior to the equator of the radial head/neck or the radiocapitellar joint (i.e., anterior to a line drawn along the long axis of the radial neck) to preserve the posterior sling of the LUCL complex.

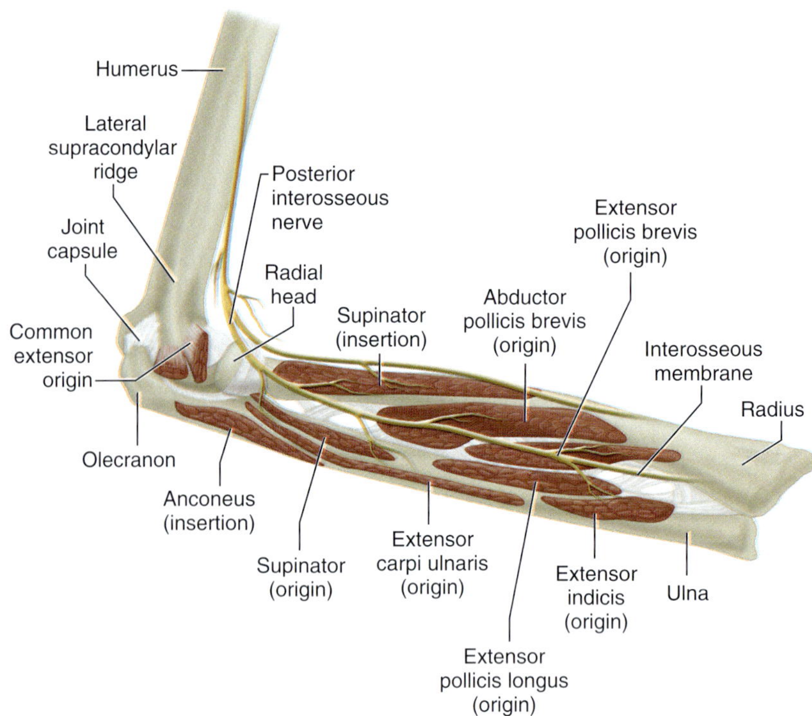

FIGURE 3

Pearls

- *After the patient is positioned, fluoroscopy should be performed prior to arm preparation to ensure adequate visualization of the elbow and radial head.*
- *A sterile tourniquet applied to the proximal brachium will significantly aid visualization.*

Positioning

- General anesthesia or regional block
- Supine position with arm table (preferred)
- Other options:
  - Supine with arm across chest
  - Lateral decubitus position with arm bolster

Pearls

- *The Kocher intermuscular interval is best identified distally, as the muscles share a common aponeurosis proximally.*
- *The Kocher interval is more posterior than the Kaplan, and therefore the LUCL complex can be inadvertently injured if the dissection is carried too far anteriorly.*
- *Because of the proximity of the PIN, the forearm is kept in a pronated position to carry the nerve out of the surgical field.*

Portals/Exposures

- The Kaplan interval, located between the extensor digitorum communis and the extensor carpi radialis longus and brevis, is used for simple radial head fractures without concomitant coronoid/olecranon fractures or collateral ligament injuries (Fig. 4).
- The Kocher interval, located between the anconeus and the extensor carpi ulnaris (ECU), is used for cases associated with complex elbow fracture-dislocations (Fig. 5A). A fat stripe is frequently seen between the anconeus and ECU (Fig. 5B, *blue arrow*).
- Alternatively, a posterior midline skin incision with full-thickness skin flaps can be used to address proximal ulna fractures while incorporating lateral and/or medial approaches to the elbow.

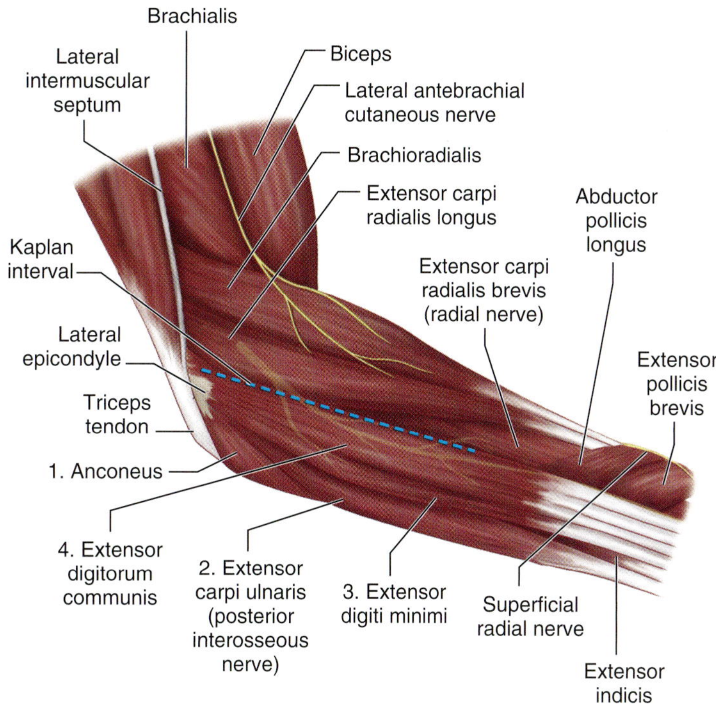

FIGURE 4

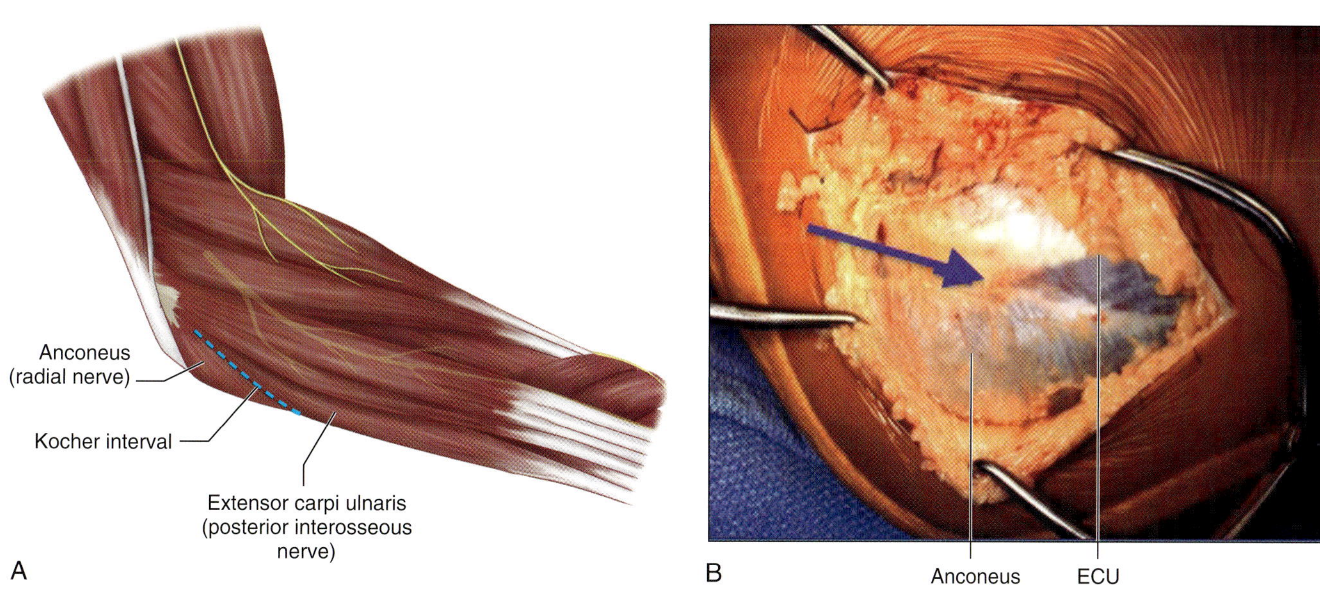

FIGURE 5

Pearls

- *In associated elbow-fracture dislocations, the LUCL is avulsed proximally, resulting in a "bald" lateral humeral epicondyle (Fig. 8).*
- *Additionally there is often a defect in the common extensor tendon. In this setting, exposure of the fractured radial head is greatly simplified.*

Procedure

Step 1

- A lateral curvilinear incision is made from the lateral epicondyle to a point distally centered over the radial neck (see Incision video).
- Alternatively, a midline posterior incision centered over the olecranon is made with elevation of full-thickness skin flaps.
- The radial head is approached via the Kaplan (preferred for simple radial head fractures) or Kocher intermuscular interval (preferred for complex radial head fractures with lateral collateral ligament injuries [Fig. 8]). Care is taken to dissect the muscular layer from the underlying capsule (Fig. 6) (see Arthrotomy 1 video).
- The capsule is incised longitudinally anterior to the LUCL, preserving the LUCL complex posteriorly (Fig. 7).
- An incision in the annular ligament can be used when distal exposures are required.

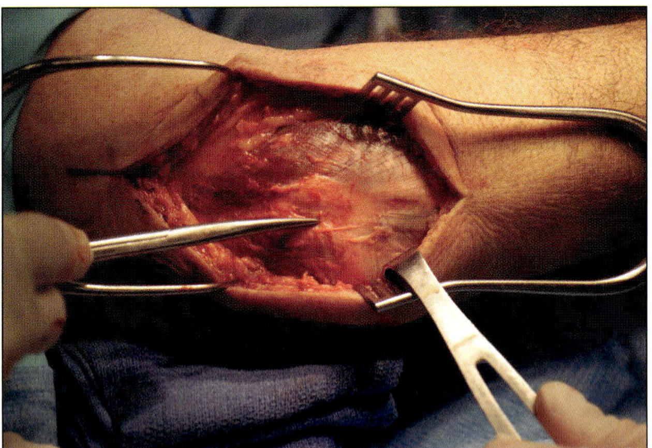

FIGURE 6

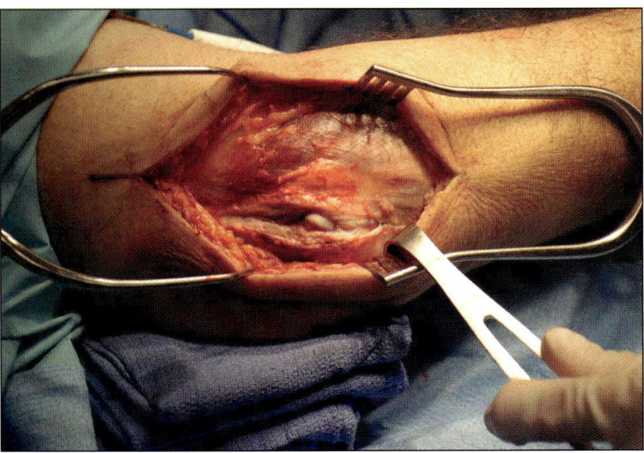

FIGURE 7

Pitfalls

- *In cases with LUCL disruption, failure to repair (acute setting) or reconstruct (chronic setting) the LUCL may result in posterolateral rotatory instability.*
- *Dissection of the elbow posterior to the long axis of the radiocapitellar joint may result in disruption of the LUCL.*

Pearls

- *A nondisplaced radial neck fracture should be cabled prior to broaching in order to avoid fracture propagation.*

Pitfalls

- *"Overstuffing" of the radiocapitellar joint should be avoided. Choose the narrower head diameter of the two implants if between sizes.*
- *When using a radial head implant with a collar or platform, the height of that collar should be calculated into the height of the resected radial head For example, if the height of the resected radial head measures 12 mm, and the width of the implant collar is 2 mm, a 10-mm radial head implant is used.*
- *Plasma coating on some implant stems effectively increases the stem diameter when compared to the trial component. Insertion of a final component into a tight canal may result in a fracture of the proximal radial neck. Downsizing of the final component may be desirable.*

Step 2

- The fracture site is exposed (Fig. 9) (see Arthrotomy 2 video).
- Radial head fragments are excised and reassembled on the back table.
  - The radial head arthroplasty is sized appropriately from the fracture fragments.
  - Both the head diameter (Fig. 10A) and length (height) (Fig. 10B) are critical to re-create with the implant (see Head Sizing video).
- The radial neck is cut with an oscillating saw perpendicular to the radial shaft if necessary (see Radial Neck Resection video).
- The proximal radius is broached and the shaft diameter of the implant is determined (Fig. 11) (see Broach video).
- The trial implant is inserted (Fig. 12) (see Trial Stem Insertion, Trial Head Insertion, and Set Screw

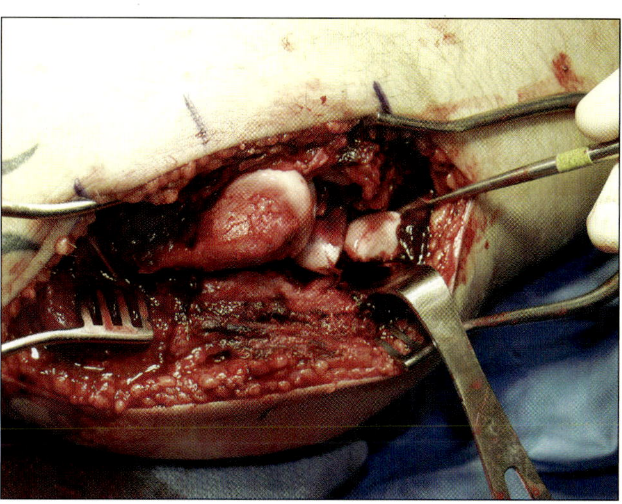

FIGURE 8

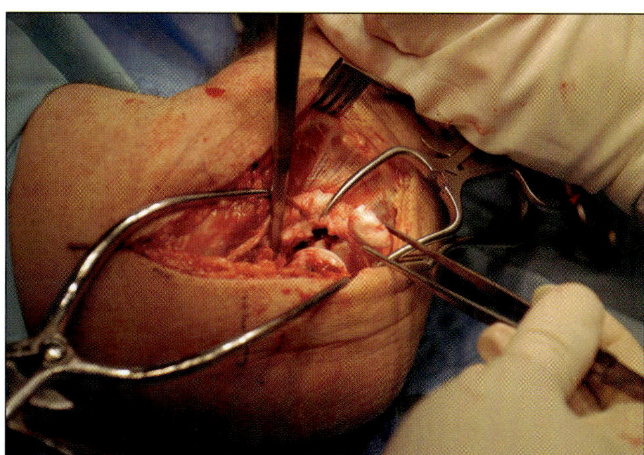

FIGURE 9

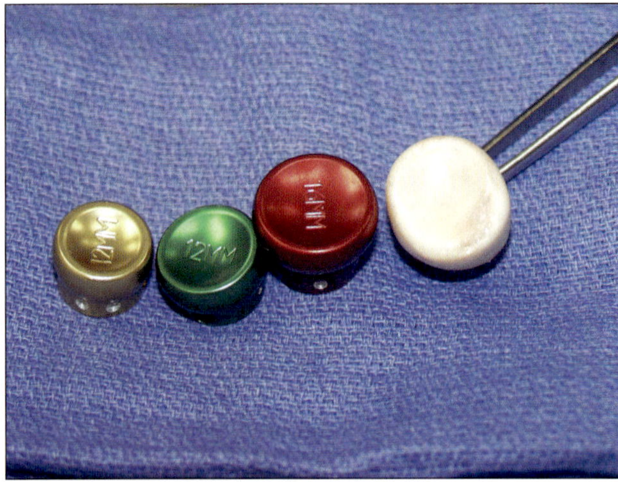

A

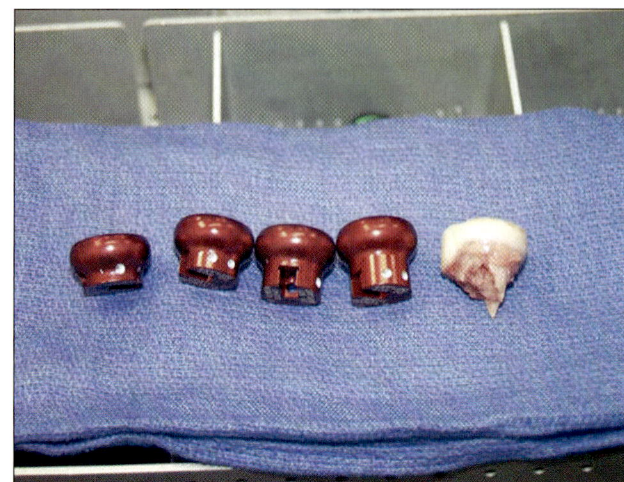

B

FIGURE 10

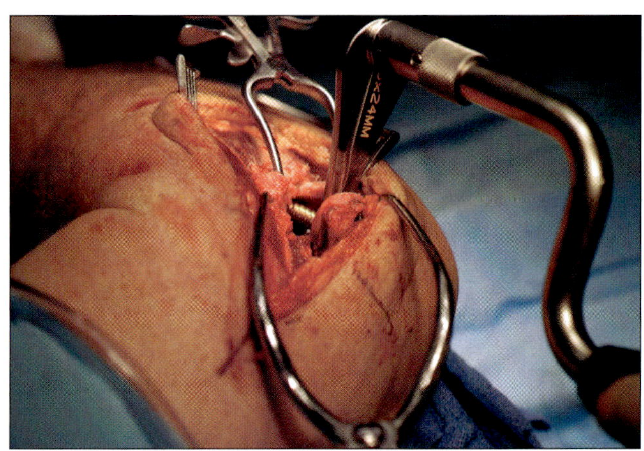

FIGURE 11

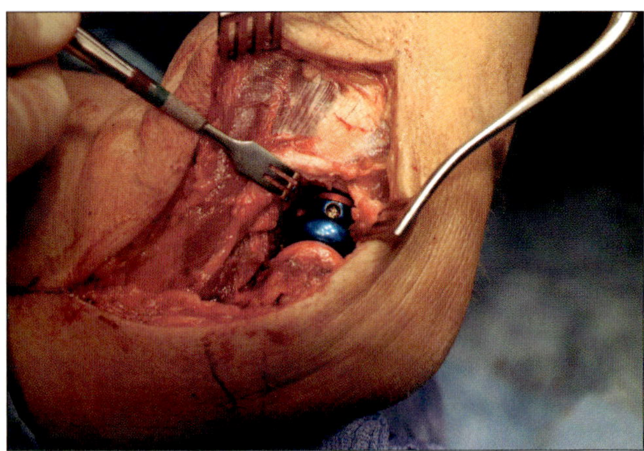

FIGURE 12

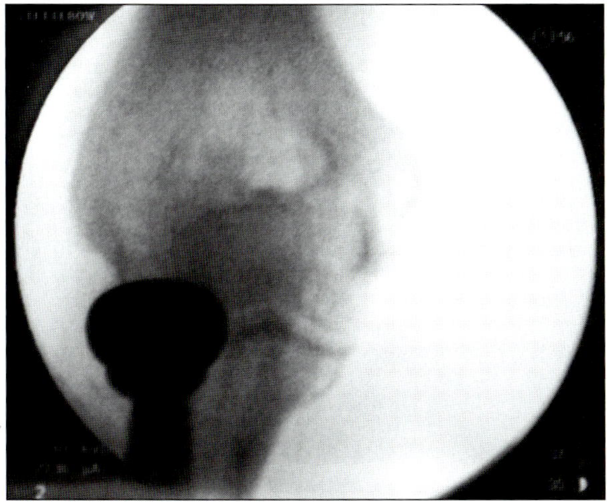

A

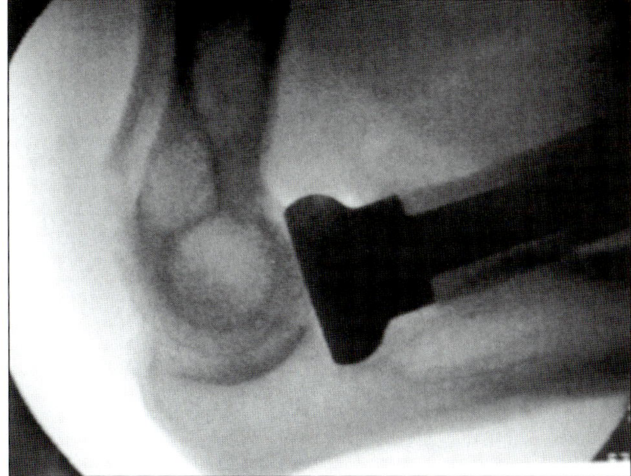

B

FIGURE 13

Instrumentation/ Implantation

- The prosthetic radial head often appears larger than the native radial head on fluoroscopy as the articular portion of the native head is radiolucent.

Controversies

- Radial head excision should be avoided, particularly in the setting of a capsuloligamentous injury to the elbow or forearm.
- Radial head resection is associated with delayed complications, including valgus and posterolateral rotatory elbow instability, longitudinal forearm instability, and osteoarthrosis.

Insertion videos), and the elbow and forearm are taken through a full range of motion using live fluoroscopy (Fig. 13A and 13B) (see Intraoperative Fluoroscopy video). The elbow is flexed and extended and the forearm pronated and supinated, and motion, stability, and joint congruency are assessed.

- Additionally, a congruent ulnohumeral articulation should be sought on the AP view to avoid "overstuffing" the radiocapitellar joint (see Fig. 13A).
- The final prosthesis is implanted via cementing or press-fit techniques (Fig. 14), and the result is checked on AP (Fig. 15A) and lateral (Fig. 15B) radiographs (see Final Stem Insertion and Final Head Insertion videos).

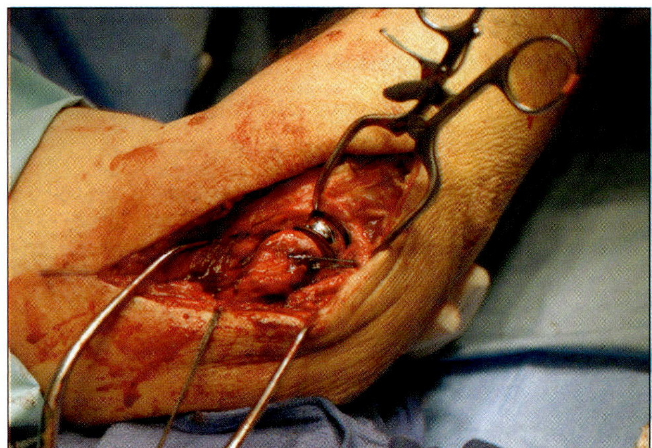

FIGURE 14

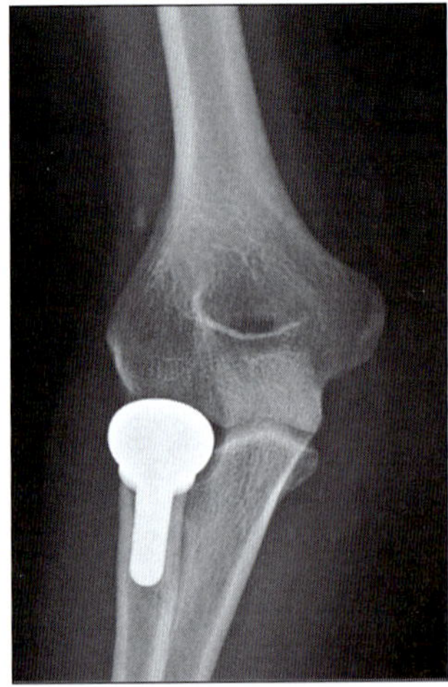

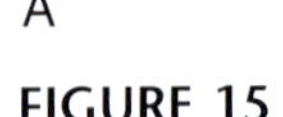

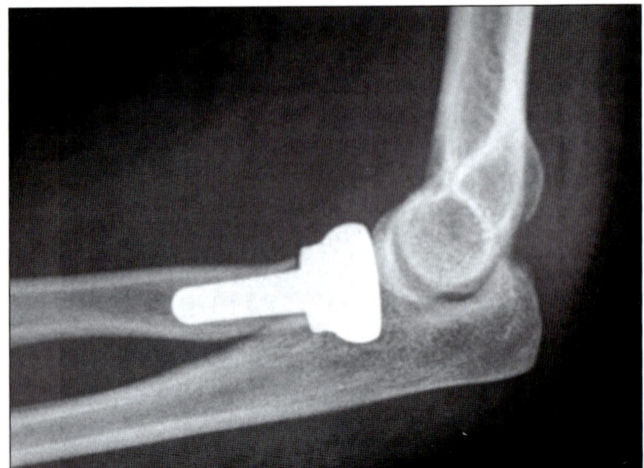

A B

FIGURE 15

Pitfalls

- *Anatomic repair of the LUCL complex is critical (see Procedure 57).*
- *Fixation of the ligamentous complex posterior to the isometric point can lead to subluxation of the ulnohumeral joint in extension.*

Instrumentation/ Implantation

- In cases of elbow fracture-dislocation, a hinged external fixator should be available in the event that elbow reduction cannot be maintained after bony and soft tissue repair.

Controversies

- Repair of the medial/ulnar collateral ligament is typically not necessary unless the elbow remains unstable after bony and lateral ligamentous repair.

- Range of motion and stability are reassessed using fluoroscopy (see Final Fluoro video).

Step 3

- The lateral collateral ligament complex is repaired to the lateral humeral epicondyle using heavy (#2) nonabsorbable sutures. Transosseous lateral epicondylar bone tunnels (see Fig. 14) or commercially available suture anchors (see Procedure 57) can be used.
- Using fluoroscopy, the ulnohumeral joint is confirmed to be congruent throughout the range of motion. Forearm pronation and elbow flexion typically improves the stability of the radiocapitellar joint and ulnohumeral joint, respectively.
- In cases of complex elbow fracture-dislocations, with residual instability of the elbow in extension, an anterior capsulodesis can be performed (see Procedure 57).
- One may choose to repair the annular ligament (see Annular Ligament Repair video).
- The fascia and skin are closed in standard fashion (see Fascial Repair video).
- A sterile dressing is incorporated into a well-padded long-arm splint.

Pearls

- *The intraoperative assessment of elbow stability is critical for determining the postoperative therapy regimen, particularly in elbow fracture-dislocations.*
- *If there is residual posterolateral sagging of the radiocapitellar joint, postoperative rehabilitation is performed with the forearm in pronation.*

Pitfalls

- *Splinting the elbow for more than a few days will lead to elbow stiffness and a potential poor outcome.*

Controversies

- Indomethacin and/or irradiation can be used to reduce the incidence of heterotopic ossification in high-risk patients.

Postoperative Care and Expected Outcomes

- Patients are instructed in immediate digital and shoulder range of motion.
- The long-arm splint applied at the end of surgery is removed 3–5 days postoperatively, a removable long-arm Thermoplast splint is applied, and the patient is instructed in gentle passive and active-assisted elbow range of motion (see Procedure 57).
- Skin sutures are removed at 8–10 days postoperatively.
- Complications include loss of elbow motion, particularly terminal extension; heterotopic ossification; loss of fixation; infection; and osteoarthrosis.

Evidence

Ashwood N, Bain GI, Unni R. Management of Mason type III radial head fractures with a titanium prosthesis, ligament repair, and early mobilization. J Bone Joint Surg [Am]. 2004;86:274-80.

A review of 16 patients with Mason type III radial head fractures and collateral ligament injuries treated with a titanium radial head prosthesis and soft tissue reconstruction. Good to excellent results were seen in 13 of 16 patients.

Morrey BF, Tanaka S, An KN. Valgus stability of the elbow: a definition of primary and secondary constraints. Clin Orthop Relat Res. 1991;(265):187-95.

This classic biomechanical study demonstrated the importance of the radial head as a secondary stabilizer of the elbow.

Ring D, Quintero J, Jupiter JB. Open reduction and internal fixation of fractures of the radial head. J Bone Joint Surg [Am]. 2002;84:1811-5.

The authors retrospectively reviewed 56 patients who underwent open reduction and internal fixation of radial head fractures. Thirteen of 14 patients with Mason III fractures of more than three articular fragments had a poor result, and therefore the authors recommended excision or radial head replacement in such patients.

PROCEDURE 44

Total Elbow Arthroplasty: Discovery Minimally Constrained Linked System

Hill Hastings II

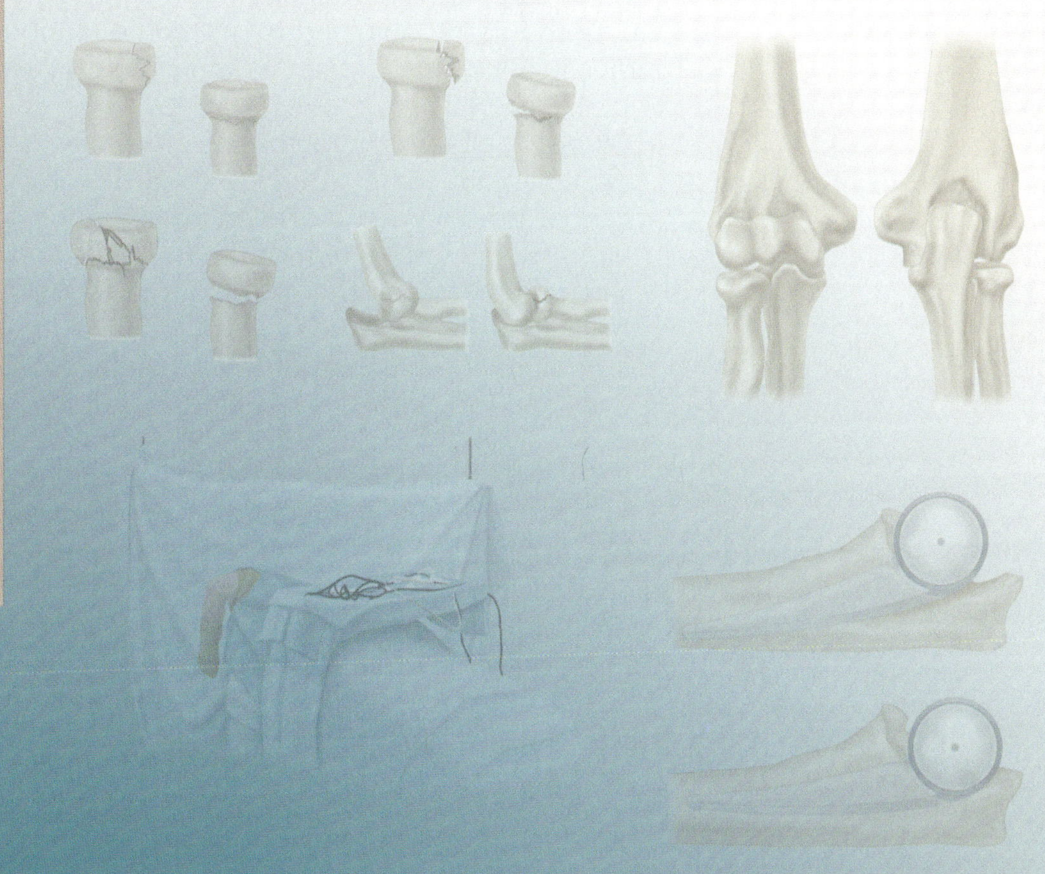

Pitfalls

- *Avoid elbow replacement arthroplasty in cases of infection.*
- *Avoid implant arthroplasty when not assured that the patient will restrict or limit his or her elbow from repetitive forceful lifting of more than 7–10 pounds, sports such as golf, and the like.*
- *There should be an adequate and healthy soft tissue envelope about the elbow.*

Controversies

- Both age of the patient and anticipated level of force exposure to the elbow are important. Avoid elbow implant arthroplasty in patients younger than age 60–65 unless no other reasonably predictable options exist. Anticipated results are better in patients with diffuse arthritic conditions such as inflammatory rheumatoid arthritis and are most guarded in posttraumatic or osteoarthritis cases in which, once the joint is replaced, the patient will have little incentive or perceived need to limit force exposure to the elbow.

Indications

- Diffuse inflammatory arthropathy of the elbow
- Diffuse severe osteoarthritis of the elbow in elderly patients
- Low comminuted fractures of distal humerus in elderly, low-demand patients
- Chronic unreconstructable instability of the elbow
- Segmental bone loss of the elbow from tumor or severe trauma

Examination/Imaging

- Anteroposterior (AP) and lateral radiographs of the elbow should be obtained to assess the ulnohumeral, radiocapitellar, and proximal radioulnar articulations (Fig. 1A and 1B).
  - When an elbow contracture of more than 30° exists, an adequate anterior and posterior view cannot be obtained of the entire elbow on one film. Instead, an AP film of the humerus and a separate AP film of the proximal ulna should be ordered.
  - If additional evaluation of the proximal radioulnar joint and radial head is required, a radiocapitellar (Coyle) view (Fig. 1C) should be ordered.
  - Routine computed tomography scanning and magnetic resonance imaging are not indicated.
- When forearm rotation is deficient, the distal radioulnar joint should be evaluated by zero-rotation posteroanterior (Fig. 1D) and lateral radiographs. Correction of deficient forearm rotation may require radial head resection and at times concomitant treatment of distal radioulnar pathology.

Treatment Options

- Handle isolated radiocapitellar arthritis by arthroscopic partial resection of the radial head. When radiocapitellar arthritis coexists with arthritis of the proximal radioulnar joint, consider radial head resection with or without radial head implant arthroplasty.
- Primary osteoarthritis may be handled by radical capsular release and débridement with partial excision of the coronoid, partial excision of the olecranon, and restoration of the coronoid and olecranon fossae. Inflammatory arthropathy may respond to arthroscopic synovectomy. In the young or high-demand posttraumatic or osteoarthritic patient, consider débridement arthroplasty with or without soft tissue interposition (resurfacing).

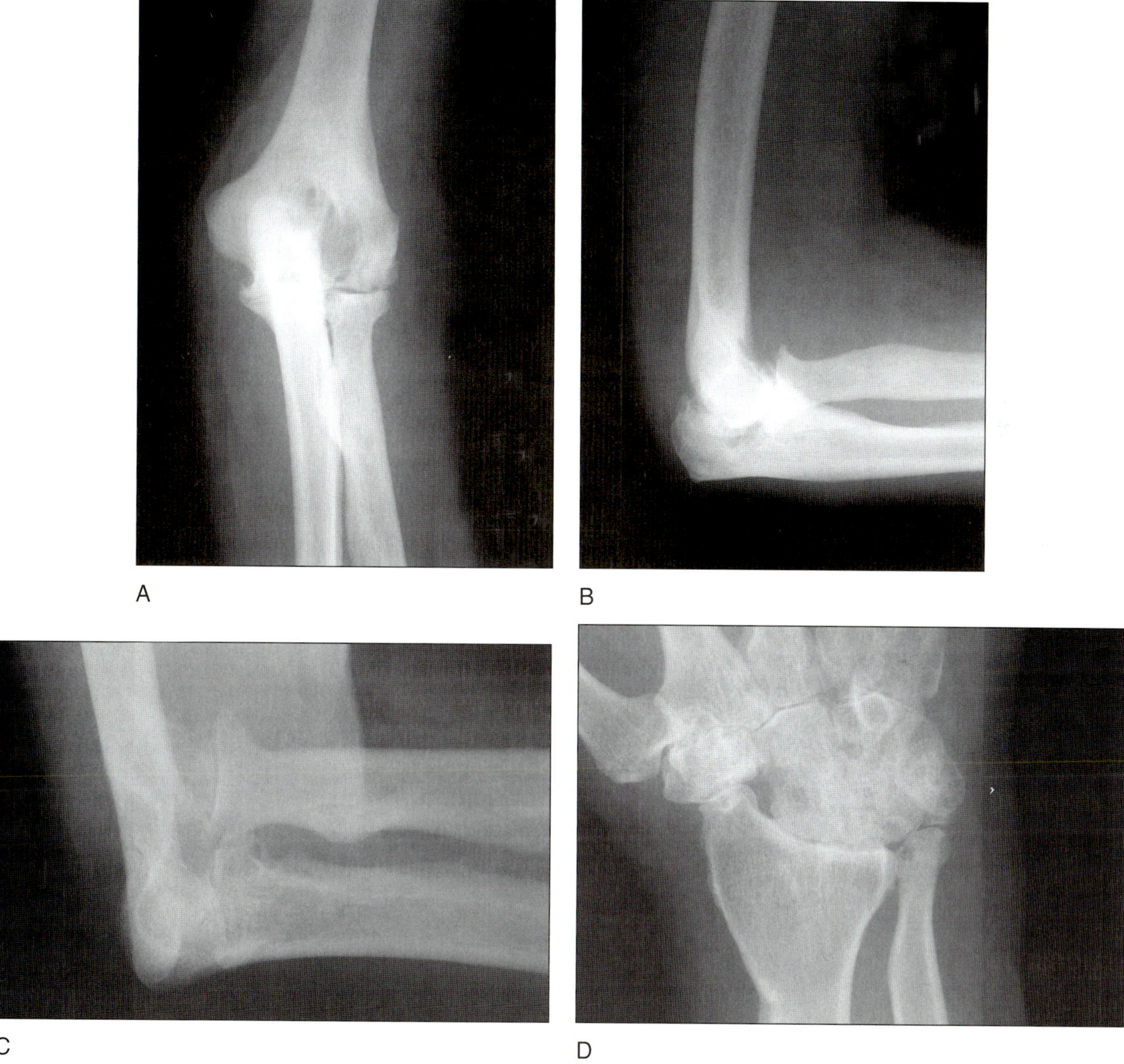

FIGURE 1

PEARLS

- *When the patient is rolled less than 40° toward the lateral decubitus position, an axillary roll is not usually required.*

PITFALLS

- *Carefully protect the lower extremities with pillows and padding underneath and between the legs. Place the opposite upper extremity on an arm support with the arm resting in external rotation and partial elbow flexion. Insert foam padding underneath the elbow.*

Equipment

- Suction beanbag
- Pillows, foam padding
- Use of a sterile brachial tourniquet allows for preparation of the arm all the way to the shoulder and a larger brachial sterile field.

Controversies

- Some surgeons prefer a lateral decubitus position with an axillary roll and the arm draped over a sterilely draped supporting armholder.

Surgical Anatomy

- The elbow joint is constrained, stabilized by the closely matching articular surfaces and tightly opposed lateral collateral annular complex, ulnar collateral ligament, and triceps expansion. The ulnar nerve passes through the cubital tunnel where it is susceptible to compression by bony deformity or alteration of soft tissue tension. It always requires at least decompression for protection against undue compression or traction during the course of the surgical procedure. The radial nerve passes directly anterior to the radiocapitellar joint. Dissection anterolaterally must respect the nerve which lies on or close to anterior capsule. Osteophytes that may have formed over time may limit motion of the elbow and must be removed to restore a functional arc of motion. The anterior capsule can be thick and tight when associated with prolonged elbow flexion contracture.

Positioning

- The patient is positioned in partial lateral decubitus position rolled 30–40° toward one side and held by a beanbag.
- The opposite upper extremity and both lower extremities are carefully protected by appropriate padding.

Portals/Exposures

- A straight posterior incision is made that deviates either medial or slightly lateral to the olecranon. The incision should start over the subcutaneous border of the ulna distally, pass adjacent to the olecranon, and end over the central posterior humerus.
- In most cases of primary arthroplasty and in all cases of revision arthroplasty, a "triceps-off" or triceps takedown approach is utilized.
- In the case of distal humerus fracture, a paratricepital approach is utilized without detachment of the triceps from the olecranon.

Procedure

STEP 1: SETUP

- A general or regional block with light general anesthesia is administered to the patient.
- A stockinette is applied over the wrist and distal forearm and a sterile proximal brachial tourniquet is

Pearls

- *The patient should be pretreated for 5 days with nasal antibiotic swabs and should shower with chlorhexidine antiseptic.*
- *A sterile brachial tourniquet affords a larger field of sterility.*
- *Marking the incision prior to applying Ioban draping assures that the incision will be properly situated. If marked after Ioban application, the incision will often lie in an unintended position, the skin having shifted during the Ioban application.*
- *A rolled sheet secured by sterile Coban can serve as a bolster underneath the draped extremity elbow.*

Pitfalls

- *Carefully assess any previous incisions or areas of skin abnormality.*
- *Previous incisions should be incorporated where possible. When previous incisions are not appropriately situated, new incisions should cross, if needed, old incisions at greater than a 30° angle.*

Instrumentation/ Implantation

- Impervious stockinette for wrist and hand.
- Coban to secure stockinette and to cover brachial tourniquet for easier removal after Ioban application.
- Surgical antibiotic-impregnated steri-drape (Ioban™).
- Sterile skin marker.
- For skin preparation, use chlorhexidine–alcohol, which has been shown to be significantly more effective than iodine-based skin preparation.
- Administer prophylactic intravenous antibiotics prior to patient preparation and draping.

Controversies

- Administration of regional anesthetic block assures comfort for the first 12 hours or so after surgery but does not allow for immediate postoperative neurologic evaluation. With routine total elbow arthroplasty, this is not of concern. It may be an issue in cases of complex deformity where proximal or anterior difficult dissections might have placed the radial nerve and/or median nerve at risk.
- The procedure can be done strictly under regional block, but for positioning and comfort during the procedure, most patients benefit from a supplemental light general anesthetic.

placed. The surgical incision is drawn prior to applying an 3M™ Ioband™ drape over the rest of the extremity (Fig. 2).

- The operative arm is elevated and exsanguinated, with the brachial tourniquet inflated to 50 mm Hg above the patient's systolic pressure.

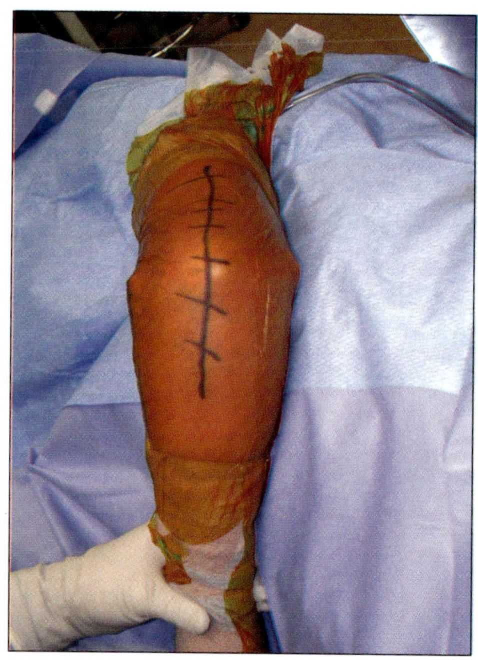

FIGURE 2

Pearls

- *Keep accompanying vessels attached to the ulnar nerve when present down to the level of the cubital tunnel to maintain optimum vascularity to the ulnar nerve.*
- *Avoid the use of a Penrose drain or other such fixed retractor on the ulnar nerve, which might create tension or stress on the nerve through the remainder of the procedure.*
- *Transposition of the ulnar nerve may require neurolysis of one or two muscular branches to the posterior FCU musculature.*

Pitfalls

- *Deformity may alter ulnar nerve position at the elbow and at times create intense scarring or entrapment of the nerve at that location. Frequently elbow arthritis leads to subclinical ulnar nerve pathology. A careful preoperative examination of the ulnar nerve is mandatory.*
- *Many patients who have previously been on steroid therapy will have thin skin and subcutaneous tissue. Be careful to keep flaps as thick as possible with elevation directly off the fascial plane. Raise the flaps laterally only as far as the lateral triceps and medially as far as required for ulnar nerve transposition.*

Instrumentation/ Implantation

- A self-retaining Gelpi retractor is helpful in skin retraction.

Step 2: Exposure and Handling of Ulnar Nerve

- The skin is incised down to fascia. Thick flaps are elevated medially and laterally to expose the triceps expansion and ulnar nerve (Fig. 3).
- The arcade of Struthers is released to expose the ulnar nerve proximal to the elbow. Release is continued up to the midbrachial level and distally down to the cubital tunnel. The ulnar nerve is decompressed through Osborne's ligament, and through the superficial and deep flexor carpi ulnaris (FCU), aponeurosis, and proximal flexor digitorum superficialis origins when present (Fig. 4).

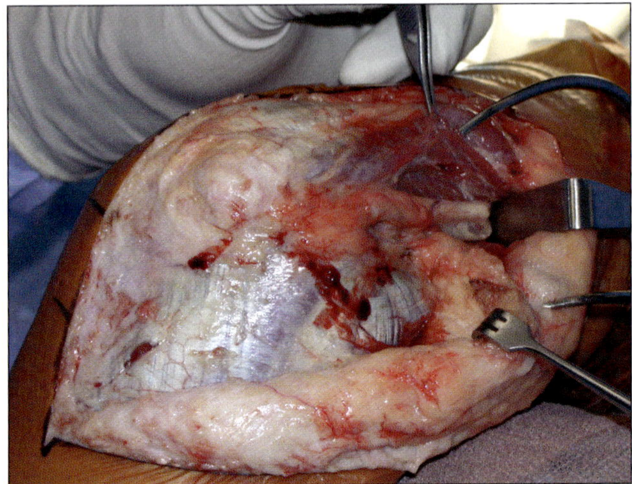

FIGURE 3

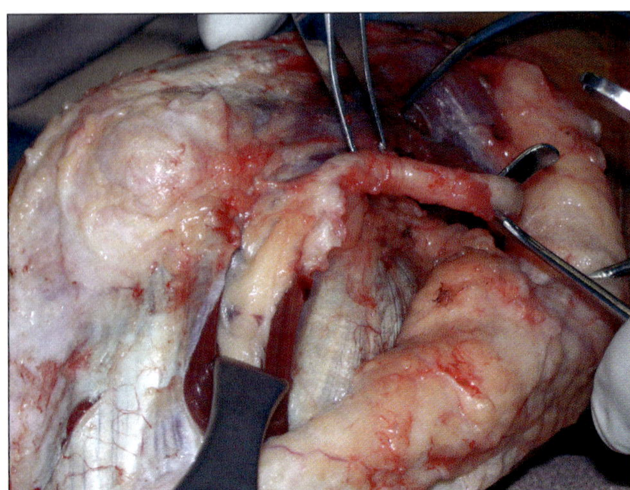

FIGURE 4

Controversies

- Total elbow replacement can be accomplished without ulnar nerve transposition if or when the entire flexor pronator origin and ulnar collateral origin as a group are elevated off of the proximal ulna.
- In most instances, decompression and transposition of the ulnar nerve protects it from undue torque retraction during the dislocation portion of the total elbow arthroplasty.

Pearls

- *Preplace suture for reattachment of the triceps as the triceps is taken off its insertion to the olecranon.*
- *Release the lateral collateral ligament from the humerus by inserting a scalpel blade deep to the lateral collateral origin and sweeping the blade proximally.*
- *In cases with significant flexion contracture, release and excise the entire anterior capsule. This is most easily done after release of the lateral collateral and extensor origin from lateral condyle with anterior dissection from the lateral side.*

Pitfalls

- *As the triceps and anconeus are released from medial to lateral, stay superficial to the annular ligament, passing over the radial head and attaching to the ulna.*
- *Anterior to the radiocapitellar joint, be careful to not stray off the anterior capsule, as the radial nerve lies immediately adjacent.*

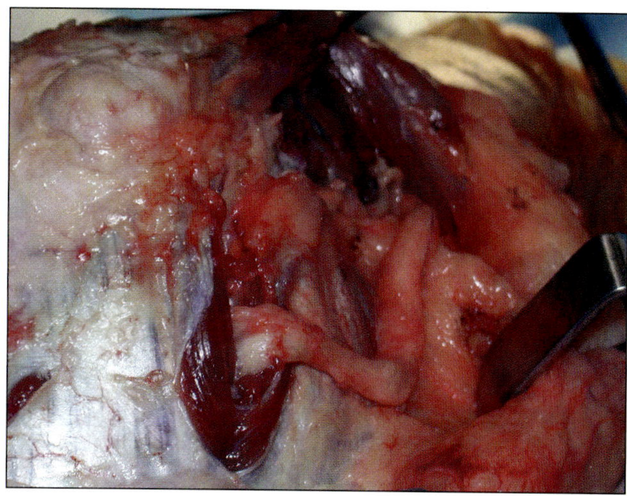

FIGURE 5

- In most all instances, anterior subcutaneous transposition of the ulnar nerve is recommended.
  - To do so, the intermuscular septum is excised. The ulnar nerve is mobilized by electrocauterization and division of small vascular branches to the triceps. The nerve is reflected or transposed ulnarly with its accompanying vasa nervorum (Fig. 5).
  - Usually at the end of the procedure, a formal stabilization sling is not required; however, the stability of the ulnar nerve should be assessed at completion of the surgical procedure.

Step 3: Exposing the Elbow Joint: Triceps-off Approach

- For a triceps-off approach, the fascia is incised over the ulnar head of the FCU muscle from the cubital tunnel proximally to a point 7–10 cm distal to the olecranon (Fig. 6). The fascia is elevated to expose the subcutaneous border of the ulna (Fig. 7).
- Having exposed the ulnar nerve anteriorly, the triceps is now elevated from the humerus starting posterior to the medial intermuscular septum. From medial to lateral, the triceps fibers of insertion into the ulna are sharply detached from the ulna. These fibers should be secured with a #2 braided Kevlar and polyester suture by Krackow technique for reattachment at the end of the procedure (Fig. 8A–C).
  - A suture is placed from deep to superficial through the most medial portion of the triceps released, run proximally in the Krackow technique for three to four passes, then laterally, and then back down

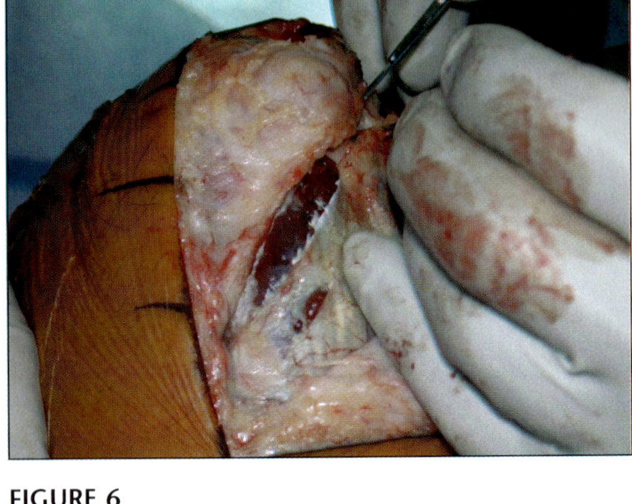

FIGURE 6

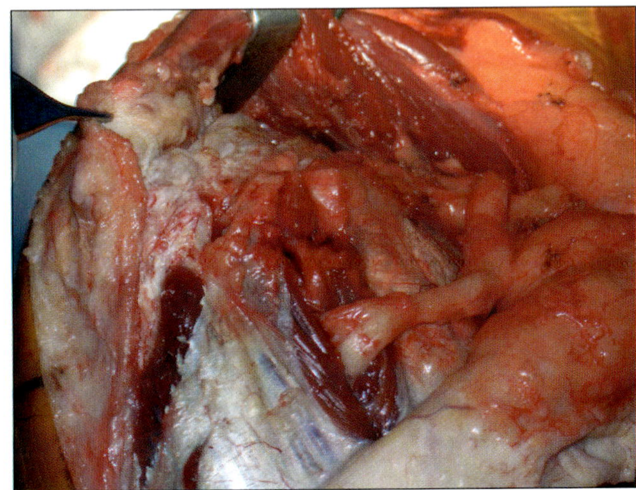

FIGURE 7

Instrumentation/ Implantation

- #2 braided polyester/Kevlar suture for reattachment of the triceps

Controversies

- Alternatively, the elbow can be approached by detaching the triceps as a distally based fascial flap (Van Gorder technique). Subluxation can be facilitated by subperiosteal release of the entire flexor pronator and ulnar collateral ligament attachments from the medial ulna.
- In cases of fracture, a "triceps-on" approach can be utilized as described in Procedure 46.

laterally to the lateral portion of the triceps attachment.

- Release of the triceps from the olecranon is continued and the triceps suture completed by passing the suture needle back to the triceps at its most lateral attachment.

- Reflection of the triceps and anconeus is continued until the lateral condyle is reached. The posterior capsule, synovium, and any pannus or scar are excised (Fig. 9).
- With an oscillating saw, the proximal-most portion of the olecranon posterior to the triceps insertion is removed (Fig. 10A and 10B). Any marginal osteophytes of the olecranon and coronoid should be trimmed away with a rongeur.

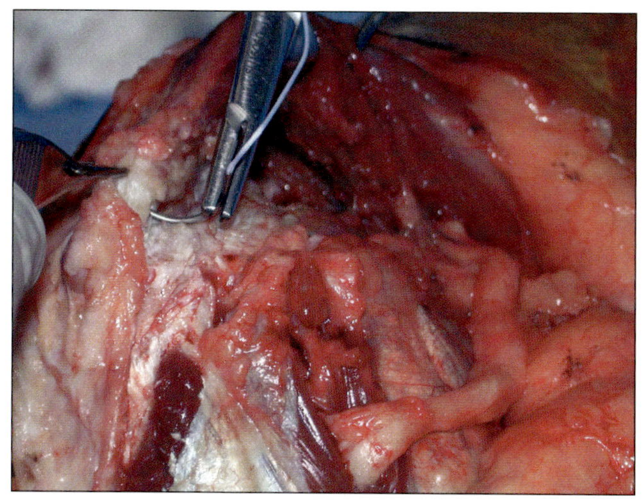

A

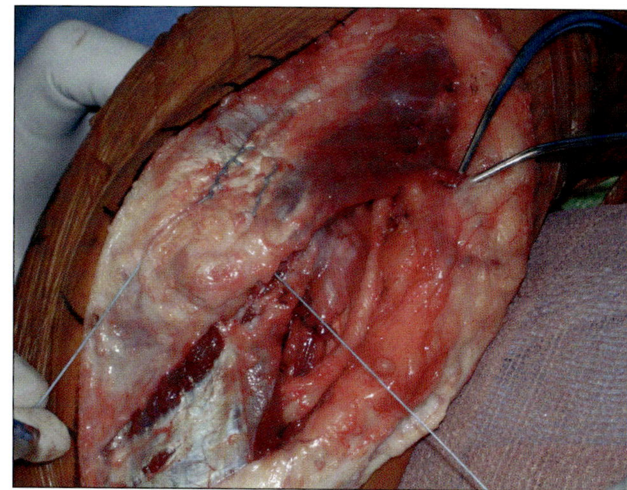

B

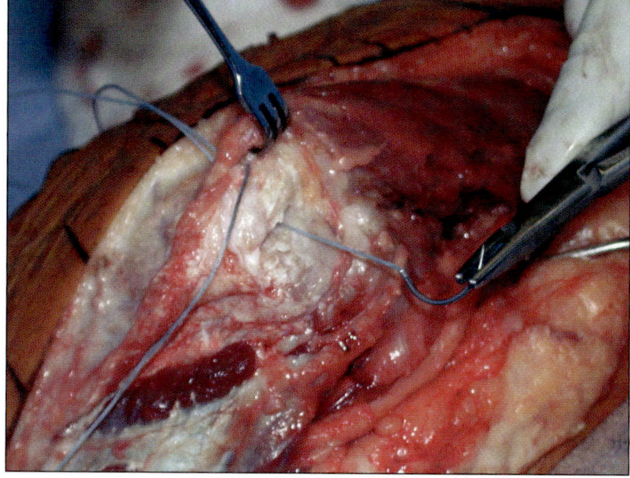

C

FIGURE 8

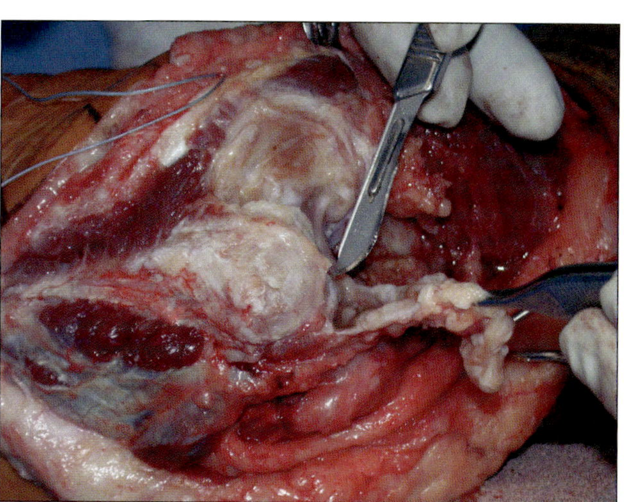

FIGURE 9

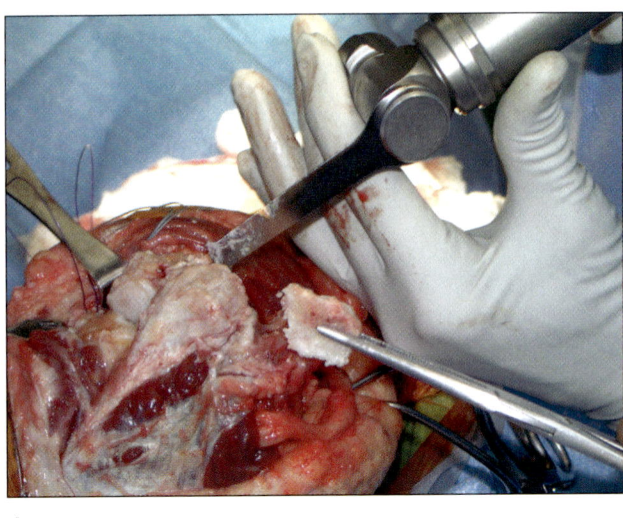

A

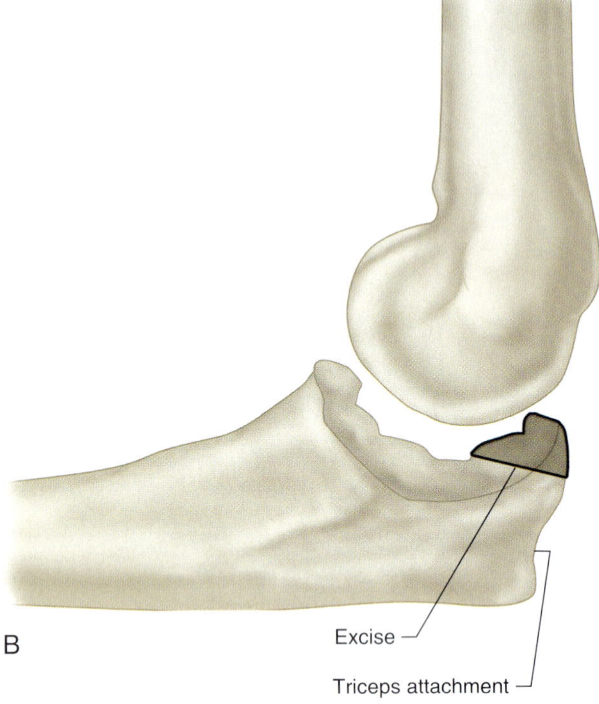

B

FIGURE 10

- Subperiosteally, the proximal origin of the lateral collateral ligament is released from the humerus (Fig. 11), and the anterior capsule released/excised from lateral to medial. This allows the elbow to be dislocated by flexion and supination of the forearm with respect to the humerus. The ulnar collateral ligament and flexor pronator origin are left intact.
- When deformity involves the radial head, the radial head is exposed with Hohmann retractors, a saw cut

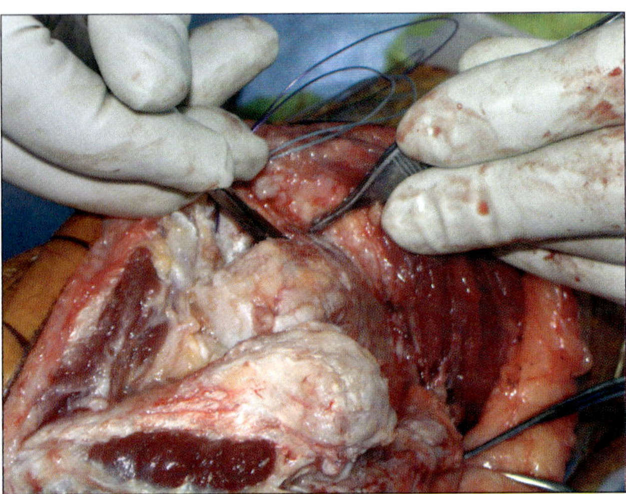

FIGURE 11

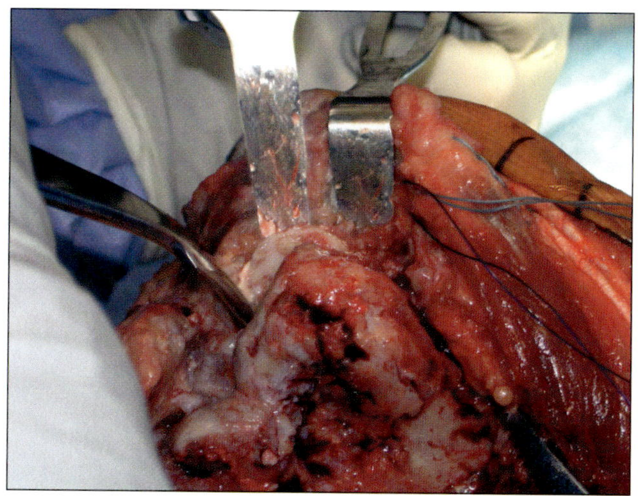
A

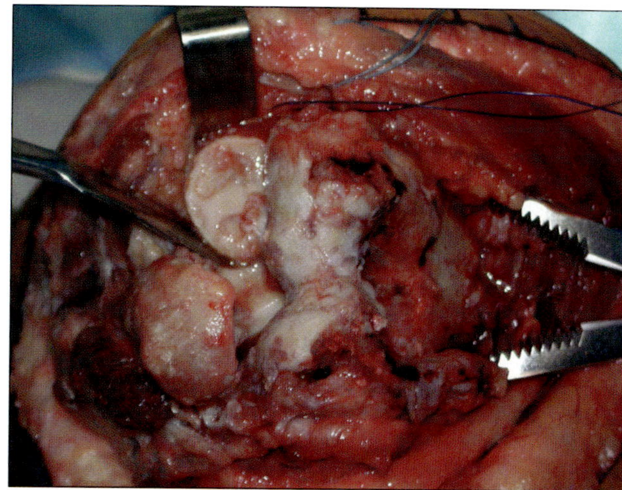
B

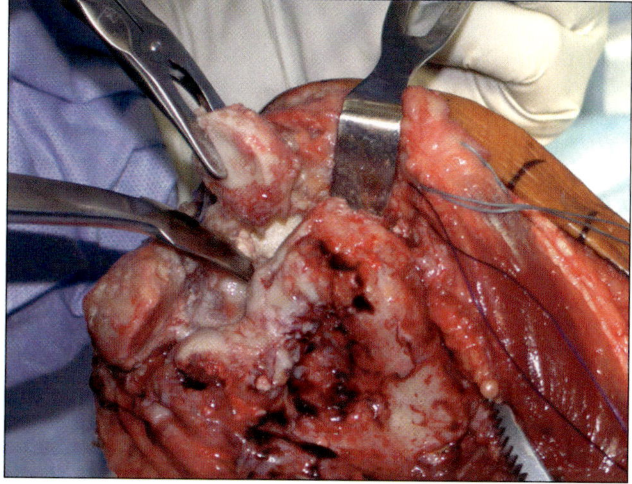
C

FIGURE 12

is made through the neck just distal to the head, and the radial head is excised (Fig. 12A–C).

Step 4: Humeral Preparation—Resection of Intercondylar Area of Distal Humerus

- Extramedullary resection method
  - The external fossa guide is positioned over the distal humerus and the medial border of guide aligned with the medial extent of the trochlea. The proximal stem is aligned over the midline of the humeral shaft (Fig. 13A and 13B). The axis marking of the external guide is aligned with the inferior-most aspect of the medial epicondyle.
    - Drilling is done through the hole of the fossa guide into the humeral fossa perpendicular to the slightly internally rotated plane of the

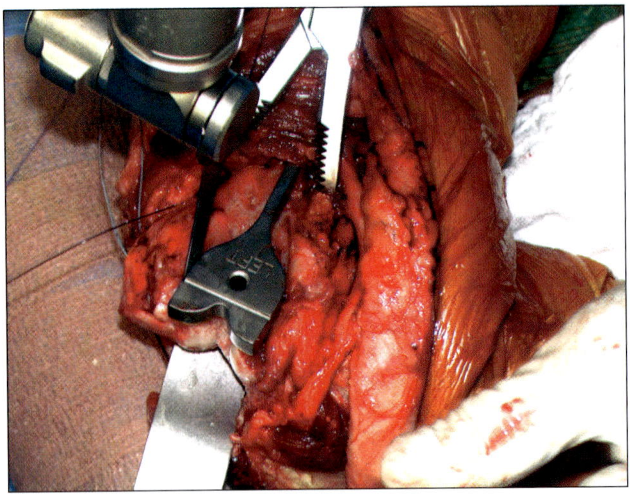

A

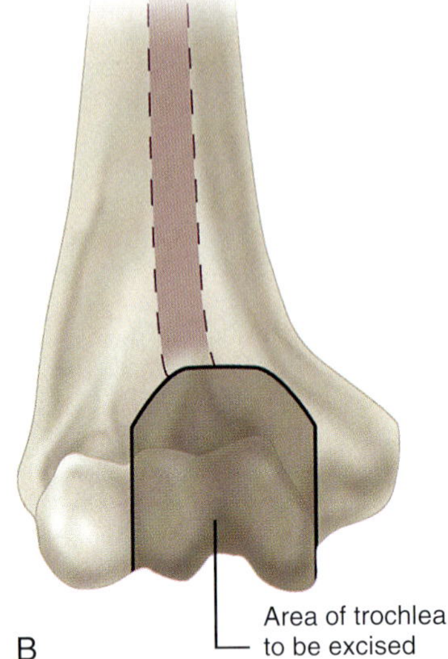

B

FIGURE 13

> **Pearls**
>
> - *Place a malleable retractor anterior to the humerus to protect the anterior soft tissues while making the humeral trochlear cuts.*
> - *Resect a wide enough slot in the trochlea so that the margins of the cut do not constrain the rasps from following the canal of the humerus*
>
> **Pitfalls**
>
> - *Be sure the oscillation of the saw blade does not encroach into the medial and lateral condyles and humeral columns, which could lead to weakening and condylar fracture.*
> - *When using the extramedullary resection guide, be sure the medial aspect distally is aligned with the most medial edge of the trochlea and the stem proximally is centered on the humerus.*

flexion-extension axis. With the drill bit in place, the medial and lateral-most aspects of the external guide are marked with electrocautery.

- The external guide is removed. A five-step fossa reamer is inserted into the drill hole of the olecranon fossa and the fossa is reamed until the outermost teeth start to engage the humeral fossa.
- The resection area is completed with use of a saw through the remnants of the trochlea previously marked by electrocautery. The trochlea is removed and a barrel reamer used to round out the proximal part of the resection area.

- A high-speed burr is used to gain access into the humeral canal through the proximal-most aspect of the olecranon fossa. The access is enlarged with a rasp or burr to allow for insertion of the 3.0-mm proximal starter rasp.
  - The humerus is rasped with progressively enlarging rasps until cortical resistance is met. Finally, a distal humerus broach corresponding to the last proximal humeral rasp utilized is used to broach the humerus. The axis mark on the broach should align with the inferior portion of the medial epicondyle.

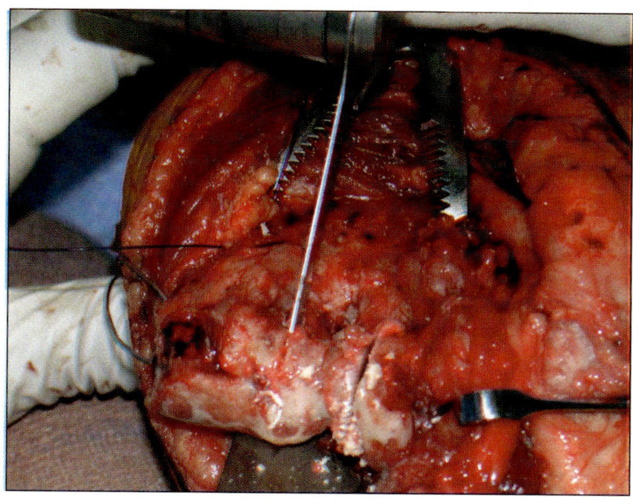
A

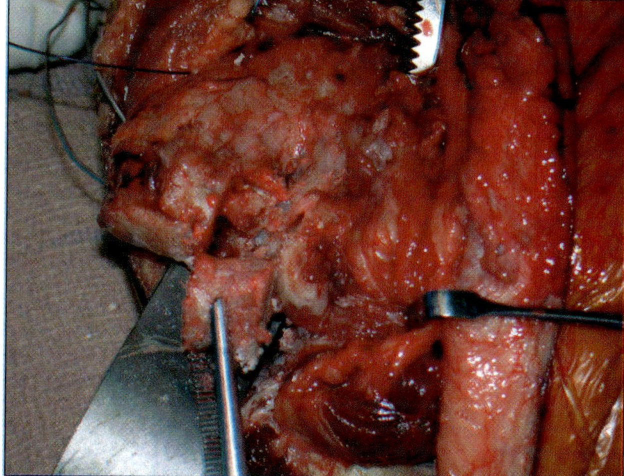
B

FIGURE 14

Instrumentation/ Implantation

- High-speed drill
- Oscillating saw
- Discovery extra- and intramedullary cutting guide
- Discovery barrel reamer
- Malleable retractor ($1^1/_2$ inch)
- Discovery humeral rasps
- Mallet

- Intramedullary resection method
  - With an oscillating saw, a small section in the center of the trochlea is resected (Fig. 14A and 14B).
    - A high-speed burr is used to enter the humeral canal at the proximal aspect of the olecranon fossa (Fig. 15). The humerus is sequentially rasped with progressively larger rasps until cortical resistance is met (Fig. 16A and 16B).
    - With the last rasp in place, the resection guide boom is applied to the rasp handle and the

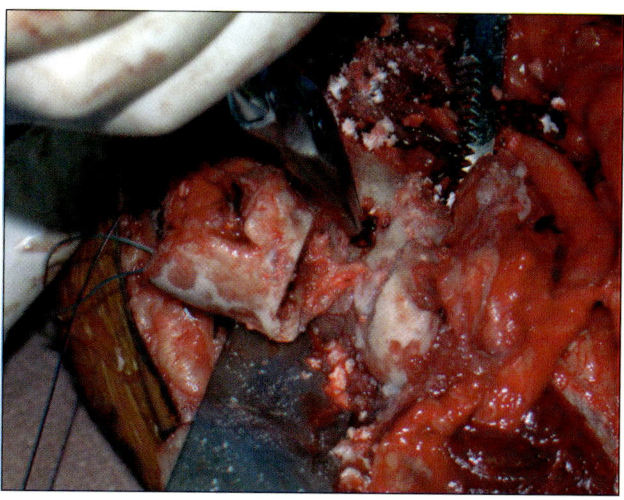

FIGURE 15

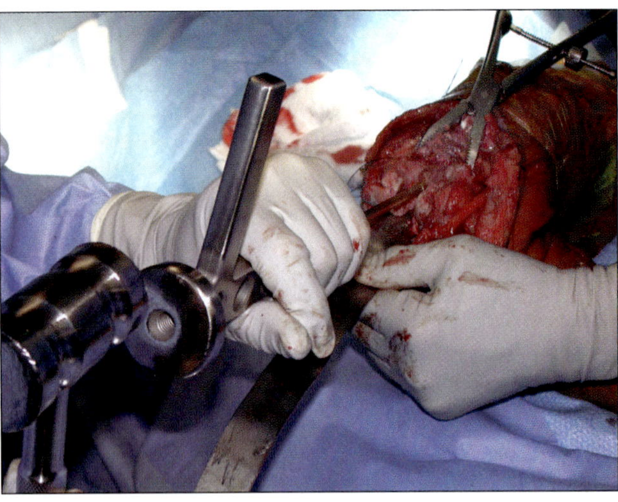
A

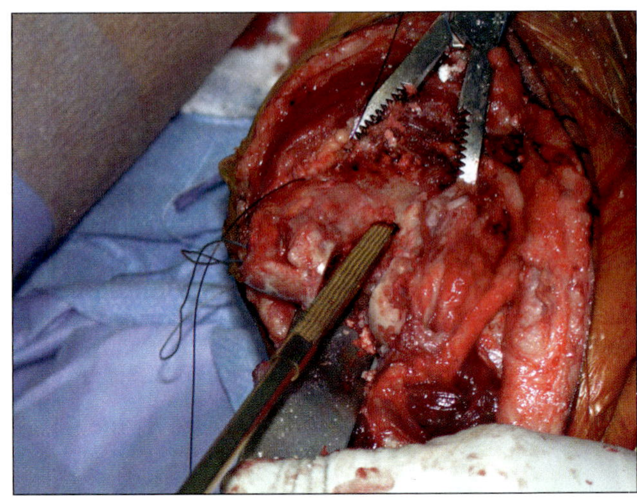
B

FIGURE 16

Controversies

- Some surgeons prefer use of the external guide for humeral intercondylar resection as this can be faster. Use of the intramedullary resection guide on the rasps assures that the resected intercondylar area will accurately match the implant since its alignment is set by the stem of the rasp, which mirrors that of the implant.

guide adjusted so that the axis rods of the resection guide are just proximal to the distal edge or inferior edge of the medial epicondyle (Fig. 17A and 17B). The resection guide is locked into place with the embedded screws. Two 0.062-inch Kirschner wires can be placed through the pinholes on either side of the resection guide to maintain it in position.

- Four saw cuts are made through the resection guide (Fig. 18). The rasp and resection guide are removed and the saw cuts completed through the anterior cortex (Fig. 19A and 19B). The surgeon must take care that the oscillation of

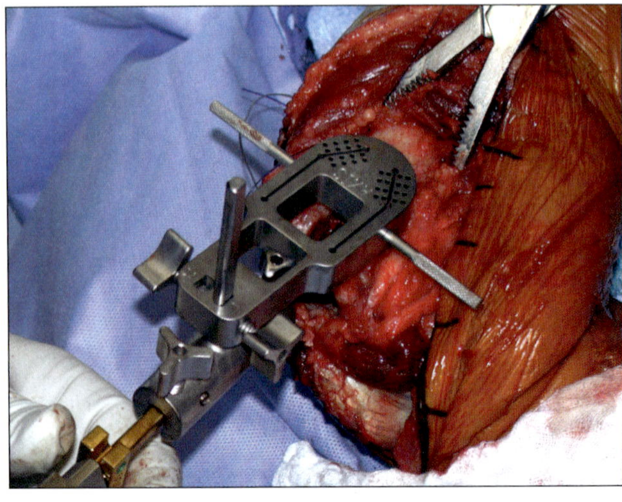
A

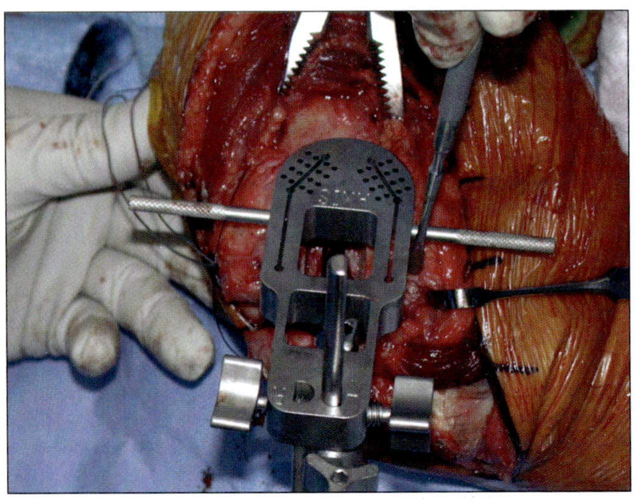
B

FIGURE 17

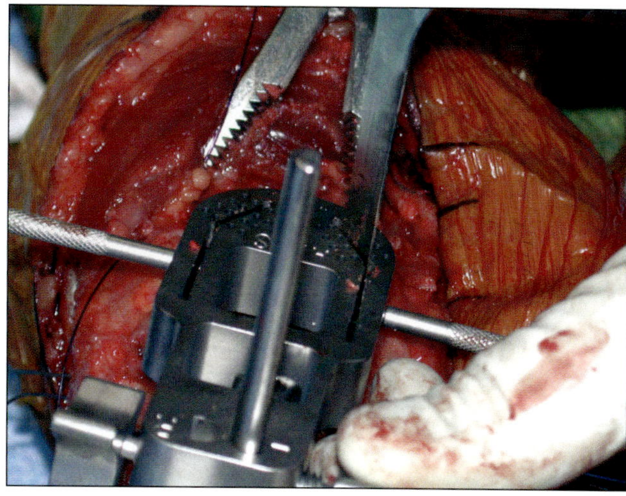

FIGURE 18

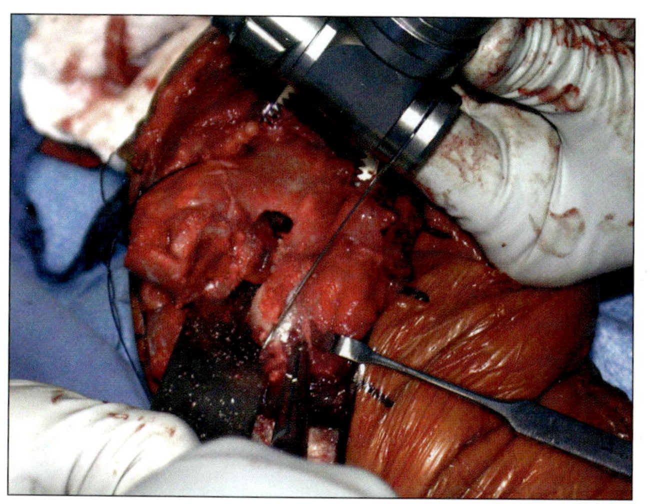

A

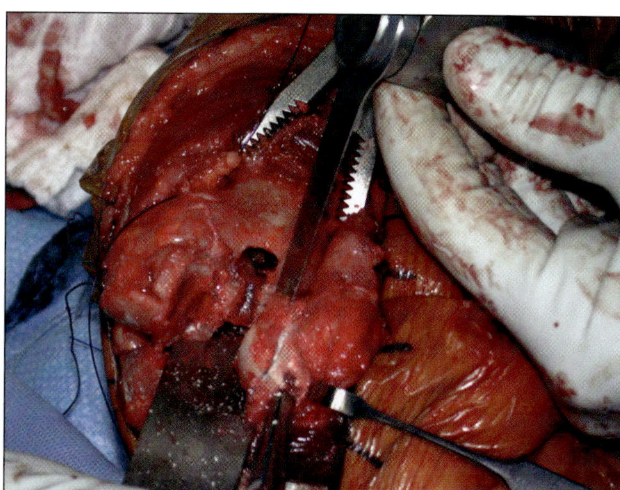

B

FIGURE 19

the blade does not compromise the condyles on either side.

- The central section cutout is removed. A barrel reamer is used to smooth out the proximal contour of the resected area (Fig. 20).

- One of the three color-coded distal humeral broaches is chosen corresponding to the size of the last rasp used. The broach is inserted or impacted into the canal until the axis mark corresponds to the inferior aspect of the medial epicondyle (Fig. 21). If undue resistance is met, a small burr can be used to widen the entrance to the humeral canal.
- The provisional humeral implant that corresponds to the size of the last rasp used is selected and inserted into the canal to check fit. Usually a small

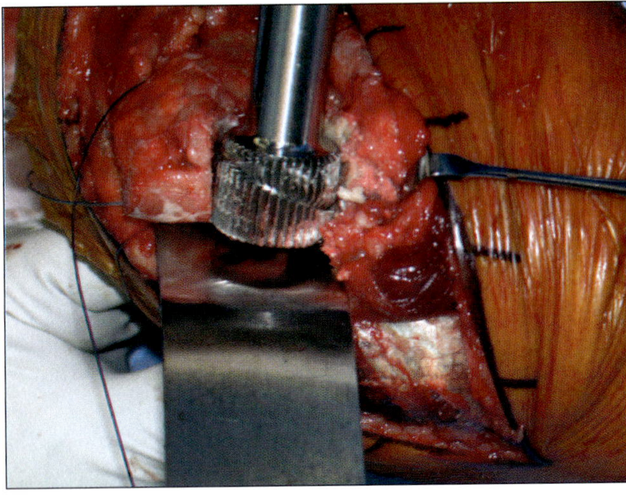

FIGURE 20

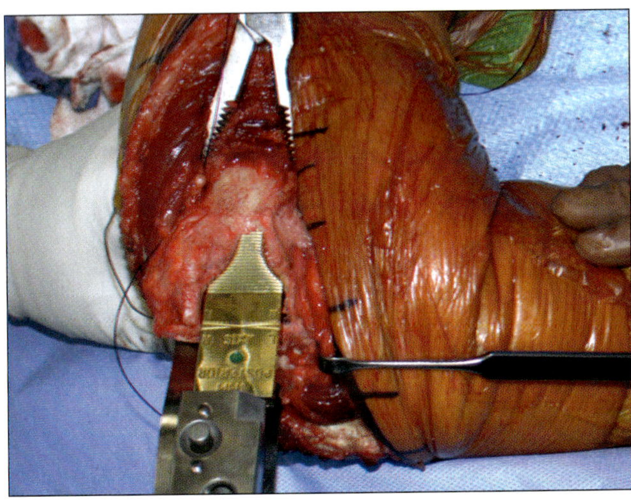

FIGURE 21

> **Pearls**
>
> - *The olecranon may have eroded asymmetrically in cases in which the humerus over time has subsided into the ulna. Use the location of the coronoid process to determine the center of the medial/lateral ulnar width in determining where to enter the ulnar canal.*
> - *When there is significant subsidence of the humerus into the ulna, with erosive loss of bone from the olecranon, a deep trough in the olecranon may not be required.*
> - *Keep the handle of the ulnar rasp aligned with the posterior surface of the proximal ulna to ensure proper rotational alignment during rasping of the ulna.*

burr is required to remove further a small area of anterior cortex to allow the anterior flange to seat fully proximally (3–4 mm of central anterior humeral cortex). The provisional trial is fine-tuned as needed with a small burr to areas of bone that need to be further removed (Fig. 22).

Step 5: Ulnar Preparation

- A canal is opened into the proximal ulna with a small burr directed 55° anterior to posterior (Fig. 23). Progressively larger flexible reamers are used to remove soft cancellous bone from within the ulnar canal (Fig. 24A and 24B). It is not necessary to remove cortical bone. The flexible reamer is advanced down to one of the two etched lines that corresponds to the length of the ulnar implant stem to be used (75 mm or 115 mm).

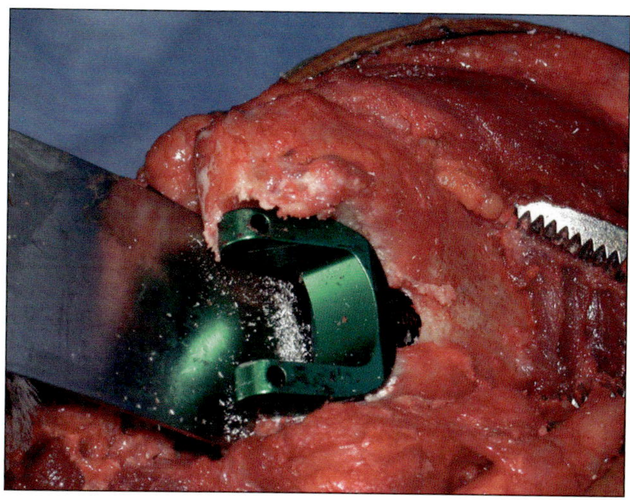

FIGURE 22

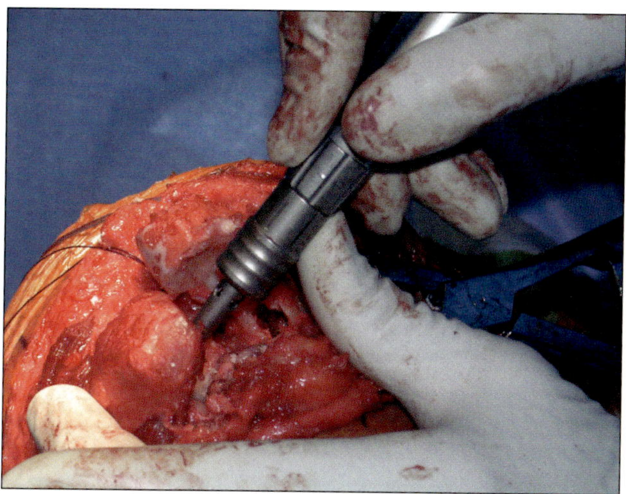

FIGURE 23

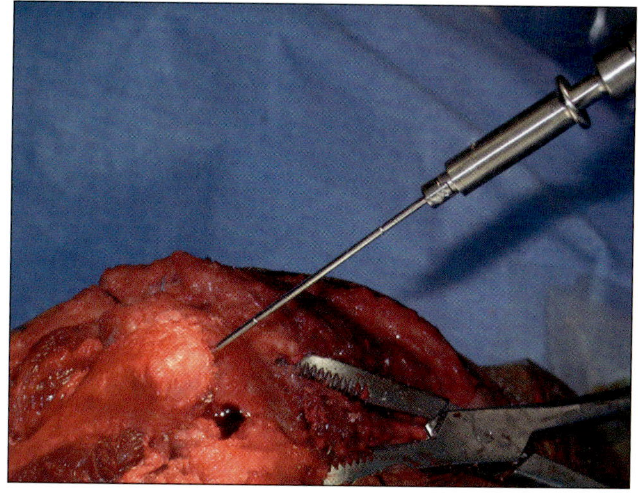

A

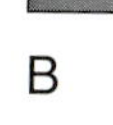

B

FIGURE 24

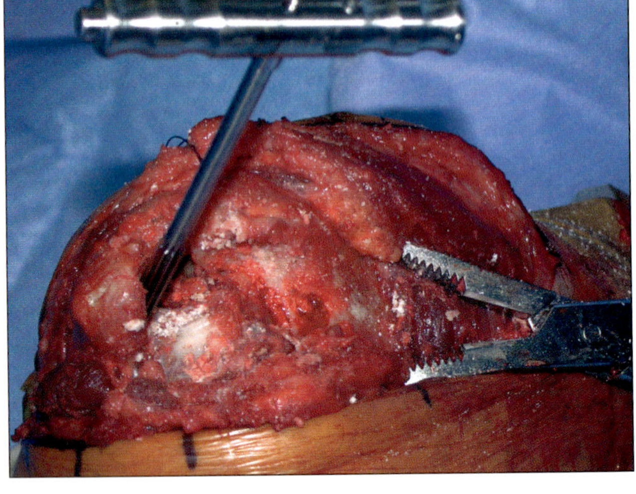

FIGURE 25

Instrumentation/ Implantation

- High-speed burr
- Discovery flexible reamer
- Discovery slot reamer
- Discovery ulnar rasps
- Discovery barrel reamer
- Mallet

- A trough is made in the proximal ulna with a burr or with an olecranon trough reamer (Fig. 25).
  - If using the latter, the smooth tip of the reamer is inserted into the ulnar canal and used as a pivot point to progressively drive the side-cutting reamer into a posterior direction. The width of the resected groove should match that of the subsequently used rasps.
  - It is essential to make an adequate trough in the olecranon to ensure that the ulna is reamed straight down the canal (Fig. 26).
- Progressively larger ulnar rasps are used to prepare the ulna. In doing so, the surgeon must continually work to seat the rasp posteriorly such that it aligns with the longitudinal canal of the ulna (Fig. 27).

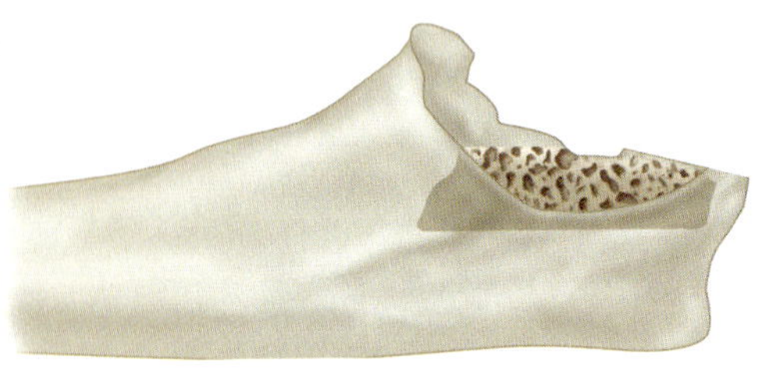

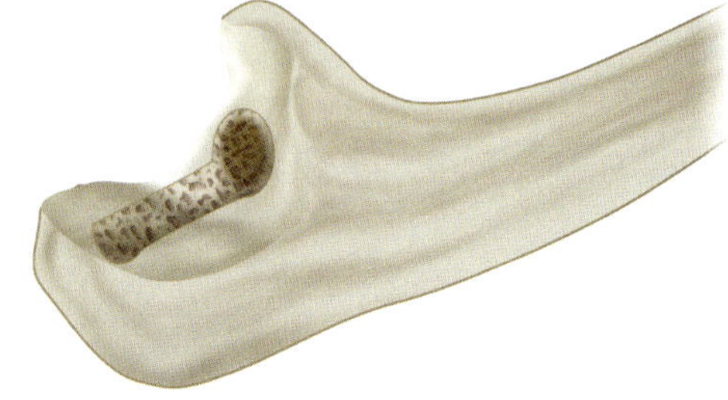

FIGURE 26

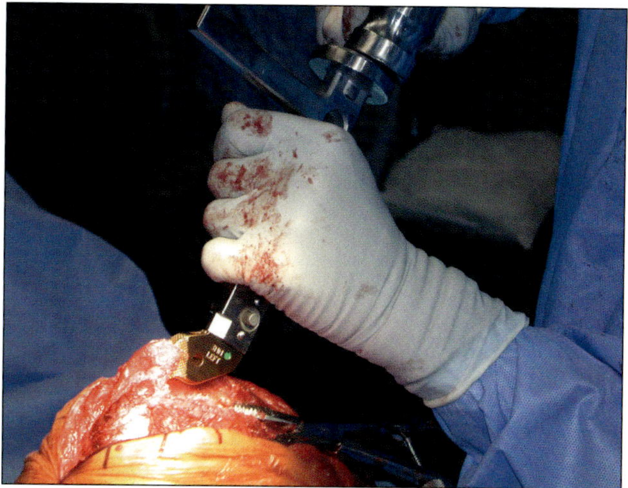

FIGURE 27

Controversies

- Ulnar exposure and preparation can be done with the triceps intact but is more difficult. In most instances, takedown of the triceps assures perfect exposure of the ulna for its preparation.

  - In most cases of ulnar implant malalignment, the implant has not been set down posteriorly far enough into the proximal ulna. This can predispose to perforation of the posterior ulnar canal cortex during rasping and also will place the central axis of the articulation too far anterior (Fig. 28A and 28B).
- The proximal coronoid and olecranon can then be rounded out with a barrel reamer. The appropriate sized provisional ulnar implant is checked for fit and fine-tuned by additional rasping or removal of bone with a high-speed burr.

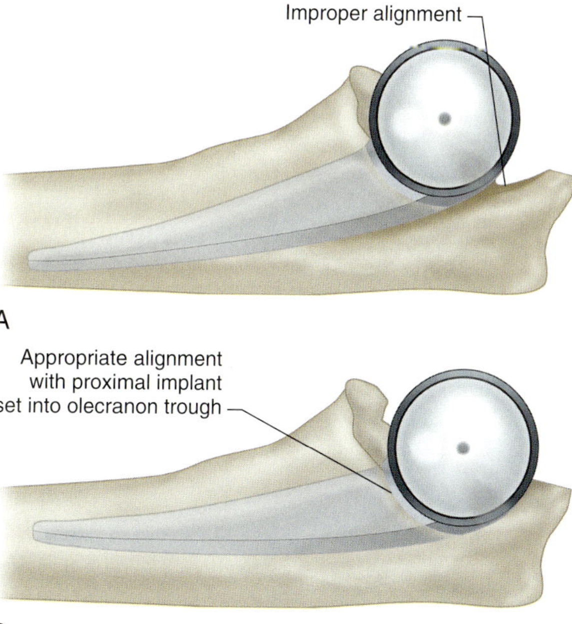

FIGURE 28

Pearls

- *It is necessary to remove 3–4 mm of the central anterior humeral cortex for the width of the anterior flange to allow the flange to sit in proper position and for the humeral implant to fully seat proximally.*
- *Make sure there is no bone overlapping the posterior or anterior surfaces of the humeral distal flanges that will interfere later with insertion of the condyles onto the flanges.*

Pitfalls

- *If the elbow does not extend fully, do not force it into extension as this may drive the humeral implant more deeply into the humerus and, in doing so, fracture the condyles.*

Instrumentation/ Implantation

- Humeral and ulnar trials
- Trial bearings

Controversies

- When elbow extension is insufficient, it may be necessary to work on static progressive bracing postoperatively. First be sure that the anterior capsule has been fully released and or excised and that the humerus has been fully seated with its axis aligned with the inferior aspect of the medial epicondyle. Seating the ulnar implant more deeply is not helpful, but seating or recessing the humeral implant more proximally may help.

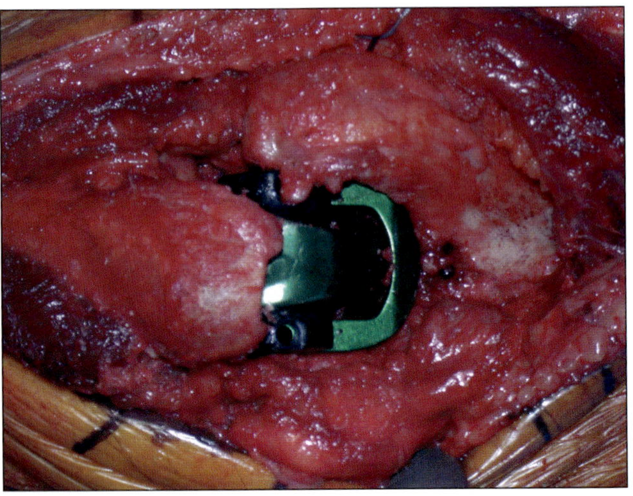

FIGURE 29

Step 6: Trial Reduction

- The provisional humeral and ulnar trials are reinserted. The provisional hemispherical condyles are assembled on the ulna and the condyles reduced onto the humerus (Fig. 29). The range of motion is trialed and that the olecranon and/or coronoid are assessed to ensure that they do not impinge in extremes of flexion and extension.

Step 7: Cementing Implants

- The humeral canal is brushed with the Discovery brush to clean up the medullary surfaces (Fig. 30).
- Polyethylene cement plugs of appropriate size are applied to the humerus and ulna, marking on the inserter rod the depth to which insertion should occur, at least 10–15 mm beyond the length of the humeral and ulnar implants (Fig. 31A and 31B). The canals are irrigated, sucked dry, and packed with thrombin-soaked gauze 4 × 4s (Fig. 32).
- Low-viscosity cement is mixed with antibiotics. With a cement gun, the humerus is injected from proximal to distal, then the ulna from distal to proximal (Fig. 33).
  - The humeral implant is inserted first and impacted to full insertion. The surgeon must be certain that the implant is displaced posteriorly such that the anterior flange solidly contacts the anterior aspect of the humerus (Fig. 34). All extra cement is removed.
  - The ulnar component is then impacted similarly, removing extra cement (Fig. 35).

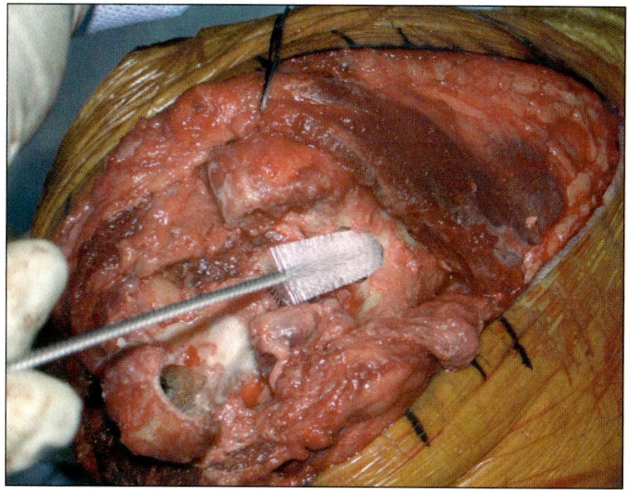

FIGURE 30

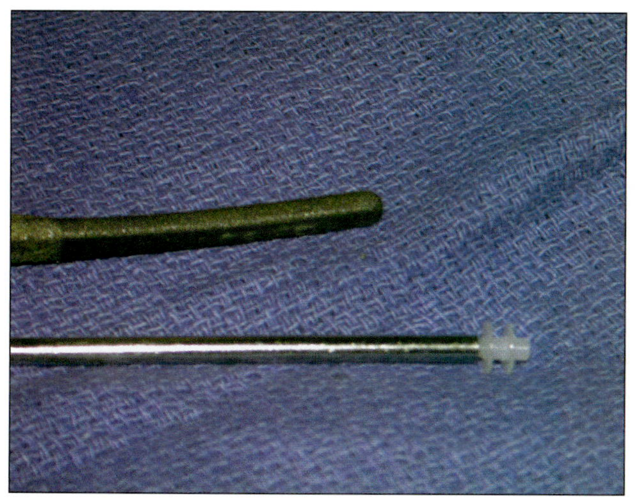

A

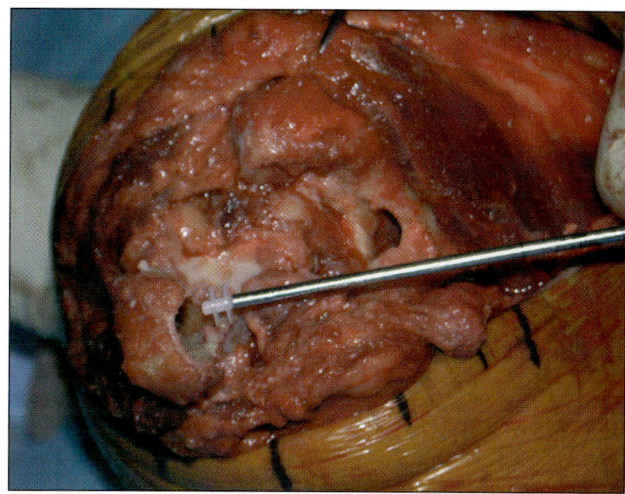

B

FIGURE 31

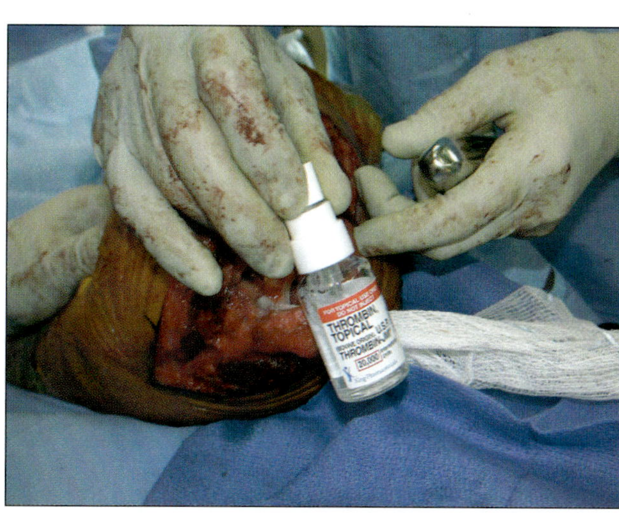

FIGURE 32

Pearls

- *Check and remove any extra cement from anterior to the humerus before inserting the ulnar component, while the exposure is optimal.*
- *Remove cement from the medial and lateral edges around of the ulnar bearing, particularly where the polyethylene meets the metal.*
- *Thoroughly irrigate with pulse lavage prior to implant articulation. This is essential to be sure that all particles of bone and cement that could lead to third-body implant wear have been removed from the joint space.*
- *There are usually small bleeders posterolaterally from the recurrent branches of the posterior interosseous artery and vein.*

Pitfalls

- *In cases in which perforations remain in the cortices of the humerus or ulna, such as following removal of plates for fracture, the cement may extrude. Fill voids in the cortices with bone graft harvested from the excised portions of the distal humerus, olecranon, or radial head.*
- *The canal diameter of the ulna is very small and will not accept cement restrictors commonly used in other joint arthroplasties. It requires restrictors as small as 3–8 mm, such as are provided with the Discovery Implant system. If small restrictors are not available, use a small plug of cancellous bone.*
- *Be sure the polyethylene bearing surfaces are clean without any residual coating of cement that could lead to early wear.*

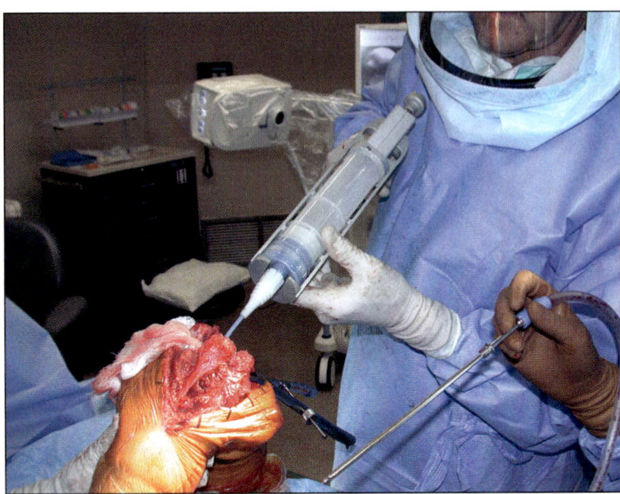

FIGURE 33

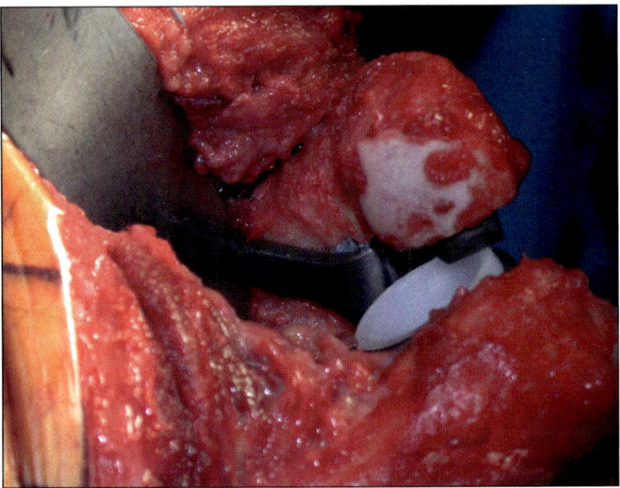

FIGURE 34

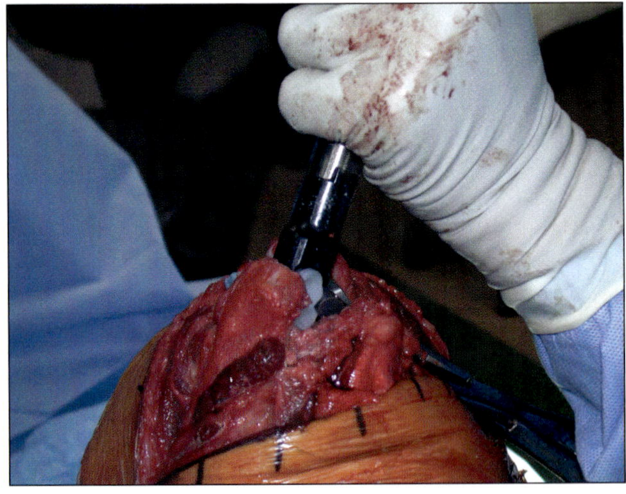

FIGURE 35

Instrumentation/ Implantation

- Medullary canal brush
- Thrombin
- Cement gun and Discovery nozzle
- Humeral and ulnar implant impactors
- Mallet
- Low-viscosity cement with premixed antibiotic

Controversies

- It is possible to articulate the humeral and ulnar implants with the condyles prior to implantation, inserting the joint as a complete unit. However, this requires a larger amount of elbow exposure/takedown and will not allow for as complete an inspection of the anterior joint for extruded cement. The Discovery system has been designed to allow for independent seating and cement fixation of the humeral and ulnar implants. Articulation with the condyles can be performed without urgency after each component is perfectly seated and extra cement removed.

Pearls

- *Minimize tension on the incision for the first 5 days by holding the elbow in 60° of flexion.*

Pitfalls

- *Patients who have been on steroid suppression usually have very thin skin. Perfect apposition of skin edges is critical. Perfect skin closure is most important about the central wound, and usually best controlled by vertical mattress sutures.*

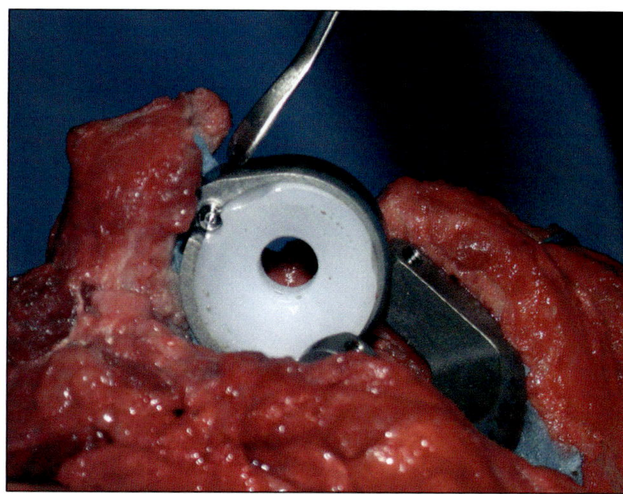

FIGURE 36

- The elbow is held immobile until the cement has fully cured (Fig. 36).

- The condyles are now applied to the ulna, ensuring that the recess for the screw heads faces posteriorly with the spheres aligned on the humerus (Fig. 37). The locking screws are inserted into the condyles and thoroughly tightened (Fig. 38). Elbow flexion and extension are rechecked to ensure that the olecranon does not impinge with the humerus in full extension.
- At this point, the tourniquet can be deflated and hemostasis obtained. Usually the tourniquet is left deflated through the remainder of the procedure.

Step 8: Wound Closure

- A $^1/_8$-inch drill is used to drill holes for reattachment of the triceps to the olecranon. The drill holes should pass through the small sulcus approximately 5 mm

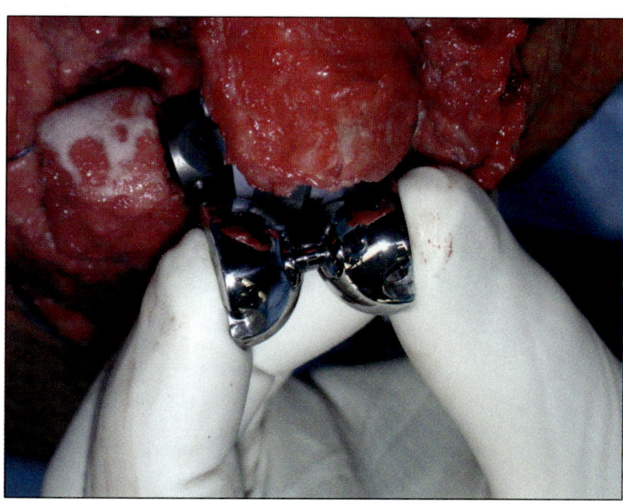

FIGURE 37

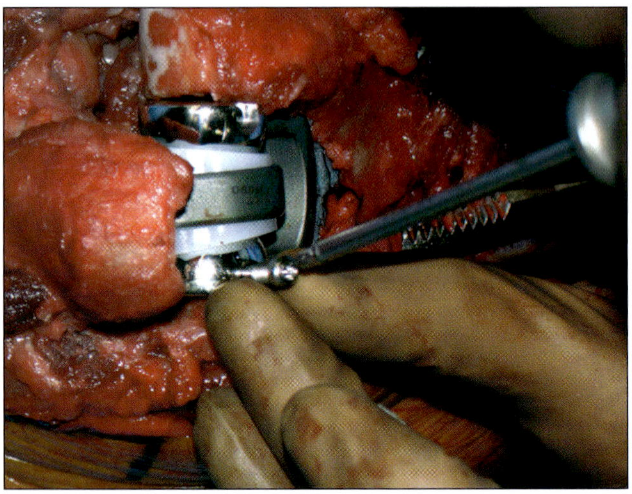

FIGURE 38

Instrumentation/ Implantation

- Medium suction drain
- 2.0 monofilament resorbable suture
- 3.0 or 4.0 resorbable suture
- 4.0 monofilament nylon suture
- Staples

proximal to the posterior surface of the olecranon, crossing and exiting with each drill medially and laterally (Fig. 39A and 39B).

- If desired, two divergent holes can be made through the lateral condyle for repair of the lateral collateral ligament and extensor origin with resorbable #0 monofilament suture (Fig. 40).
- Keith needles are used to pass the #2 braided polyester and Kevlar sutures through the ulna (Fig. 41).

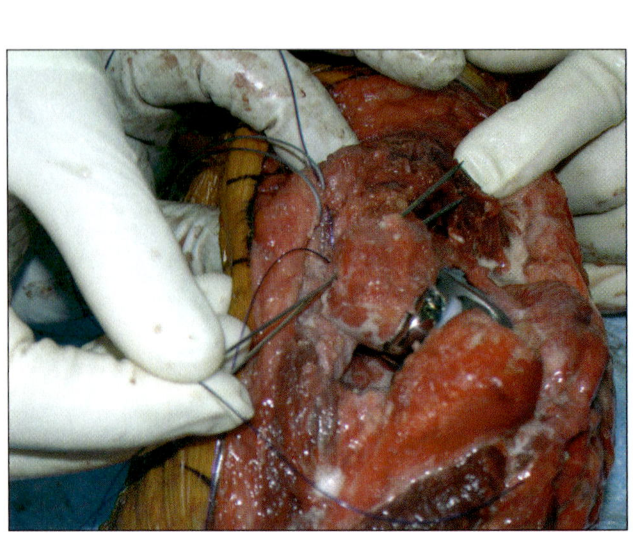

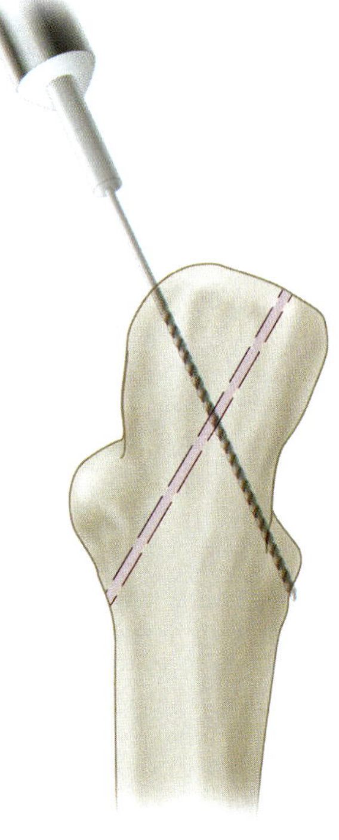

A B

FIGURE 39

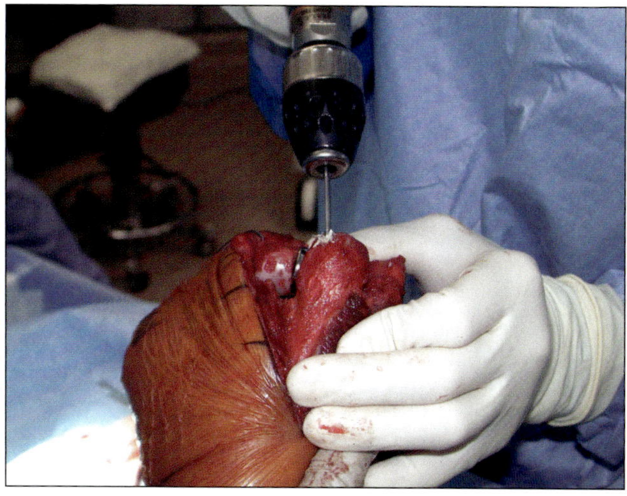

FIGURE 40

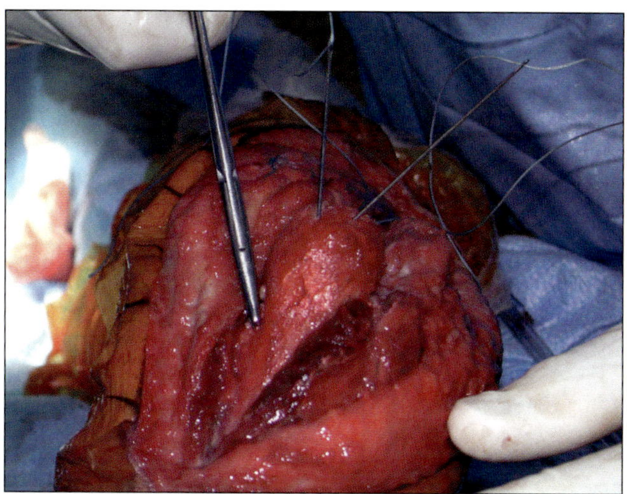

FIGURE 41

Controversies

- There remains debate as to whether postoperative antibiotics are essential. I administer preoperative antibiotics at least 20 minutes prior to skin incision and for two doses after surgery.

  - The lateral suture should then pass through the extensor sleeve and then back ulnarly and be tied to the ulnar suture at the point where the ulnar suture exits through bone (Fig. 42).
  - The surgeon must ensure that the triceps is solidly pulled to the olecranon surface prior to tying the sutures.
- The ulnar nerve should be checked for stability in its anteriorly transposed position. Usually it is stable without requirement for a fascial sling.
- The fascia of the FCU is repaired up to the level of the elbow and across the medial aspect of the elbow with 2-0 bioabsorbable sutures (Fig. 43).
- A small suction drain catheter is inserted, the dermis is approximated with 3-0 or 4-0 resorbable suture, and the skin is closed with staples or sutures (Fig. 44).

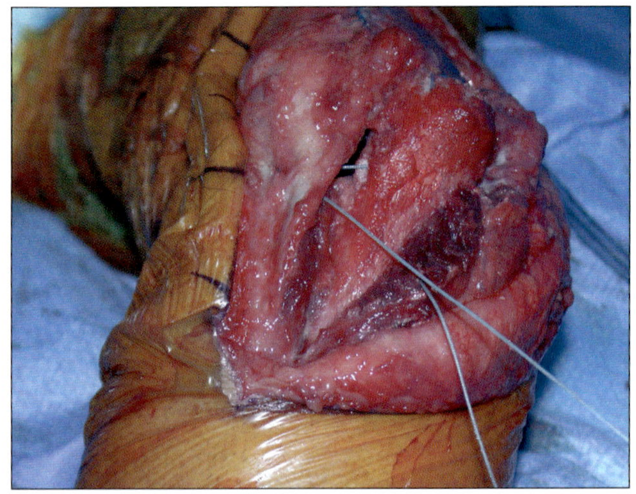

FIGURE 42

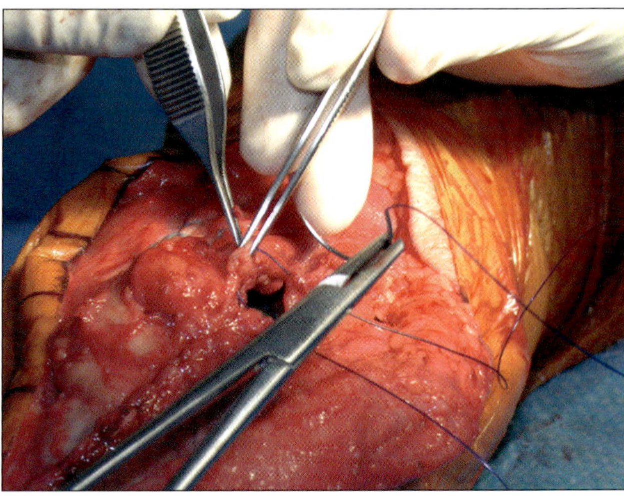

FIGURE 43

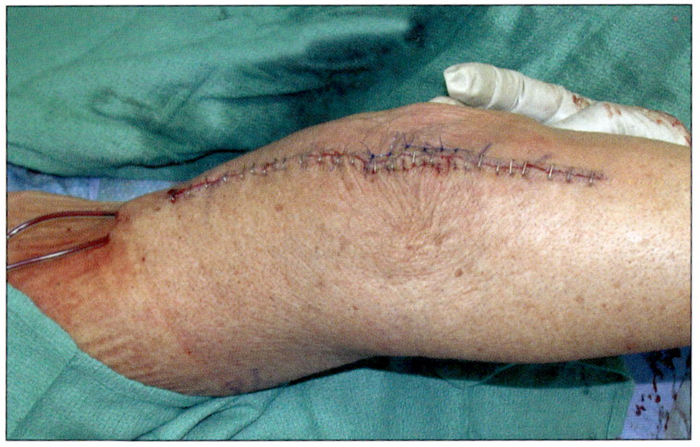

FIGURE 44

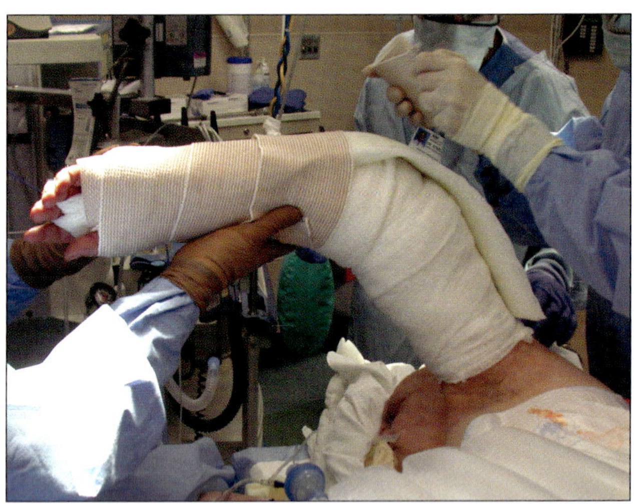

FIGURE 45

- A bulky dressing is applied and the arm is splinted with the elbow in 60° of flexion to minimize tension on the posterior incision (Fig. 45).
- Figure 46 shows postoperative AP radiographs of the humerus (Fig. 46A) and ulna (Fig. 46B) and a lateral radiograph of the elbow (Fig. 46C).

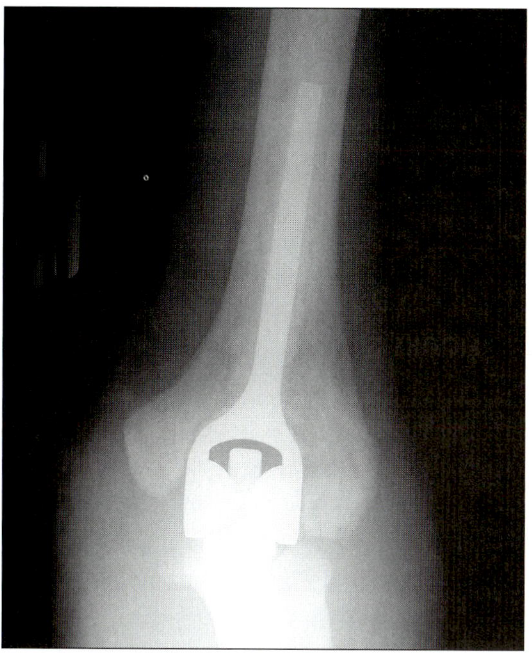
A

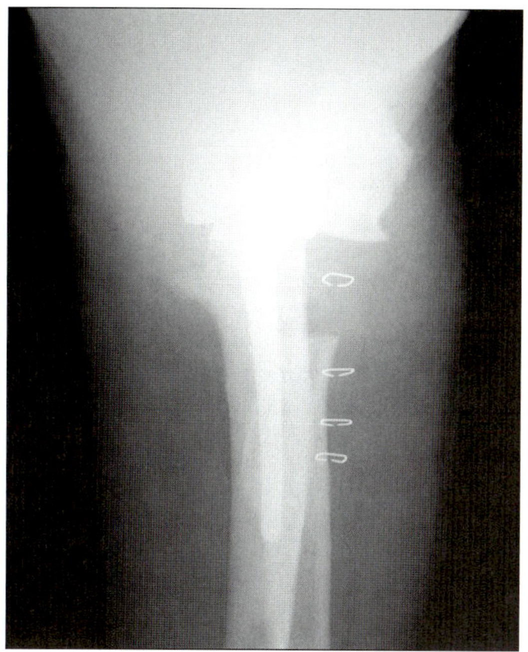
B

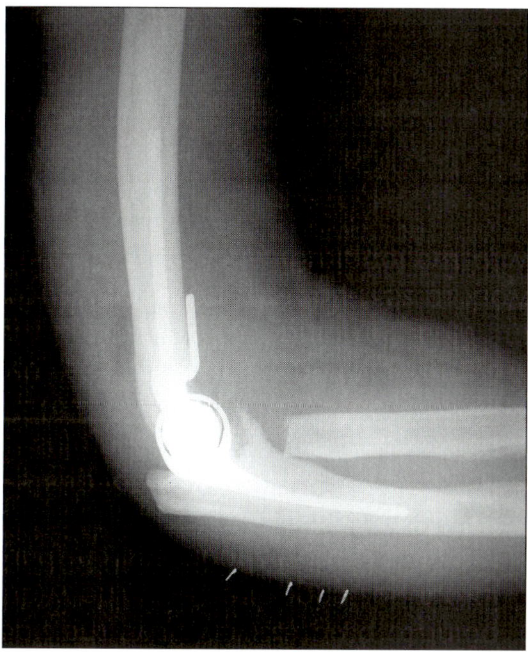
FIGURE 46 C

Postoperative Care and Expected Outcomes

Postoperative Care

- Postoperative antibiotics are employed for 24 hours. Suction drains are removed at 24 or 48 hours depending on when drainage is stopped.
- Patients are usually discharged on the second postoperative day and seen about 5 days

Pearls

- *If motion is not steadily improving by the second or third week, dynamic or static progressive splinting should be added.*

Pitfalls

- *Early infection rates remain less than 1%, with most occurring in patients with complications of delayed would healing. Be sure the wound is well sealed and without drainage prior to beginning elbow motion.*
- *Development of heterotopic ossification is rare and most commonly associated with arthroplasty for acute trauma or fracture. Be sure to débride all nonviable tissue and evacuate hematoma by débridement and wound lavage.*

postoperatively to remove the dressing, check the wound, and begin active range of motion. Motion should not be initiated until assurance that the wound is healthy and sealed.

- Active and passive flexion and extension are initiated at 5 days. Active extension against resistance is not allowed for 6 weeks. The patient is cautioned not to push with resistance against the elbow, such as when getting up out of a chair.
- Weighted stretching or extension splinting can be utilized to correct any residual tightness to extension. A long-arm splint is usually helpful at night to maintain full extension.
- Sutures or staples are removed at 10–14 days. Normal light use of the arm for activities of daily living is initiated at 5 days and strengthening at 6 weeks following surgery.

Expected Outcomes

- Results have been evaluated from a single-surgeon prospective series of 63 elbows implanted between 2003 and 2008 by an independent investigator.
- There were 46 females and 17 males with average age of 63 ± 13 years (range, 33–88 years). Diagnoses included inflammatory arthritis in 54%, osteoarthritis and posttraumatic arthritis in 12%, fracture or instability in 21%, revision replacement in 2%, and other conditions in 11%. Of the total, 93% were right hand dominant, with unilateral involvement in 57%; 51% involved the left side and 49% the right. The operative approach spared the triceps in 44% of cases, with triceps split or reflection in 56% of cases.
- Flexion/extension improved from 118° (65–150°)/46° (10–95°) to 137° (75–155°)/19° (0–90°). Preoperative pronation improved from 68° (20–90°) to 72° (45–90°). Preoperative supination improved from 46° (30–90°) to postoperative 80° (45 to 90°).
- Complications occurred in 19% of patients (12/63); 11% (7/63) required surgery, including one drainage of postoperative hematoma due to a clotting disorder, one ulnar neurolysis at 3½ months postoperative, one triceps suture foreign body granuloma excision at 2 years, one bushing exchange at 5 years, and incision and drainage of two septic elbows, both occurring at 4 years, due to septic pneumonia in one case and an infected spinal stimulator in the other. Complications not requiring surgery included two patients with delayed wound

healing, two patients with suture abscesses at 4 and 6 weeks postoperative, and one patient with a partially loose condylar screw at 5 years.

- Average preoperative to postoperative American Shoulder and Elbow Surgeons (ASES) pain score diminished from 36.9 to 3.26. ASES function improved from 14.8 to 31.6. Signs improved from 14.8 to 0.76.
- Review of eight radiologic zones for cement-prosthesis and bone-cement interfaces were evaluated for the humerus, and nine zones for the ulna, and demonstrated no progressive lucencies in follow-up.

Evidence

Duggal N, Dunning CE, Johnson JA, King GJW. The flat spot of the proximal ulna: a useful anatomic landmark in total elbow arthroplasty. J Shoulder Elbow Surg. 2004;13:206-7.

This article described that by electromagnetic tracking analysis the dorsal flat spot on the proximal ulna was found to be nearly perpendicular to the plane of the greater sigmoid notch. The flat spot therefore can be used to orient the ulnar component axially in total elbow replacement.

Goldberg SH, Omid R, Nassr AN, Beck R, Cohen MS. Osseous anatomy of the distal humerus and proximal ulna: implications for total elbow arthroplasty. J Shoulder Elbow Surg. 2007;16(3 Suppl):S39-46.

This article showed that by sequential axial sections of 27 human cadavers, the lateral x-ray view most closely approximates the minimum canal diameter for templating. Frontage lateral radial grafts can overestimate the minimal canal size for total elbow arthroplasty components.

Hastings H II, Theng CS. Total elbow replacement for distal humerus fractures and traumatic deformity: results and complications of semiconstrained implants and design rationale for the Discovery Elbow System. Am J Orthop. 2003;32(9 Suppl):20-8.

Authors found that implant elbow replacement remains a valuable tool in the treatment of traumatic and post-traumatic deformities of the elbow with predictable short term and intermediate results in low demand patients. Most complications related to failure of polythene bushings with 5 of 19 patients requiring a revision surgery for Coonrad-Morrey bushings. The authors believe that bushing failure is at higher risk when patients have absent medial or lateral column support for the collateral ligaments and flexor extensor origins.

Ikävalko M, Lehto MU, Repo A, Kautiainen H, Hämäläinen M. The Souter-Strathclyde elbow arthroplasty: a clinical and radiological study of 525 consecutive cases. J Bone Joint Surg [Br]. 2002;84:77-82.

This series evaluated 525 primary Souter elbow arthroplasties undertaken in 406 patients. Revision surgery was required in 30 instances for implant dislocation, 33 cases for revision surgery for aseptic loosening, 12 cases for deep infection, and 2 for superficial infection. Excluding aseptic loosening, the cumulative rate of success at 5 years was 96% and at 10 years 85%.

Lee DH. Posttraumatic elbow arthritis and arthroplasty. Orthop Clin North Am. 1999;30:141-62.

This review of posttraumatic elbow arthritis found elbow distraction interposition arthroplasty best advised for younger, active patients and implant arthroplasty for elderly patients. While improvements in surgical technique and implant design have improved results, reported complications with elbow implant arthroplasty average 25 to 40%.

Little CP, Graham AJ, Karatzas G, Woods DA, Carr AJ. Outcomes of total elbow arthroplasty for rheumatoid arthritis: comparative study of three implants. J Bone Joint Surg [Am]. 2005;87:2439-48.

This article compared results in prosthetic elbow arthroplasty by Souter-Strathclyde, Kudo and Coonrad-Morrey implants for rheumatoid arthritis. Function in the three groups was similar. Survival of the linked Coonrad-Morrey implant was better than the other two groups with unlinked implants yet 16% of Coonrad-Morrey ulnar components showed focal osteolysis and half of these cases progressed to frank loosening. Elbow replacement with a linked implant provides similar pain relief and range of motion compared to unlinked components and removes the risk of dislocation.

Morrey BF, Adams RA. Semiconstrained arthroplasty for the treatment of rheumatoid arthritis of the elbow. J Bone Joint Surg [Am]. 1992;74:479-90.

This article reviews 54 patients who underwent 58 modified Coonrad elbow implants for rheumatoid arthritis with a mean follow-up of 3.8 years. Excellent result was obtained in 69%, good result in 22%, fair result in 4, and poor result in 1. Reoperation was required in 6 elbows for injection, triceps insufficiency, and fractured ulnar component. No patient showed radiographic evidence of loosening.

Schneeberger AG, Adams R, Morrey BF. Semiconstrained total elbow replacement for the treatment of post-traumatic osteoarthrosis. J Bone Joint Surg [Am]. 1997;79:1211-22.

This article reports on 41 Coonrad-Morrey elbow prosthesis for post-traumatic arthrosis, 27% of patients sustained a major complication with 22% of cases requiring an additional operation mostly for mechanical failures. Ulnar component fracture occurred in 12% of cases. Polyethylene bushings wore out in 5% while linked. Linked implant arthroplasty is reliable and frequently the only option for post-traumatic joint deformity, mechanical failure seen in this study underscores the increased complication rate in this patient population. This patient group has the tendency for increased and excessive use of the previously functionless joint.

Wright TW, Hastings H II. Total elbow arthroplasty failure due to overuse, C-ring failure, and/or bushing wear. J Shoulder Elbow Surg. 2005;14:65-72.

This series of patients form two different institutions reports on 10 patients with Coonrad-Morrey implants which presented with bushing wear and C-ring failure. Time to revision averaged 60 months (range, 9-156 months). The normal Coonrad-Morrey hinge allows for 7° of motion from full varus to valgus. 7 to 10° of varus-valgus motion suggests partial wearing of bushings and when varus-valgus exceeds 10°, the bushings are entirely worn with risk of metal particulate synovitis. In high demand post-traumatic patients, there is significant edge loading of the polyethylene as the elbow is moved from varus to valgus. This may be exacerbated in patients without epicondyles and no flexor pronator and extensor supinator origins to protect against excessive loading. Authors advise early bushing exchange and synovectomy when bushing wear is diagnosed to avoid progressive osteolysis and/or implant stem failure.

Wright TW, Wong AM, Jaffe R. Functional outcome comparison of semiconstrained and unconstrained total elbow arthroplasties. J Shoulder Elbow Surg. 2000;9:524-31.

Authors compared 26 patients who had undergone linked Mayo modified Coonrad and unlinked Ewald capitellar condylar total elbow arthroplasties. One Coonrad-Morrey required removal for aseptic loosening and one Ewald unlinked implant for chronic dislocation. Excluding the two failures, no significant differences in functional performance was found and no patients demonstrated progressive radiographic loosening.

PROCEDURE 45

Total Elbow Arthroplasty for the Treatment of Complex Distal Humerus Fractures

Christopher M. Stutz, Hill Hastings II, Douglas R. Weikert, and Donald H. Lee

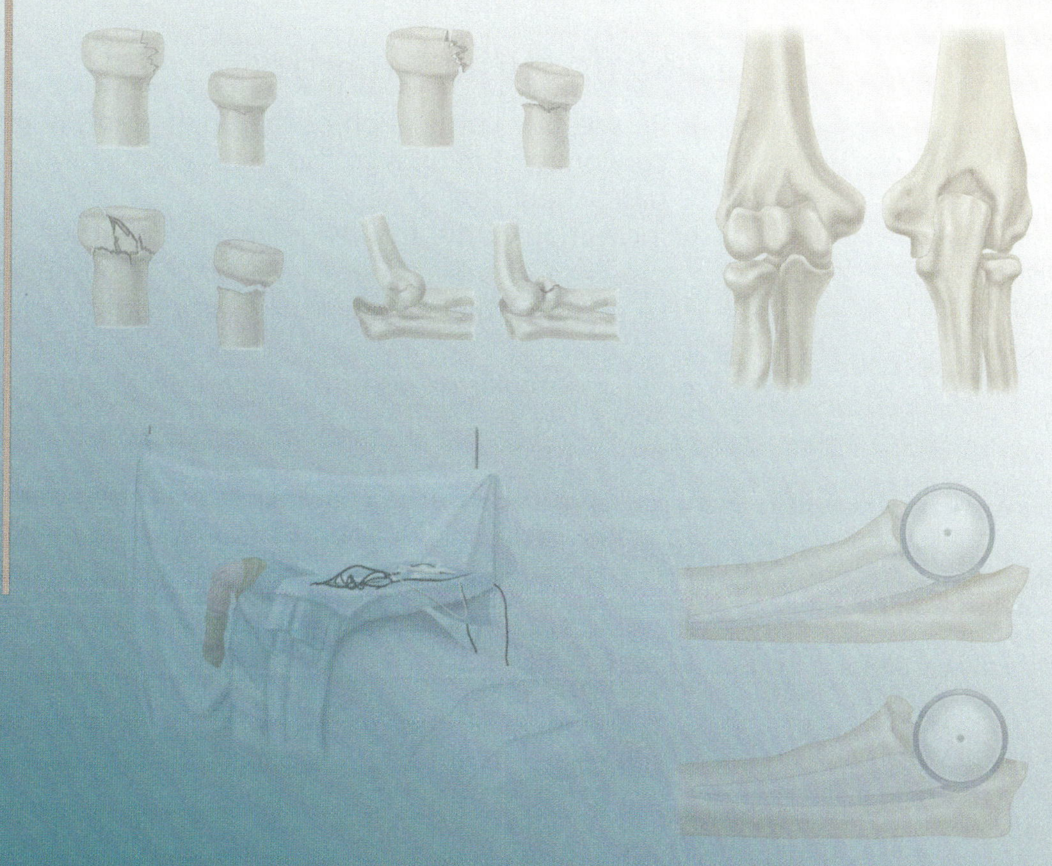

PITFALLS

- *Contraindications to the procedure include Gustilo type II and III open fractures, infection, neuropathic joint, severe impairment of limb function, and the need for weight bearing by using a cane or walker with the affected extremity.*
- *Fractures with diaphyseal extension of greater that 8 cm from the distal humeral joint line may require custom implants that may not be immediately available.*

Controversies

- Patient selection for total elbow arthroplasty requires careful consideration and discussion of postoperative activity limitations.
- Gustilo type II and III open fractures need to be appropriately débrided and have sufficient wound coverage prior to total elbow arthroplasty.

Treatment Options

- Nonoperative management: mainly reserved for patients with medical comorbidities precluding surgical intervention, those with limited extremity function (i.e., paralysis), and some nondisplaced fractures
- Open reduction and internal fixation
  - Standard of care for most displaced, intra-articular fractures of the distal humerus
  - Technically difficult, with poor outcomes in elderly patients with severe articular comminution and compromised bone quality
- Total elbow arthroplasty: reliable option for treatment of elderly patients with severe, comminuted fractures of the distal humerus

Indications

- Complex, intra-articular fractures of the distal humerus in elderly (>65 years of age), low-demand patients
- Complex, intra-articular fractures of the distal humerus in patients with poor bone quality rendering the techniques of open reduction and internal fixation unsuccessful, including fractures:
  - With bone loss (i.e., open fractures)
  - With a large number of small bone fragments
  - Involving severely osteoporotic bone
  - With pre-existing joint disease (i.e., rheumatoid arthritis, posttraumatic arthritis)

Examination/Imaging

- Preoperative evaluation of the upper extremity for concomitant injuries to the shoulder, forearm, and hand should be done.
- Inspection of the soft tissue envelope for the presence of other wounds may preclude the decision to perform total elbow arthroplasty in the acute setting.
- Neurovascular status of the extremity should be evaluated and documented.
- Plain radiographs
  - Anteroposterior (AP) and lateral views should be obtained (Fig. 1A and 1B)
  - Traction views of the injury can help to define fracture anatomy by revealing fragments that may be impacted or collapsed.
- Computed tomography
  - Two-dimensional images can be helpful in defining fracture anatomy as long as the images are formatted in the correct plane.
  - Three-dimensional reconstructions can be obtained to compensate for oblique scans but are rarely necessary for preoperative planning.

Surgical Anatomy

- The humerus terminates distally into two condyles, medial and lateral, with their respective articular surfaces, the trochlea and the capitellum, forming the superior portion of elbow joint (Fig. 2A and 2B).
- The trochlea is a spool-shaped structure that is covered by articular cartilage in a 300° arc that articulates with the olecranon process of the proximal ulna.

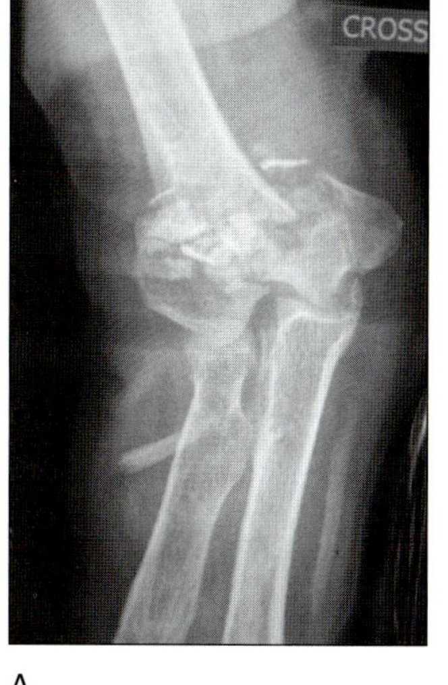

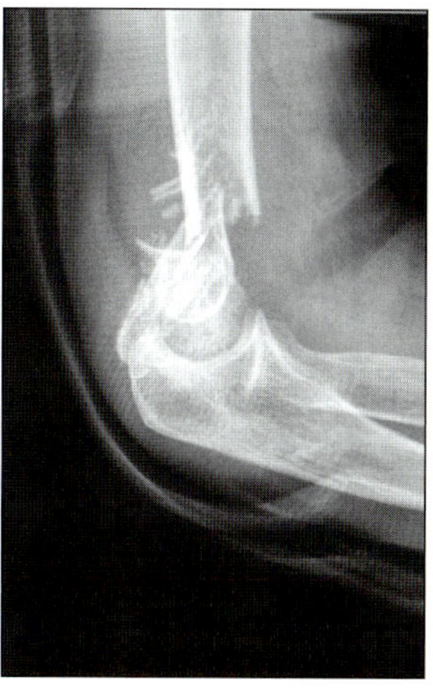

A B

FIGURE 1

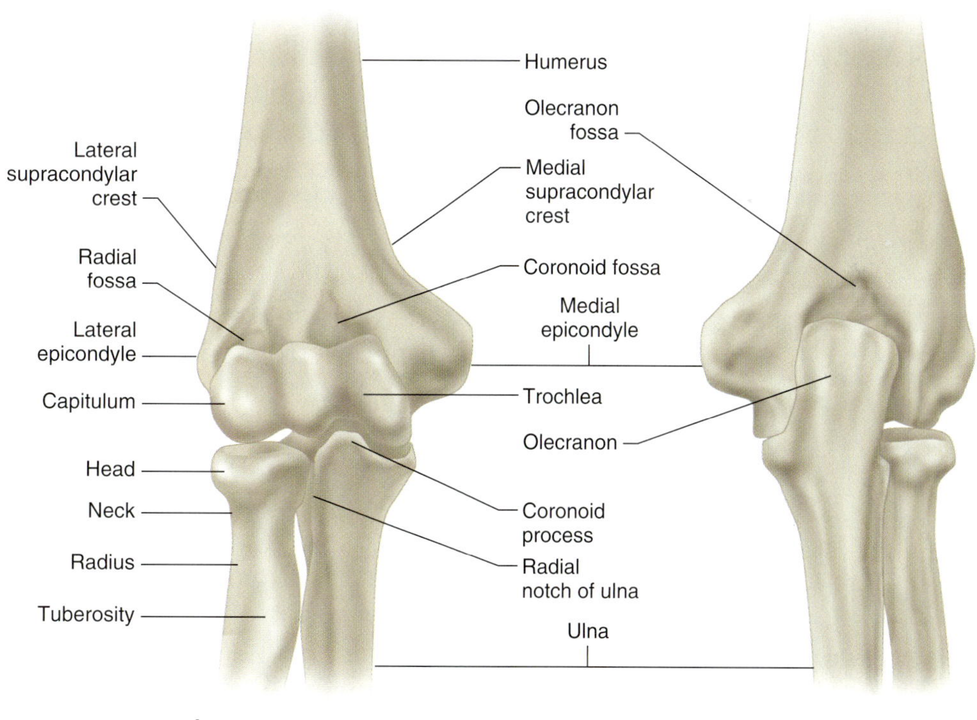

FIGURE 2

- The ulnohumeral joint is essentially a hinge joint that lies in 3–9° of external rotation and 4–8° of valgus in relation to the humeral shaft.
- The convex surface of the capitellum articulates with the concave surface of the radial head.
  - The unconstrained nature of the radiocapitellar joint allows for forearm pronation and supination.
- The medial column terminates as the medial epicondyle.
  - The medial epicondyle serves as the origin of the anterior and posterior bundles of the medial collateral ligament and the flexor/pronator mass.
- The lateral column terminates as the lateral supracondylar ridge and the lateral epicondyle.
  - The lateral supracondylar ridge and lateral epicondyle serve as the origin of the lateral collateral ligament and the extensor mass.
- The coronoid and olecranon fossae accommodate their corresponding portions of the proximal ulna during flexion and extension of the elbow joint.
- The radial nerve exits the spiral groove of the humerus approximately 10–14 cm above the lateral epicondyle and courses anterior through the lateral intermuscular septum at an average of 10 cm above the elbow joint line.
  - The radial nerve lies in the plane between the brachioradialis and the brachialis at the level of the elbow joint prior to dividing into the posterior interosseous nerve and the superficial radial nerve at the level of the supinator.
- The ulnar nerve travels anterior to the medial intermuscular septum until approximately 8 cm proximal to the medial epicondyle, where it pierces the intermuscular septum to enter the posterior muscular compartment of the arm and course distally posterior to the medial epicondyle through the cubital tunnel.
  - The ulnar nerve enters the forearm between the two heads of the flexor carpi ulnaris.
- The median nerve and brachial artery course anterior to the elbow joint and enter the forearm between the pronator teres and the distal tendon of the biceps brachii muscle.
  - The median nerve and brachial artery are rarely injured in adult distal humerus fractures and rarely encountered in surgical dissections used for management of these injuries.

Pearls

- *Regional anesthetic block may be helpful in reducing the need for general anesthetic and may facilitate postoperative pain control.*
- *Confirmation of fluoroscopy position for proper intraoperative radiographs should be completed prior to sterile preparation.*
- *A sterile, padded Mayo stand, brought in laterally, can be used to support the posterior humerus.*

Pitfalls

- *Previous incisions should be incorporated when possible.*

Equipment

- Impervious stockinette secured with Coban for the wrist and hand
- Ioban steri-drape over exposed skin

Positioning

- The patient is placed in supine position with a bump beneath the scapula of the injured extremity.
- A bolster or bump is placed on the patient's chest for supporting the arm in the over-the-top position.
- The surgical arm is prepped free with a sterile tourniquet placed high on the brachium (Fig. 3).
- Operative fluoroscopy is placed at the head of the bed to facilitate gaining AP and lateral radiographs intraoperatively.

Portals/Exposures

- The surgical incision begins directly posterior over the triceps approximately 7–9 cm proximal to the distal tip of the olecranon and extends distally, curving slightly medial or lateral around the tip of the olecranon before returning to midline over the subcutaneous border of the ulna (Fig. 4).

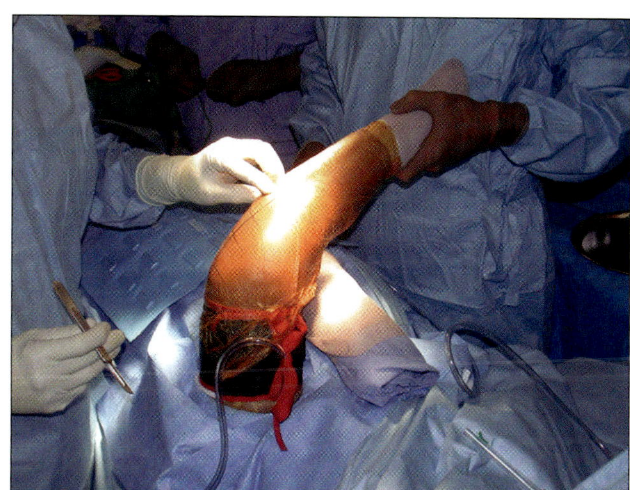

FIGURE 3

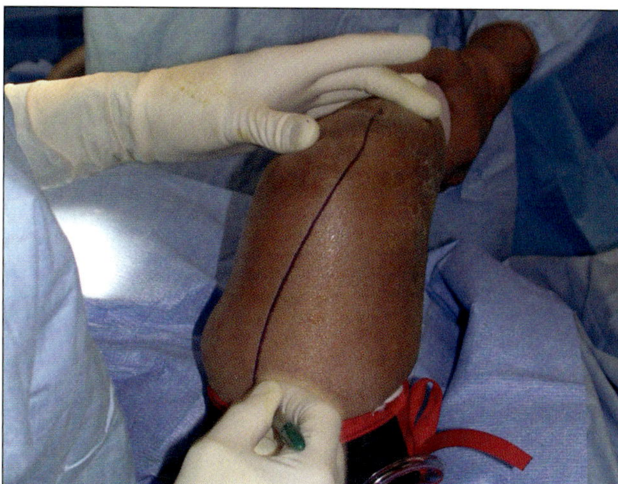

FIGURE 4

Controversies

- Some surgeons prefer positioning the patient in the lateral decubitus position with the operative arm placed over a sterile draped crutch or armholder.
- Regional anesthetic does not allow for immediate postoperative neurologic evaluation.

- Full-thickness fasciocutaneous flaps are developed medially and laterally along the entire length of the incision.
- The ulnar nerve is identified in the epineurial fat at the medial border of the triceps and dissected free from the cubital tunnel distally to its first motor branch between the two heads of the flexor carpi ulnaris (Fig. 5).
- "Triceps-off" approach (Fig. 6)
  - The medial aspect of the triceps is elevated bluntly from the humeral shaft along the intermuscular septum.
  - The superficial fascia of the forearm is incised distally approximately 6 cm to the periosteum of the medial aspect of the olecranon and proximal ulna.

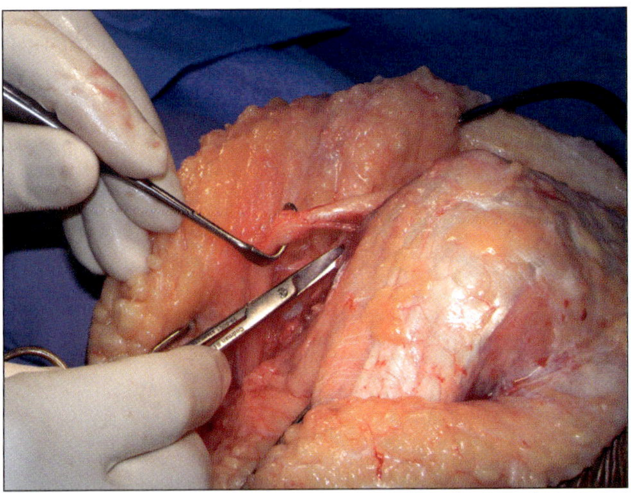

FIGURE 5

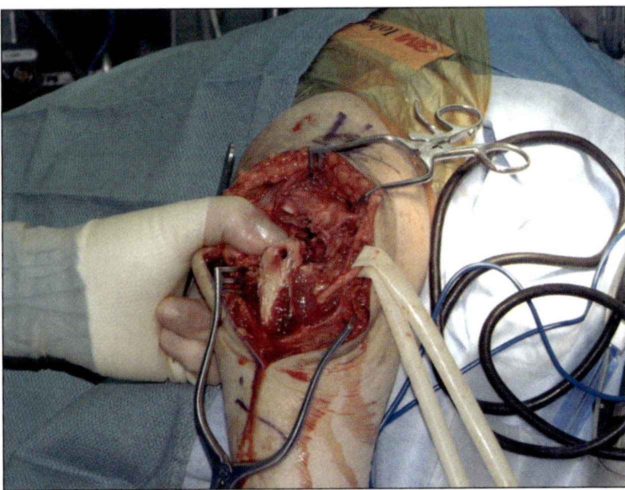

FIGURE 6

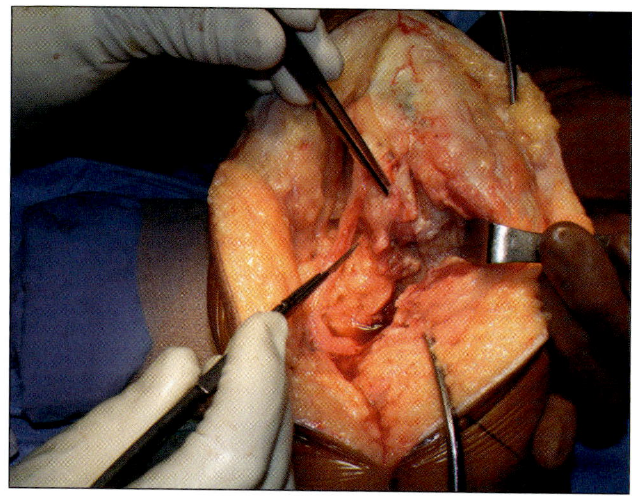

FIGURE 7

Pearls

- *Keep accompanying vessels attached to the ulnar nerve to maintain optimum vascularity.*
- *Transposition of the ulnar nerve may require neurolysis of one or two of the muscular branches to the flexor carpi ulnaris musculature.*

Pitfalls

- *Avoid use of a Penrose drain or Vesi-loop retractor on the ulnar nerve to prevent inadvertent tension or stress on the nerve during the surgical procedure.*

Controversies

- Use of the triceps-on versus triceps-off approach is dependent on surgeon preference.

Pearls

- *Fractures that have diaphyseal extension greater than 8 cm from the distal humeral joint line are not amenable to noncustom total elbow arthroplasty.*

    - The periosteum and fascia are reflected from medial to lateral sharply from the posterior aspect of the olecranon, releasing the Sharpey's fibers of the triceps insertion as a single unit.
    - The dissection is then continued lateral to release the anconeus from the lateral aspect of the olecranon subperiosteally to expose the radial head and neck.
- "Triceps-on" approach (Fig. 7)
    - The triceps is left intact on its olecranon insertion and the humeral and ulnar canals are made through medial and lateral windows after resection of the condylar fracture fragments as detailed below.
    - The ulna is most appropriately exposed from the medial aspect of the triceps.
    - Twenty percent to 25% of the triceps insertion on the medial aspect of the olecranon is released sharply, allowing the medial margin of the triceps to be reflected.
    - Flexing and rotating the forearm allows exposure of the olecranon and coronoid.

Procedure

Step 1

- The flexor pronator attachment to the medial epicondylar fragment is sharply released.
    - All medial fragments are then removed by releasing all soft tissue attachments, including the capsule.

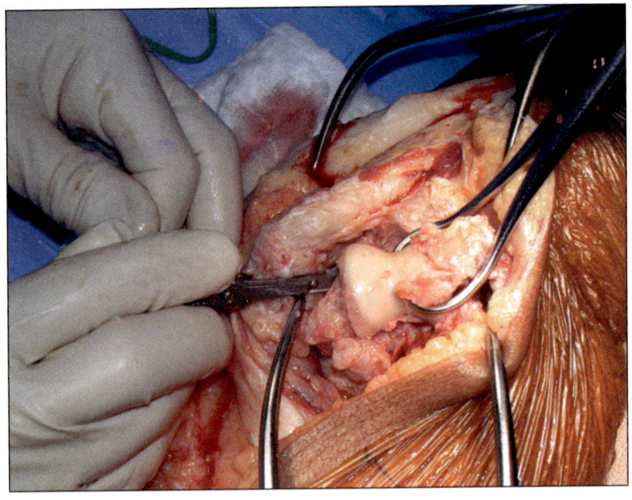

A

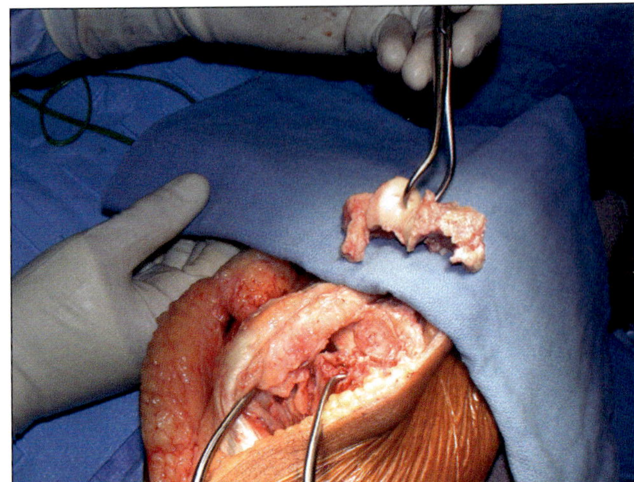

B

FIGURE 8

PEARLS

- *Do not constrain the rasps from following the canal of the humerus.*
- *Very distal fractures may require additional resection of the humeral condyles to accommodate the humeral prosthesis; use humeral cutting guides to determine the need for additional bony resection.*

- The extensor muscle components are released sharply from the lateral epicondylar fragment.
  - All lateral fragments are then removed by releasing all soft tissue attachments, including the capsule (Fig. 8A and 8B).

STEP 2

- The distal humerus is delivered into the surgical field through the window medial to the triceps muscle (Fig. 9).
- The humeral canal is enlarged with the use of serial humeral broaches to the appropriate size (Fig. 10).
- A distal humerus trial of appropriate size is inserted into the humeral canal (Fig. 11).

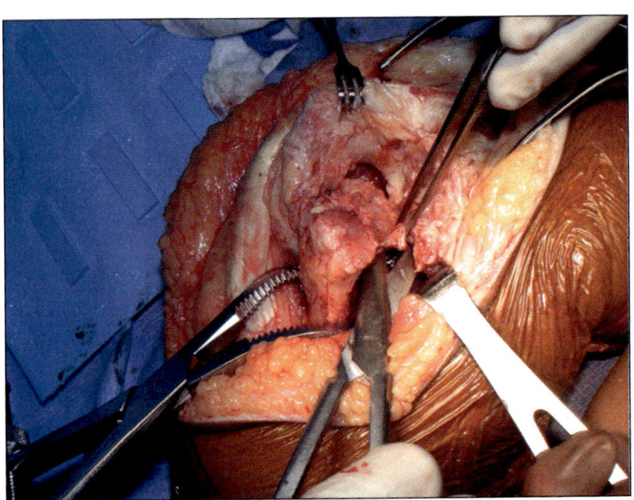

FIGURE 9

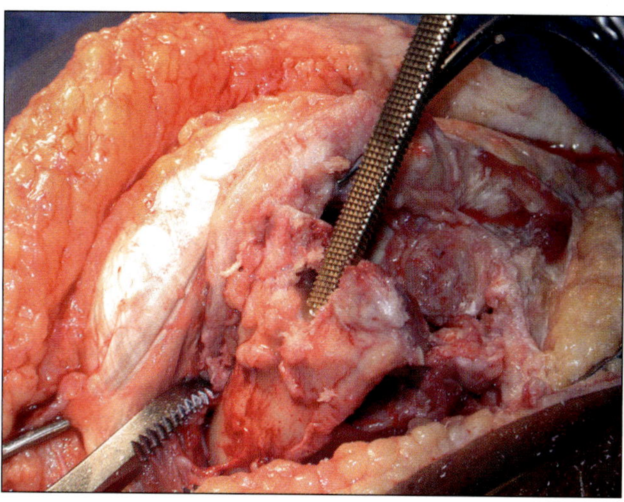

FIGURE 10

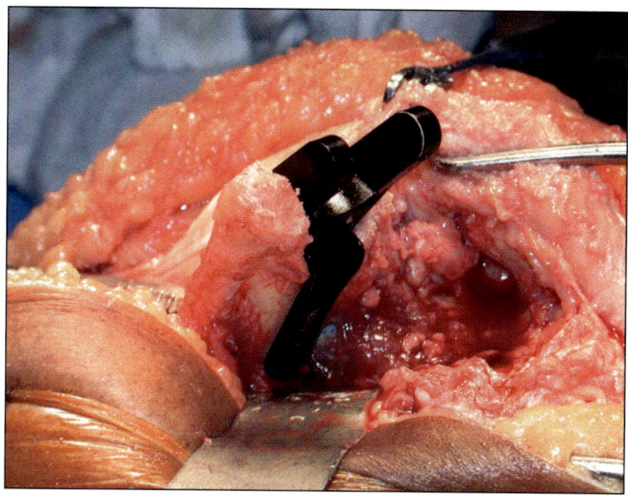

FIGURE 11

Instrumentation/ Implantation

- Oscillating saw
- Extramedullary/intramedullary cutting guides
- Barrel reamer
- Humeral rasps
- Mallet

Instrumentation/ Implantation

- Oscillating saw

Controversies

- Some surgeons leave the radial head intact rather than proceeding with radial head resection.

- Residual bone interfering with proper seating of the humeral implant trial is trimmed accordingly.
  - Typically no humeral cuts are necessary after excision of the fracture fragments.
- The depth of insertion of the humeral component is determined by the flange of the implant resting on the roof of the coronoid fossa.
  - In cases in which the fracture is proximal to this landmark, the depth of the humeral component is determined by placing an axial load on the forearm after placement of the ulnar trial component.

Step 3

- Radial head resection is carried out prior to the preparation of the ulnar canal.

Pearls

- *Use the coronoid process to determine the center of the medial/lateral ulnar width in determining where to enter the ulnar canal.*
- *Keep the handle of the ulnar rasp aligned with the posterior surface of the proximal ulna to ensure proper rotational alignment.*

Pitfalls

- *Make an adequate trough in the olecranon to ensure that the ulna is reamed straight down the canal to avoid breaching of the ulnar cortex.*
- *The ulnar trough must be deep enough to allow the ulnar component to sit appropriately posterior, ensuring proper placement of the central axis of articulation.*

Instrumentation/ Implantation

- High-speed burr
- Oscillating saw
- Ulnar reamers/rasps
- Mallet

- The annular ligament is released from the rim of the radial head, and the radial neck is exposed subperiosteally, taking care to protect the posterior interosseous nerve.
- An oscillating saw is used to resect the radial head at the junction of the radial head and neck.

Step 4

- The tip of the olecranon and a portion of the greater sigmoid notch matching the contour of the olecranon component are removed with an oscillating saw.
- The proximal portion of the ulnar canal is accessed with a high-speed burr at the base of the coronoid (Fig. 12).
- The ulnar canal is enlarged with serial reamers and broaches to the appropriate sized to accommodate the ulnar component.
- A trial ulnar component is inserted to assure proper fit and alignment (Fig. 13).

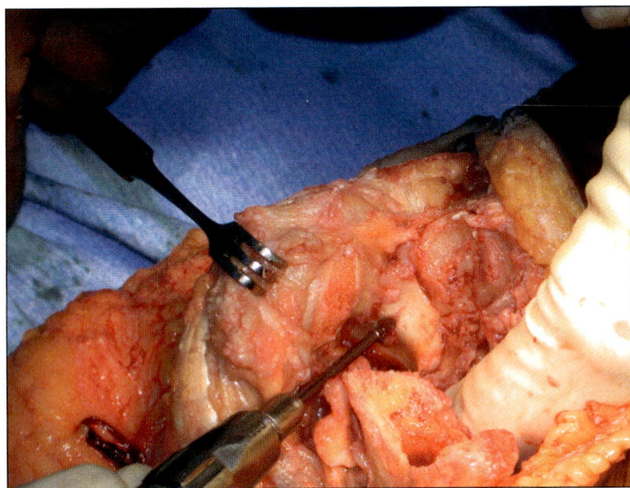

FIGURE 12

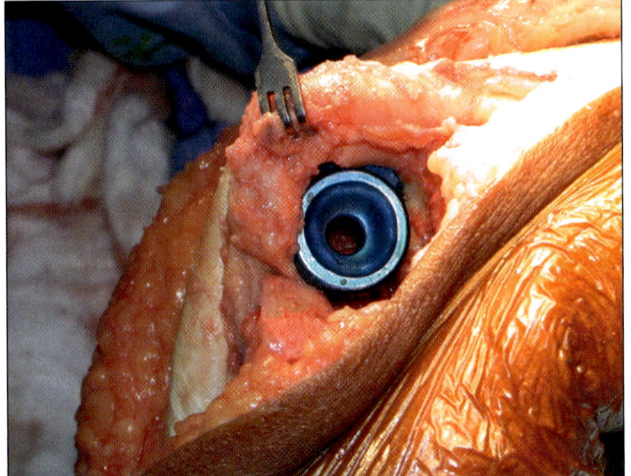

FIGURE 13

Pearls

- *Depending on fracture pattern, it may be necessary to remove 3–4 mm of central anterior humeral cortex to allow the anterior humeral flange to sit in proper position and allow the humeral implant to seat properly.*
- *If needed, bone graft can be contoured from one of the previously removed larger fracture fragments.*

Pitfalls

- *If the elbow does not extend fully, do not force it into extension as this may drive the humeral implant deeper into the humeral canal and potentially propogate the humeral fracture.*

Instrumentation/ Implantation

- Humeral and ulnar trials
- Trial bearings

Instrumentation/ Implantation

- Medullary canal brush
- Pulse lavage irrigation
- Cement restrictors

Controversies

- Some surgeons employ the use of epinephrine-soaked sponges or thrombin during canal preparation to assist in medullary hemostasis.

Step 5

- Trial humeral and ulnar components are inserted and linked.
- The elbow should be taken through a full range of motion to ensure proper seating of trial components and assess for proper size.
- The coronoid and/or olecranon are assessed to ensure that they do not impinge at the extremes of flexion and extension, respectively.
- Determination of the need for bone graft beneath the anterior humeral flange is made at this time.

Step 6

- Both the humeral and ulnar canals are prepared for methylmethacrylate cementing of the final components.
- The canals should be brushed and irrigated with copious amounts of normal saline.
- Cement restrictors are placed in both canals at a depth approximately two stem diameters longer than the final implant length to allow for an appropriate cement mantle and complete seating of the final components (Fig. 14).
- The canals are dried with 4 × 8-inch sponges.

Pearls

- *Fill any voids in the cortices with bone graft from excised fracture fragments to prevent cement extrusion.*
- *Use a small plug of cancellous bone as a cement restrictor for the ulna if cement restrictors of appropriate size are not available.*

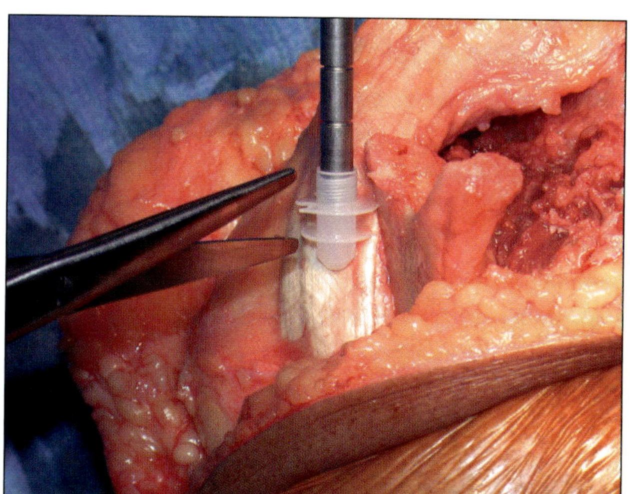

FIGURE 14

Pearls

- *Remove excess cement from the anterior humeral component prior to coupling of the implants, while exposure is optimal.*
- *Irrigate the wound copiously prior to implant articulation to remove small residual fragments of cement and bone.*
- *Intraoperative cultures are taken in cases of open fractures or previous surgery.*

Pitfalls

- *Meticulous removal of residual bone and cement particles will prevent third-body implant wear.*

Instrumentation/Implantation

- Methylmethacrylate cement with gun
- Humeral and ulnar implant impactors
- Mallet
- Final components: humeral, ulnar, and bearing components

Controversies

- Antibiotics are often added to the cement prior to mixing; vancomycin and tobramycin are most commonly utilized.
- Some surgeons prefer to insert the humeral and ulnar components after they have been coupled on the back table. This practice makes meticulous removal of excess cement anterior to the components difficult and is often unnecessary.

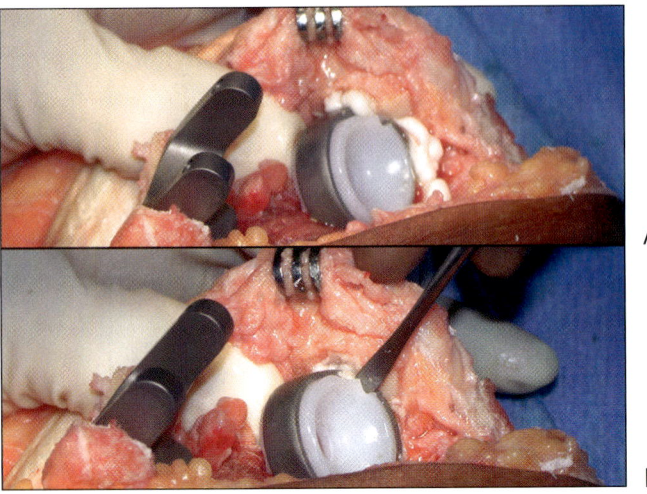

FIGURE 15

Step 7

- The methylmethacrylate cement is injected into the humeral and ulnar canals.
  - Antibiotic cement should be considered, particularly for open fractures.
- The final components are seated within their respective canals (Fig. 15A and 15B), and the coupling device is inserted to join the components (Fig. 16).
- The bone graft is placed beneath the anterior humeral flange at this point, if needed.
- Care should be taken to remove any excess cement.
- The components are held in place until the methylmethacrylate has had sufficient time to dry (approximately 12–15 minutes).

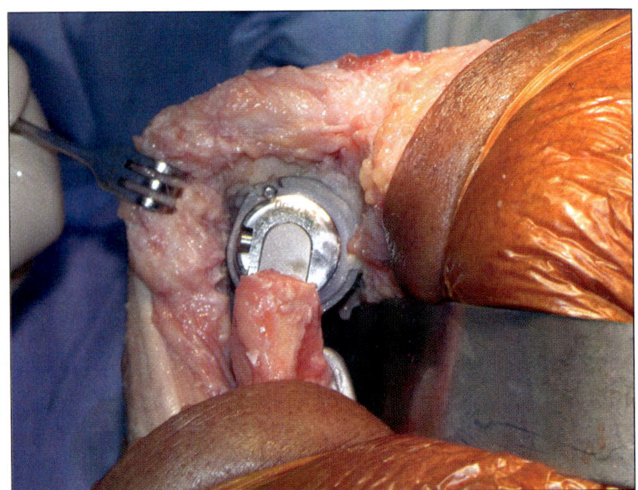

FIGURE 16

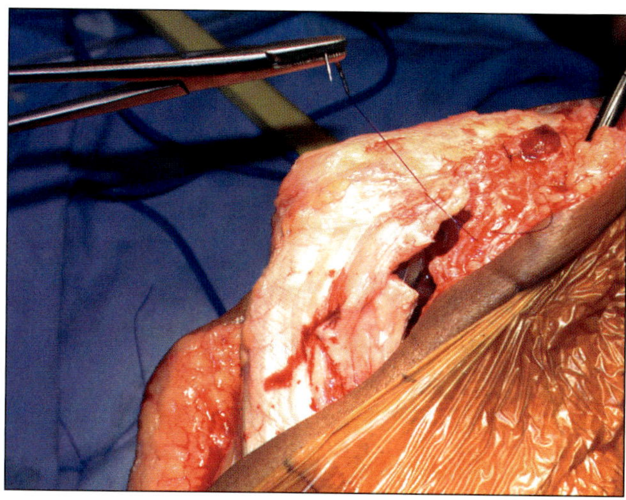

FIGURE 17

PEARLS

- *Perfect apposition of skin edges is critical whether suture or staples are used for final closure.*
- *The suction drain is removed postoperatively, usually within 48 hours.*

PITFALLS

- *The ulnar nerve should be evaluated for impingement/ instability through the full range of motion. A fascial sling may be required to maintain anterior transposition of the ulnar nerve following total elbow arthroplasty.*

Instrumentation/ Implantation

- Small suction drain
- #2 braided suture for triceps repair

- Fluoroscopic images are obtained to confirm proper placement of final components.

Step 8

- The wound is copiously irrigated with normal saline prior to closure.
- The triceps mechanism is meticulously repaired as sleeve in continuity with the ulnar periosteum if the triceps-off technique has been used.
  - Transosseus sutures may be used to repair the triceps mechanism to the olecranon using a figure-of-8 suture pattern.
- The triceps fascia is repaired as far proximally as possible (Fig. 17).
- The ulnar nerve is formally transposed anteriorly at the time of triceps closure.
- A suction drain is placed subcutaneously.
- The medial and lateral fasciocutaneous flaps are then reapproximated, finalizing the closure of the wound.
- A bulky soft dressing is applied in addition to a plaster splint to protect the triceps mechanism with the elbow in approximately 60° of flexion to full extension (to protect a repaired triceps with the triceps-off technique).
- Figure 18 shows postoperative lateral (Fig. 18A) and anteroposterior (Fig. 18B) radiographs.

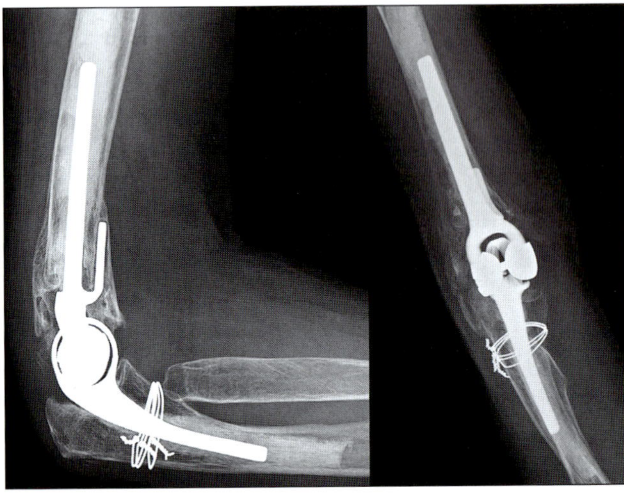

FIGURE 18

Postoperative Care and Expected Outcomes

- Postoperative empirical antibiotics are administered for 24 hours postsurgically.
- The patient is usually discharge in 24–48 hours and then seen in the clinic in 5–7 days to begin active/passive flexion and passive extension exercises.
- The sutures are removed at 2 weeks.
- No active extension is permitted until 6 weeks in order to protect the extensor mechanism repair (with the triceps-off technique).
- Night splinting in extension for 6 weeks may be useful to overcome flexion contracture.
- Strengthening exercises are begun at 6 weeks postoperatively. The patient is limited to a 4.5-kg lifting restriction with the extremity and is discouraged from repetitively lifting greater than 1.0 kg.

Expected Outcomes

- A multicenter, randomized trial comparing total elbow arthroplasty (TEA) with open reduction and internal fixation (ORIF) found complication rates to be similar. Disability of the Arm, Shoulder and Hand scores were significantly improved in TEA patients at 6 weeks and 6 months but were similar between groups at 12 months and 2 years (McKee et al., 2009).
- There was no significant difference in mean flexion, extension, or arc of motion at 2 years between TEA and ORIF. Mean values were 26° of extension and 133° of flexion, with a mean arc of motion of 107°.

Pearls

- *If motion is not steadily improving by the second or third week postoperatively, dynamic or static progressive splinting should be used.*

Pitfalls

- *Be sure the wound is well sealed and without drainage prior to initiating elbow range of motion.*

Complications

- Potential complications include infection, heterotopic ossification, implant failure, ulnar nerve symptoms, hematoma, and wound healing problems.

Evidence

Bryan RS, Morrey BF. Extensive posterior exposure of the elbow: a triceps sparing approach. Clin Orthop Relat Res. 1982;(166):188-92.

The authors provided a detailed description of the posterior approach to the elbow joint. The paper detailed the release of the triceps as a single unit from the posterior aspect of the olecranon. In addition, the technique of triceps repair through drill holes in the proximal ulna was described.

Chalidis B, Dimitriou C, Papadopoulos P, Petsatodis G, Giannoudis PV. Total elbow arthroplasty for the treatment of insufficient distal humeral fractures: a retrospective clinical study and review of the literature. Injury. 2009;(40):582-90.

This paper reported the results of 11 patients over 75 years of age who underwent semiconstrained sloppy-hinge total elbow arthroplasty due to comminuted intra-articular fractures of the distal humerus. The authors concluded that total elbow arthroplasty remains a viable option for treatment of complex distal humerus fractures in elderly and medically compromised patients. (Level IV evidence)

Frankle MA, Herscovici D, DiPasquale TG, Vasey MB, Sanders RW. A comparison of open reduction and internal fixation and primary total elbow arthroplasty in the treatment of intraarticular distal humerus fractures in women older than age 65. J Orthop Trauma. 2003;7:473-80.

This paper compared open reduction and internal fixation with total elbow arthroplasty for intra-articular distal humerus fractures in women older than 65 years of age. The retrospective review of 24 patients concluded that the results of fractures treated with total elbow arthroplasty were superior to those treated with open reduction and internal fixation. (Level III evidence)

Galano GJ, Ahmad CS, Levine WN. Current treatment strategies for bicolumnar distal humerus fractures. J Am Acad Orthop Surg. 2010;18:20-30.

This article reviewed the treatment current strategies used when managing bicolumnar fractures of the distal humerus. The authors present total elbow arthroplasty as an acceptable option for treating comminuted fractures of the distal humerus in the elderly, low-demand patient.

Goldberg SH, Omid R, Nassr AN, Beck R, Cohen MS. Osseous anatomy of the distal humerus and proximal ulna: implications for total elbow arthroplasty. J Shoulder Elbow Surg. 2007;16(3 Suppl):39s-46s.

This article provided a detailed description of the anatomy of the elbow as it pertains to total elbow arthroplasty. Precise measurements of anatomic angles and intramedullary diameters were reported in 27 human cadavers. On the basis of these data, a cylindrical humeral stem and a tapered ulnar stem may be optimal for total elbow arthroplasty.

Kalogrianitis S, Sinopidis C, El Meligy M, Rawal A, Frostick SP. Unlinked elbow arthroplasty as primary treatment for fractures of the distal humerus. J Shoulder Elbow Surg. 2008;17:287-92.

This article was a retrospective review of complex, intra-articular fractures of the distal humerus treated with unlinked elbow arthroplasty. The authors noted that there was postoperative mediolateral laxity of 5-10° in all patients. Despite this laxity, none of the patients complained of instability. No postoperative dislocations were reported. (Level IV evidence)

Kamineni S, Morrey BF. Distal humeral fractures treated with noncustom total elbow replacement. J Bone Joint Surg [Am]. 2004;86:940-7.

This article provided a detailed description of the surgical technique used by the authors for treatment of distal humeral fractures with total elbow arthroplasty. They used a triceps-on technique that accomplishes the operation through medial and lateral windows on either side of the triceps insertion.

McKee MD, Veillette CJH, Hall JA, Schemitsch EH, Wild LM, McCormack R, Perey B, Goetz T, Zomar M, Moon K, Mandel S, Petit S, Guy P, Leung I. A multicenter, prospective, randomized, controlled trial of open reduction-internal fixation versus total elbow arthroplasty for displaced intra-articular distal humeral fractures in elderly patients. J Shoulder Elbow Surg. 2009;18:3-12.

This prospective, randomized, controlled trial compared functional outcomes, complications, and reoperation rates in elderly patients with displaced intra-articular distal humerus fractures treated with open reduction and internal fixation or primary semiconstrained total elbow arthroplasty in patients older than 65 years of age. Forty-two patients were included in the study. The authors concluded that total elbow arthroplasty is a preferred alternative to open reduction and internal fixation for elderly patients with complex distal humerus fractures that are not amenable to stable fixation. (Level I evidence)

Prasad N, Dent C. Outcome of total elbow replacement for distal humeral fractures in the elderly: a comparison of primary surgery and surgery after failed internal fixation or conservative treatment. J Bone Joint Surg [Br]. 2008;90:343-8.

This article was a retrospective review of the outcomes of distal humerus fractures in elderly patients treated with total elbow arthroplasty in an immediate or delayed fashion. No significant difference in outcomes or complications was found between the two groups. (Level III evidence)

Prokopis PM, Weiland AJ. The triceps-preserving approach for semiconstrained total elbow arthroplasty. J Shoulder Elbow Surg. 2008;17:454-8.

This article described a triceps-sparing technique used for total elbow arthoplasty. Using a posterior incision, the authors used an approach in which the triceps is only dissected from the medial side, leaving the tendon insertion on the olecranon and the lateral soft tissue envelope undisturbed.

PROCEDURE 46

Hemiarthroplasty of the Distal Humerus

Rick F. Papandrea

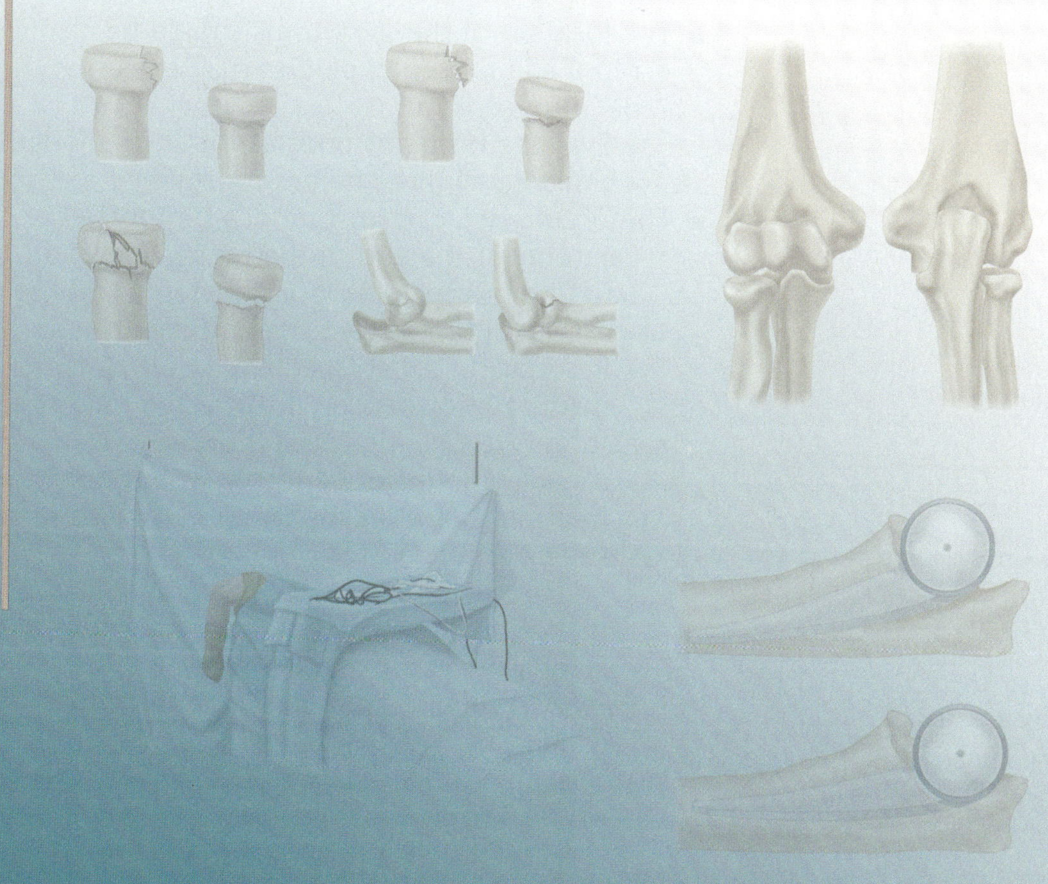

PITFALLS

- *Infection must be ruled out prior to implantation.*
- *Use of any available prostheses in the United States is considered "off-label" by the Food and Drug Administration.*
- *Ability and ease of conversion to a total elbow arthroplasty (TEA) will depend upon both the approach and the implant used for the hemiarthroplasty*
- *If the epicondyles and/or columns are fractured or absent, they must be reconstructed. If a nonflanged device is used without column support, it will fail.*
- *Treatment of the ulnar nerve will be dependent on the pathology encountered and approach undertaken.*
- *Use in inflammatory arthropathies is not advised.*

Controversies

- Use with loss of cartilage or deformity of the proximal radius and/or ulna may lessen effectiveness.
- Longevity of implants is uncertain and unproven.
- The best surgical approach is unknown.

Indications

- Failed distal humeral fracture fixation
- Failed articular débridement procedures of the distal humerus too large to resurface with alternative methods
- Irreparable distal humerus fractures (loss of subchondral support for cartilage, or loss of cartilage)
- Avascular necrosis (AVN) of the distal humerus that fails conservative management and débridement
- Posttraumatic loss of the distal humerus articulation

Examination/Imaging

- The location of the symptoms should be clarified.
  - More common pathologies may coexist with joint derangement.
    - Evaluate both epicondyles for ensthenopathies.
    - Evaluate all three nerves for signs of entrapment.
- The occurrence of pain can localize the cause.
  - Pain only at the end of the range of motion is often from impinging osteophytes.
    - These respond well to débridement.
    - Resurfacing or replacement of the distal humerus is usually not needed if this is the only pain.
  - Pain at rest may indicate synovitis.
    - If this is the major concern, synovectomy and treatment of the cause of the synovitis may be sufficient for relief.
    - There may be rest pain with AVN, but this diagnosis should be readily made with a standard workup.
  - Pain with midarc motion is thought to be mediated by the damaged articular surface.
    - This pain may require resurfacing or replacement of the damaged articulation.
    - Depending on severity, débridement alone or partial resurfacing may suffice.
- Stability of the elbow must be assessed.
  - Hemiarthroplasty will not address instability unless reconstruction of the stabilizing structures is also done.
  - Instability that includes significant bone loss may not be best treated with hemiarthroplasty.
    - The proximal radius and ulna must be normal or near normal.

- The epicondyles and columns must be intact or reconstructable.
- Standard radiographs
  - Routine radiographs in anteroposterior (AP), lateral, and oblique views are often sufficient to determine the need for a hemiarthroplasty of the elbow.
  - Anteroposterior radiographs can be used to diagnose AVN of the trochlea (Fig. 1A), chronic nonunion of a low distal humerus fracture (Fig. 1B), and failed (twice) fixation of distal humeral shear fracture (Fig. 1C).
  - Radiographs should be evaluated for osteophytes, loose bodies, joint space narrowing, and posttraumatic heterotopic ossification.

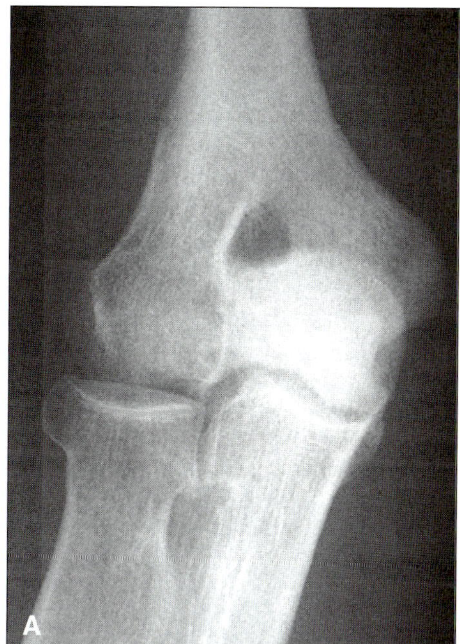

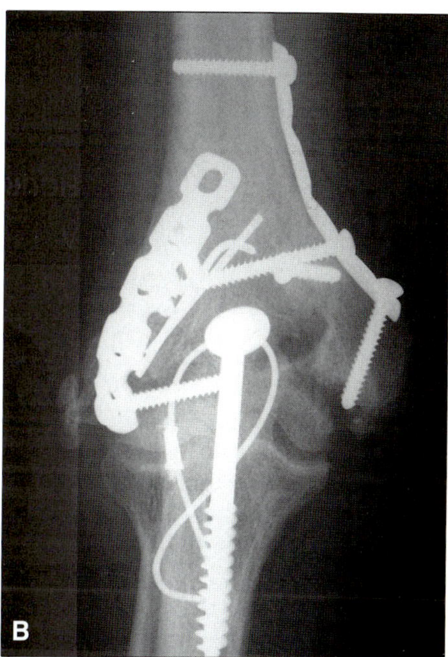

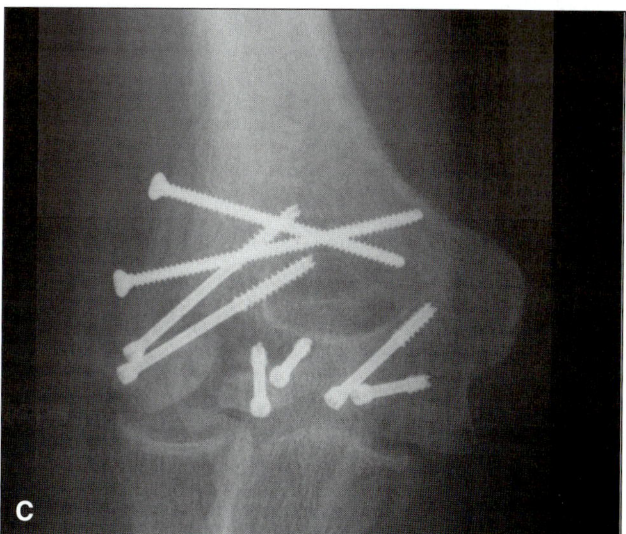

FIGURE 1

- The proximal radius and ulna should be evaluated. Deformity and/or loss of cartilage may diminish the benefit of distal humeral resurfacing.

- Computed tomography (CT) scan
  - CT scans, especially three-dimensional reconstructions, may define the distal humeral anatomy with more clarity than simple radiographs.
  - Three-dimensional reconstructions make the assessment more meaningful.
    - This can be done with raw DICOM data by the surgeon using free, open-source programs (Rosset et al., 2004).
    - Reconstruction of a CT scan of the same patient as in Figure 1C demonstrates additional information such as the extent of bone loss, especially at the lateral condyle (Fig. 2A and 2B).
  - CT scans can be used to assess the olecranon, coronoid, and radial head and their corresponding fossae for proper articulation, and cause for impingement pain.
  - joint narrowing or focal damage from AVN or other isolated conditions such as osteochondritis dissecans can be localized on CT scans.
  - When a fracture is present, a CT scan may lend insight into the probability of successful repair.

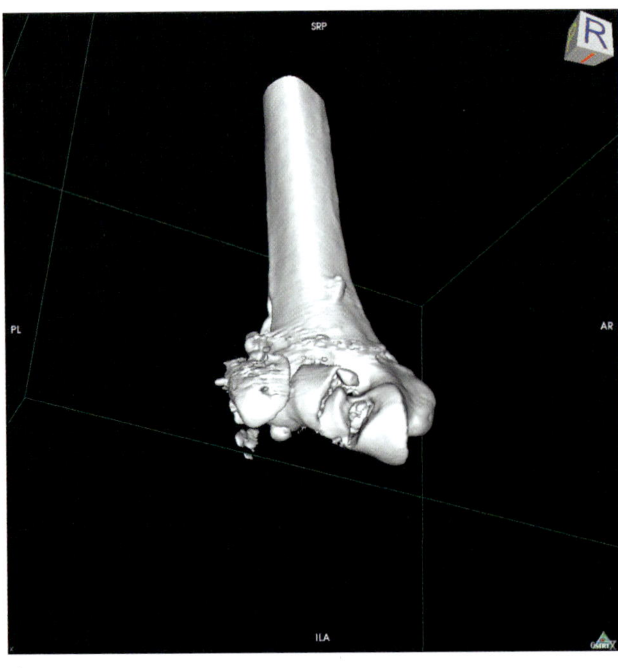

A

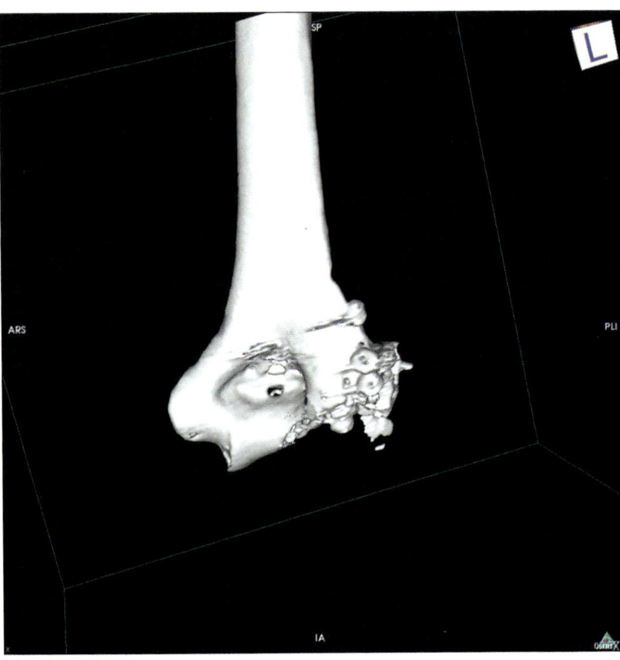

B

FIGURE 2

Treatment Options

- Less invasive procedures should be considered first.
  - Débridement of loose bodies, isolated cartilage damage, and osteophytes can be treated with an open or arthroscopic procedure.
  - Treatment of nerve entrapment or epicondylitis should be undertaken if these symptoms appear to be dominant.
- If the cartilage lesion is more focal, complete resurfacing of the distal humerus may not be needed.
  - Autologous cartilage transplantation has been described for osteochondritis dissecans lesions.
  - Partial distal humerus resurfacing is possible; however, this off-label procedure uses different implants and a different approach.
  - In a sedentary patient, a painful radiocapitellar joint may be treated with a radial head resection. Caution should be excercised because ulnohumeral stress will increase and, if this articulation is abnormal, pain may increase medially. This may exacerbate or uncover instability.
- If the joint derangement is diffuse, the patient may be better served with a TEA. However, more restrictions are placed on the postoperative TEA than a hemiarthroplasty

- Depending on the condition, and the information from other sources, CT scans may not be necessary.

- Magnetic resonance imaging (MRI)
  - MRI may allow for better delineation of cartilage loss/damage, both the location and extent.
  - MRI is useful for following AVN.
  - Similar to CT scans, MRI may not be necessary for every patient in whom a hemiarthroplasty is considered.
- Previous documented intraoperative information is important.
  - Location of the ulnar nerve
  - Previously placed implants
  - Prior approaches
  - Location and severity of cartilage damage
  - Stability and status of the collateral ligaments/epicondyles
- Arthroscopy may allow for final planning when there is uncertainty regarding the appropriateness of a hemiarthroplasty.

Surgical Anatomy

- Epicondyles (Fig. 3A and 3B)
  - The relationship of the epicondyles to the center of rotation (COR) and ligaments needs to be understood and maintained with the hemiarthroplasty.
  - The COR is the isometric point of the lateral collateral ligament. The anterior band of the medial collateral ligament is slightly posterior to the COR.
    - The COR should be left intact or reconstructed if deficient.

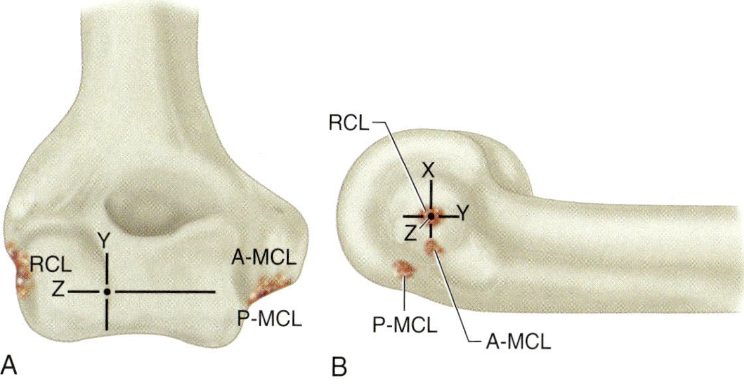

FIGURE 3

PEARLS

- *Commercially available positioners decrease the need for additional assistants. If not available, a bolster on the chest, with a weight on the opposite side of the table connected to the wrist, will minimize the support needed from an assistant.*
- *Supine position allows for easier access for fluoroscopic imaging. The arm may be readily abducted away from the body for both lateral and AP radiographs.*

PITFALLS

- *Nonsterile tourniquets should be placed proximal as possible.*
- *A sterile tourniquet should be used if the possibility of high radial nerve exposure is anticipated. This would be more likely in a revision surgery, especially if mid to proximal humeral hardware would need to be removed.*

Equipment

- Commercially available supports are optional.
  - Supine, suspended
  - Lateral decubitus, supported

    - Failure to maintain the COR with the hemiarthroplasty will lead to decreased range of motion and possibly early failure.
- If not previously transected, the anconeus may be left attached to the olecranon during osteotomy (Fig. 4).

Positioning

- Supine position
  - Aided by using a bolster to support the forearm; requires constant traction or support
  - Using commercially available positioner (see Fig. 6), suspending arm over torso
- Lateral decubitus position
  - Supported by positioner (Fig. 5)

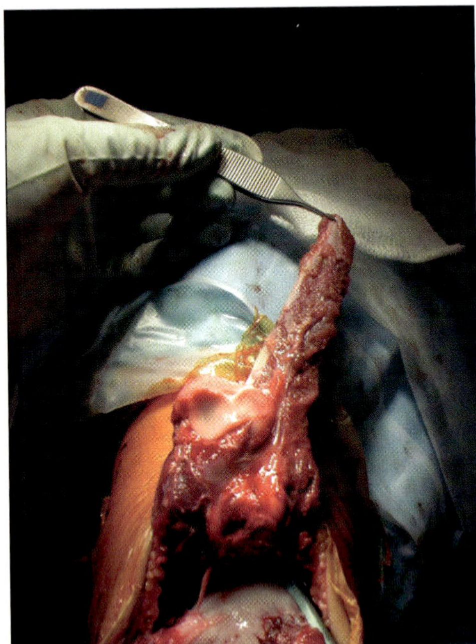

FIGURE 4

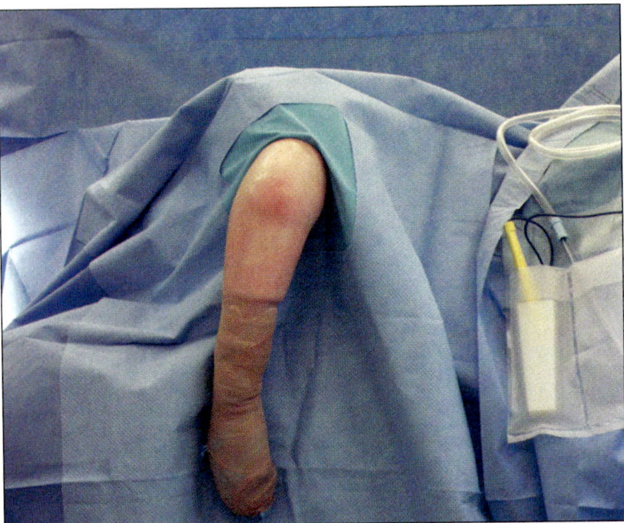

FIGURE 5

Portals/Exposures

- Posterior incision (Fig. 6).
  - Watershed cutaneous innervation allows for fewer paresthesias.
- Ulnar nerve release and subcutaneous transposition (Fig. 7)

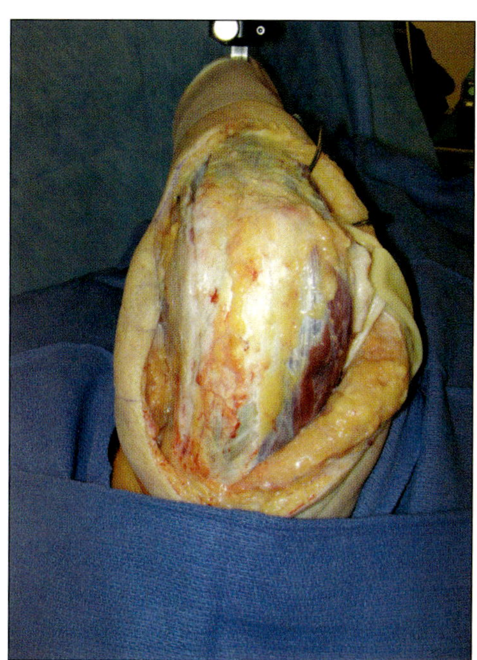

FIGURE 6

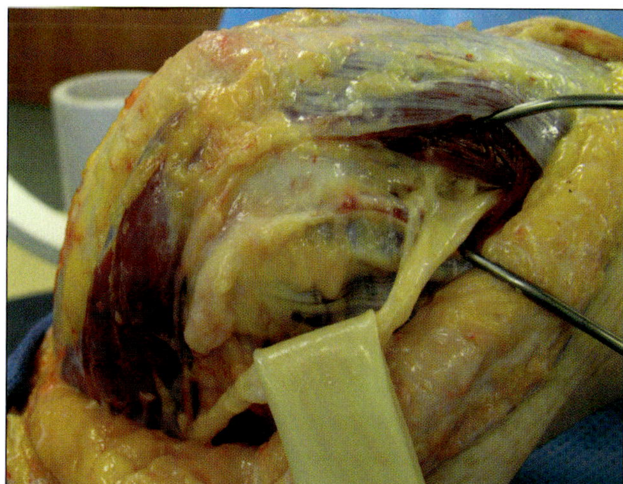

FIGURE 7

Pearls

- *Identify the ulnar nerve initially, and minimize trauma to it by manipulating it with a wide Penrose drain.*
- *A posterior incision allows for larger cutaneous nerves to stay with the flaps.*
  - *Avoid incising directly over the tip of the olecranon.*
  - *Previous surgeries may alter location of the skin incision.*
- *Preserve the collateral and flexor/extensor origins at the epicondyles.*

Pitfalls

- *Hemiarthroplasty is an off-label procedure; the implants used are not designed for implantation through an osteotomy.*
  - *Supporting documentation from the implant manufacturer does not demonstrate hemiarthroplasty via any approach.*
  - *Review the use of instrumentation prior to the procedure.*

Instrumentation

- If using a commercially designed cutting block, the location and design of the olecranon osteotomy are important.
  - A proximal cut, or too deep of a V in the chevron, will impede the cutting block.
  - The osteotomy should be transverse, or a shallow V, with the proximal extent of the cut at the bare spot in the olecranon.

Controversies

- Exposure can be obtained via more traditional total elbow exposure, with detachment of the triceps. This introduces triceps weakness as a potential complication. The collaterals are usually also released in these exposures; however, this will introduce the potential for instability. Overall stability will be jeopardized, and rehabilitation will have to be curtailed compared to osteotomy.

- Olecranon osteotomy
  - A transverse or shallow chevron is used (Fig. 8).
  - The anconeus (if not previously violated) may be kept in continuity with the olecranon and triceps. This preserves innervation and allows for soft tissue coverage of implants.
  - If the anconeus will not be preserved, it is transected and devitalized; the transected ends may impede visualization.

Procedure

Step 1

- The ulnar nerve is controlled.
  - It is released or identified (if previously released).
  - A subcutaneous pocket is created for transposition.
- The anconeus is dissected and released.
- Osteotomy of the olecranon is performed (Fig. 9).
  - The surgeon should ensure that the cutting blocks will fit appropriately.
  - Use of a transverse or shallow chevron should be considered.

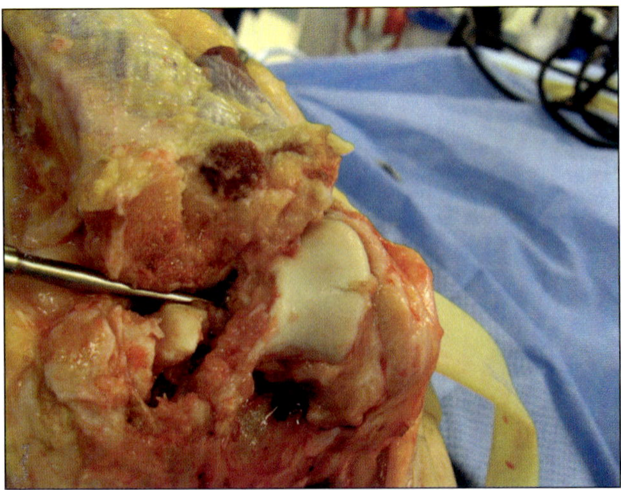

FIGURE 8

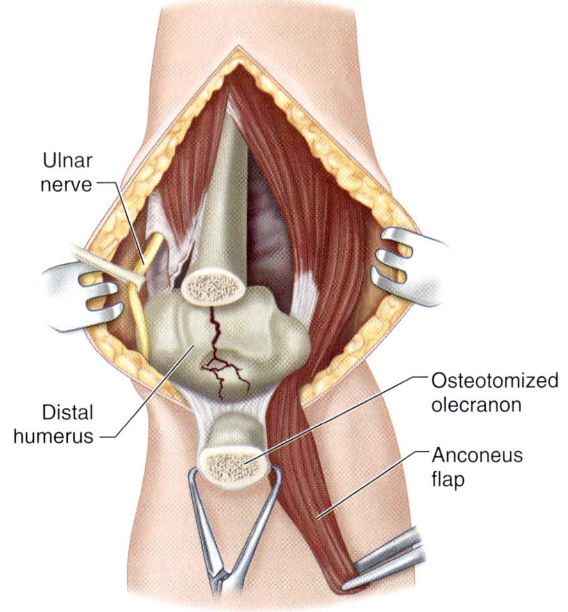

FIGURE 9

PEARLS

- *Identify the ulnar nerve proximal or distal to zones of previous surgery to expedite the dissection and minimize trauma.*
- *Releasing the aconeus from distal to proximal allows for reliable separation from the lateral capsule and lateral collateral ligament.*
- *Complete osteotomy with an osteotome allows for interdigitation of the repaired osteotomy. The saw "kerf" does not remove cartilage if it does not go through it.*

PITFALLS

- *If previous surgery was done, the ulnar nerve must be identified, even if previously released.*
  - *Never assume the nerve will be out of harm's way due to a previous transposition.*
  - *The nerve may take unexpected turns, even coming back upon itself after a previous transposition.*
- *If the epicondyles are intact, the olecranon osteotomy cut may impede the cutting jig for some systems.*

  - Release of the olecranon and triceps will serve as any necessary posterior capsular release (Fig. 10).
- The capsule is released off the anterior distal humerus as needed for full extension.
- The existing trochlea or capitellum is utilized to estimate the appropriate size of implant (Fig. 11).

STEP 2

- Access to the intramedullary (IM) canal is needed for the cutting jig system.
  - If there is no distal humeral fracture up into the fossae:

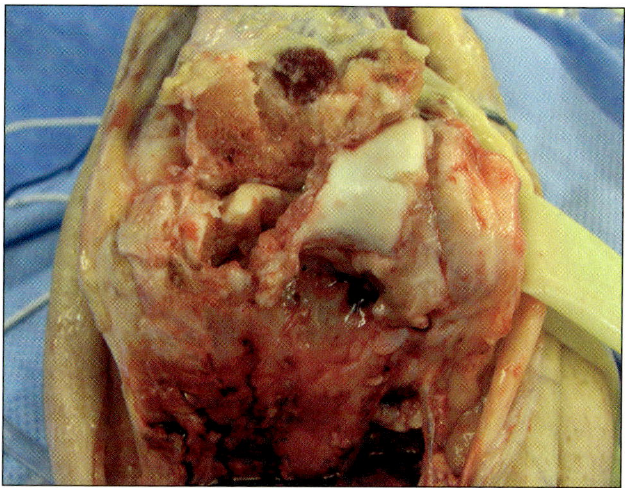

FIGURE 10

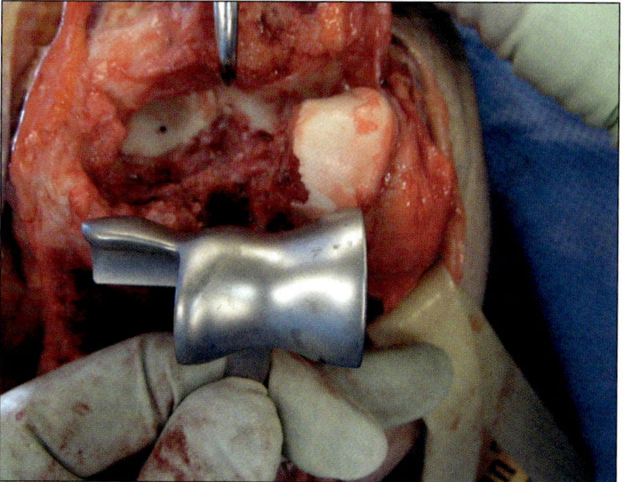

FIGURE 11

Instrumentation/ Implantation

- Oscillating saw for osteotomy.
- A wide Penrose drain around the ulnar nerve allows for atraumatic retraction of the nerve.

Controversies

- Some surgeons advocate creating a fascial sling for the ulnar nerve. This is done to prevent the nerve from sliding posterior. Some believe this will only create a point of scarring and potential compression of the nerve.

    - Bone will be blocking the access to the IM canal (Fig. 12A).
    - The cutting guide from the implant is utilized, or the portion of the trochlear spool distal to the IM canal is freehand cut (Fig. 12B).
  - If a fracture exends into the trochlea:
    - Only enough fracture fragments are removed to gain access to the canal.
    - Do not remove medial or lateral subcondral bone, or any columnar bone; this is necessary for support of the implant.
- The epicondyles are repaired provisionally if fractured.
  - Location of the epicondyles will determine the COR for the distal humeral replacement.
  - Provisional fixation can usually be accomplished with Kirschner wires (K-wires).
  - An alternative is to rigidly fix the fracture with unicortical plate and screw fixation.
- If bone is missing (see the distal lateral condyle in Figs. 10 and 11), utilize the IM canal and existing COR point to align the cutting jig.
  - The stylus may not engage bone on the side where the fracture extends proximally (Fig. 13).
- Distal humeral cuts are made (Fig. 14).

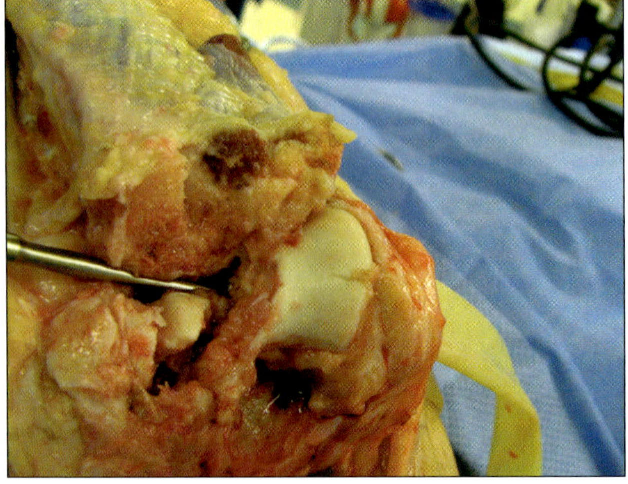
A

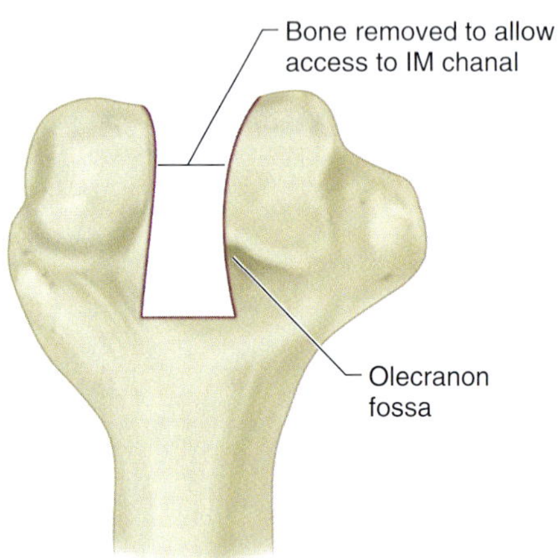

B

FIGURE 12

STEP 3: TRIALING

- The distal humerus is assessed for size (Fig. 15).
  - The center of the radial head is referenced on the center of the capitellum while the coronoid is reduced in the trochlear notch.
  - The implant should be sized down when measurements are between sizes.

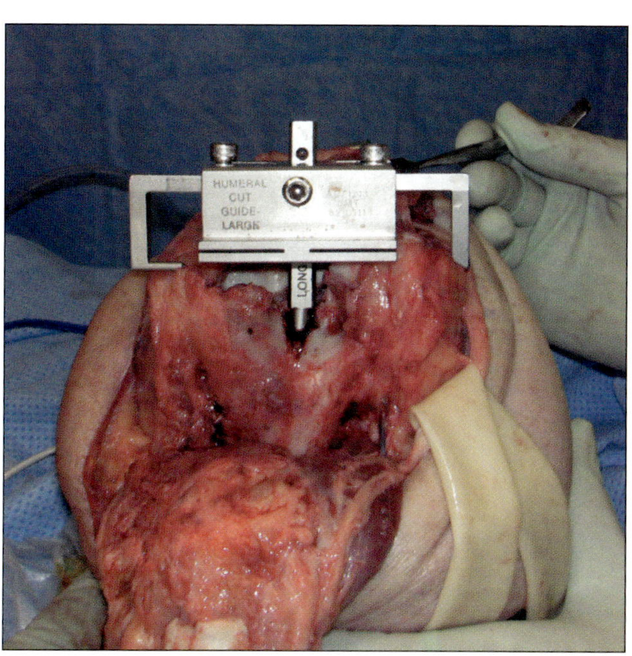

FIGURE 13

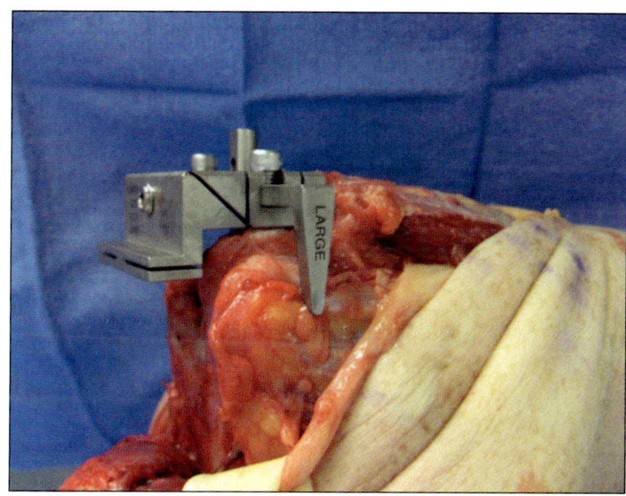

FIGURE 14

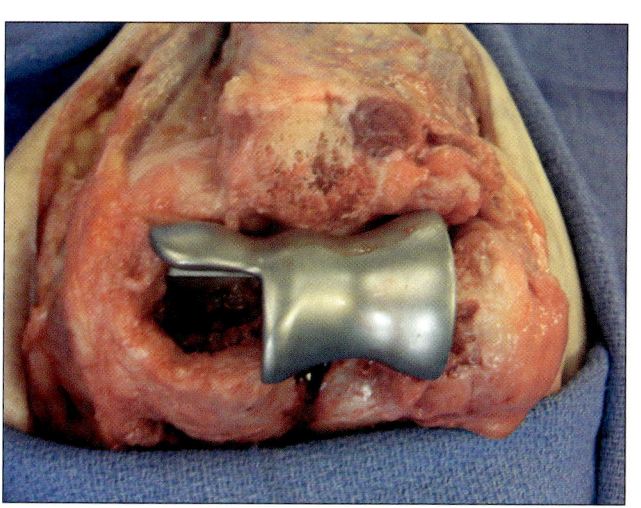

FIGURE 15

Pearls

- *The distal humeral medullary canal tapers in the sagittal plane.*
  - *If the dense cortical bone is left anterior and/or posterior, an IM alignment rod may be flexed or extended inadvertently.*
  - *Remove adequate bone to allow the true IM canal to align the rod.*

Pitfalls

- *Bone loss from previous surgery may hamper fixation or proper location of the epicondyles.*
- *Soft tissue should not be removed from the epicondyles despite technique guides showing otherwise (see Fig. 14).*

Instrumentation/ Implantation

- Guide rod and cutting jig
- Fixation for fractured epicondyles and/or columns
  - K-wires (preferred)
  - Plates (optional; hardware may make implanting arthroplasty more difficult)

Controversies

- Freehand cutting of the distal humerus
  - Obviates use of a cutting jig
  - May be less technically challenging
  - Most likely less accurate than the jig
- Plate fixation versus more cost-effective methods for repairing columns:
  - K-wires
  - Tension bands
  - Suture or wire to prosthesis

- An assessment is made for bone loss.
  - Small distal incongruities may be cemented.
  - Structural support of a column should be obtained from structural bone graft (Fig. 16) using an iliac crest autograft or an allograft.
- Fractured epicondyles are reduced, and a check is made for isometry.
- The surgeon must ensure that the device "captures" some native bone in the AP plane.
  - Resurfacing implant: rotational and posterior vector stability will be obtained from this "cupping" of the distal humerus.
  - Implant with flange:
    - The flange will provide stability for the posterior vector and rotation.
    - Condylar support may be less important; however, results of implantation without condylar support are unknown, and loss of condylar support from around the implant may leave a painful prominence subcutaneously.

Step 4: Implantation

- Cement restrictor
  - Revision of a hemiarthroplasty is a valid concern.
  - Limiting cement to the region of the implant is imperative.
  - Choice for restrictors
    - Commercially available restrictors often are too large and may lose fixation, because the IM canal widens proximally.
    - Bone packed to the level of the implant may become incarcerated prematurely. If this heals, it

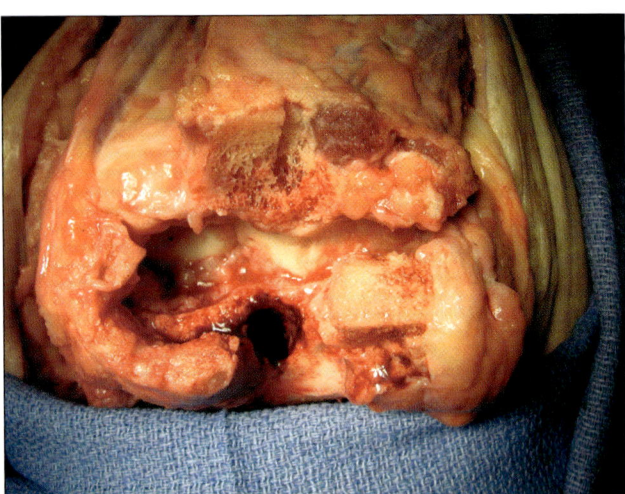

FIGURE 16

PEARLS

- *If measurements are between sizes of implant, use the smaller size.*
  - *Try not to undersize in the coronal (medial/lateral) plane.*
  - *Use fluoroscopy with trialing to ensure that the device aligns properly and the epicondyles are located appropriately.*

PITFALLS

- *Previous surgery may weaken the cortical bone.*
  - *The implant may not stay intraosseous.*
  - *Use fluoroscopy to confirm IM location of the implant.*

may make revision more difficult because it obliterates the IM canal.
- Oxidized cellulose (Surgicel, Johnson & Johnson) can be cut into small squares and packed into the IM canal at appropriate distance until resistance it felt. It will resorb, simplifying revision.

- Final fixation for any graft or fracture (Fig. 17A and 17B)
  - The surgeon must ensure that a graft interdigitates as much as possible with host bone.
    - The distal aspect is shaped to allow capture by the implant.
    - The graft is held with K-wires to stabilize it. The wires must not impede implantation of the device, and the trial device must insert easily.
  - Final fracture fixation may be completed after cementing of the implant; however, provisional fixation must align in the proper position.
- Cementing of implant
  - Narrow-nozzel cement delivery is needed. Most standard hip/knee systems will not have a nozzel that fits up the humeral canal.
  - Commercially available dyed cement aids in removal if revision is necessary. Methylene blue is added to undyed cement at mixing.

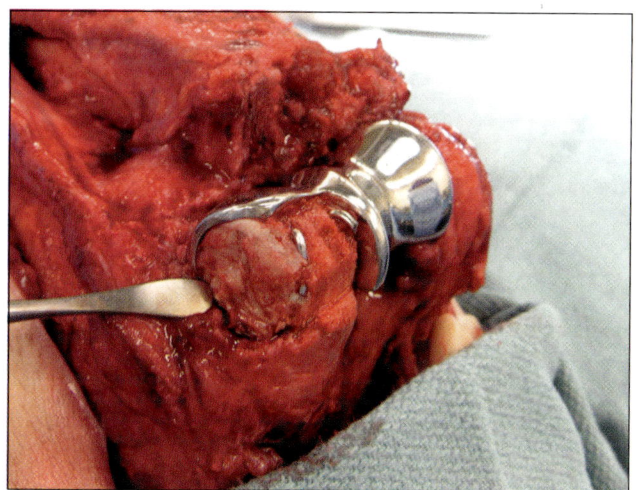
A

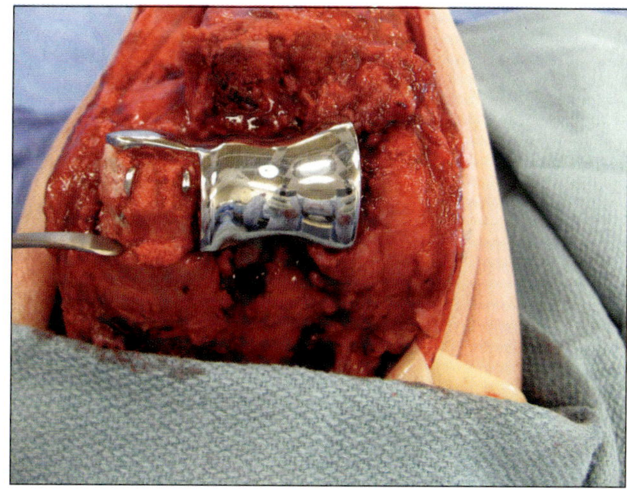
B

FIGURE 17

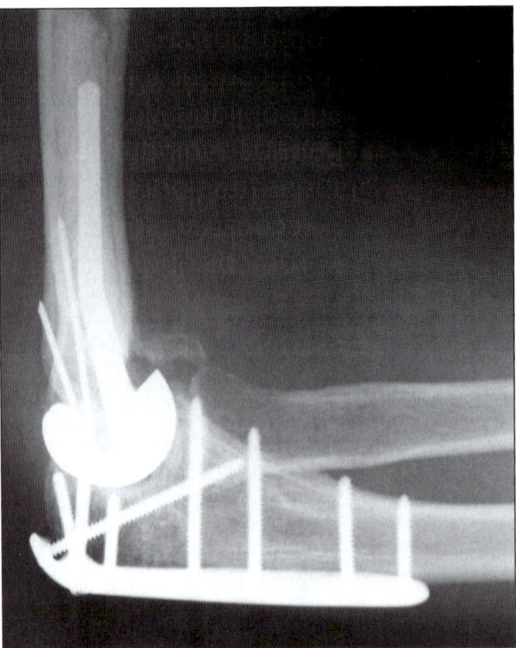
A

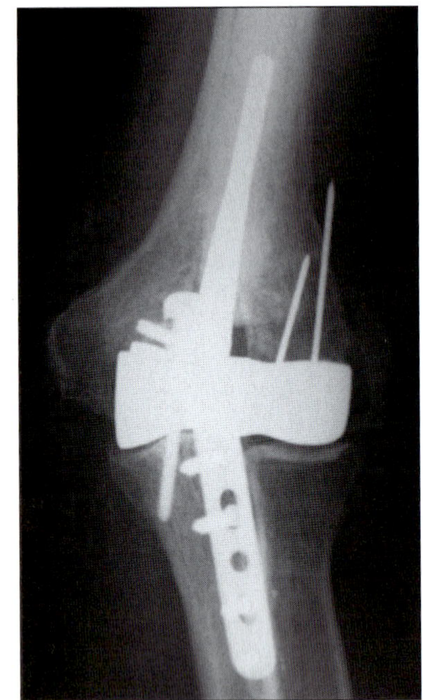
B

FIGURE 18

Instrumentation/Implantation

- Trial implants
  - Systems that utilize a custom component will not have trial components. Custom implants must be ordered based on preoperative radiographs.
- Bone graft
  - Autograft vs. allograft
  - Instrumentation to shape graft

Controversies

- A flanged implant may allow for implantation without column support.

Step 5: Closure

- The osteotomy is repaired (Fig. 18A and 18B) utilizing a technique that will not hamper aggressive rehabilitation.
- Skin closure should allow for high stress during flexion and postoperative swelling.
  - Consider leaving staples or sutures in place for longer than usual, especially if the incision is one that was used previously.

Postoperative Care and Expected Outcomes

Immediate

- Splint
  - A splint should be used if preoperative contracture exists.
  - Use 24–48 hours of splinting to maximize any capsular release.
- Robert-Jones compression
  - Use compression in a resting flexed position if no significant contracture existed preoperatively.

Pearls

- *Using oxidized cellulose as a cement restrictor will make potential revisions easier.*
- *Using dyed polymethylmethacrylate will aid revision.*

Pitfalls

- *If bony defects exist from previous surgery, care must be taken.*
  - *Ensure that cement is not extruded from defects or screw holes; this can cause radial nerve burns.*
  - *The implant stem can exit through a defect, even if the trial stem did not. Use fluoroscopy for both the trial and implant stems to ensure intraosseous placement.*

Instrumentation/ Implantation

- Cement system with nozzle small enough for distal humerus
- Cement restrictor
  - Commercial
  - Bone from trochlea
  - Oxidized cellulose (Surgicel)

Controversies

- Flange: will it improve implant longevity?
- Modular implant
  - Revision without stem removal
  - Requires custom implant ordered prior to surgery
- Ease of removal of stem; monoblock stem removal at time of revision to TEA may be difficult
- Fixation of graft or fracture with K-wires/wire versus plates and screws

  - Maintain for 24–48 hours to minimize swelling.
- Drains
  - Use drains as indicated by the surgical field after tourniquet release.
  - Exiting a drain through the triceps prevents prolonged drainage.
  - Drains may limit seroma/hematoma formation.

Early

- Range of motion (ROM)
  - With rigid fixation of the olecraonon, early active, active-assisted, and passive ROM are started.
  - Continuous passive motion is rarely needed.
- Protection of the collaterals is not usually necessary as they are typically not violated during reconstruction.

Intermediate

- Stretch and strengthen (Fig. 19A–D)
  - These exercises are allowed as soon as tolerated.
  - If the olecranon osteotomy fixation is tenuous, limit flexion stretch and extension strengthening until bony healing.
- Splint
  - Consider splinting if progression to intraoperative motion is delayed at 6–8 weeks.
  - Current research suggests no difference in dynamic versus static adjustable splinting.

Long-Term

- Restrictions
  - Native cartilage of the radius and ulna will certainly be subjected to increase stress from the metallic articulation.
  - Patients with these devices should avoid contact sports and high-stress occupations such as plumbings, pipefitting, and ironwork.
  - Currently the author does not restrict golf, tennis, or other noncontact sports.

Pearls

- *Final placement/advancement of K-wires or placement of other hardware can be done during cement curing.*
- *Suture the flaps to fascia in multiple locations to limit the potential space for hematoma and/or seroma. Avoid sutures around cutaneous nerves in the flap.*

Pitfalls

- *Tenuous osteotomy repair will hamper rehabilitation.*
- *Poor tissue closure will increase the chances for prolonged drainage or postoperative wound dehiscence.*

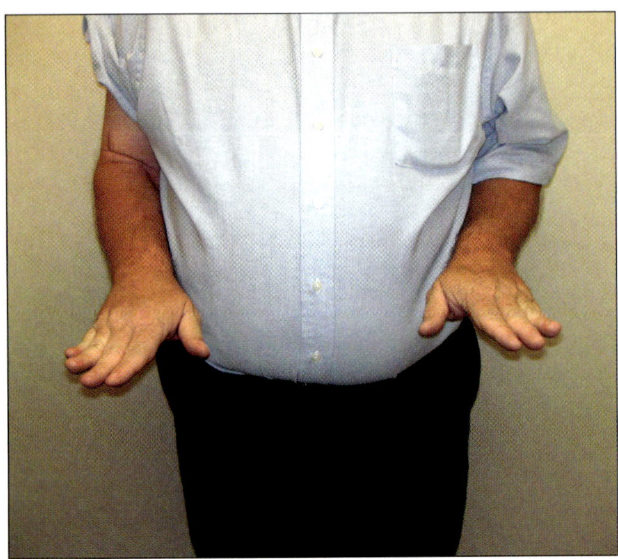
A

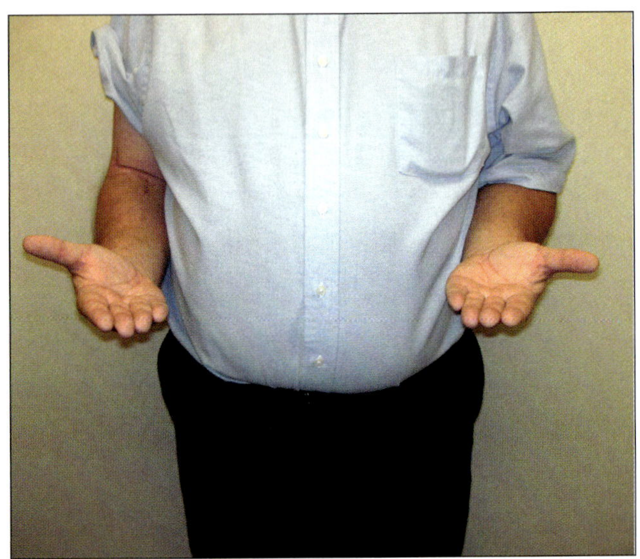
B

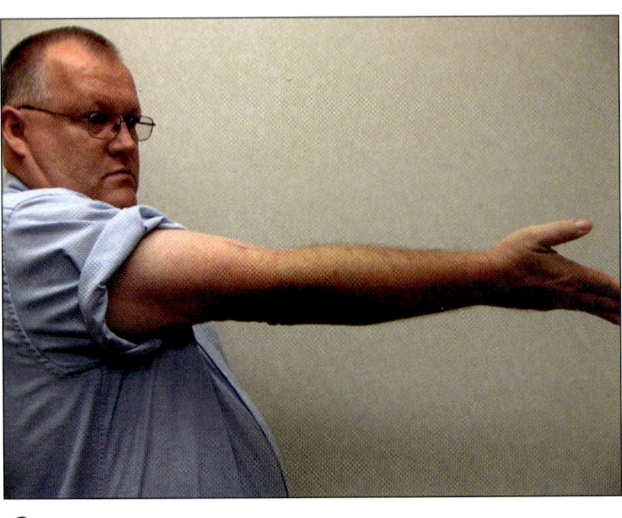
C

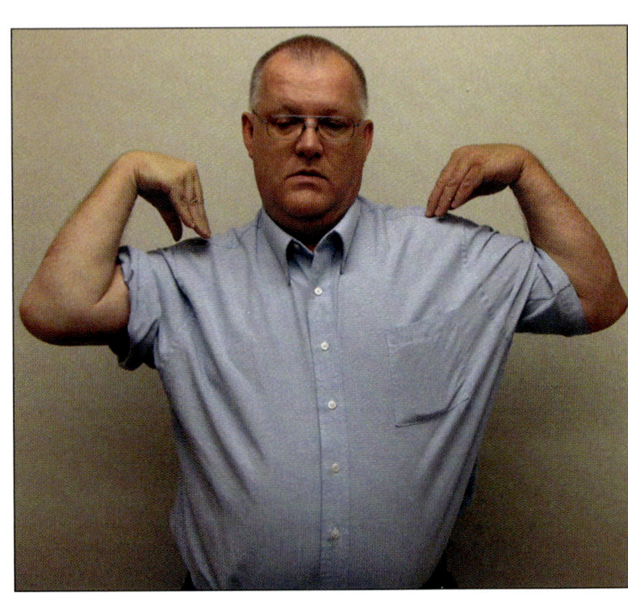
D

FIGURE 19

Instrumentation/ Implantation

- Osteotomy fixation of choice

Controversies

- Method of closure of osteotomy: screw, screw plus tension band, pins and tension band, or plate
- Subcutaneous ulnar nerve transposition: need for or importance of fascial sling, which may add a point of scarring or compression

Pearls

- *Stop all ROM, reapply a compressive bandage, and elevate the limb with skin concerns.*
- *Drain large hematomas or seromas to decrease pressure on the incision with elbow flexion.*

Pitfalls

- *Early removal of staples or sutures may lead to dehiscence of the wound. Consider leaving them in for at least 2 weeks.*

- Joint narrowing has been demonstrated at intermediate follow-up but is asymptomatic.
- The longevity of hemiarthroplasty is unknown.
  - Shifrin and Johnson (1990) have reported a 20+ year follow-up.
  - In this author's experience, excellent results can be expected at intermediate follow-up (4–8 years).

Evidence

There is no strong evidence (level I or II) for hemiarthroplasty of the distal humerus.

Adolfsson L, Hammer R. Elbow hemiarthroplasty for acute reconstruction of intraarticular distal humerus fractures: a preliminary report involving 4 patients. Acta Orthop. 2006;77:785-7.

This is a case series using a nonanatomic device with short-term follow-up of 3–14 months.

Gramstad GD, King GJ, et al. Elbow arthroplasty using a convertible implant. Tech Hand Upper Extrem Surg. 2005;9:153-63.

The authors presented a technique description of a flanged implant with a modular spool. Custom, off-label anatomic spools may be ordered to utilize as a hemiarthroplasty. Later conversion to a TEA can be accomplished without removing the cemented, flanged stem.

Parsons M, O'Brien RJ, et al. Elbow hemiarthroplasty for acute and salvage reconstruction of intra-articular distal humerus fractures. Tech Shoulder Elbow. 2005;6:87-97.

In this short-term follow-up of hemiarthroplasty utilizing a stemmed, anatomic device without a flange, results were promising in both acute and chronic indications, although slightly better in acute reconstructions.

Rosset A, Spadola L, et al. OsiriX: an open-source software for navigating in multidimensional DICOM images. J Digit Imaging. 2004;17:205-16.

This paper provided a description of open-source software that can be utilized by the surgeon to create three-dimensional reconstructions from routine two-dimensional CT images.

Shifrin PG, Johnson DP. Elbow hemiarthroplasty with 20-year follow-up study: a case report and literature review. Clin Orthop Relat Res. 1990;(254):128-33.

Long-term follow-up of a custom device in this case report demonstrated that hemiarthroplasty has the potential for long-term survival.

Swoboda B, Scott RD. Humeral hemiarthroplasty of the elbow joint in young patients with rheumatoid arthritis: a report on 7 arthroplasties. J Arthroplasty. 1999;14:553-9.

The authors noted poor results using a nonanatomic distal humerus prosthesis in patients with inflammatory arthritis. This report highlights the concept that hemiarthroplasty should be done with an anatomically shaped device and not in patients with inflammatory disease.

PROCEDURE 47

Radiocapitellar Replacement

Rick F. Papandrea

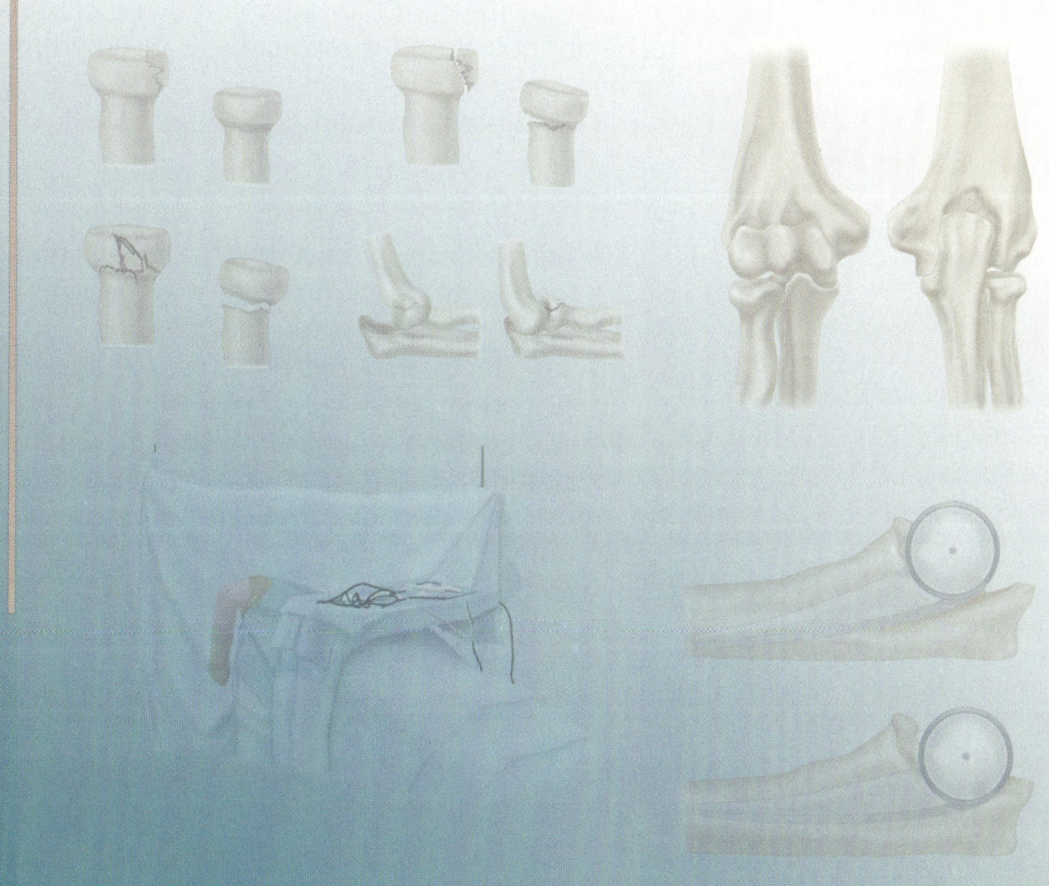

Pitfalls

- *Radiocapitellar replacement cannot be utilized with active or suppressed infection.*
- *The joint must have ligaments intact, or they must be reconstructable.*
- *If this procedure is being contemplated in a patient who has already had a radial head resection, the shaft of the radius must point to the center of the capitellum in all views. A malaligned radial shaft is unlikely to allow a radial head component to articulate properly.*
- *If only the capitellum is being replaced, the radial head must be normal, or near normal.*

Controversies

- Best technique for implantation is unknown. The technique described herein is preferred by the author.
  - Exposure is wide.
  - Repair is anatomic and secure.
- Implant manufacturers recommend leaving the lateral collateral ligament attached. However, this limits exposure.
  - With attempts at increased exposure, the ligament can be avulsed. Ligament release, intentional or otherwise, is more difficult to repair anatomically and rigidly than an osteotomy.
- Longevity of implants is unknown.
- Use is off-label in the United States if only the capitellum is replaced.
- Published information is sparse and consists only of case reviews.

Indications

- Isolated lateral joint damage to both capitellum and radial head (complete radiocapitellar replacement)
  - Unreconstructable isolated capitellar fractures
  - Posttraumatic degenerative changes of the capitellum
  - Failed internal fixation of capitellar fractures
  - Large osteochondritis dissecans lesions in less active patients
  - Essex-Lopresti lesions in lower demand patients (this is a potential indication, with no published results)
- Damage to the capitellum alone may be considered to be an indication for replacement of only the capitellum.
  - This is "off-label" use in the United States.

Examination/Imaging

- The location of the symptoms should be clarified, since more common pathologies may coexist with joint derangement.
  - Both epicondyles should be evaluated for enthesopathies.
  - All three nerves should be evaluated for signs of entrapment.
- The occurrence of pain can localize the cause
  - Pain only at the end of the range of motion is often from impinging osteophytes.
    - These respond well to débridement.
    - Resurfacing or replacement is usually not needed if this is the only pain.
  - Pain at rest may indicate synovitis.
    - If this is the major concern, synovectomy and treatment of the cause of the synovitis may be sufficient for relief.
    - There may be rest pain with avascular necrosis (AVN), but this diagnosis should be readily made with a standard workup.
  - Pain with midarc motion is thought to be mediated by the damaged articular surface.
    - This pain may require resurfacing or replacement of the damaged articulation.
    - Depending on severity, débridement alone or partial resurfacing may suffice.

Treatment Options

- Less invasive procedures should be considered first.
  - Open or arthroscopic débridement of loose bodies, isolated cartilage damage, and osteophytes
  - Treatment of nerve entrapment or epicondylitis if these symptoms appear to be dominant
- If the cartilage lesion is more focal, complete resurfacing of the capitellum may not be needed.
  - Autologous cartilage transplantation has been described for osteochondritis dissecans lesions.
  - Partial capitellar resurfacing is possible (HemiCap, metatarsal implant, Arthrosurface). This technique uses different implants and a different approach, and is considered off-label.
  - In a sedentary patient, a painful radiocapitellar joint may be treated with a radial head resection. Caution should be excercised because ulnohumeral stress will increase and, if this articulation is abnormal, pain may increase medially. This may exacerbate or uncover instability.
- If the joint derangement is diffuse, the patient may be better served with a total elbow athroplasty (TEA).
  - More restrictions are placed on the postoperative TEA than a partial arthroplasty.
  - This should be reserved for less active and older patients.

- Stability of the elbow must be assessed.
  - Arthroplasty will not address instability unless reconstruction of the stabilizing structures is also done.
  - Instability that includes significant bone loss may not be best treated with a capitellar replacement (with or without a radial head component).
    - Current implants require significant lateral-column bone.
    - The epicondyles and columns must be intact, or reconstructable.
- Standard radiographs
  - Anteroposterior (AP), lateral, and oblique views are obtained. In the AP view of the elbow with posttraumatic degenerative joint changes in Figure 1A, note the relative sparing of the ulnohumeral joint. In a lateral view of the same elbow (Fig. 1B), a fragmented capitellum is noted anterior and posterior. An oblique radiograph (Fig. 1C) emphasizes the focus of damage to the capitellum.
  - Radiographs are evaluated for osteophytes, loose bodies, joint space narrowing, and posttraumatic heterotopic ossification.
  - The radial head must be evaluated; deformity and/or loss of cartilage may diminish benefit of isolated (hemiarthroplasty) capitellar resurfacing.
  - Radiocapitellar alignment must be ensured. Malignment will lead to failure after replacement.
- Computed tomography (CT) scan (Fig. 2)
  - Three-dimensional reconstructions make the assessment more meaningful.
    - This can be done with raw DICOM data by the surgeon using free, open-source programs (Rosset et al., 2004).
  - The olecranon, coronoid, and radial head and their corresponding fossae are assessed for proper articulation, and cause for impingement pain.
  - Joint space narrowing or focal damage from AVN or other isolated conditions such as osteochondritis dissecans is localized.
  - When a fracture is present, it may lend insight into the probability of successful repair.
  - Depending on the condition, and the information from other sources, CT scans may not be necessary.
- Magnetic resonance imaging (MRI)
  - MRI may allow for better delineation of cartilage loss/damage, both location and extent.

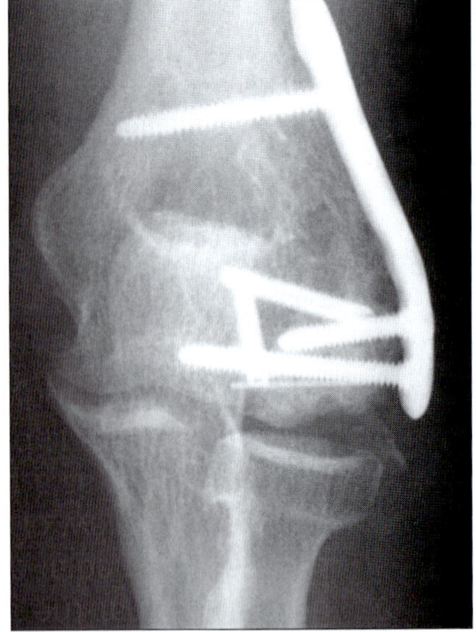

A

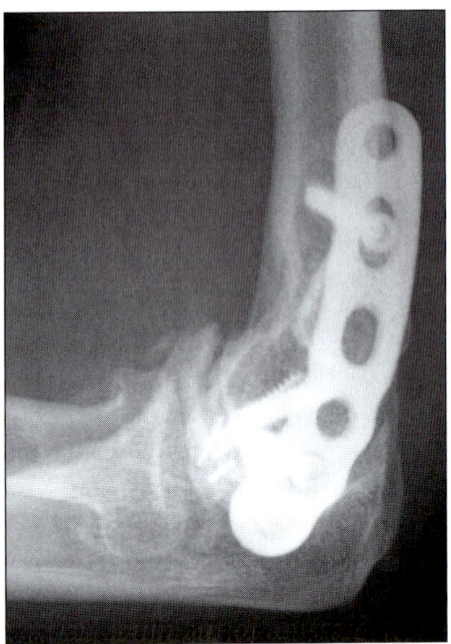

B

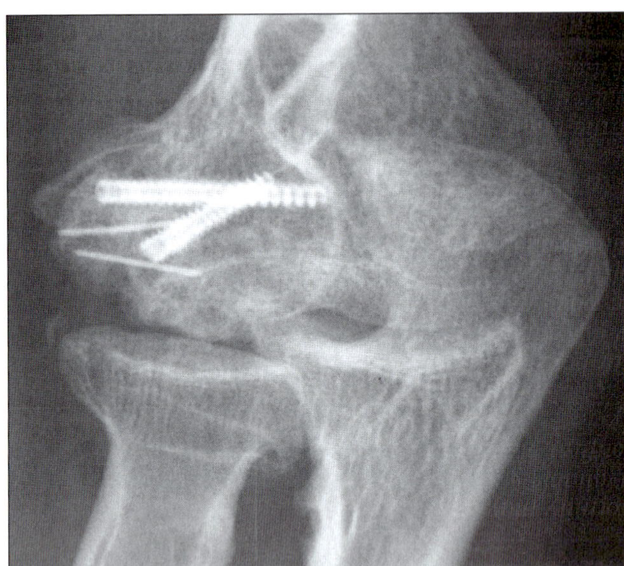

C

FIGURE 1

- It is useful for following AVN.
- As with CT scans, MRI may not be necessary for every patient in whom an arthroplasty (hemi or total) is considered.

■ Previous documented intraoperative information is important.
  - Location of the ulnar nerve
  - Previously placed implants
  - Prior approaches
  - Location and severity of cartilage damage
  - Stability and the status of the collateral ligaments/ epicondyles

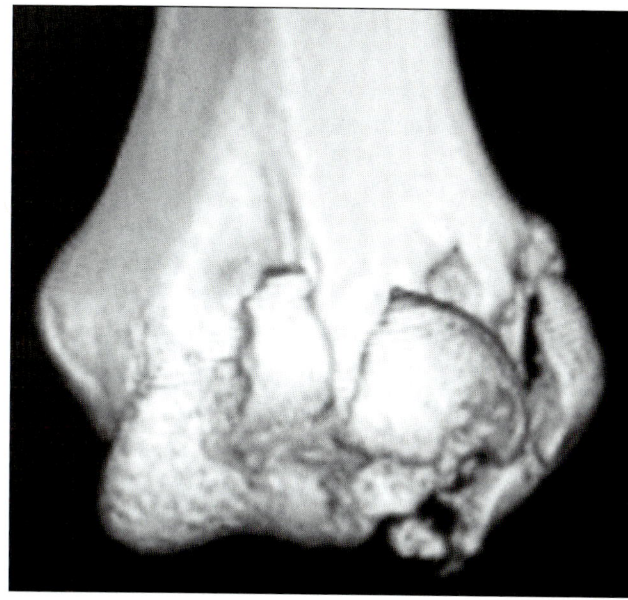

FIGURE 2

- Arthroscopy may allow for final planning when there is uncertainty regarding the appropriateness of an arthroplasty.

Surgical Anatomy

- The relationship of the epicondyles to the center of rotation (COR) and ligaments needs to be understood and maintained with the arthroplasty (Fig. 3A and 3B).
  - The epicondyles and collaterals should be left intact or reconstructed if deficient.
  - A lateral epicondylar osteotomy may be utilized for exposure.
  - Failure to maintain the COR with the arthroplasty will lead to decreased range of motion and possibly early failure.

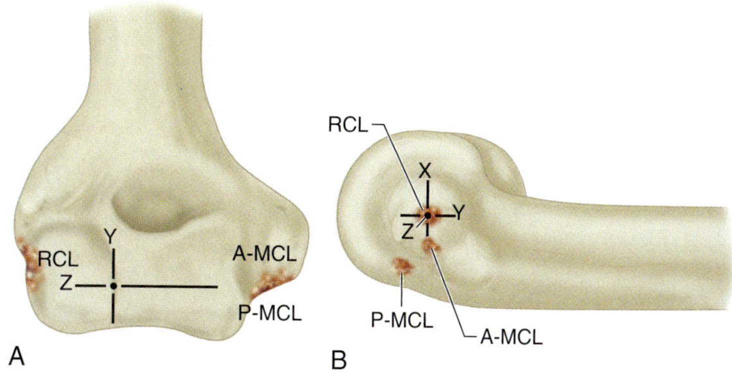

FIGURE 3

PEARLS

- *A proximal nonsterile tourniquet is typically used.*

PITFALLS

- *Large body habitus may make intraoperative imaging difficult.*
  - *Trial imaging should be completed prior to sterile prepping and draping.*
  - *A sterile tourniquet should be considered, such that it can be removed if access is limited.*

- Center of rotation
  - The COR is the isometric point of the lateral collateral ligament (LCL).
  - The anterior band of the medial collateral ligament is slightly posterior to the COR.

Positioning

- The patient is placed in the supine position.
- Use of an arm table is optional.
  - Supports the arm, limits the need for an assistant or device to keep the arm across the body
  - May limit access for image fluoroscopy

PEARLS

- *A direct lateral approach is typically sufficient but may limit access to other areas.*
- *If concern exists for the need for a more extensile exposure, a posterior superficial (skin) incision can be done, with a deep (muscular) lateral approach to the capitellum. Posterior incision may allow for fewer paresthesias due to the watershed cutaneous innervation of this approach.*

PITFALLS

- *Consider previous incisions. Less than ideal skin incisions may be used, so long as full-thickness flaps are developed.*
  - *If full-thickness flaps are created, care should be taken to avoid hematoma or seroma formation.*
- *If work must also be done medially, consider a single posterior incision.*
  - *Two separate incisions may be utilized.*
  - *Minimal undermining of the dual incisions should be carried out.*

Portals/Exposures

- A straight lateral skin incision is made from the lateral epicondyle in line with Lister's tubercle for approximately 4–6 cm. The deep, muscle-splitting dissection will be in line with the skin incision (Fig. 4, *straight line*).
  - Kocher's interval (Fig. 4, *dotted line*) will be too posterior and will compromise the LCL.
- Once the extensors are split, the supinator can be identified. The radial nerve may be palpated, and if necessary dissected at the arcade of Frohse as indicated by the elevator in Figure 5.
  - If a lateral epicondylar osteotomy is used, dissection usually does not need to go this distal.

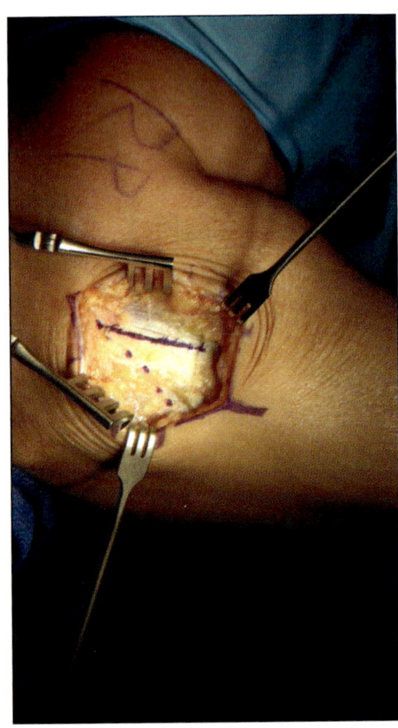

FIGURE 4

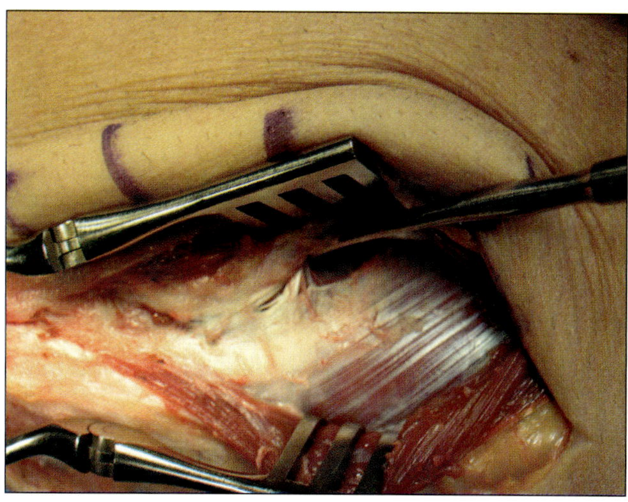

FIGURE 5

Procedure

Step 1: Performing Deep Lateral Dissection

- The radial head is exposed to the neck. In Figure 6, capsular dissection has proceeded proximally up the column. The rake retractor is on the posterior extensor musculature and LCL complex.
- The LCL attachment to the lateral epicondyle is kept intact.

Step 2: Osteotomizing Lateral Epicondyle with LCL and Exensor Musculature

- Figure 7 shows the location of the bony cuts for lateral epicondylar osteotomy.
- The blade of the osteotome is placed inside the LCL/ extensor musculature.

Pearls

- *If further dissection is needed distal to the radial neck, the radial nerve should be palpated and/or dissected.*
- *If flexion contracture is present, capsular release or excision up the lateral column may be performed at this time.*
  - *Release of the anterior capsule will also allow for visualization of the medial joint.*

Pitfalls

- *Too posterior of an incision will violate the LCL.*

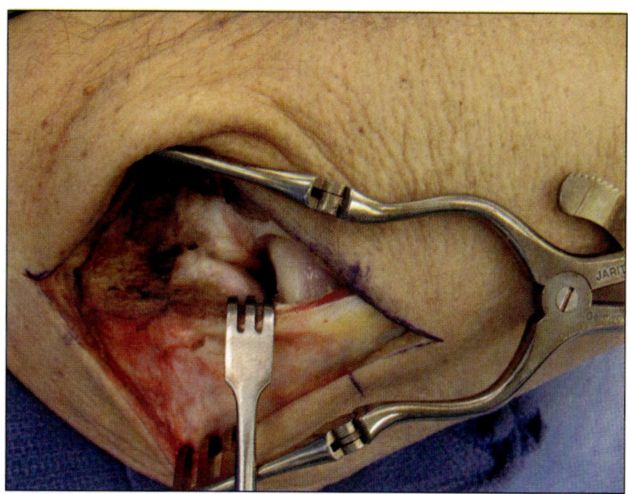

FIGURE 6

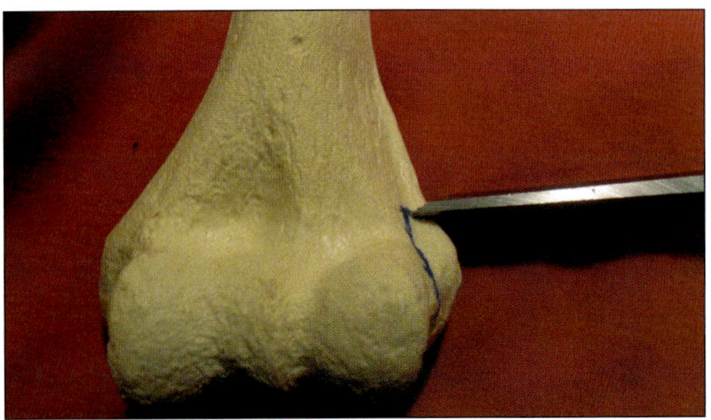
A

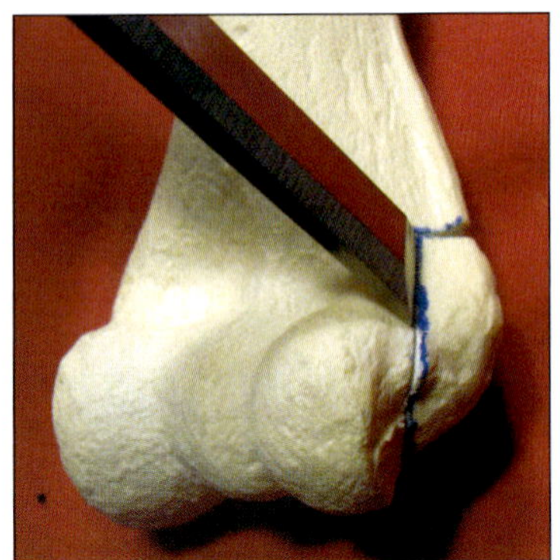
B

FIGURE 7

Pearls

- *A sharp, disposable osteotome or chisel is most effective. Standard osteotomes often are too thick or dull, and will fracture the epicondyle or take too thin a segment of bone.*

Instrumentation/ Implantation

- A sharp, double-bevelled osteotome

Controversies

- The implant manufacturer's procedure utilizes a "ligament-sparing" technique that this author finds difficult to do in a manner that allows for both adequate exposure and rigid collateral fixation postoperatively.

  - A sharp, double-bevelled single-use osteotome simplifies osteotomy completion (Fig. 8).
  - A countercut should be made superiorly to prevent propagation of the osteotomy.
- When 80–90% of the osteotomy is completed, the osteotome is levered posteriorly to free the lateral epicondyle and create a posteriorly fractured cortical margin (Fig. 9).
- Wide exposure is gained by releasing the lateral epicondylar fragment (located behind the elevator in Fig. 10). Access to the posterior and anterior elbow is gained.

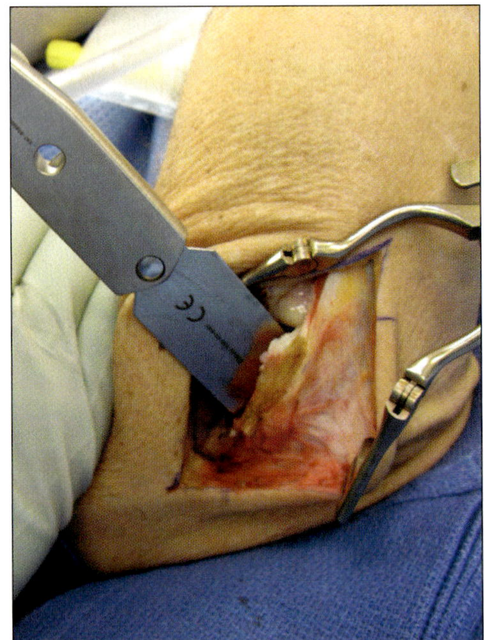

FIGURE 8

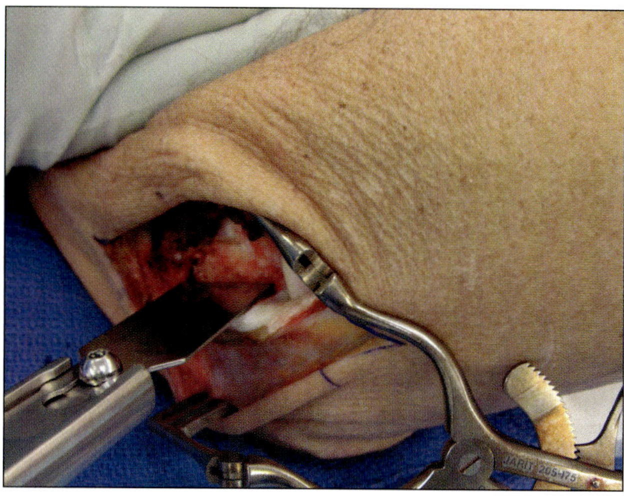

FIGURE 9

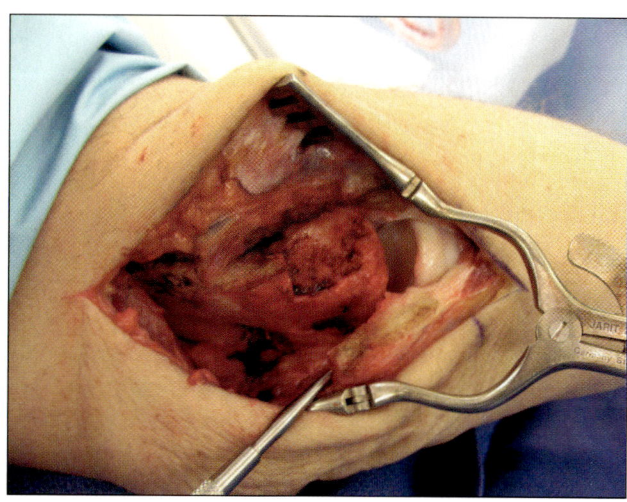

FIGURE 10

PEARLS

- *The COR should exist at a point that sits on a line from the lateral epicondyle to the inferior medial epicondyle on an AP radiographic view.*
- *On a lateral radiographic view, the guidewire should appear as a point in the center of the capitellum (if it were not deformed).*

PITFALLS

- *Pre-existing deformity may make commercially available guides less effective; confirm placement radiographically.*
- *Loss of capitellar bone will alter the lateral view. Accommodation should be made when assessing for the center of the capitellum; the "center" point should be chosen as if the capitellum were not deformed.*
- *The location of the ulnar nerve should be considered regardless of wire implantation technique.*
  - *If a guide is utilized, the medial anchor point of the guide should not apply pressure to the ulnar nerve.*
  - *The guidewire should approach the medial epicondyle, but should not penetrate the medial cortex.*

STEP 3: FINDING COR FOR DISTAL HUMERUS

- A guidewire is placed down the COR of the distal humerus.
- Entry is lateral, at the location of the LCL's attachment to the lateral epicondyle, as seen in the AP view of the guidewire in Figure 11. The epicondyle and LCL have been released with the osteotomy, leaving a flat, cancellous bed for wire entry. The wire is advanced medial enough to determine that the trajectory is properly aimed to the inferior medial epicondyle.
- On a lateral view of the guidewire (Fig. 12), the wire should appear as a point if the axis is properly aligned. If there is bone loss, the wire may be positioned anteriorly within the capitellum.

Instrumentation/ Implantation

- Commercial guides are available from multiple manufacturers.
  - It is imperative that the surgeon understand the landmarks that the guide utilizes, since deformity may alter their accuracy.
  - Some guides designed for other purposes are sometimes useful. Anterior cruciate ligament guides are utilized by some surgeons. The smaller guidewire utilized for the capitellar guide may target less accurately than the pin for which the guide was designed.
- Kirschner wires (K-wires)

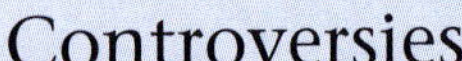

Controversies

- Some surgeons prefer freehand placement of the guidewire.

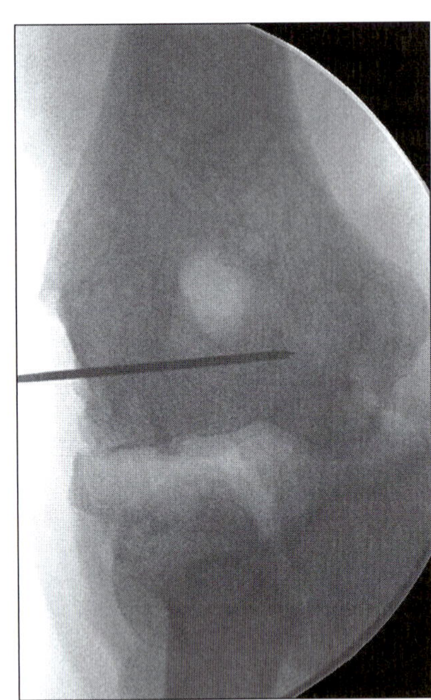

FIGURE 11

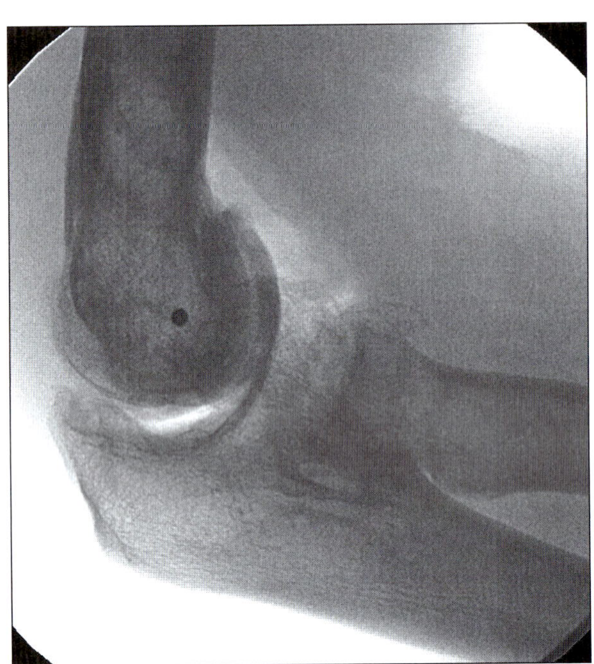

FIGURE 12

Step 4: Making Capitellar Cuts for Resurfacing

- The capitellar cutting guide is applied to the guidewire and the cuts are made for the resurfacing.
- The guide rod should be aligned with the humeral shaft to properly rotate the cutting guide (Fig. 13).
- The size of implant is determined by sizing the guide to the capitellum (Fig. 14). There are two cutting surfaces to choose from.

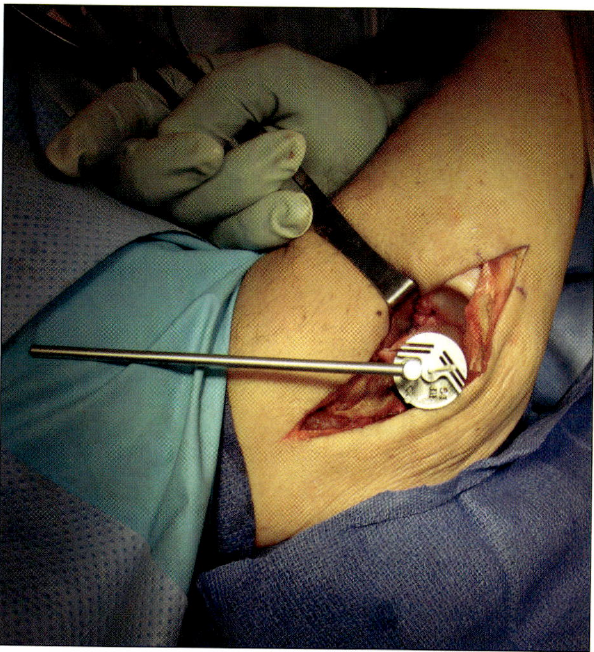

FIGURE 13

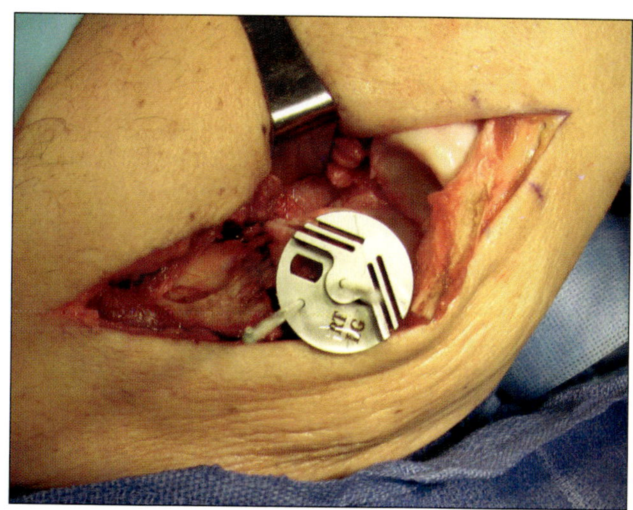

FIGURE 14

Pearls

- *If there is doubt about which cutting surface to use, the distal cut should be made first.*
- *The increased exposure afforded by utilizing the epicondylar osteotomy in comparison to a "ligament-sparing" approach advocated by some allows an enhanced view of the trochlea during capitellar cutting.*

Pitfalls

- *An improperly placed guidewire will cause malrotation of the capitellar implant in one or more planes.*
- *Sclerotic bone from osteoarthritis may cause the saw blades to deflect during cutting.*
  - *Cut surface should be checked before proceeding on to the next step.*
  - *Free hand cutting of the surfaces may be necessary if the cuts are oblique.*
- *Capitellar resurfacing systems are in early generations of development. There is currently little adjustment available in implantation.*

Instrumentation/ Implantation

- Capitellar cutting guide
- Micro-sagittal saw

  - If there is significant capitellar bone loss, the distal cuts are used to "build up" the capitellar surface.
  - If more bone removal is necessary, the more proximal cuts may be utilized.
- A countercut should be made at the medial-most capitellum to prevent cutting into the trochlea when removing the capitellar surface.
- Cuts are then made in the chosen slot to the medial-most capitellum.

Pearls

- *Temporary reduction of the lateral epicondylar osteotomy allows for assessment of soft tissue tension and elbow stability as well as range of motion.*

Pitfalls

- *Uneven cuts will cause the trial implant to shift. Provisional pin fixation may not eliminate this toggle.*

Instrumentation/ Implantation

- Trial implants
- K-wires

Step 5: Trialing the Capitellar Component

- Provisional pin fixation allows the capitellar component to be trialed
  - Cut surfaces should be evaluated, and gaps should be noted.
  - Cementing the final implant on the surface will accommodate imperfections in the cut surface.
- The capitellar relationship to the trochlea and radial head should be evaluated at this time.
  - Figure 15 shows the trial capitellar implant in position with the joint distracted. Assessment of capitellar relationship to the trochlea is optimized.
  - Figure 16 shows the reduction of the joint with the trial capitellar implant in place. Radiocapitellar alignment and fit can be evaluated.
  - Adjustments are best made prior to measuring and cutting for the radial head component.

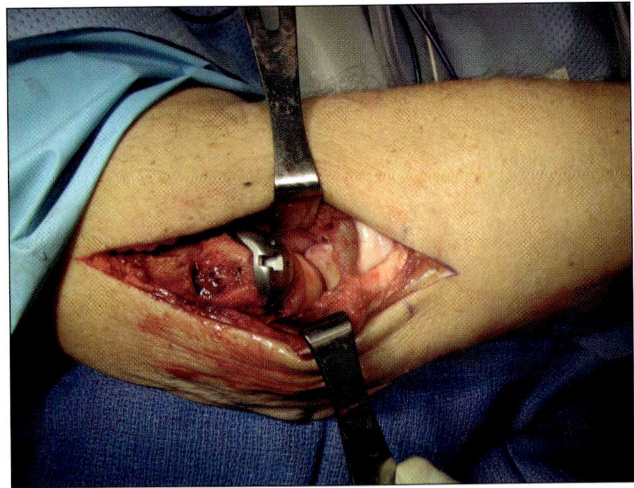

FIGURE 15

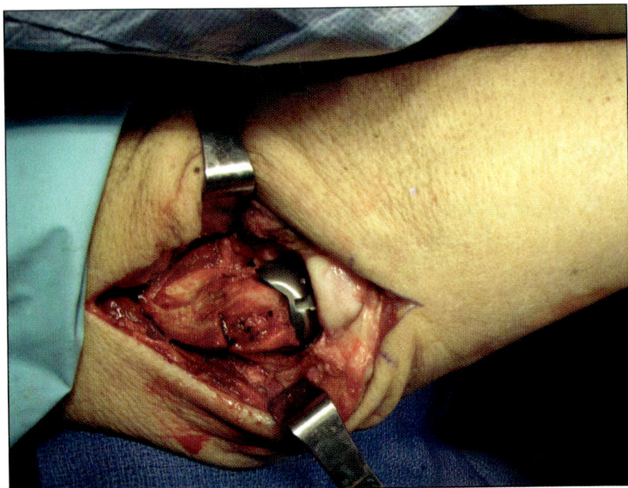

FIGURE 16

Pearls

- *The trial implant should be aligned optimally and held in this position while placing the guidewire.*
- *The guidewire should be imaged to ensure that the stem of the implant will have adequate bone support.*
  - *The wire should be placed at a depth greater than the drill to prevent accidental removal prior to rasping.*

Pitfalls

- *Drilling at an angle off of the wire may lead to shearing of the pin.*

Instrumentation/ Implantation

- Guide pin
- Drill for stem hole
- Cannulated rasp

Step 6: Preparing Intramedullary Distal Humerus for Stem of Capitellar Implant

- A guidewire is placed in the trial capitellar implant for drilling the stem hole for the final implant (Fig. 17).
- The cannulated drill is utilized to create the pilot hole for the stem on the final implant (Fig. 18).
- The cannulated rasp is used to finalize preparation of the stem's hole.
  - Proper orientation of the rasp is ensured by use of the outrigger.
  - Fluoroscopic imaging of the rasp is done to ensure that there is adequate bone around the rasp/stem (Fig. 19).

Step 7: Implanting the Final Capitellar Component

- Use of cement should be considered based on the trial and bone stock.

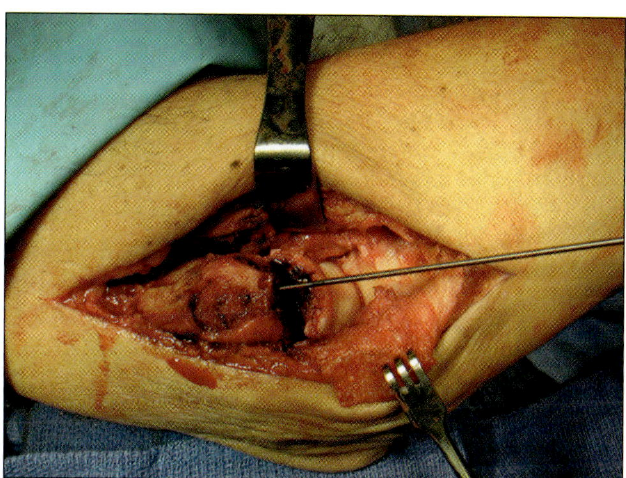

FIGURE 17

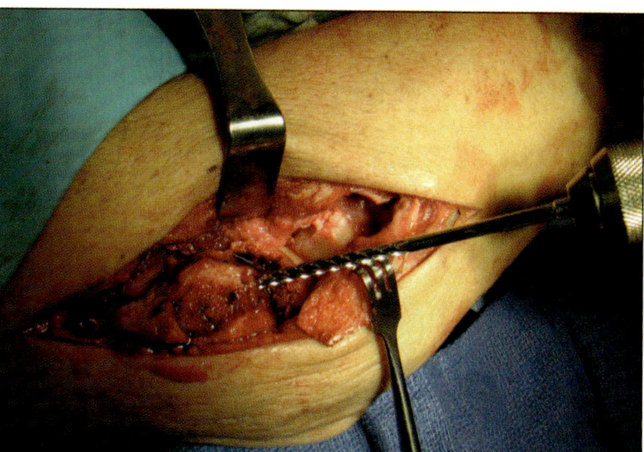

FIGURE 18

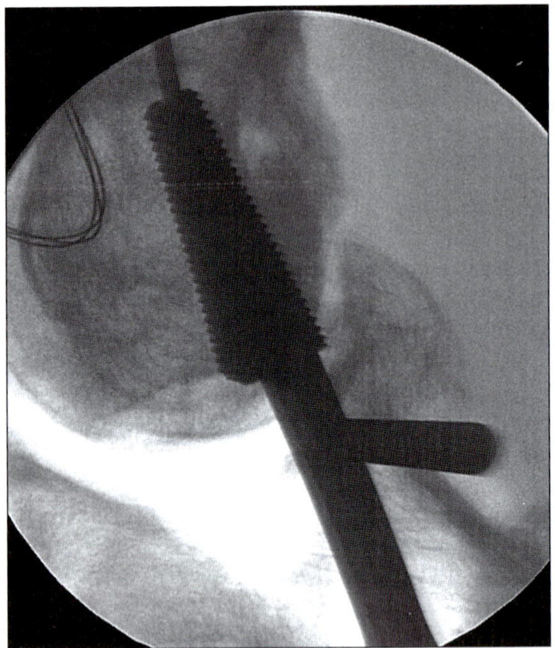

FIGURE 19

Pearls

- *Cement should be allowed to cure enough to not adhere to the surgeon's gloves. This prevents inadvertent cement proximally up the stem.*

Pitfalls

- *Rasping such that the intramedullary hole is expanded, combined with uneven cuts at the distal humerus, will allow the final implant to toggle its position.*
  - *The surgeon must have an understanding of the intended alignment if this is the case, such that the implant can be cemented into the proper orientation.*

Instrumentation/ Implantation

- Final implant
- Cement
- Impactor

- If there are gaps beneath the implant and the cut surface, the undersurface of the implant should be cemented.
- If the bone is adequate up the column, the stem may be left uncemented and press-fitted.
  - Poor bone quality, or an intramedullary hole up the column that is not tight, should be considered indications for cementing the stem of the implant.
- Figure 20 shows the final implant in placed. Cement was utilized on the undersurface only, to accommodate for imperfections.

Step 8: Preparing the Radius for Implantation

- If a decision has been made to utilized a hemiarthroplasty of the capitellum with the native radial head, the surgeon may proceed to Step 9. If the radial head is being replaced, the radius is prepared for the implant. Radial preparation is best done prior to placing the final capitellar component.
- The guide is utilized to remove the radial head at the neck.
- The intramedullary canal is prepared.
- Trial radial heads are checked for articulation with the final capitellar implant.
  - Sizing should be done throughout a full arc of flexion, extension, supination, and pronation.

Pearls

- *The articular surface of the capitellum with the trochlea and the radial head with the coronoid can be evaluated by distracting the joint.*
- *Assess the coronoid-to–lateral trochlea articulation for proper length of the radial head implant.*
  - *The joint should be reduced with the radial head trial in place. A thin nonabrasive material should be placed between the trial radial head (if metallic) and final capitellar component to prevent scratching.*
  - *With adequate soft tissue retraction proximally, when the joint is reduced, the lateral coronoid should articulate with the lateral trochlea.*
- *At the same time, the radial head should be articulating with the capitellum.*
  - *If there is a gap between the coronoid and trochlea, more radial neck needs to be resected.*
  - *If there is a gap between the radial head and capitellum, the radial head needs to be placed proud.*

Pitfalls

- *A recessed capitellar component may require the radial head to be implanted proud to articulate properly.*
- *A proud capitellum will require the radial head to be recessed.*

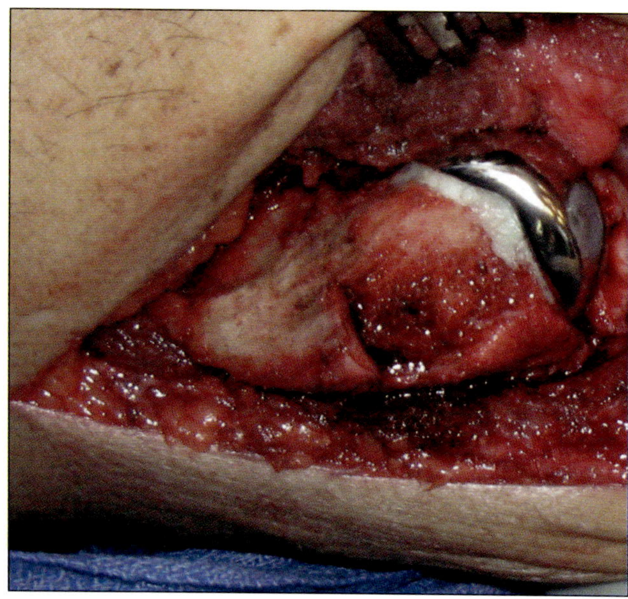

FIGURE 20

- ◆ Placing the device so that it is recessed in some of its arc is preferred to placing it proud in any position.
- When between sizes, the smaller implant should be chosen.
- Length as well as diameter should be assessed; however, length is more critical than diameter.

- ▪ The final radial head implant is placed press-fitted or cemented depending on surgeon preference and trial fitting.
- ▪ Due to the wide access afforded by the epicondylar osteotomy, the radial head can be impacted without impediment from adjacent soft tissues (Fig. 21).

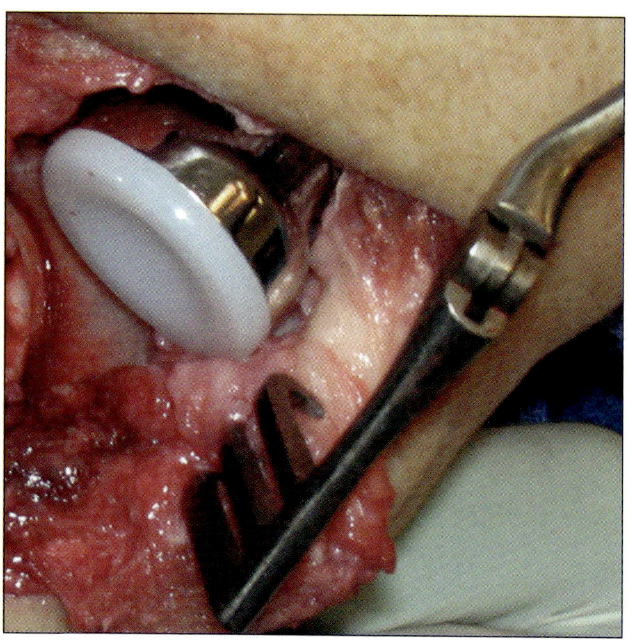

FIGURE 21

Instrumentation/ Implantation

- Radial neck cutting guide
- Trial radial heads

Controversies

- There are not enough data to determine if cement use in the radius is advantageous.

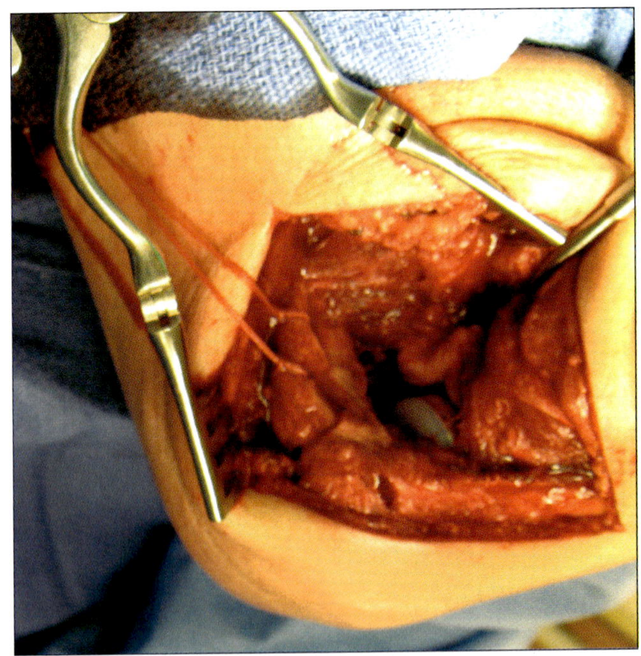

FIGURE 22

Pearls

- *The transverse portion of the osteotomy, combined with the posterior fractured portion, ensures that reattachment will occur in the anatomically correct location.*
- *If the lateral epicondylar fragment is too thin to hold a screw, or fractures when placing a screw, alternative techniques should be used.*
  - *Plate fixation augmented with sutures throught the plate in the LCL*
  - *Cerclage fixation through bone, encircling the epicondyle; wire or suture can be used*

Pitfalls

- *Tenuous fixation may fail under the typical varus stress applied to the elbow in activities of daily living.*

Step 9: Closure of the Lateral Epicondylar Osteotomy and Soft Tissues

- The lateral epicondylar fragment is rotated back into place and held provisionally with K-wires. This should restore stability to the joint.
- Final assessment of the components is made prior to secure fixation of the osteotomy.
- Fixation can be gained by screws, plates, or cerclage wire/suture.
  - If cannulated screws are used, they may be placed over the guidewires for temporary fixation.
  - In Figure 22, the lateral epicondylar fragment is repaired with two cannulated, headless screws. Note the radial head now sits posterior to the LCL and adjacent soft tissue sleeve.
- The superior portion of the lateral extensor mass can be closed to the supracondylar ridge.
- Figure 23A shows a lateral image of final implants with the epicondyle repaired. The AP view in Figure 23B demonstrates anatomic repair of the lateral epicondyle and LCL.

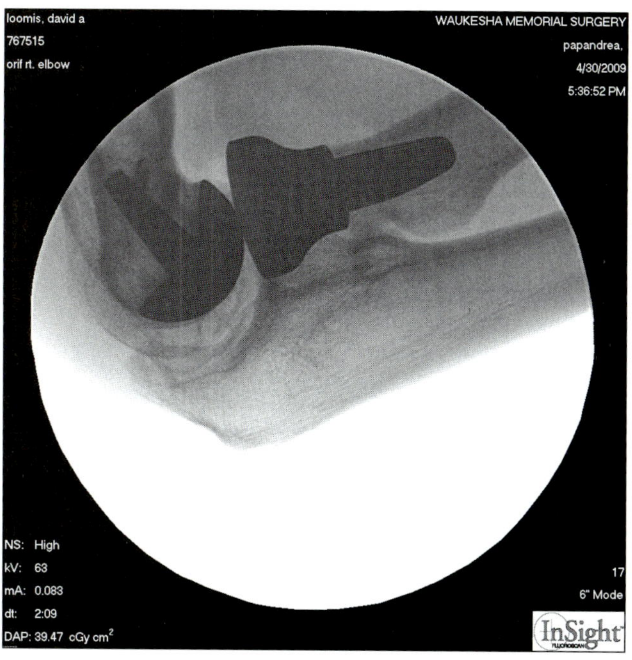

A

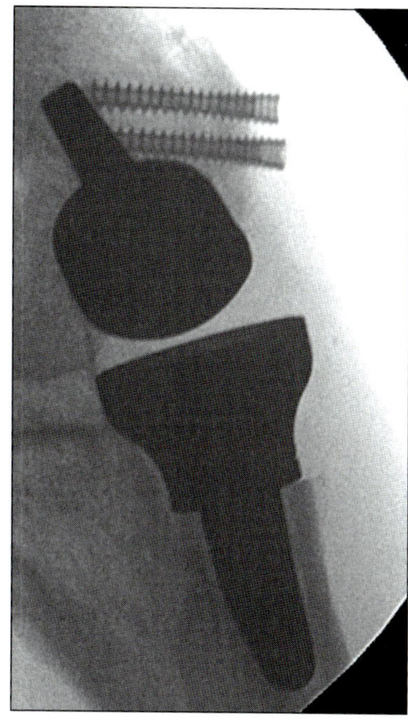
B

FIGURE 23

Instrumentation/ Implantation

- K-wires
- Implants for fixation of the epicondyle
  - Cannulated screws
  - Anatomic plates: rarely needed; bulkier than other options
  - Cerclage wire or suture

Controversies

- Alternative methods of exposure, without osteotomy, will not allow the access that was gained with the osteotomy unless extensive soft tissue release was done.
  - Repair of a soft-tissue-only release is more difficult to judge as to isometry. Repair methods are not as rigid as bone fixation.

Postoperative Care and Expected Outcomes

Immediate

- Splint
  - Support from varus stress if the LCL repair is tenuous or if patient compliance is questionable.
  - Splint in extension if preoperative contracture exists; 24–48 hours of splinting is necessary to maximize any capsular release.
- Robert-Jones compression
  - In resting flexed position if no significant contracture existed preoperatively
  - For 24–48 hours to minimize swelling
- Use drains as indicated by the surgical field after tourniquet release.
  - An exit drain is placed through the triceps (prevents prolonged drainage).
  - Drains may limit seroma/hematoma formation.

Early

- Range of motion
  - With rigid fixation of the LCL and/or lateral epicondyle, early active, active-assistive, and passive range of motion are started.
  - Continuous passive motion is rarely needed.
- Protection of the collaterals
  - Obligatory varus stress during shoulder abduction should be avoided.
  - Frequent reinforcement to the patient is necessary, as this common position in activities of daily living is often difficult to limit.

Intermediate

- Stretch and strengthen
  - Stretching and strengthening exercises are allowed once the lateral repair is sufficiently healed.
  - If lateral stability is tenuous, shoulder abduction should be avoid and a hinged orthosis considered if it would fit well.
- Splint
  - Consider splinting if progression to intraoperatively determined range of motion is delayed at 6–8 weeks.
  - Current research suggests no difference in dynamic versus static adjustable splints.
  - The author prefers static adjustable splints.

Long term

- Restrictions
  - If any native cartilage of the radius is articulating with the prosthesis, it will certainly be subjected to increased stress.
  - Patients with these devices should avoid contact sports and high-stress occupations such as plumbing, pipefitting, and ironwork.
  - Currently the author does not restrict golf, tennis, or other noncontact sports.
- Joint space narrowing
  - This has been demonstrated on intermediate follow-up in elbow hemiarthroplasty. However, there is not enough follow-up on capitellar replacement.
  - It is asymptomatic at intermediate follow-up in hemiarthroplasty.
- Longevity
  - Longevity of radiocapitellar replacement is unknown.

Pitfalls

- *Early removal of staples or sutures may lead to dehiscence of the wound. Consider leaving these in for at least 2 weeks.*

- Complete lateral replacement would be expected to have the highest failure rate.
    - Essex-Lopresti lesions would be expected to have increased frequency of failure in comparison to a stable joint with arthritis.

Evidence

Heijink A, Morrey BF, Cooney WP, 3rd. Radiocapitellar hemiarthroplasty for radiocapitellar arthritis: a report of three cases. J Shoulder Elbow Surg. 2008;17(2):e12-5.

This case series is presented by the developers of the device described.

Pooley J. Unicompartmental elbow replacement: development of a lateral replacement elbow (LRE) arthroplasty. Tech Shoulder Elbow. 2007;8(4):204-12.

This technique article describes a device not presented in the preceeding chapter.

Rosset A, Spadola L, Ratib O, Osiri X. An open-source software for navigating in multidimensional DICOM images. J Digit Imaging. 2004;17(3):205-16.

Open source software description which can be utilized by the surgeon to create 3D reconstructions from routine 2D CT images.

PROCEDURE 48

Revision Total Elbow Arthroplasty

Donald H. Lee

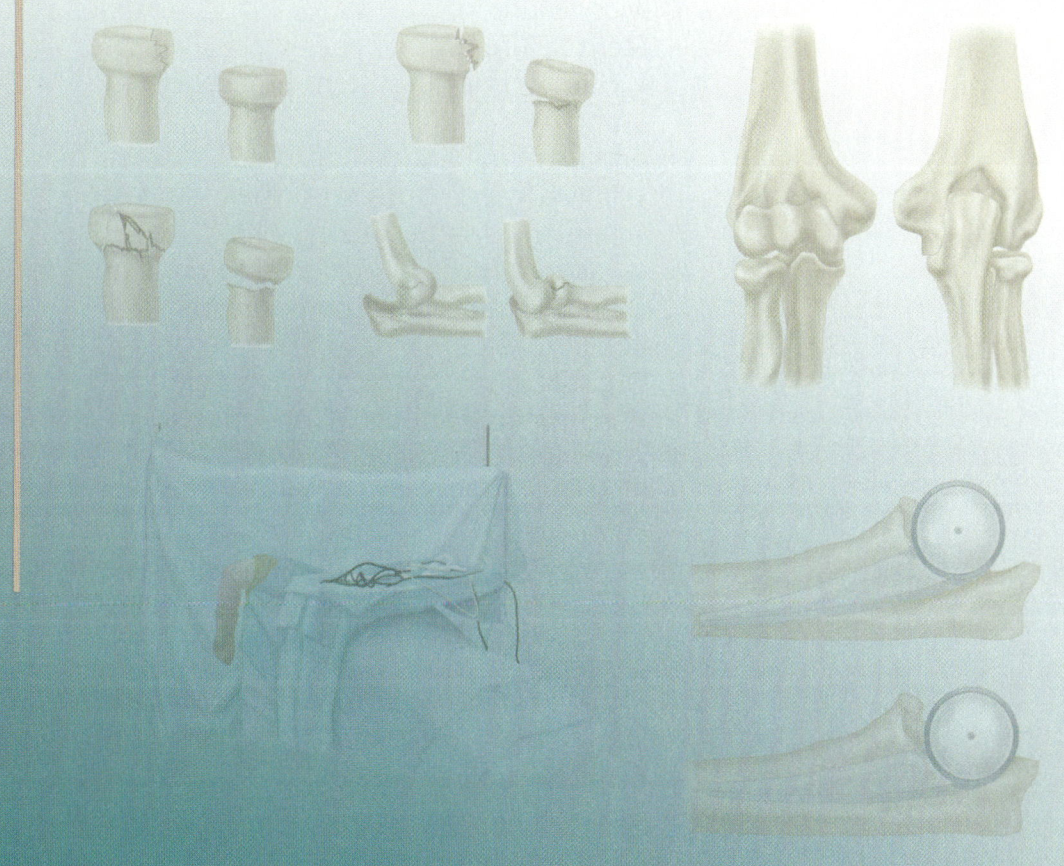

Indications

- Failed total elbow arthroplasty

Modes of Failure

- Nonseptic loosening
  - At bone-cement interface, cement-implant interface, or both
  - With or without bone resorption
  - With bone destruction (cortical thinning and enlargement ["ballooning"] of humeral or ulnar canals or both)
- Septic failure (findings similar to those found with nonseptic loosening)
- Device failure
  - Stem failure
    - Humeral or ulnar stem breakage (Fig. 1A and 1B)
  - Articular coupling failure
    - Polyethylene bushing or bearing wear (Fig. 2)
    - Implant disarticulation
    - Failure of axis pin or bearing apparatus between humeral and ulnar components
- Instability
  - Disarticulation of unconstrained implant
- Periprosthetic fracture
- Massive bone loss secondary to
  - Failure of previous total elbow implant
  - Tumor resection: Figure 3 shows massive bone loss of proximal ulna and distal humerus secondary to tumor.

Revision Options

- For failed total elbow implant with adequate bone stock:
  - Semiconstrained implant
  - Unconstrained implant (less commonly used, requires adequate joint stability)
- For failed total elbow implant with inadequate bone stock:
  - Semiconstrained implants: standard, with long anterior flange, placed with impaction allografting, with strut allografts, or combined with humeral or ulnar structural allograft (alloprosthesis)
  - Custom semiconstrained implant (humeral, ulnar, or both components)
  - Allograft

Pitfalls

- *Septic failure of implant will need to be assessed.*
- *Laboratory assessment includes looking for elevated levels of:*
  - *Complete blood count with white blood cell count differential count*
  - *C-reactive protein*
  - *Erythrocyte sedimentation rate*
  - *Joint aspiration with Gram stain and culture*
- *Positive bone scintigraphy will not differentiate between aseptic loosening and an infected implant.*

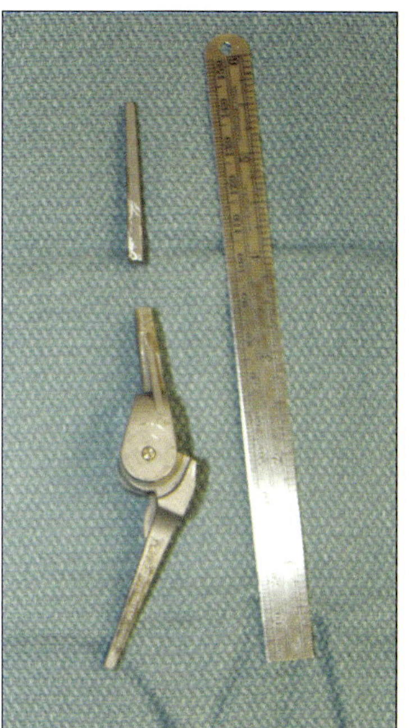

A

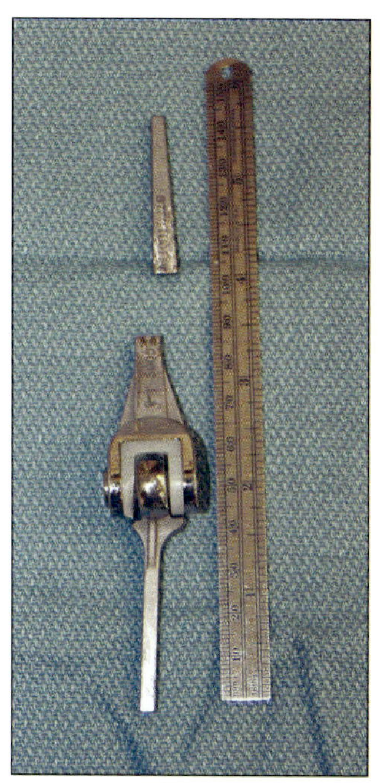

B

FIGURE 1

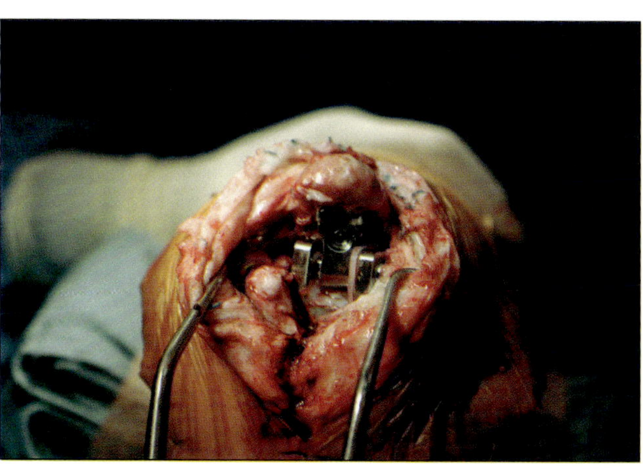

FIGURE 2

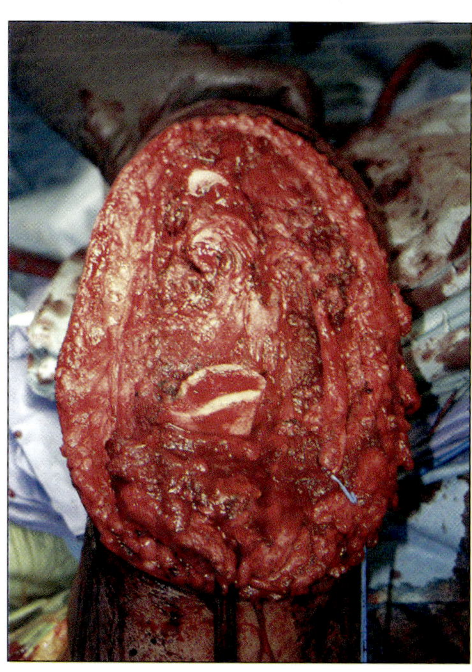

FIGURE 3

Treatment Options

- Alternative treatment options for failed total elbow implant include:
  - Elbow arthrodesis
  - Interposition arthroplasty
  - Resection arthroplasty

Examination/Imaging

- Physical examination should evaluate:
  - Skin and soft tissue envelope
    - Previous skin incisions
    - Insufficient soft tissue envelope (may require soft tissue coverage)
  - Nerve dysfunction
    - Ulnar nerve
    - Radial nerve (associated with humeral shaft fractures)
  - Triceps function
  - Collateral ligament status
    - Joint instability (particularly with unconstrained implant)
  - Joint capsular contractions limiting elbow flexion and extension
  - Status of osseous structures
    - Associated fractures or pending fractures
    - Bone loss
- Operative reports from the previous operative procedure should be obtained to determine:
  - The manufacturer of the previously used implant and whether extracting devices are available
  - The size of previously placed implants
  - If the ulnar nerve has been previously transposed
  - Any previous complications (cortical perforations, etc.)
- Anteroposterior and lateral radiographs of the elbow, showing the entire length of both the humeral and ulnar stems, should be obtained.
  - The radiographs should be reviewed for:
    - Implant loosening with (Fig. 4A and 4B) or without (Fig. 5A and 5B) bone resorption
    - Bone destruction: cortical thinning and canal enlargement (Fig. 6A and 6B)
    - Implant disarticulation (Fig. 7A and 7B)
    - Periprosthetic fracture (Fig. 8)
    - Massive bone loss secondary to failure of previous total elbow implant (Fig. 9) or tumor resection (see Fig. 3)
  - On the anteroposterior view, an increased angle between lines drawn along the long axes of the humeral and ulnar components may show evidence of bushing wear.
  - Radiographs of the entire humerus and forearm may be needed (e.g., cases with a shoulder implant or previous fractures of the humerus and ulna).

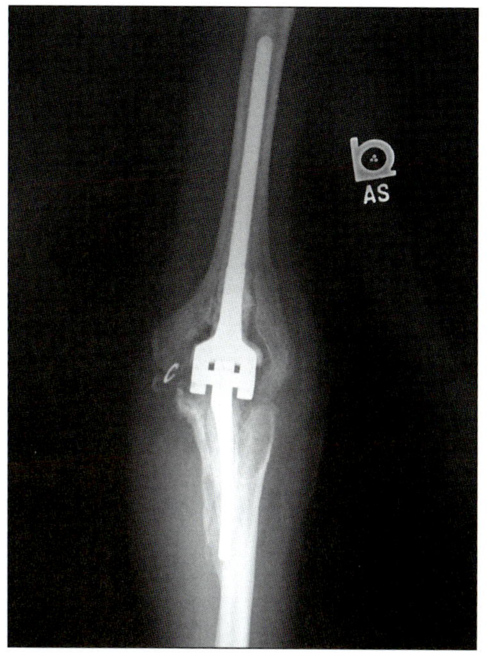

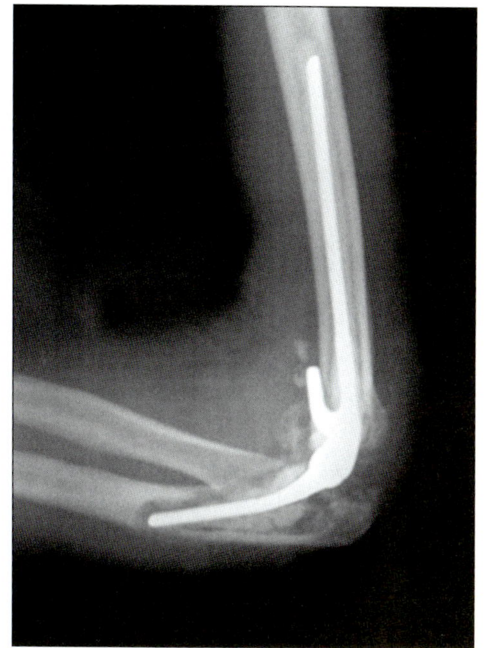

A B

FIGURE 4

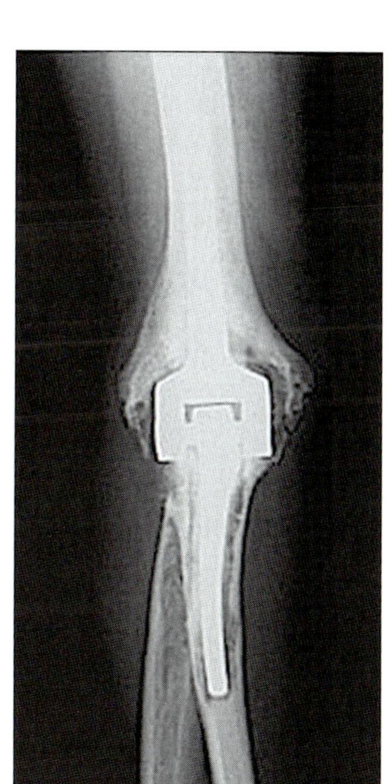

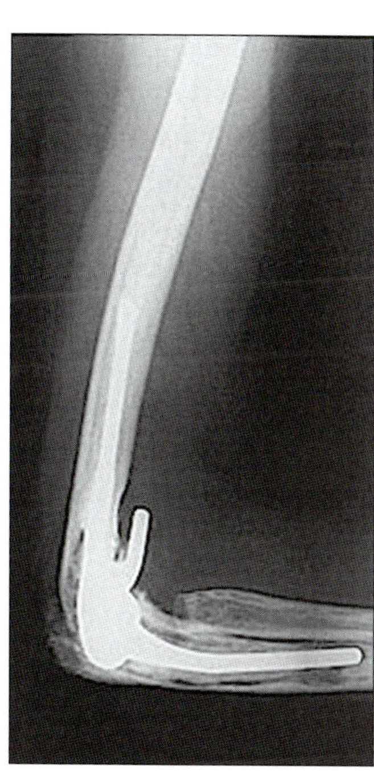

A B

FIGURE 5

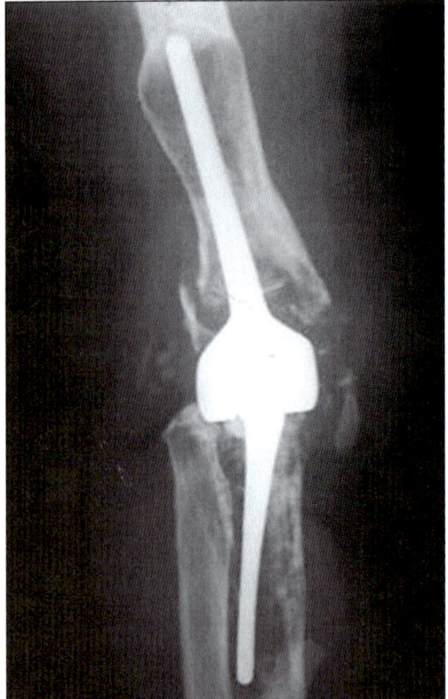

A

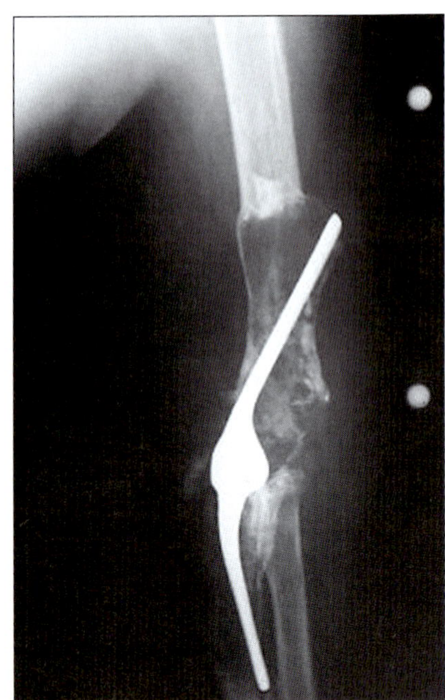

B

FIGURE 6

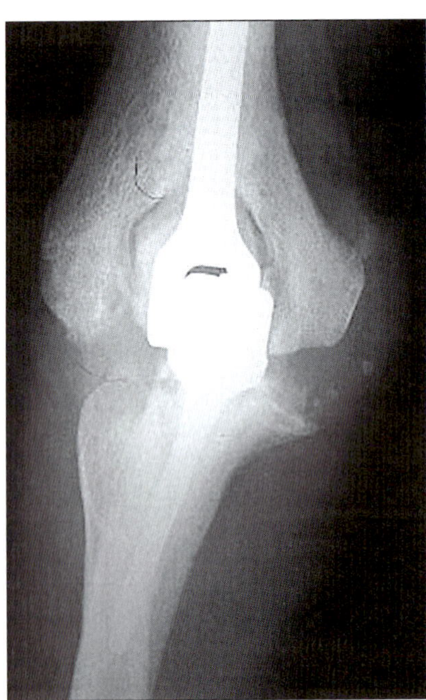

A

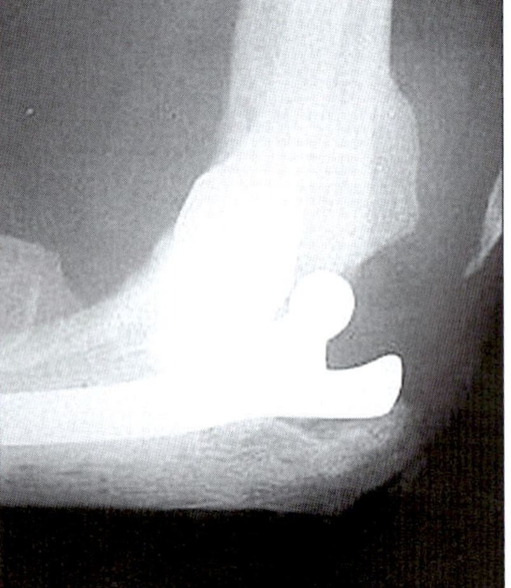

B

FIGURE 7

- Radiographs should include sizing markers for possible custom implants (Fig. 10A and 10B).
- Standard and custom humeral and ulnar templates are used to determine if standard implants, noncustom long-stemmed implants, or custom long-stemmed implants may be needed.

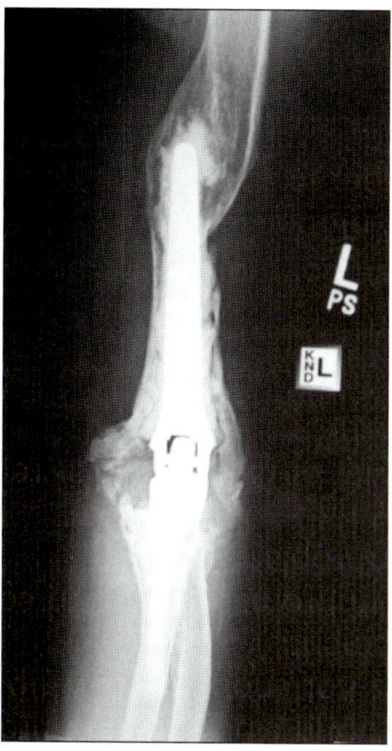

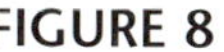
FIGURE 8

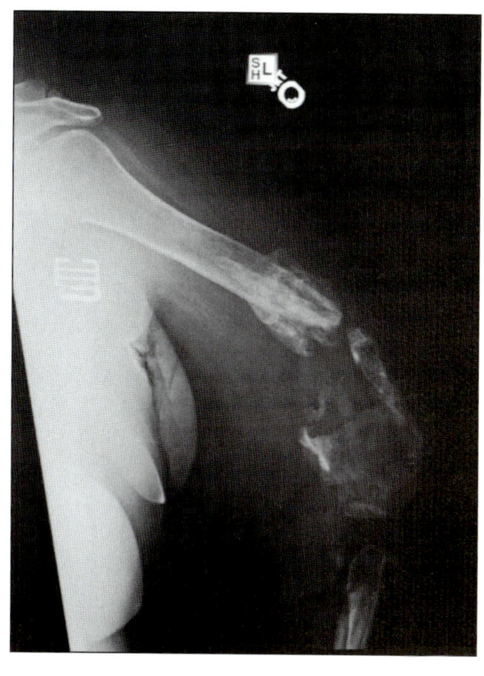

FIGURE 9

- Figure 11 shows a template for a custom humeral component.
- Preoperative radiographs used for templating for a custom ulnar component are shown in Figure 12A and 12B.

■ Preoperative computed tomography scans with three-dimensional reconstruction are also needed for custom implants (Fig. 13A and 13B).

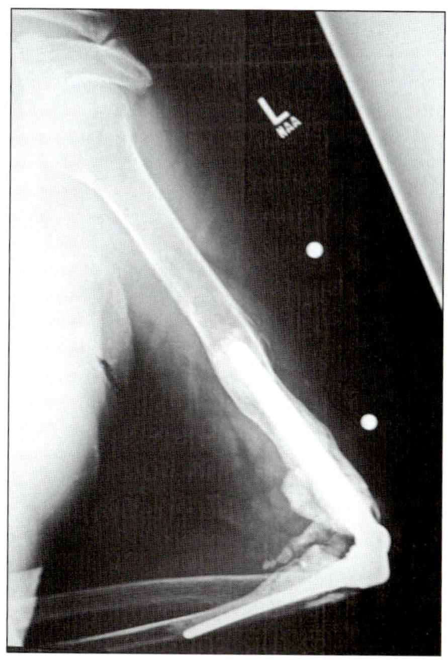

A

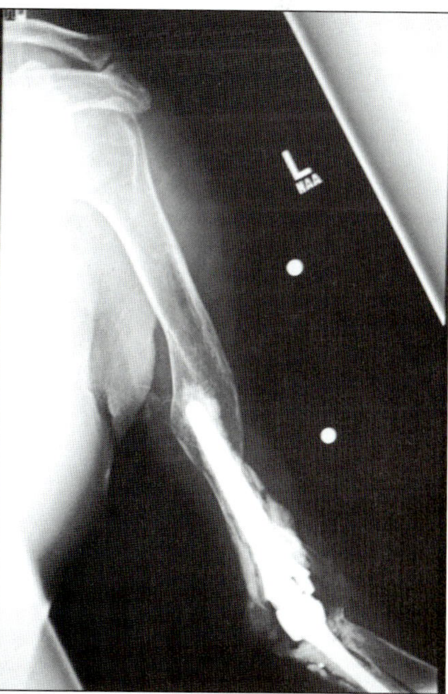

B

FIGURE 10

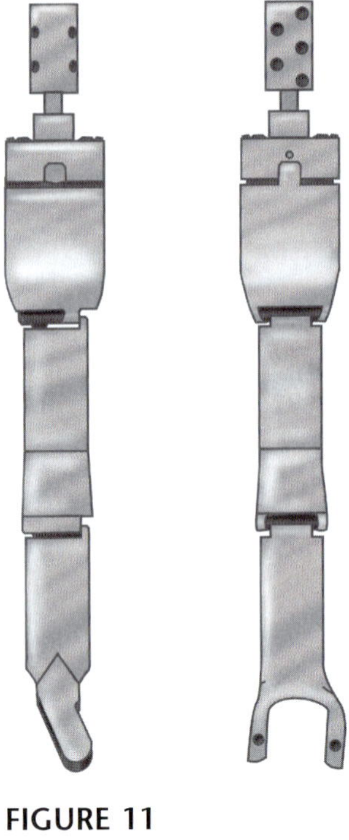

FIGURE 11

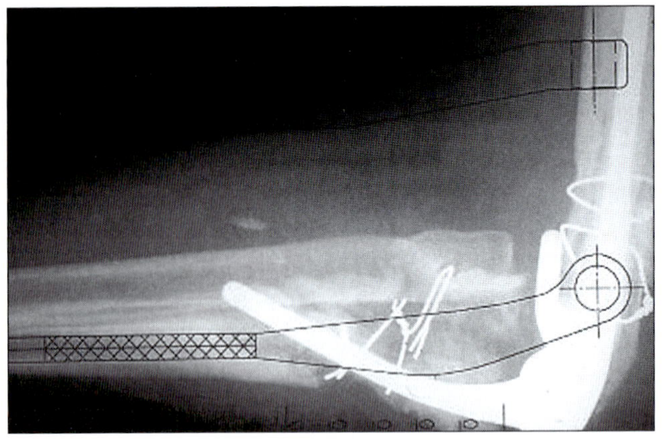

A

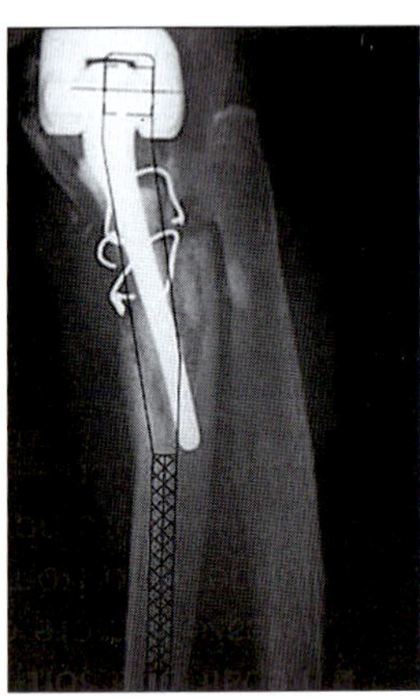

B

FIGURE 12

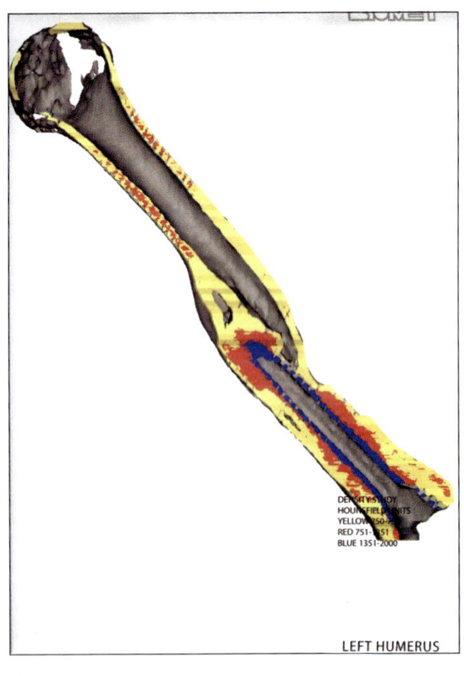

A

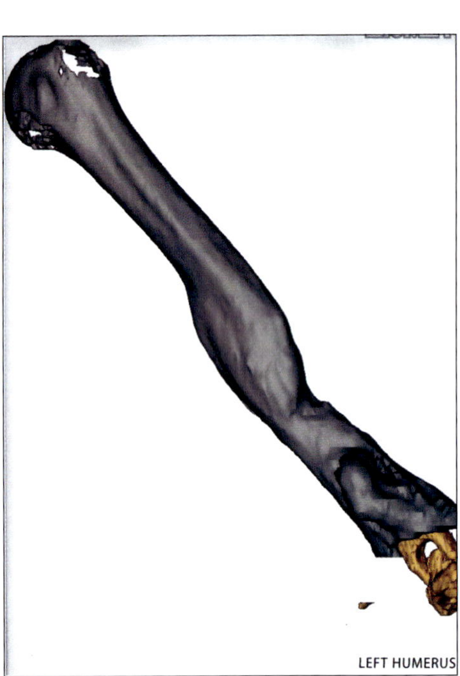

B

FIGURE 13

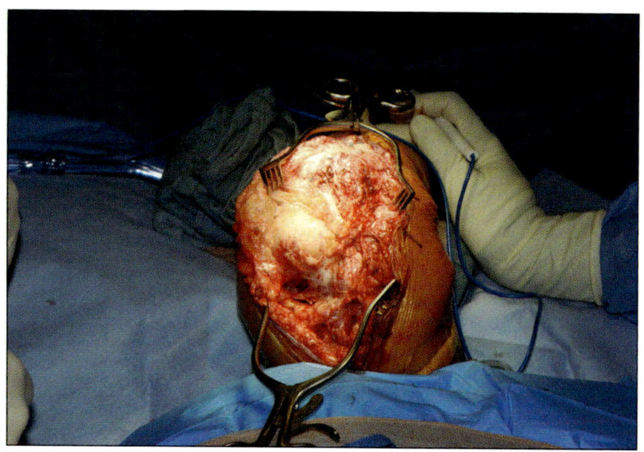

FIGURE 14

Pearls

- *A padded Mayo stand is placed along the posterior aspect of the humerus to help support the arm across the chest (Fig. 14).*
- *A bolster is used to support the forearm on the chest.*

Equipment

- Sterile tourniquet
- Padded Mayo stand
- Bolster

Controversies

- An alternative positioning option is a lateral decubitus position with a beanbag and the affected arm supported on a bolster.

Pitfalls

- *Flaps (e.g., random rotation flaps or pedicle flaps) may be needed if there is poor wound coverage (Fig. 16).*

Surgical Anatomy

- The ulnar nerve will need to be identified, dissected, and protected. The dissection can start either at the level of the cubital tunnel or proximally in a relatively unscarred area. If the ulnar nerve has been previously anteriorly transposed, then the nerve may not need to be dissected.
- With dissection of the humerus proximally, at approximately the midhumerus level (the level of spiral groove), the radial nerve and profunda brachii artery will need to be identified and protected.

Positioning

- The patient is placed supine with the arm across the chest.
- The entire arm is prepped and draped to the shoulder level.
- A sterile tourniquet is used for dissection about the elbow. It may need to be removed for dissection more proximally along the humerus.
- Ioban drapes can be used to cover the extremity during the procedure.

Portals/Exposures

- Previous skin incisions should be used to minimize wound healing problems (Fig. 15)
- Elevation of skin flaps should be minimized.
- The ulnar nerve is identified (either at the cubital tunnel or more proximally), dissected, and protected. If the ulnar nerve has not been previously transposed anteriorly, the nerve should be transposed.

Controversies

- A sliver or wafer of the posterior olecranon can be elevated with the triceps in cases in which elevation of the triceps off the posterior olecranon may result in significant thinning of the triceps tendon insertion.
- Alternative approaches for the elbow (see Procedure 40: Surgical Approaches Surgical Approaches for Open Treatment of the Elbow II–IV)
  - Extended Kocher posterolateral approach: between the ECU and anconeus
  - Campbell (van Gorder) approaches: triceps-splitting or triceps tendon–reflecting approach
  - Olecranon osteotomy

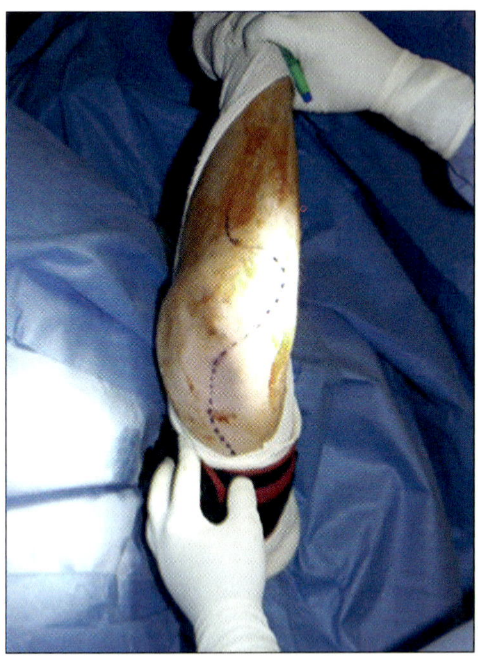

FIGURE 15

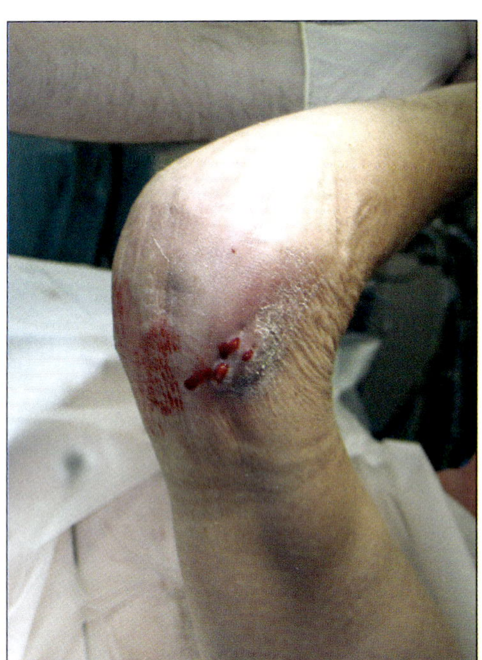

FIGURE 16

- The triceps is reflected subperiosteally off the posterior olecranon process, usually in a medial-to-lateral direction, and the triceps muscle is elevated off the posterior aspect of the humeral shaft (Bryan-Morrey approach; see Procedure 40: Surgical Approaches for Open Treatment of the Elbow I).
- Alternatively, the triceps is elevated medially and laterally from the humerus and left attached to the olecranon process (triceps mobilization approach).

- For dissection involving the proximal half of the humerus, the radial nerve and profunda brachii artery are identified in the spiral groove and protected.

Procedure

Step 1: Joint Exposure and Implant Removal

- Joint exposure
  - Soft tissue is removed around the articulation between the humeral and ulnar components (Fig. 17).
  - Periprosthetic soft tissue is sent for an intraoperative frozen section. A finding of five neutrophils or more per high-power field is indicative of a probable infected implant.
  - Intraoperative cultures are sent.
- The elbow implant coupling mechanism is removed and the humeral and ulnar components are dissociated (Fig. 18).
- Depending on the type of elbow implant, a portion of one or both humeral condyles may be osteotomized or removed to undo and remove the coupling mechanism.
- If an infection is suspected, both the humeral and ulnar components and cement mantles are removed.

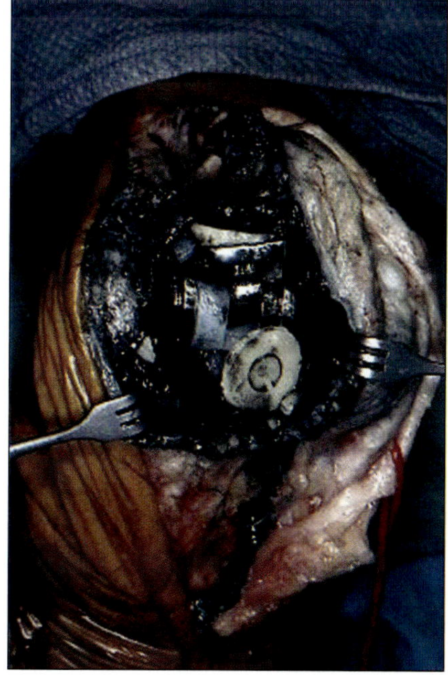

FIGURE 17

Instrumentation/ Implantation

- Extraction device, provided by implant manufacturer or universal type
- Cerclage wire (18 gauge) or cable
- High-speed burrs, oscillating saw with narrow-width blade
- Long angled curettes, flexible reamers, flexible and curved osteotomes and gouges
- Pulsed lavage system

Controversies

- High-frequency ultrasonic equipment for cement removal must be used with caution due to potential thermal injury to the ulnar and particularly the radial nerve.
- In cases in which infection is not suspected, a firmly adherent cement mantle may be left in situ, if the cement mantle will not interfere with cement fixation of a new component.

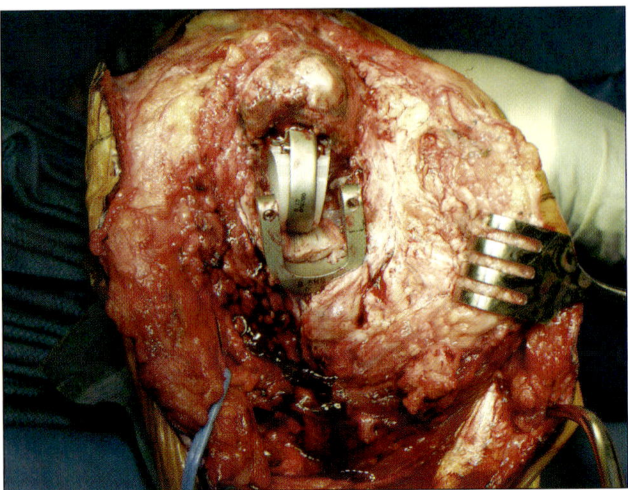

FIGURE 18

- An extraction device, either provided by the manufacturer or a universal type (with or without attachment to a slap hammer) is used to attempt removal of the humeral and ulnar implants.
  - Loose implants are easily removed (Fig. 19).
  - Well-fixed implants will require removal of the visible cement mantle.
    - A longitudinal slot can be made through the posterior humeral cortex and cement mantle down to the humeral implant with an oscillating saw. Flexible osteotomes can be used to further loosen the cement mantle.
    - A similar slot can be made in the proximal ulna. The loosened implant may then be removable with an extractor.

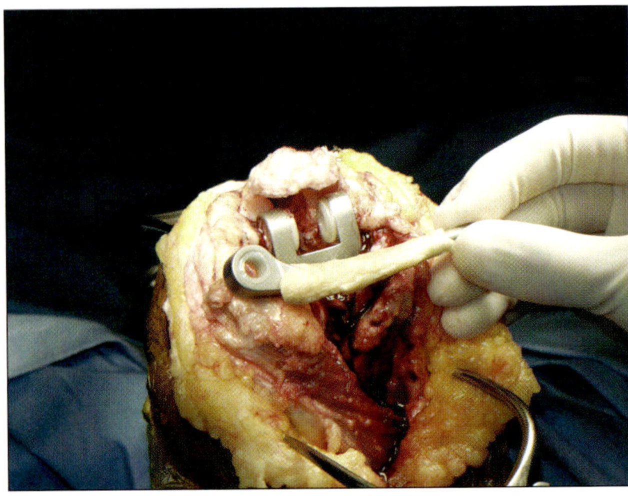

FIGURE 19

- Alternatively, cortical windows may be needed to facilitate implant and cement mantle removal.
  - The proximal edge of the humeral cortical window (Fig. 20A) should be proximal to the humeral implant and cement mantle, and the distal edge of the ulnar cortical window (Fig. 20B) distal to the ulnar implant and cement mantle.
  - An oscillating saw with a narrow-width blade is used to create the cortical windows. The cortical window edges should be bevelled 45° inward to prevent the window from falling into the canal at the time of cerclage wiring.
  - The implant can be tapped out of the medullary canal (see Fig. 20B), and the cement plugs are removed with osteotomes, gouges, curettes, or a high-speed burr. The humeral and ulnar medullary canals should be curetted and brushed, removing all debris.
  - Following removal of the implant and cement mantle, cerclage wires are carefully placed around the humeral and ulnar shafts. Care is taken not to entrap soft tissue with the wires. The cortical windows are closed with two or more cerclage wires.

Instrumentation/ Implantation

- Polymethylmethacrylate
- Antibiotics
- Steinmann pins

Step 2: Placement of Antibiotic Spacers

- If an infection is suspected or known, antibiotic impregnated spacers are used following removal of the implant and cement mantle. Options include:

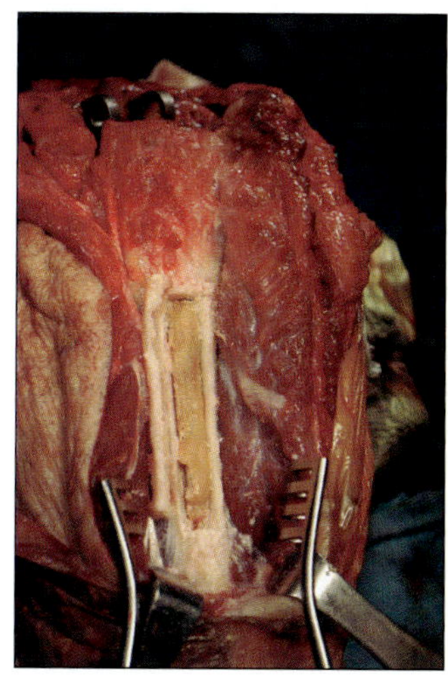

A

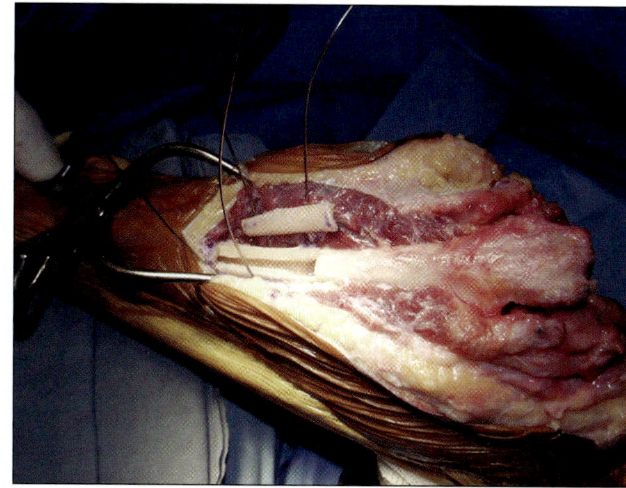

B

FIGURE 20

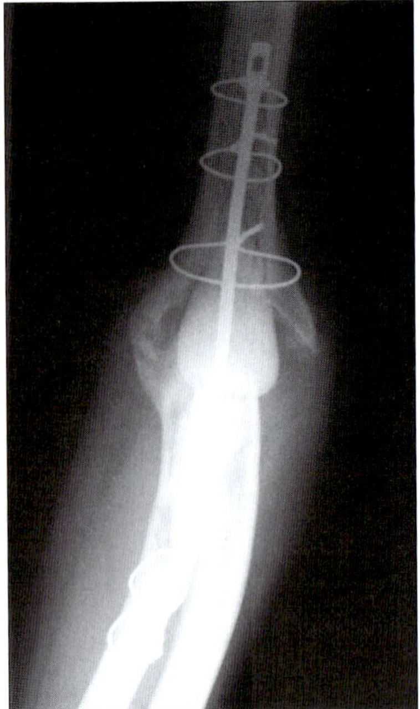

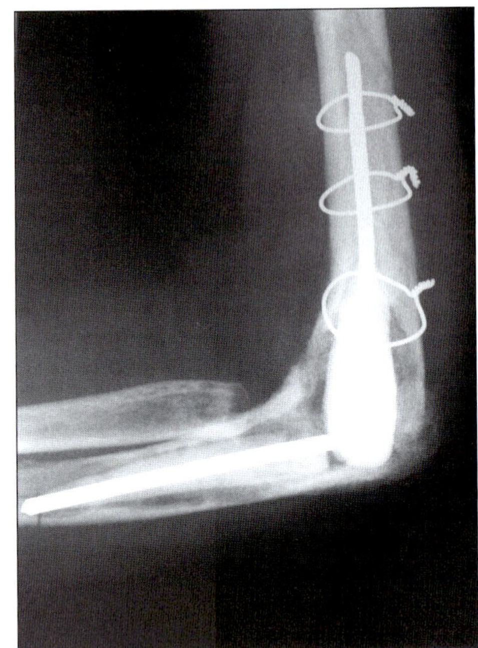

A B

FIGURE 21

- Elongated humeral and ulnar antibiotic spacers with (Fig. 21A and 21B) or without (Fig. 22A and 22B) an intramedullary metal rod are placed within the medullary canal.
- The recommended antibiotics and dosages vary, but the most common antibiotics used are

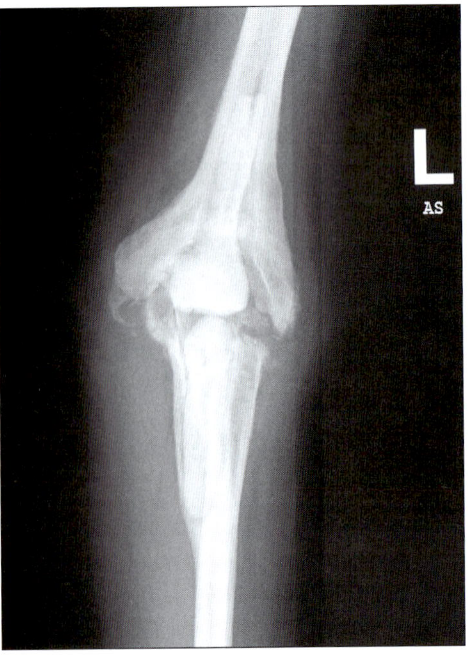

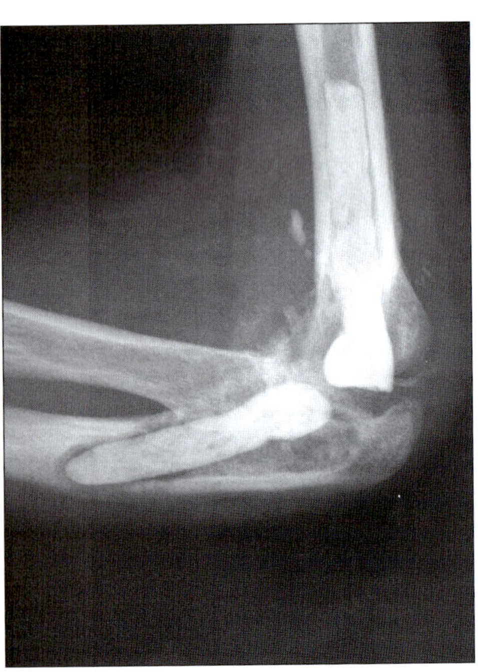

A B

FIGURE 22

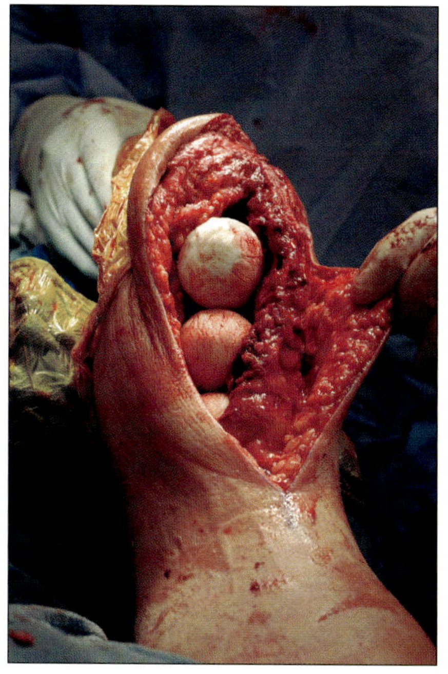

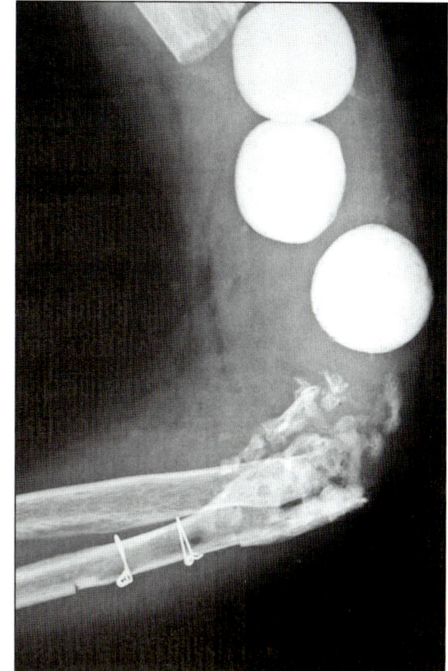

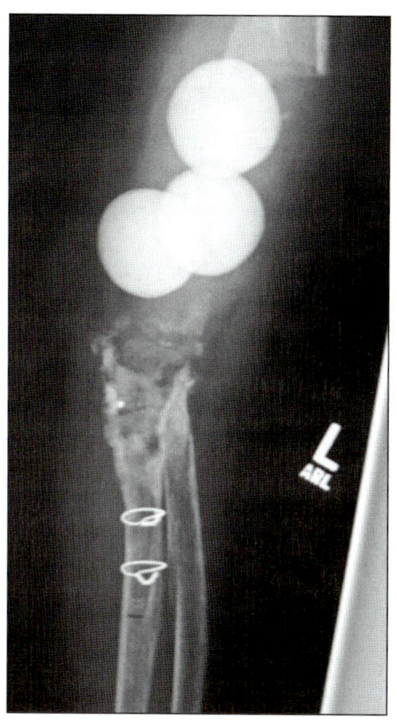

A B C

FIGURE 23

Controversies

- In cases of massive bone loss with an infection, an alternative method uses several large antibiotic-impregnated beads ("cue ball technique") to maintain an open space for implantation of a subsequent implant (Fig. 23A–C).

gentamicin (1–4.8 g/40 g polymethylmethacrylate [PMMA] cement) or tobramycin (1–4.8 g/40 g PMMA cement) and vancomycin (1–4 g/40 g PMMA cement).

Step 3A: Revision Arthroplasty Implant Options

- Nonseptic loosening without bone resorption: semiconstrained standard long-stemmed implants
- Nonseptic loosening with
  - Humeral bone loss (mild to moderate)
    - Humeral implant with long anterior flange
    - Supplemental allograft struts
    - Custom humeral implant
  - Ulnar bone loss (mild to moderate)
    - Long-stemmed ulnar implant
    - Custom ulnar implant
- Nonseptic loosening with bone destruction (cortical thinning and enlargement ["ballooning"] of humeral canal): impaction allografting (see below)
- Device failure
  - Stem failure: semiconstrained long-stemmed implant
  - Articular coupling failure
    - Polyethylene bushing or bearing wear: revision of polyethylene bushing, or revision with semiconstrained long-stemmed implant

    - Implant disarticulation: revision with semiconstrained long-stemmed implant
    - Failure of axis pin or bearing apparatus between humeral and ulnar components: revision of axis pin or bearing apparatus with polyethylene bushing, or revision with semiconstrained long-stemmed implant
  - Instability: revision with semiconstrained long-stemmed implant
- Periprosthetic fracture
  - Closed treatment
  - Revision with semiconstrained long-stemmed implant
  - Open reduction and internal fixation
- Revision of implant with massive bone loss
  - Custom semiconstrained implant
  - Semiconstrained implant placed with impaction allografting
  - Semiconstrained implant combined with humeral or ulnar structural allograft (alloprosthesis)
  - Custom semiconstrained implant (humeral, ulnar, or both components)
  - Allograft

Step 3B: Revision of Failed Implant with Nonseptic Loosening Without Bone Resorption

- Preoperative templating is performed to determine if standard long-stemmed components available from the manufacturer can be used or if custom long-stemmed implants may be needed.
  - The implants should preferably extended two stem diameters proximal to any cortical windows that have been created or areas of cortical thinning (Fig. 24A and 24B).
- The old components are removed as described in Steps 1 and 2 (if needed).
- The joint is exposed.
- The humeral and ulnar components are placed in a manner similar to a primary total elbow arthroplasty (see Procedure 45).
  - The collateral ligaments and capsule are released as needed.
  - The humeral and ulnar canals are reamed and broached as needed.
  - Cement restrictors are placed in the humeral and ulnar canals.

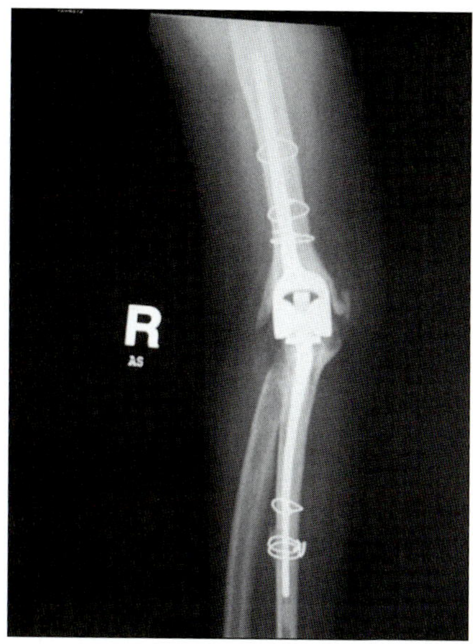

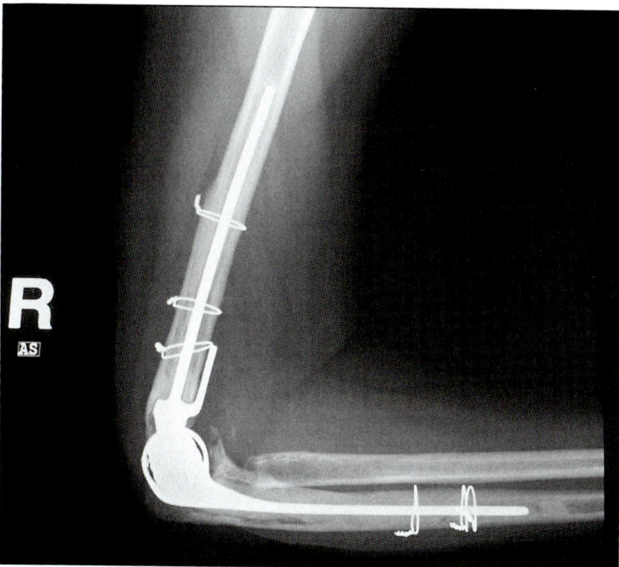

A B

FIGURE 24

- The components are cemented using antibiotic-impregnated cement.
- Closure is performed (see Step 4).

Step 3C: Revision of Failed Implant with Nonseptic Loosening with Humeral or Ulnar Bone Loss

- In cases with only mild distal humeral or proximal ulnar bone loss, standard long-stemmed implants can be used.
- Humeral bone loss in cases in which standard long-stemmed implants cannot be used
  - In cases with humeral bone loss limited to approximately 2–3 cm proximal to the olecranon fossa, a standard or custom humeral implant with a long anterior flange (Fig. 25A and 25 B) can be used.
    - Following preparation of the humeral canal, a cement restrictor is placed.
    - The humeral component is cemented in placed in a standard fashion, with or without bone graft behind the anterior flange depending on how the humeral component fits within the humeral canal and the anterior flange fits along the anterior humeral cortex.
  - In cases with weakening of the humeral cortex or periprosthetic fractures, the distal portion of the humerus can be strengthened using allograft struts secured to the shaft using cerclage wires (Fig. 26A and 26B).

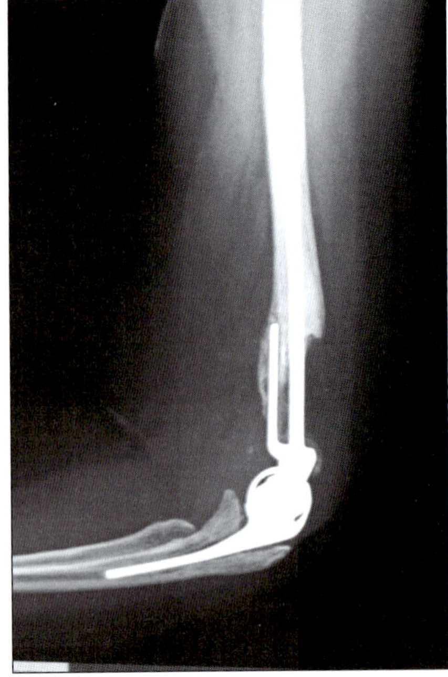

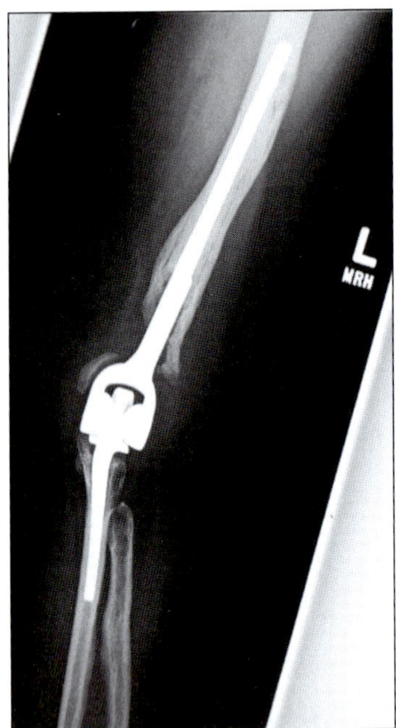

A B

FIGURE 25

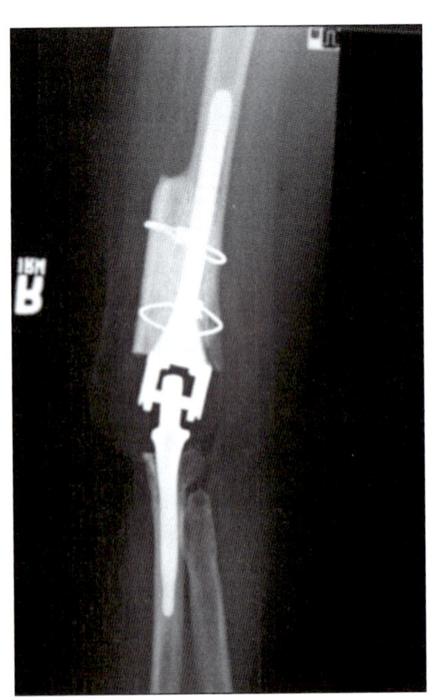

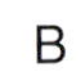

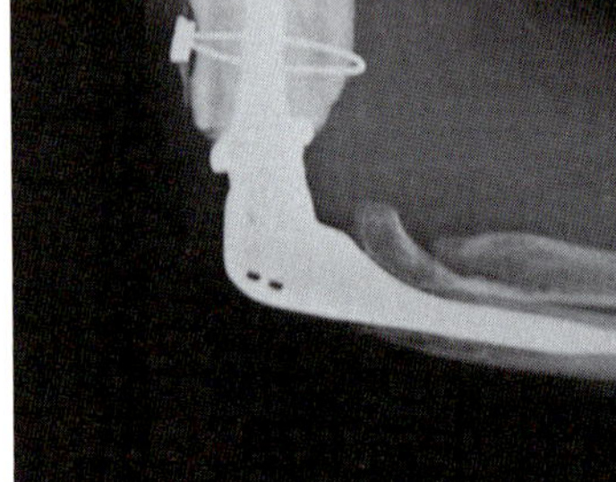

A B

FIGURE 26

- The distal humerus is carefully dissected of soft tissue, including identification and protection of the radial nerve (if needed).
- The humeral canal is prepared.
- If a fracture is present, the fracture is reduced.
- Allograft strut grafts are placed, generally one anterior and one posterior, over the area of cortical weakness or across the fracture site.
- In general, two sets of 18-gauge wires are used to stabilize the allograft, one set proximal and the other set distal to the area of cortical weakness or fracture site.
- Care is taken not to overtighten the wires to hinder placement of the humeral component.
- Care is taken to ensure that the humeral stem passes the area of cortical weakness or fracture by at least two stem diameters.
- Care is taken to ensure that there is sufficient room for the anterior flange of the humeral component on either the native anterior distal humeral cortex or allograft bone.
- A humeral cement restrictor is placed.
- The humeral component is cemented with antibiotic-impregnated cement.

• Alternatively, a custom humeral implant may be used (Fig. 27A and 27B). In general, an implant with an anterior flange is preferred (see Fig. 25A and 25B).

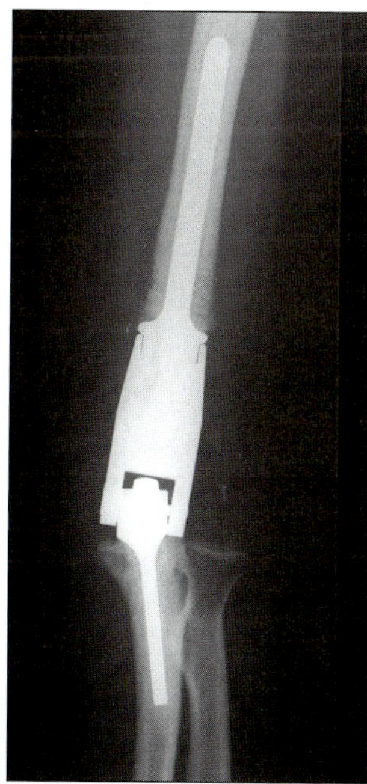

A

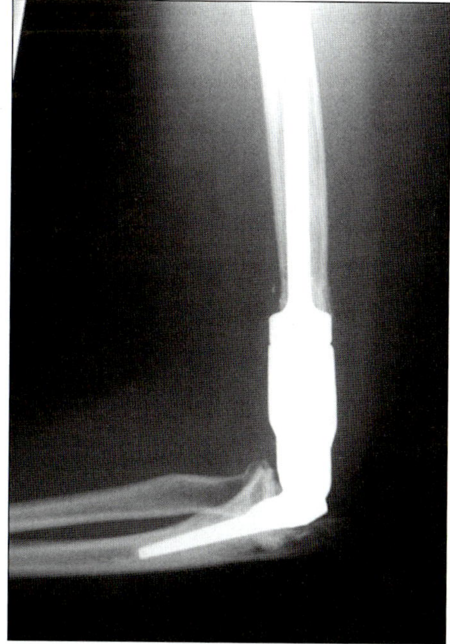

B

FIGURE 27

- Ulnar bone loss in cases in which standard long-stemmed implants cannot be used
  - A custom implant is used (Fig. 28).
    - Figure 29 shows a custom ulnar implant for massive proximal ulnar bone loss.
    - Following placement of a cement restrictor, the ulnar component is cemented into position in a standard fashion (Fig. 30A and 30B).
  - In cases with weakening of the proximal ulnar cortex or periprosthetic fractures, the proximal portion of the ulna can be strengthened using allograft struts secured to the ulnar shaft using

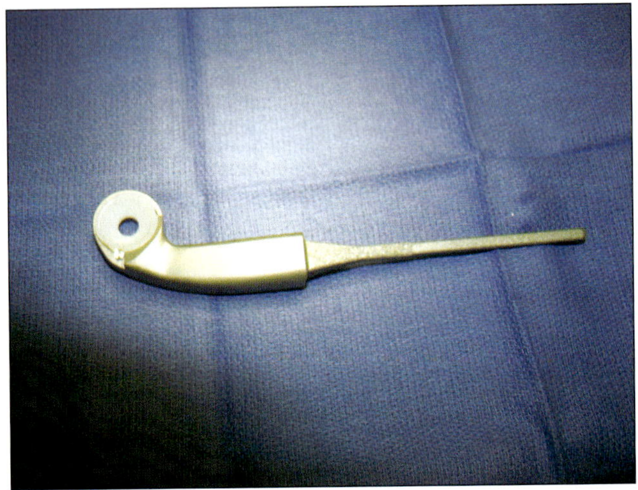

FIGURE 28

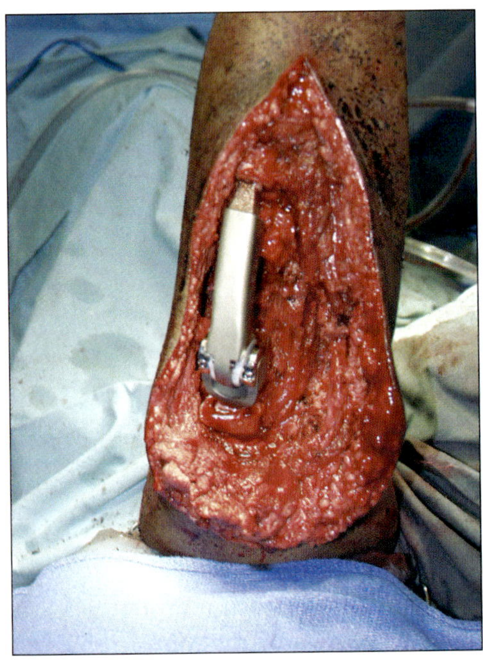

FIGURE 29

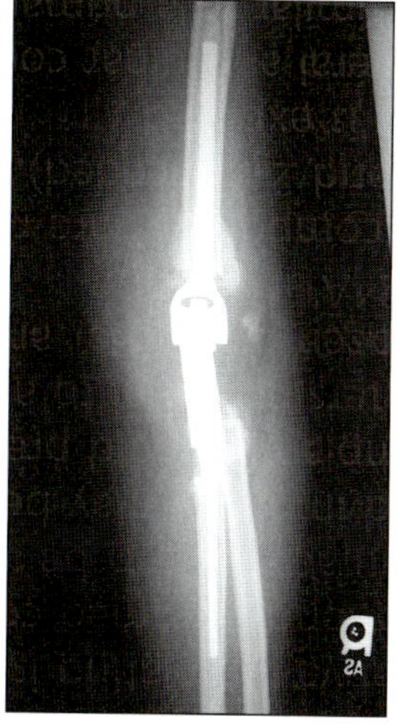

A

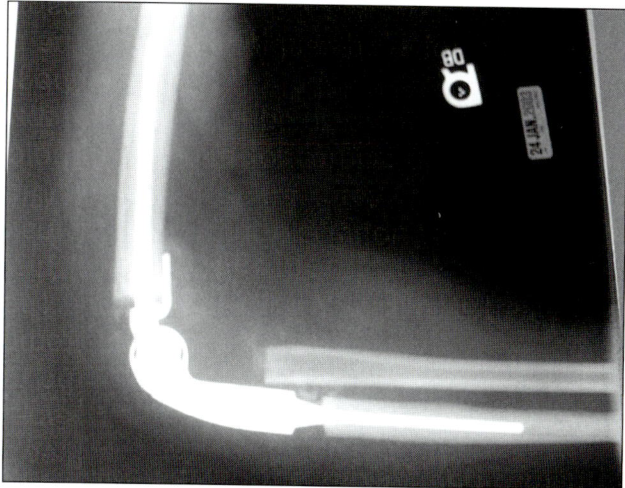

B

FIGURE 30

cerclage wires (see technique above for humeral strut allografts).

- Allograft strut grafts can be used to:
  - Contain discrete areas of cortical defects
  - Support periprosthetic fractures
  - Supplement a deficient olecranon to provide a site for triceps attachment
  - Supplement areas of cortical weakness treated with impaction grafting (see below)

Step 3D: Revision of Device Failure

- Stem failure
  - The joint is exposed and the implant and cement mantle are removed (see above).
  - A long-stemmed semiconstrained implant is used (see above).
- Articular coupling failure
  - Polyethylene bushing or bearing wear
    - The joint is exposed.
    - Biopsy of the soft tissues should be sent for frozen section and cultures (see above).
    - The polyethylene bushing and bearing apparatus or mechanism is removed. Depending on the type of implant used, this may require removal/osteotomy of one or both condyles.
    - Complete joint débridement and lavage are performed.
    - A new polyethylene bushing and bearing apparatus is placed.
    - Joint closure is performed (see below).

- Implant disarticulation
  - With an unconstrained implant, a custom coupling mechanism may be available from the implant manufacturer.
  - With a semiconstrained implant, the coupling mechanism can be exchanged (see above).
  - Alternatively, the implant is revised with a semiconstrained implant (see above).
- Failure of axis pin or bearing apparatus between humeral and ulnar components (see above)
  - Revision of axis pin or bearing apparatus with polyethylene bushing
  - Revision with semiconstrained implant

- Instability
  - Revision with a long-stemmed semiconstrained implant (see above)

Step 3E: Revision of Periprosthetic Fractures

- Type I—periarticular fractures (epicondylar, condylar, coronoid, olecranon fractures) with a stable implant
  - These fractures can be treated nonoperatively.
  - With persistent pain/nonunion, the fracture fragment(s) can be removed.
- Type II—diaphyseal fractures involving the bone-implant composite region
  - Stable implant
    - Cerclage wiring, plate and screw fixation, or combined fixation
  - Unstable implant
    - Revision with long-stemmed implant with fracture stabilization (see above).
    - The stem of the new implant should bypass the fracture site.
- Type III—fractures proximal to the humeral stem tip and distal to the ulnar stem tip
  - Stable implant
    - Nonoperative treatment: Sarmiento-type brace
    - Cerclage wiring, plate and screw fixation, or combined fixation
  - Unstable implant
    - Revision with long-stemmed implant with fracture stabilization

Step 3F: Revision of Failed Implant with Massive Bone Loss

- Custom semiconstrained implants (see above)
- Semiconstrained implant with impaction allografting
  - This revision can be performed with standard or custom long-stemmed implants.

Pearls

- *When using an allograft as an alloprothesis or as allograft replacement alone, care must be taken to ensure that there is enough space within the soft tissue envelope to cover the allograft.*

- A shell of humeral and ulnar cortical bone is needed. Radiographs should be reviewed to determine this.
  - Figure 31A and 31B show preoperative radiographs of a failed ulnar implant.
  - In the preoperative radiographs shown in Figure 32A and 32B, both the humeral and ulnar components have failed.
- The ulnar and humeral shafts are circumferentially exposed.
- Cortical perforations in the humerus and ulna are identified and exposed.

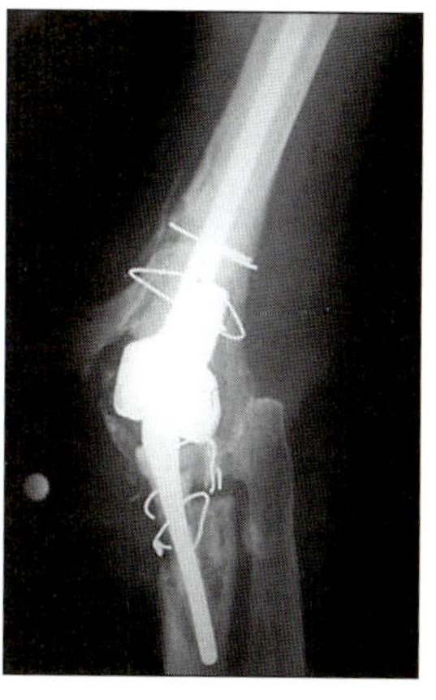
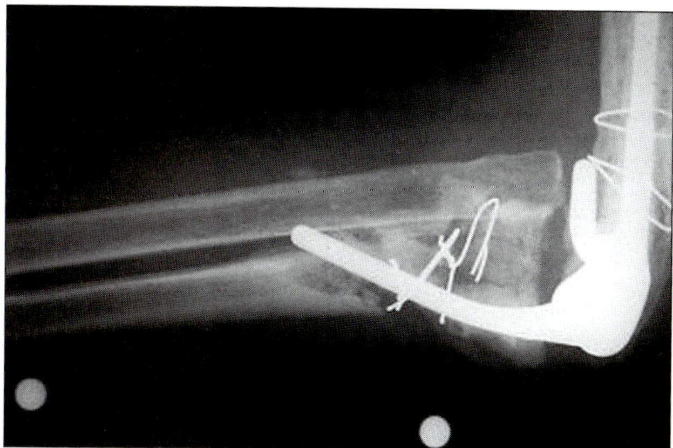
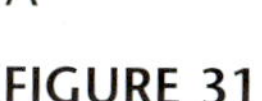

A B

FIGURE 31

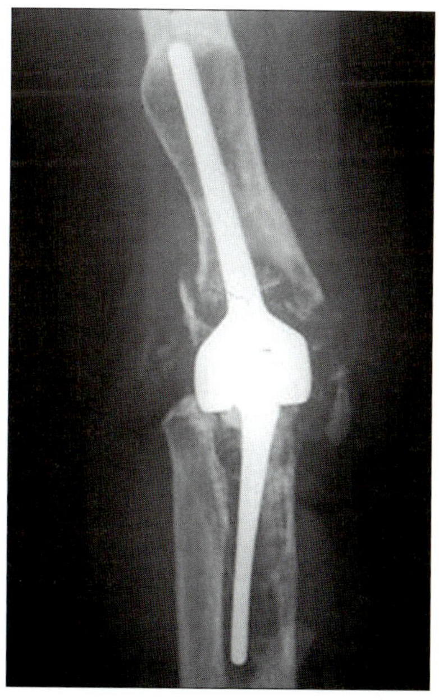
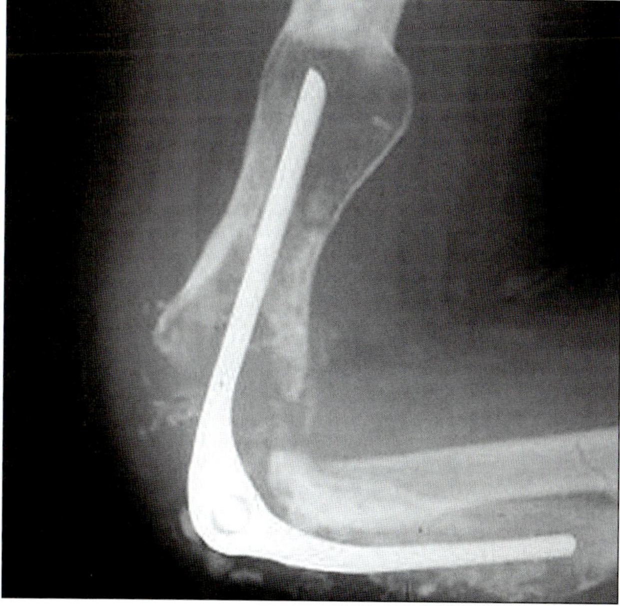

A B

FIGURE 32

Instrumentation/ Implantation

- Implants
  - Standard and long-stemmed elbow implants
  - New bearing apparatus (as needed)
  - Custom elbow implants (as needed)
- Allograft: struts, cancellous, humeral and/or ulnar allografts (as needed)
- Plating systems
  - Small- and large-fragment plating sets
  - Combination plates allowing for screw-and-wire fixation
- Wire mesh
- Humeral and ulnar cement restrictors
- 18-gauge wire
- PMMA with injection systems

Controversies

- The use of press-fit, noncemented customs implants has been described.
- In cases in which the ulnar component cannot be placed into the ulnar canal, another option is placement of the ulnar component into the radial canal (Fig. 45A and 45B).

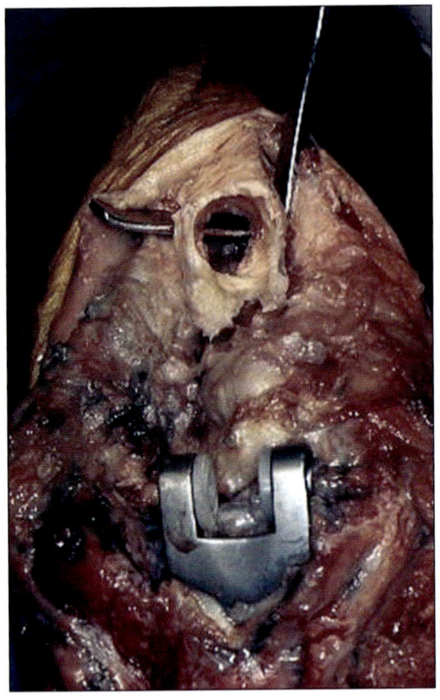

FIGURE 33

- Figure 33 shows an exposed ulna with cortical perforation.
- Figure 34 shows an exposed ulna with multiple perforations.
- Figure 35 shows an exposed humerus with perforation.
- The ulnar nerve and radial nerves will need to be identified and protected.

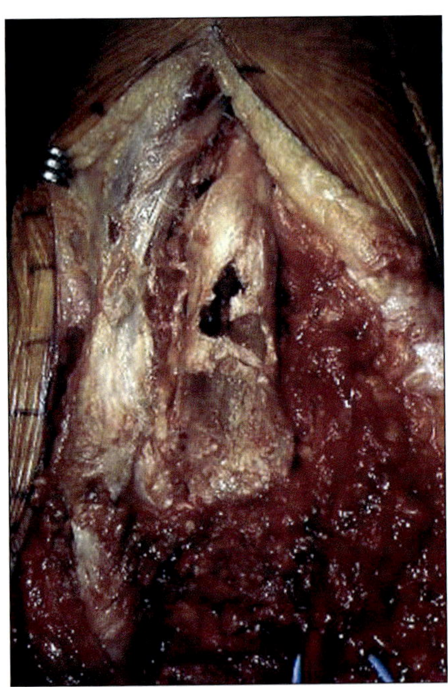

FIGURE 34

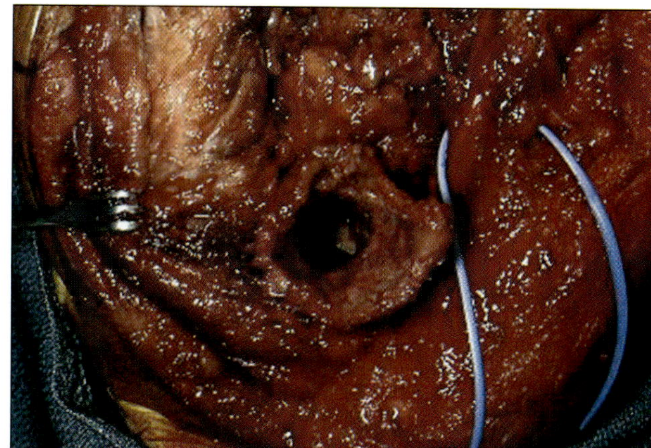

FIGURE 35

- Wire mesh is placed circumferentially around the humerus or ulna (Fig. 36).
- Alternatively, strut allografts can be wired around the cortical defects (see Fig. 26A and 26B).
- Following placement of the wire mesh, a long-stemmed implant is temporarily placed into the medullary canal.
- Cancelleous allograft, usually combined with autogenous cancellous iliac crest graft, is carefully impacted around the implant.
- The graft is tightly compacted distally on the stem and gradually toward the elbow joint, creating a new medullary canal (Fig. 37).

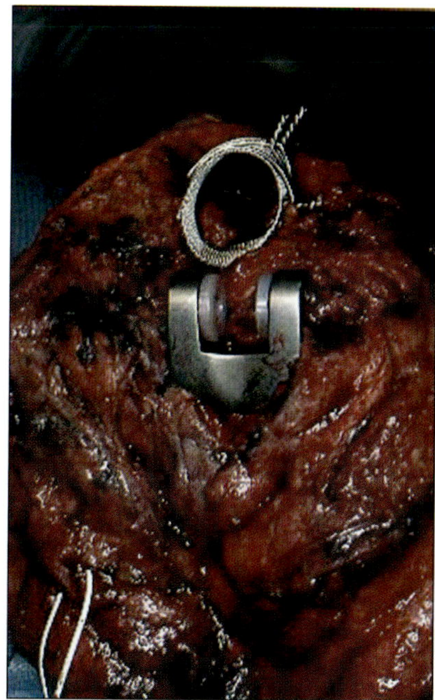

FIGURE 36

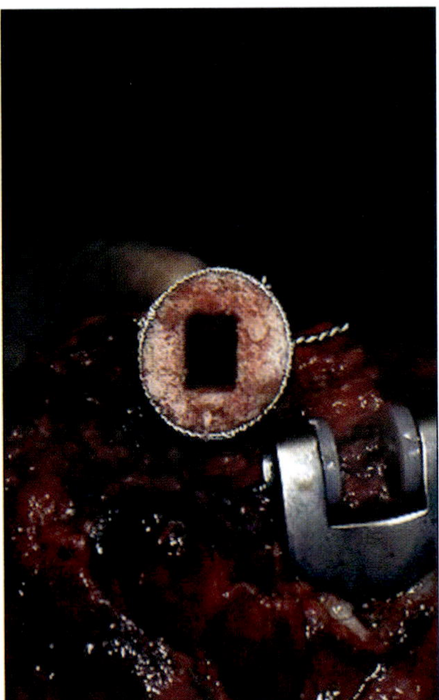

FIGURE 37

- Figure 38 shows prepared humeral and ulnar canals with wire mesh, new medullary canals, and implants.
- The new component, either standard or custom (Fig. 39A), is cemented into the new medullary canal (Fig. 39B).
  - Figure 40A and 40B show radiographs taken following placement of custom ulnar implant with impaction grafting.
  - Figure 41 shows new humeral and ulnar implants.

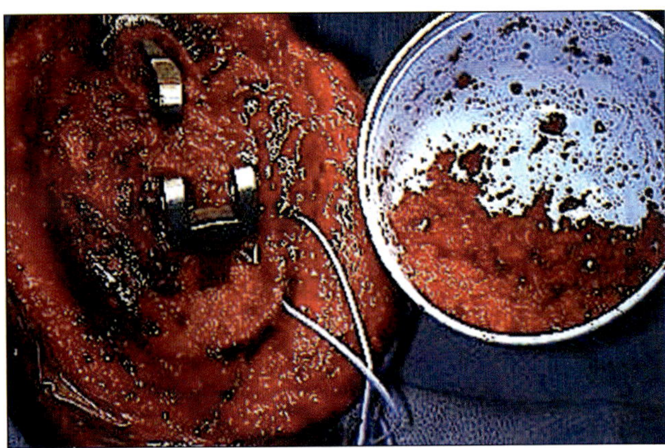

FIGURE 38

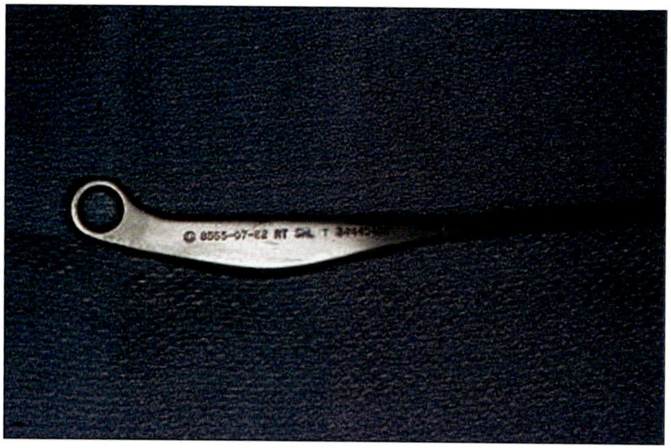

A

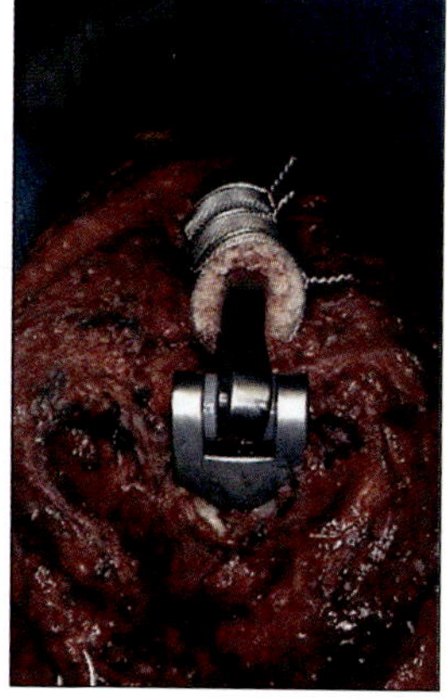

B

FIGURE 39

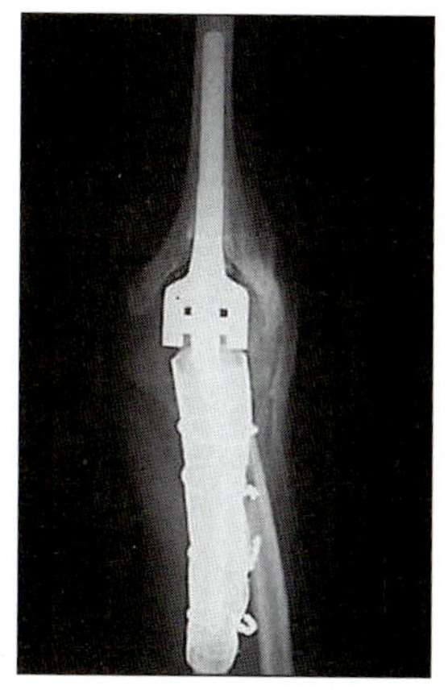

A

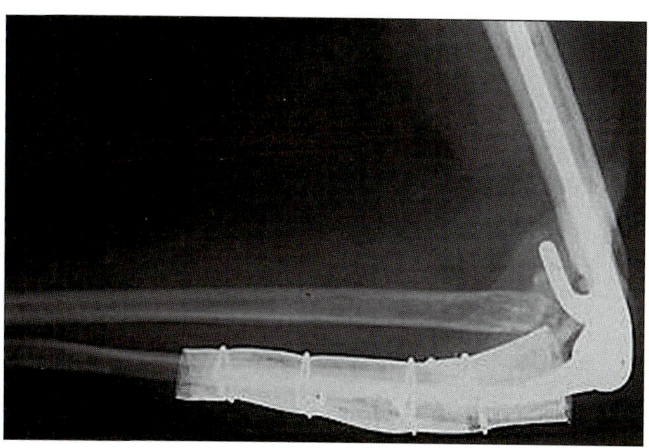

B

FIGURE 40

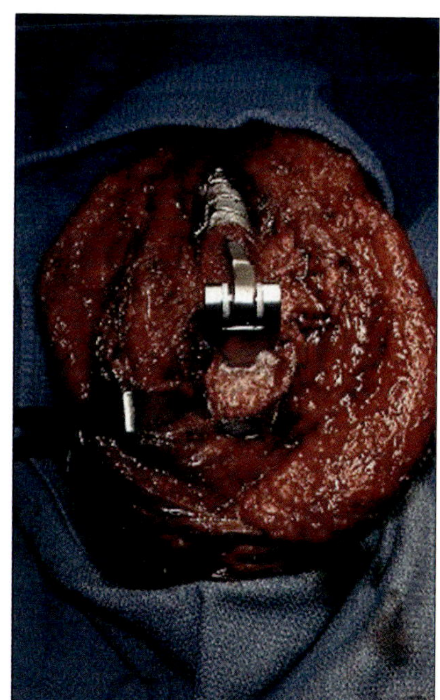

FIGURE 41

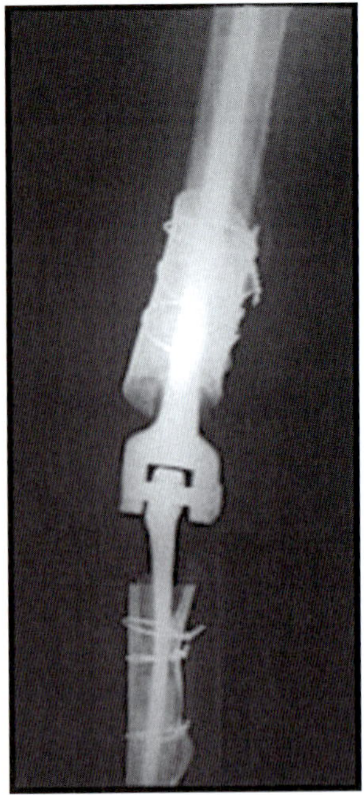
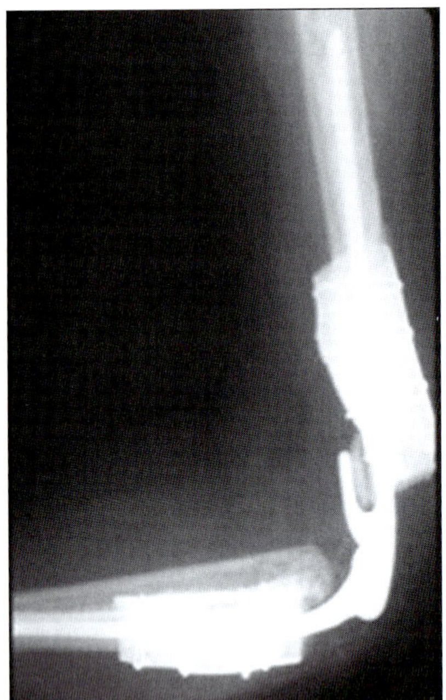

A B

FIGURE 42

- Radiographs of revised implants are shown in Figure 42A and 42B.
- An alternative method includes the use of a double-tube technique for impaction grafting.
  - A larger outer, cut-to-length femoral cementation tube with a smaller inner, humeral cementation tube is used.
  - Cancellous graft is packed around the larger outer tube, which substitutes for the implant.
  - Cement is injected using the smaller inner tube, which is placed farther into the medullary canal than the larger outer tube.
  - As the inner tube is withdrawn to the level of the outer tube, more cement is injected as both tubes are withdrawn from the medullary canal.
  - The implant is then inserted into the canal.

- Semiconstrained implant combined with humeral or ulnar structural allograft-prosthesis composite (alloprosthesis)
  - This type of revision is usually reserved for younger patients (<50 years of age).
  - Following exposure of the humeral and ulnar shafts, the canals are prepared for the new implant.
  - An adequate length of humerus/ulna is needed to allow for plate fixation.
  - This technique require bony union to occur at the host-allograft junction.

- The humeral and/or ulnar allograft shaft diameters should closely match the host bone shaft diameters (preoperative sizing should be performed).
- The host bone is trimmed with a saw to relatively healthy bleeding bone.
- The allograft is cut to the appropriate length depending on the amount of bone loss and the degree of soft tissue contracture that will allow for wound closure around the final construct.
- The allograft canal is brushed and lavaged to remove the majority of bone marrow.
- A step-cut osteotomy (preferred) or transverse osteotomy is used.
- Double plating is used for fixation of the allograft to host bone; locking plates should be considered.
- Autogenous corticocancellous iliac crest bone graft should be used across the host-allograft junction, generally using cerclage wires.
- PMMA can be use to augment screw fixation in osteoporotic bone.
- When an allograft-prosthesis (alloprosthesis) is used:
  - The allograft canal is prepared using cutting guides, reamers and broaches to accept the new implant.
  - A long-stemmed implant, of sufficient length, is used that passes the allograft-host junction by a minimum of two stem diameters. Failure of the implant to bypass the allograft-host junction

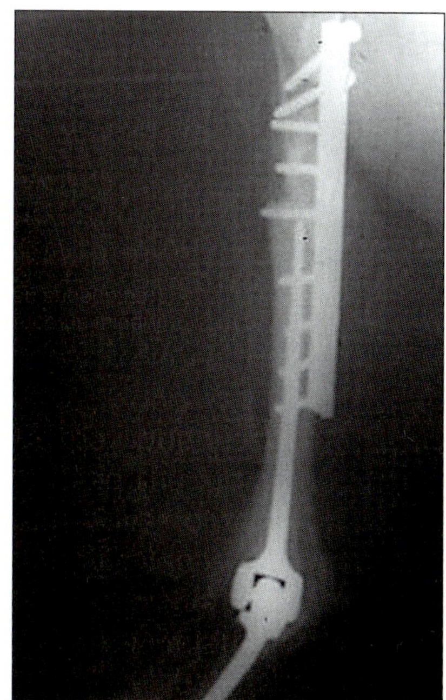

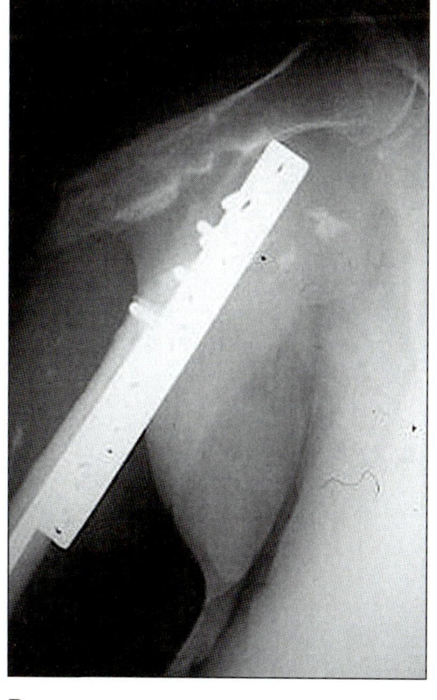

FIGURE 43 A B

may result in early failure of the composite (Fig. 43A and 43B).
  - Plate fixation can be performed prior to cementing the humeral/ulnar component(s) by using a trial implant (if available) or final long-stemmed implant.
  - The implant is first placed, then screws are placed around the implant (if locking compression plates are used, unicortical screws can be used).
  - An attempt is made to compress across the allograft-host junction.
  - Following fixation of the allograft component, the long-stemmed implant(s) are cemented into the canal(s). Care is taken to minimize extravasation of cement into the host-allograft junction.
  - Alternatively, the implant can be cemented through the allograft canal, followed by cementing the remaining stem into the host canal.
  - Plate fixation is then performed at the allograft-host junction. Autogenous iliac corticocancellous graft is added as previously described.
- Custom semiconstrained implant (humeral, ulnar, or both components)
  - Following exposure of the humeral and ulnar shafts, the canals are prepared for the new implant.
  - The type of fixation of the new implant will depend on the type of implant used (Fig. 44A–C).
- Allograft replacement (see above)

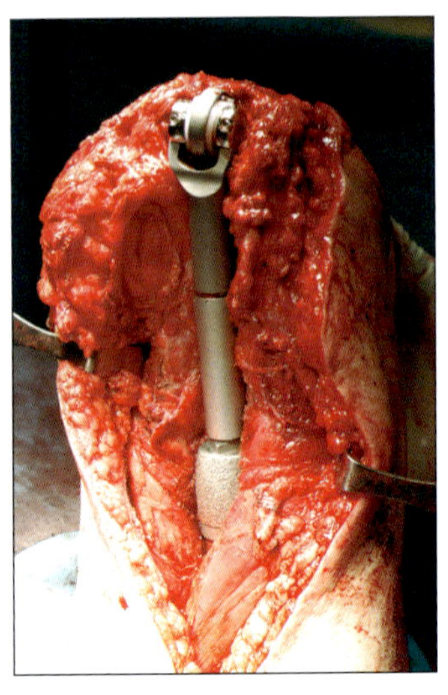
A

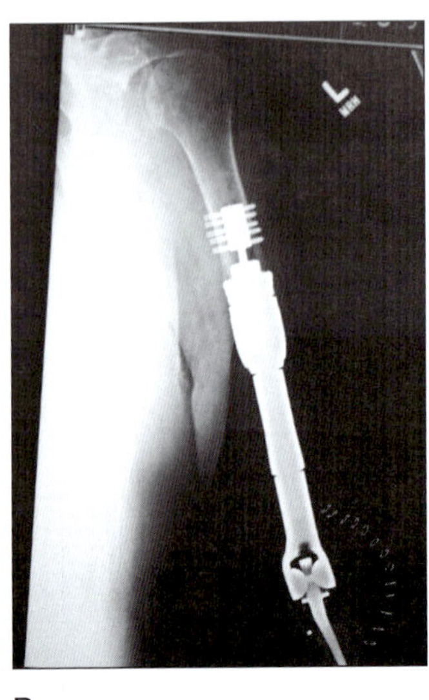
B

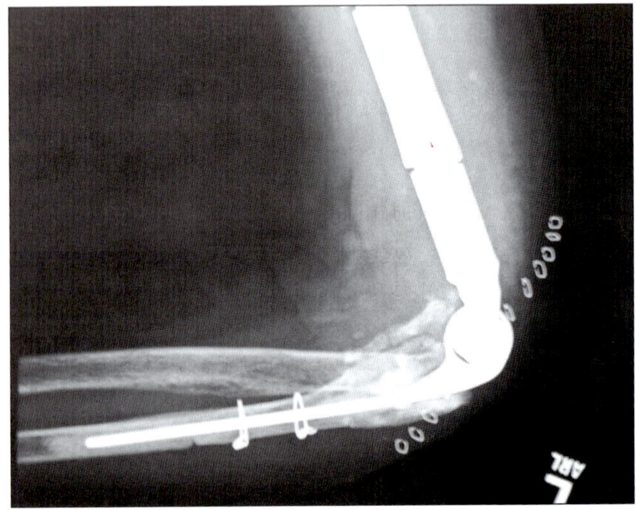
C

FIGURE 44

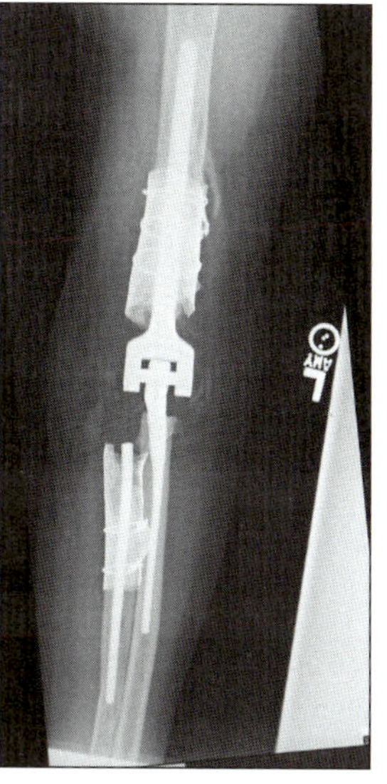

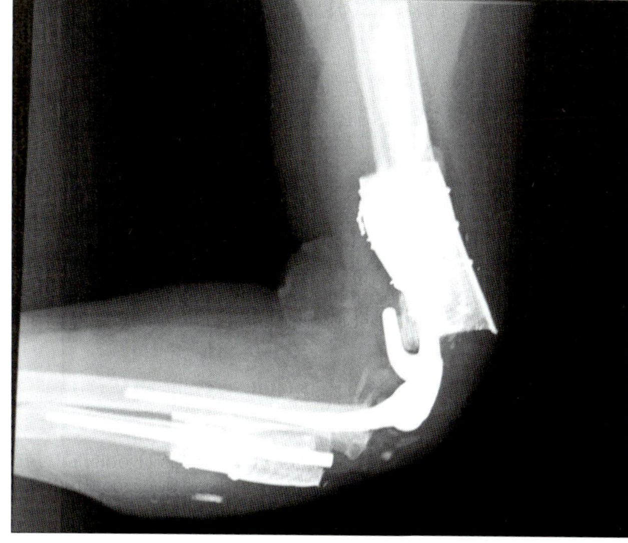

A B

FIGURE 45

PEARLS

- *Splint options include a long-arm splint with the elbow in full extension to protect the triceps repair or a splint with the elbow flexed to 90°.*

STEP 4: CLOSURE

- The tourniquet is generally released once the implant has been cemented and hemostasis obtained.
- The triceps is meticulously repaired with or without transosseous sutures placed into the olecranon process.
- The ulnar nerve is formally transposed anteriorly (if not previously performed).
- A suction drain is placed as needed.
- The skin is closed in layers.
- A long-arm splint is applied.

Postoperative Care and Expected Outcomes

- Postoperative rehabilitation will vary depending on the type of revision arthroplasty performed.
  - Revision with standard or custom implants with good fixation
    - Early active range of motion is permitted within a few days.
  - Revision with alloprosthesis or allograft
    - Cast immobilization is used for approximately 6 weeks to allow for the allograft-host junction to heal followed by splint immobilization for an additional 6 weeks.
    - Active motion is started when healing appears to have occurred.

Evidence

Kamineni S, Morrey BF. Proximal ulnar reconstruction with strut allograft revision total elbow arthroplasty. J Bone Joint Surg. 2004;86:1223-9.

This study reviewed patients with aseptic failure of a total elbow replacement and proximal ulnar bone deficiencies that were treated with allograft bone struts. (Level IV evidence)

King GJW, Adams RA, Morrey BF. Total elbow arthroplaty: revision with use of a non-custom semiconstrained prosthesis. J Bone Joint Surg. 1997;79:394-400.

This study reviewed revision elbow arthroplasty in 41 patients with a semiconstrained implant. (Level IV evidence)

Lee DH. Impaction allograft bone-grafting for revision total elbow arthroplasty—a case report. J Bone Joint Surg [Am]. 1999;81:1008-12.

The technique of impaction allograft bone grafting for revision total elbow arthroplasty was described in this paper. (Level IV evidence)

Lodenberg MI, Adams R, O'Driscoll SW, Morrey BF. Impaction grafting in revision total elbow arthroplasty. J Bone Joint Surg. 2005;87:99-106.

This study reviewed 12 patients who had undergone revision total elbow arthroplasty with impaction grafting. (Level IV evidence)

Mansat P, Adams RA, Morrey BF. Allograft-prosthesis composite for revision catastrophic failure of total elbow arthroplasty. J Bone Joint Surg. 2004;86:724-35.

This study reviewed 13 patients undergoing revision elbow arthroplasty with use of an allograft-prosthesis composite. (Level IV evidence)

Ring D, Kocher M, Koris M, Thornhill TS. Revision of unstable capitellocondylar (unlinked) total elbow replacement. J Bone Joint Surg. 2005;87:1075-9.

This study reviewed 12 patients who underwent revision of an unlinked to a linked total elbow prosthesis. (Level IV evidence)

Sanchez-Sotelo J, O'Driscoll S, Morrey BF. Periprosthetic humeral fractures after total elbow arthroplasty: treatment with implant revision and strut allograft augmentation. J Bone Joint Surg. 2002;84:1642-50.

This study reviewed patients undergoing implant revision and strut allograft augmentation for the treatment of humeral periprosthetic fractures that occurred around a loose humeral component. (Level IV evidence)

Shi LL, Zurakowski D, Jones DG, Koris MJ, Thornhill TS. Semiconstrained primary and revision total elbow arthroplasty with use of the Coonrad-Morrey Prosthesis. J Bone Jones Surg. 2007;89:1467-75.

This study reviewed 37 primary arthroplastes and 38 revision arthroplasties using a semiconstrained implant. (Level IV evidence)

Yamaguichi K, Adams RA, Morrey BF. Infection after total elbow arthroplasty. J Bone Joint Surg. 1998;80:481-91.

This study reviewed 25 patients with infection after total elbow arthroplasty. (Level IV evidence)

SECTION II

Elbow

Soft Tissue Pathology

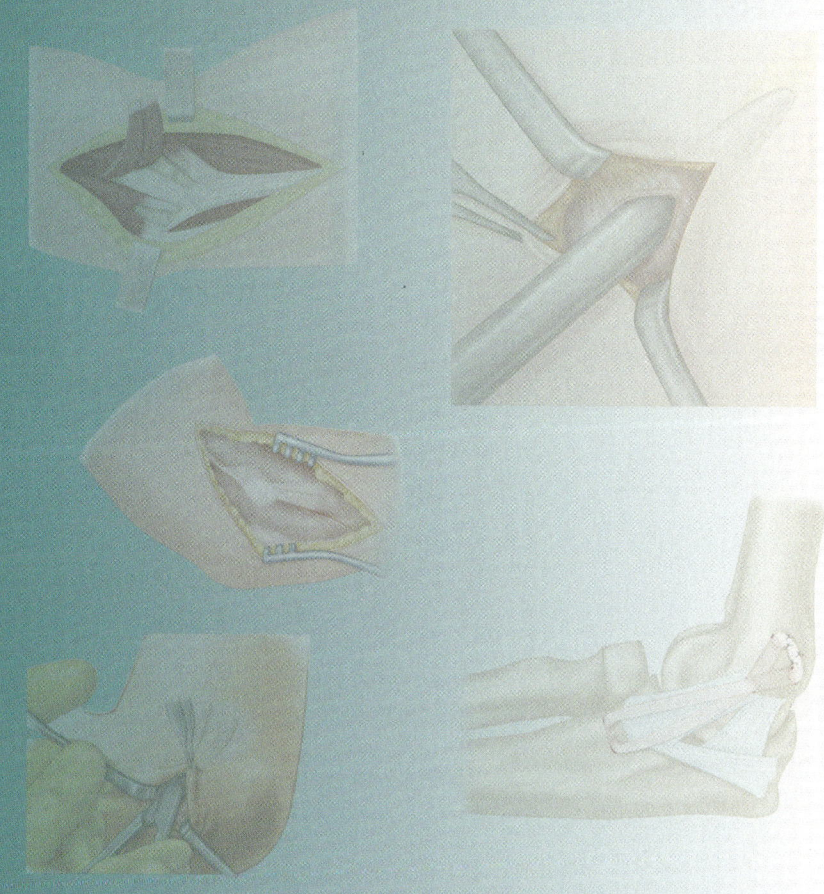

PROCEDURE 49

Medial Epicondylitis: Open Treatment

Milford H. Marchant, Jr. and Frank W. Jobe

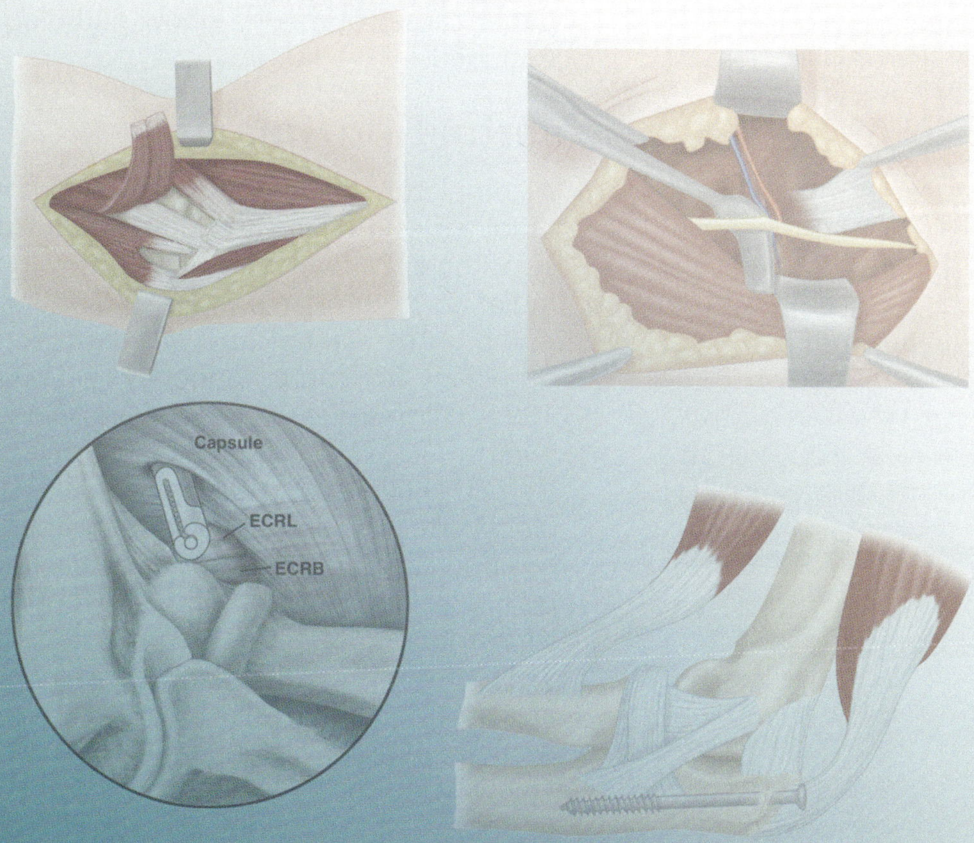

Figure 3 from Park GY, Lee SM, Lee MY. Diagnostic value of ultrasonography for clinical medial epicondylitis. Arch Phys Med Rehabil. 2008;89:738-42.

PITFALLS

- *A focused physical examination and appropriate imaging studies must be performed to avoid unrecognized medial elbow instability, especially in the throwing athelete (Chen et al., 2001).*

Controversies

- The duration of attempted nonoperative care and the timing of surgical intervention remain controversial.
- Professional throwing athletes with tendinosis unresponsive to physiotherapy may require early operative treatment.
- Acute tears or tendon disruption diagnosed on clinical or radiologic examination may also prompt early operative intervention, particularly in elite overhead athletes (Chen et al., 2001).

Indications

- Medial epicondylitis, also known as "golfer's elbow," is characterized by medial elbow pain, and may be a persistant source of discomfort in patients who participate in repetitive occupations or sporting activities.
- The indications for operative intervention include persistent epidondylar pain at the medial side of the elbow despite a well-coordinated nonoperative treatement program including modalities, physiotherapy, and associated work or sport modifications for 3–6 months.
- Other causes of medial elbow pathology should be excluded.

Examination/Imaging

- A complete athletic or work history should be obtained as it relates to duration and onset of symptoms. Patients may also complain of pain radiating to the forearm. Hand dominance should be noted, as medial epicondylitis tends to affect the dominant arm more frequently (O'Dwyer and Howie, 1995; Ollivierre et al., 1995; Vangsness and Jobe, 1991).
- Certain activities that generate valgus stress at the elbow place participants at risk for medial epicondylitis. Common sporting activities include golf, tennis, raquetball, baseball, football, javelin throwing, and bowling. Common occupations include carpentry, plumbing, food industry work, and assembly line work.
- A complete elbow examination for medial epicondylitis includes inspection of the medial epicondyle for musculotendinous defects, as well as palpation of the medial epicondyle and the origin of the flexor-pronator mass distal and anterior to the epicondyle.
  - Patients may demonstrate a mild flexion contracture, particularly baseball pitchers. Tenderness to palpation is often present from the medial epicondyle to approximately 5 mm distal and anterior along the flexor-pronator mass (Fig. 1).
  - Provocative tests include pain with resisted wrist flexion and forearm pronation. It is crucial to evaluate the patient for other sources of pain on

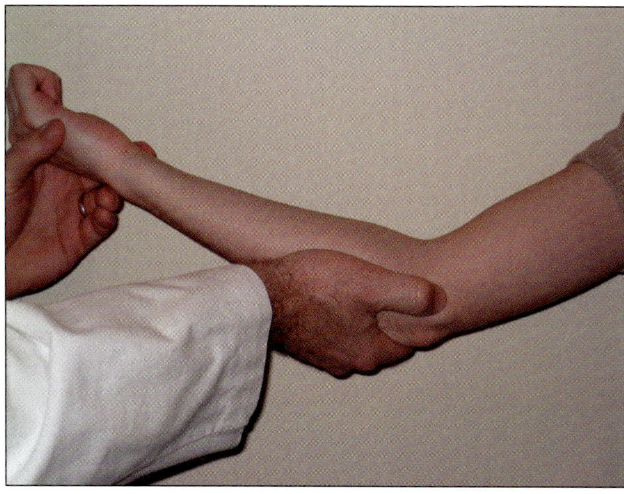

FIGURE 1

Treatment Options

- Nonoperative treament includes a period of rest and cessation of inciting maneuvers, followed by an organized rehabilitation program and slow return to normal activities (Ciccotti et al., 2004).
- Corticosteroid injections may be performed as a means of providing short-term pain relief and acceleration of early rehabilitative efforts (Stahl and Kaufman, 1997).
- Several other nonoperative modalities have also been described, including bracing, shock-wave therapy, low-intensity laser therapy, and iontophoresis treatments (Ciccotti et al., 2004).

the medial side of the elbow, including injury to the ulnar collateral ligament, ulnar neuritis or subluxation, and a snapping medial triceps tendon.

- A thorough neurovascular examination, including examination of the cervical spine, should also be performed to rule out radicular symptoms.

- Medial epicondylitis is a clinical diagnosis; however, in certain instances radiographic imaging is warranted.
  - Plain radiographs are often normal. In youth baseball pitchers, medial epicondylar hypertrophy and fragmentation may also be present. Also, 18–25% of patients may have soft tissue calcifications or osseous spurs off of the medial epicondyle (Ciccoti et al., 2004; Kurvers and Verhaar, 1995; Vangsness and Jobe, 1991).
  - The plain radiograph in Figure 2 demonstrates soft tissue calcifications in a golfer with isolated medial epicondylitis (*solid arrow*). An ossicle is also present at the origin of the ulnar collateral ligament (*dashed arrow*).
- Recent evidence regarding the diagnostic capability of ultrasound demonstrated 95% sensitivity and 92% specificity when prospectively evaluating patients with medial epicondylitis (Park et al., 2008). Ultrasound may be useful as an initial diagnostic tool.
  - Figure 3 is a longitudinal ultrasonographic image of the common flexor tendon of the left elbow in a 56-year-old woman with medial epicondylitis. The tendon had a focal hyperechoic area (*arrow*) that was consistent with tendinosis.

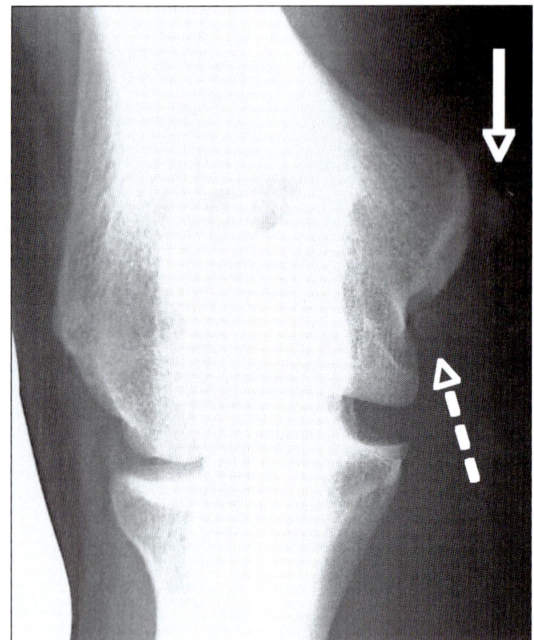

FIGURE 2

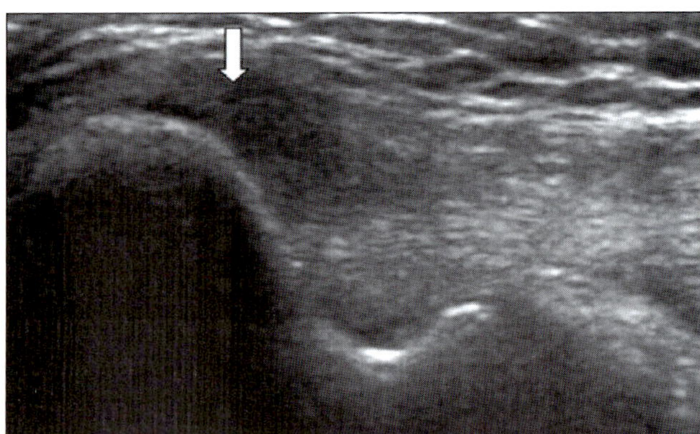

FIGURE 3

- Magnetic resonance imaging (MRI) is not necessary to diagnose medial epicondylitis.
  - MRI findings consist of thickening and increased T_1- and T_2-weighted signal intensity of the flexor-pronator mass. In Figure 4, axial (Fig. 4A) and coronal (Fig. 4B) T_2-weighted MRI images demonstrate edema of the common flexor origin.
  - Paratendinous soft tissue edema and high T_2-weighted signal are the most specific findings (Kijowski and De Smet, 2005). Tendon tears, complete or partial, may also be visualized. The coronal T_2-weighted image in Figure 4C demonstrates a partial tear of the common flexor origin.

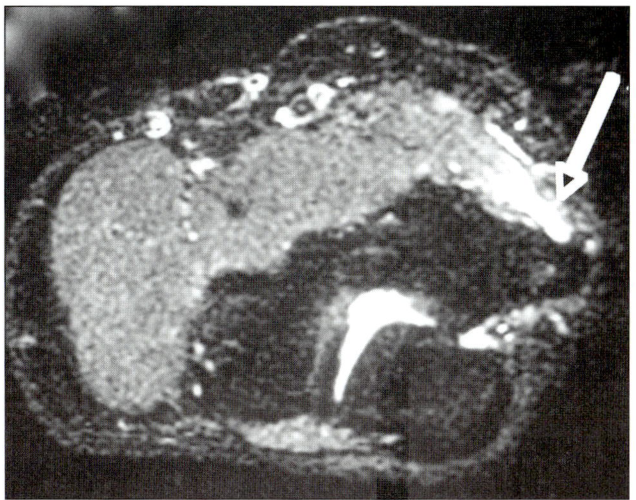

A

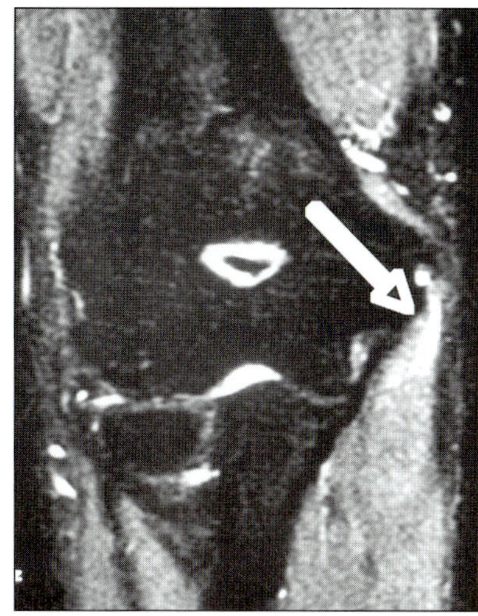

B

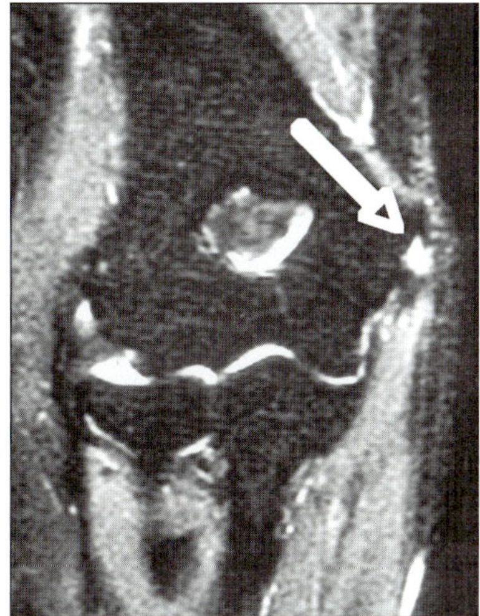

C

FIGURE 4

- MRI is useful in throwing athletes when there is concern for medial elbow instability, and can identify partial- and full-thickness tears of the ulnar collateral ligament as well as avulsion fractures of the medial epicondyle not seen on plain radiographs.

- Electrodiagnostic studies, although not used routinely, can assist in diagnosing compressive ulnar neuropathy and cervical radiculopathy.

Surgical Anatomy

- Superfical dissection will identify the medial antebrachial cutaneous nerve, which must be protected to avoid complications secondary to neuroma formation.

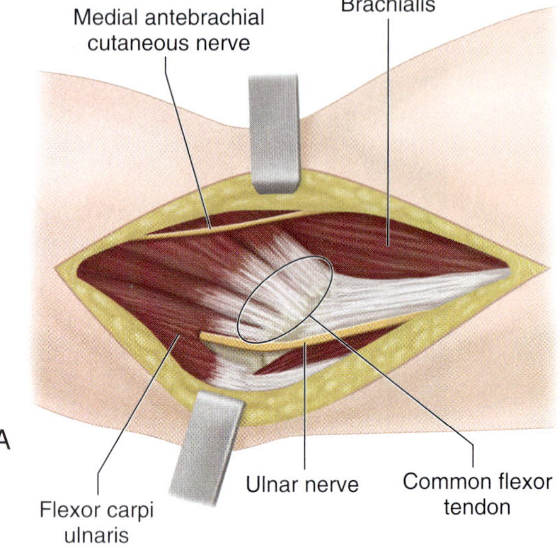

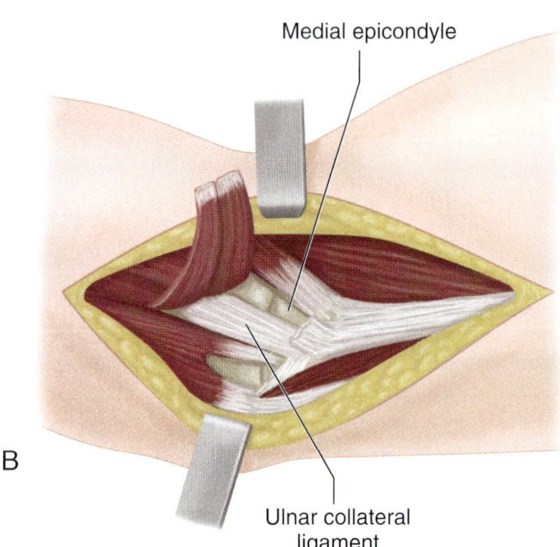

FIGURE 5

- The common flexor tendon originates from the anteromedial border of the distal humerus and extends from the medial epicodyle proximal along the medial supracondylar ridge approximately 3–4 cm (Fig. 5A).
- The flexor-pronator mass consists of the pronator teres, flexor carpi radialis, palmaris longus, and flexor digitorum superficialis, innervated by the median nerve, and the flexor carpi ulnaris, innervated by the ulnar nerve.
- Degenerative tissue within the tendon origin, consistent with enthesopathy, is characterized macroscopically by gray friable tissue. Microscopically, this alteration in the normal collagen network has been termed *angiofibroblastic hyperplasia* (Nirschl and Pettrone, 1979). Degenerative tissue is

Equipment

- A small stack of towels may be used to help level the operative field.

Pearls

- *Exposure of the ulnar nerve is not required to gain exposure or carry out the necessary procedure. However, if the ulnar nerve transposition is to accompany tendon débridement, then the incision may be moved behind the epicondyle. The ulnar nerve should then be identified and protected first.*
  - *The various techniques for submuscular ulnar nerve transposition are described in Procedure 54.*

Pitfalls

- *Careful posterior retraction is necessary to avoid injury to the ulnar nerve.*

most often found in the pronator teres and flexor carpi radialis portions of the common flexor tendon, and is often on the deep surface of the tendon.

- Posterior to the medial epicondyle lies the ulnar nerve (see Fig. 5A).
- Deep to the common flexor origin is the medial elbow capsule and the ulnar collateral ligament (Fig. 5B).

Positioning

- The patient is positioned supine on the operating table with an armboard extension for the injured elbow (Fig. 6).
- A tourniquet should be placed high on the arm, or a sterile tourniquet may be used.

Portals/Exposures

- A 5- to 8-cm longitudinal skin incision is made slightly anterior and centered in relationship to the medial epicondyle (Fig. 7).

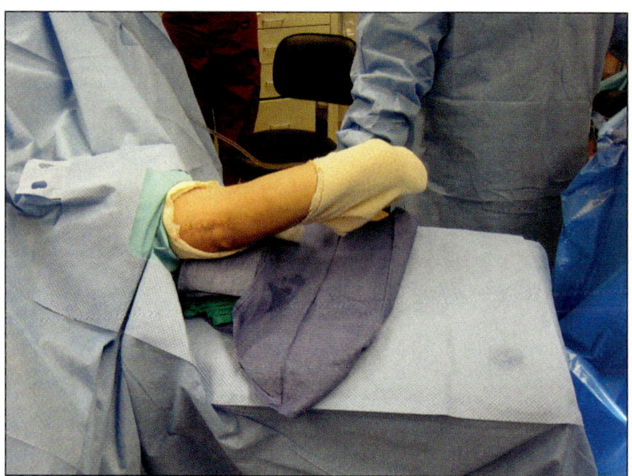

FIGURE 6

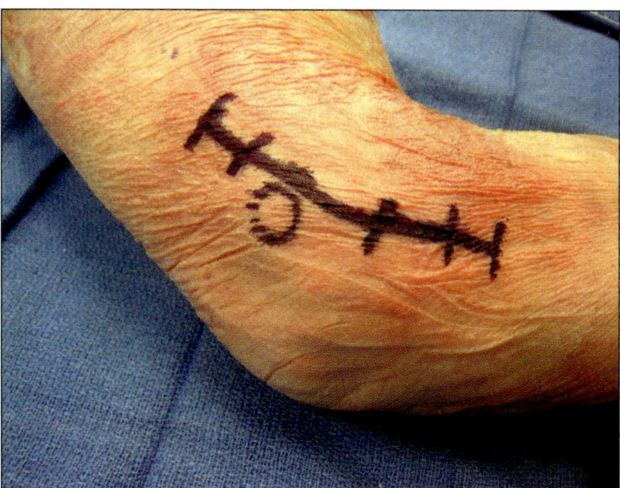

FIGURE 7

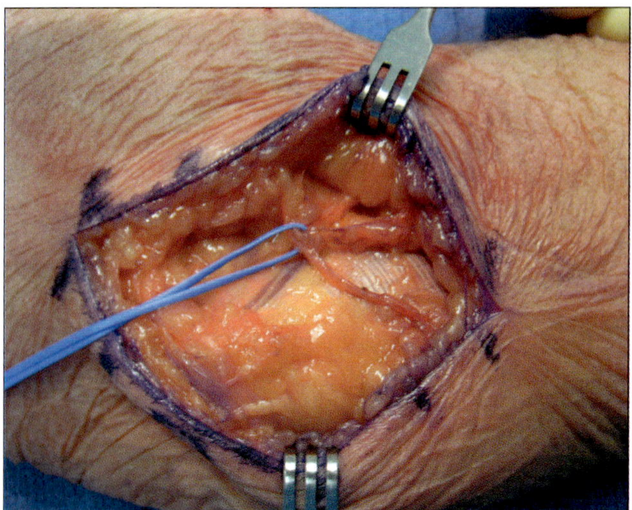

FIGURE 8

- Care should be taken to avoid damage to the medial antebrachial cutaneous nerve, which may cross the distal portion of the incision (Fig. 8).

- Blunt dissection through the subcutaneous tissue is performed down to the fascia of the common flexor origin.
- The plane above the fascia should be developed to expose the common flexor origin and its insertion on the medial supracondylar ridge and epicondyle (Fig. 9).
- Once the origin of the flexor-pronator mass is exposed, the surgeon can address the tendonopathy through one of two methods, depending on surgeon preference and the extent of disease (Ciccotti et al., 2004).
  - Option 1: Longitudinal split and reapproximation (Ollivierre et al., 1995)

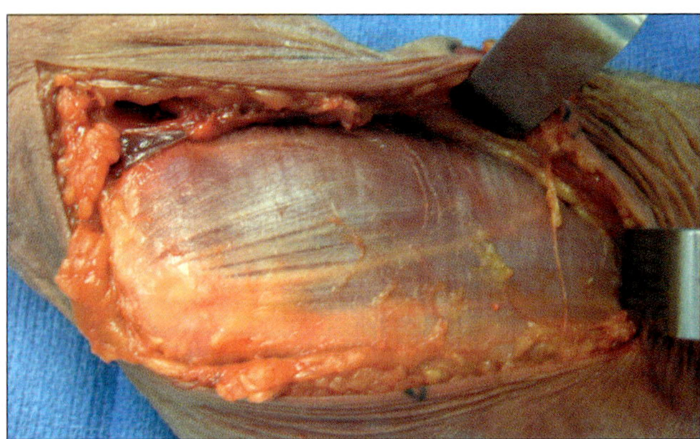

FIGURE 9

Controversies

- Up to 60% of patients requiring operative treatment for medial epicondylitis also have signs and symptoms of ulnar neuropathy. Patients with ulnar neuritis had less favorable outcomes (Gabel and Morrey, 1995; Kurvers and Verhaar, 1995).
- We perform concomitant ulnar nerve transposition only in those patients with moderate to severe preoperative symptoms and electromyographic evidence of ulnar neuropathy.

Pitfalls

- *Care must be taken not to dissect sharply through the musculature or plunge deeply during tendon elevation so as to avoid injury to the underlying ligament and elbow capsule.*

Pitfalls

- *Failure to inspect the deep portion of the common flexor origin may cause incomplete removal of diseased tissue.*

- Option 2: Transverse tendon takedown and reattachment (Ciccotti et al., 2004; Vangsness and Jobe, 1991)

- Release of the flexor-pronator muscles has been described, but is not favored by the authors secondary to the persistence of painful degenerative tissue in the common flexor origin, tendon weakness, and the projected loss of wrist flexion and pronation strength, particularly in overhead athletes. Percutaneous release has also been described but is also discouraged to to the risks related to iatrogenic ulnar nerve and/or ulnar collateral ligament injury, in addition to those mentioned above.

Procedure: Longitudinal Split and Reapproximation

Step 1

- The fascia and tendon of the common flexor origin is split in line with the muscle fibers just anterior to the medial raphe, as marked in Figure 10.
- Blunt dissection using a round or key elevator is performed to dissect through the common muscle origin.
- The tendon origin is identified and elevated off of the bony surface of the medial epicondyle.

Step 2

- Diseased tissue is removed with sharp dissection or a rongeur (Fig. 11).
- The bony surface of the medial epicondyle is then prepared for muscle reattachment. Using a 2.0-mm

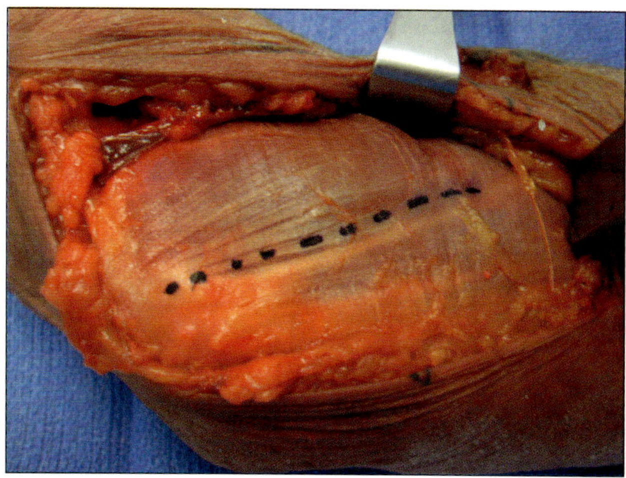

FIGURE 10

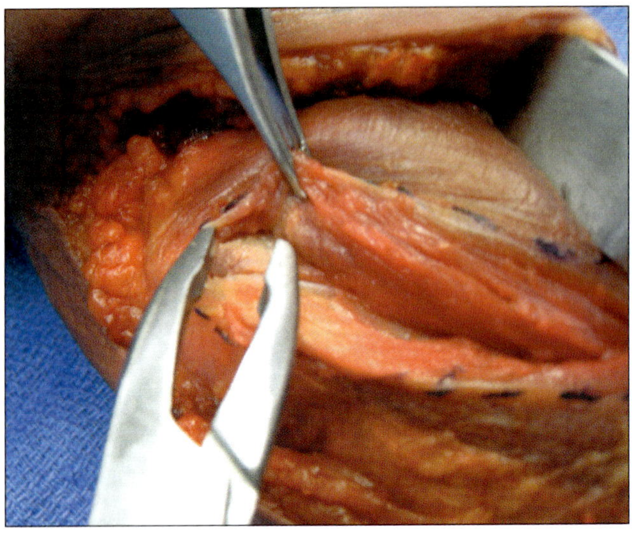

FIGURE 11

drill bit, three to four shallow unicortical drill holes are created on the epicondylar surface to facilitate bleeding in the tendon healing zone and tendon reattachment to the bony surface (Fig. 12).

Instrumentation/ Implantation

- Suture anchor (2.4-mm Micro Bio-Suture Tak, Arthrex Inc., Naples, FL) (see Fig. 15)

Step 3

- The common flexor tendon is then reapproximated and reattached to the prepared medial epicondylar surface.
- If the muscle tendon edges can be reapproximated easily, then two to three nonabsorbable interrupted sutures are placed to reapproximate the tendon edges. The remaining muscle fascia can be reapproximated using a running absorbable suture (Fig. 13).

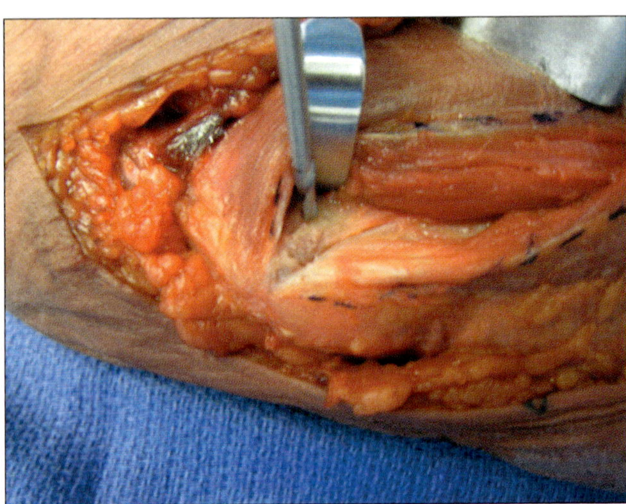

FIGURE 12

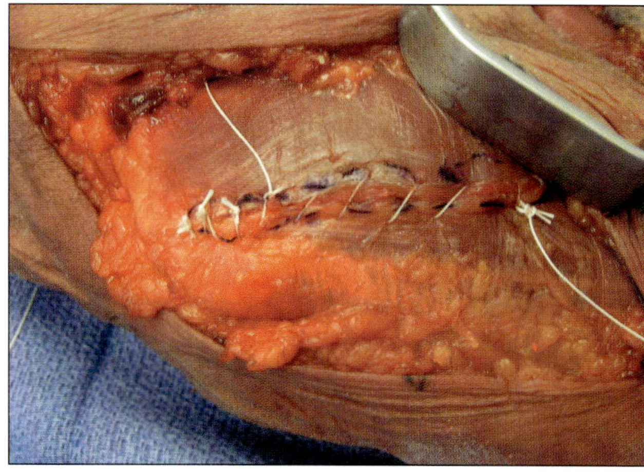

FIGURE 13

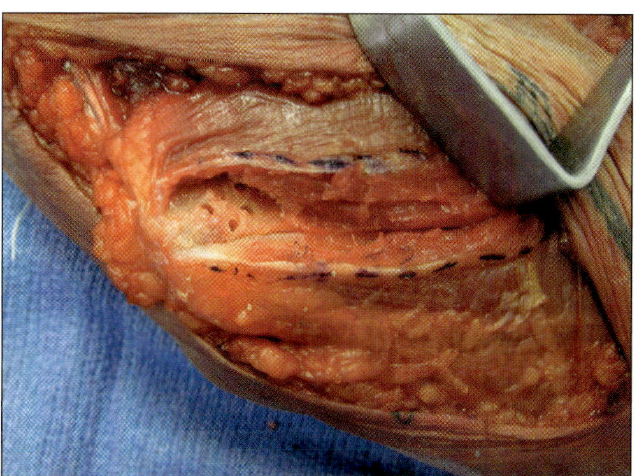

FIGURE 14

- Large débridement using the longitudinal split may make reapproximation difficult using suture alone (Fig. 14). If a larger dissection is necessary to remove the diseased tissue, a small bioabsorbable suture anchor may be used to facilitate closure and reattachment. A small suture anchor is placed in the medial epicondyle to allow suture passage through both tendon edges (Fig. 15A). The sutures are then tied to augment tendon reattachment (Fig. 15B).

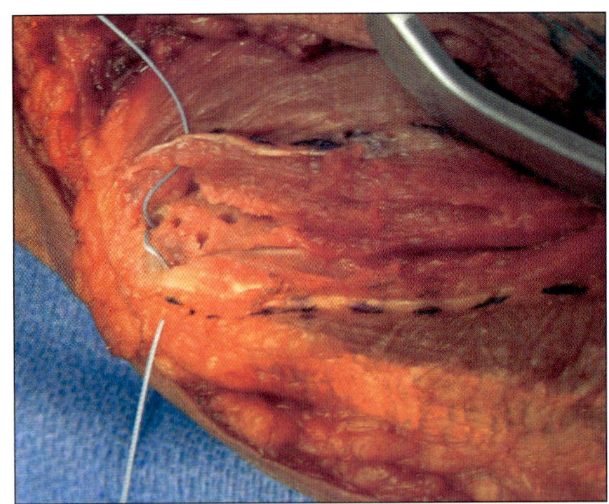

A

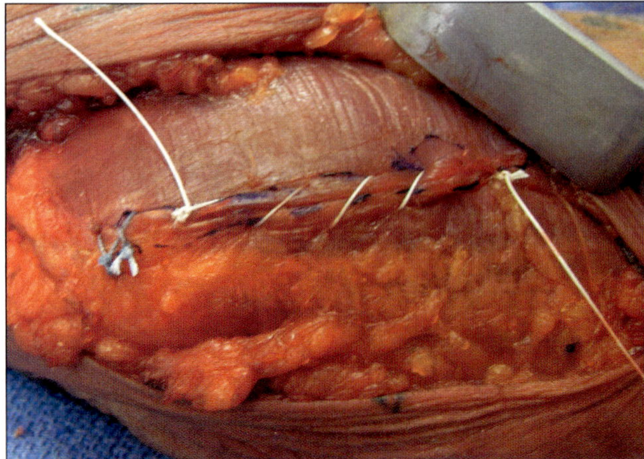

B

FIGURE 15

PEARLS

- *A small cuff of tissue should be left on the humerus to provide tissue for reattachment.*

PITFALLS

- *Care must be taken not to dissect sharply through the musculature or plunge deeply during tendon elevation so as to avoid injury to the underlying ligament and elbow capsule.*

Procedure: Transverse Tendon Takedown and Reattachment

STEP 1

- The portion of common flexor tendon origin proximal to the medial muscular raphe is elevated off of the medial column of the distal humerus, and the muscle fibers are split longitudinally to create a small flap.
- In Figure 16A, the flap is marked prior to dissection. Figure 16B shows the transverse flap and elevation of the common extensor origin.

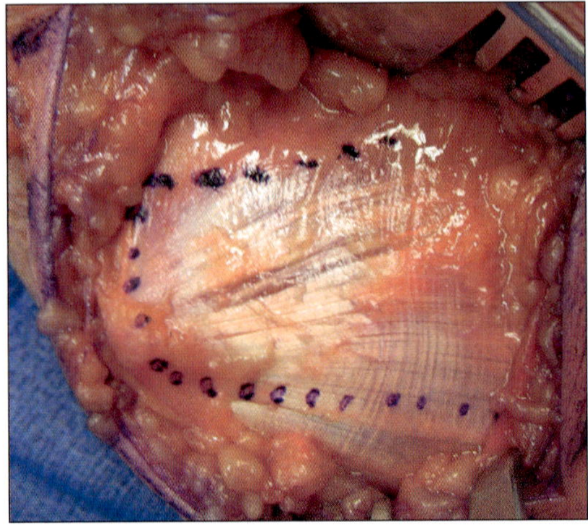

A

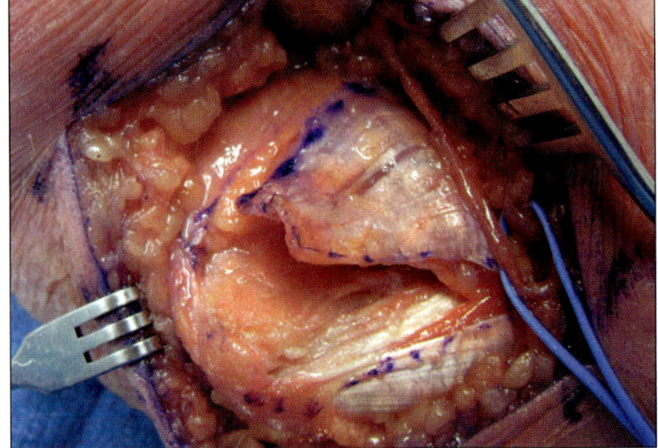

B

FIGURE 16

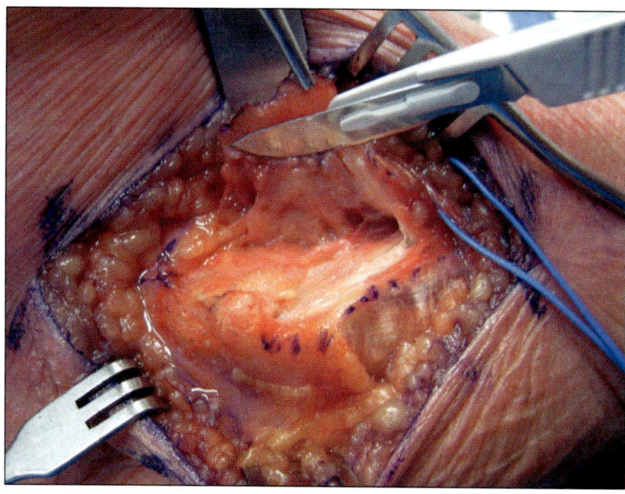

FIGURE 17

Step 2

- Similar to the longitudinal split procedure, a rongeur is used to remove degenerative pathologic tissue on the tendon origin on the medial epicondyle.
- A #10 blade may also be used to remove the pathologic tissue from the undersurface of the tendon (Fig. 17).

Pearls

- *The mattress suture is placed in such a fashion as to allow a cuff of tissue to sew back to the epicondylar cuff.*

Step 3

- A 2.0-mm drill bit is used to make two bicortical holes in the medial column of the distal humerus (Fig. 18).
- Using nonabsorbable suture, a horizontal mattress suture is placed in the common flexor origin, and each limb of the suture is passed through the drill holes.

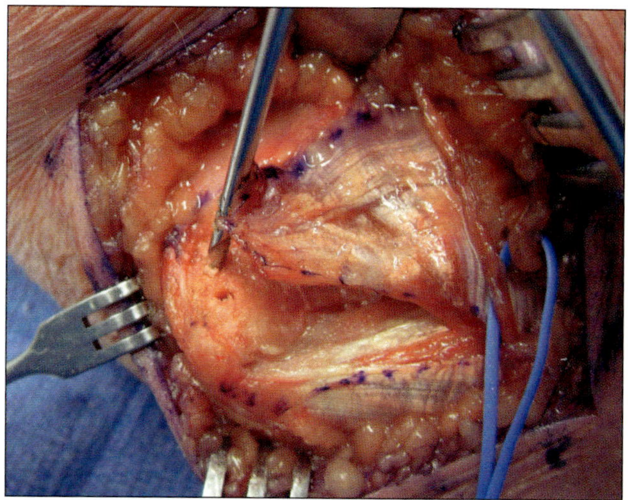

FIGURE 18

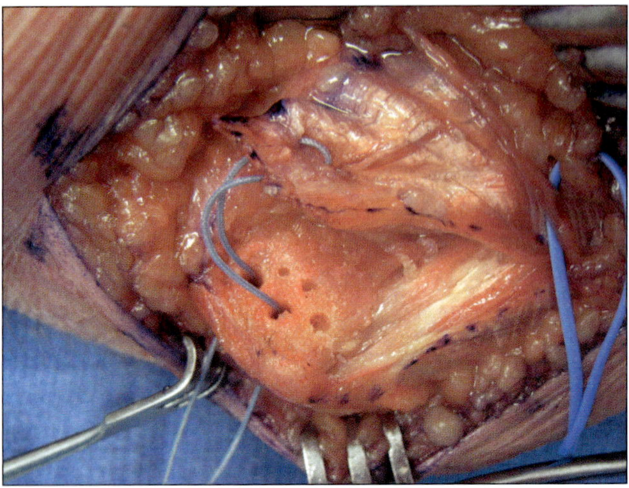

FIGURE 19

- The 2.0-mm drill bit is then used to make several small unicortical holes on the anterior surface of the medial epicondyle to prepare the bone bed for tendon reattachment (Fig. 19).

Step 4

- The tendon is reattached to the epicondyle first by tying the bone tunnel suture over the bone bridge along the posterior humerus using a mattress suture (Fig. 20).
- Interrupted simple absorbable suture is then used to close the fascia and complete the tendon reattachment (Fig. 21).
- The wound is then closed in a layered fashion.

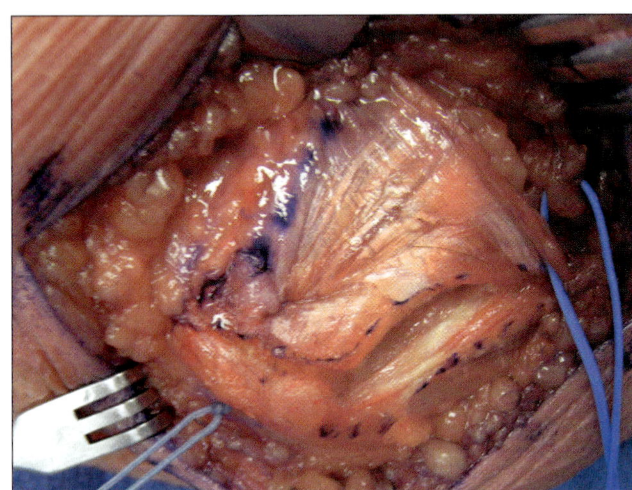

FIGURE 20

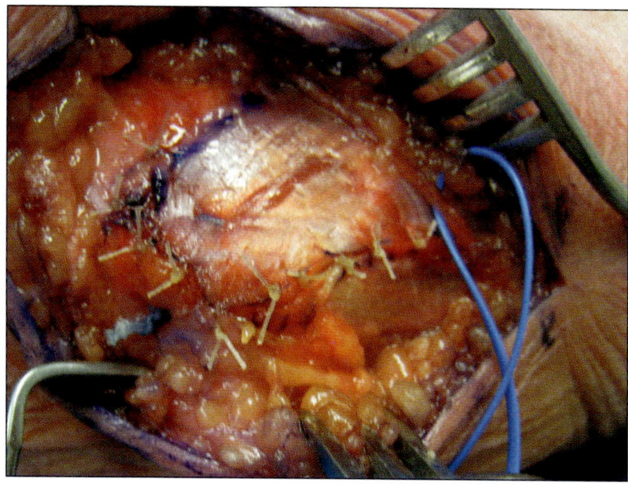

FIGURE 21

Complications

- Potential complications include, but are not limited to, hematoma; infection; and iatrogenic injury to the ulnar nerve, medial antebrachial cutaneous nerve, or ulnar collateral ligament. The incidence of these complications is rare in most reported series in the literature.
- Persistent ulnar neuritis in patients with preoperative ulnar nerve symptoms is another complication that is unpredictable, yet seems to occur more frequently in patients with moderate to severe preoperative neuropathy.

Postoperative Care and Expected Outcomes

- A posterior plaster splint is used postoperatively to provide initial protection against wrist flexion and pronation, and to provide comfort for the patient. Finger and shoulder motion are encouraged.
- The splint and sutures are removed in 7–10 days and passive wrist and elbow exercises are intitiated under the guidance of a physiotherapist.
- Active range-of-motion and isometric exercises are initiated at 3–4 weeks, and more vigorous concentric and eccentric exercises are begun at 6–8 weeks postsurgery.
- Modalities such as ultrasound and electrical stimulation may also be incorporated by the physiotherapist to aid in recovery.
- Return to sports or the inciting activity may be initiated at approximately 8 weeks in a controlled, graduated fashion.
- Depending on the activity, full recovery can be expected in 3–6 months.

Evidence

Chen FS, Rokito AS, Jobe FW. Medial elbow problems in the overhead-throwing athlete. J Am Acad Orthop Surg. 2001;9:99-113.

This comprehensive review described the interconnection of injuries that can occur at the medial elbow in an overhead athlete. Evaluation and treatment strategies for medial epicondylitis and injuries to the flexor-pronator musculature were described.

Ciccotti MC, Schwartz MA, Ciccotti MG. Diagnosis and treatment of medial epicondylitis of the elbow. Clin Sports Med. 2004;23:693-705.

This comprehensive review of medial epicondylitis described the medial elbow anatomy, pathophysiology, clinical evaluation, and nonoperative and operative treatment strategies. Rationale and technique for longitudinal split and transverse takedown operative approaches were discussed. Transverse takedown technique was emphasized.

Gabel GT, Morrey BF. Operative treatment of medical epicondylitis: influence of concomitant ulnar neuropathy at the elbow. J Bone Joint Surg [Am]. 1995;77: 1065-9.

The authors presented a retrospective review of 30 elbows treated operatively for medial epicondylitis, 16 of which had concomitant ulnar neuropathy (53.3%). Débridement of the origin of the flexor-pronator mass and ulnar nerve decompression or transposition resulted in 87% good to excellent results at a minumum 2-year follow-up. Outcomes in patients with no or mild ulnar neuropathy were significantly better than in those with moderate or severe ulnar nerve symptoms.

Kijowski R, De Smet AA. Magnetic resonance imaging findings in patients with medial epicondylitis. Skeletal Radiol. 2005;34:196-202.

MRI findings in patients with epicondylitis were compared to those in a control group. Patients with medial epicondylitis demonstrated thickening and increased T_1- and T_2-weighted signal intensity of the common flexor origin, and adjacent soft tissue edema.

Kurvers H, Verhaar J. The results of operative treatment of medial epicondylitis. J Bone Joint Surg [Am]. 1995;77:1374-9.

In this retrospective review of 40 elbows treated operatively for medial epicondylitis, 24 patients (60%) had concomitant ulnar neuropathy. Overall results indicated only 63% good to excellent outcomes. Eleven of 16 patients (69%) treated for medial epicondylitis were symptom free at follow-up, compared to only 3 of 24 patients with combined pathology ($p < .01$).

Nirschl RP, Pettrone FA. Tennis elbow: the surgical treatment of lateral epicondylitis. J Bone Joint Surg [Am]. 1979;61:832-9.

This classic paper on lateral-sided disease described the incomplete healing response and microscopic pathology of epicondylitis–angiofibroblastic hyperplasia.

O'Dwyer KJ, Howie CR. Medial epicondylitis of the elbow. Int Orthop. 1995;19:69-71.

This study was a retrospective review of the treatment course of 95 cases of medial epicondylitis. Eleven (12%) patients required operative intervention; 8 of the 10 patients treated with open release were completely cured at an average of 3 months after the operation. One patient with percutaneous release had partial relief.

Ollivierre CO, Nirschl RP, Pettrone FA. Resection and repair for medial tennis elbow: a prospective analysis. Am J Sports Med. 1995;23:214-21.

This prospective study analyzed the operative treatment of medial epicondylitis in 50 elbows (48 patients) using the longitudinal split approach. Operative treatment significantly benefited patients in regard to grip strength and pain relief. Ten patients did not return to their previous sporting or occupational activities. Pathologic analysis of ressected tissue revealed no inflammatory cells, but confirmed microscopic findings similar to lateral epicondylitis–angiofibroblastic hyperplasia.

Park GY, Lee SM, Lee MY. Diagnostic value of ultrasonography for clinical medial epicondylitis. Arch Phys Med Rehabil. 2008;89:738-42.

This prospective, single-blind study evaluated the diagnostic use of ultrasound for medial epicondylitis. Results demonstrated 95% sensitivity, 92% specificity, and 93.5% accuracy. The most common abnormality seen was a focal hypoechoic or anechoic abnormality of the tendons.

Stahl S, Kaufman T. The efficacy of an injection of steroids for medial epicondylitis: a prospective study of sixty elbows. J Bone Joint Surg [Am]. 1997;79:1648-52.

This prospective, randomized, double-blind study analyzed the short-term and long-term effects of methylprednisolone injection for medial epicondylitis compared with concomitant physical therapy and nonsteroidal anti-inflammatory use. A significant benefit in regard to symptom relief was seen in the steroid group at 6 weeks, but not at 3 months or 1 year, postinjection.

Vangsness CT Jr, Jobe FW. Surgical treatment of medial epicondylitis: results in 35 elbows. J Bone Joint Surg [Br]. 1991;73:409-11.

This study was a retrospective review of 35 cases of medial epicondylitis treated operatively with the transverse takedown approach. Thirty-four of 35 cases (97%) demonstrated good to excellent results, with 86% having no limitations regarding daily or sporting activities. One patient failed to return to the previous level of athletics.

PROCEDURE 50

Lateral Epicondylitis: Arthroscopic and Open Treatment

Mark S. Cohen

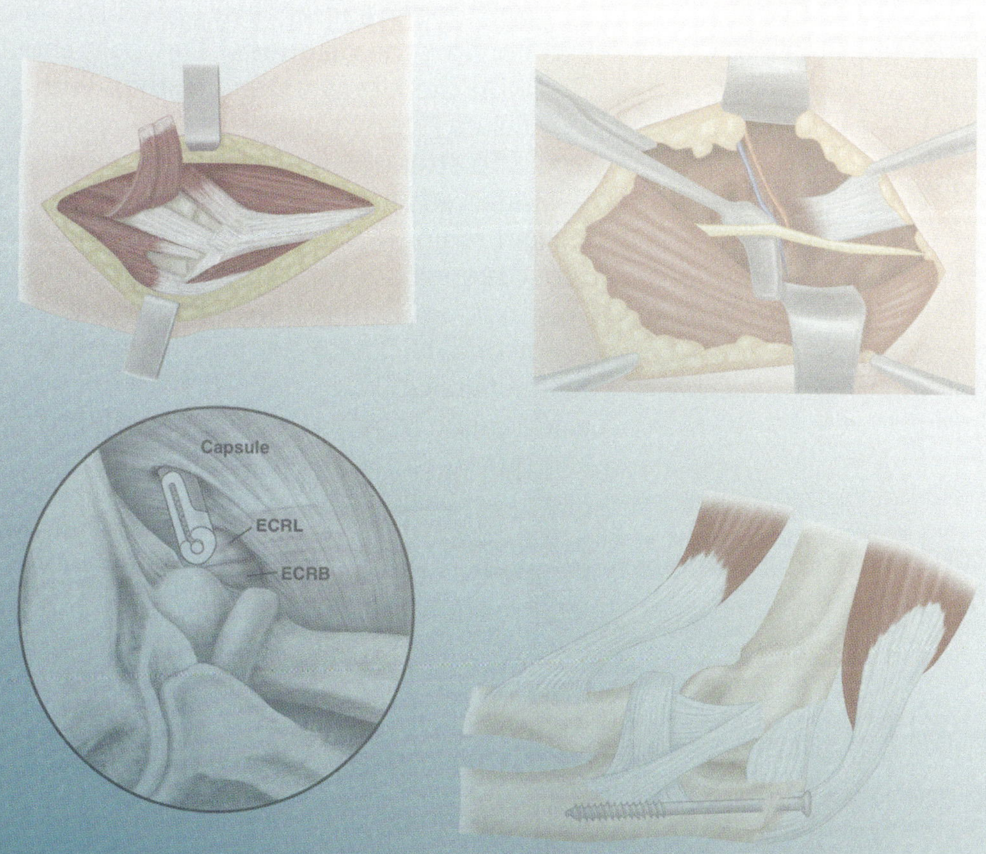

PITFALLS

- *Lateral epicondylitis is the most common affliction of the elbow. The condition is self-limiting in the vast majority of cases. It can take 9–12 months for symptoms to resolve with conservative care. Thus, patient selection for surgery is important.*
- *One must confirm the proper diagnosis, which typically is not difficult.*
- *Although rare, one must rule out lateral ligament involvement, which manifests as lateral joint insufficiency. A simple varus stress anteroposterior radiograph should suffice when there is a question regarding lateral instability of the elbow. The radiocapitellar joint should not gap during applied varus stress.*
- *Surgery for epicondylitis is less predictable than other procedures around the elbow, regardless of technique. All series have a documented failure rate, and even cases with a favorable outcome can have persistent symptoms with certain activities. Preoperative education is thus essential.*

Treatment Options

- Nonoperative measures are successful in the vast majority of cases of lateral epicondylitis.
- Surgery for epicondylitis can be performed by open or arthroscopic methods. At present, there are no data to suggest superiority of one technique over the other.

Indications

- Clinical examination and history consistent with lateral epicondylitis
- Failed conservative measures, including education, counterforce bracing, therapy modalities, injections, and the like, for at least 6–9 months

Examination/Imaging

- Patients with epicondylitis will have tenderness directly over the epicondyle.
  - Pain at the epicondyle is accentuated by active wrist extension against resistance. This helps confirm the diagnosis. This pain should be greater with the elbow extended than with the elbow flexed.
  - Grip strength should also be diminished on the affected side.
- Plain radiographs are typically normal, but occasionally one can see calcification or other benign-appearing bony changes at the lateral epicondyle. These findings have no prognostic significance.
- Magnetic resonance imaging (MRI) is not typically required to make the diagnosis and it does not dictate treatment, as there is no evidence to date that the MRI provides prognostic information. The only exception would be in the rare case involving disruption of both the tendinous and ligamentous origins from the humeral epicondyle with resultant instability.

Surgical Anatomy

- The extensor carpi radialis longus (ECRL) is entirely muscular along the lateral supracondylar ridge of the humerus. The muscle origin has a triangular configuration with the apex pointing proximally (Fig. 1).
- The extensor carpi radialis brevis (ECRB) origin is entirely tendinous.
  - While it blends with the origin of the extensor digitorum communis (EDC), when dissected from a distal-to-proximal direction and using the tendon undersurface, it can be separated from the EDC back to the humerus.

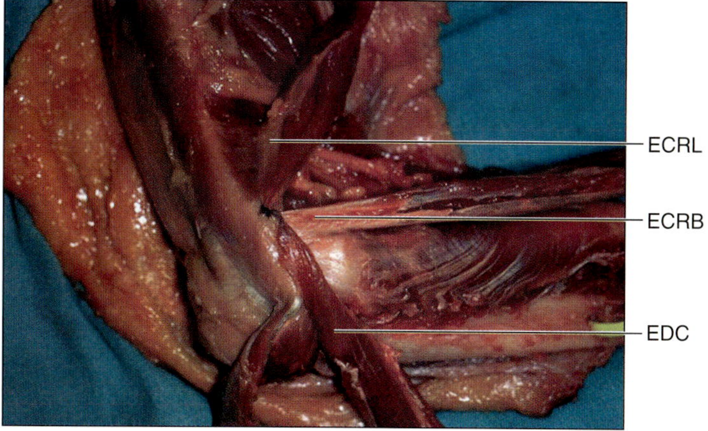

FIGURE 1

- The tendinous origin of the ECRB is the most commonly identified source of pathology. Surgery is typically directed to this tendon.

■ The anatomic origin of the ECRB is located just beneath the distal-most tip of the lateral supracondylar ridge. The footprint is diamond shaped, measuring approximately 13 by 7 mm (Fig. 2).
  - At the level of the radiocapitellar joint, the ECRB is intimate with the underlying anterior capsule of the elbow joint, but it is easily separable at this level.
  - The tendon origin does not originate on the epicondyle specifically (Fig. 3).

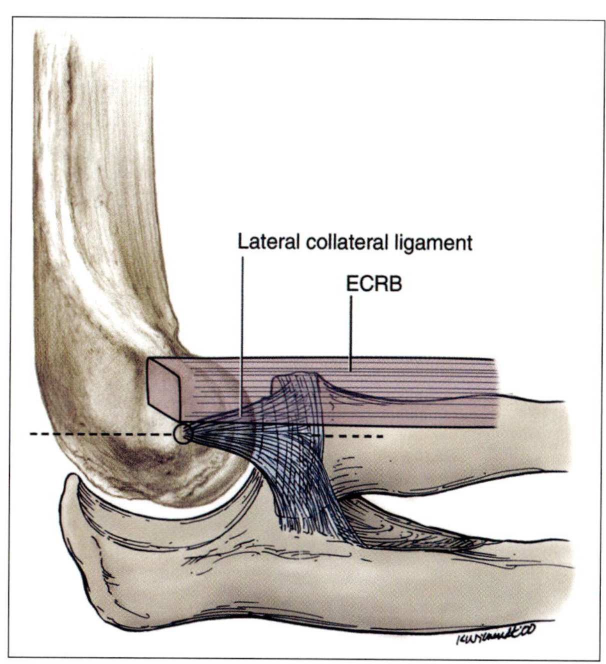

FIGURE 2

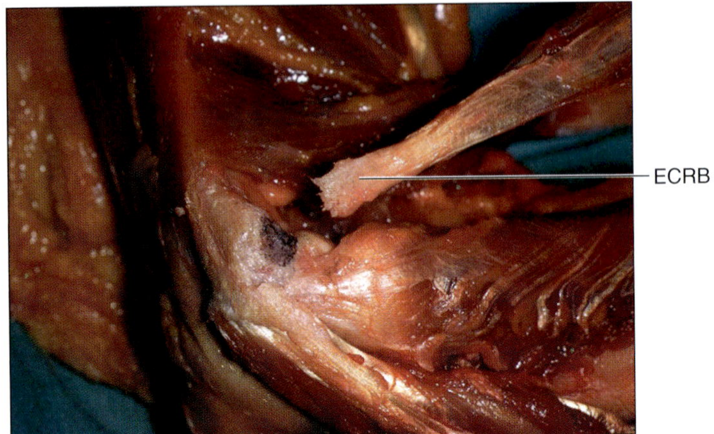

FIGURE 3

Positioning

Arthroscopic Treatment

- Patients are placed either in the lateral decubitus position or prone. The elbow is placed over a bump supporting the humerus and leaving as much of the elbow free as possible.
- Bony landmarks are drawn out, and special attention must be given to the path of the ulnar nerve.
- A regional block is most commonly used with a sterile tourniquet.
- Arthroscopic treatment requires a familiarity with arthroscopic instrumentation and techniques as applied to the elbow joint.

Open Treatment

- Patients are typically positioned supine with the arm resting on an armboard or table. A sterile tourniquet is applied.
- A bump under the elbow with the shoulder internally rotated helps expose the lateral joint region.

Pearls

- *Arthroscopy of the elbow is most commonly performed with the joint flexed over a bolster or a bump. Care must be taken to stabilize the patient and the elbow. Tilting the table slightly toward the surgeon can help keep the elbow supported and give the surgeon free room in which to operate.*

Portals/Exposures

Arthroscopic Treatment

- A standard anteromedial portal is established (Fig. 4). This is started several centimeters proximal and anterior to the medial epicondyle and well anterior to the palpable intermuscular septum. Care is taken to slide along the anterior humerus, and the joint is entered with a blunt introducer or a switching stick.
- This medial portal allows one to view the lateral joint, including the radial head, capitellum, and lateral capsule (Fig. 5).

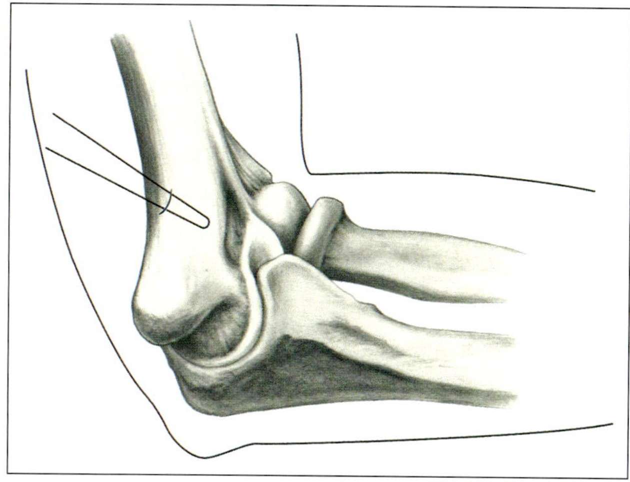

FIGURE 4

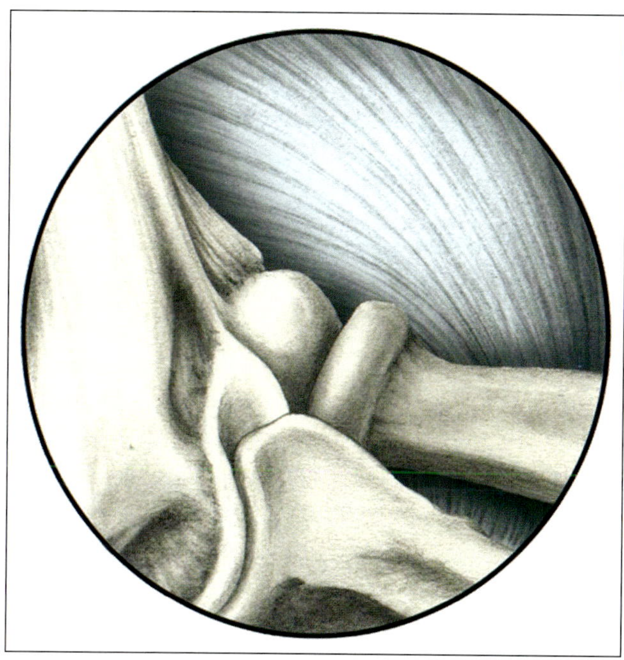

FIGURE 5

- It is often helpful at this point to open the inflow to allow distention of the capsule.
- If visualization is a problem, a retractor can be introduced through a proximal anterolateral portal 2–3 cm proximal and just anterior to the lateral supracondylar ridge. A simple Freer elevator is useful for this purpose. By tensioning the capsule anteriorly, improved visualization of the lateral capsule and soft tissues can be achieved (Fig. 6).

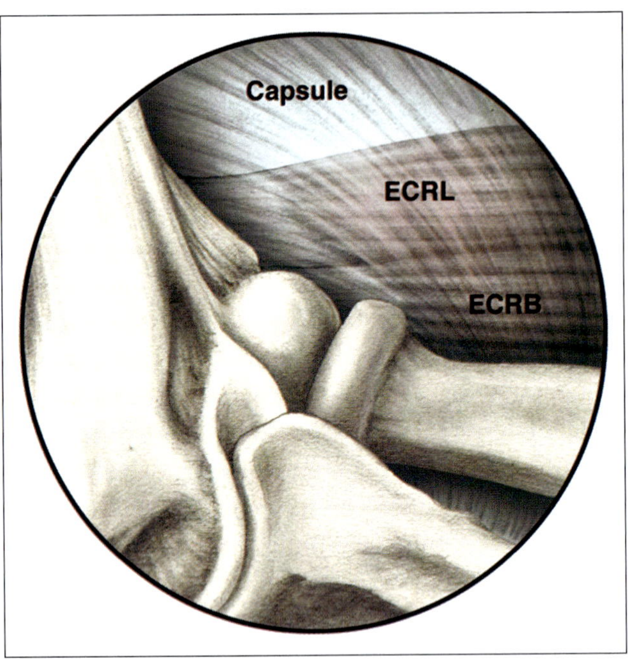

FIGURE 6

- A modified anterolateral portal is established using an inside-out technique (Fig. 7). This is started 2–3 cm above and anterior to the lateral epicondyle.
  - The portal is slightly more proximal than a standard anterolateral portal. This allows instrumentation down to the tendon origin rather than entering the joint through the ECRB tendon itself.

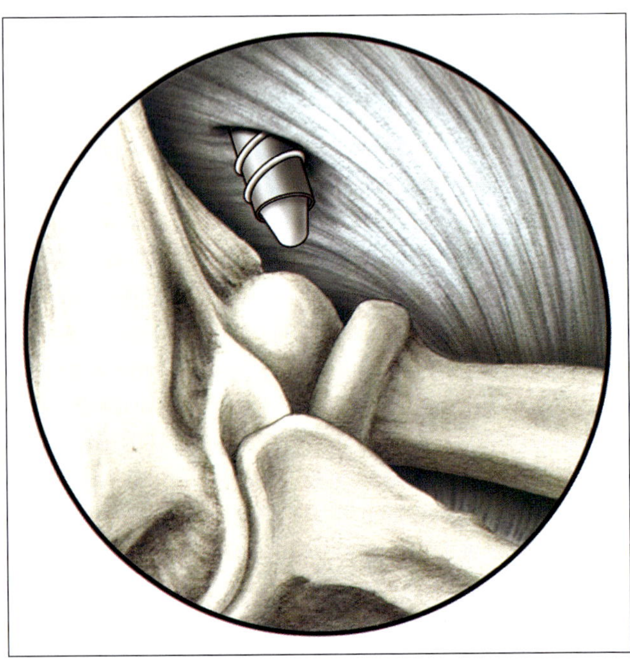

FIGURE 7

- If lateral synovitis is present, this can be débrided with a resector.

Open Treatment

- Exposure of the lateral epicondyle and extensor tendon origin is straightforward.
- There are no important sensory nerves located about the lateral epicondyle. The incision can thus be taken directly down to the tendon level using full-thickness skin flaps.

Procedure: Arthroscopic Treatment

Step 1

- Once a view is present and a lateral portal established, the capsule is next released. Occasionally in epicondylitis, one can find a disruption of the underlying capsule from the humerus (Fig. 8). Most commonly, the capsule is intact, although small linear tears can be present.
- It is easier to release the lateral soft tissues in layers using a monopolar thermal device.
  - With this method, the capsule is first incised or released from the humerus (Fig. 9).
  - When it retracts distally, one can recognize the ECRB tendon posteriorly and the ECRL, which is principally muscular, more anterior (Fig. 10).

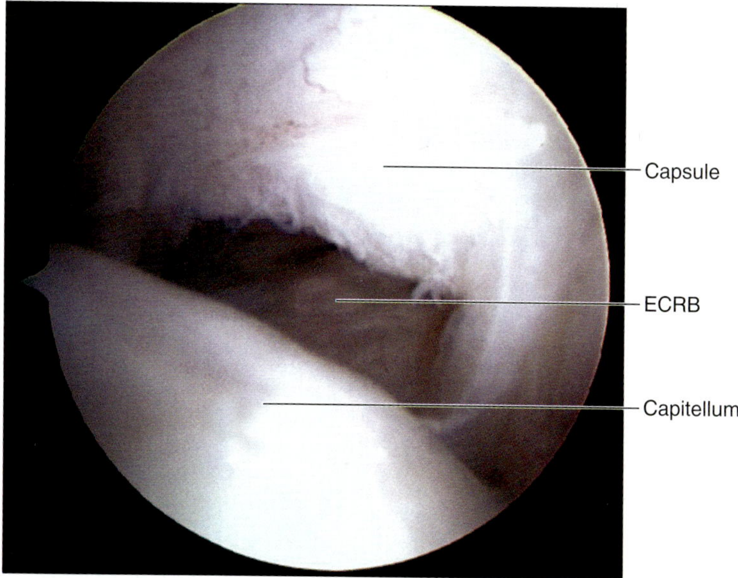

FIGURE 8

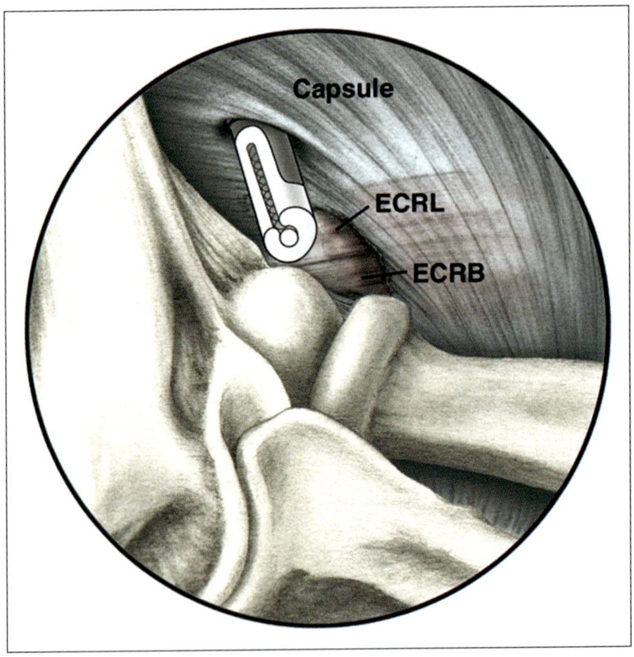

FIGURE 9

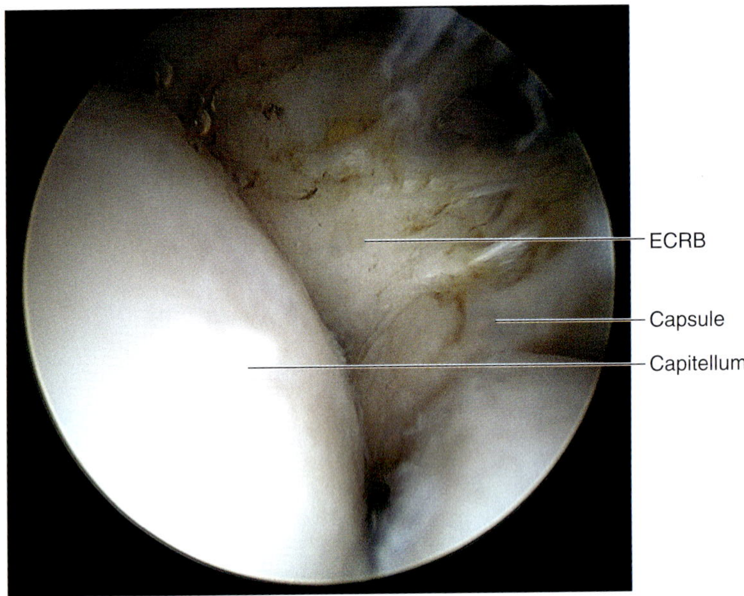

FIGURE 10

Step 2

- Once the capsule is adequately resected, the ECRB origin is released from the epicondyle (Fig. 11). This is started at the top of the capitellum and carried posteriorly. The lateral collateral ligament is not at risk if the release is kept anterior to the midline of the radiocapitellar joint.
  - On average, adequate resection of the ECRB must include approximately 13 mm of tendon origin from anterior to posterior.

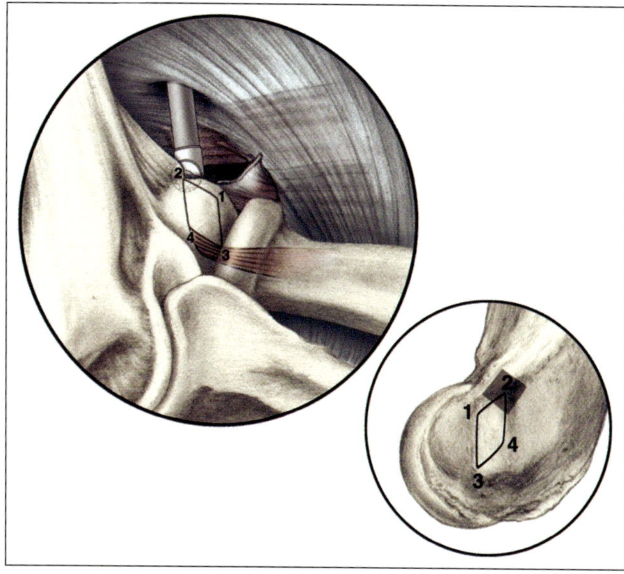

FIGURE 11

- Care is taken to drive the scope in adequately to view the release down to the midline of the radiocapitellar joint. Typically, the entire ECRB retracts distally away from the humerus (Fig. 12).

■ After the ECRB is detached, one should be careful not to release the extensor apponeurosis, which lies behind the ECRB tendon.
  - This can be visualized as a striped background of longitudinally oriented tendon and muscle fibers much less distinct than the ECRB (Fig. 13, *asterisk*). It is located posterior to the ECRL, which again is principally muscular in origin.

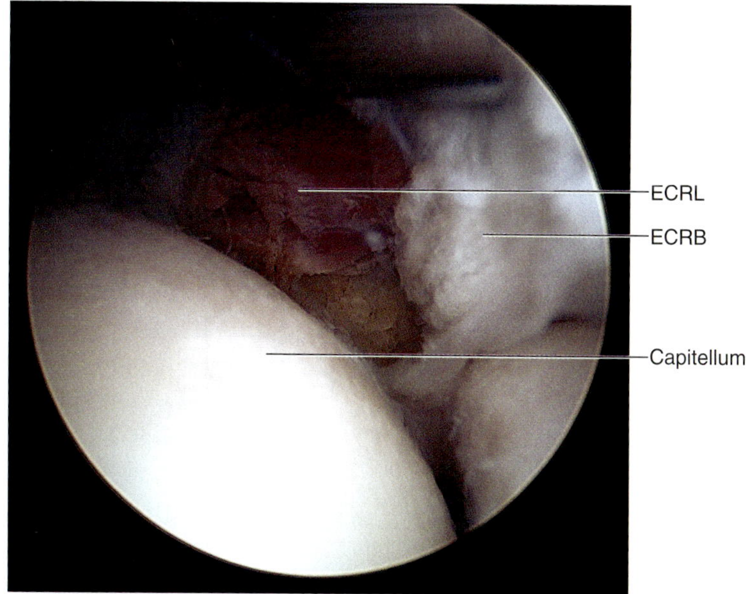

FIGURE 12

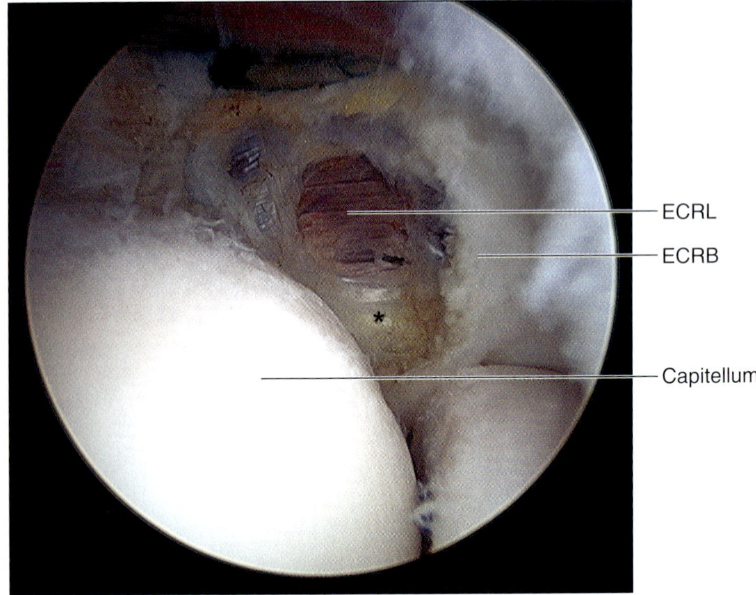

FIGURE 13

- If the aponeurosis is violated, one will débride into the subcutaneous tissue about the lateral elbow.

Procedure: Open Treatment

Step 1

- The most common technique for open treatment utilized currently involves identification and excision of any abnormal tissue identified at the extensor tendon origin, with creation of a bony bed to promote healing, followed by reapproximation of the overlying aponeurosis. The procedure requires identification of the ECRB tendon.
  - The bony origin of the ECRB is beneath the lateral epicondylar prominence, along a longitudinally oriented ridge coursing from the top of the capitellum to the midline of the radiocapitellar joint.
  - Distal to the epicondyle, the ECRB tendon lies beneath the EDC and its aponeurosis. It can most easily be identified by dissecting in an anterior-to-posterior direction, beginning at the junction between the ECRL and EDC aponeurosis (Fig. 14). The distinction is made by the ECRL anteriorly, which is purely muscular.
- The undersurface of the brevis tendon can be elevated from the longus muscle in oblique fashion (Fig. 15). The aponeurosis of the EDC lies on top of the brevis and is tightly apposed.

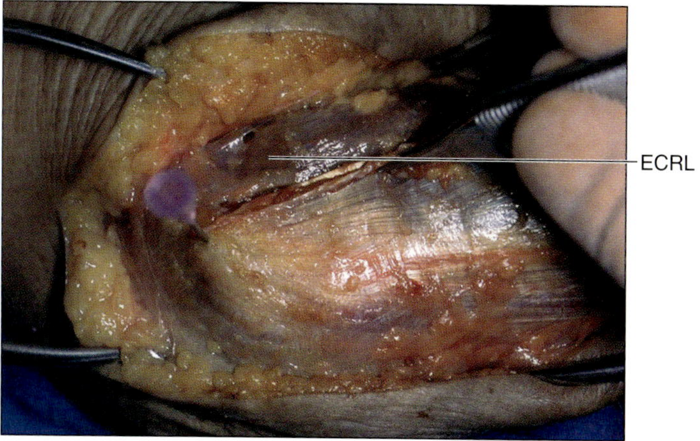

FIGURE 14

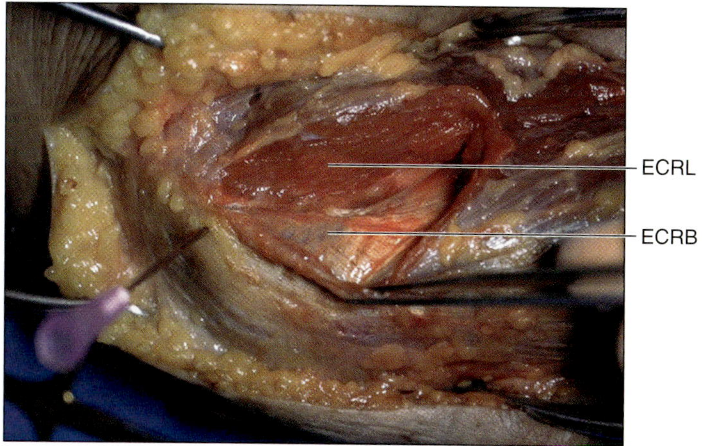

FIGURE 15

- By dissecting the EDC off of the underlying ECRB, the anterior and posterior margins of the ECRB tendon can be identified (Fig. 16).

Step 2

- An alternative method of brevis tendon identification involves anterior elevation of the common tendon origin beginning at the midline of the radiocapitellar joint (Fig. 17). This marks the posterior margin of the brevis tendon.
- Elevation posterior to the midline of the joint is unnecessary and puts the collateral ligament complex origin in jeopardy.

Step 3

- The brevis undersurface is débrided, and the epicondylar origin can be denuded or drilled.
- The fascia is then closed to seal the joint.

Pearls

- *The midline of the radiocapitellar joint marks the border between the ECRB anteriorly and the EDC posteriorly. This is most easily identified by palpation and by looking for the center of the white tendinous origin at the epicondyle. The muscle anteriorly located is the ECRL and the muscle posteriorly located is the anconeus.*

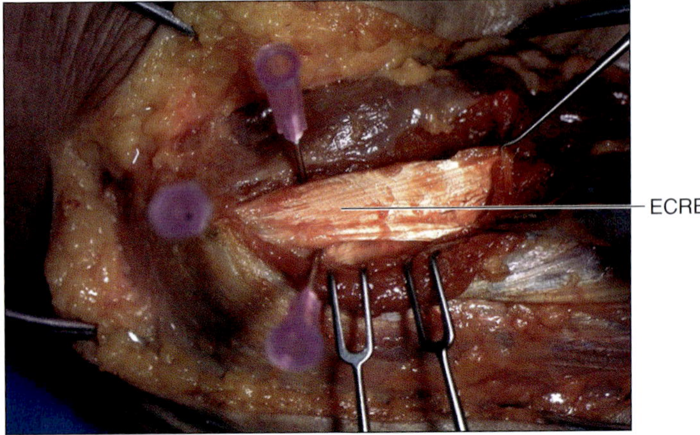

FIGURE 16

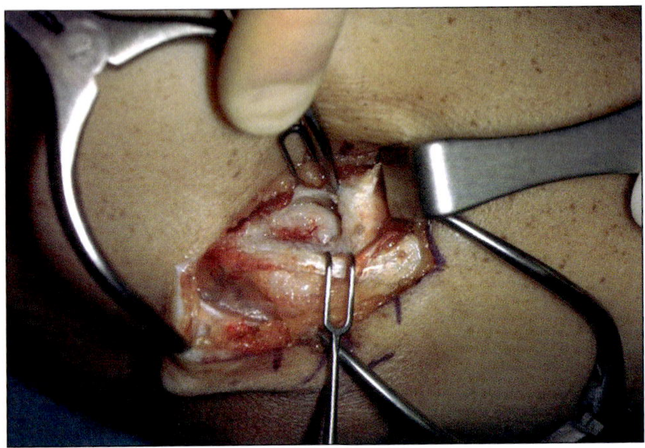

FIGURE 17

Postoperative Care and Expected Outcomes

- The elbow is typically placed in a compressive dressing with or without a splint postoperatively for comfort and support.
- An early rehabilitation program can be initiated regardless of the surgical technique chosen. Patients should be counseled on the need to protect the elbow from loading for at least 4–6 weeks. A too-rapid return to loading can be detrimental to the recovery following surgery.
- The majority of retrospective studies report successful outcomes following surgical intervention, with 80–90% good and excellent results.
  - The largest prospective series, however, consisting of 57 patients followed for approximately 5 years after an open procedure, revealed continued

symptoms in many patients. At 5 years, although the majority of surgically treated patients were improved, 9% continued to experience moderate to severe pain and 28% reported persistent low-grade symptoms.
- The results of results of arthroscopic treatment of epicondylitis have been variable but similar to open methods.

- It is clear that surgical intervention for lateral epicondylitis is somewhat less predictable than other operative procedures about the elbow. Unfortunately, no variables predictive of success have been identified, including time between the onset of symptoms and surgery, occupation, grip strength, pain severity, limitation of motion, tenderness, age, number of cortisone injections, and the use of preoperative therapy. When surgery is offered, patients must be counseled on the possibility of a long recovery period with some continued symptoms about the lateral elbow. Arthroscopic release may offer a more rapid return of function, but this has yet to be proven scientifically. Knowledge of the anatomy, including the extensor tendon origins, is essential for effective surgical release regardless of the technique utilized.

Evidence

Assendelft WJ, Hay EM, Adshead R, Bouter LM. Corticosteroid injections for lateral epicondylitis: a systematic overview. Br J Gen Pract. 1996;46:209-16.

Baker CL. Arthroscopic versus open techniques for extensor tendinosis of the elbow. Tech Shoulder Elbow Surg. 2000;1:184-91.

Baker CL, Murphy KP, Gottlob CA, Curd DT. Arthroscopic classification and treatment of lateral epicondylitis: two-year clinical results. J Shoulder Elbow Surg. 2000;9:475-82.

Boyer MI, Hastings H. Lateral tennis elbow: "Is there any science out there?" J Shoulder Elbow Surg. 1999;8:481-91.

Cohen MS, Romeo AA, Hennigan SP, Gordon M. Lateral epicondylitis: anatomic relationships of the extensor tendon origins and implications for arthroscopic treatment. J Shoulder Elbow Surg. 2008;17:954-60.

Cummins CA. Lateral epicondylitis: in vivo assessment of arthroscopic debridment and correlation with patient outcomes. Am J Sports Med. 2006;34:1486-91.

Galloway M, DeMaio M, Mangine R. Rehabilitation techniques in the treatment of medial and lateral epicondylitis. Orthopaedics. 1992;15:1089-96.

Gruchow HW, Pelletier D. An epidemiologic study of tennis elbow: incidence, recurrence and effectiveness of preventive strategies. Am J Sports Med. 1979;7:234-8.

Hay EM, Paterson SM, Lewis M, Hosie G, Croft P. Pragmatic randomized controlled trial of local corticosteroid injection and naproxen for treatment of lateral epicondylitis of elbow in primary care. BMJ. 1999;319:964-8.

Ho CP. MR imaging of tendon injuries in the elbow. Magn Reson Imaging Clin N Am. 1997;5:529-43.

Kalainov DM, Cohen MS: Posterolateral rotatory instability of the elbow in association with lateral epicondylitis. J Bone Joint Surg [Am]. 2005;87:1120-5.

Kraushaar BS, Nirschl RP. Tendinosis of the elbow: clinical features and findings of histological, immunohistochemical and electron microscopy studies. J Bone Joint Surg [Am]. 1999;81:259-78.

Kuklo TR, Taylor KF, Murphy KP, Islinger RB, Heekin RD, Baker CL. Arthroscopic release for lateral epicondylitis: a cadaveric model. Arthroscopy. 1999;15:259-64.

Labelle H, Guibert R, Joncas J, Newman N, Fallaha M, Rivard CH. Lack of scientific evidence for the treatment of lateral epicondylitis of the elbow: an attempted meta-analysis. J Bone Joint Surg 1992;74B:646-51.
Lattermann C, Romeo AA, Anbari A, Meininger AK, McCarty LP, Cole BJ, Cohen MS. Arthroscopic debridement of the extensor carpi radialis brevis for recalcitrant lateral epicondylitis. J Shoulder Elbow Surg. 2010;19(5):651-6.
Martin CE, Schweitzer ME. MR imaging of epicondylitis. Skeletal Radiol. 1998;27:133-8.
Morrey BF. Surgical failure of tennis elbow. In Morrey BF (ed). The Elbow and Its Disorders, ed 3. Philadelphia: WB Saunders, 2000:543-8.
Nirschl RP, Pettrone FA. The surgical treatment of lateral epicondylitis. J Bone Joint Surg [Am]. 1979;61:832-9.
Peart RE, Strickler SS, Schweitzer ME. Lateral epicondylitis: a comparative study of open and arthroscopic lateral release. Am J Orthop. 2004;33:565-7.
Pienimaki T, Karinen P, Kemila T, Koivukangas P, Vanharanta H. Long-term follow-up of conservatively treated chronic tennis elbow patients: a prospective and retrospective analysis. Scand J Rehabil Med. 1998;30:159-66.
Posch JH, Goldberg VM, Larrey R. Extensor fasciotomy for tennis elbow: a long-term follow-up study. Clin Orthop Relat Res. 1978;(135):179-82.
Regan W, Wold LE, Coonrad R, Morrey BF. Microscopic histopathology of chronic refractory lateral epicondylitis. Am J Sports Med. 1992;20:746-9.
Smith AM, Castle JA, Ruch DS. Arthroscopic resection of the common extensor origin: anatomic considerations. J Shoulder Elbow Surg. 2003;12:375-9.
Stapleton TR, Baker CL. Arthroscopic treatment of lateral epicondylitis. Arthroscopy. 1996;12:365-6.
Tseng V. Arthroscopic lateral release for treatment of tennis elbow. Arthroscopy. 1994;10:335-6.
Verhaar J, Walenkamp G, Kester A, van Mameren H, van der Linden T. Lateral extensor release for tennis elbow: a prospective long-term study. J Bone Joint Surg [Am]. 1993;75:1034-43.

PROCEDURE 51

Repair of Distal Biceps Tendon Ruptures

William Thomas Payne and Jeffrey A. Greenberg

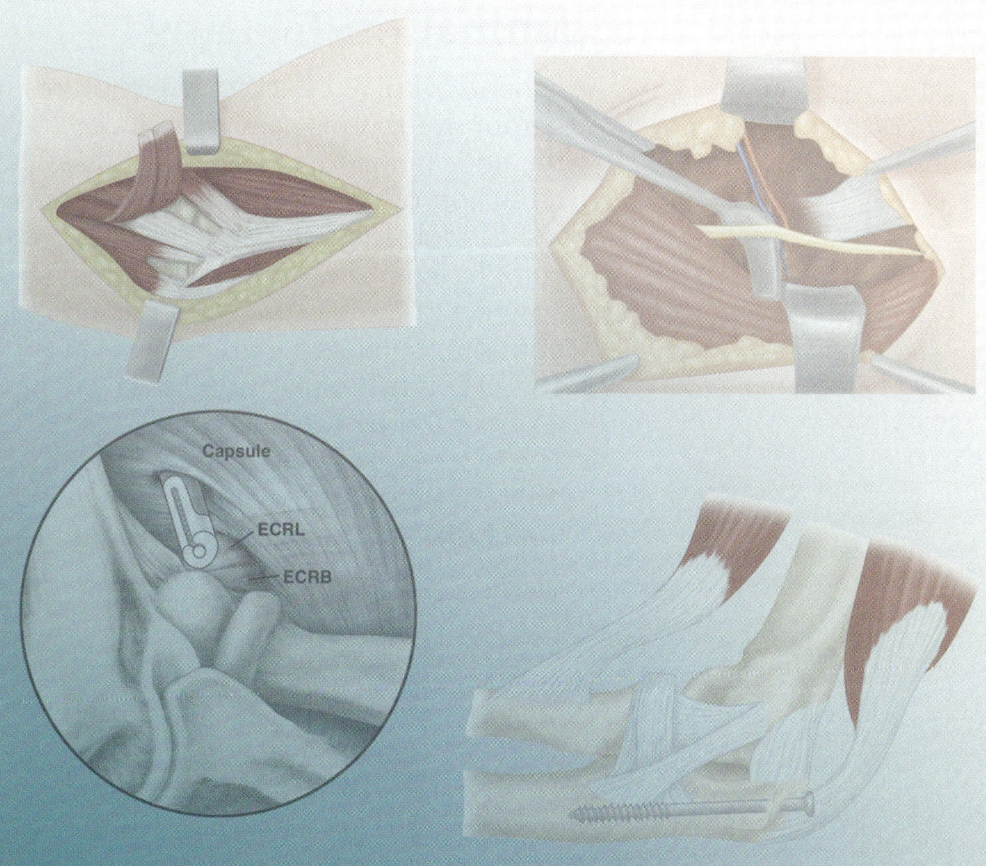

PITFALLS

- *Patients should fully understand the postoperative rehabilitative protocol and be willing to comply with activity limitations to avoid compromising the reconstruction.*
- *Patients must have the capability for full recovery and should not have associated musculoskeletal or neurologic deficits that would compromise full functional recovery of biceps reconstruction.*
- *Nonoperative management should be considered for low-demand, sedentary patients who would not benefit from biceps reconstruction.*

Controversies

- The decision to proceed with operative management for any type of distal biceps rupture is patient specific and is dependent upon the patient's symptoms and unique functional demands.

Indications

- Acute rupture of distal biceps tendon.
- Subacute rupture of distal biceps tendon.
- Chronic rupture of distal biceps tendon.
- Persistently symptomatic partial distal biceps ruptures failing conservative management.
- Repair is indicated for active, healthy patients who desire or require recovery of full strength and endurance in the injured extremity. Patients must be willing and able to participate in appropriate postoperative protective bracing and rehabilitation.

Examination/Imaging

- Patients with acute, complete ruptures usually demonstrate significant ecchymosis, tenderness in the antecubital fossa, a deformity associated with retraction of the biceps, and pain and weakness with resisted forearm supination (Fig. 1). Patients with complete ruptures frequently demonstrate palpable absence of the biceps tendon when compared to the opposite, uninjured extremity.
- The O'Driscoll hook test (Fig. 2) will demonstrate laxity of the biceps tendon.
- The biceps crease interval (BCI) is a measurement using the distance between the antecubital crease of the elbow and the cusp of the musculotendinous

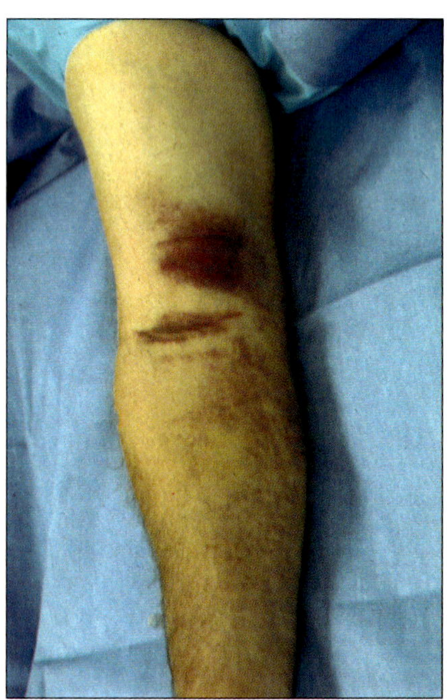

FIGURE 1

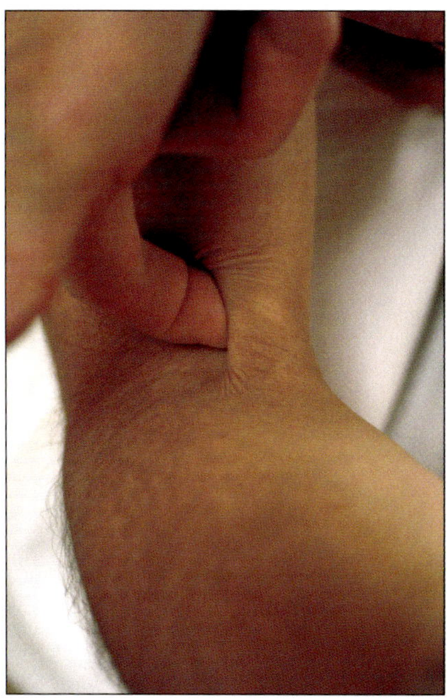

FIGURE 2

junction at the "distal descent" of the biceps tendon. The biceps crease interval is 4.8 ± 0.6 cm in normal uninjured subjects with a side-to-side biceps crease ratio (BCR) of 1.0 ± 0.1. A BCI of greater than 6.0 cm or a BCR greater than 1.2 is associated with a complete biceps rupture with a sensitivity of 96% and a diagnostic accuracy of 93%.

- Patients with chronic ruptures may not manifest significant pain; however, they frequently will have a positive hook test, a positive BCI, and weakness with supination.
- Patients with chronic partial ruptures will frequently demonstrate pain with palpation over the biceps tendon and significant pain and reduced strength with resisted forearm supination.
- Plain radiographs are frequently normal in appearance; however, occasionally hypertrophic changes and bony abnormalities at the bicipital tuberosity may be evident.
- Magnetic resonance imaging (MRI) evaluation is not indicated for the clearly diagnosed cases of acute rupture; however, it is helpful in cases of chronic rupture in demonstrating the location and amount of retraction of the biceps tendon.
  - In partial ruptures, MRI can show fluid accumulation, tendonosis and partial detachment of the tendon at the tuberosity.

Treatment Options

- Nonoperative management is an option for sedentary patients or patients who do not feel they would benefit from surgical reconstruction. Patients can expect to lose 21–55% of supination strength and 86% of supination endurance along with 8–13% loss in flexion strength and 62% loss in flexion endurance with nonoperative management.
- Operative techniques include anatomic and nonanatomic reconstructions. Nonanatomic repair of the biceps tendon to the brachialis has been recommended for chronic and non-reconstructible cases. It is felt to restore biceps contour for cosmetic purposes only. This nonanatomic repair does not restore supination, flexion strength or endurance.
- An alternative technique to a single anterior incision repair is an anatomic two-incision repair. The Boyd Anderson technique popularized in 1961 retrieves the tendon through an anterior incision and delivers it using blunt dissection between the proximal radius and ulna to deliver the tendon posteriorly. A posterior incision exposes the bicipital tuberosity, and the tendon is then anchored to the tuberosity using a bone trough with drill holes or bone anchors.
- Single-incision, anterior techniques have been facilitated by the use of various tendon-bone anchors. In multiple studies, the Endobutton technique has been demonstrated to have the highest peak load to failure. Suture anchors, biotenodesis screws, variations of the Endobutton®, and combinations have all been described for single-incision anterior repairs.

- The FABS (flexion-abduction-supination) view is obtained with specific positioning of the patient in the MRI gantry (Fig. 3). The patient lies prone with the shoulder abducted, the elbow flexed, and the forearm supinated. This view frequently produces a sagittal section through the entire length of the tendon, including the insertion (Fig. 4), enhancing visualization and detection of distal bicipital tendon pathology.

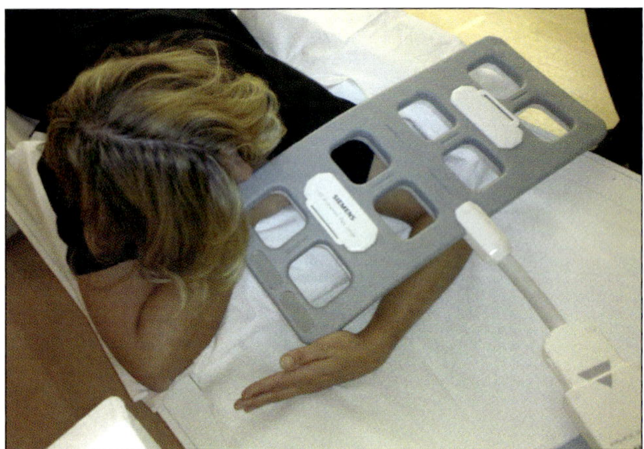

FIGURE 3

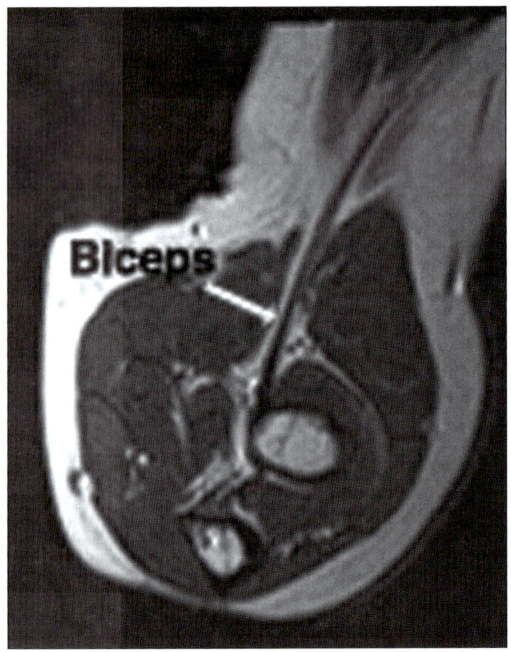

FIGURE 4

Surgical Anatomy

- The biceps tendon lies between the brachioradialis and pronator teres (Fig. 5).
- The biceps inserts on the bicipital tuberosity of the proximal radius approximately 23 mm distal to the articular cartilage of the radial head.
- The size of the biceps insertion is approximately 21 mm long by 7 mm wide on the radial tuberosity.
- The lateral antebrachial cutaneous nerve emerges lateral to the biceps tendon and is at risk of injury with the approach and lateral retraction (Fig. 6).

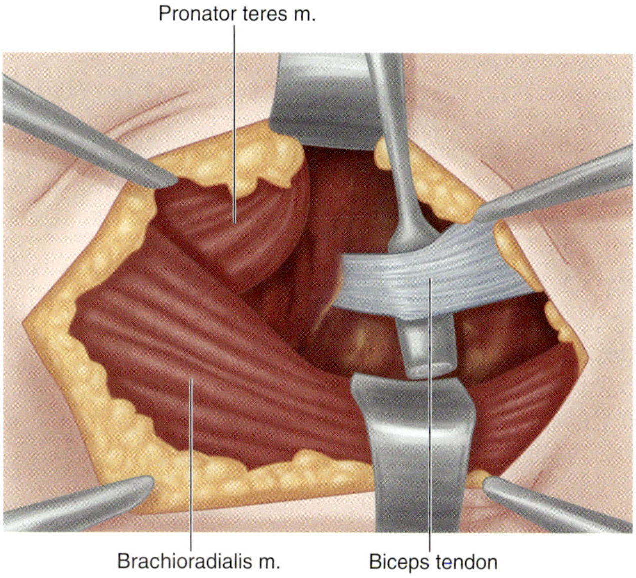

Pronator teres m.
Brachioradialis m.
Biceps tendon

FIGURE 5

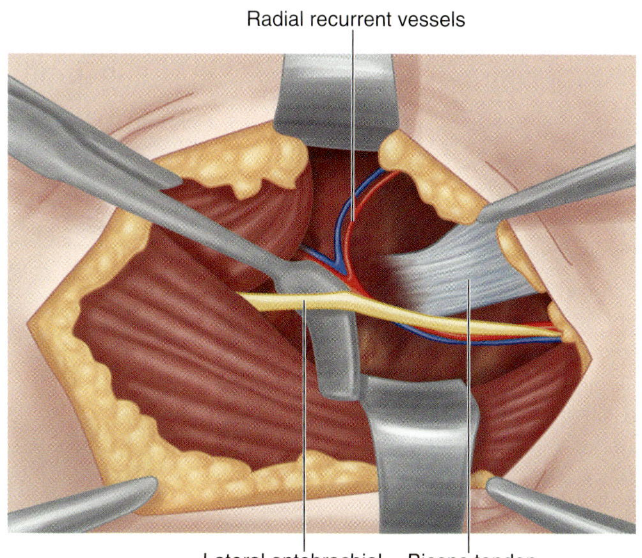

FIGURE 6

PEARLS

- *In cases in which it is difficult to retrieve the biceps tendon proximally or, in chronic cases, reach the bicipital tuberosity, it is occasionally necessary to deflate the tourniquet as this may impede biceps muscle excursion.*

PITFALLS

- *With significant retraction of the biceps, tourniquet use may not be possible. Surgical draping must expose enough of the arm to allow proximal dissection, especially in cases of chronic ruptures and retraction.*

Equipment

- An armboard or hand table that can support the extremity and allow access for intraoperative fluoroscopy
- A sterile upper arm tourniquet

PEARLS

- *With significant biceps retraction, an additional transverse incision proximal to the antecubital flexion crease may be necessary to access, mobilize, and prepare the biceps stump (see Fig. 8).*
- *During the approach, care should be taken to minimize trauma to the periosteum of the proximal radius.*

PITFALLS

- *The lateral antebrachial cutaneous nerve should be identified and protected throughout the procedure. Excessive retraction can lead to neuritis.*

- The radial nerve crosses the elbow between the brachialis and brachioradialis muscles. It then branches, sending the posterior interosseous nerve into the supinator muscle belly to lie on the dorsal cortex of the radius.
- A leash of radial recurrent vessels overlies the proximal radius (see Fig. 6).
- The bicipital aponeurosis or lacertus fibrosus is a broad sheet of connective tissue that originates from the biceps brachii tendon and fans out medially, blending with the deep fascia that covers the anterior compartment. In some cases, if intact, the lacertus can limit proximal retraction of the ruptured biceps tendon.

Positioning

- The patient is placed supine with the affected arm extended on a table designed for hand surgery (Fig. 7).
- Enough clearance for intraoperative fluoroscopy and a sterile upper arm tourniquet is necessary.
- A sterile tourniquet is used on the proximal arm to allow access to the entire upper arm.

Portals/Exposures

- In most cases, the proximal portion of an anterior Henry approach is all that is necessary (Fig. 8).
  - Proximally, the interval is between the brachioradialis and brachialis muscles.
  - Distal to the elbow, the interval is between the brachioradialis and pronator teres.
- The incision may be longitudinal, beginning at the elbow flexion crease, or transverse, overlying the

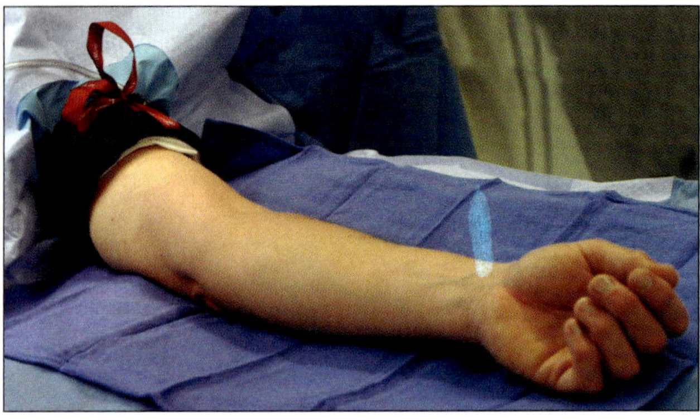

FIGURE 7

Instrumentation

- Army-Navy, Soffield, or small Richardson retractors may be used to enhance visualization of the tuberosity as the muscular interval is developed.

Controversies

- The main controversy regarding exposure involves the philosophy regarding an anterior single incision versus a two-incision technique. Some authors and surgeons feel that a more anatomic reattachment of the biceps tendon is obtained only with a two-incision technique; however, the Endobutton® construct is biomechanically superior to two-incision reconstructive constructs, and outcomes regarding recovery of motion, strength, and endurance are satisfactory using either technique.
- In acute ruptures, a transverse incision directly over the tuberosity may be utilized. This type of incision is more cosmetic, yet more difficult to extend. In cases in which easy retrieval of the ruptured tendon is not anticipated, a longitudinal approach is recommended.

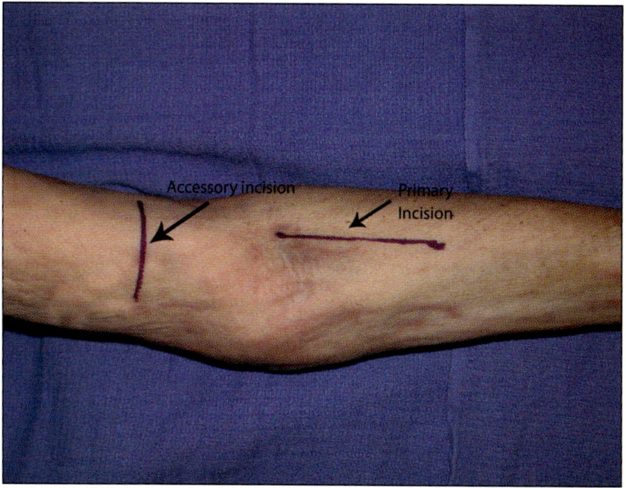

FIGURE 8

radial tuberosity, depending upon the surgeon's preference.

- Once the interval is developed, a leash of veins representing elements of the basilic and cephalic systems is often encountered. The components of the radial recurrent arterial leash frequently need to be ligated to enhance exposure to the bicipital tuberosity.

Procedure

Step 1: Procurement of the Biceps Tendon

- In acute and subacute ruptures, the tendon is frequently easily identified in the proximal portion of the wound or just proximal to the antecubital flexion crease. Scarring and adhesions usually have not matured, and the tendon can be easily mobilized with blunt dissection techniques and delivered into the surgical wound. In subacute injuries, a pseudosheath is frequently present that evaginates off the tendon as it retracts, and this can be traced distally to the biceps tuberosity (Fig. 9).
- In chronic ruptures, retraction of the tendon is occasionally limited by an intact lacertus fibrosis; in these cases, the tendon may be easily visualized and extracted through the surgical incision.
  - In cases with tendon retraction, significant scarring and adhesions develop that make recovery of the tendon difficult. In these cases, a secondary transverse incision (see Fig. 8) at the junction of the distal and middle thirds of the biceps is made and the tendon can be extracted and mobilized

Pearls

- *If the lacertus fibrosus is intact, the tendon frequently will not retract and is easily located.*
- *Do not hesitate to make a separate, more proximal incision if extraction and preparation of the tendon is difficult.*
- *Utilize the degenerative portion of the tendon to facilitate handling and preparation of the tendon for repair.*

Pitfalls

- *An incorrectly located incision may make tendon procurement difficult.*
- *Do not hesitate to make a second, more proximal incision to access the biceps tendon.*

Instrumentation/ Implantation

- A Kocher or Allis clamp is used to grasp the tendon end and helps in manipulating the tendon.

Controversies

- The main controversy in tendon procurement has to do with the debate between a one- and two-incision technique.
- In addition, surgeon preference determines whether a longitudinal or transverse incision is made.
- Some surgeons prefer to make one long S-shaped, curvilinear or zigzag incision when more proximal exposure is necessary. Two separate incisions are recommended.

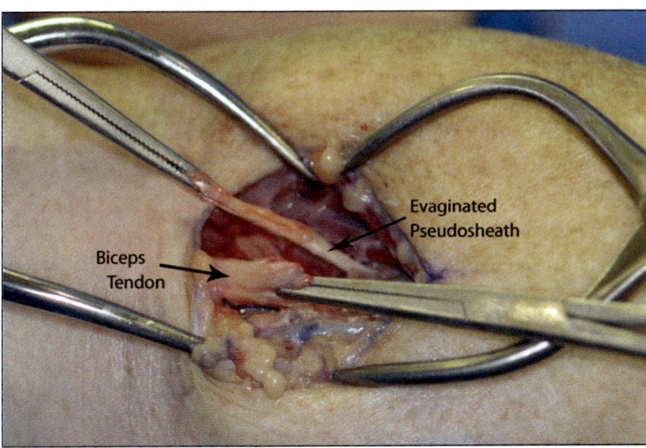

FIGURE 9

through this incision and then delivered under the skin bridge into the distal incision for passage and attachment to the bicipital tuberosity.
- In chronic cases, especially with lateral scarring and adhesions, care must be taken to avoid injury to the lateral antebrachial cutaneous nerve as it exits its muscular interval.

- In almost all cases, degeneration of the tendon is noted at its end. This degenerative tissue should be excised prior to reattachment. During preparation of the tendon, an Allis or Kocher clamp can grasp the degenerative part of the tendon, which facilitates manipulation and preparation of the tendon (Fig. 10).

Step 2: Preparation of the Bicipital Tuberosity

- It is recommended that the biceps tuberosity be prepared for passing the Endobutton® prior to attaching the Endobutton® to the tendon. This allows

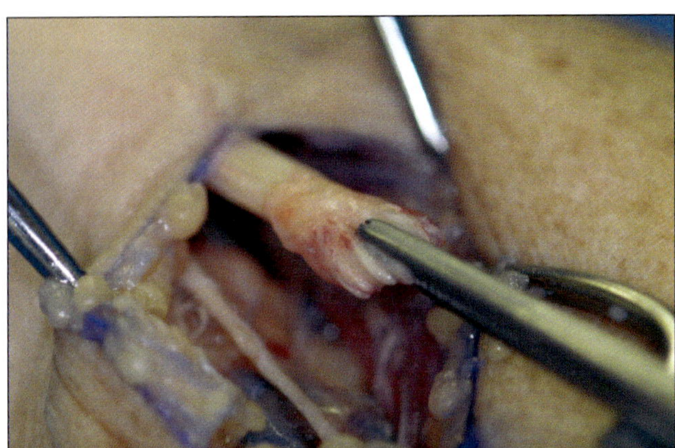

FIGURE 10

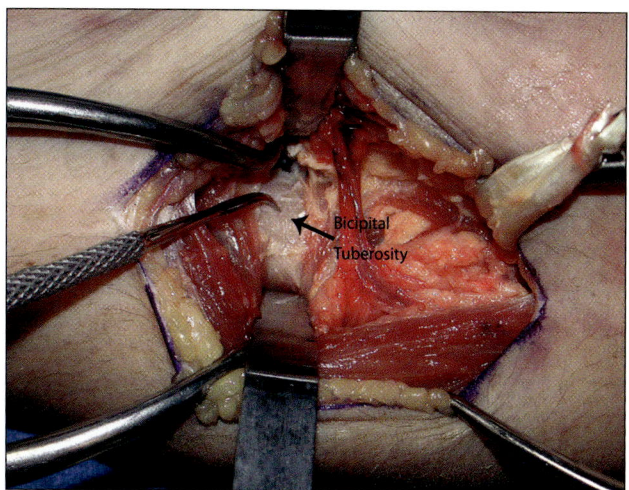

FIGURE 11

the surgeon to determine the appropriate distance from the tendon end to attach the Endobutton®.

- Deeper dissection exposes the bicipital tuberosity (Fig. 11). Frequently a pseudotendon is encountered that can be traced to the bare bicipital tuberosity. A fluid-filled bursa is often encountered at the site of the tendon rupture.
- In partial ruptures, the tuberosity is easily identified as the tendon is intact and can be traced down to the tuberosity. Frequently, in chronic ruptures, a significant portion of the biceps tendon is detached from the tuberosity and only approximately 5–10% of the deep, supinatory fibers of the biceps tendon are intact. In these cases, the remaining fibers are sharply transected, converting the partial rupture to a complete rupture and exposing the bicipital tuberosity.
- During preparation of the tuberosity, the arm is held at 90° of supination. This position places the posterior interosseous nerve at minimum risk when passing instruments through the cortex of the proximal radius. Care is taken during retraction of soft tissue to avoid injury to the lateral antebrachial cutaneous nerve.
- Once the location of the drill hole is determined, a slotted Beath pin is drilled from anterior to posterior (Fig. 12). The power drilling is stopped when the posterior cortex is penetrated. Deeper penetration of the Beath pin through the soft tissues of the posterior forearm is done by tapping with a mallet to avoid twisting vital structures in a rotating power bit.

Pearls

- *Maintain the position of supination to avoid injury to the posterior interosseous nerve when passing the Beath pin or drilling the posterior cortex with the cannulated bit.*
- *Stop drilling once the posterior cortex is penetrated*
- *Do not use power tools to prepare the anterior hole for the tendon. A Kerrison rongeur creates less bone debris.*

Pitfalls

- *Excessive retraction may injure the lateral antebrachial cutaneous nerve.*
- *Inappropriate positioning or aggressive power drilling once instruments penetrate the posterior radius can damage the posterior interosseous nerve.*
- *Excessive bone debris and periosteal injury may stimulate heterotopic bone formation.*

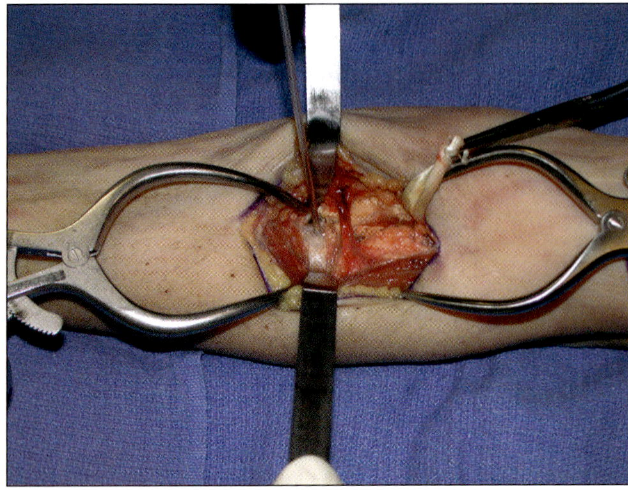

FIGURE 12

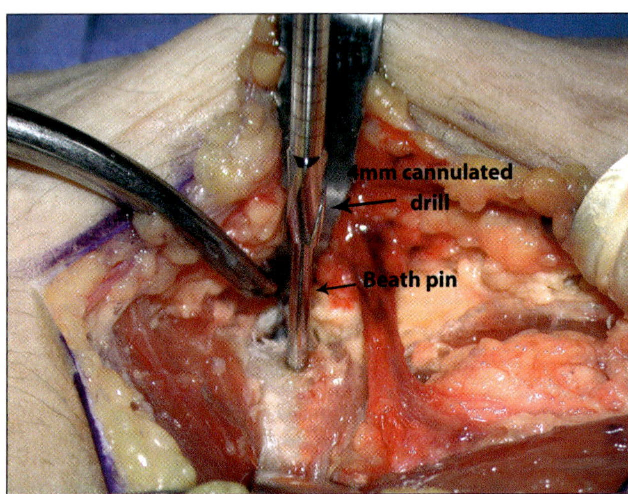

FIGURE 13

Instrumentation/ Implantation

- A slotted Beath pin is the rigid guide pin that determines the location for the cannulated bit and is also used to pass the sutures out the posterior forearm. Next, the cannulated bit drills a 4-mm-wide hole so that the Endobutton® can be passed vertically through the proximal radius.

An alternative method would be to use an oscillating drill.

- With the Beath pin in place, the cannulated 4-mm drill overdrills the anterior and posterior cortices of the radius (Fig. 13). The cannulated drill and Beath pin are now removed.
- The anterior cortex is enlarged to accept the biceps tendon using a Kerrison rongeur (Fig. 14). Care is taken during this step to minimize the amount of bone debris created and to minimize injury and trauma to the periosteum. Copious irrigation and suction are utilized to remove bony debris.
- Once the hole that will accept the tendon is created (Fig. 15), the depth is sized. The surgeon may choose to estimate the depth that will determine the

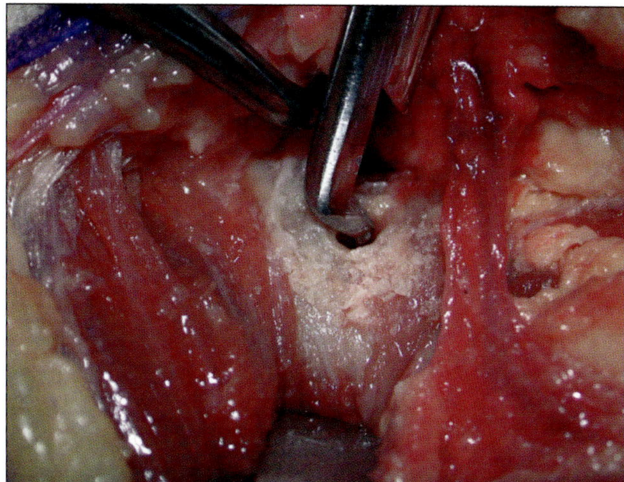

FIGURE 14

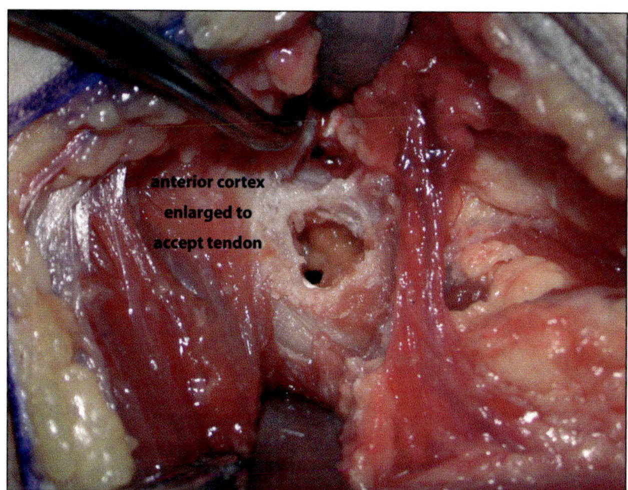

FIGURE 15

distance between the tendon and the Endobutton, or can directly measure it using Kirschner wires or a depth gauge.

Step 3: Tendon Preparation

- A heavy, braided synthetic suture is utilized for preparation of the tendon. A #2 FiberWire or similar suture is recommended.
  - The tendon is prepared using a running, locking Krakow-type suture (Fig. 16). Approximately 3–4 cm of tendon on either side are incorporated with the running Krakow suture.
  - Distally, the suture exits just proximal to the portion of the tendon that will be excised.
- Alternatively, a looped suture technique can be utilized, which creates a modified suture geometry (Fig. 17).

Pearls

- *Using a running, locking suture of heavily braided synthetic suture prevents bunching of the tendon. In grasping the tendon in a Krakow fashion, the amount of tendon that is grasped with each suture bite is varied to avoid creating a linear defect in which the suture could pull out. The distal degenerative portion of the tendon should be débrided to fresh tendon.*

Pitfalls

- *An inappropriate suture technique will allow excessive tendon collapse and "bunching" and compromise the tendon-suture strength.*
- *Leaving degenerated tendon intact will compromise the repair as devitalized, degenerative tendon will engage the proximal radius.*
- *A linear "suture stress riser" will be created if the same amount of tendon is grasped with each suture throw*

Instrumentation/ Implantation

- A heavy, braided nonabsorbable suture material is used for the repair. Kevlar-reinforced suture such as FiberWire is recommended.

Controversies

- Some surgeons prefer to use a prelooped suture that allows a looped-grasping type of suture configuration instead of a running locking configuration.

PEARLS

- *Sutures of different color and/or consistency are used in the peripheral holes of the Endobutton® to allow the surgeon to differentiate the leading and trailing "kite string" suture when the Endobutton® is guided and engaged on the proximal radius. A third rescue suture is allowed to remain anterior after the Endobutton® is engaged. This allows retrieval of the Endobutton® in cases in which the Endobutton® is not engaged properly. In most cases in which the Endobutton® needs to be retrieved, it is due to inappropriate tension in the biceps tendon after the Endobutton® is engaged.*

PITFALLS

- *An insufficient gap between the tendon and the Endobutton® will make passage of the Endobutton® through the proximal radius difficult. A gap that is too large will prevent appropriate tensioning of the biceps tendon to the proximal radius.*
- *Tying the knot on the central portion of the Endobutton® can lead to exit site irritation due to a prominent suture knot complex.*

Instrumentation/ Implantation

- The Endobutton® is a 4-mm × 12-mm titanium implant originally designed for anterior cruciate ligament reconstruction. It allows for suture fixation through two central holes as well as passage and engagement of the Endobutton® using sutures in two peripheral holes.

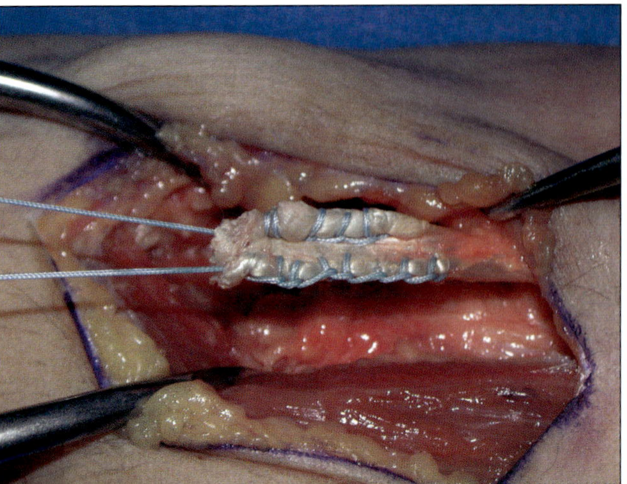

FIGURE 16

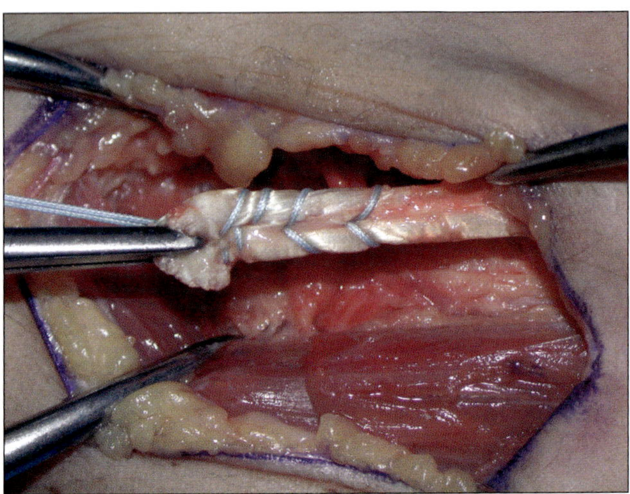

FIGURE 17

STEP 4: SECURING THE ENDOBUTTON®

- One tail of the previously placed nonabsorbable suture is placed through one of the central holes of the Endobutton® and then brought back through the second, central hole of the Endobutton®. This allows for knot tying adjacent to the tendon and avoids placing the knot over the central portion of the Endobutton®.
- Sutures of different quality/consistency are then placed in the peripheral holes of the Endobutton®. Two sutures are placed in one of the peripheral holes and one suture is placed in the other peripheral hole (Fig. 18). One suture from each peripheral hole will be delivered posteriorly and will function to guide and engage the Endobutton® on the posterior surface of the radius. The remaining suture will be

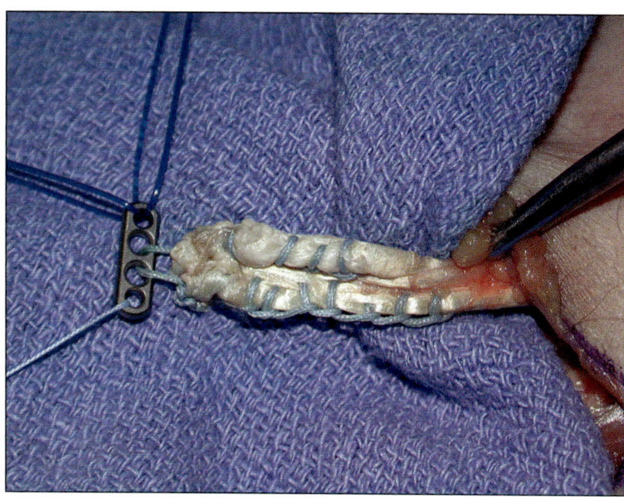

FIGURE 18

left anteriorly as a "rescue suture" in cases in which the Endobutton® needs to be retrieved.

- After the peripheral sutures are placed, these are used to support and hold the Endobutton® while the heavy, braided, nonabsorbable suture is tied. A gap between the end of the tendon and the Endobutton® of approximately 2–4 mm is left, depending upon the distance determined during bicipital tuberosity preparation.

Step 5: Passage and Deployment of the Endobutton

- The Beath pin is reinserted into the previously prepared hole. It is then bluntly passed through the soft tissues of the dorsal forearm and out through a puncture wound in the proximal dorsal forearm (Fig. 19).

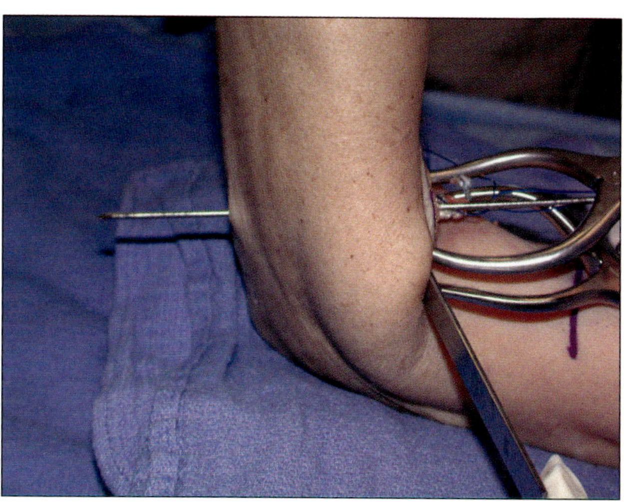

FIGURE 19

Controversies

- There are alternative devices that function similar to the Endobutton®. In addition, techniques associated with these alternative devices use a tension sliding knot technique in which the knot is tied after the Endobutton® is engaged. This technique eliminates the problem of presetting the gap between the tendon and the fixation device; however, it requires tying and anchoring sutures in the depths of the surgical wound, and setting tension can sometimes be difficult.

Pearls

- *Fluoroscopy should be utilized.*
- *Ensure that the appropriate kite string suture is being tensioned while trying to deliver the Endobutton®.*
- *Extension of the elbow should firmly engage the Endobutton® on the posterior radius, and appropriate tension should be palpated in the biceps tendon.*
- *The kite string suture should be left in the anterior wound; if the Endobutton® does not engage, then the rescue suture can be used to extract the Endobutton anteriorly and appropriate correction to the tendon-Endobutton interface can be made.*

Pitfalls

- *Ensure that the appropriate kite string suture is being tensioned when the Endobutton® is being delivered. Do not pull the Endobutton® excessively past the radius as this can increase the chance for entrapment of soft tissues on the posterior radius. This will increase the chance of damage to the posterior interosseous nerve.*

Instrumentation/ Implantation

- Intraoperative fluoroscopy is utilized to facilitate passage and confirm that the Endobutton is engaged in the appropriate position.

- One suture from each of the peripheral holes is placed in the slot in the Beath pin. The Beath pin is fully extracted, delivering the kite string sutures (Fig. 20). The rescue suture is left anteriorly (Fig. 21).
- The surgeon determines which suture is the leading and trailing suture so that appropriate tension and traction can be applied as the Endobutton® is deployed.
- Intraoperative fluoroscopy is brought into the operative field.
- The leading suture is tensioned while visualizing passage of the Endobutton® through the radius using fluoroscopy. Once the Endobutton® passes through the proximal radius, the trailing kite string suture is tensioned. This action should flip the Endobutton® 90°. The arm is then brought out into full extension, locking the Endobutton® onto the posterior radius.

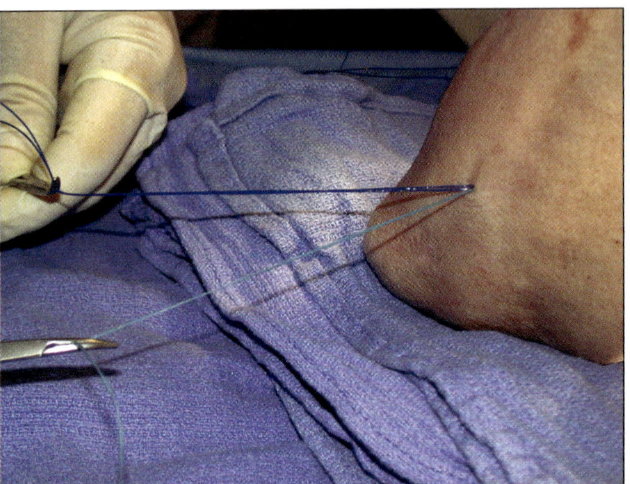

FIGURE 20

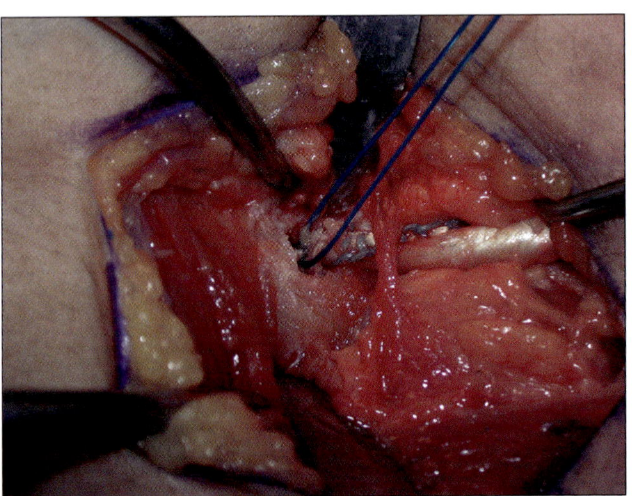

FIGURE 21

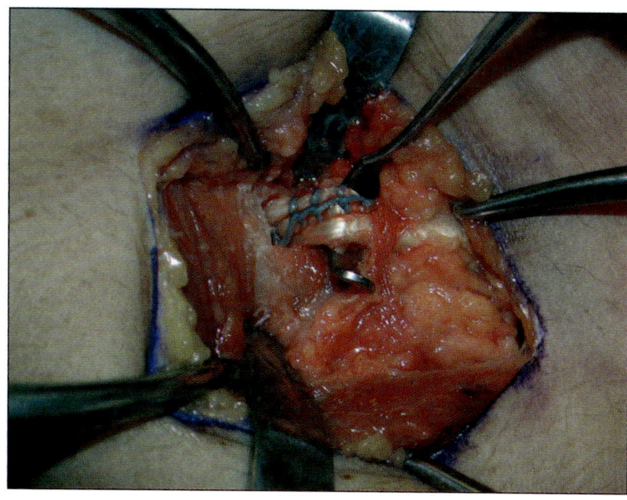

FIGURE 22

■ Next, the tendon is palpated. It should have good tension and be seated within the previously prepared hole within the anterior radius (Fig. 22).

Postoperative Care and Expected Outcomes

■ A bulky, compressive long-arm dressing is applied postoperatively. At day 5, the patient's bulky dressing is removed. A light compressive dressing is substituted and the patient's arm supported in a Bledsoe or other hinged brace. For the first 6 weeks after surgery, extension is limited to 30° but patients are encouraged to perform active, active-assisted, and passive range of motion, including extension, flexion, and especially forearm rotation.

■ At 6 weeks postsurgery, the bracing is discontinued and full terminal extension is allowed and encouraged. Strengthening and resistive exercises start at 10–12 weeks postsurgery. Expected outcomes are recovery of full range of motion with recovery of 97% of flexion strength and 82% of supination strength.

■ In many cases of chronic repairs, the biceps tendon is significantly retracted to a position that precludes primary attachment of the tendon to the tuberosity with the arm in full extension. Many authors have advocated a variety of tendon grafts to bridge the defect between the tendon and biceps tuberosity in these cases. It is these authors' experience that tendon grafts have, for the most part, been

Pearls

- *The Endobutton® construct is strong enough to allow early range of motion. Emphasis is on forearm rotation. Protection of the repair by limiting terminal extension is indicated for 6 weeks postoperatively.*

Pitfalls

- *Complications of distal biceps repair are numerous. The complications of heterotopic ossification, synostosis, and subsequent limited range of motion, common in earlier reports on biceps tendon repairs, have been mitigated but not eliminated using single anterior approaches. Lateral antebrachial neuritis is the most common complication seen after repair. It is usually due to excessive or inappropriate retraction; however, fortunately it is usually transient. Other complications include posterior interosseous nerve injuries, vascular injuries, hematoma formation, loss of motion, repair failure, proximal radius fracture, persistent pain, and complex regional pain syndromes.*

unnecessary. Using the Endobutton® construct, chronic ruptures of the biceps tendon have been repaired directly to the biceps tuberosity even in cases in which significant limitation of elbow extension is noted upon attachment of the tendon to the bone. Over the course of 4–8 weeks, myostatic contracture is overcome in these cases, and even in cases in which the limitation of elbow motion was excessive and the biceps repair was excessively tight, patients with chronic ruptures can be expected to overcome myostatic contraction and recover full elbow extension without the need for supplementary tendon grafts.

Evidence

Athwal GS, Steinmann SP, Rispoli DM. The distal biceps tendon: footprint and relevant clinical anatomy. J Hand Surg [Am]. 2007;32:1225-9.

Fifteen cadavers were evaluated to characterize the anatomic nature of the biceps tendon footprint. The average length of the biceps insertion was found to be 21 mm. The average width of the insertion was found to be 7 mm.

Bain GI, Prem H, Heptinstall RJ, Verhellen R, Paix D. Repair of distal biceps tendon rupture: a new technique using the Endobutton. J Shoulder Elbow Surg. 2000;9:120-6.

This was the first published paper describing the Endobutton technique. Satisfactory clinical results were reported for 12 patients, and anatomic studies demonstrated the safety in regard to posterior interosseous nerve injuries. (Level IV evidence)

Chavan PR, Duquin TR, Bisson LJ. Repair of the ruptured distal biceps tendon: a systematic review. Am J Sports Med. 2008;36:1618-24.

This literature review compiled data regarding biomechanical testing, complications, and clinical outcomes. The review of eight papers with biomechanical data revealed that the Endobutton construct performed best in comparative studies. Two-incision and single-incision techniques had similar incidences of complications. Nineteen papers were reviewed regarding clinical outcomes, and the single-incision repairs demonstrated superior results in regard to range of motion and rotational strength. (Level III evidence)

Greenberg JA, Fernandez JJ, Wang T, Turner C. Endobutton-assisted repair of distal biceps tendon ruptures. J Shoulder Elbow Surg. 2003;12:484-90.

This paper described the clinical, anatomic, and biomechanical characteristics of the Endobutton technique. In cadaver studies, the safety of the procedure relative to posterior interosseous nerve injuries was demonstrated. Biomechanical studies demonstrated the strength of the repair construct, and comparative biomechanical testing demonstrated the superior strength of the Endobutton repair. In clinical review and biomechanical assessment, patients who had their tendon repaired using the Endobutton technique recovered 97% of flexion and 82% of supination strength. (Level IV evidence)

Hetsroni I, Pilz-Burstein R, Nyksa M, Back Z, Barchilon V, Mann G. Avulsion of the distal biceps brachii tendon in the middle-aged population: is surgical repair advisable? A comparative study of 22 patients treated with either non-operative management or early anatomic repair. Injury 2008;39:753-60.

Surgical repair of distal biceps ruptures was found to be subjectively and objectively superior in this study that followed a group of 22 patients prospectively. However, the nonoperated group also had good to excellent outcomes, supporting nonoperative treatment in patients who are sedentary or poor candidates for surgical reconstruction. (Level III evidence)

Karunakar MA, Cha P, Stern P. Distal biceps ruptures: a follow-up of Boyd and Anderson repair. Clin Orthop Relat Res. 1999;(363):100-7.

At an average 44-month follow-up of patients undergoing two-incision repairs of the distal biceps tendon, weakness in supination was found in 48% of patients and flexion weakness in 14%. Despite this, all 20 patients were felt to have a good or excellent outcome. (Level IV evidence)

Kettler M, Lunger J, Kuhn V, Mutschler W, Tingart MJ. Failure strengths in distal biceps tendon repair. Am J Sports Med. 2007;35:1544-8.

This cadaver study tested 13 different fixation techniques of distal biceps tendon repairs. Mode of failure and single load-to-failure data were collected. The Endobutton construct had the highest load-to-failure of any of the repair techniques.

McKee MD, Hirji R, Schemitsch EH, Wild LM, Waddell JP. Patient oriented functional outcome after repair of distal biceps tendon ruptures using a single incision technique. J Shoulder Elbow Surg. 2005;14:302-6.

The DASH score was used to assess patient-oriented outcomes in a large group of patients who had distal biceps ruptures repaired using a single anterior incision. The results indicated efficacy in restoration of near-normal upper extremity function with low morbidity. (Level IV evidence)

Nesterenko S, Domire ZJ, Morrey BF, Sanchez-Sotelo J. Elbow strength and endurance in patients with a ruptured distal biceps tendon. J Shoulder Elbow Surg. 2010;19:184-9.

Nine patients with unilateral complete distal biceps ruptures were assessed using isokinetic strength and endurance testing. A substantial decrease in both flexion and supination strength was noted when compared to the uninjured extremity.

Sutton KM, Dodds SD, Ahmad CS, Sethi PM. Surgical treatment of distal biceps rupture. J Am Acad Ortho Surg. 2010;18:139-48.

This paper presented a contemporary review of the anatomy and pathomechanics of distal biceps tendon ruptures. In addition, it presented a good review of treatment options for patients with distal ruptures as well as a review of outcomes following surgical repair of distal ruptures.

PROCEDURE 52

Repair and Reconstruction of the Ruptured Triceps

Robert M. Baltera

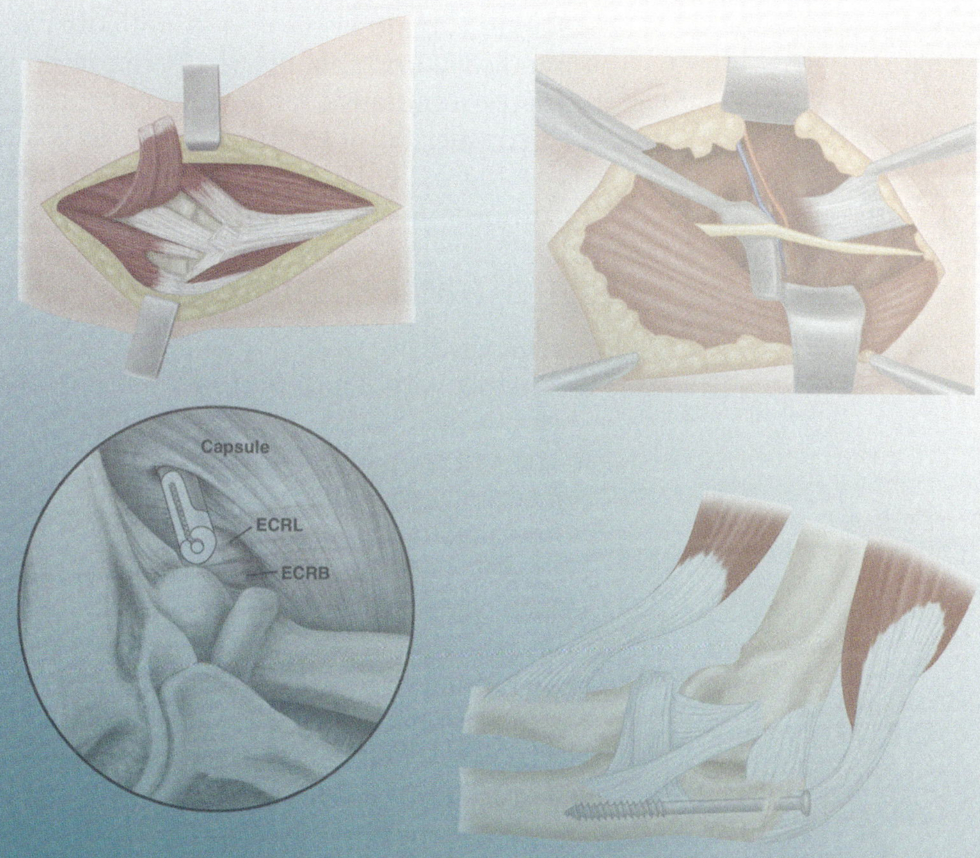

PEARLS

- *Anabolic steroid use should be considered in body builders or other athletes with triceps ruptures.*
- *Ruptures have also been associated with local steroid injections.*

Controversies

- Nonoperative treatment may be an option for patients with magnetic resonance imaging (MRI)—or ultrasound-confirmed partial ruptures when there is no significant loss of extension power.

Indications

- Acute rupture of the triceps tendon is rare and the least common of all upper extremity tendon injuries. It is seen in a broad spectrum of age groups.
- The patient usually gives a history of a fall or other type of decelerating force applied to an actively contracting triceps. Ruptures can also be seen following surgical release and reattachment after total elbow arthroplasty.
- Repair of acute complete ruptures is indicated in healthy, active patients in order to restore power of elbow extension.
- Repair is contraindicated in patients who are medically unstable or are unable to cooperate with the postoperative rehabilitation program.
- Reconstruction of chronic ruptures is indicated in healthy patients in whom weakness has compromised their function.

Examination/Imaging

PHYSICAL EXAMINATION

- Patients with acute ruptures present with posterior elbow pain, swelling, and ecchymosis.
- The site of failure is usually at the olecranon insertion, and this may be partial or complete. Ruptures of the musculotendinous junction and muscle belly have also been reported.
- Two thirds of patients have a palpable defect immediately proximal to the olecranon.
- All complete ruptures have weakness of elbow extension, but only 20% have complete loss.
  - Some active elbow extension may be maintained through the continuity of the lateral fascia between the triceps and anconeus.
- With a partial rupture, motion and extension against resistance are maintained.
- Associated injuries may include fractures of the radial head as well as wrist injuries.
- The modified Thompson test, described by Viegas, can be performed to assess the integrity of the triceps tendon. With the patient prone and the elbow flexed over the edge of the table, firm compression of the triceps muscle should result in some elbow extension if the tendon is intact (Fig. 1).

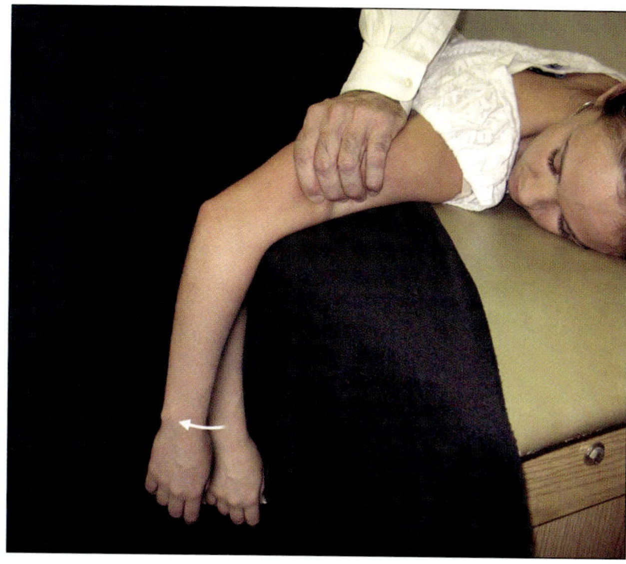

FIGURE 1

Imaging

- Anteroposterior and lateral plain radiographs of the elbow should be obtained.
  - About 70% will have a "flake sign," which represents a small olecranon avulsion fragment.
- For equivocal cases or suspected partial injuries, MRI without contrast or ultrasound (Fig. 2) is indicated.

Surgical Anatomy

- The triceps tendon represents the confluence of the long, lateral, and medial heads of the triceps.
  - The tendon attaches broadly upon the posterior surface of the olecranon (Fig. 3).

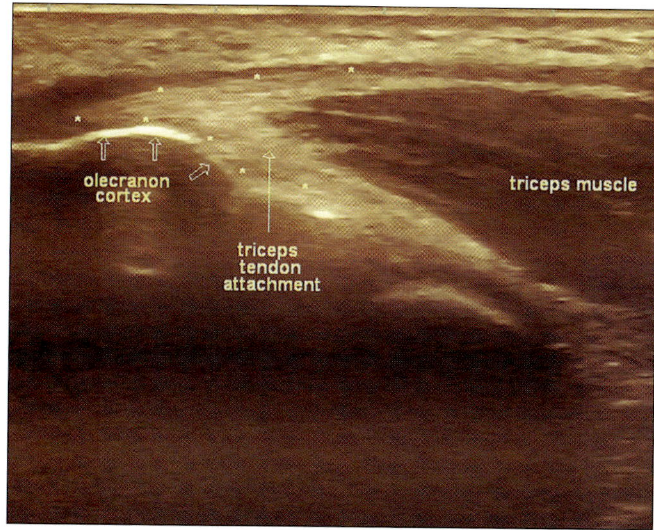

FIGURE 2

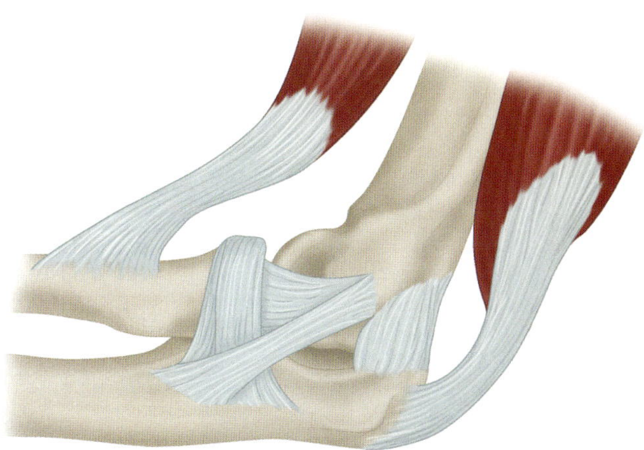

FIGURE 3

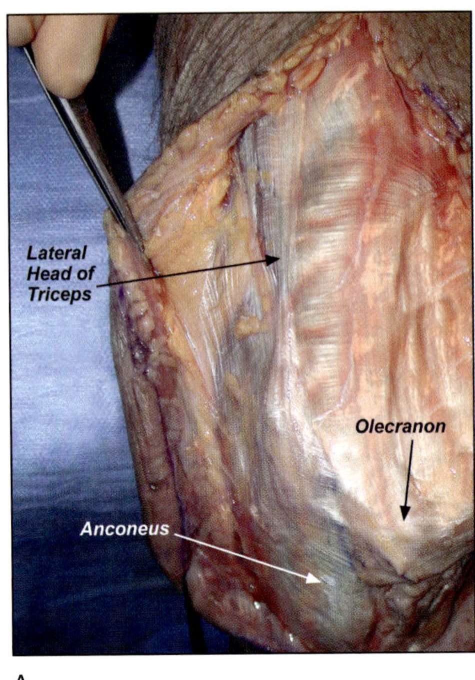

A

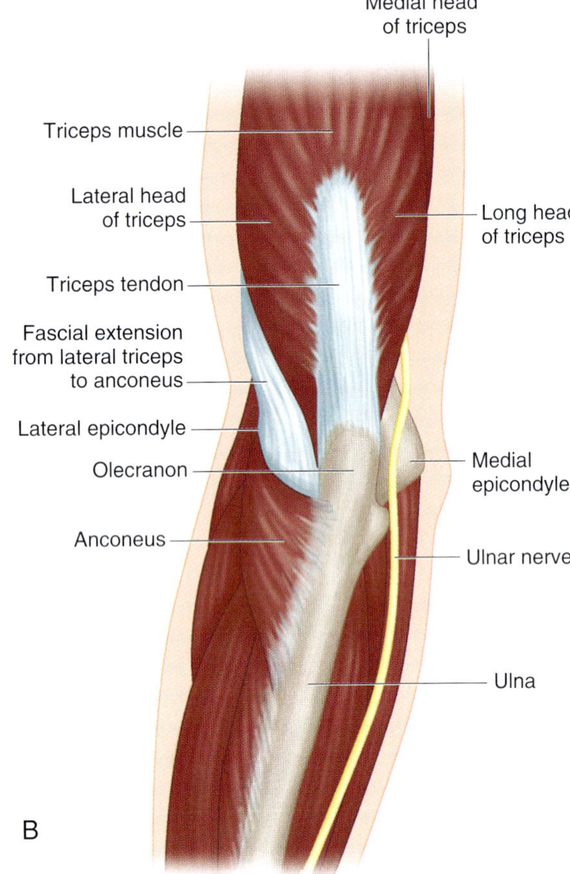

B

FIGURE 4

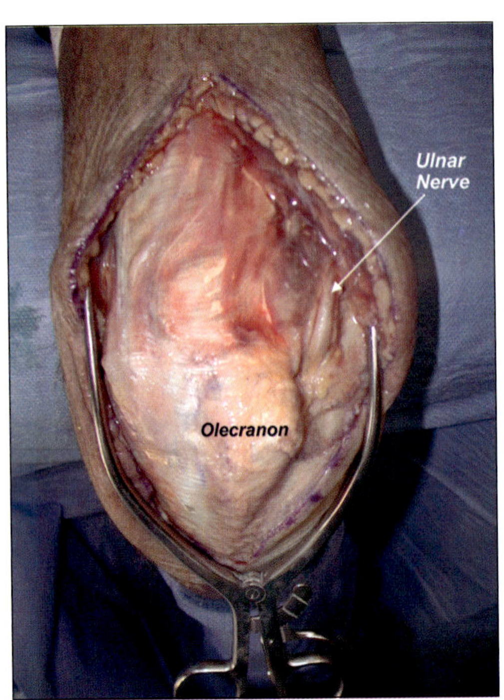

FIGURE 5

- A lateral fascial band passes from the triceps tendon to the anconeus, which can allow for some active elbow extension in the face of a complete tendon avulsion (Fig. 4A and 4B).
- The ulnar nerve lies directly anterior to the medial head of the triceps and immediately behind the medial intermuscular septum (Fig. 5).

Positioning

- The patient is placed supine with the arm and elbow folded over the body.

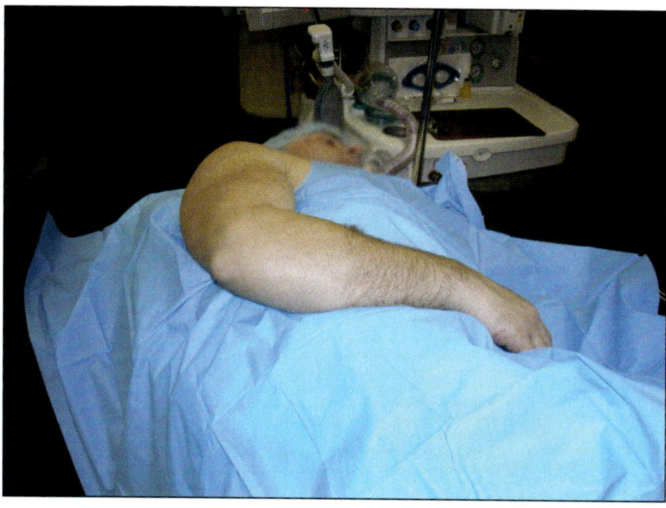

FIGURE 6

Equipment

- Sterile tourniquet high on the arm
- Beanbag

- Rotating the body 30–45° with a bolster or beanbag under the ipsilateral side allows easier visualization of the posterior arm (Fig. 6).
- Alternatively, the contralateral-side-down lateral decubitus position can be used. In this position, a bump or custom crutch that attaches to the operating table is helpful to support the upper arm, leaving the forearm to hang freely (Fig. 7).

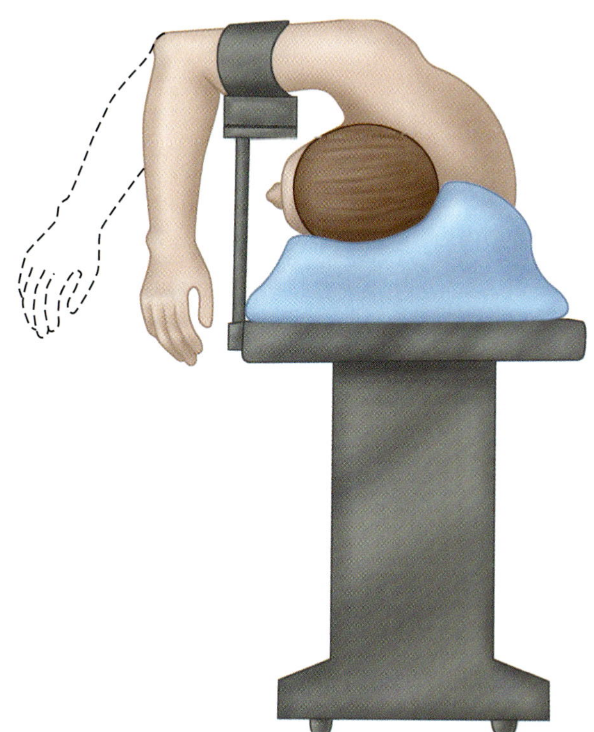

FIGURE 7

Portals/Exposures

- A straight or gentle curvilinear incision is made through the skin and subcutaneous tissue just lateral to the midline (Fig. 8).
- Skin flaps are elevated off of the triceps, ulna, anconeus, and flexor carpi ulnaris.
- The ulnar nerve is identified and protected but typically not formally decompressed or transposed.
- The ulna is exposed several centimeters distal to the olecranon for exit of the drill holes and repair sutures (Fig. 9).

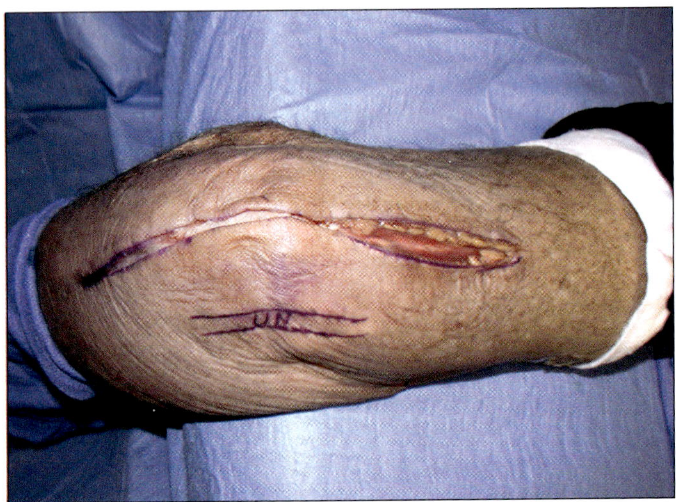

FIGURE 8

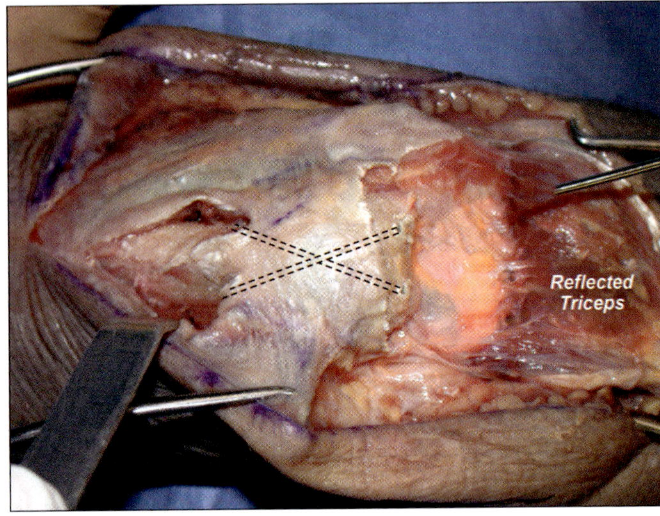

FIGURE 9

PITFALLS

- *A completely ruptured triceps tendon can invert into the triceps muscle proximally. It is important to identify this to maximize tendon length for repair.*

Instrumentation/Implantation

- High-speed burr

Procedure: Primary Repair—Anatomic Reattachment of the Triceps Tendon to Bone through Drill Holes

STEP 1

- The stump of the avulsed tendon is identified and débrided back to normal-appearing tendon. Small avulsed bony fragments are excised (Fig. 10).
- The lateral aponeurotic extension to the anconeus is often intact, preventing significant proximal migration of the tendon.
- The insertion site on the posterior olecranon is partially decorticated with a burr (Fig. 11).

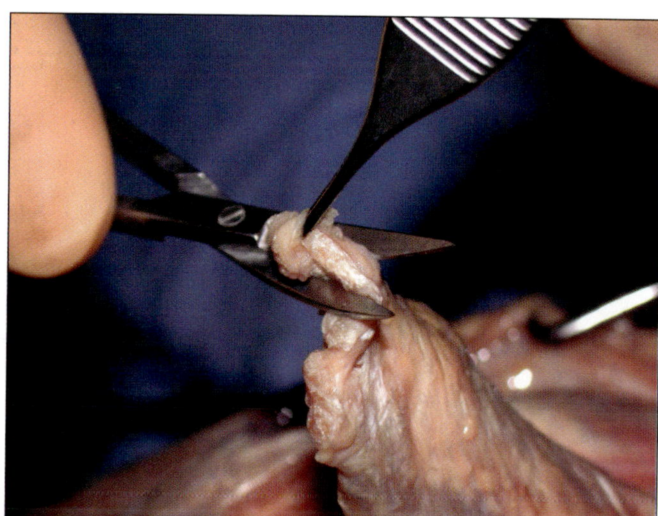

FIGURE 10

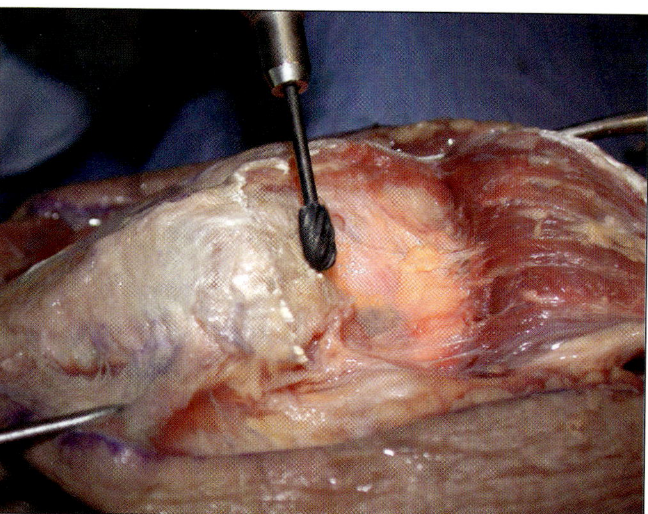

FIGURE 11

STEP 2

- Cruciate 2.5-mm drill holes are made starting at the triceps insertion site and exiting the ulna distal to the olecranon (Fig. 12).
- A #2 or #5 high-strength suture is passed in a running locked fashion into the stump of the tendon starting at the distal end, working proximally for 4–6 cm and then back distally (Fig. 13).

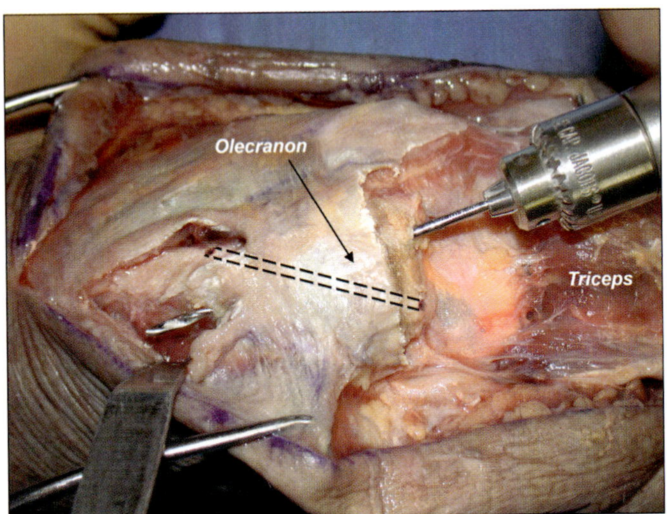

FIGURE 12

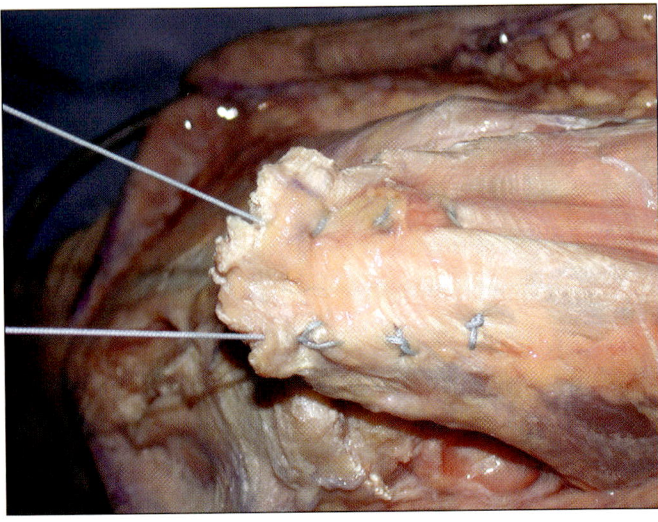

FIGURE 13

Pearls

- *If there is a sufficiently large bony avulsion, it can be reattached with a screw, affording bone-to-bone rather than tendon-to-bone healing (Fig. 14A and 14B).*

Instrumentation/ Implantation

- High-speed drill
- High-strength #2 or #5 nonabsorbable suture

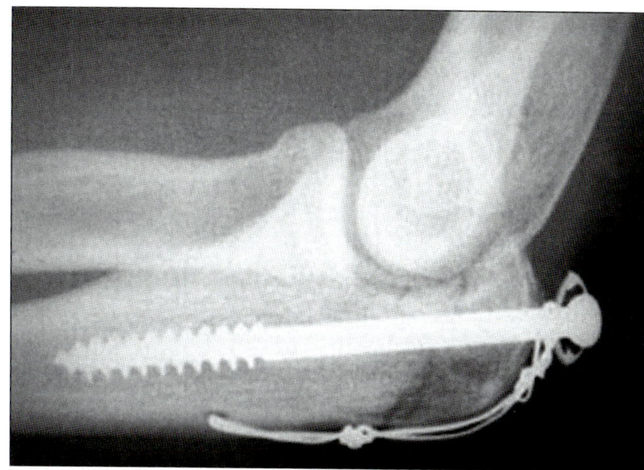

A

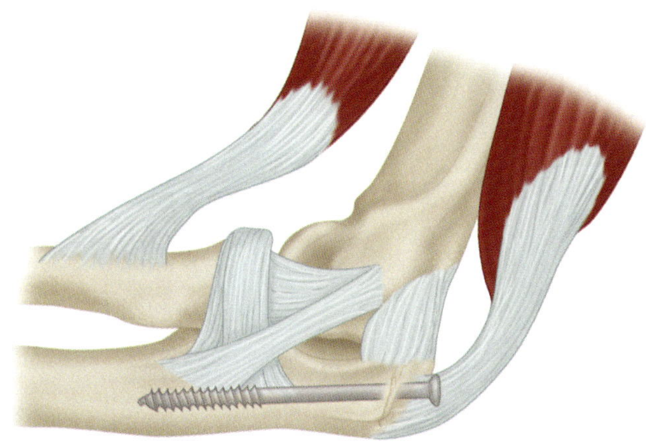

B

FIGURE 14

Pearls

- *Consider augmenting the repair with a proximally based flap of forearm fascia or a distally based partial-thickness flap of triceps fascia if there is excessive tension on the repair in 90° of flexion (see Procedure: Tendon Graft for Chronic Triceps Ruptures below).*

Step 3

- The sutures are passed through the drill holes using Keith needles (Fig. 15).
- With the elbow in extension, the tendon is advanced to the olecranon and the sutures are tied with the knot placed laterally to avoid irritation of the ulnar nerve (Fig. 16).
- Once repaired, flexion to 90° should be obtainable.

Step 4

- The wound is irrigated. If exposure required significant elevation of skin flaps, creating potential dead space, consideration should be given to the use of a subcutaneous drain for 24 hours.
- Skin and subcutaneous tissue are closed in the standard fashion.
- A bulky compressive dressing is applied as well as a long-arm splint in 30–40° of flexion depending on the tension on the repair site.

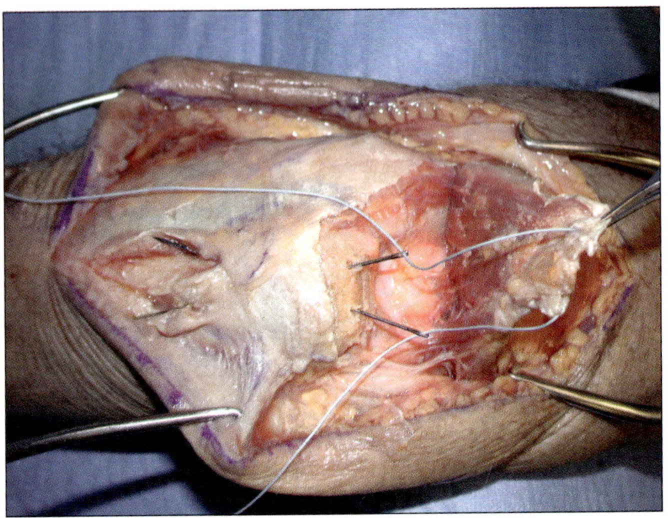

FIGURE 15

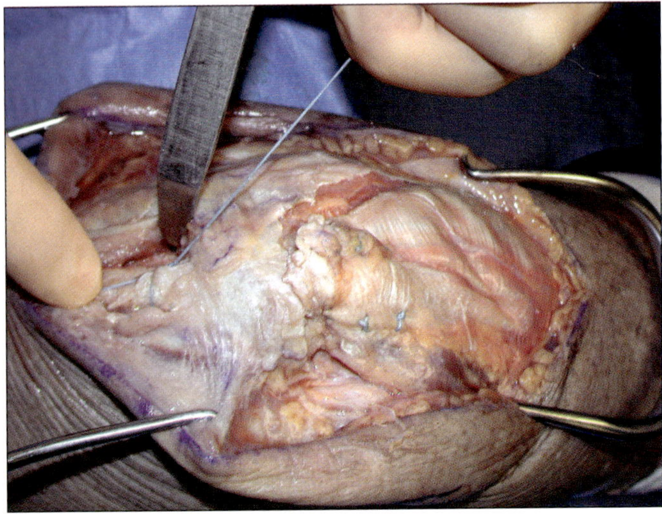

FIGURE 16

Procedure: Tendon Graft for Chronic Triceps Ruptures

Instrumentation/ Implantation

- Tendon stripper (Fig. 18)

Step 1

- If the tendon quality is good and there is minimal tendon retraction, a delayed primary repair can be achieved.
- In the face of poor tendon quality with significant retraction:
  - Small defects can be reconstructed with a palmaris longus, plantaris, or flexor carpi radialis autograft.
  - Larger defects require a hamstring autograft or an Achilles or hamstring allograft.
- Triceps and olecranon preparation are identical to the technique for a primary repair.
- To maximize length, the triceps tendon is tenolysed superficially and deep up to the level of the spiral groove.
- The tendon graft is harvested with a tendon stripper and woven through the stump of the triceps tendon (Fig. 17).

Step 2

- High-strength #2 or #5 suture is used to sew the tendon graft to the triceps tendon and also to itself (Fig. 19).

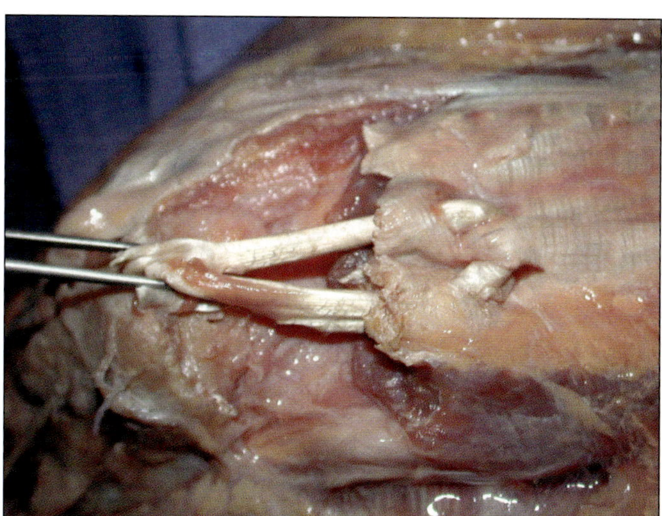

FIGURE 17

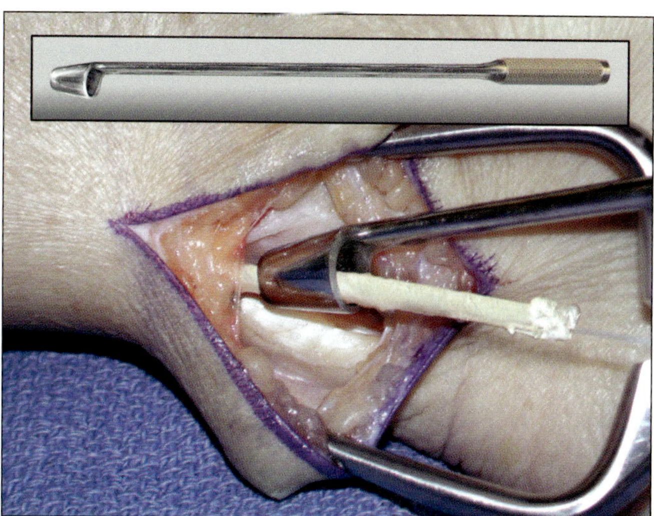

FIGURE 18

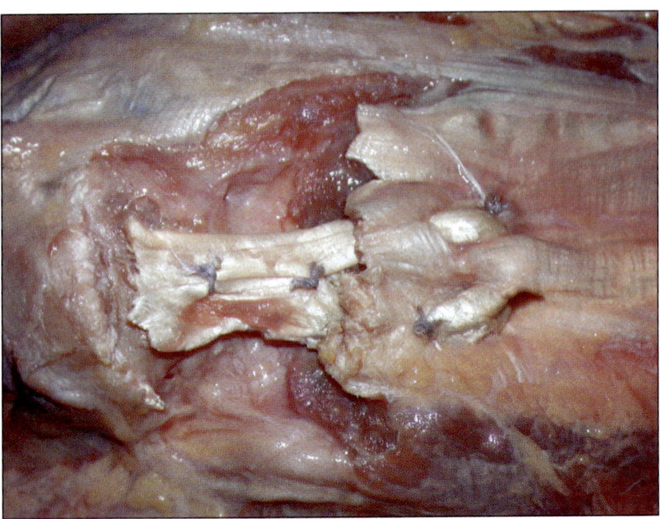

FIGURE 19

- The same suture is passed through the graft and triceps tendon in a running locked fashion and then passed through cruciate bone tunnels in the olecranon similar to that for a primary repair (Fig. 20).

STEP 3

- The repair is secured such that there is moderate tension on the repair site at 90° of flexion.
- The repair can be augmented with a proximally based flap of forearm fascia (Fig. 21) (Bennett, 1962) or a distally based partial-thickness flap of triceps fascia (Fig. 22A–C) (Clayton and Thirupathi, 1984).

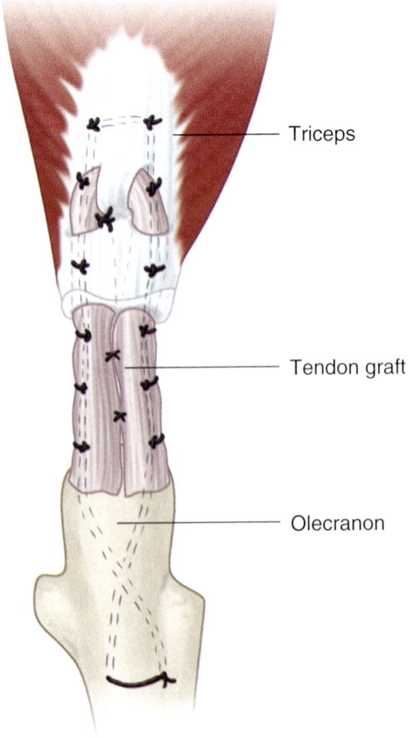

FIGURE 20

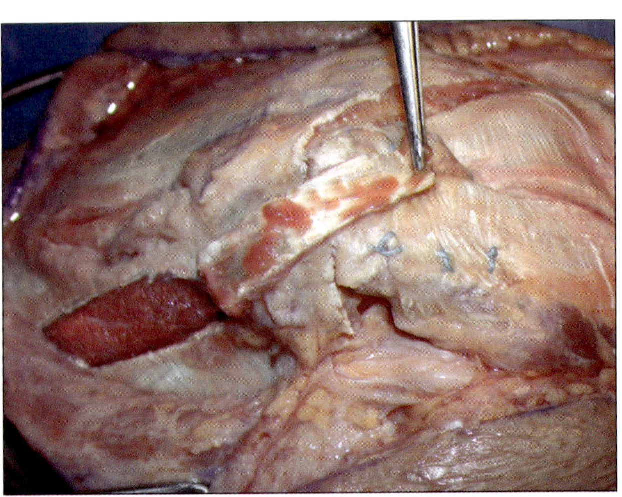

FIGURE 21

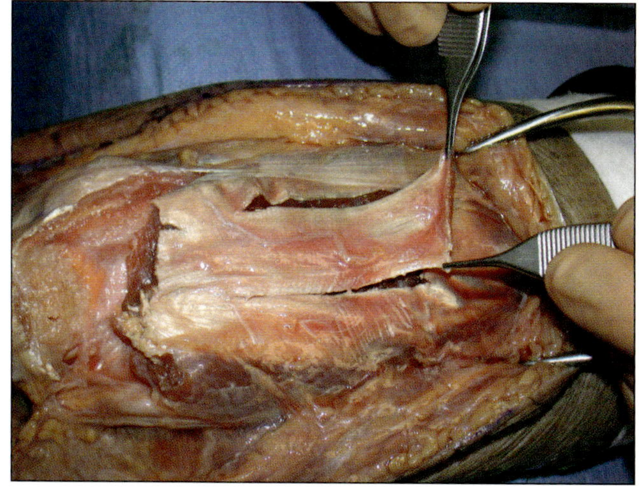
A

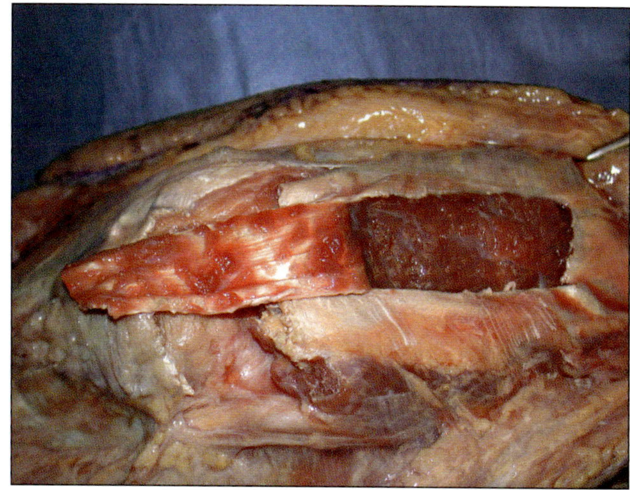
B

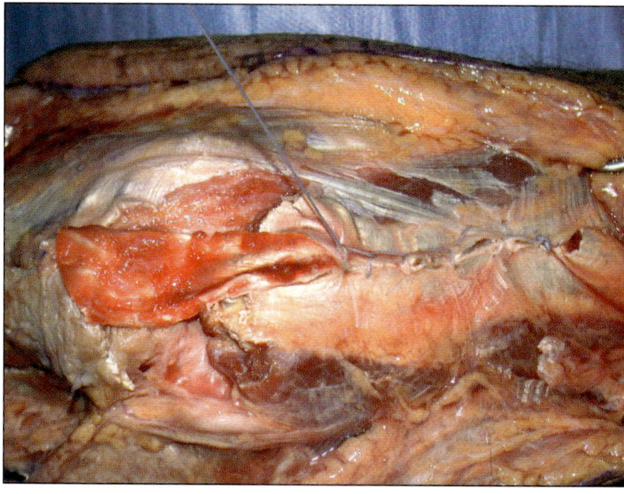
C

FIGURE 22

- A drain is used as needed and the wound is closed in the standard fashion.
- The elbow is immobilized in 30–40° of elbow flexion.

Procedure: Anconeus Rotation Flap

Step 1

- An anconeus rotation flap is indicated for chronic ruptures in which the anconeus muscle and lateral triceps fascia are preserved and the triceps defect is relatively small (Morrey, 2008).
- Tendon and olecranon preparation are identical to that for a primary repair.
- To maximize length, the triceps tendon is tenolysed superficially and deep up to the level of the spiral groove.

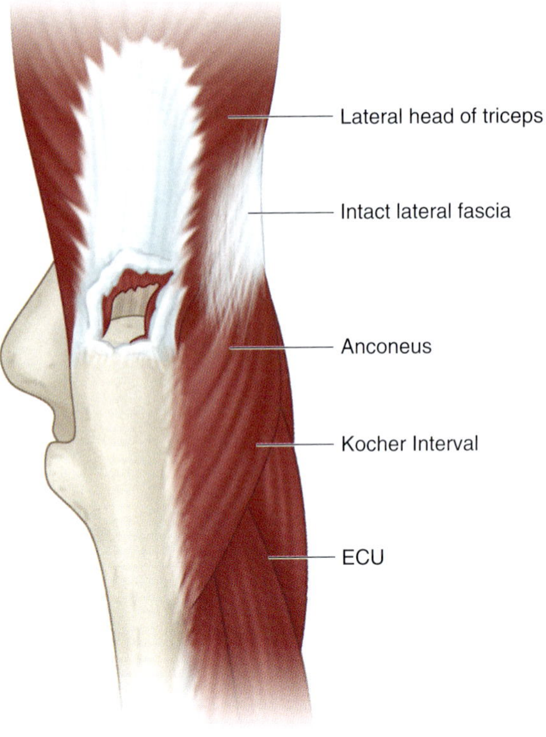

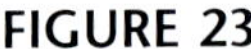

FIGURE 23

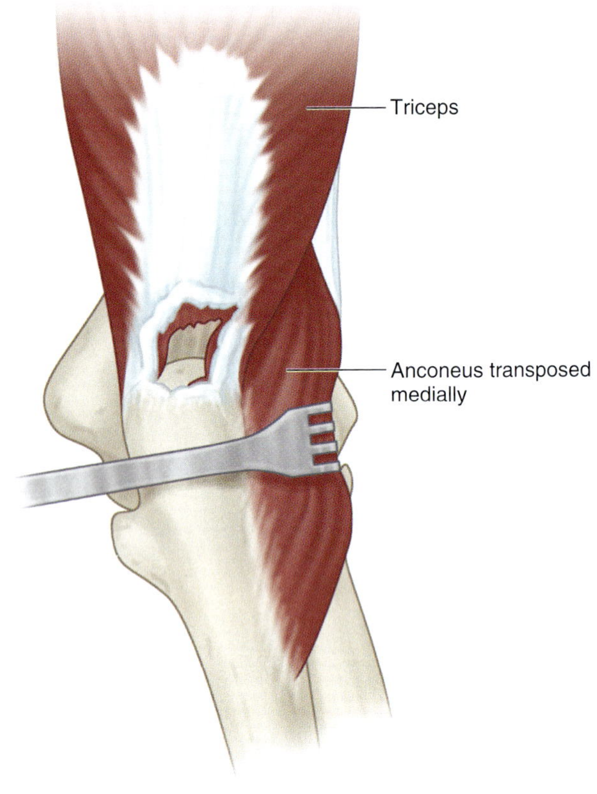

FIGURE 24

Step 2

- If the triceps defect is small, the Kocher interval between the anconeus and the extensor carpi ulnaris is entered (Fig. 23).
- The anconeus is mobilized off of the ulna and the humerus, care being taken to preserve its superficial fascial connection to the lateral triceps.
- Ideally the anconeus distal attachment is left intact and the entire muscle and lateral triceps are translated medially to close the triceps defect (Fig. 24).

Step 3

- The anconeus is secured to the olecranon through drill holes.
- The stump of the triceps is sutured to the medial fascia of the anconeus (Fig. 25).
- The wound is closed in the standard fashion and the elbow is immobilized in 30–45° of flexion.

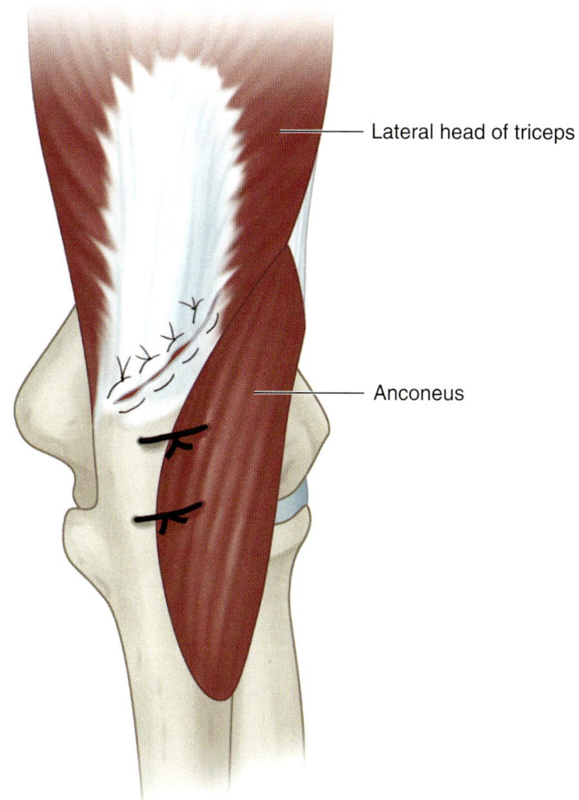

FIGURE 25

> **Pitfalls**
>
> - *Adequate lateral fascial release must be done to prevent the triceps from slipping back laterally with elbow flexion.*

Procedure: Achilles Tendon Allograft

Step 1

- Chronic triceps rupture with significant muscle retraction and a large tendon defect requires allograft repair (see Fig. 5)
- Tendon and olecranon preparation are identical to that for primary repair.
- The Achilles tendon is detached from the calcaneus (Fig. 26) and repaired directly to the olecranon through drill holes as described for a direct repair (see Fig. 15).

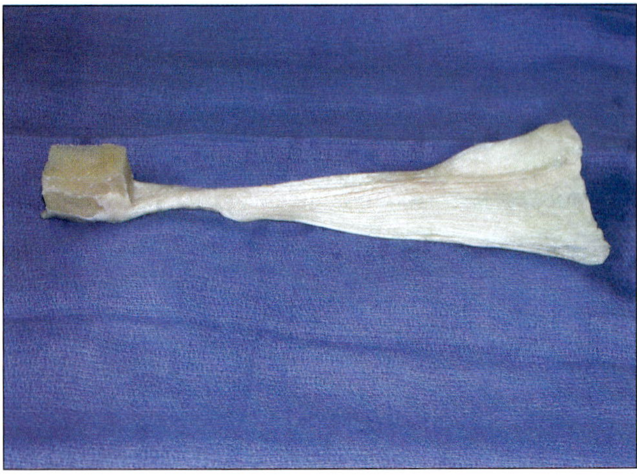

FIGURE 26

- In cases of total elbow arthroplasty with loss of bone stock, the calcaneal portion of the allograft (Fig. 27A) can be fixed to the remaining olecranon (Fig. 27B) with a tension-band wire to improve the mechanical advantage of the triceps (Fig. 28) (Celli et al., 2005).

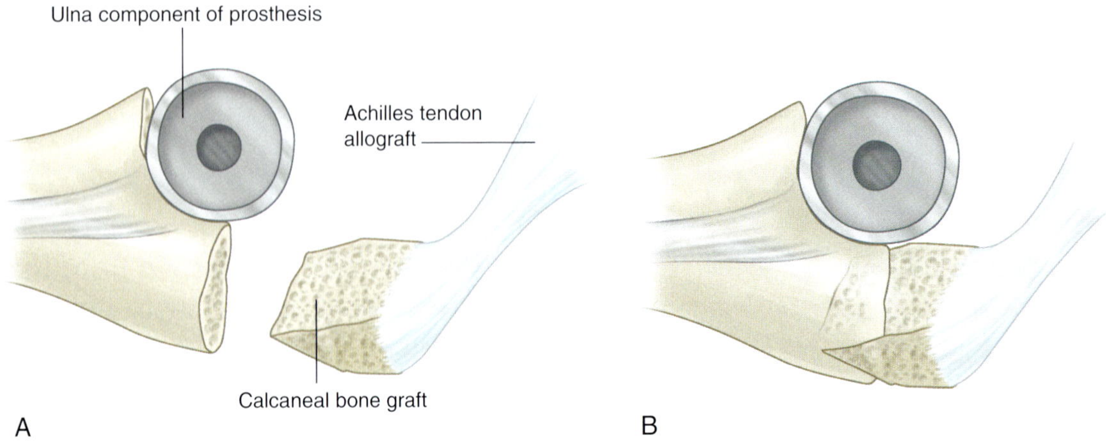

FIGURE 27

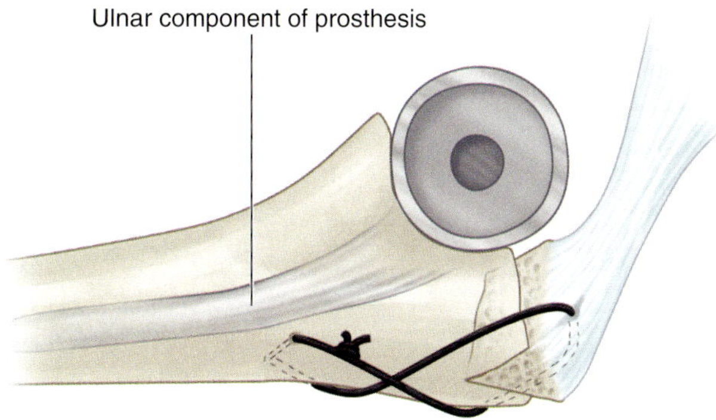

FIGURE 28

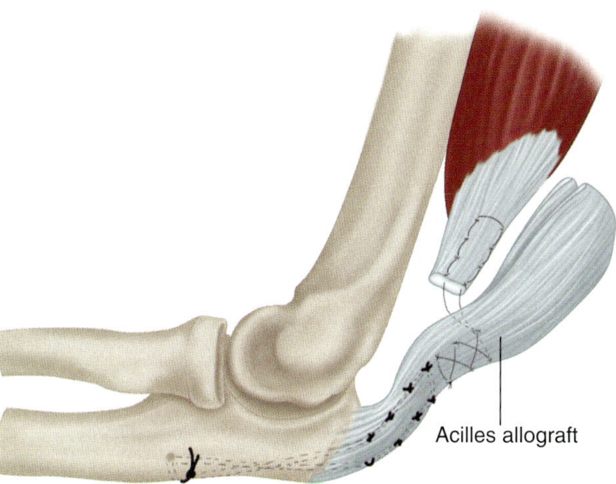

FIGURE 29

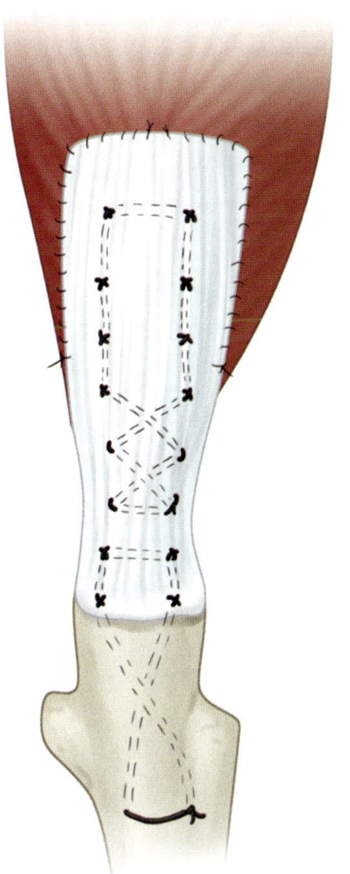

FIGURE 30

Step 2

- A #2 or #5 high-strength suture is placed in the distal triceps stump in a running locked fashion and passed through and tied to the Achilles allograft under moderate tension in 40–60° of elbow flexion (Fig. 29).
- The proximal portion of the graft is wrapped around and sutured to the remaining triceps tendon (Fig. 30).
- The wound is closed and the elbow immobilized in 30–45° of flexion.

PITFALLS

- *Excessive bulk of the allograft might make wound closure difficult.*

Postoperative Care and Expected Outcomes

PRIMARY REPAIR

- The postoperative splint is removed at 10–14 days and a hinge brace is applied with a flexion block at 30–45° (Fig. 31).
- Active flexion and passive extension are allowed.
- If full passive extension is difficult to achieve, then a night splint in full extension is used.
- The flexion block is gradually decreased between weeks 3 and 6 (see Fig. 31), allowing full active flexion at 6 weeks.
- Active extension is allowed at 6 weeks and passive flexion is allowed at 8 weeks.
- Isometric triceps strengthening is started at 10–12 weeks, progressing to full strengthening.
- Unrestricted activity is allowed at 5 months postoperative (Blackmore et al., 2006).

OTHER REPAIRS

- Tendon autograft and allograft for chronic triceps ruptures: The postoperative protocol is the same as that for primary repair but all steps are delayed by 2 weeks to allow for adequate graft revascularization.
- Anconeus rotation flap: The postoperative protocol is similar to that for acute repairs.

EXPECTED OUTCOMES

- Primary repair is usually achievable within the first 3–4 weeks of injury in the majority of patients.
- A 5–10° loss of terminal extension can be expected, with strength returning to approximately 90% of normal (Van Riet et al., 2003).
- Recovery can be slow, with continued improvement seen between the third and sixth months.

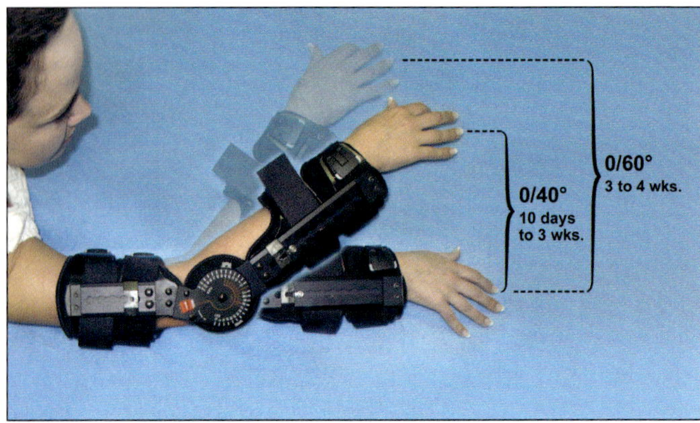

FIGURE 31

Evidence

Bennett BS. Triceps tendon rupture. J Bone Joint Surg [Am]. 1962;44:741-4.

This case report described the repair of an acutely ruptured triceps tendon using a proximally based sleeve of forearm fascia. A flap of fascia was raised from the posterior aspect of the forearm, leaving its base attached to the medial and lateral epicondyles and the olecranon.

Blackmore SM, Jander RM, Culp RW. Management of distal biceps and triceps ruptures. J Hand Ther. 2006;19:154-68.

The authors presented an extensive review of the postoperative rehabilitation following distal triceps repairs. The protocol was broken down into phases: protected, progressive motion, and strengthening.

Celli A, Arash A, Adams RA, Morrey BF. Triceps insufficiency following total elbow arthroplasty. J Bone Joint Surg [Am]. 2005;87:1957-64.

This study was a retrospective review of 16 elbows with tricep insufficiency after total elbow arthroplasty. The results of a direct repair, anconeus rotation flap, and Achilles tendon allograft were reported. A good treatment algorithm was presented. (Level IV evidence [case series])

Clayton ML, Thirupathi RG. Rupture of the triceps tendon with olecranon bursitis, a case report with a new method of repair. Clin Orthop Relat Res. 1984;(184):183-5.

The authors presented a description of the use of the distally based triceps fascia/ tendon turndown flap to reconstruct a chronically ruptured triceps tendon.

Morrey BF. Open treatment of acute and chronic triceps tendon ruptures. In: Yamaguchi K, ed., Advanced reconstruction elbow. Rosemont, IL: American Academy of Orthopaedic Surgeons, 2007;107-13.

The author described his technique and rehabilitation protocol for direct repair of triceps ruptures. Anconeus rotation flap and Achilles tendon allograft reconstruction were also described and illustrated. (Level V evidence)

Van Riet RP, Morrey BF, Ho E, O'Driscoll SW. Surgical treatment of distal triceps ruptures. J Bone Joint Surg [Am]. 2003;85:1961-7.

This study was a retrospective review of the results of 14 direct repairs and 9 reconstructions of various types. When comparing the two groups, the total arc of motion was similar; however, isokinetic peak strength averaged 92% of that in the uninvolved extremity in the direct repair group compared to 66% in the reconstruction group. (Level IV evidence [case series])

SECTION II

Elbow Nerves

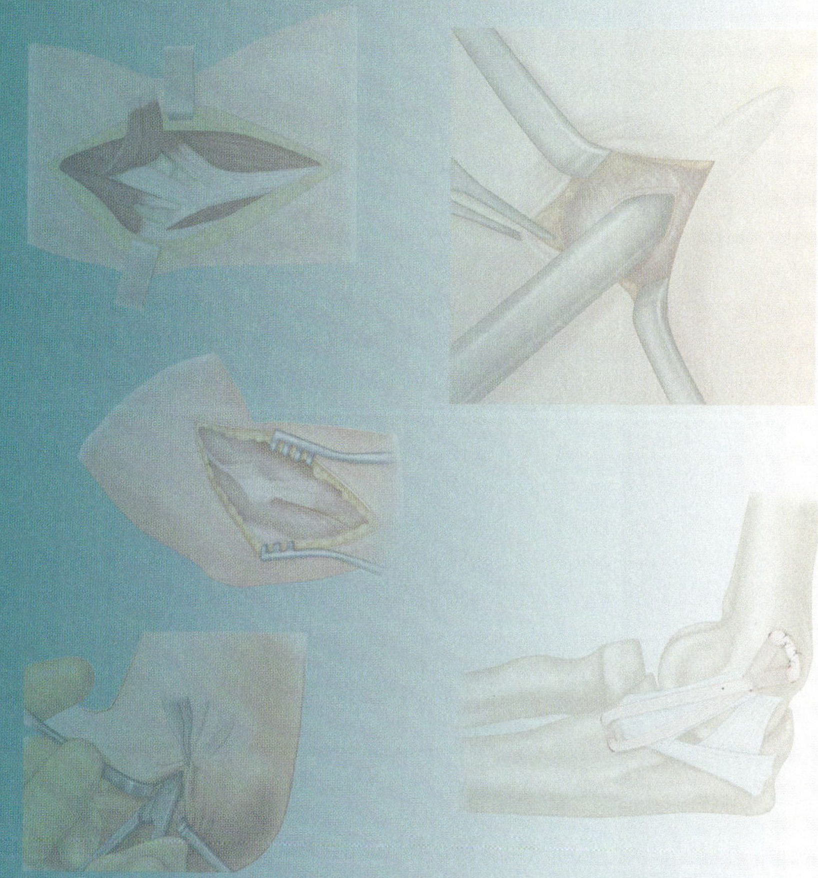

PROCEDURE 53

Endoscopic Cubital Tunnel Release

Tyson Cobb

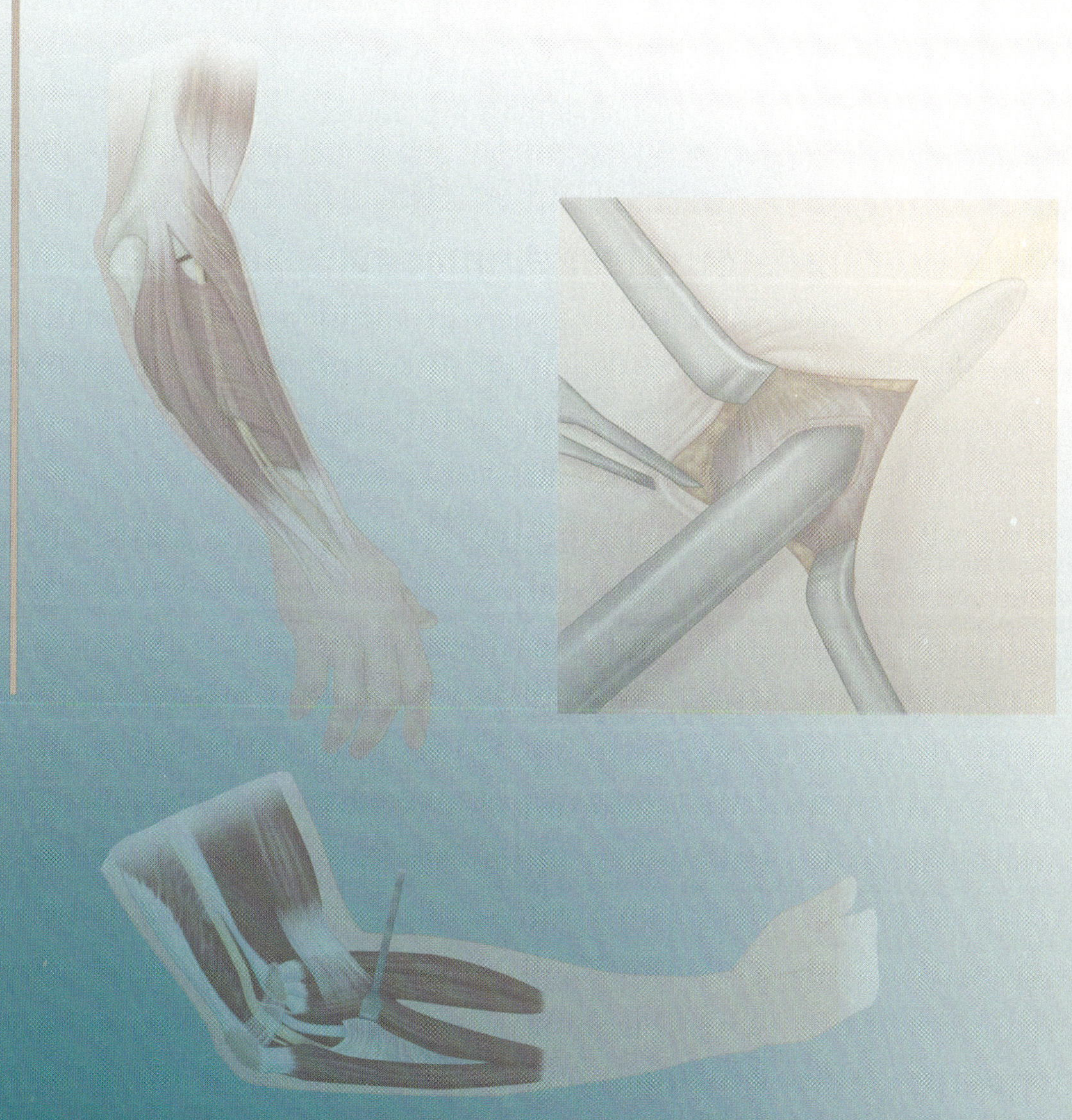

Figures 4B, 5B, 6B, 10, 12B, 13B, 14, and 15 courtesy of Integra LifeSciences Corporation, Cincinnati, Ohio.

Pitfalls

- *Contraindications*
  - *Masses or space-occupying lesions*
  - *Severe and long-standing elbow contractures requiring release*
  - *Conditions necessitating anterior transposition, such as humeral malunions with cubitus valgus*
  - *Prior surgery or trauma with a scarred and adherent nerve*
  - *Dislocating ulnar nerve and concomitant prominent ulnar neuritis with symptoms reproduced during elbow flexion*

Controversies

- Patients with a subluxing ulnar nerve are a relative contraindication.
- Patients with cubital tunnel in which symptoms predominate in the hand (as opposed to prominent medial-sided elbow pain) in association with a subluxing ulnar nerve will respond favorably to endoscopic cubital tunnel release.
- Patients with medial epicondylosis tend to have a more protracted course postoperatively, particularly if concomitant medial epicondylectomy is performed.

Treatment Options

- Conservative treatment includes elbow splinting at night. The author typically uses pillow splints to maintain some degree of elbow extension (at night), job/activity modification, and steroid and nonsteroidal medications.

Indications

- Idiopathic cubital tunnel in patients failing conservative treatment

Examination/Imaging

- Patients are evaluated for the presence of Tinel's sign over the ulnar nerve at the elbow, subjective diminution, atrophy, and the presence of a mass over the ulnar nerve. Additional assessments include flexion-compression and two-point discrimination tests.
- Magnetic resonance imaging is indicated if a palpable mass is present.
- Anteroposterior and lateral radiographs may be obtained if necessary to rule out bony abnormalities.

Surgical Anatomy

- The ulnar nerve, comprising the ventral rami of the C8 and T1 nerve roots, exits the brachial plexus as the terminal branch of the medial cord. It passes through the medial aspect of the anterior compartment of the brachium.
  - The ulnar nerve then passes through the intermuscular septum and enters the posterior compartment of the arm. It passes through a band of deep brachial fascia attached to the intermuscular septum—the arcade of Struthers—approximately 8 cm proximal to the medial epicondyle (Fig. 1, Med. epi.).
  - The ulnar nerve passes posterior to the intermuscular septum and deep to the deep brachial fascia. It courses under the cubital tunnel retinaculum, where it lies posterior to the medial epicondyle. The cubital tunnel retinaculum or Osborne's ligament serves as the roof of the cubital tunnel proper, attaching to the medial epicondyle and the olecranon (Olec. in Fig. 1). The floor of the cubital tunnel is composed of the elbow joint, its capsule, and the medial collateral ligament.
  - The ulnar nerve continues distally in the forearm deep to the deep layer of the aponeurosis of the two heads of the flexor carpi ulnaris (FCU) muscle (Osborne's fascia). Proximally this fascia comprises two layers that invest the FCU muscle. The more superficial layer continues as the deep fascia of the

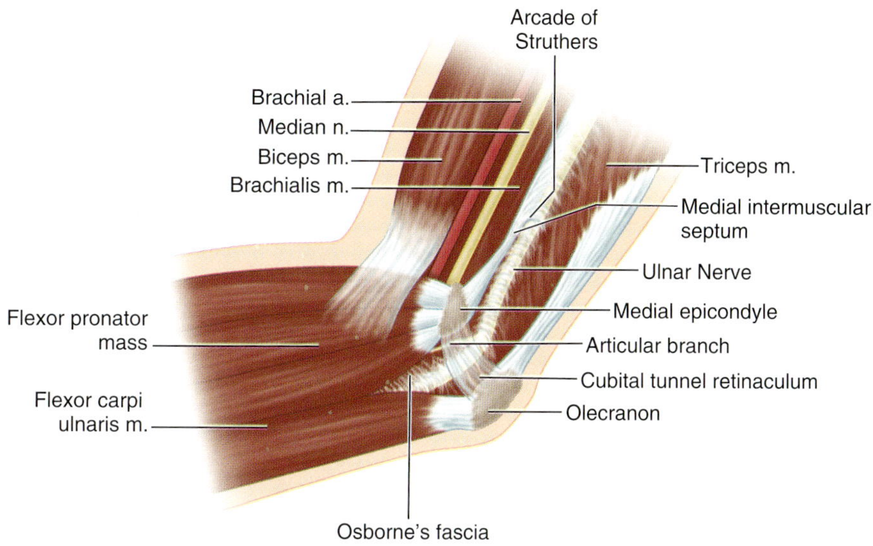

FIGURE 1

forearm. The deeper layer continues distally as the deep fascia of the FCU muscle.

- The structures implicated in the compression of the ulnar nerve at the elbow are often described and depicted in drawings as isolated and distinctly separate anatomic structures. In reality, they represent a continuous or contiguous layer forming a tunnel both proximally and distally.
- The proximal portion of the release includes the cubital tunnel retinaculum (Osborne's ligament) and the deep brachial fascia, which is said to be thickened proximally (arcade of Struthers). The significance of the latter is questionable. The deep brachial fascia and arcade of Struthers are seldom a significant source of ulnar nerve compression. The author has never seen convincing morphologic ulnar nerve changes suggesting compression at this level.
- The distal portion of the release includes the distal portion of the cubital tunnel retinaculum (Osborne's ligament), the aponeurosis of the two heads of the FCU muscle (Osborne's fascia), and more distally the fascia deep to the FCU muscle (Fig. 2). During open release, the deep fascia of the forearm and FCU muscle tissue must also be opened and separated. This is not necessary with endoscopic cubital tunnel release.
- The medial antebrachial cutaneous nerve passes through the brachial fascia along with the basilic vein (Fig. 3). Several branches of the medial antebrachial cutaneous nerve extends distally and posteriorly to

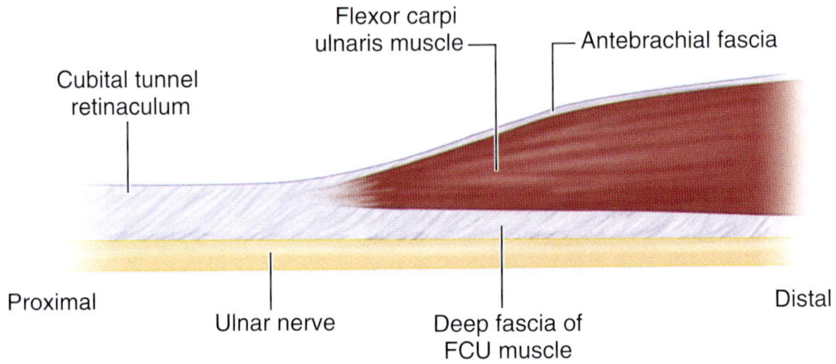

FIGURE 2

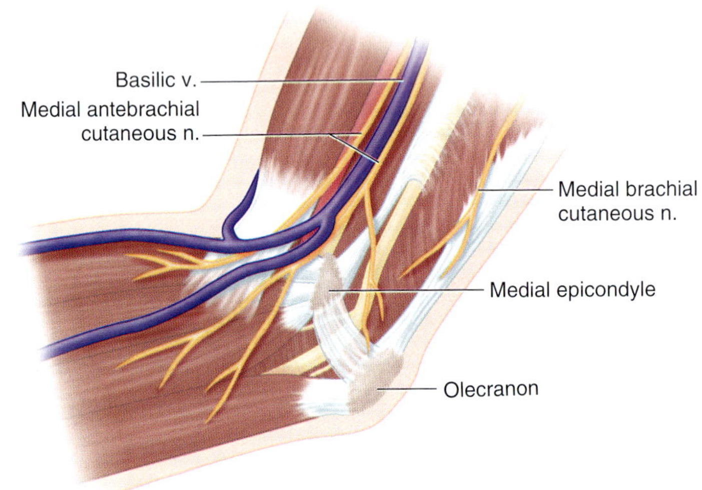

FIGURE 3

innervate the skin overlying the site of endoscopic cubital tunnel release. These branches are often injured during open exposures, resulting in sensitive scar problems postoperatively. During endoscopic cubital tunnel release, these branches are elevated and held out of harm's way by the retractor attached to the cannula.

Positioning

- The patient is placed supine on the operating room table with the shoulder abducted and externally rotated, with the arm on an arm table.
- A nonsterile tourniquet is placed high on the brachium.

Pearls

- *The arm is placed on a bath blanket so as to elevate it off of the arm table sufficiently to facilitate instrumentation of the cubital tunnel.*
- *The nonsterile tourniquet should be placed sufficiently high on the brachium so as not to interfere with release.*

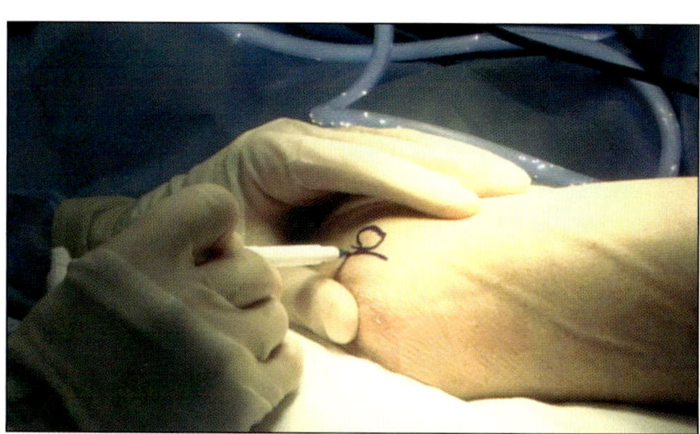
A

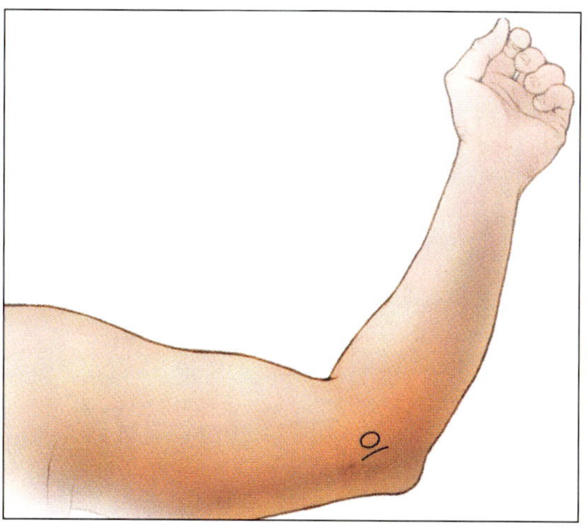
B

FIGURE 4

Pearls

- *The incision can be placed in the skin crease to improve cosmesis.*

Pitfalls

- *For the first few cases, it is recommended to use a longitudinal incision larger than 2 cm until the surgeon is comfortable with the dissection and exposure.*

Portals/Exposures

- A 2-cm incision is made over the cubital tunnel just posterior to the medial epicondyle (Fig. 4A).
- A slightly larger incision is used in obese patients, very large patients, or patients with an anconeus epitrochlearis muscle.
- The incision is made just through the skin (Fig. 4B).

Procedure

Step 1

- Scissors are utilized to dissect directly down to the medial epicondyle (Fig. 5A). Superficial nerves are not intentionally dissected out, but they are protected as they are encountered (Fig. 5B).

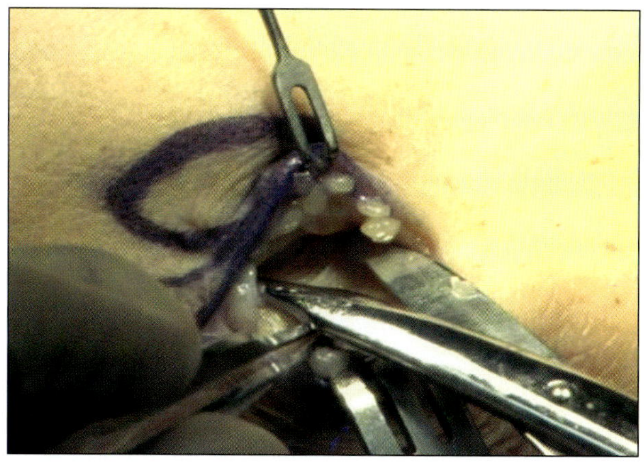
A

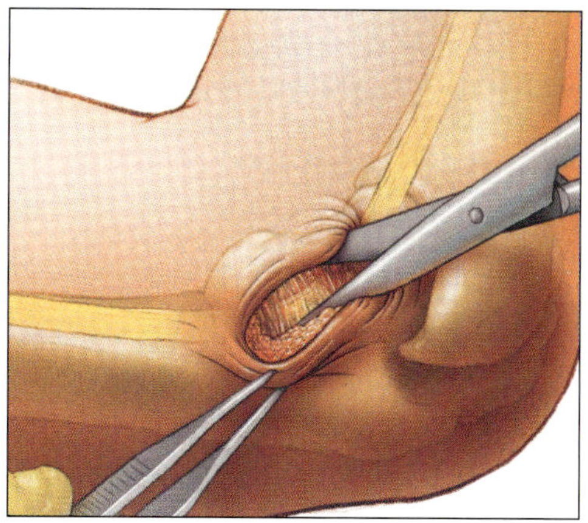
B

FIGURE 5

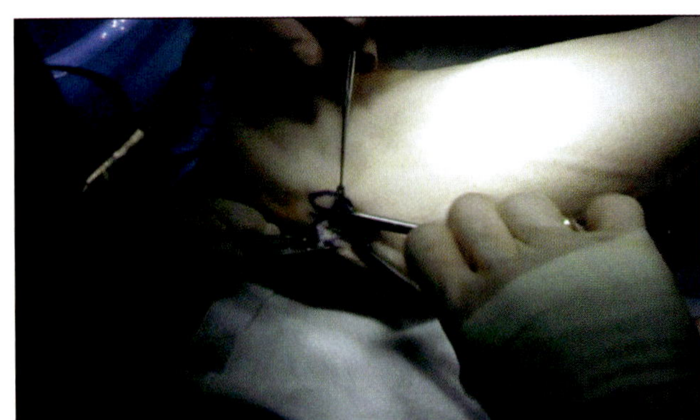
A

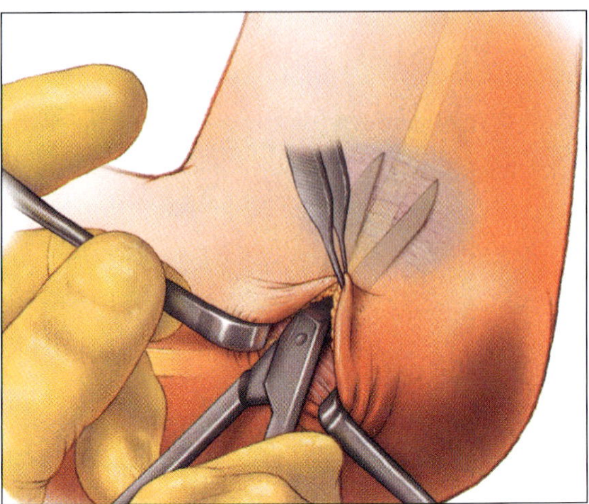
B

FIGURE 6

Pearls

- *Do not violate the deep fascia during the initial exposure.*
- *Narrow retractors are helpful during this portion of the procedure.*
- *Do not dissect through, but rather dissect under the adipose tissue, developing the potential space between the adipose tissue and superficial nerves and the deep fascia.*

Pitfalls

- *Avoid developing multiple layers through the adipose tissue.*
- *Do not open the deep fascia during this portion of the procedure.*

- Once the medial epicondyle is identified, blunt scissors are utilized to dissect the adipose tissue and superficial nerves off the deep fascia over the course of the ulnar nerve both proximally and distally (Fig. 6A and 6B).

Step 2

- The palpating finger is placed directly on the medial epicondyle. Pressure is applied, and the finger is brought posteriorly over the course of the ulnar nerve, and the ulnar nerve is palpated. In some patients this may require fairly deep palpation with the tip of the index finger.

Pearls

- *The canal needs to be open sufficiently to allow instrumentation to be placed without binding.*
- *If an anconeus epitrochlearis muscle is encountered, it is incised directly over the cubital tunnel, and the procedure continues as otherwise described.*

Pitfalls

- *If the canal is not opened sufficiently to prevent binding, or if the elbow is flexed too much in combination with a small opening, there will be risk of violating the canal with instrumentation.*
- *The canal should not be opened beyond the skin incision so as to make layer identification and instrumentation difficult to visualize.*

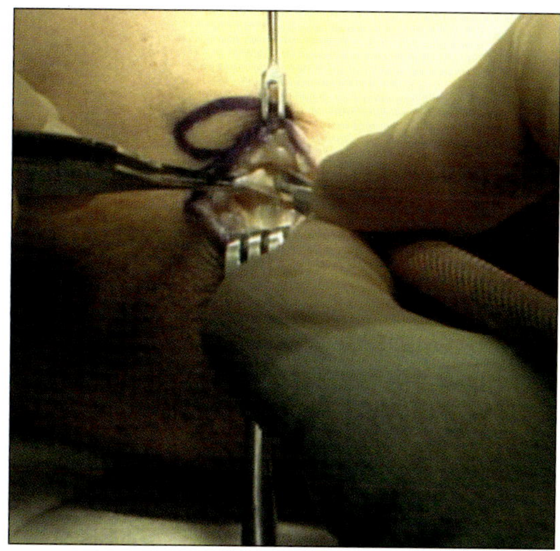

FIGURE 7

PEARLS

- *The spatula, once in the potential space between the ulnar nerve and the roof of the canal, allows the surgeon to confirm the course of the ulnar nerve.*
- *Confirm that the adipose tissue and superficial nerves have been sufficiently elevated off of the fascia throughout the course of the ulnar nerve both proximally and distally.*

PITFALLS

- *If the spatula is placed against resistance, one runs the risk of potentially violating the wall of the canal and complicating the release, or potentially injuring the ulnar nerve.*

Instrumentation/ Implantation

- EndoRelease™ set (Integra LifeSciences Corporation, Cincinnati, OH)

- Once the ulnar nerve position is confirmed, pickups are utilized to place tension on the roof of the cubital tunnel, which is open with a #15 blade (Fig. 7).
- Once the initial fibers are divided and areolar-appearing tissue is visible, scissors are utilized to open the canal several centimeters, exposing the ulnar nerve, which is identified and protected (Fig. 8).

STEP 3

- The author utilizes an EndoRelease set for cubital tunnel release (Fig. 9). Spatulas are included in the set that facilitate placement of instrumentation into the canal.
- The spatula is moistened with saline and inserted in the potential space between the ulnar nerve and the roof of the canal.

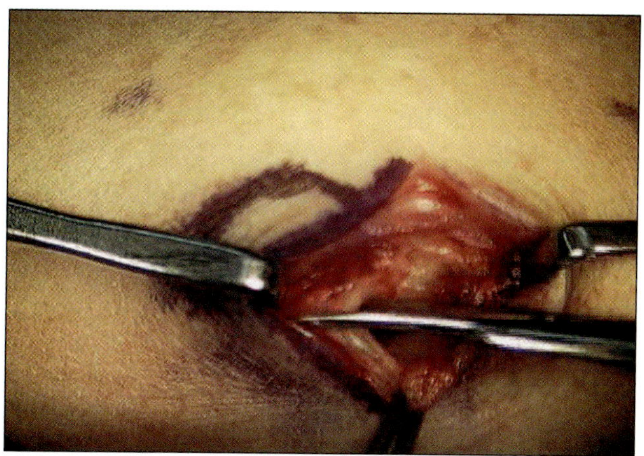

FIGURE 8

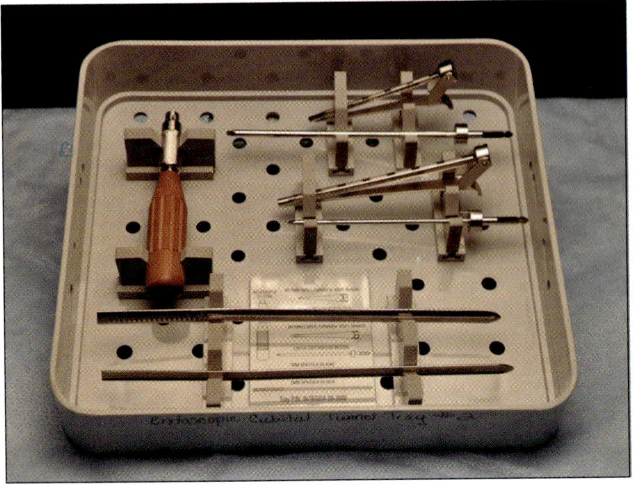

FIGURE 9

Pearls

- *Wet the trocar prior to placement to minimize resistance. If resistance is encountered as the cannula is placed, remove the cannula and confirm that the adipose tissue is not adherent to the deep fascia and therefore binding on the retractor.*
- *The canal may need to be opened slightly with scissors if the instrumention appears to be binding. Extending the elbow will help if the cannula is binding as the canal bends around the medial epicondyle.*

- The spatula is then advanced without resistance. The spatula is placed both proximally and distally (Fig. 10).

Step 4

- The EndoRelease set includes a cannula specifically designed for cubital tunnel release. The cannula has a flat undersurface that helps hold the nerve under the cannula and slots on the inferior surface that allow visualization of the ulnar nerve during the release (Fig. 11).

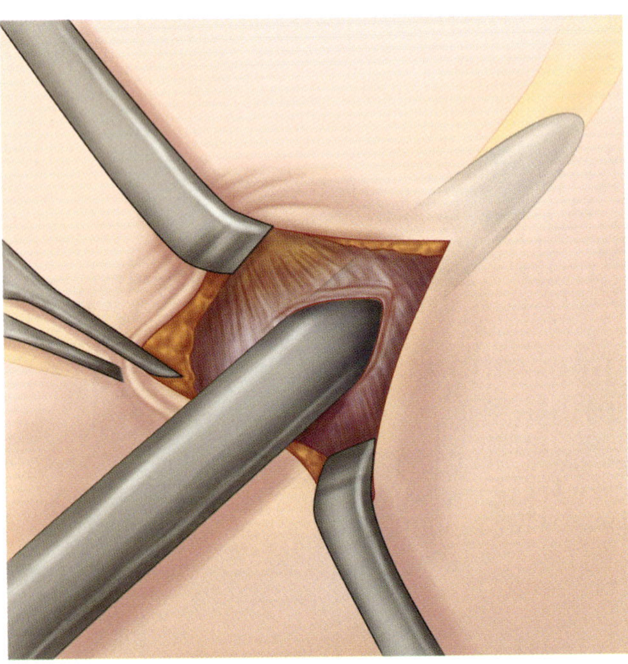

FIGURE 10

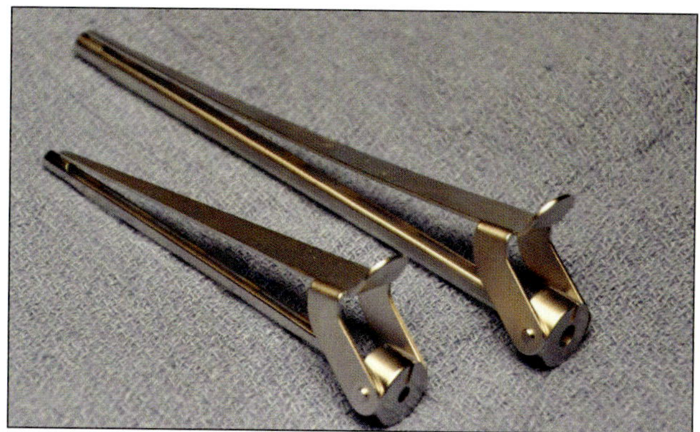

FIGURE 11

Instrumentation/ Implantation

- A standard 30° 4-mm endoscope is used. This is a dry endoscopy, and therefore no fluid is required.

- The cannula/trocar is placed into the canal and advanced proximally between the ulnar nerve and the roof of the canal (Fig. 12A).
- The attached retractor is placed on the external surface of the fascia and allowed to slide on the fascia as the trocar is advanced. The retractor therefore elevates the adipose tissue and superficial nerves out of harm's way (Fig. 12B).
- The trocar is removed from the cannula. The scope is placed initially between the cannula and the retractor to confirm that there are no superficial nerves in harm's way (Fig. 13A and 13B).
- The scope is then placed into the cannula and turned to view the inferior slots to identify the ulnar nerve (Fig. 14).
- The ulnar nerve should be identified throughout the entire course of the cannula. Rotation of the cannula may help identify the nerve as it pops under the flat surface of the cannula.

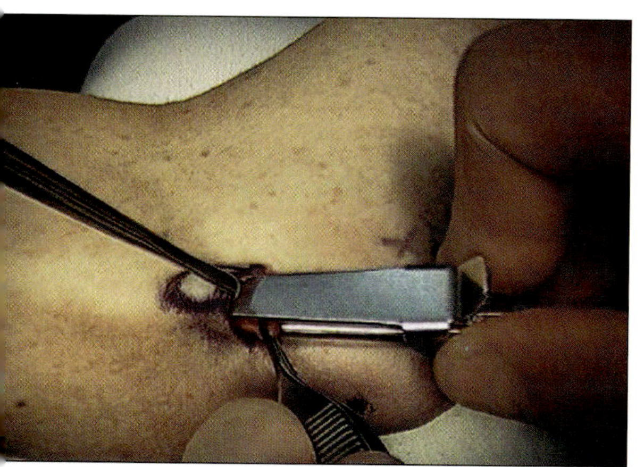

A

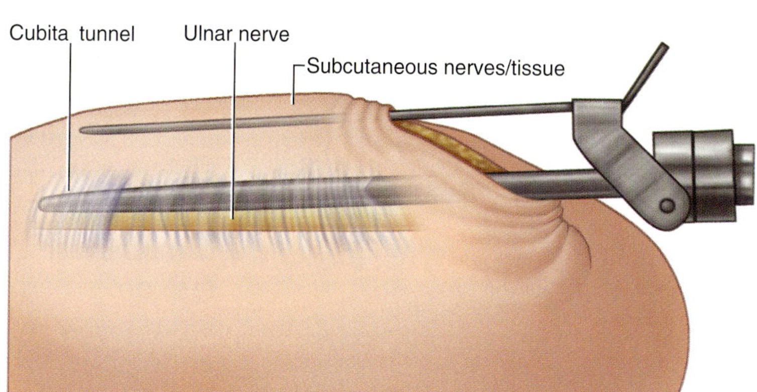

B

FIGURE 12

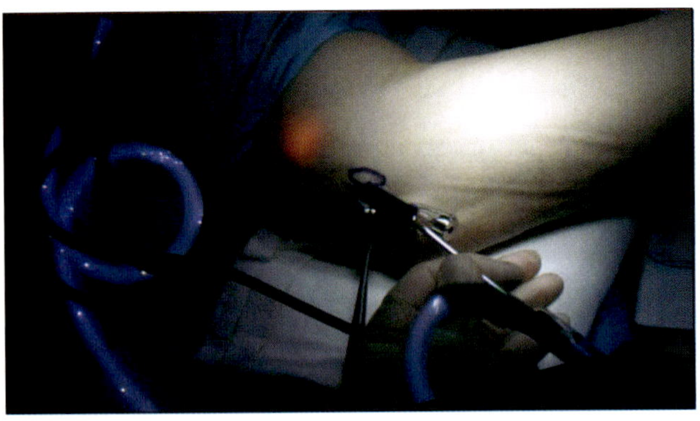
A

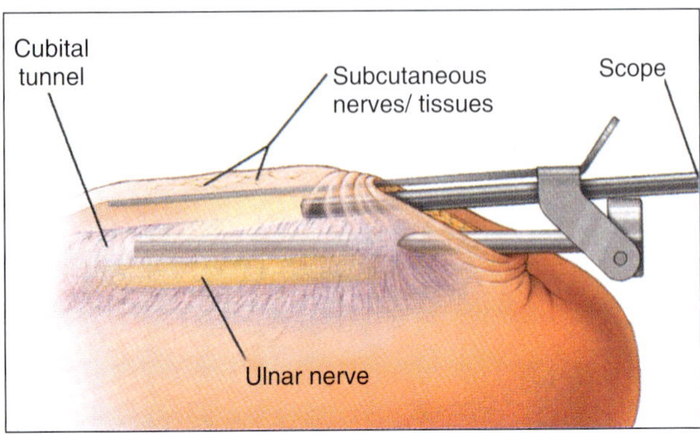

B

FIGURE 13

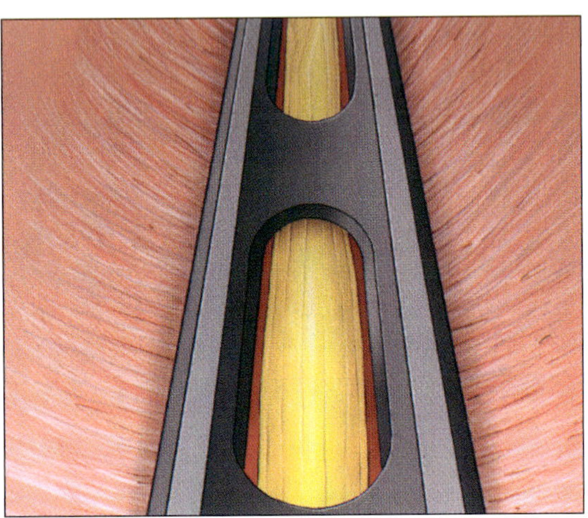

FIGURE 14

- After the nerve is clearly identified, the fascia (roof of the canal) is divided with a push knife along the superior slot of the cannula (Fig. 15).

STEP 5

- The cannula is removed and release is checked with the endoscope to confirm complete release. This can be done by pulling the cannula back on the scope and out of the canal.
- If the release cannot be confirmed visually in this fashion, a narrow retractor is placed exposing the ulnar nerve, which is then visualized with the endoscope, which is held under the retractor.
- The scope is then slowly withdrawn, confirming complete release.

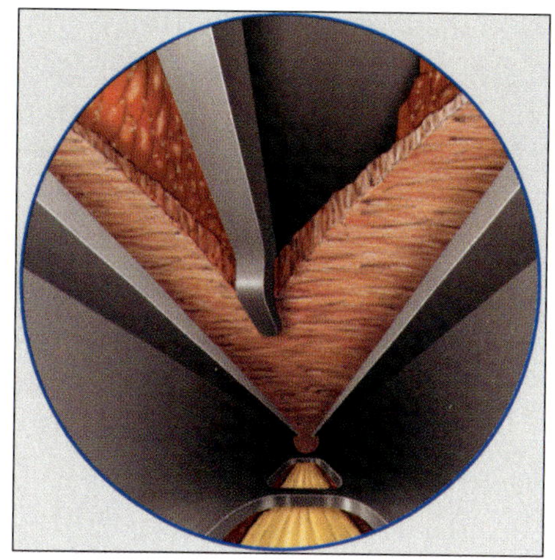

FIGURE 15

PITFALLS

- *Never force the cannula into the canal. This may result in injury to the ulnar nerve or rupture through the wall of the fascia.*
- *Do not release the fascia with the knife if the ulnar nerve is not clearly visible below the cannula. The ulnar nerve may rotate superiorly into harm's way. Therefore, it must be identified visually throughout the course of the entire cannula prior to release of any tissue.*
- *If resistance is encountered, it is usually one of several things:*
  - *Friction has developed because the instrumentation was not wet prior to placement.*
  - *The adipose tissue is not elevated off the fascia and is binding the retractor.*
  - *The canal is not open sufficiently enough, and the instrumentation is binding.*
  - *The elbow is flexed too much, causing the instrumention to bind in the canal.*
  - *The trocar is not being placed in the correct orientation and is hitting either the ulnar nerve or the wall of the canal. Orientation should be confirmed when the spatula is placed, and the trocar should be placed in the exact same orientation.*

STEP 6

- The cannula/trocar are then placed into the canal and advanced distally. The procedure is performed using the same technique as described above.
- After the distal release, the muscle of the flexor-pronator mass will be seen through the superior slot of the cannula. This tissue does not need to be released and may result in unnecessary bleeding if released.

STEP 7

- The tourniquet is dropped and pressure is applied.
- A retractor is then placed into the incision, and the endoscope is utilized to visualize the operative field both proximally and distally to confirm that excessive bleeding is not present. Typical generalized punctuate bleeding is handled easily with direct pressure and a compressive dressing.
- Excessive bleeding may occasionally occur from division of large vessels. These should be cauterized with bipolar cautery. This is facilitated by placement of a retractor while the endoscope is held directly under the retractor, allowing the bipolar cautery to be advanced. Obviously the ulnar nerve needs to be visualized and protected if bipolar cautery is required.

PEARLS

- *Most bleeding can be controlled with direct pressure.*

PITFALLS

- *Hematoma formation is one of the more common complications following endoscopic cubital tunnel release. Therefore, hemostasis should always be obtained prior to closure.*

PEARLS

- *Use of an Angiocath allows for Marcaine with epinephrine to infiltrate throughout the course of the release so as not to be potentially compartmentalized in the adipose tissue, which can occur if this drug is injected with a hypodermic needle after closure.*
- *Furthermore, the Angiocath facilitates placement without fear of potentially injuring the ulnar nerve with hypodermic needle.*

PEARLS

- *Defining expectations for range of motion and return to work with the patient preoperatively will greatly facilitate meeting postoperative goals.*

PITFALLS

- *Wound dehiscence can and will occur during the postoperative range of motion if tight closure is not obtained.*

STEP 8

- A 20-gauge Angiocath is placed through the skin and into the wound. The needle is withdrawn after placement. Placement of the Angiocath is in line with the incision so that the Angiocath does not interfere with placement of Steri-Strips after closure.
- The wound is closed tightly with subcuticular absorbable suture such as 3-0 Monocryl. The closure is supplemented with Steri-Strips.
- If not contraindicated, 15 to 20 ml of 0.5 Marcaine with epinephrine is infiltrated through the Angiocath and directly into the wound.
- The Angiocath is then removed, and a compressive dressing is applied.

Postoperative Care and Expected Outcomes

- Patients are instructed to work on range of motion with the expectation of full range of motion by the first postoperative visit (postoperative day 5–7). They are instructed to debulk the dressing as necessary to facilitate full range of motion.
- Patients can expect to go back to sedentary/office type activity on the first postoperative day. Manual labors are typically restricted for a week, and then advanced as tolerated, with most patients returning to full activity by 1 week.

Evidence

Ahcan U, Zorman P. Endoscopic decompression of the ulnar nerve at the elbow. J Hand Surg [Am]. 2007;32:23-9.

Thirty-six cases of endoscopic cubital tunnel release were reported demonstrating 58% excellence, 33% good, and 8% fair. A hematoma occurred in 1 case. Thirty-two patients returned to full duty/activity by 3 weeks. One hundred percent were satisfied and would have the surgery again.

Bain G, Bajhau A. Endoscopic release of the ulnar nerve and the elbow using the Agee device: a cadaveric study. J Arthroscopic Relat Surg. 2005;21:691-5.

Bruno W, Tsai T. Minimally invasive release of the cubital tunnel. Oper Tech Plast Reconstr Surg. 2002;9:131-7.

Cobb TK, Sterbank P. Comparison of return to work: endoscopic cubital tunnel. Hand. 2007;2:73.

Comparison of return to work: endoscopic cubital tunnel release versus anterior subcutaneous transposition of the ulnar nerve. The authors compare return to work in a retrospective analysis for anterior subcutaneous transposition of the ulnar nerve versus endoscopic cubital tunnel release. The average return to work time for anterior subcutaneous transposition was 70 days compared to 7 days for endoscopic cubital tunnel release.

Cobb TK, Sterbank P. Five year review of endoscopic cubital tunnel release. (Abstract Publication SP41). J Hand Surg [Br]. 2008;33E(Suppl 1):49.

Five-year review of endoscopic cubital tunnel release. Authors reviewed the outcome of 127 consecutive cases of endoscopic cubital tunnel release. The overall outcome as reported by the patients was acceptable and consistent with outcome from open techniques. Complications were minor including cellulitis, wound dehiscence and hematomas. No nerve injuries occurred. There were 75% excellent, 21% good, and 4% fair or poor results.

Cobb TK, Tyler J, Sterbank P, Lemke J. Efficacy of endoscopic cubital tunnel release. Hand. 2008;3:191.

Efficacy of endoscopic cubital tunnel release. The authors compare 113 cases of endoscopic cubital tunnel release to literature controls to evaluate the efficacy. The efficacy was defined as resolution of preoperative paresthesias in the ulnar nerve distribution. The endoscopic release was found to be as efficacious as open releases.

Hoffman R, Siemionow M. The endoscopic management of cubital tunnel syndrome. J Hand Surg [Br]. 2006;31:23-9.

The authors report 76 cases of endoscopic cubital tunnel release. Good to excellent outcome was reported in 94%. Fair to poor outcome was reported in 6%. They reported 4 cases of hematoma, 1 case of CRPS and 9 cases of antebrachial cutaneous nerve abnormality most of which resolved within the first 3 months.

Tsai TM, Chen IC, Majd ME, Lim BH. Cubital tunnel release with endoscopic assistance: results of a new technique. J Hand Surg 1999;24A:21-29.

Eighty-five cases of endoscopic cubital tunnel release were reported. Good to excellent outcome was reported in 97%, and fair to poor in 13%. They reported 4 hematomas. They concluded that the operation was safe and reliable.

Watts AC, Bain GI. Patient rated outcomes of ulnar nerve decompression: a comparison of endoscopic and open in situ decompression. J Hand Surg. 2009;34A:1492-98.

Nineteen cases of endoscopic cubital tunnel release were compared to 15 cases of open in situ release. There was no difference in the preoperative McGowan Score (P = 0.31). The patient's satisfaction was significantly better for endoscopic release (90%) versus open in situ (60%) (P = 0.02). Complications were significantly higher for open release (40%) compared to the endoscopic release (11%) (P = 0.04).

PROCEDURE 54

Submuscular Ulnar Nerve Transposition

Kevin J. Malone, Thanapong Waitayawinyu, and Thomas E. Trumble

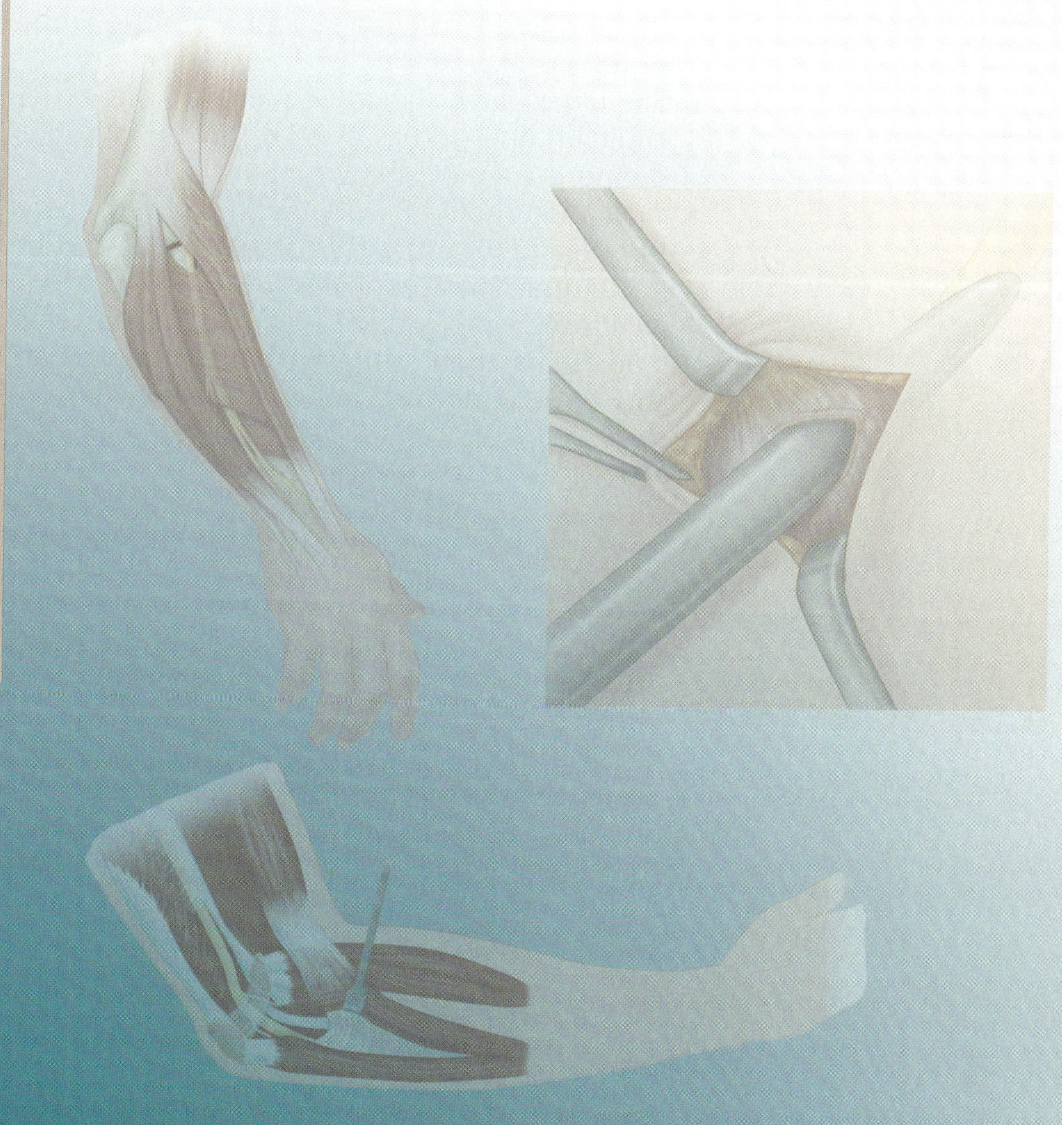

Figures 3, 4, and 6A reprinted from Fitzgerald BT, Hofmeister EP, Shin AY. Ulnar nerve transposition. In Reider B (ed). Operative Techniques: Sports Medicine Surgery. Philadelphia: Elsevier, 2009:276, 278, 279.

Differential Diagnosis

- Cervical radiculopathy
- Thoracic outlet syndrome
- Peripheral neuropathy
- Amytrophic lateral sclerosis
- Guillain-Barré syndrome
- Ulnar nerve compression at Guyon's canal

Treatment Options

- Mild cases can be treated with elbow pads to prevent external compression when resting the elbow on a hard surface, and nighttime splinting that prevents elbow flexion greater than 45°.
- At least a 2- to 3-month trial of nonoperative management is recommended before considering surgical decompression.

Indications

- Ulnar nerve compression at the elbow not relieved by conservative measures

Examination/Imaging

- A positive Tinel's sign and/or decreased sensation in ulnar nerve distribution, including the dorsal side of the ulnar border of the hand will be noted at the cubital tunnel. Severe cases can develop intrinsic weakness and atrophy in the hand with clawing of the ring and small fingers and a positive Froment's sign (Fig. 1).
- The ulnar nerve should be palpated within the cubital tunnel and assessed for potential subluxation during the arc of elbow motion.
- Evaluation should include radiographs of the elbow to evaluate for excessive cubitus valgus and/or posteromedial osteophytes.
- Electromyography and nerve conduction velocity studies can confirm the site of compression and should be performed prior to surgical intervention.

Surgical Anatomy

- Sites of potential compression that need to be addressed include the medial intermuscular septum (arcade of Struthers), the ligament of the cubital tunnel (Osborne's ligament), the anconeus epitrochlearis muscle within the epicondylar groove (when present as an anatomic variant), the superficial fascia of the flexor carpi ulnaris (FCU) muscle, and the deep fascia of the FCU muscle (Fig. 2).
- The ulnar nerve is under tension and compression in the cubital tunnel. Decompression alone will not alter the tension component and often needs to be accompanied by an anterior transposition.

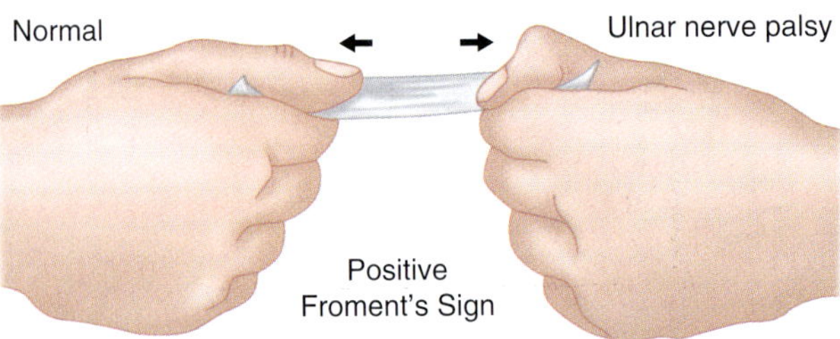

FIGURE 1

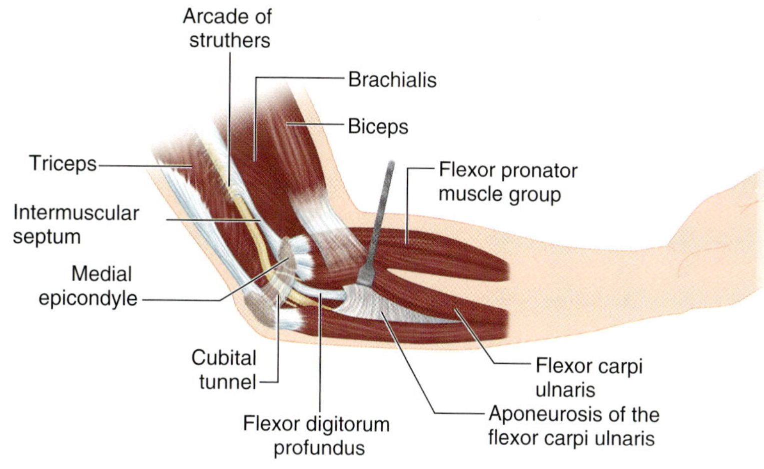

FIGURE 2

> **PEARLS**
>
> - *If using a pneumatic tourniquet, it must be placed high in the axilla to preserve the surgical field. A sterile tourniquet can be considered, but it is often easier to place a nonsterile tourniquet higher.*

> **PITFALLS**
>
> - *Branches of the medial brachial cutaneous and medial antebrachial cutaneous nerves lie in the subcutaneous tissue and cross the surgical field. These nerves are vulnerable to injury and prone to forming painful neuromas. They must be identified early and protected during the procedure.*

Positioning

- The patient is place supine on the operating table with the arm abducted on a hand table.

Portals/Exposures

- A curved medial incision is made along the posterior border of the medial intramuscular septum, extending posteriorly to the medial epicondyle and over the proximal aspect of the FCU muscle.
- The incision must extend at least 10 cm proximal to the medial epicondyle to allow for adequate exposure and release of the intramuscular septum.
- Distally the incision needs to provide enough exposure to trace the ulnar nerve through the deep fascia of the FCU.

Procedure

Step 1

- The ulnar nerve is identified deep to the brachial fascia immediately posterior to the medial intermuscular septum above the elbow. The nerve and any associated vessels are carefully mobilized from the septum, extending proximally at least 10 cm from the medial epicondyle (Fig. 3).
- The septum should then be removed from the distal humerus down to the epicondyle. Palpation of the intermuscular interval should reveal that the septum has been completely excised and that there are no sharp margins that the nerve will lie against when it is transposed anteriorly.

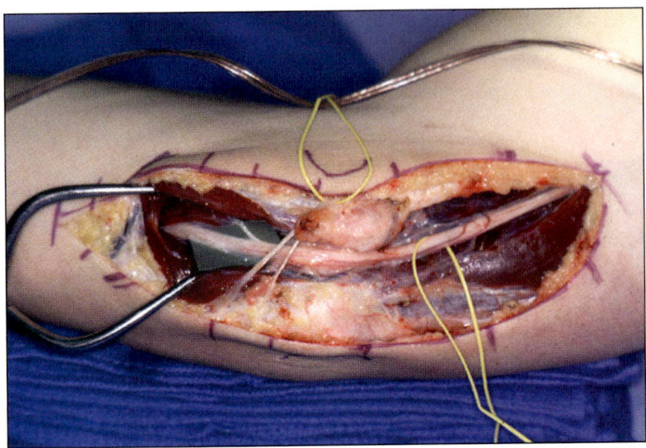

FIGURE 3

Pearls

- *Use of bipolar electrocautery will allow for accurate and precise cauterization of smaller vessels around the intermuscular septum, medial epicondyle, and FCU origin.*

Pitfalls

- *Avoid performing a neurolysis as this can compromise the blood supply to the ulnar nerve and lead to poor outcomes.*
- *The use of a Penrose drain or vessel loop around the nerve can reduce the possibility of injury to the nerve with metal retractors. Be careful to avoid vigorous retraction on the nerve.*

Instrumentation/ Implantation

- Bipolar electrocautery
- Penrose drain

- Distally, the nerve and associated vessels should be mobilized from the cubital tunnel.
  - The first branch of the ulnar nerve is to the elbow joint, and it should be divided to allow for easier mobilization of the nerve. The superficial fascia over the FCU muscle should be divided, and the nerve can be traced distally between the ulnar and humeral heads of the muscle.
  - The motor branches to the two heads of the FCU should be identified and protected. They can be bluntly traced into the muscle bellies to reduce the tension on the nerve when it is transposed anteriorly.
  - The main trunk of the ulnar nerve should be traced distally as it exits through the deep fascia of the FCU to enter the forearm in its dorsal position relative to the FCU.

Step 2

- The origin of the flexor-pronator mass from the medial epicondyle is identified. A plane is developed deep to this muscle group, and a blunt curved clamp can be placed in this plane to protect the median nerve.
- The flexor-pronator mass is then incised 1–2 cm distal to its origin to leave a cuff for repair. An elevator is used to reflect the muscle distally. Be careful to not disrupt the deeper ulnar collateral ligament. There are often vertical septae from the flexor-pronator group to the ulna that need to be divided so as to not kink the ulnar nerve when it has been transposed.

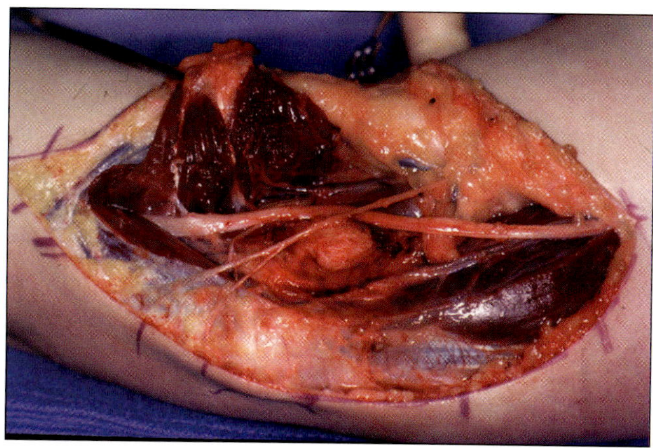

FIGURE 4

Pearls

- *Prior to advancing to repair of the flexor-pronator mass, place the ulnar nerve next to the median nerve and bring the retracted muscle origin back to its anatomic location. Take the elbow through a full range of motion and observe the ulnar nerve for any evidence of tension or kinking along its course. These should be addressed prior to proceeding to the next step.*

Pitfalls

- *Be careful to protect the first branch of the median nerve (nerve to the pronator teres) when reflecting the flexor-pronator mass.*

- The muscle group should be reflected distally and medially until the ulnar nerve can be placed adjacent to the median nerve (Fig. 4).
- There may be tension from the motor branch to the ulnar head of the FCU muscle. In this situation, the motor branch can be dissected out further into the muscle belly to reduce tension or the FCU can be elevated from its ulnar origin and repaired anterior to the humeral head of the FCU and the flexor-pronator mass in the next step.
- This step can be skipped when performing a subcutaneous transposition which also avoids the need to divide the flexor-pronator origin.
  - In this scenario, a fascial sling can be created from a distally based flap of the superficial fascia of the flexor-pronator muscles that is sutured to the subcutaneous tissue to prevent the ulnar nerve from returning to the cubital tunnel (Fig. 5).

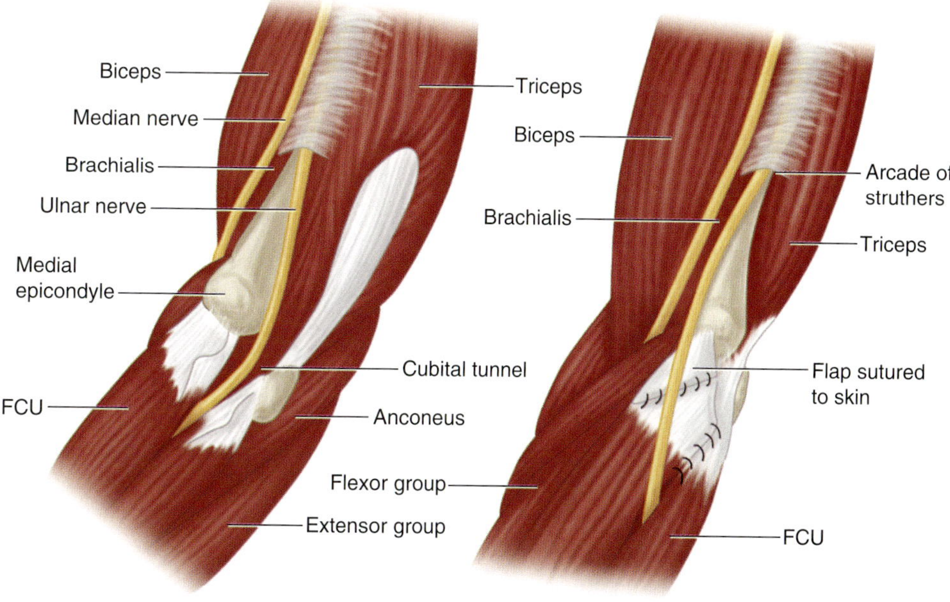

FIGURE 5

Controversies

- There is no consensus as to the most appropriate form of anterior ulnar nerve transposition and many options exist, including simple decompression, medial epicondylectomy, subcutaneous transposition, transmuscular transposition, and submuscular transposition. Many authors advocate subcutaneous transposition for simple and mild ulnar nerve compression at the elbow, while others have demonstrated that submuscular transposition is most appropriate for moderate to severe cases of ulnar nerve compression, for posttraumatic cubital tunnel syndrome, or in the revision setting. It is our preferred approach to perform the submuscular transposition as most of the patients that we treat have severe compression or present for revision surgery.

- Additionally, the cubital tunnel can be closed by suturing the two heads of the FCU together.

Step 3

- The flexor-pronator mass should be reattached with nonabsorbable sutures (Fig. 6A and 6B).
- A step-cut and lengthening of the flexor-pronator muscle group is often used to treat concomitant epicondylitis or to decrease the compression on the transposed nerve caused by the repair of the flexor-pronator origin.
- Prior to wound closure, the nerve should be inspected for potential kinking along its new course during elbow motion.

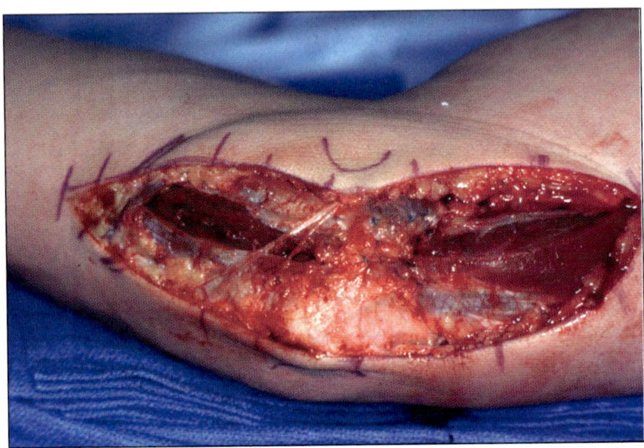

A

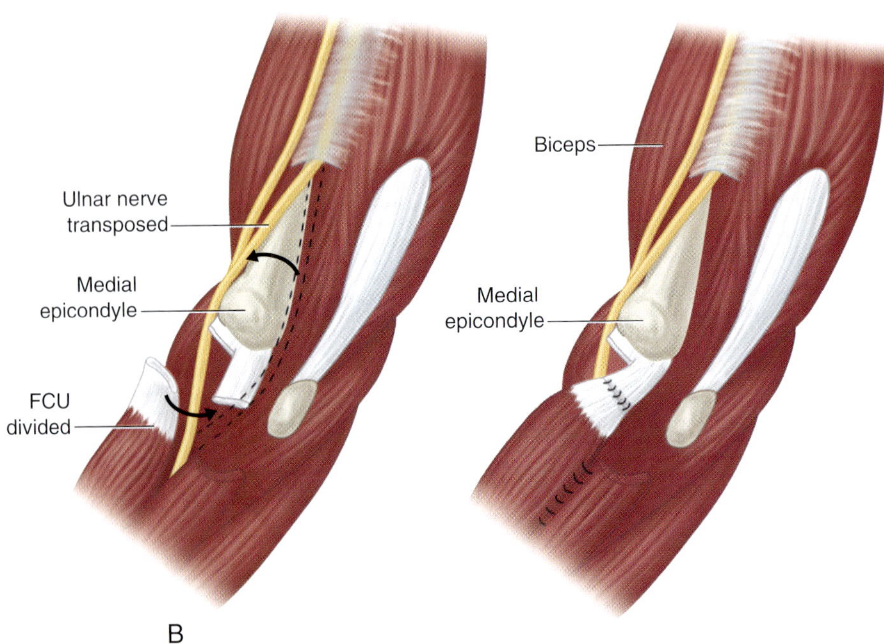

B

FIGURE 6

- The tourniquet should be released to achieve hemostasis, and the wound should be closed in layers over a drain. The arm should be placed in a well-padded splint with the elbow in 90° of flexion, the wrist in neutral, and the forearm in pronation to protect the repair of the flexor-pronator group.

Postoperative Care and Expected Outcomes

- The drain can be removed when output is minimal.
- The patient should return for follow-up within 1 week to have the splint removed and be initiated into an early motion protocol with a physical therapist. The focus should be to restore full extension and forearm rotation early. Nerve gliding exercises can be initiated at this time to minimized adhesions around the nerve in its new location. Strengthening is avoided for 4 weeks.

Evidence

Dellon AL. Review of treatment results for ulnar nerve entrapment at the elbow. J Hand Surg [Am]. 1989;14:688-700.

A review of 50 published reports between 1898 and 1988, comprising more than 2000 patients treated for ulnar nerve compression at the elbow, demonstrated that little more than personal bias is available for guidance in selecting treatment. This analysis suggests that for a minimal degree of compression, excellent results can be achieved in 50% of the patients by nonoperative techniques and in almost 100% of patients by any of five surgical techniques. For a moderate degree of compression, the anterior submuscular technique yields the most excellent results with the fewest recurrences. For a severe degree of compression, the anterior intramuscular transposition yielded the fewest excellent and the most recurrent results. This review suggests that an internal neurolysis, combined with an anterior submuscular transposition, may be the best approach when the ulnar nerve is severely compressed.

Learmonth JR. A technique for transplanting the ulnar nerve. Surg Gynecol Obstet. 1942;75:792-3.

This is the classic description of the submuscular technique by Learmonth.

Leffert RD. Anterior submuscular transposition for ulnar neuropathy at the elbow. J Hand Surg [Br]. 1982;7:147-55.

Thirty-eight patients with progressive post-traumatic ulnar neuropathy at the elbow underwent anterior submuscular transposition of their nerves. Fourteen patients had undergone previous surgery for ulnar neuropathy, while 24 had not. Postsurgical follow-up averaged 23.1 months. The operative technique is described and illustrated in detail. Complications attributable to surgery were minimal. No absolute prognostic factors could be identified, and even those patients with significant muscular atrophy or time delay before operation were generally benefited. If prior surgery had induced significant scarring and neural damage, the prognosis for recovery was considerably worse, as it also was for patients who had severe preoperative dysesthesia or pain. Four patients thought to represent examples of double crush or compression syndrome were identified.

Mowlavi A, Andrews K, Lille S, et al. The management of cubital tunnel syndrome: a meta-analysis of clinical studies. Plast Reconstr Surg. 2000;106:327-34.

Despite extensive clinical experience in treating cubital tunnel syndrome, optimal surgical management remains controversial. A meta-analysis of 30 studies with accurate preoperative and postoperative staging was undertaken. Patients were staged preoperatively into minimum, moderate, and severe groups on the basis of clinical presentation. Treatment modalities included nonoperative management, surgical decompression, medial epicondylectomy, anterior subcutaneous transposition, and anterior submuscular transposition. For minimum-staged patients, all modalities produced similar degrees of satisfaction. However, total relief occurred most after medial epicondylectomy and least after anterior subcutaneous transposition. Patients treated nonoperatively had the highest rate of recurrence. For moderate-staged patients, submuscular transposition was most efficacious, whereas patients with nonoperative management fared the worst. Finally, for severe-staged patients, current therapeutic modalities were not consistently effective, with medial epicondylectomy producing the poorest operative result.

Pasque CB, Rayan GM. Anterior submuscular transposition of the ulnar nerve for cubital tunnel syndrome. J Hand Surg [Br]. 1995;20:447-53.

Forty-eight patients with 50 involved limbs were retrospectively analyzed to determine factors influencing the outcome of surgical treatment for cubital tunnel syndrome. All patients were treated by anterior submuscular transposition of the ulnar nerve with Z-lengthening of the flexor-pronator origin. There were 24 men and 24 women with an average age of 42 years +/– 16.4 years (range, 5-75 years). The average follow-up time was 58 months (range, 12-156 months). Ninety-two percent of the patients were satisfied, or satisfied with some reservations, and only 8% were dissatisfied. All patients had either fair or poor pre-operative grades. Eighty-four percent had excellent or good postoperative grades and only 16% had fair grades. There were no recurrences or poor post-operative grades in our series. Workers' compensation status had no statistically significant adverse effect on postoperative patient satisfaction or postoperative grade. Anterior submuscular transposition of the ulnar nerve in this series provided satisfactory subjective outcome, relief of symptoms and adequate decompression of the ulnar nerve at the elbow.

PROCEDURE 55

Surgical Decompression for Radial Tunnel Syndrome

Eric S. Stuffmann, Zinon T. Kokkalis, and Dean G. Sotereanos

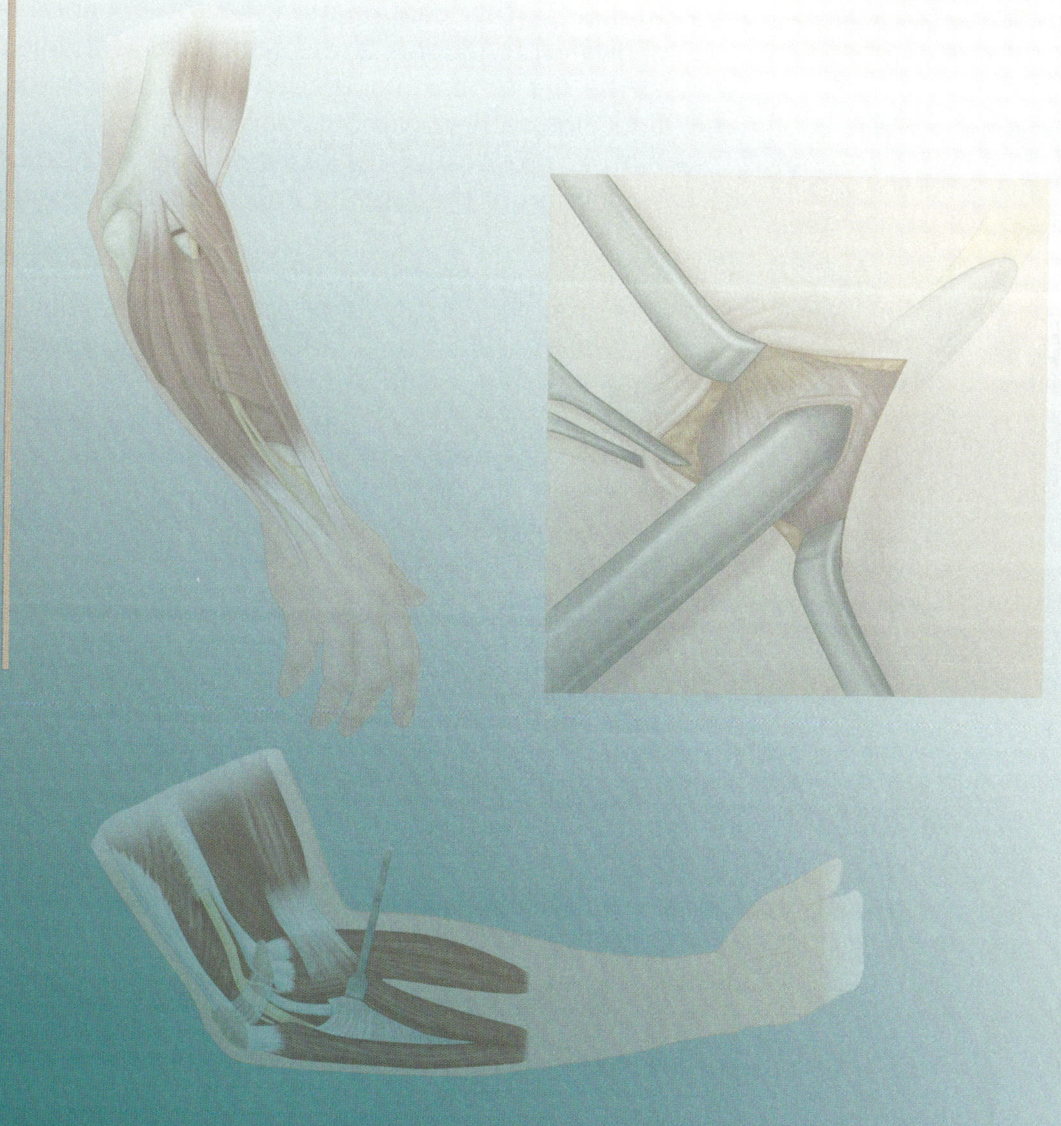

PITFALLS

- *Failure to recognize alternative sources of arm pain, such as lateral epicondylitis*
- *Inability of patient and surgeon to clearly localize anatomic site of pain and tenderness*
- *Surgical treatment prior to adequate course of conservative treatment, including therapy and possibly injections*

Controversies

- A double crush syndrome with cervical nerve root entrapment in addition to radial tunnel syndrome must be distinguished from posterior interosseous nerve (PIN) syndrome. PIN syndrome presents with associated weakness and/or atrophy of the dorsal forearm compartment and may or may not be associated with pain.

Treatment Options

- Two to 3 months of physical therapy consisting of ergonomic retraining, stretching, and strengthening of the wrist and finger extensors and supinator
- Injections with either cortisone or local anesthetic

Indications

- Presence of arm pain with the characteristics of radial tunnel syndrome as described below, the exclusion of the associated differential diagnoses, and failure of conservative treatment

Examination/Imaging

- The diagnosis of radial tunnel syndrome can be made by reproduction of the patient's symptoms with palpation of the radial nerve within the radial tunnel. Further confirmation may be obtained by achieving resolution of the symptoms with injection at the site of maximal tenderness using 2 ml of lidocaine with or without triamcinolone.
- Further provocative tests include pain with resisted supination of the forearm and resisted extension of the middle finger (Fig. 1).
- Plain radiographs of the elbow (posteroanterior, lateral, oblique) can show bony abnormalities such as malunion and chronic radial head dislocation/subluxation in posttraumatic cases.
- In rare cases, the radial nerve and its posterior interosseous branch may be compressed by a mass such as a ganglion, lipoma, inflamed bursa, or proliferative rheumatoid synovitis. In such cases, magnetic resonance imaging (MRI) may be useful to elucidate the pathology preoperatively. In a 43-year-old female with persistent forearm pain, axial (Fig. 2A) and sagittal (Fig. 2B) MRI views of the left elbow indicated a large ganglion cyst around the proximal radius, seen intraoperatively in Figure 2C.
- Electrodiagnostic testing is not particularly helpful with this condition.

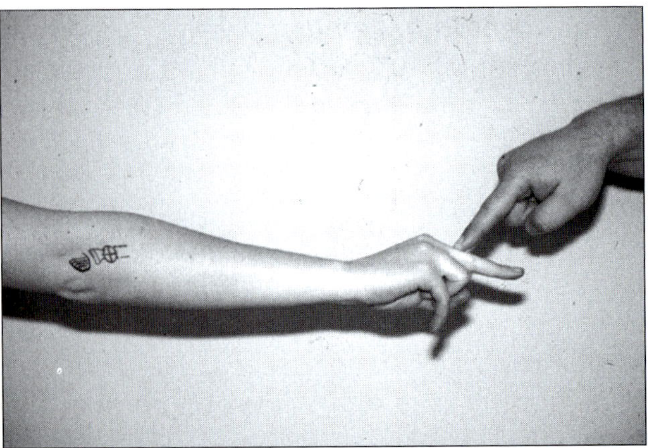

FIGURE 1

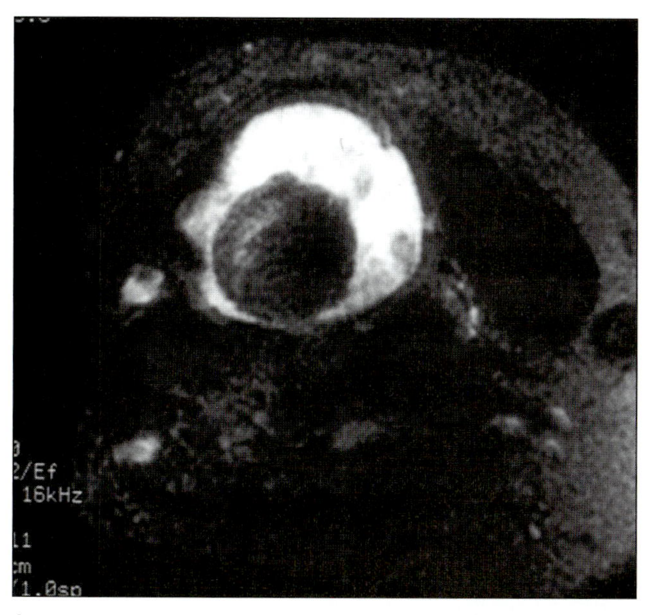

A

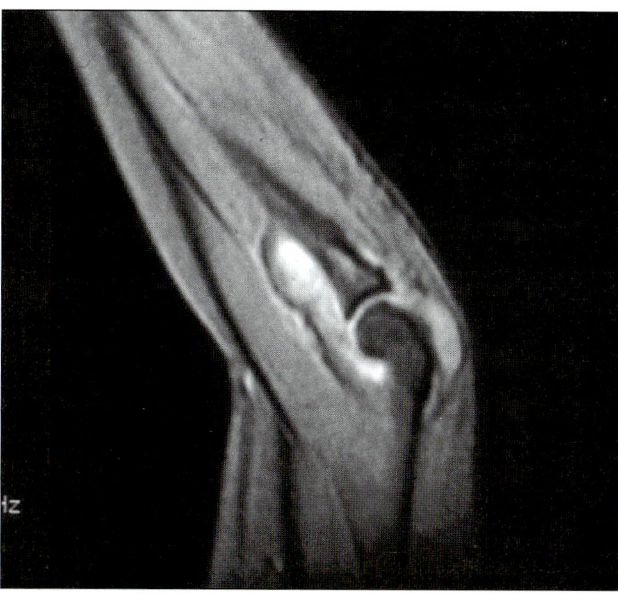

B

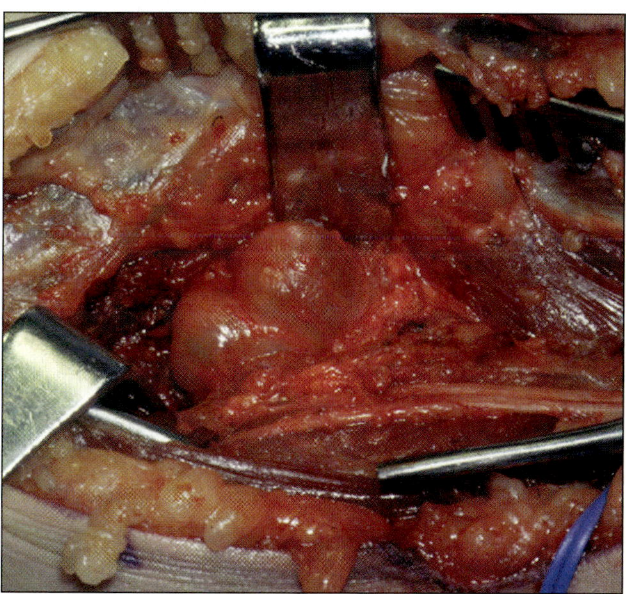

C

FIGURE 2

Surgical Anatomy

- The radial tunnel is a potential space traversed by the radial nerve and its posterior interosseous branch (Fig. 3).
  - It is defined by the lateral epicondyle of the humerus proximally, the distal edge of the supinator distally, the brachioradialis and extensor carpi radialis longus and brevis tendons laterally, and the brachialis muscle and biceps tendon medially.
  - The floor of the tunnel is the anterior capsule of the radiocapitellar joint and the deep portion of the supinator muscle. The roof is formed by the brachioradialis muscle and the superficial portion of the supinator muscle and fibrous bands traversing between the medial and lateral walls.
- After entering the anterior compartment of the arm, and before crossing the elbow joint line, the radial nerve innervates the brachialis, brachioradialis, anconeus, and extensor carpi radialis longus (ECRL). The radial nerve then enters the forearm anterior to the lateral epicondyle, where it branches into the superficial radial nerve and the PIN. Either the superficial radial nerve or the PIN innervates the extensor carpi radialis brevis (ECRB) before passing under the arcade of Frohse.

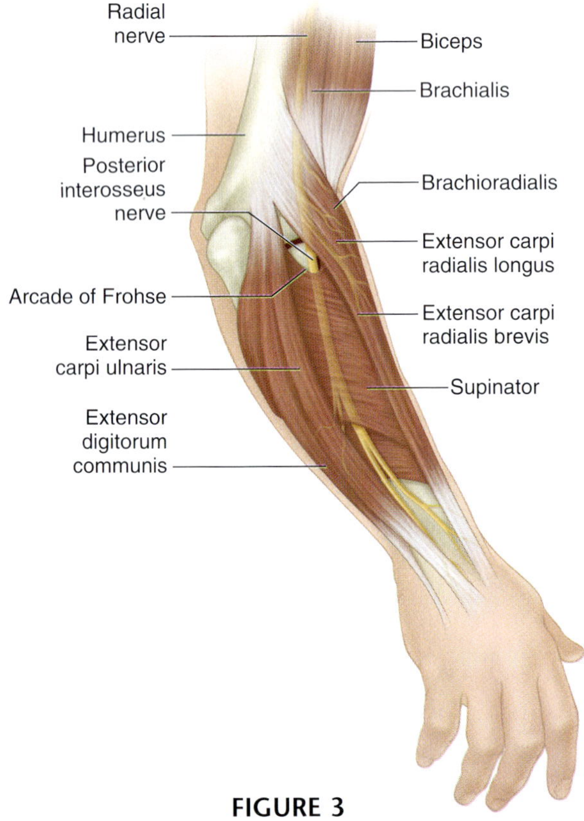

FIGURE 3

- The structures known to cause compression of the radial nerve and its posterior interosseous branch are, from proximal to distal:
  - The proximal fibrous border of the supinator muscle known as the arcade of Frohse
  - Fascial bands within the supinator
  - The superomedial border of the ECRB muscle, and the inferior border of the superficial layer of the supinator muscle
  - Fibrous bands anterior to the radiocapitellar joint, the recurrent radial vessels, and their tributaries
- The ECRB tendon may be implicated in both radial tunnel syndrome and lateral epicondylitis.

PEARLS

- *The planned interval may be identified preoperatively by asking the patient to flex the elbow against resistance with the forearm in neutral rotation. This will help to identify the brachioradialis muscle.*
- *The correct interval may be identified by having the patient flex the elbow against resistance preoperatively, thus identifying the brachioradialis muscle.*

PITFALLS

- *If a previous procedure has been performed (i.e., lateral epicondylectomy), the surgeon may want to use an alternate approach.*

Positioning

- The patient is placed in the supine position with the arm on a hand table.
- A nonsterile tourniquet is applied to the upper arm.

Portals/Exposures

- Multiple approaches have been described.
- These include the dorsal approach of Thompson between the extensor digitorum communis (EDC) and ECRB, the interval between the brachioradialis and ECRL, and the brachialis-splitting approach.

Procedure

Step 1: Approach

- Thompson's approach (EDC/ECRB)
  - A 10-cm incision is made along the imaginary line from the lateral epicondyle to Lister's tubercle.
  - The interval between the EDC and ECRB is identified (Fig. 4). The EDC muscle may be

PEARLS

- *Intraoperatively the color of the fascia gives a clue as to the correct interval. The brachioradialis muscle appears redder than the adjacent ECRL, due to the relative thickness of the fascia.*

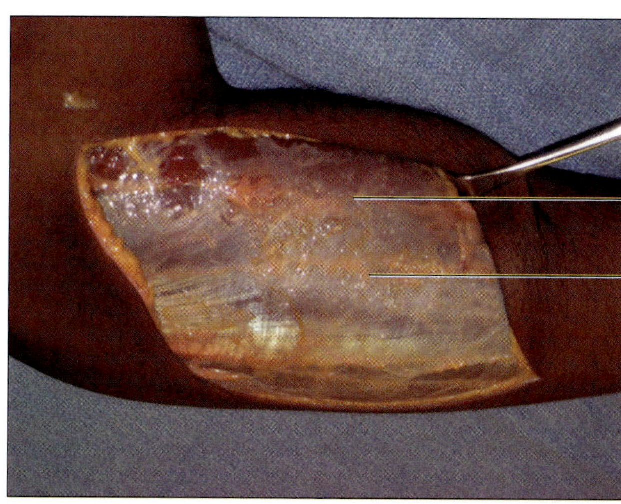

FIGURE 4

identified by the striated appearance of its muscle fascia. The antebrachial facsia over this interval is incised, and dissection proceeds in this interval until the supinator muscle is reached. The radial nerve and its branches can be identified at this level. The PIN can be identified entering deep to the supinator under the arcade of Frohse.
  - The radial nerve is identified lying within fat deep to the mobile wad muscle fibers (Fig. 5).
  - If necessary, the ECRB can be released to gain more proximal exposure to the radial nerve.
- Brachialis splitting
  - An incision is made extending from just proximal to the radiocapitellar joint to 3 cm lateral to the biceps tendon. The brachialis fascia is incised and the brachialis muscle is bluntly dissected with scissors aiming toward the radial head.
  - Care is taken upon encountering the fat that surrounds the radial nerve.
- Interval between brachioradialis and ECRL
  - A 10-cm incision is made over the interval between the brachioradialis and ECRL as identified preoperatively. The posterior antebrachial cutaneous nerve is identified over this interval and protected. Intraoperatively, this interval is identified by the relative color of the muscles, with the brachioradialis appearing redder than the ECRL due to the relative thicknesses of the fascia overlying these muscles (see Fig. 4).
  - The fascia overlying this interval is sharply incised, and blunt dissection leads directly to the radial tunnel and its contents.

Step 2: Decompression

- The radial nerve and its branches, the superficial radial nerve and the PIN, are clearly identified (Fig. 6).
- All transverse structures overlying the radial nerve are released, including vessels, fibrous bands, and the fibrous edge of the ECRB (Fig. 7).
- The release proceeds distally, ligating the recurrent radial vessels and releasing the arcade of Frohse. The course of the PIN is followed, dissecting it out of the supinator and releasing it from any fascial bands that may exist, until the distal edge of this muscle is reached (Fig. 8).

Pearls

- *It is imperative to dissect the nerve under loupe magnification with ample light.*
- *The recurrent radial vessels should be ligated carefully to avoid postoperative bleeding.*

Pitfalls

- *The most significant complication inherent to this procedure is iatrogenic damage to the PIN.*
- *It is imperative to avoid direct handling of the nerve.*
- *Temporary superficial radial nerve neurapraxia is not uncommon after surgery.*

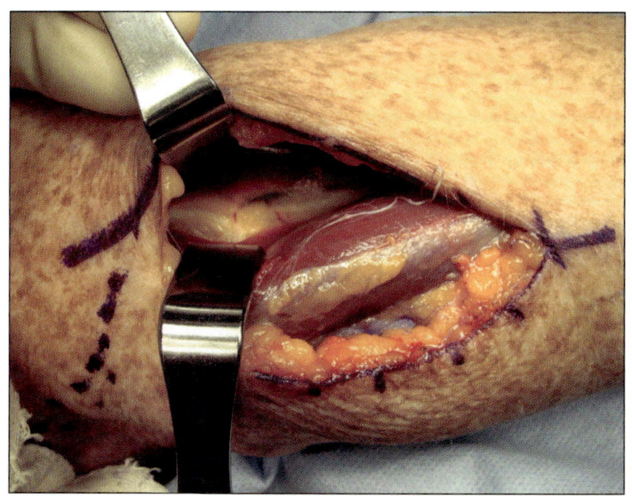

FIGURE 5

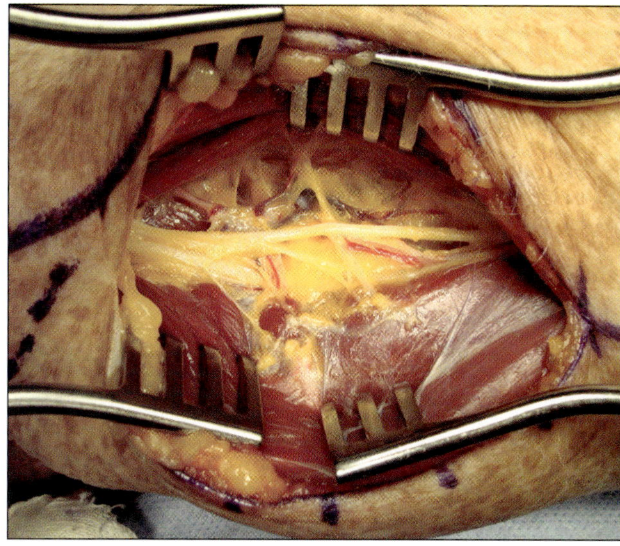

FIGURE 6

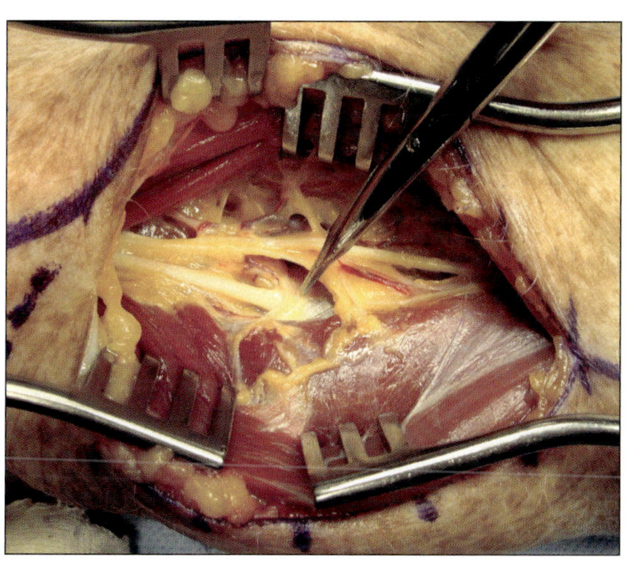

FIGURE 7

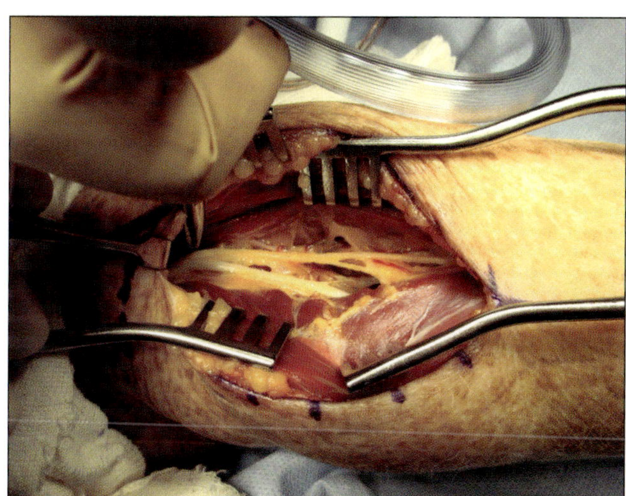

FIGURE 8

Step 3: Wound Closure

- Before closing, the tourniquet is released and meticulous haemostasis performed.
- Wound is closed by layers.

Postoperative Care and Expected Outcomes

- The patient is placed in a soft dressing, and motion is allowed immediately.
- Stretching exercises are performed several times daily for 4–6 weeks, emphasizing the wrist and finger extensors and supinator.

- After 4–6 weeks, progressive strengthening of these muscles begins as the patient gradually returns to his or her usual activities.
- In our series with 28 patients (Sotereanos et al., 1999), the reported complications included 11 (31%) temporary superficial radial nerve neurapraxias and 1 (3.6%) transient PIN palsy in a revision case.

Evidence

Jebson PJ, Engber WD. Radial tunnel syndrome: long-term results of surgical decompression. J Hand Surg [Am]. 1997;22:889-96.

This study reported outcomes in 31 patients (33 extremities) undergoing radial tunnel decompression; 67% of extremities had excellent or good results, and 33% had fair or poor results based on the criteria of Roles and Maudsley. This study found no significant difference in outcomes in patients with and without workers' compensation. (Level IV evidence [retrospective review])

Lee JT, Azari K, Jones NF. Long term results of radial tunnel release—the effect of co-existing tennis elbow, multiple compression syndromes and workers' compensation. J Plastic Reconstr Aesthetic Surg. 2008;61:1095-9.

In this study of outcomes of 33 extremities in 31 patients who underwent decompression of the radial tunnel, 27 extremities in 25 patients were available for long-term follow-up (avg. 57 months). By the criteria of Ritts, 18 of 27 extremities (67%) had a good outcome, 4 extremities (15%) had a fair outcome, and 5 extremities (18%) had a poor outcome. Patients with simple radial tunnel syndrome had a better outcome than those with additional nerve compression syndromes, coexisting lateral epicondylitis, or patients receiving workers' compensation. (Level IV evidence [retrospective review])

Sotereanos DG, Varitimidis SE, Giannakopoulos PN, Westkaemper JG. Results of surgical treatment for radial tunnel syndrome. J Hand Surg [Am]. 1999;24:566-70.

This study reported outcomes in patients undergoing radial tunnel decompression for radial tunnel syndrome. Only 39% of patients had excellent or good results based on objective criteria, although 64% subjectively rated their results as excellent or good. Workers' compensation patients had significantly worse results. (Level IV evidence [retrospective review])

SECTION II

Elbow

Trauma

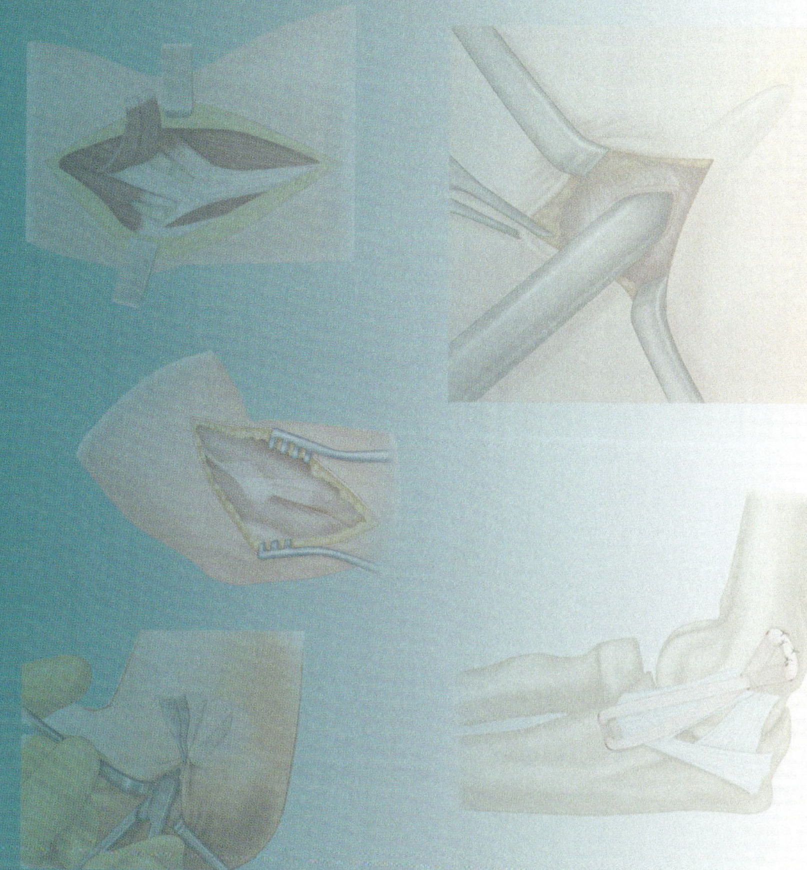

PROCEDURE 56

Distal Humerus Fractures, Including Isolated Distal Lateral Column and Capitellar Fractures

Jeffry T. Watson

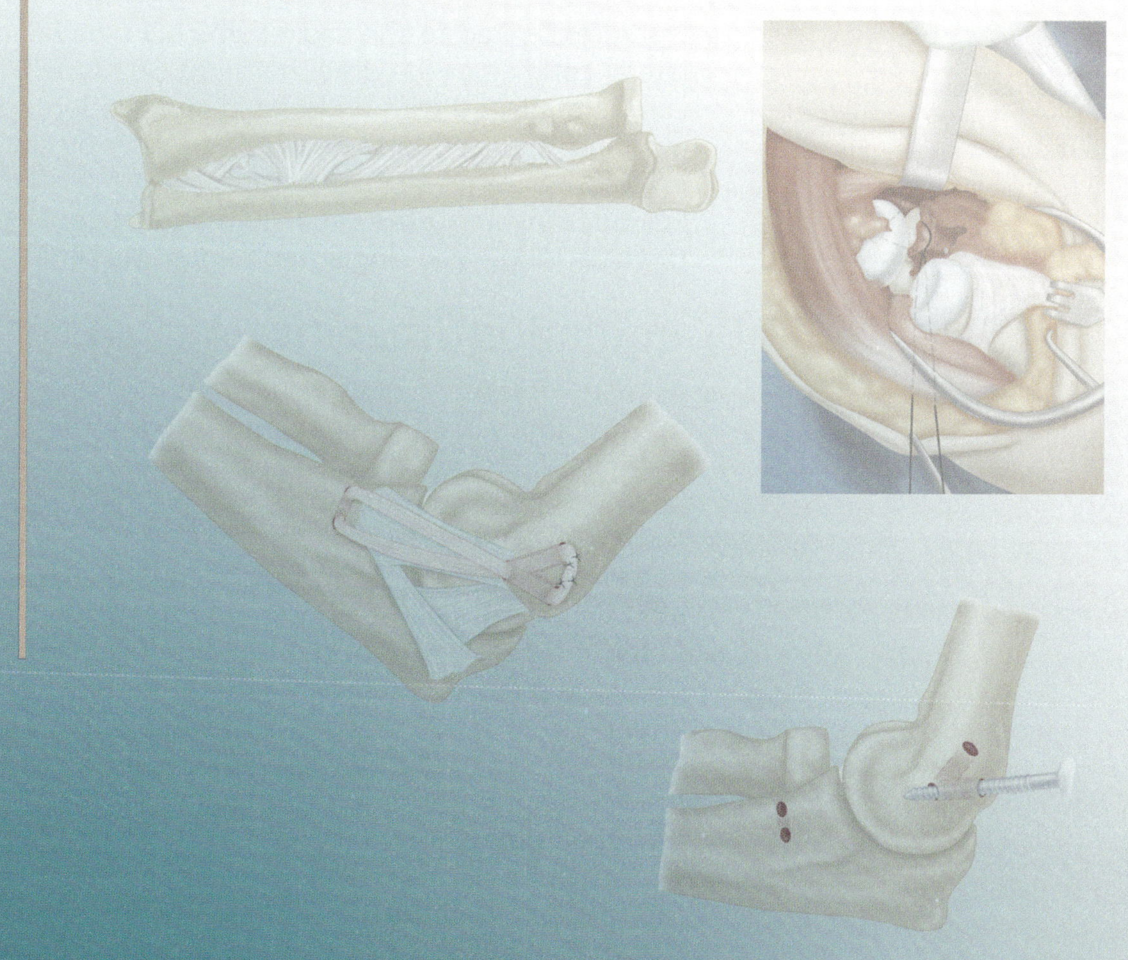

Pitfalls

- *In isolated distal lateral column and capitellar fractures, if the fracture pattern involves the medial column or has more complex involvement of the trochlea, a lateral approach will be insufficient.*

Controversies

- Reasonable function and motion can be achieved with functional bracing for extra-articular distal third fractures. Plate fixation, while possessing some risk for infection or iatrogenic nerve injury, offers more predictable alignment and quicker return of function.
- The "bag of bones" method of nonsurgical splint management of comminuted patterns should be reserved for minimal-demand, medically unfit patients with the goal being a minimally painful, functional pseudarthrosis.
- Very distal or comminuted fracture patterns in osteoporotic bone may be better managed with total elbow arthroplasty instead of open reduction and internal fixation (ORIF) (Fig. 1).

Treatment Options

- For distal humerus fractures
  - Splint immobilization
  - ORIF
  - Primary total elbow arthroplasty
- For isolated distal lateral column and capitellar fractures
  - ORIF for displaced or unstable patterns
  - Nonoperative management (temporary immobilization followed by protected motion at a 3- to 4-week window) for nondisplaced fractures

Indications

Distal Humerus Fractures

- Displaced fractures of the distal humeral articular surface
- Displaced extra-articular fractures in which alignment cannot be maintained with external splinting techniques
- Open intra- or extra-articular fractures
- Fractures with associated vascular injury

Isolated Distal Lateral Column and Capitellar Fractures

- Fractures limited to the capitellum (AO type B3.1) or lateral condyle of the distal humerus (AO type B1) can be managed with an isolated lateral approach, avoiding the need for triceps reflection or olecranon osteotomy.
- Fractures involving the capitellum and lateral trochlear ridge as a single fragment.

Examination/Imaging

- As many of these injuries result from high-energy mechanisms, circumferential inspection of the elbow is required. The proximal shaft fragment is especially prone to penetrate the triceps and posterior soft tissues.
- Associated ipsilateral injuries (wrist, hand) are easy to miss due to pain and deformity at the elbow.
- Anterior displacement of the proximal fragment should raise concern about injury to the brachial artery and/or median or radial nerves.
- The ulnar nerve is more vulnerable to injury with the more common posterior displacement of the proximal fragment.
- Quality of distal pulses and sensorimotor function of the three main nerve groups must be determined and documented.
- Standard anteroposterior (AP) and lateral radiographic views are routine.
  - Figure 2 shows a bicolumnar, intra-articular comminuted distal humerus fracture in anteroposterior (Fig. 2A) and lateral (Fig. 2B) views.
  - Overlapping fragments may obscure visualization in comminuted patterns, and traction views under anesthesia may help in determining fracture pattern and fixation strategy.

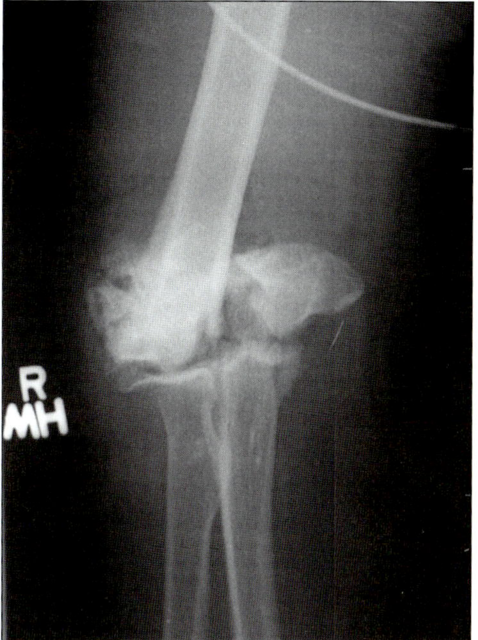

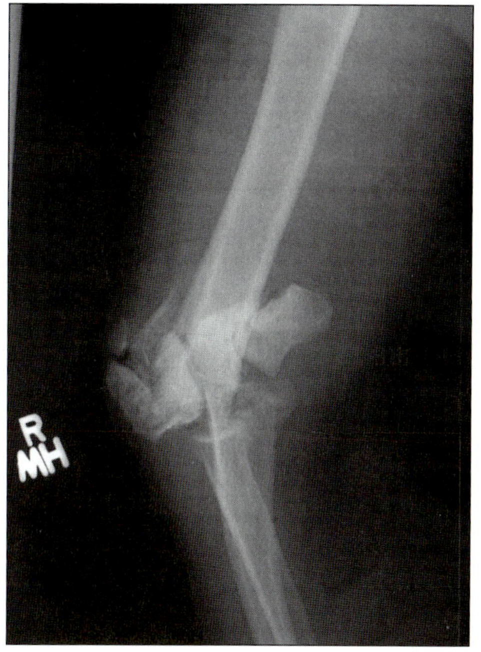

FIGURE 1 A B

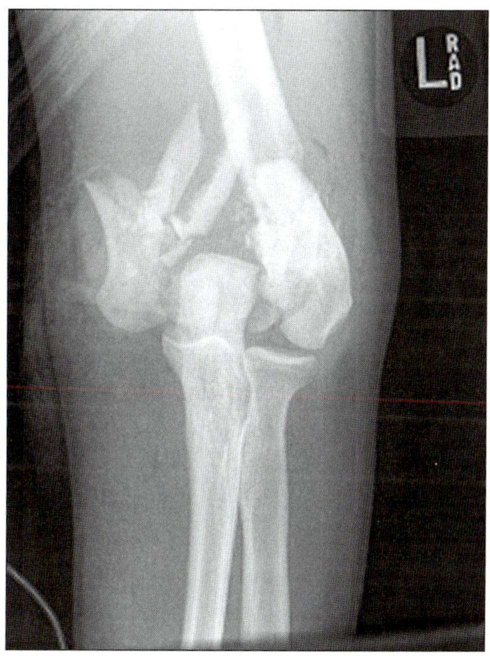

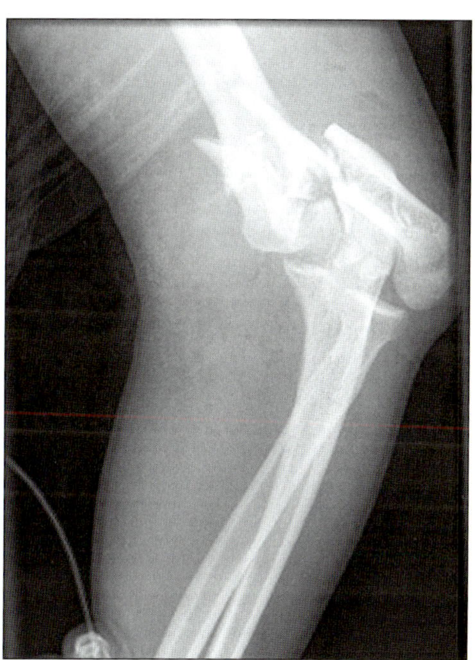

FIGURE 2 A B

- Computed tomography (CT) is unlikely to affect surgical decision making in most complex patterns, as the same approach will be utilized in most such cases. However, a capitellar fracture with significant medial involvement of the trochlea may not be adequately exposed and managed through a lateral approach. If the pattern appears limited to the lateral articular surface (isolated distal lateral column or capitellar fractures), CT scanning may offer pertinent

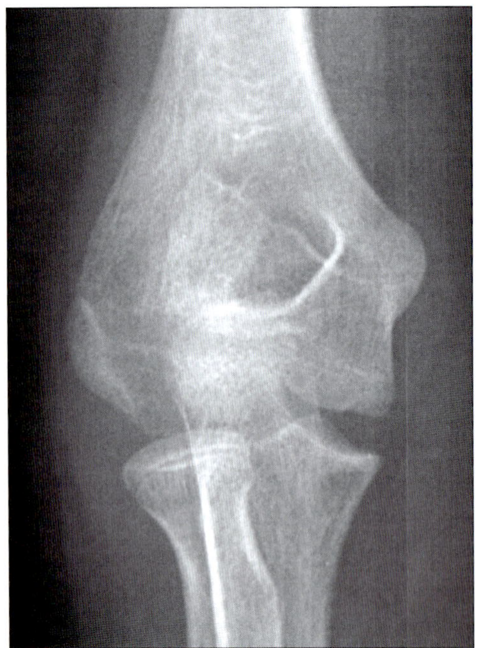

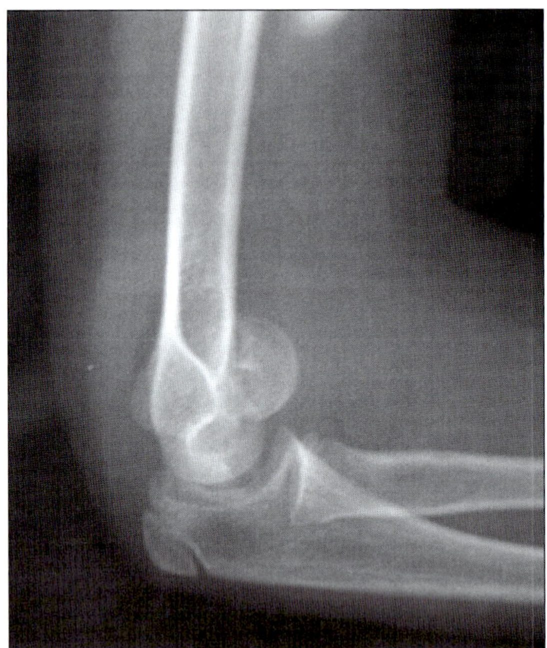

A B

FIGURE 3

detail regarding the displacement and medial extent of fracture involvement. Isolated capitellar fractures should be reviewed by CT scan to verify that the fracture does not involve the trochlea or medial column.

- In Figure 3, AP (Fig. 3A) and lateral (Fig. 3B) radiographs show an isolated capitellar fracture that can be managed through a lateral approach.
- In Figure 4, the apparent capitellar fracture seen in AP (Fig. 4A) and lateral (Fig. 4B) plain radiographs is revealed by CT scanning (Fig. 4C) to have medial extension into trochlea.

Surgical Anatomy

- Trochlea
  - The medial and lateral eminences (medial is larger) are separated by an intervening sulcus or groove. Figure 5 shows anterior (Fig. 5A), distal (Fig. 5B), and posterior (Fig. 5C) perspectives of a cadaveric distal humerus stripped of soft tissue attachments. Note the contours, and the relationship of the medial and lateral ridges of the trochlea to the groove.
  - The trochlea has an articular arc of 270°.
  - The coronoid and olecranon fossae reside at the terminations of the groove anteriorly and posteriorly, respectively.

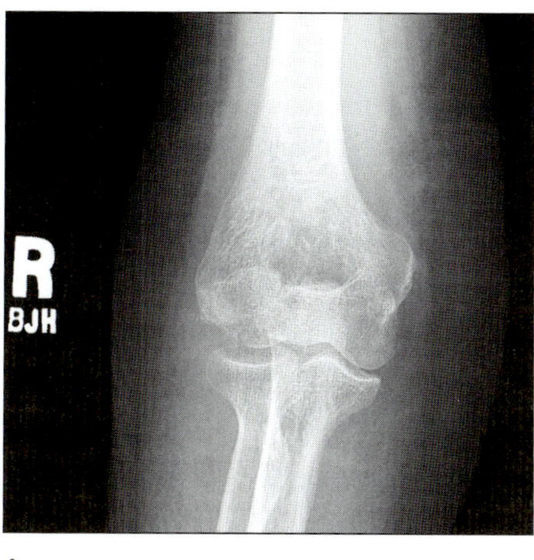

A

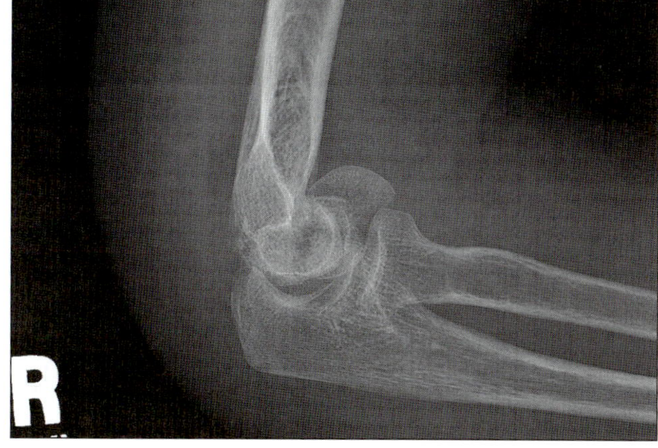

B

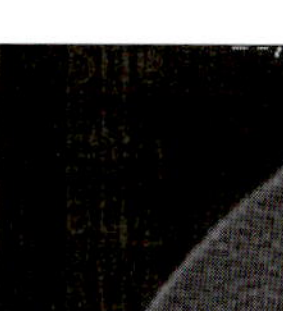
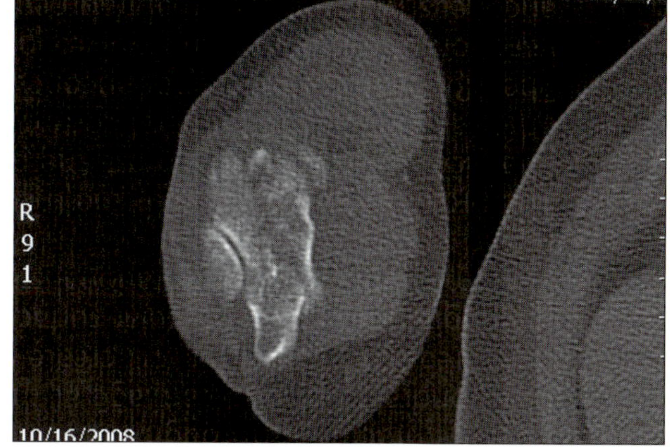

FIGURE 4 C

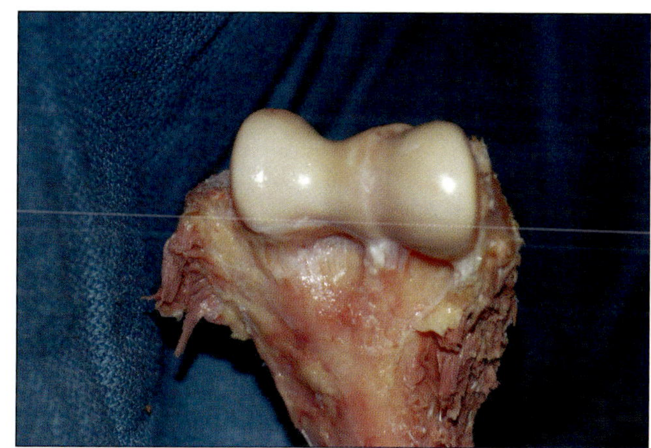

A

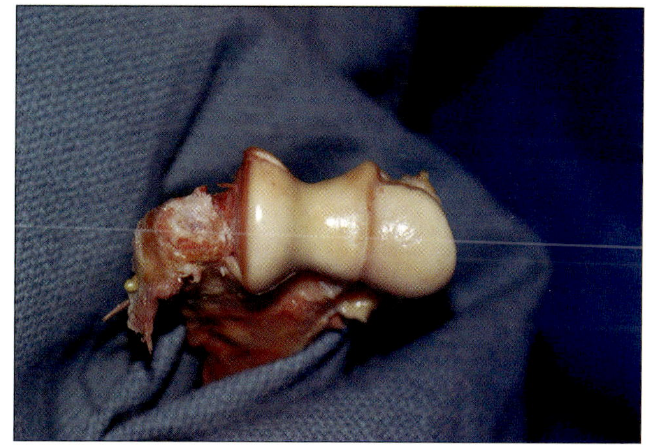

B

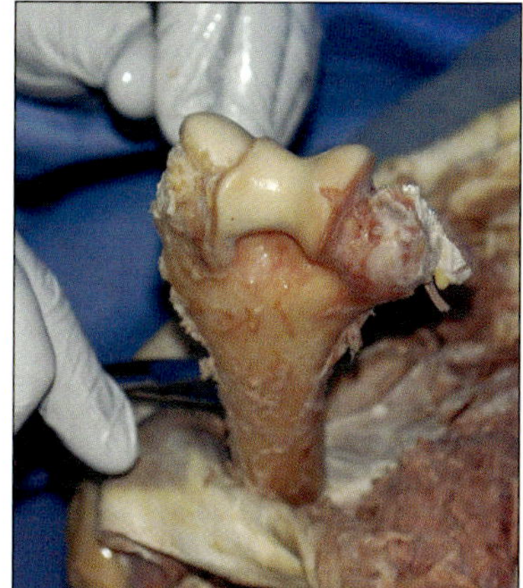

C

FIGURE 5

- Ulnotrochlear articulation
  - The guiding ridge of the proximal ulna's semilunar notch glides within the ulnar groove.
  - This articulation contributes to varus/valgus stability of the elbow.
  - Anteriorly, the contact of the coronoid process against the trochlea resists posterior subluxation of the joint. Therefore, every effort should be made to restore at least the anterior portion of the trochlea.
- Radiocapitellar joint
  - This joint is the platform for forearm rotation.
  - It is a critical stabilizer for valgus instability if the medial collateral ligament (MCL) or lateral trochlea is deficient.
  - If the coronoid process of the ulna is compromised, an intact radiocapitellar articulation will resist posterior subluxation.
- Medial and lateral metaphyseal "columns" (see Fig. 5C)
  - These columns straddle the olecranon and coronoid fossae to provide a platform for the articular bearing.
  - The medial column terminates as the medial epicondyle, which is nonarticular and is a useful platform for medial fixation.
  - The lateral column ends at the capitellum, whose nonarticular posterior surface allows for more distal hardware placement.
- Keeping the fossae for the coronoid, olecranon, and radial head clear of hardware or displaced bone is essential for normal elbow motion.
- Lateral collateral ligament (LCL) complex: consists of
  - Annular ligament
  - Lateral collateral ligament
  - Lateral ulnar collateral ligament (LUCL)
    - This ligament is a critical stabilizer for posterolateral stability and must be preserved.
    - It originates from the central portion of the capitellum, along the axis of elbow rotation, and inserts along the crista supinatoris (supinator crest) of the proximal ulna.
- Medial collateral ligament
  - This ligament originates from the lateral inferior portion of the medial epicondyle.
  - It is composed of anterior, posterior, and transverse bands.

- The anterior band contributes to valgus stability and inserts along the sublime tubercle of the proximal ulna.

- Ulnar nerve
  - The ulnar nerve pierces the medial intermuscular septum to enter the posterior compartment of the brachium about 8 cm from the medial epicondyle.
  - It enters the cubital tunnel along the dorsal aspect of the medial epicondyle, then passes superficial to the posterormedial ulnohumeral joint capsule and the posterior band of the MCL.
  - Within the cubital tunnel, it gives off expendable short articulating branches to the joint capsule.
  - Mobilization and anterior transposition of the ulnar nerve is usually recommended with hardware placement along the medial epicondyle.
- Radial nerve
  - The radial nerve runs with the profunda brachii artery along the posterior portion of the humeral diaphysis in the groove between the medial and lateral heads of the triceps muscle.
  - It pierces the lateral intermuscular septum about 10 cm proximal to the lateral epicondyle.

Isolated Distal Lateral Column and Capitellar Fractures

- The lateral collateral ligament originates just anterior and distal to the lateral epicondyle, along the axis of rotation. If detached, it must be repaired at the conclusion of the procedure.
- Fractures limited to the capitellum articular surface (AO type B3.1) and the lateral portion of the trochlea (some B3.3 patterns) can be stabilized with screws placed in either an anterior-to-posterior or a posterior-to anterior orientation.
- Isolated lateral column fractures (AO types B1.1 and B1.2) can be managed with either direct lag screw placement or single lateral column plating.

Positioning

- Optimal positioning depends on the desired approach.
  - For lateral approaches (used in management of isolated lateral condyle or capitellum fractures), supine position with the elbow flexed on an armboard is usually sufficient.

- Most distal humerus fixation procedures will require a posterior approach, which may be performed with the patient in either the supine or lateral decubitus position.

Distal Humerus Fractures

- Supine positioning
  - The injured arm will need to be placed across the chest. A bump behind the ipsilateral scapula will help keep the arm across the chest while allowing more "working room" for elbow flexion. Figure 6 shows the flexed elbow projecting upward, with a padded Mayo stand supporting the humerus from falling back.
  - If iliac crest bone grafting will be necessary, a bump is placed behind the desired hip.
  - The surgical team is on the side of the injured arm.
  - Tilting the operating table slightly away from the surgical team will assist in maintaining arm position across the chest, which will aid in presentation of that field.
  - Supine position allows the involved limb to be placed on a short armboard at the side, should easier access to the medial elbow be required. This armboard may be removed during any portion of the procedure to place the limb back across the chest.
  - Supine positioning also allows for easier airway access for the anesthesia team.
- Lateral decubitus positioning
  - The lateral decubitus position allows for easy visibility along the posterior humerus.

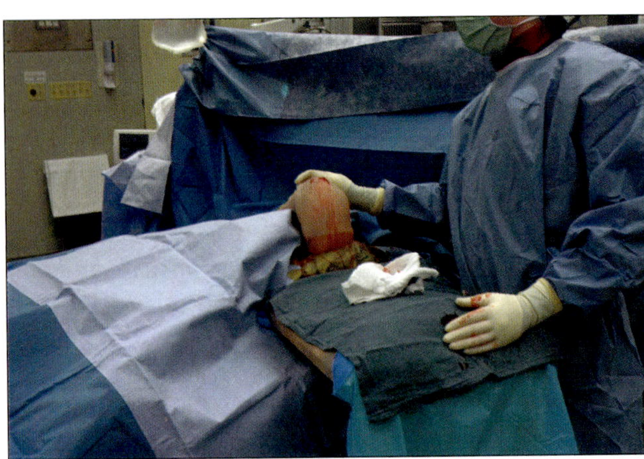

FIGURE 6

- The arm may be draped over an armholder or bolster, which offers some stability for the brachium during surgery.
- The use of a beanbag with an axillary roll and appropriate protection for the contralateral peroneal nerve is preferred.

- In all but the most distal patterns, the use of a sterile tourniquet that may be removed to accommodate proximal exposure is advised over nonsterile tourniquets.
- Adequate access to the airway for the anesthesiologist must be ensured before draping.

Isolated Distal Lateral Column and Capitellar Fractures

- Supine positioning with an armboard is sufficient for exposure and fixation of the lateral column and capitellum. A towel bump placed under the medial elbow is helpful.

Pearls

- *Prior to prepping and draping, verify adequate fluoroscopic visualization of the humeral shaft and elbow with current patient position.*
- *A sterile draped Mayo stand from the contralateral side may be used to stabilize the forearm across the chest. A wrapped forearm sleeve clamped to the stand with a nonpenetrating clamp can stabilize the limb onto the tray. Alternatively, a gauze roll wrapped around the wrist and stabilized with traction weights on the contralateral side of the stand can also be used.*
- *A magnetic strip, adhesive pouch, or stable platform on the patient can be used for placement of instruments during the surgery, which usually requires a high volume of instrument passage.*

Pitfalls

- *Insufficient protection of the contralateral axilla and peroneal nerve.*
- *Inadequate access for fluoroscopic visualization, which may be more difficult in the lateral decubitus position.*
- *Lateral positioning with an armboard may impede elbow hyperflexion, limiting access to more anterior articular fragments.*

Portals/Exposures

- The "universal" approach for elbow fracture or instability management is through a posterior skin incision with full-thickness skin flaps to allow for circumferential access. The plane of elevation is deep to the cutaneous nerves along the brachium, so potential painful neuromas can be avoided. Potential disadvantages are dead space, hematomas, and seromas created with such large flaps. Furthermore, access to medial, lateral, or anterior elements may require significant retraction efforts, particularly in obese patients or with the elbow in extension.
- Separate medial and/or lateral incisions may be used for focal medial or lateral pathology, respectively. Although this avoids the creation of such large skin flaps, full articular access through either the triceps-reflecting or olecranon osteotomy pathways (see below) will be hindered.

Posterior Approaches

- Posterior approaches differ based on how they navigate around the extensor mechanism. Each technique offers different levels of articular exposure and potential postoperative drawbacks. Common methods include
  - Olecranon osteotomy
  - Triceps-splitting approach
  - Triceps-reflecting approach (Bryan-Morrey)

Equipment

- Beanbag, axillary roll, and armholder or bolster for the lateral position.
- Towel bump, sterile Mayo stand for supine position.
- Possible ipsilateral armboard for supine position.
- For isolated distal lateral column and capitellar fractures, a short armboard provides support of the elbow while allowing both surgeons access to the elbow.

  - Triceps-reflecting anconeus pedicle flap (TRAP)
  - Paratricipital (triceps-sparing) approach
- The initial skin and subcutaneous approach is similar among all posterior approaches.
  - A posterior midline skin incision is made over the triceps to the tip of the olecranon, at which point it is carried either just medial or lateral to it. Distally, the incision passes along the proximal ulnar subcutaneous border.
  - Full-thickness flaps are developed deep to the triceps fascia proximally and deep to the forearm fascia distally.
  - The ulnar nerve can be palpated along the medial edge of the triceps, posterior to the medial septum, where it can be visualized following release of the superficial fascia (Fig. 7A).
    - If the nerve is to be transposed (recommended for posteriomedial capsulotomy or placement of hardware along the medial epicondyle), it should be mobilized from the cubital tunnel. The fascia overlying the cubital tunnel (often referred to as Osborne's bands) is divided along with the aponeurosis between the two heads of the FCU distally.
    - Proximal-to-distal dissection and mobilization of the nerve will allow identification of the motor branch to the FCU, which should be preserved. Short, articular branches entering the posteromedial joint capsule (Fig. 7B) can be divided to mobilize the nerve, and the multiple venous branches in the distal portion of the tunnel can be ligated with bipolar electrocautery forceps.

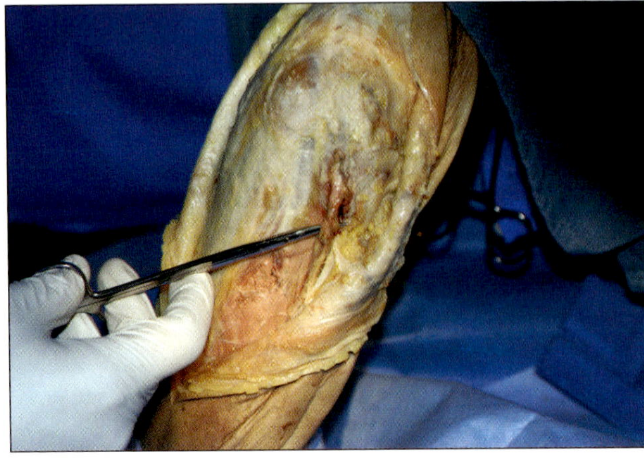

A

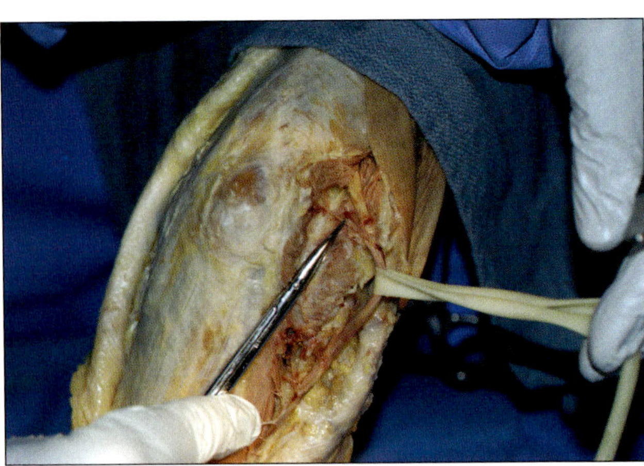

B

FIGURE 7

- The distal portion of the medial intermuscular septum is excised, as it will tether or compress the anteriorly transposed nerve.
- A full-thickness subcutaneous flap over the medial flexor-pronator origin is created for placement of the nerve at the conclusion of the procedure.
- The medial and lateral borders of the triceps are visualized and the distal portion is sharply separated from the posterior humeral cortex. The muscle can be elevated from the bone proximally, leaving it tethered distally at its olecranon insertion (Fig. 8). Recall that the radial nerve resides in the groove between the medial and lateral heads of the triceps. It penetrates the lateral intermuscular septum approximately 10 cm from the lateral epicondyle, whose normal anatomic distance is likely to be shortened in the fracture situation.

- Olecranon osteotomy
  - The olecranon osteotomy offers the widest exposure for both fracture reduction and hardware placement. Full access to the humeral metadiaphysis and all but the most anterior portion of the articular surface is available through this approach (Fig. 9A and 9B). Furthermore, as the osteotomized fragments "fall away" from the distal humeral surface, there is less need for an assistant delegated to full-time retraction of the proximal ulna throughout the procedure.
  - Potential drawbacks include olecranon nonunion and compromise of ulnar component placement in subsequent total elbow arthroplasty, if necessary. Furthermore, hardware used for fixation of the osteotomy is frequently symptomatic, requiring removal.

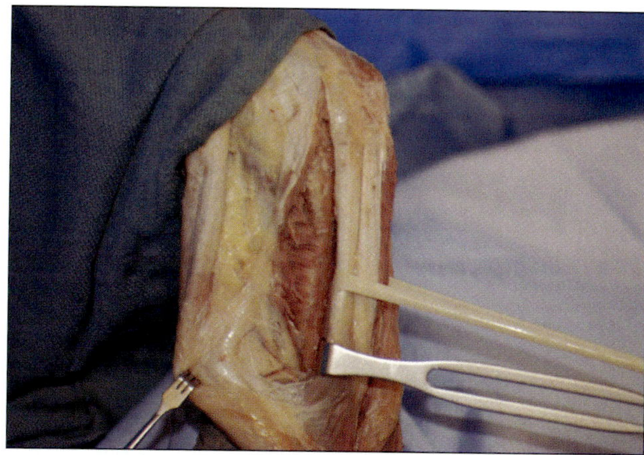

FIGURE 8

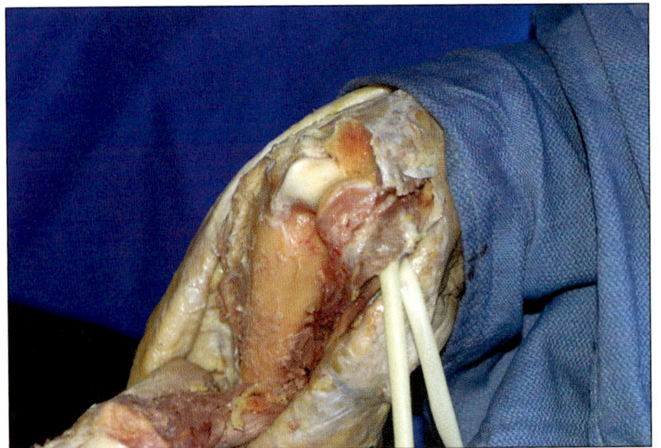

A

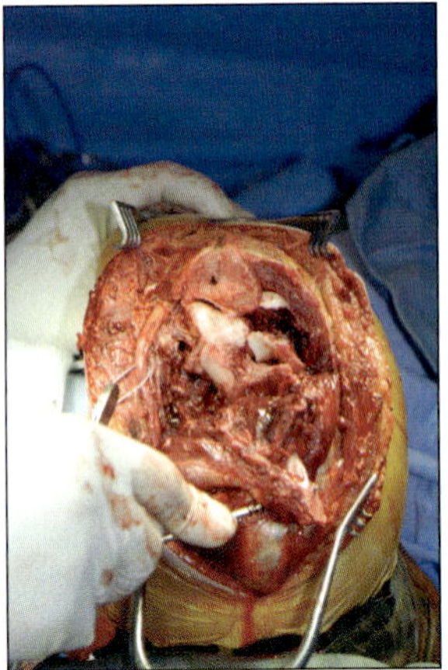

B

FIGURE 9

- Following the previously described posterior approach and ulnar nerve mobilization, a posterior capsulotomy is completed on the medial and ulnar aspects of the ulnohumeral joint, exposing the central "bare area" of the ulnar sigmoid notch. The osteotomy is to broach the articular surface at this level.
- Before actually performing the osteotomy, it is useful to temporarily apply whatever fixation method is preferred: Kirschner wires (K-wires), intramedullary compression screws, or a posterior plate. This allows the fixation device to assist with anatomic reduction at the time of closure.
- An osteotomy is performed with a thin oscillating saw blade in an apex-distal chevron configuration through the posterior cortex, stopping short of penetrating the articular surface (Fig. 10A).
- The osteotomy is completed with osteotome leverage, fracturing through the remaining subchondral bone and cartilage at the level of the bare area (Fig. 10B). This will create small interdigitations at the articular surface, enhancing anatomic reduction and rotational stability upon repair.
- The proximal fragment, with the triceps still attached, is reflected to expose the posterior articular surface and humeral cortex.
- The TRAP (triceps-reflecting, anconeus-preserving) variation of this approach involves inclusion of the anconeus with the proximal fragment, which avoids denervation of this dynamic stabilizing muscle.

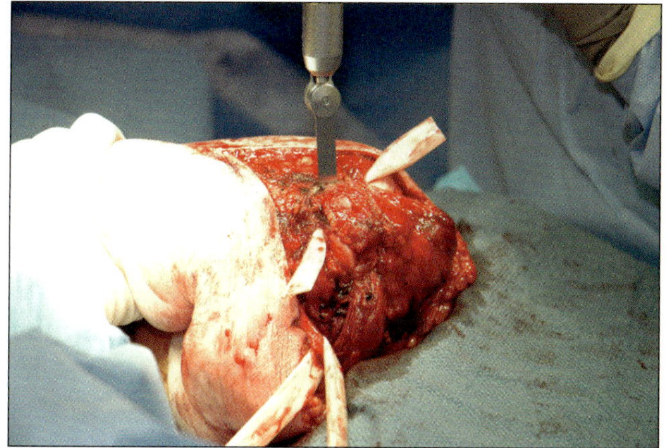
A

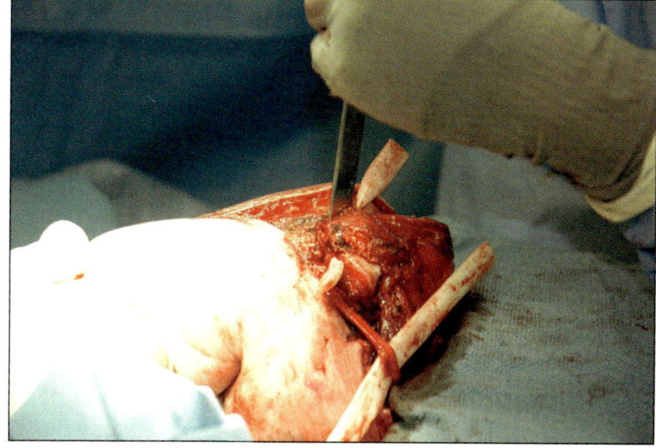
B

FIGURE 10

- Following posterior capsulotomy, the fascia is divided between the anconeus and extensor carpi ulnaris to the level of the anconeus insertion on the ulna (Fig. 11A).
- The anconeus is separated from its ulnar insertion, leaving the proximal origin intact, just proximal to the level of the osteotomy (Fig. 11B).

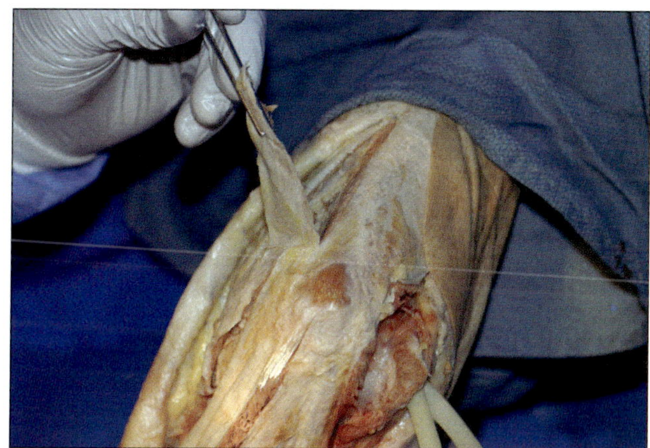
A

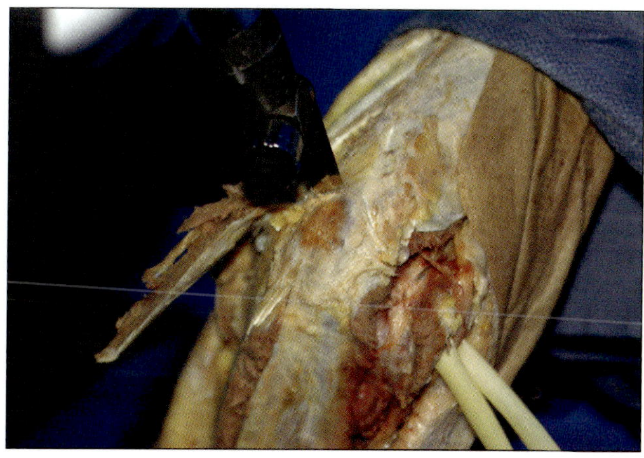
B

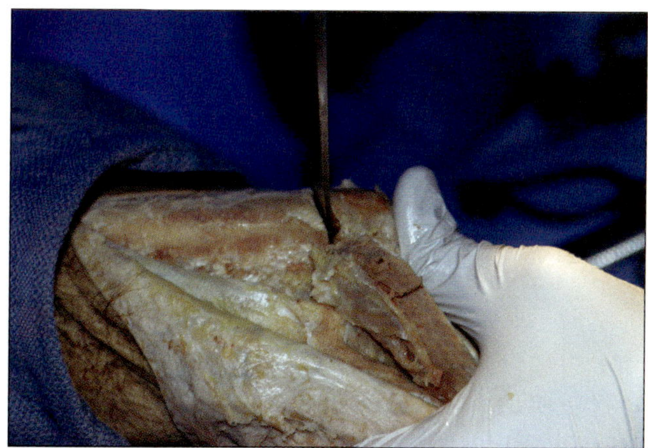
C

FIGURE 11

    - After muscle detachment from the ulna and underlying joint capsule, the osteotomy is completed and the muscle reflected proximally with the triceps and proximal ulnar fragment (Fig. 11C).
  - Exposure and access for fixation of anterior articular surface fragments may require release of the collateral ligament (medial or lateral) (Fig. 12A–C), followed by anatomic reattachment with suture anchors or drill tunnels at the conclusion of the procedure.
- Triceps-splitting approach
  - This approach is a full-thickness, midline split of the triceps tendon down to the ulnar insertion, allowing adequate exposure of the posterior capsule and proximal ulna.
  - The muscle is divided proximally to expose the posterior humeral cortex, but the proximal

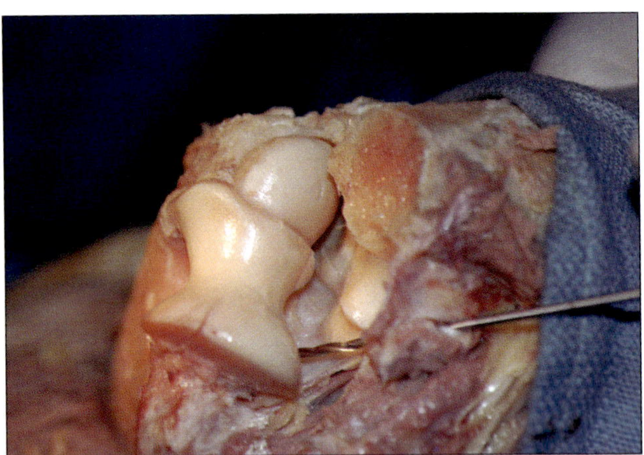

A

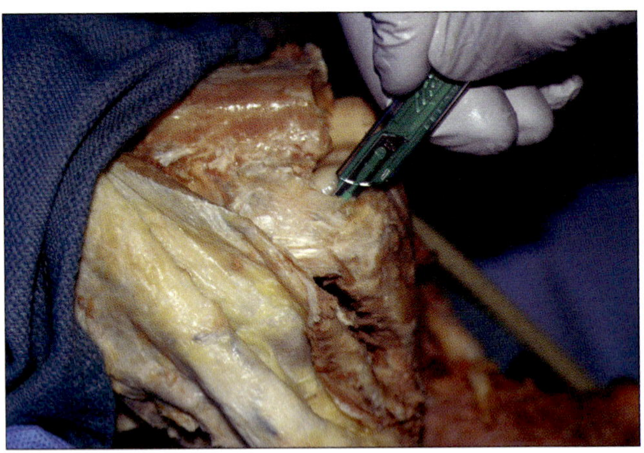

B

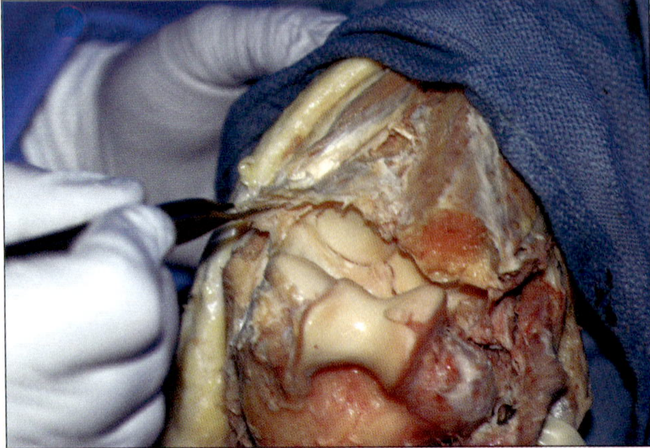

C

FIGURE 12

extension of this approach is limited by the radial nerve.

- Distally, the tendinous split is extended over the proximal ulna, elevating both sleeves subperiosteally.
  - The ulnar nerve must be identified and protected as the medial sleeve is reflected.
- Any ligamentous detachment from the epicondylar fragments to improve articular exposure mandates anatomic repair with bone tunnels or suture anchors with nonabsorbable suture (#0 or #2) upon closure.
- The tendon is repaired with nonabsorbable suture at the end of the procedure. Traversing drill tunnels for suture placement through the proximal ulna may help stabilize the repair onto the ulna.
- Postoperatively, the patient will need to refrain from elbow hyperflexion (>90°) or resisted extension for at least 6 weeks.

■ Triceps-reflecting approach
- This approach entails reflection of the entire extensor mechanism from the proximal ulna following the medial capsulotomy.
- Following ulnar nerve mobilization and reflection of the distal triceps from the posterior humeral cortex, the triceps tendon, ulnar periosteum, and forearm facscia are sharply reflected from the olecranon as a contiguous sleeve from the proximal ulna with the fascia along the ulnar forearm (Fig. 13A and 13B). (Division of Sharpey's fibers from the ulnar insertion must be done carefully with a sharp blade to avoid buttonholing

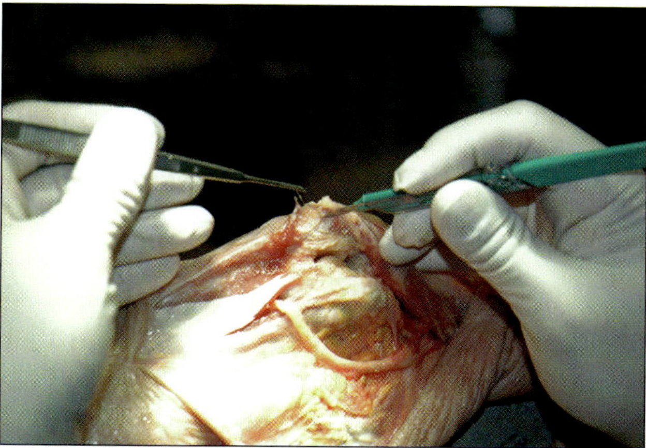

A

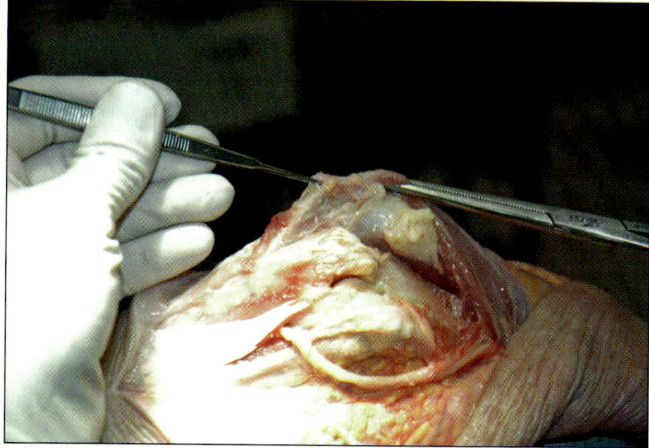

B

FIGURE 13

Pearls

- *Tourniquet use is helpful during the approach and fracture exposure, particularly for dissection and mobilization of the median nerve. It may then be deflated for more proximal exposure or fracture fixation work.*
- *Olecranon osteotomy negates the diverging "wedge" effect of the intact proximal ulna on the trochlear groove, thus facilitating reapproximation of the medial and lateral fragments. Otherwise, collateral ligament detachment will be needed to reflect the proximal ulna, or an assistant will be required to support the forearm and eliminate the pressure of the ulna on the trochlear groove.*
- *The radial nerve may also be located posterolaterally by following the lateral brachial cutaneous nerve, which branches from the radial nerve and emerges on the posterior aspect of the lateral intermuscular septum.*
- *If greater access to the articular surface is required for an isolated distal lateral column or capitellar fracture, sharp detachment of the LUCL origin may be beneficial. The ligament origin will need to be anatomically restored with #2 or #5 braided suture either through drill tunnels or with a suture anchor at the conclusion of the procedure.*

through the triceps tendon.) The entire extensor sleeve is reflected laterally, exposing the entire proximal ulna and distal humerus.

- Alternatively, a thin wafer of bone from the olecranon tip may be elevated with the tendon to minimize the likelihood of inadvertent perforation and enhance the subsequent repair by allowing bone-to-bone healing.
- Detachment of collateral ligament origins may be required to reflect the proximal ulna and enhance articular exposure. Again, however, the collateral ligament origin must be repaired upon closure.
- Following fracture fixation, the tendon is repaired to the proximal ulna with nonabsorbable suture (I prefer #2 or #5 FiberWire) passed through ulnar drill tunnels created with a 2-mm drill bit.
- The repair must be protected against resisted elbow extension or hyperflexion for at least 6 weeks.

■ Paratricipital approach
- Aside from elevation of the medial and lateral aspects of the muscle from the posterior humeral cortex, the triceps is left undisturbed. The central portion of the muscle may be elevated proximally off the humerus, taking care to avoid injury to the radial nerve.
- Although this approach avoids the potential disadvantages of triceps insufficiency, osteotomy nonunion, or symptomatic posterior ulnar hardware, visualization of the articular surface is significantly limited.
- This approach is indicated for the most simple fracture patterns, such as an extra-articular or simple intercondylar split configuration.
- Collateral ligament origin detachment will allow for reflection of the triceps-forearm unit and exposure of the humeral metaphysis and articular surface, if necessary.
- Anatomic repair of the collateral ligament origin and subsequent protection of repair are required at the conclusion of the procedure.

Lateral Approaches

■ For isolated fracture patterns of the lateral condyle or capitellum, lateral incision and joint exposure with any necessary extension up the lateral humeral column should provide adequate access for lateral articular hardware and lateral column plate placement.

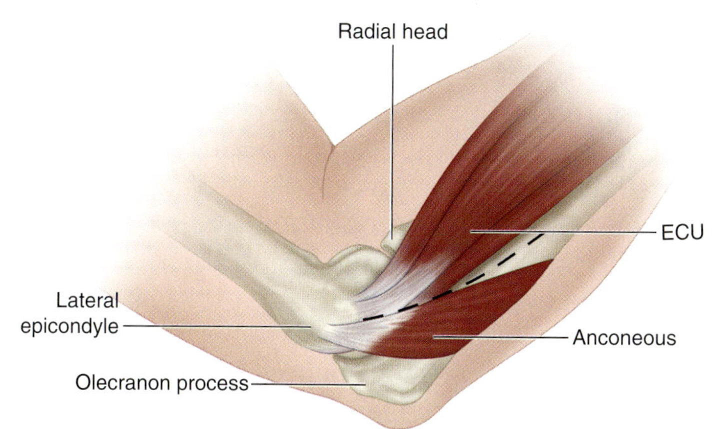

A

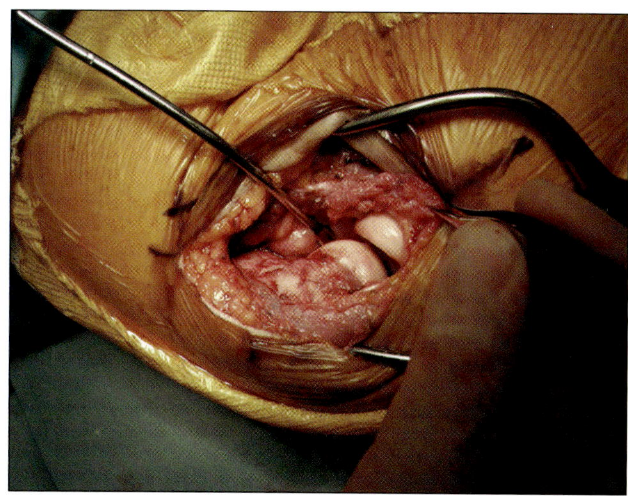
B

FIGURE 14

PITFALLS

- *Allowing a thick oscillating saw blade with a wide kerf to penetrate the articular surface may result in bone loss at the osteotomy site. Upon repair, this may result in narrowing of the ulnar sigmoid notch and incongruity of the ulnohumeral articulation.*
- *In isolated distal lateral column and capitellar fractures, avoid inadvertent detachment of the LUCL origin just anterior and distal to the lateral epicondyle, unless it is deemed necessary for greater medial articular access.*

- Kocher approach
  - The interval for the Kocher approach is between the extensor carpi ulnaris and the anconeus (Fig. 14A and 14B), sometimes indentified by a subtle fat stripe between the two muscles. The supinator muscle fibers are found traversing the radial neck in the distal portion of the interval. The fascia is incised from the lateral epicondyle toward the distal border of the anconeus insertion on the ulna.
  - To avoid disruption of the LUCL origin (Fig. 15; marked in red), the capsulotomy begins proximally at the midcoronal line of the radiocapitellar joint, extending from the lateral collateral ligament origin toward the radial neck. The annular ligament can be divided, if necessary, for greater exposure.

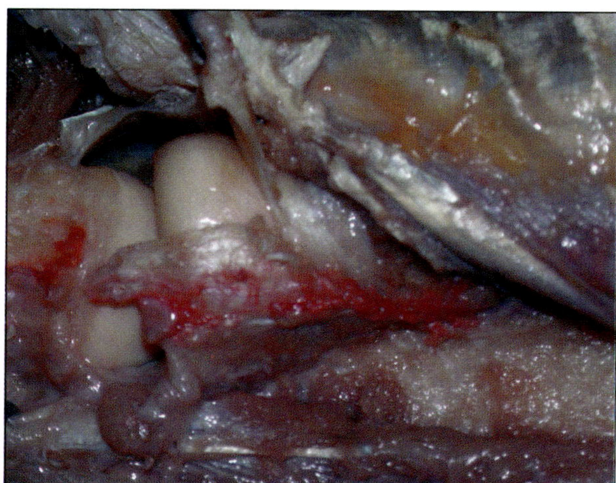

FIGURE 15

Instrumentation

- Thin oscillating saw blade, osteotomes for olecranon osteotomy
- Hardware for eventual osteotomy repair: 6.5- or 7.3-mm cannulated screw with washer, 18-gauge tension band wire, 0.045-inch K-wires, or precontoured olecranon plate
- 2.0-mm drill bit, looped suture passer, and #2 or #5 nonabsorbable suture for triceps tendon reattachment or collateral ligament repair
- Possible suture anchor with #2 or #5 nonabsorbable suture for collateral ligament repair

  - Forearm pronation will maximize the distance between the scalpel and the posterior interosseous nerve (PIN), lying between the bellies of the supinator muscle along the radial neck.
  - The lateral portion of the anterior joint capsule can be sharply reflected from the lateral humerus to expose the lateral articular surface. Further access to the lateral column can be obtained by extending the incision proximally along the lateral supracondylar ridge.
- Kaplan approach
  - The Kaplan approach offers an exposure to the lateral epicondyle and articular surface similar to that of the Kocher approach, but splits the extensor musculature more anterior, providing greater exposure of radial neck than the Kocher interval, if needed (Fig. 16A).
  - A skin incision is made from the lateral epicondyle toward Lister's tubercle with the forearm in neutral rotation for a distance of 4 cm.
  - As with the Kocher interval, the incision basically bisects the radiocapitellar joint, but uses the interval between the extensor carpi radialis longus (ECRL) and the extensor digitorum communis (EDC). This interval can be identified by the muscular ECRL originating from the supracondylar ridge and the more tendonous EDC just posterior. The extensor carpi radialis brevis (ECRB) is just deep to this interval, overlying the joint capsule (Fig. 16B).
  - The interval may be incised as one layer down through the joint capsule, keeping the forearm

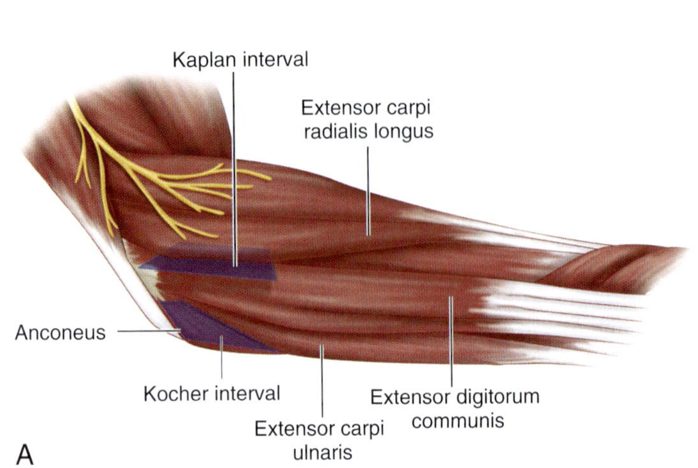

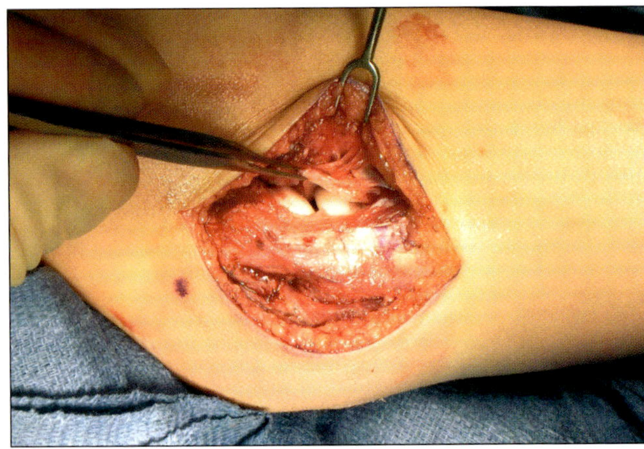

FIGURE 16

pronated to avoid injury to the PIN. Distally, divide the annular ligament for exposure of the radial neck. The supinator may also be divided, but be aware of the PIN, which can usually be palpated within the muscle.

- As with the Kocher interval, the Kaplan approach may be extended proximally up the lateral supracondylar ridge to provide proximal exposure of the lateral column.

Instrumentation/ Implantation

- As inadequate distal fixation is a commonly cited reason for failure, modern precontoured distal humerus plates available from a variety of implant manufacturers offer more distal screw holes, both locking and nonlocking (Fig. 17).
- If such plates are not available, 3.5-mm recon plates (preferably locking) can be contoured along the medial and lateral columns. However, they do not usually offer as many distal fixation holes.

Procedure: Distal Humerus Fractures

Step 1

- The strategy for repair of distal humerus fractures is restoration and stabilization of articular congruity with stable proximal fixation to the medial and lateral columns to allow for early motion.
  - Historically, distal comminution, osteoporotic bone, and limited fixation options have made this a difficult objective. Fixation failure usually occurs at the supracondylar level, where the bone is thinner and stable distal fixation is difficult to obtain.
  - Prolonged immobilization to protect marginal fixation leads to joint contracture.
  - The most common strategy for fracture management entails initial assembly and provisional fixation of the distal platform, then "docking" of the articular platform to the humeral metadiaphysis with definitive distal fixation and compression columnar plating.

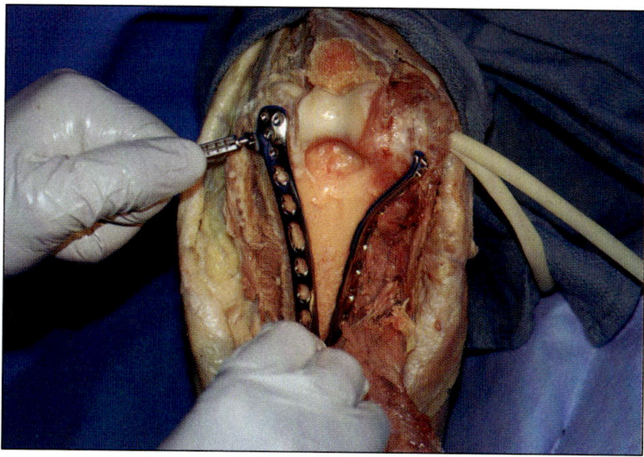

FIGURE 17

Controversies

- "90-90" fixation, in which columnar plates were oriented perpendicular to each other along the humerus (medial plate in the sagittal plane and lateral plate in the coronal plane), has been the formal recommendation of the AO/ASIF group. However, the distal humerus undergoes internal rotational forces each time the flexed elbow is abducted from the body, pulling the lateral column away from any posterior-to-anterior fixation. Alignment of the lateral column plate more in the sagittal plane with screws traversing to the medial side of the distal fragment confers greater stability. It should be noted that, while some systems offer posteriorly positioned lateral column plates, the distal locking screw holes are oriented to provide obliquely oriented rigid fixation.

- O'Driscoll (2005) has offered useful guidelines for the management of distal humerus bicolumnar fractures. Although not every recommendation may be met when addressing a given fracture, the principles are useful to keep in mind throughout the procedure:
  - Every screw engaging the distal fragments should pass through a plate.
  - Screws should engage a fragment on the opposite side that is also fixed to a plate.
  - As many screws as possible should be placed through plates into the distal fragments.
  - Each screw should be as long as possible.
  - Each screw should engage as many articular fragments as possible.
  - Screws in the distal fragments should interdigitate from each side.
  - Columnar plates should be used to achieve compression fixation of the articular segment at the supracondylar level.
  - Plates must be strong enough to resist failure prior to fracture union.
- The remaining description of the repair technique assumes posterior exposure of bicolumnar patterns through one of the posterior approaches described above. For more complex patterns, the olecranon osteotomy approach will provide the most versatile exposure.

Step 2

- Plain radiographs often underestimate the degree of articular comminution. The surgeon must avoid the temptation to immediately remove the loose fragments and begin reassembling them on the back table. Before mobilizing (or removing) the fragments, their relationship in situ to the other fragments and columns should be noted.
- A dental pick or small curette is used with irrigation to débride hematoma from the joint and among articular fragments.
- Provisional K-wires are used to assemble fragments in their native anatomic position relative to each other and to the epicondyles.
- Following olecranon osteotomy, the forearm pulls the medial and lateral epicondylar fragments apart through the collateral ligaments as it falls away from the humerus. This force may need to be neutralized by an assistant or by temporarily securing the forearm to the Mayo stand until the joint platform is provisionally reassembled.

Pitfalls

- *Avoid use of traversing lag screw fixation across comminuted articular fragments, as this may compress and alter the anatomic contours of the joint surface (do not narrow the articular groove) (Fig. 19).*
- *Avoid using screw fixation for initial reassembly of the articular surface. Distal screws that are not placed through columnar plates potentially impede space for placement of essential fixation components later.*

Instrumentation/ Implantation

- Temporary smooth or permanent threaded 0.035-inch or 0.045-inch pins
- Small countersunk or headless compression screws

- In situations of severe comminution, every effort should be made to restore at least the anterior articular surface. At a minimum, the medial trochlear eminence and either the lateral eminence or capitellum is required for stability. If the MCL is deficient, an intact radiocapitellar articulation is necessary. The radial head or osteotomized olecranon/coronoid fragment can be held against the articular surface as a reduction template.
- Smaller or thin osteochondral fragments that cannot eventually be captured by screw fixation through plates may require fixation through countersunk threaded pins or compression screws. However, these should be applied sparingly, as excessive permanent hardware in the distal platform will obscure passage of vital screws placed through the distal portions of the columnar plates to stabilize the articular block to the proximal fragments. Either headless or standard compression screws, in particular, have a larger profile that may hinder subsequent screw placement. If possible, it is better to delay such countersunk hardware placement until after distal screws have been placed through plates.
- Countersunk threaded pins may be used as permanent fixation to stabilize small or thin osteochondral fragments. Use of 0.045-inch or 0.062-inch K-wires is generally preferred.
  - While the fragment is held in place, the pin is drilled antegrade through the articular surface at such an angle that it will exit outside of the joint cavity and not under a plate (Fig. 18A; fracture lines drawn in black ink). The threaded pin is advanced across the fracture, exiting in a safe location that will not impede motion or injure neurovascular structures.
  - When the pin exits the opposite cortex, it is drilled retrograde (recall that the pin driver must be switched to the "reverse" setting for threaded pins) until it is well seated under the articular surface, while still maintaining purchase of the thin subchondral articular bone fragment (Fig. 18B; fracture lines drawn in black ink).
  - The pin is then cut, leaving enough length exposed to allow instrument purchase for removal, if necessary (Fig. 18C). I prefer to cut the pin with *at least* 5 mm protruding from the cortex to allow for potential eventual removal with a needle driver. Such a scenario may arise in the setting of infected

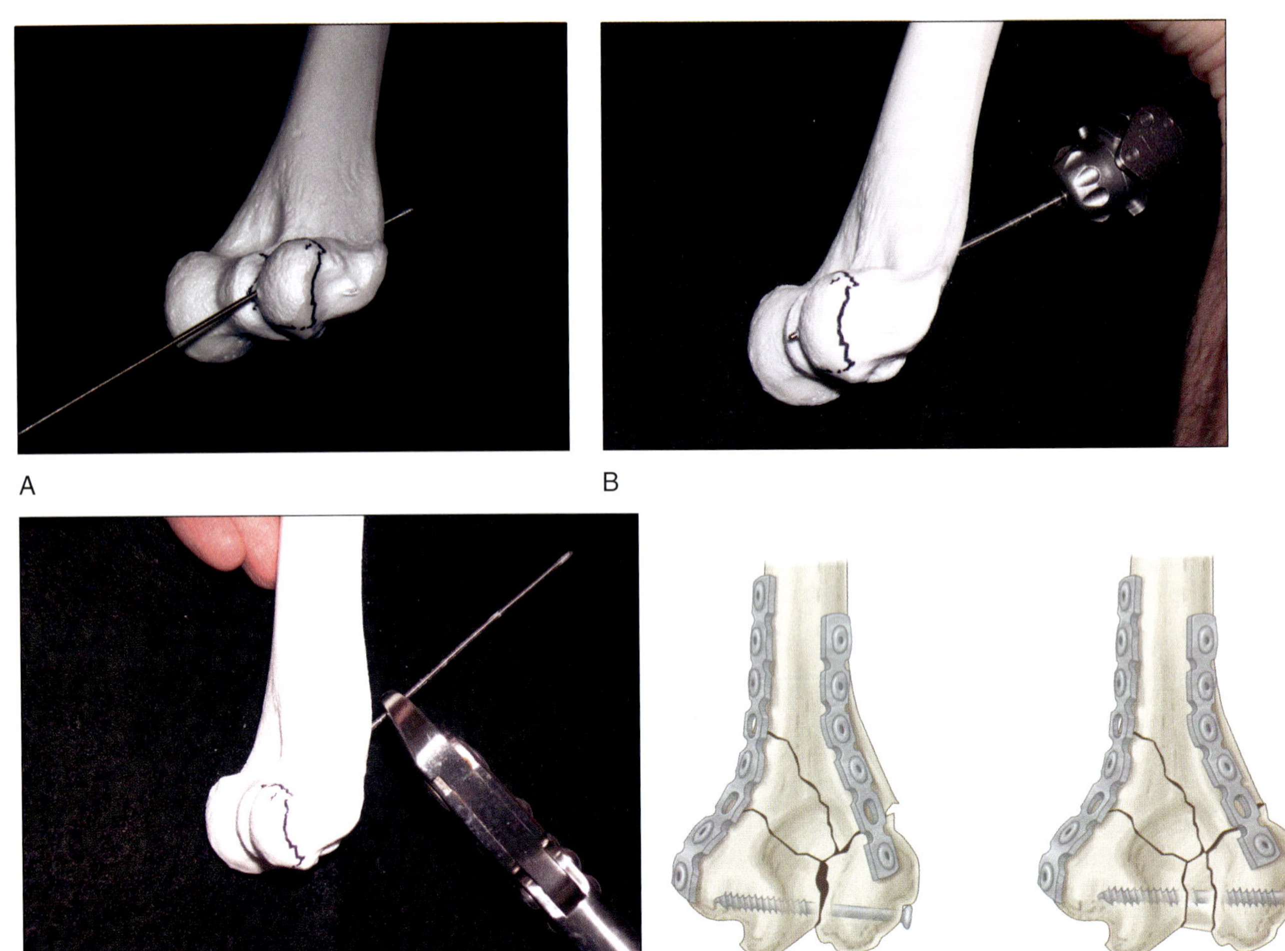

FIGURE 18

FIGURE 19

or symptomatic hardware, conversion to total elbow arthroplasty, or articular settling that results in the distal portion of the pin protruding into the joint.

- In situations with articular comminution, avoid altering the medial-lateral joint dimensions with compression fixation (Fig. 19)

Instrumentation/ Implantation

- Medial and lateral columnar plates with the maximum number of distal screw holes for purchase of the articular platform

Step 3

- Following articular surface restoration and provisional fixation, the distal segment is "docked" to the proximal metadiaphysis. This entails selecting, contouring, and positioning plates so that they will obtain as many traversing screws as possible in the distal segment while compressing it to the proximal columns.
- If there is significant metaphyseal comminution, the surgeon should proceed from proximal to distal using smaller lag screws and perhaps temporary smooth K-wires.

- Metadiaphyseal bone loss is not uncommon in open metadiaphyseal high-energy injuries in which the proximal bone penetrates the posterior soft tissues and strikes the pavement. In these situations, primary shortening is used to close the gap and provide compression of the remaining shaft to the distal segment. This is preferred over primary bone grafting to maintain length, as union will be slower and such injuries are more prone to infection.
  - Preoperative radiographs of such an open injury (Fig. 20A and 20B) reveal obvious bone loss of the distal metaphysis.

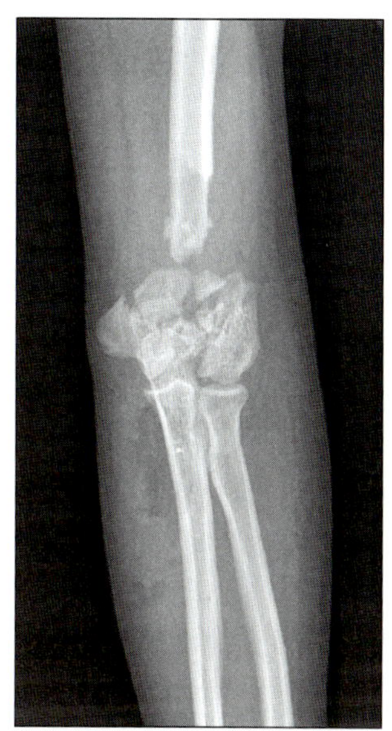

A

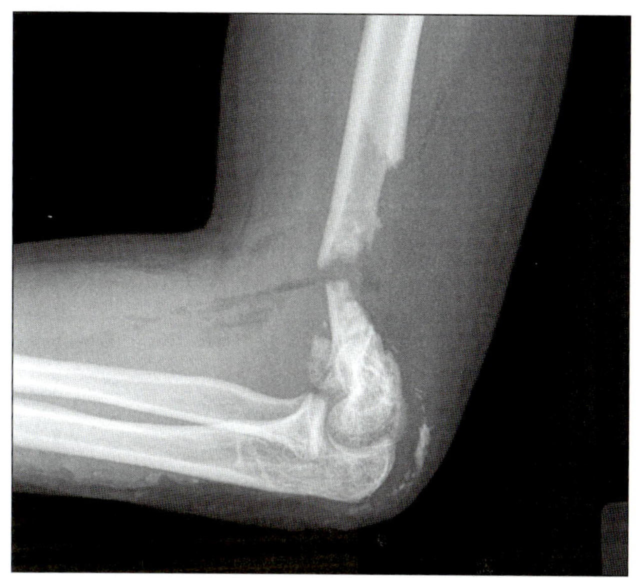

B

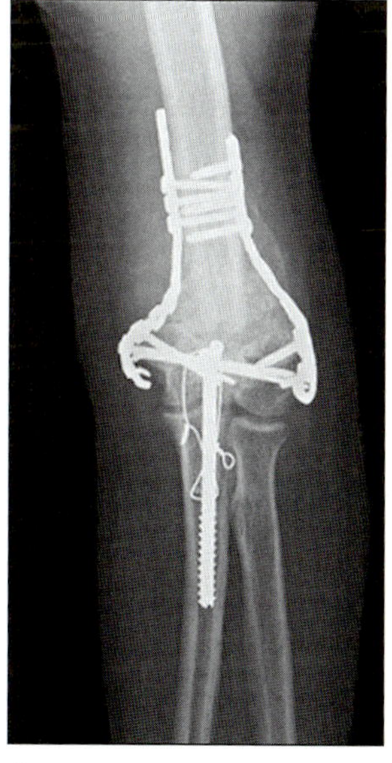

C

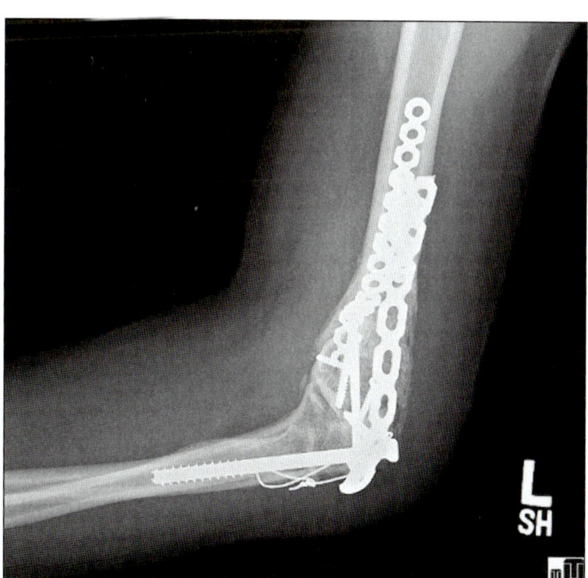

D

FIGURE 20

  - Postoperative radiographs following a subsequent bone grafting procedure at a later date (Fig. 20C and 20D) demonstrate primary shortening to obtain bone contact. When soft tissues had stabilized without features of infection, subsequent cancellous autograft was placed.
- The distal segment can be either held in the reduced position by an assistant or provisionally secured with 0.062-inch smooth pins placed down the medial and lateral columns. Even with the pins, someone usually needs to neutralize the weight of the forearm, which is pulling the distal segment anteriorly through the collateral ligaments.
- Columnar plates are selected that:
  - Provide the maximum number of holes for fixation in the distal segment (preferably three from each side).
  - Provide at least three holes for purchase in a stable, noncomminuted metaphysis or diaphysis proximally.
  - Contact (or can be contoured for a low profile fit on) the distal segments. This is especially important if nonlocking fixation is to be used, as it will pull the distal fragment to the plate, potentially displacing it.
  - Preferably do not end at the same level proximally, which would theoretically create a stress riser at that level.
- The plates are then provisionally applied to the distal and proximal segments, employing either temporary pin holes in some systems, screws placed in slotted holes in the proximal or distal fragments, or clamps holding the plates onto the bone.
- The medial column plate should be more in the sagittal plane, reaching distally to the inferior portion of the medial epicondyle.
- The lateral column plate should ideally be placed posterolaterally, so that the distal screws project distally, anteriorly, and medially across the lateral condyle, capturing trochlear components (Fig. 21). As noted earlier, some precontoured lateral column plates “wrap around” the distal portion of the lateral column, so that their distal screws project medially instead of straight anterior.
- The distal screws are placed in an alternating sequence (medial, lateral) to ensure that at least some screws from each side are able to traverse to the far side of the distal fragment to obtain optimal

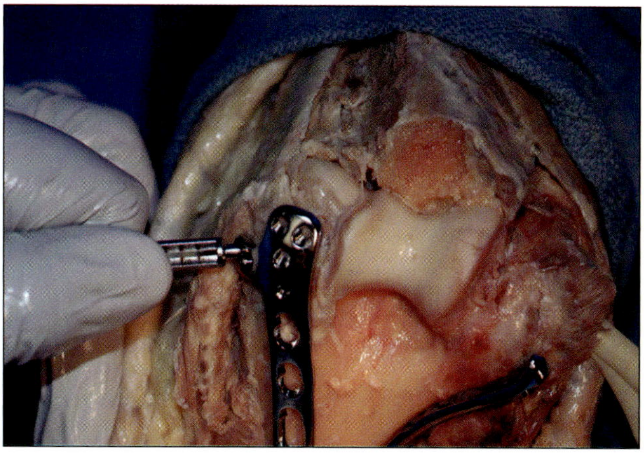

FIGURE 21

Pitfalls

- *Some surgeons do not transpose the ulnar nerve if there is no hardware infringing upon the ulnar groove by the medial epicondyle. In my opinion, this only invites problems. The surgical manipulation of the nerve and subsequent swelling alone can induce postoperative sensory or motor changes, which are usually transient. Leaving the nerve in the groove not only subjects the surgeon to significant self-reproach, it may also result in a return to the operating room for a transposition. Also, the pain from flexion-induced traction on the nerve left in the groove can significantly hamper motion exercises.*
- *Inadequate length of intramedullary screw fixation of the osteotomy can result in failure. It is probably safe to at least have thread contact with the endosteum of the ulnar canal (usually 85–100 mm). Supplementation with an 18-gauge wire tension band construct is advised.*
- *Excessively long K-wires used as an alternative to intramedullary screw fixation risk injury to the anterior interosseous nerve.*

stability before the trochlear intersection gets too crowded. Locking screws, if available, can provide more rigid fixation in distal osteoporotic bone.
  - Recall that, ideally, each screw should pass through a plate, be as long and traverse as many fragments as possible, and capture a fragment on the opposite side that is also attached to a plate.
- Verify that no screws traverse or obstruct the coronoid, olecranon, or radial head fossae of the distal humerus.
- The columnar plates are then definitively fixed to the proximal fragment with at least three bicortical nonlocking or three unicortical locking screws. If possible, the surgeon should work to place at least one nonlocking screw in compression mode through each plate to promote union at the supracondylar level.

Step 4

- The wound is irrigated, removing articular debris.
- The olecranon osteotomy, if performed, is repaired. Interdigitations along the articular surface are used to verify rotational orientation of fragments.
  - If an intramedullary compression screw has been predrilled and preplaced prior to the osteotomy, the screw (with a washer) is placed back into the fragments and tightening is stopped just before contact with the triceps tendon. This may be supplemented with a tension band (Fig. 22A and 22B).
    - For tension band wire passage, a transverse bone tunnel is drilled with a 1.5- to 2.0-mm drill bit in the dorsal half of the proximal ulna, distal to the

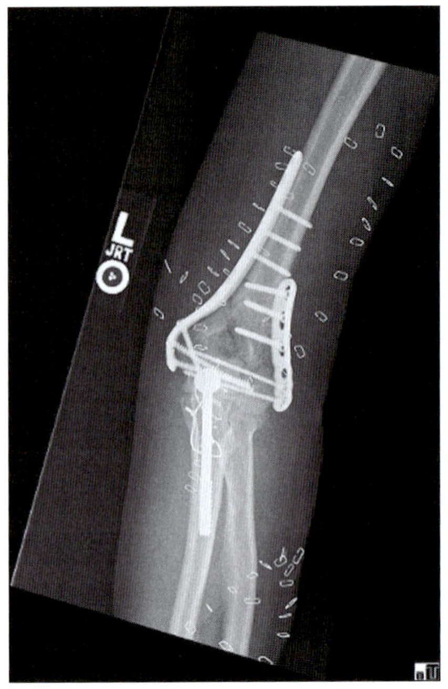

A

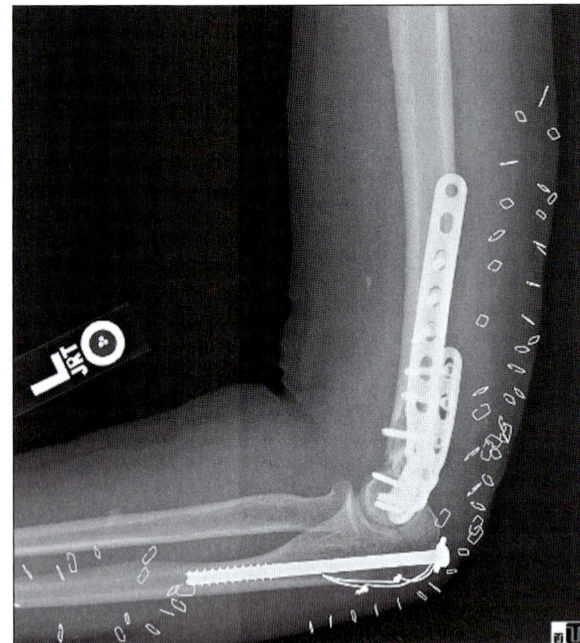

B

FIGURE 22

Controversies

- Postoperative splinting of the elbow in extension may help with hemostasis and also help the patient in regaining extension postoperatively. Extension splinting also minimizes tension along the olecranon incision line and should be considered if posterior flap perfusion appears tenuous.

osteotomy site. The distance of the drill tunnel from the osteotomy should equal the distance from the osteotomy to the tip of the olecranon.

- The 18-gauge wire is placed through the tunnel, crossing each limb of the wire over the osteotomy site, and passing one arm under the shaft of the screw, distal to the washer.
- As the screw is tightened, the surfaces of the osteotomy site should align and compressed.
- The ends of the wire are twisted together while a loop is twisted into the other arm of the wire to create a double-twist configuration to the tension band. Both twists are continued until the wire is taut. The wire is then cut so that at least four twists remain in each bundle, and the bundles are then folded down and seated with a tamp until flush with the surrounding tissue.

- An alternative to intramedullary screw fixation is the use of two parallel K-wires crossing the osteotomy site as the proximal anchor point for the tension band wiring. However, the K-wires should not be directed down the medullary canal. They should obtain purchase in the anterior ulnar cortex along the base of the coronoid process, as seen in the transverse olecranon fracture pattern in Figure. 23A and 23B.

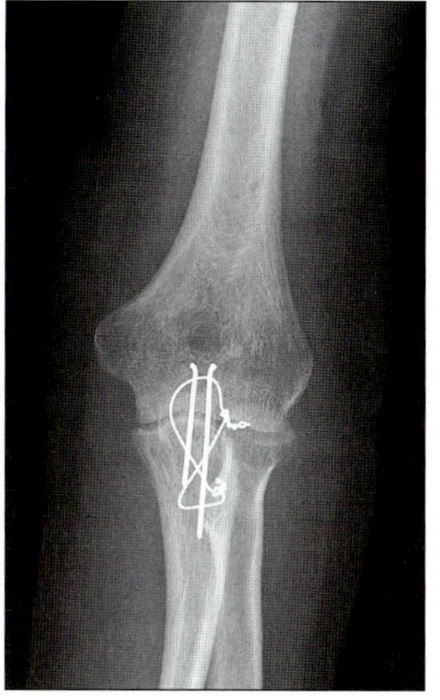

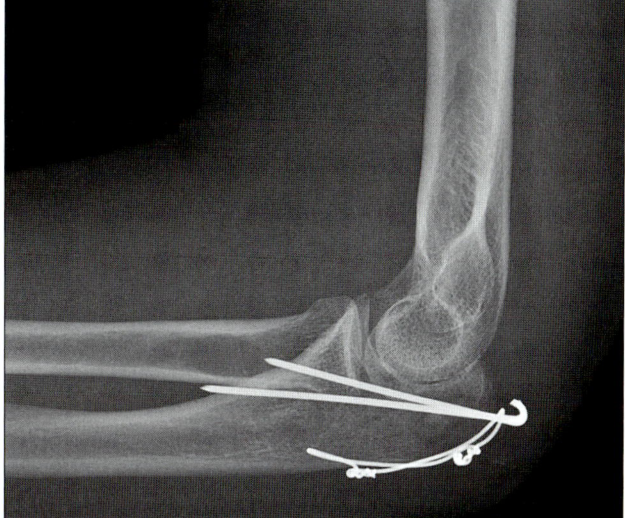

A B

FIGURE 23

- Precontoured olecranon plates may also be used for osteotomy repair.
- The joint is flexed, extended, supinated, and pronated to verify that there is no crepitus or hardware protruding into the articular surface.
- Fracture, olecranon, and hardware position are verified with fluoroscopy or plain radiographs before proceeding further.
- If a triceps-reflecting approach was utilized, 2.0-mm drill tunnels are placed in a cruciate manner for reattachment of the triceps to the olecranon with #2 nonabsorbable suture. A transverse drill tunnel just distal to the cruciate holes is placed to supplement the repair with a separate #2 suture.
- Triceps-splitting approaches are repaired with #2 nonabsorbable suture in figure-of-8 fashion. Two transverse tunnels in the proximal ulna can be used to further anchor the repair to the bone with nonabsorbable suture.
- The medial and lateral joint capsule can be repaired with #0 Vicryl suture.
- If used, the tourniquet should be deflated to verify hemostasis prior to further closure. The surgeon should not hesitate to place a drain if there is significant oozing of the wound.
- The ulnar nerve is placed in the previously prepared subcutaneous pocket anterior to the medial epicondyle. The nerve may be secured anteriorly with a fascial sling elevated and sutured to the subcutaneous tissue or by a direct suture from the

subcutaneous tissue to the medial epicondyle. Prior to placing the stitch in the medial subcutaneous layer, the surgeon must verify that it is not being passed through or around the medial antebrachial cutaneous nerve. Following suture placement, the nerve is subjected to a gentle proximal-distal "glide" test to verify that it is not incarcerated.

- The subcutaneous layers are closed with absorbable suture. Nylon or staples can be safely used for skin, but I prefer mattress 4-0 nylon directly over the thinner layer at the olecranon, as staples may apply more tension than is needed for skin edge approximation at that level.
- A sterile padded dressing is applied and the arm is splinted in either extension or 90° of flexion (see Controversies). An antecubital splint may be more effective in obese patients.

PROCEDURE: Isolated Distal Lateral Column and Capitellar Fractures

Step 1

- The surgical approach is as described earlier for either the Kaplan or Kocher interval.
- The fracture site is cleared of hematoma and smaller articular fragments with irrigation and a dental pick. Smaller, free fragments that cannot be captured with hardware may need to be excised.
- The fragment(s) are reduced with a dental pick or small reduction clamp.
- Smooth 0.035-inch or 0.045-inch K-wires are used for provisional fixation (Fig. 24).

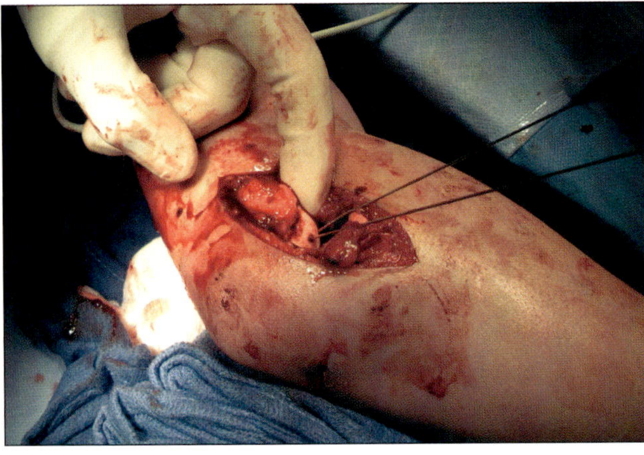

FIGURE 24

Step 2

- Carefully scrutinize the reduction, verifying its relation to the lateral trochlear ridge. For capitellar fractures, the articular fragment must not be fixed with any proximal displacement, which would obstruct the radial head during elbow flexion.
- Anterior articular surface fractures (Fig. 25A) can then be fixed with screws placed either anteriorly or posteriorly. Headless compression screws (Fig. 25B and 25C) or 2.0-mm countersunk headed screws can be placed through the articular surface. Countersunk headed screws, however, are more prone to protrude into the joint with articular fragment settling.
- More complex patterns may have involvement of the lateral epicondyle and posterior aspect of the lateral column. This posterior involvement may include the posterior portion of the trochlea. If the epicondyle is fractured, it may be reflected distally with the common extensor origin and LCL to provide reasonable exposure to the articular surface. The posterior fragments are often impacted, which should be addressed in order to restore proper alignment.
- Fractures involving the entire lateral condyle may be better stabilized with a lateral column plate. The capitellar fracture seen in Figure 26A was found to have posterior extension through the lateral condyle on CT imaging (Fig. 26B), necessitating lateral column plate fixation (Fig. 26C and 26D).
    - Either precontoured lateral column plates or a manually contoured recon plate can be applied.

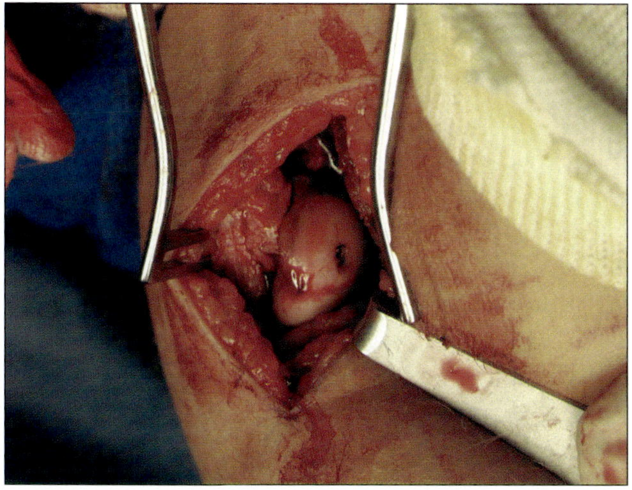

A

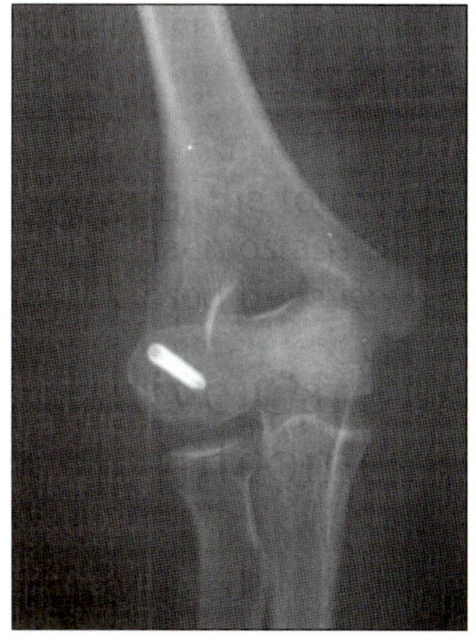

B

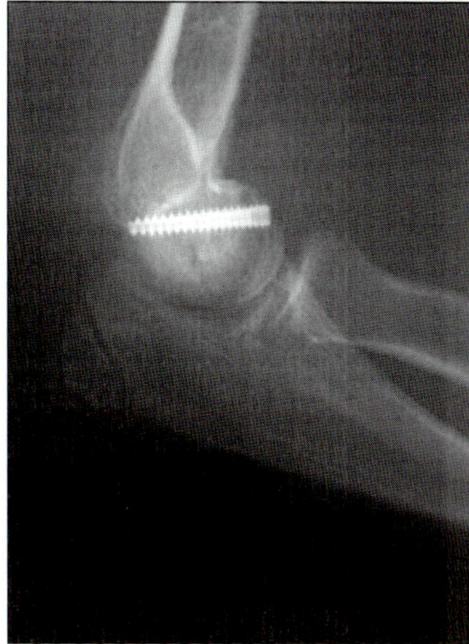

C

FIGURE 25

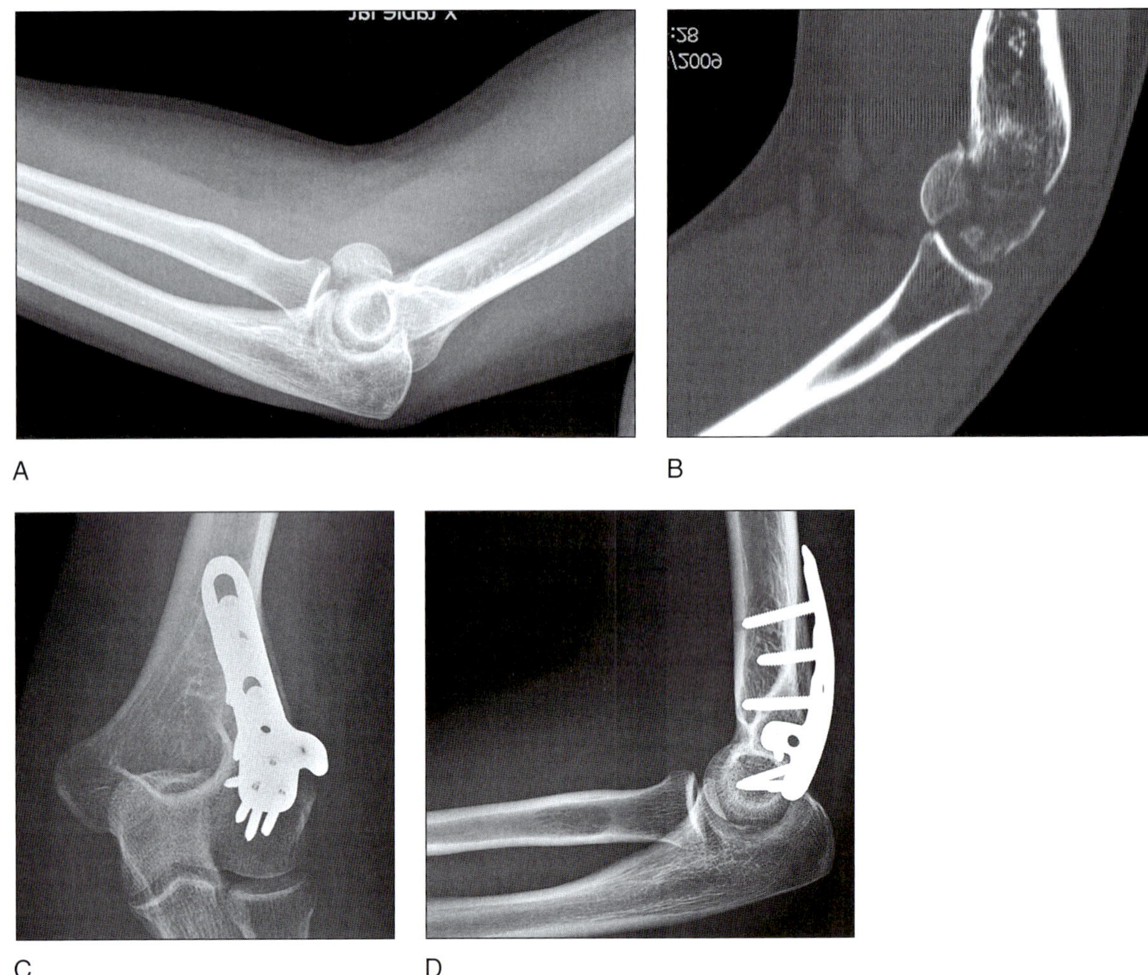

FIGURE 26

For optimal stability, three screws in the proximal fragment and as many as possible in the distal fragment are advised.

- Smaller, 2.7-mm screws in the distal fragment may allow for a greater number of screws to be placed at variable angles. If possible, distal fragment screws should pass through the plate and condylar fragment, and into the stable medial column.

Step 3

- Along with verifying reduction and hardware placement with fluoroscopy, the joint should be passively ranged through flexion, extension, supination, and pronation.
- If the capitellum is severely comminuted and cannot be anatomically restored, excision is an option *only if* the lateral trochlear ridge and the medial collateral ligament are intact. Also, the bony origin of the LUCL must be stable.

- If necessary, the LCL origin is repaired. This may be accomplished with either suture anchors or drill tunnels exiting the posterior lateral condylar cortex. With either technique, the suture must enter the bone at the anatomic origin of the LCL.

Step 4

- The wound is irrigated and the common extensor origin and capsule are reapproximated as a single layer with #0 absorbable suture.
- Subcutaneous and skin closure is performed with 3-0 absorbable and 4-0 nylon sutures, respectively.

Pitfalls

- *In capitellar fragments with only a thin rim of subchondral bone attached (such as in the Kocher-Lorenz-type fragment), there is little room for screw thread purchase. Avoid screw overpenetration.*
- *Avoid hardware protrusion into the olecranon fossa.*

Instrumentation/ Implantation

- Headless, cannulated compression screws or 2.0-mm screws to be used with countersink for management of isolated articular surface fractures.
- Either 3.5-mm recon or precontoured lateral column plates for management of isolated lateral column fractures.
- If reattachment of LUCL origin is needed, suture anchors with #2 or #5 braided suture are useful.

Postoperative Care and Expected Outcomes

Distal Humerus Fractures

- The wound should be checked within the first few days, and any hematoma that may be compromising posterior skin flaps evacuated.
- Postoperative mobilization depends on stability of fracture fixation. A recognized advantage of rigid, stable fixation of these fractures is early pursuit of motion with hopes of avoiding debilitating stiffness. Therefore, we strive to have these patients working in a supervised therapy program on flexion and extension within 5–10 days.
  - *However,* one should not staunchly adhere to the principle of early mobilization in the presence of marginal fixation. It is better to achieve a stiff union than an unstable nonunion. Eventual contracture release carries less morbidity and effort than revision ORIF with potential bone grafting.
- Professional therapist supervision and guidance are essential during the early postoperative phases. Pain, swelling, and uncertainty regarding appropriate level of discomfort during exercises complicate the initial motion recovery initiative. Patients also need to be directed to maintain motion and function of surrounding joints (digits, shoulder).
- Swelling is an omnipresent foe in the early and middle phases of recovery, hindering efforts at motion and placing significant tension on the wound. Therefore, I prefer to leave the sutures/ staples in for about 3 weeks. The patient has enough difficulty with motion without the added concern of wound dehiscence following early suture removal.

- Weekly radiographic follow-up is advised in the first 2–3 weeks, especially if the patient is in an aggressive motion regimen.
- Complications
  - Fixation failure or nonunion averages 6% with modern methods. Risk factors include more distal fracture patterns, inadequate fixation ($^1/_3$ tubular plates, K-wires, or screws to fix columns). This may be less common with better bicolumnar plate options with multiple distal locking and nonlocking screw holes. It can be minimized by following the principles mentioned above for bicolumnar patterns.
  - Malunion: mild degrees of procurvatum, recurvatum, and varus or valgus deformity are usually well tolerated.
  - Infection: Superficial infections can be difficult to distinguish from mild wound hematoma or erythema, and usually subside with oral antibiotics. Deep wound infections, detected early, should be promptly surgically débrided with retention of hardware. Intravenous antibiotic therapy is also recommended. At times, suppressive therapy until fracture union is required, at which point hardware can be removed.
  - Nerve complications: The ulnar nerve is most commonly injured, both upon injury and during surgery. Most injuries are transient and can be followed expectantly if the nerve was transposed. If the nerve was left in situ, re-exploration and transposition may need to be considered. While the ulnar nerve is more at risk with triceps-reflecting approaches, the radial nerve is more vulnerable during triceps-splitting exposures.
  - Olecranon osteotomy complications: Prominent, symptomatic hardware is common and may necessitate removal. A 6% nonunion rate that requires treatment has been reported.
  - Stiffness: Some motion loss in virtually inevitable following fractures with articular involvement. More than 30° flexion contracture or flexion restriction beyond 120° may result in significant impairment. Risk factors for stiffness include advanced age, more severe soft tissue or bone injury, delayed surgery, and prolonged immobilization following surgery. Risk factors for heterotopic ossification include head injury, delayed intervention, and severe bone or soft

tissue trauma. The routine use of prophylactic measures against heterotopic ossification (i.e., low-dose irradiation) is controversial.
- Degenerative arthritis may result from failure to restore articular anatomy, osteonecrosis from free bone fragments, loose fragments, or hardware protruding into the joint. Salvage with linked (versus unlinked) total elbow arthroplasty (TEA) is a reasonable measure in older patients. However, younger individuals undergoing TEA for posttraumatic osteoarthritis have more problems, particularly early loosening.

- Outcomes
  - The published literature on distal humerus fractures is mostly composed of Level IV case series with heterogeneous fracture patterns and patient populations. For example, the results of extra-articular or noncomminuted patterns are likely to differ considerably from those of more complicated patterns. Also, different outcome measurement tools with varying scoring weights on specific domains (motion, pain, activities of daily living) permeate the reports to date. Earlier series also utilized fewer of the modern fixation options available today (precontoured plates with a greater number of distal fixation points, locking hardware, etc.). Despite difficulties in making direct comparisons among studies, patterns do emerge that can help guide treatment and patient expectations:
    - Despite acknowledged complications from surgery, rigid ORIF of bicolumnar distal fracture patterns is superior to nonoperative treatment in medically competent individuals.
    - Age is a significant variable when comparing treatment outcomes for comminuted or very distal fracture patterns. In the elderly population, there is evidence supporting the use of primary TEA over ORIF, but controversy persists.
    - Recovery of flexion is usually more rapid than extension.
    - Greater recovery occurs in the first 6 months, although modest gains may continue through 2 years.
    - Even in apparently successfully treated comminuted distal humeral fracture patterns (the majority of published reports of bicolumnar patterns reveal "excellent or good" outcomes in

over 75% of patients, albeit with variable groups and injury patterns), the elbow is rarely normal. Continued long-term weakness and moderate range-of-motion deficits (often flexion contractures of 20–30°) can be expected relative to the contralateral normal elbow.

Isolated Distal Lateral Column and Capitellar Fractures

- Early, active postoperative motion is the ideal. However, this effort must be tempered by fracture and ligament stability. In cases of significant osteoporosis or marginal fixation, motion may need to be delayed for 3–4 weeks while the elbow is protected with a splint.
- The most common complication following ORIF of capitellar fractures is stiffness from capsular contracture. Intra-articular incongruity or hardware impingement are less common causes.
    - Settling or separation of fracture fragments may occur as a result of osteonecrosis, at times requiring delayed fragment excision.
    - Delayed osteoarthrosis has been described, but this is not always progressively symptomatic and may not require further intervention.
- Results following ORIF are based on a number of smaller clinical series, but in general reflect good functional outcomes. Excision of irreparable capitellar fractures usually produces satisfactory short-term results, but delayed stiffness or instability is common.

Pearls

- *Final range of motion may not be determined for months. Many patients will quietly make significant gains once swelling subsides, although they may have seemed to have plateaued beforehand.*
- *Maintain motion of joints proximal and distal to the elbow. Shoulder pain and stiffness are frequent problems for patients who keep the limb at their side during elbow surgery convalescence.*

Pitfalls

- *Any postoperative motion regimen must be tempered by the stability of fracture fixation. Delaying aggressive motion work, especially passive stretching modalities, may be necessary in cases of marginal distal fixation.*
- *Protect triceps repair by avoiding resisted extension in the first 6 weeks following triceps-splitting or -reflecting approaches.*

Controversies

- Static progressive splinting may be a useful adjunct to motion work in the early stages, alternating between phases of flexion and extension.

Evidence

Anglen J. Distal humerus fractures. J Am Acad Orthop Surg. 2005;13:291-7.

This paper presented an excellent review of epidemiology, fracture patterns, fixation principles, and pitfalls. The author did not discuss fixation with newer precontoured locking plates, but the applied principles and approaches remain noteworthy. The journal also offers video supplementation on the AAOS website. (Level V evidence)

Frankle MA, Herscovici D, Pasquale TF, et al. A comparison of open reduction and internal fixation and primary total elbow arthroplasty in the treatment of distal humeral fractures in women older than age 65. J Orthop Trauma. 2003;17:473-80.

This retrospective review compared the results of ORIF and primary TEA of AO types C2 or C3 fractures in women older than 65 years. There were 12 patients in each group, and follow-up was a minimum of 2 years. Eight of the 12 patients in the arthroplasty group had rheumatoid arthritis, compared to none in the osteosynthesis group. Mayo Elbow Performance Scale (MEPS) results in the ORIF group were 4 excellent, 4 good, 1 fair, and 3 poor. The three "poor" results all required conversion to TEA. Of the arthroplasty group, there were 11 excellent and 1 good result in a patient who was noted to have symptomatic radiolucency of her ulnar component before dying 5 years postoperatively. (Level III evidence)

Jawa A. Extra-articular distal third diaphyseal fractures of the humerus: a comparison of functional bracing and plate fixation. J Bone Joint Surg [Am]. 2006;88:2343-7.

Although ORIF is generally recommended for management of distal humeral fractures, this retrospective study compared ORIF (19 patients) to functional bracing (21 patients) of extra-articular distal third fractures. ORIF demonstrated better radiographic alignment and quicker return of function, but complications included loss of fixation, postoperative infection, and permanent radial nerve palsy in 3 of 19 patients. Of the 21 splinted patients, 2 required conversion to ORIF, 2 had problems with skin breakdown, and 2 lost more than 20° of shoulder or elbow motion. Although operative treatment can provide more predictable alignment, significant complications can occur. Nonoperative splinting, despite poorer radiographic alignment, can provide acceptable functional results. (Level III evidence)

McKee MD, Veillette CJH, Hall JA, et al. A multicenter, prospective, randomized, controlled trial of open reduction—internal fixation versus total elbow arthroplasty for displaced intra-articular distal humeral fractures in elderly patients. J Shoulder Elbow Surg. 2009;18:3-12.

This paper presented a prospective, randomized, controlled trial to compare functional outcomes, complications, and reoperation rates in elderly patients with displaced intra-articular, distal humeral fractures treated with open reduction—internal fixation (ORIF) or primary semiconstrained total elbow arthroplasty (TEA). Forty-two patients were randomized by sealed envelope. Inclusion criteria were age greater than 65 years; displaced, comminuted, intra-articular fractures of the distal humerus (Orthopaedic Trauma Association type 13C); and closed or Gustilo grade I open fractures treated within 12 hours of injury. Both ORIF and TEA were performed following a standardized protocol. The Mayo Elbow Performance Score (MEPS) and Disabilities of the Arm, Shoulder and Hand (DASH) score were determined at 6 week, 3 months, 6 months, 12 months, and 2 years.

O'Driscoll SW. Optimizing stability in distal humeral fracture fixation. J Shoulder Elbow Surg. 2005;14:186S-94S.

The author provided an excellent description of the biomechanical principles of bicolumnar fracture management. Although the work emphasized the benefits of the parallel plating concept, the author outlined a logical and biomechanically sound approach to stabilization of these difficult injuries with any plate system. (Level V evidence)

This paper is the only prospective, randomized series comparing ORIF TEA of displaced, intra-articular fractures. The authors presented minimum 2-year follow-up on 21 patients randomized to each group with similar baseline demographics, fracture types, comorbidities, and activity level. Five of the ORIF elbows were converted to TEA intraoperatively secondary to inability to obtain stable fixation. The findings indicated slightly improved MEPS and DASH scores for the TEA group over the ORIF group at 3, 6, 12, and 24 months postoperatively

Wilkinson JM, Stanley D. Posterior surgical approaches to the elbow: a comparative anatomic study. J Shoulder Elbow Surg. 2001;10:380-2.

This cadaver study compared triceps splitting, triceps reflecting, and olecranon osteotomy for exposure of the distal humeral articular surface. The triceps-splitting approach provided the least exposure, while the osteotomy seemed to provide the best. However, even the osteotomy did not provide visualization of the anterior trochlear or radial head. (Level V evidence)

Isolated Distal Lateral Column and Capitellar Fractures

Elkowitz SJ, Polatsch DB, Egol KA, Kummer FJ, Koval KJ. Capitellum fractures: a biomechanical evaluation of three fixation methods. J Orthop Trauma. 2002;16:503-6.

This cadaver study compared anterioposterior against posteroanterior (PA) placement of cancellous lag screws in 12 matched elbow pairs, with PA placement proving to be significantly more stable. However, headless compression Acutrak screws placed in the anteroposterior direction proved to be more stable than both lag screw techniques. (Level V evidence)

Ruchelsman DE, Tejwani NC, Young WK, Egol KA. Open reduction and internal fixation of capitellar fractures with headless screws. J Bone Joint Surg [Am]. 2008;90:1321-9.

This paper presented a case series of 16 adult capitellar fractures (Bryan and Morrey types I, III, and IV) treated with ORIF using headless compression screws. Fourteen of sixteen patients had functional motion with a mean Mayo Elbow Performance Index score of 92 points. Type IV patterns exhibited decreased overall motion. Although five patients had concomitant radial head fractures, this did not appear to impact functional score or outcome. (Level IV evidence)

PROCEDURE 57

Radial Head Fractures: Open Reduction and Internal Fixation

Donald H. Lee and John M. Erickson

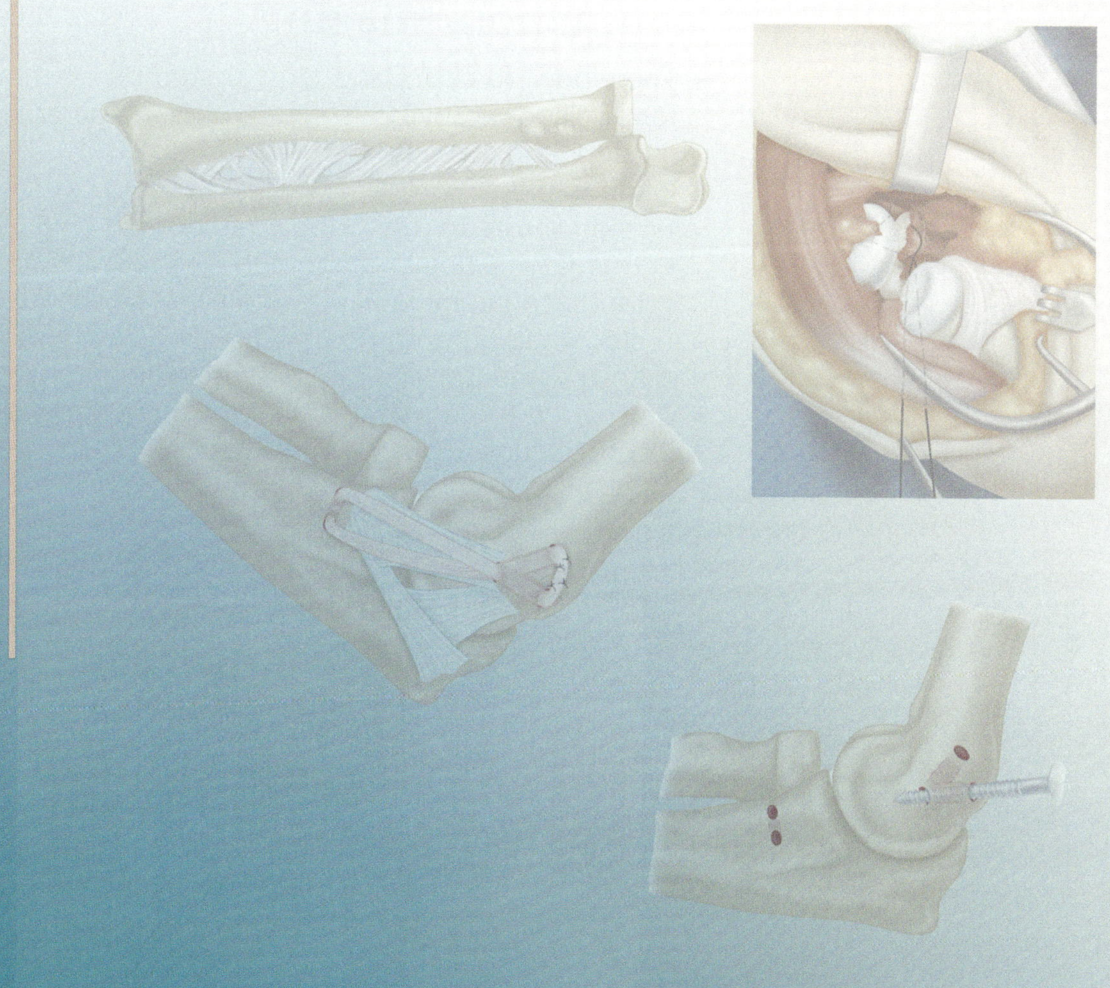

Indications

- Mason type II radial head fracture with mechanical block to elbow motion
- Mason type III radial head fracture
- Mason type IV radial head fracture associated with elbow dislocation
- Complex or complicated radial head fracture associated with concomitant injury, including fracture of the coronoid and/or olecranon or associated ligamentous injuries (Fig. 1)

Pitfalls

- *Internal fixation of radial head fractures is generally indicated in fractures with three or fewer fragments.*
- *Radial head fractures with more than three fracture fragments, especially associated with a radial neck fracture, will be difficult to internally fix, and radial head arthroplasty may be indicated.*

Controversies

- Mason type II radial head fractures without a mechanical block to forearm rotation or elbow motion may be treated nonoperatively.
- In the setting of a comminuted radial head fracture, patients should be assumed to have a complex injury pattern in which elbow instability is common.

Examination/Imaging

- The elbow, forearm, and wrist should be examined for swelling, ecchymosis, tenderness, range of motion, and stability.
- Radiographs
  - Anteroposterior (AP) elbow radiograph (Fig. 2A)
  - True lateral elbow radiograph (Fig. 2B)
  - Modified lateral radial head view (45° oblique elbow radiograph) (Fig. 2C)
  - Posteroanterior and lateral wrist radiographs
- Computed tomography scan with three-dimensional reconstructions (Fig. 3A and 3B)

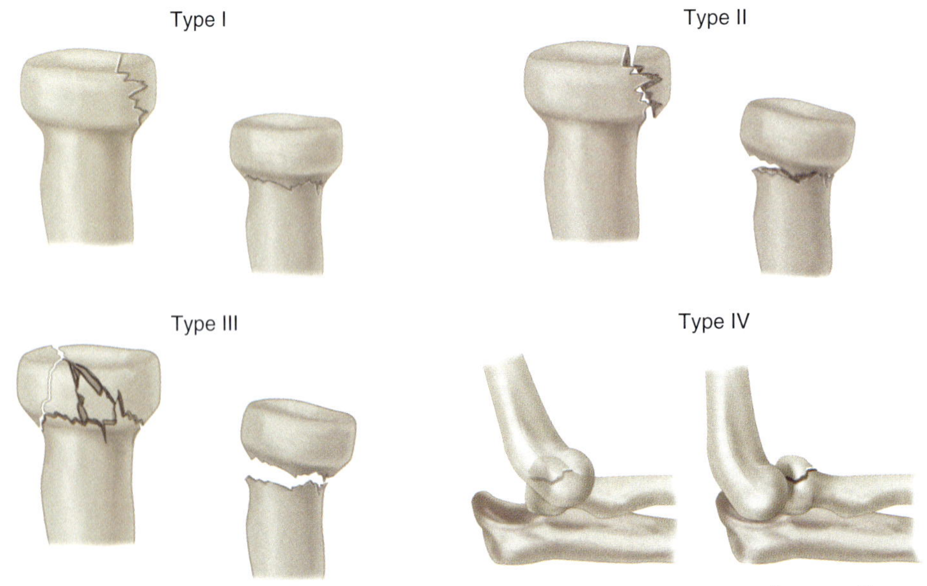

FIGURE 1

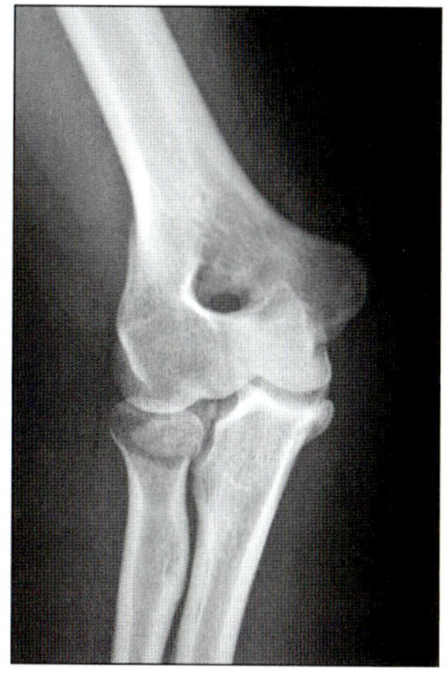
A

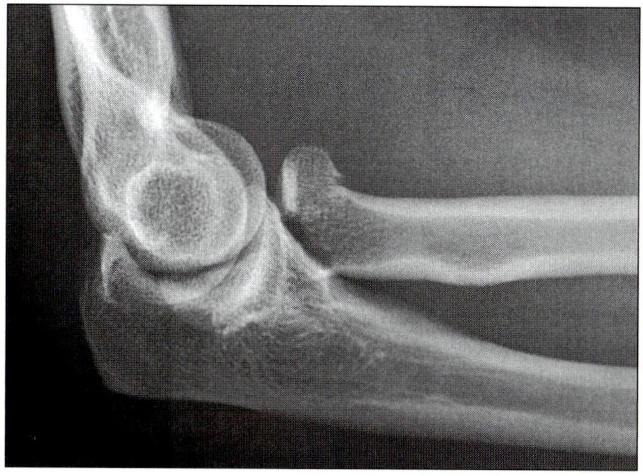
B

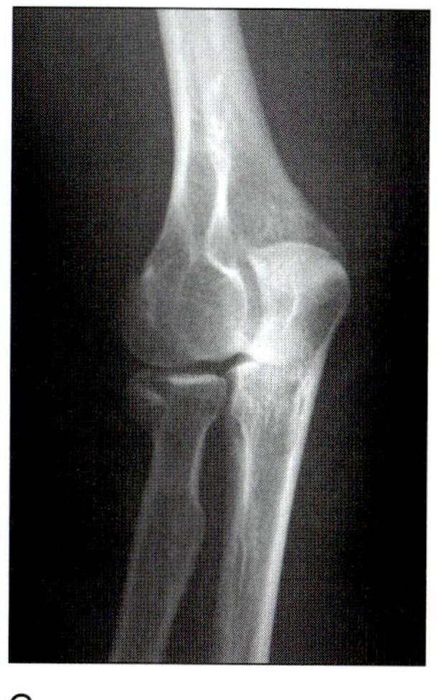
C

FIGURE 2

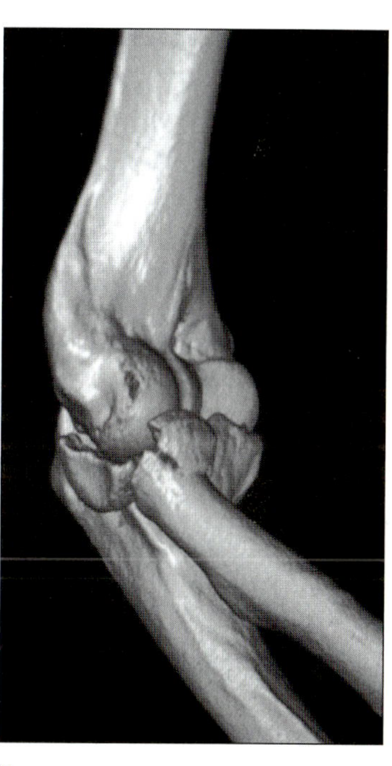
A B

FIGURE 3

Treatment Options

- Open reduction and internal fixation
- Metallic radial head replacement
- Radial head resection (rarely indicated in the acute setting)

Surgical Anatomy

- The proximal radius is important for valgus and posterolateral rotatory stability of the elbow and longitudinal stability of the forearm. The radiocapitellar joint transmits approximately 50–60% of the load across the elbow.
- Every attempt should be made to repair or replace the radial head, particularly in cases of elbow or longitudinal forearm instability.

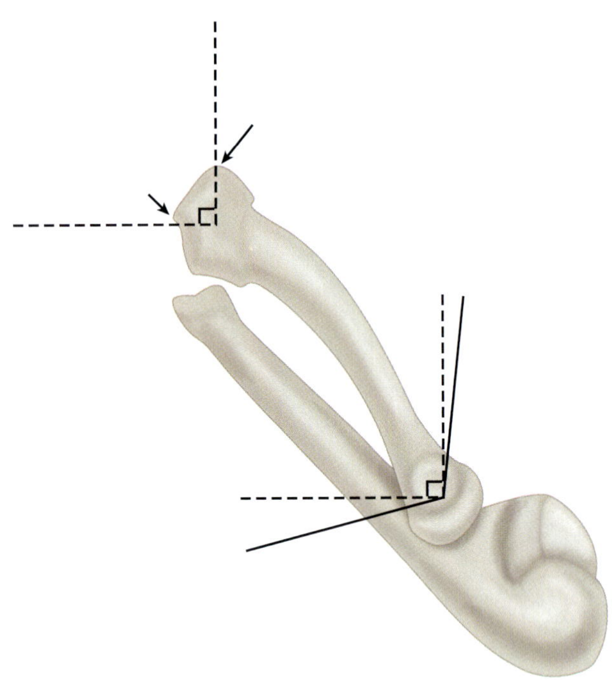

FIGURE 4

- The proximal radius articulates with the sigmoid notch of the ulna in an arc of approximately 270°. Therefore, implants should be placed on the nonarticular "safe zone" of the proximal radius to avoid impingement. This is defined as a 90° arc centered between the radial styloid and Lister's tubercle (Fig. 4).
- The posterior interosseus nerve (PIN) is intimately associated with the proximal radius as it passes through the supinator in its course from the anterior to the posterior aspect of the forearm (Fig. 5). Pronation of the forearm delivers the PIN medially and further from the surgical field. Placement of retractors around the radial neck should be minimized or such retractors used judiciously to avoid injury to the PIN.
- The lateral ulnar collateral ligament (LUCL) complex is at risk with lateral approaches to the elbow and is critical for elbow stability. It is important to remain anterior to the equator of the radial head/neck or the radiocapitellar joint (i.e., anterior to a line drawn along the long axis of the radial neck) to preserve the posterior sling of the LUCL complex.

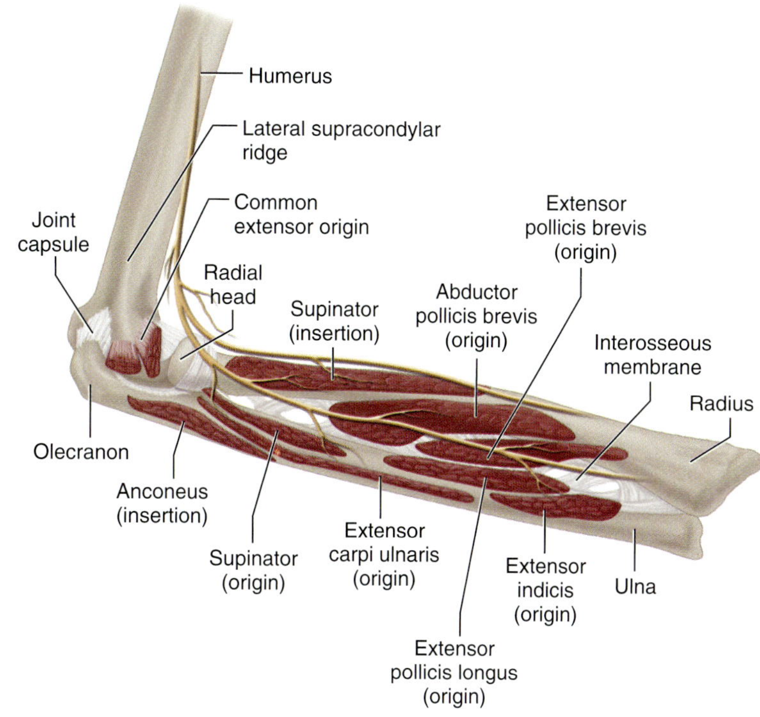

FIGURE 5

PEARLS

- *After the patient is positioned, fluoroscopy should be performed prior to arm preparation to ensure adequate visualization of the elbow and radial head.*
- *A sterile tourniquet applied to the proximal brachium will significantly aid visualization.*

Positioning

- General anesthesia or regional block
- Supine position with arm table (preferred)
- Other options:
  - Supine with arm across chest
  - Lateral decubitus position with arm bolster

PEARLS

- *The Kocher intermuscular interval is best identified distally, as the muscles share a common aponeurosis proximally.*
- *The Kocher interval is more posterior than the Kaplan, and therefore the LUCL complex can be inadvertently injured if the dissection is carried too far anteriorly.*
- *Because of the proximity of the PIN, the forearm is kept in a pronated position to carry the nerve out of the surgical field.*

Portals/Exposures

- The Kaplan interval, located between the extensor digitorum communis and the extensor carpi radialis longus and brevis, is used for simple radial head fractures without concomitant coronoid/olecranon fractures or collateral ligament injuries (Fig. 6).
- The Kocher interval, located between the anconeus and the extensor carpi ulnaris (ECU), is used for complex radial head fracture associated with elbow-fracture dislocations (Fig. 7A). A fat stripe is frequently seen between the anconeus and ECU (Fig. 7B, *blue arrow*).
- Alternatively, a posterior midline skin incision with full-thickness skin flaps can be used to address proximal ulna fractures while incorporating either lateral and/or medial approaches to the elbow.

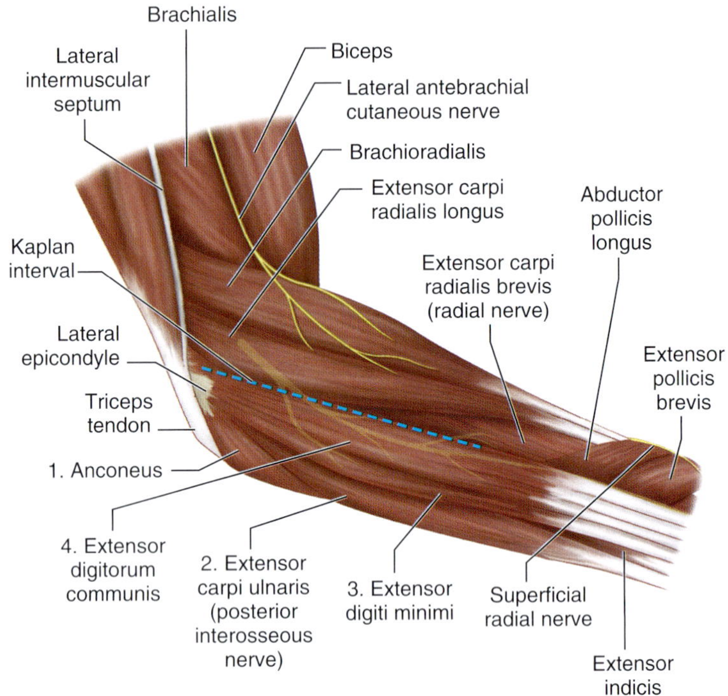

FIGURE 6

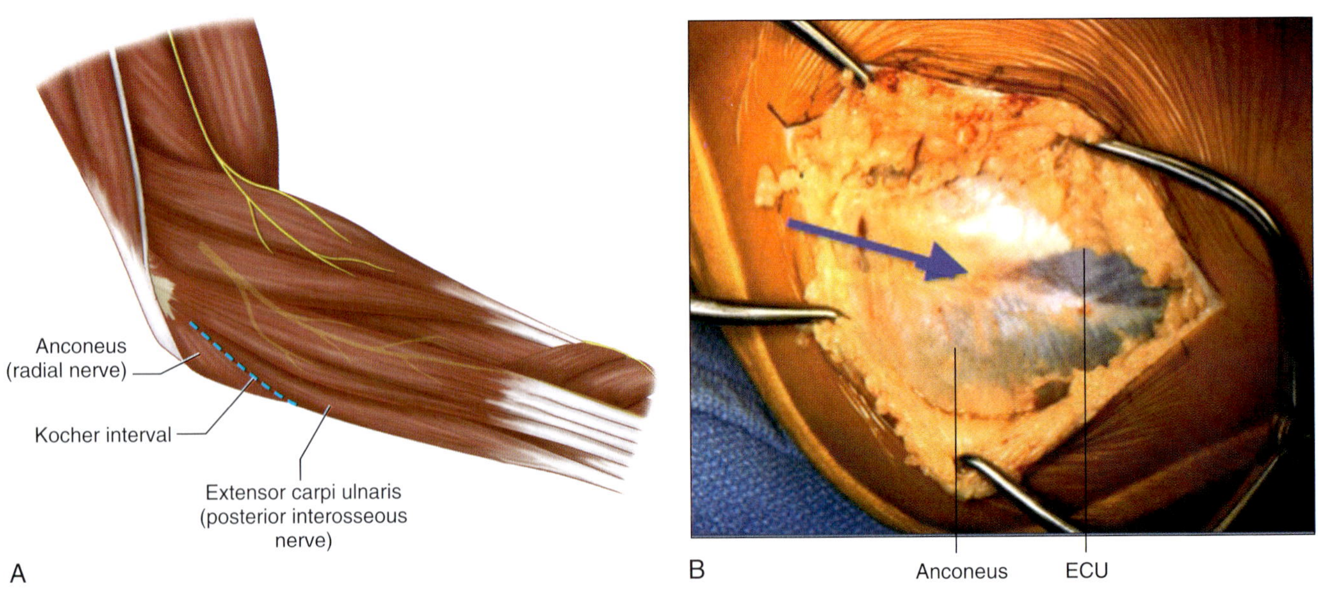

FIGURE 7

Procedure

Step 1

- A lateral curvilinear incision is made from the lateral epicondyle to a point distally centered over the radial neck (see RH Fx Drawing Incision and RH Fx Incision videos).
- Alternatively, a midline posterior incision centered over the olecranon is made with elevation of full-thickness skin flaps.
- The radial head is approached via either the Kaplan (preferred for simple radial head fractures) or Kocher intermuscular interval (preferred for complex radial head fractures with left lateral collateral ligament injuries [Fig. 9]). Care is taken to dissect the muscular layer from the underlying capsule (Fig. 8) (see RH Fx Fascial Incision video).
- The capsule is incised longitudinally anterior to the LUCL, preserving the LUCL complex posteriorly (see RH Fx Arthrotomy video).
- An incision in the annular ligament can be used when distal exposures are required.

Pearls

- *In associated elbow-fracture dislocations, the LUCL is avulsed proximally, resulting in a "bald" lateral humeral epicondyle (Fig. 9).*
- *Additionally, there is often a defect in the common extensor tendon. In this setting, exposure of the fractured radial head is greatly simplified.*

Pitfalls

- *In cases with LUCL disruption, failure to repair (acute setting) or reconstruct (chronic setting) the LUCL may result in posterolateral rotatory instability.*
- *Dissection of the elbow posterior to the long axis of the radiocapitellar joint may result in disruption of the LUCL.*

Step 2

- The fracture site is exposed (Fig. 10) and reduced under direct visualization, and held provisionally with Kirshner wires (see RH Fx Fracture Fragment Identification and RH Fx Fracture Reduction videos).
- Fractures of the radial head without extension into the neck can be internally fixed with a variety of 1.5- to 2.5-mm screws.
- Traditional headed screws may be used but must be countersunk below the articular surface (Fig. 11A). Interosseous headless screws may also be used in some cases (Fig. 11B) (see RH Fx Tripod Screw video).

Pearls

- *Articular fragments can be removed and pieced together with Kirschner wires on the back table.*
- *The surgical hardware should be placed in the nonarticular safe zone to avoid radioulnar impingement (see Fig. 4) (see RH Fx Safe Zone video).*

Pitfalls

- *Noting the concavity of the proximal radial head, care is taken to avoid extra-articular placement of subchondral screws.*
- *The surgical hardware should not extend distal to the bicipital tuberosity; doing so places the PIN at risk.*

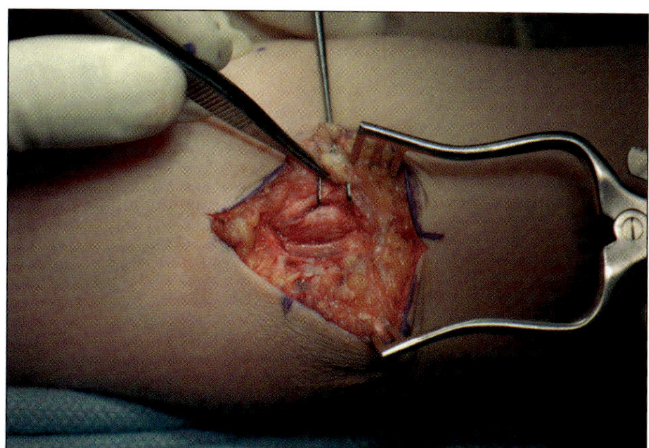

FIGURE 8

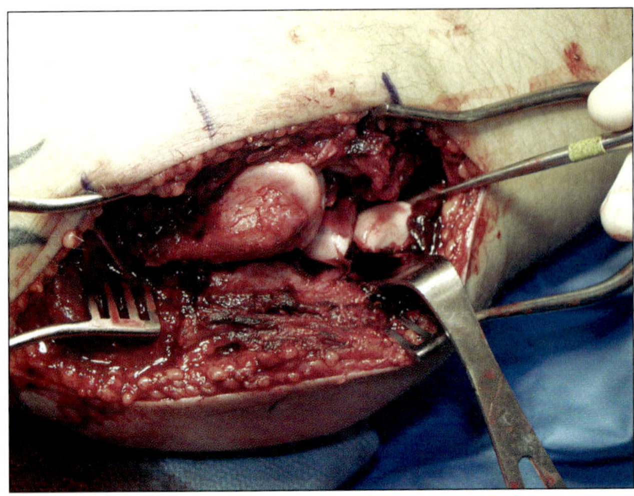

FIGURE 9

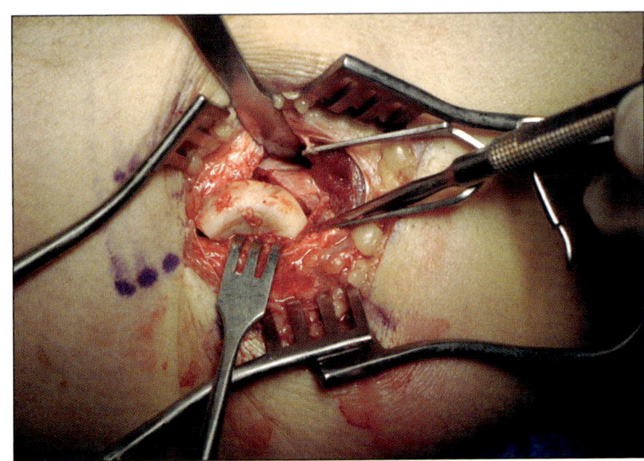

FIGURE 10

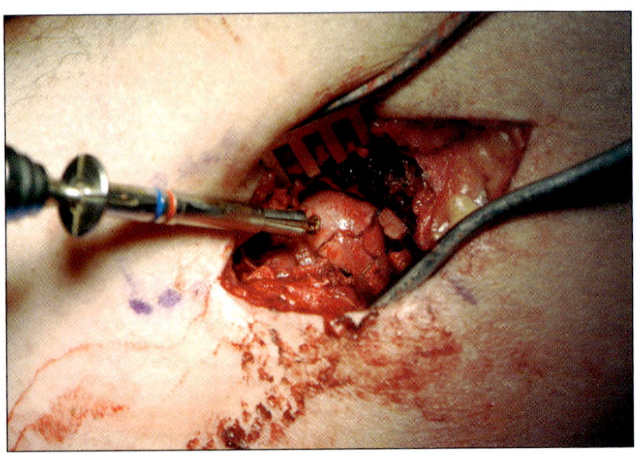

A

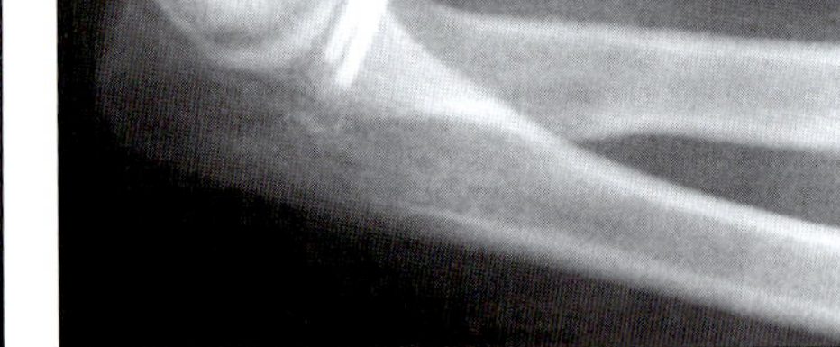

B

FIGURE 11

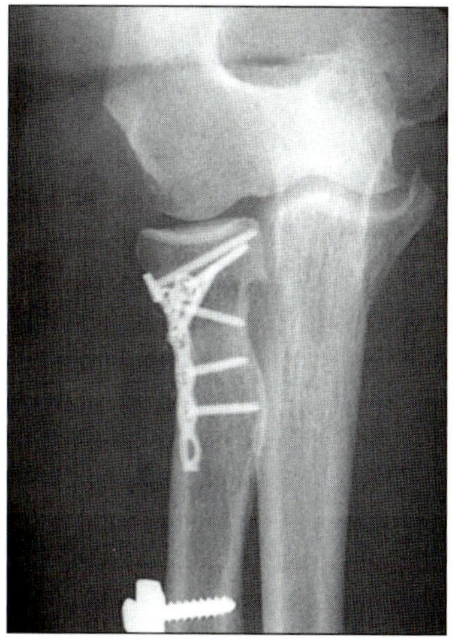

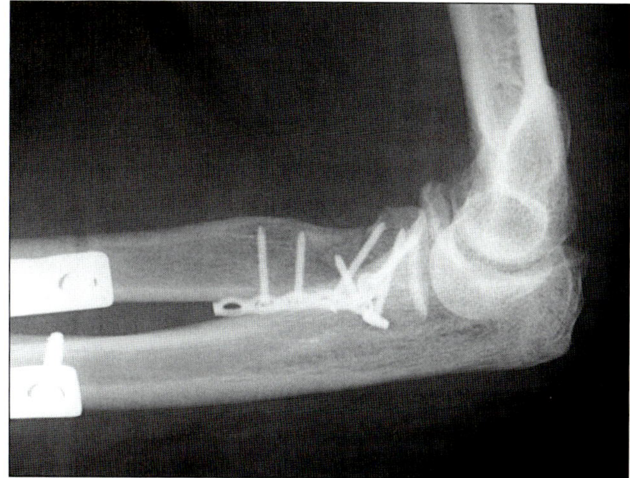

A B

FIGURE 12

Instrumentation/ Implantation

- Available implant options for internal fixation of the radial head should include:
  - Kirshner wires
  - Mini-fragment internal fixation set (1.5- to 2.5-mm screws)
  - Headless interosseous screws
  - Reconstruction plates (e.g., precontoured proximal radial plates, malleable locking plates, mini-T or Y plates)
- Radial head replacement system

Controversies

- Radial head excision should be avoided, particularly in the setting of a capsuloligamentous injury to the elbow or forearm.
- Radial head resection is associated with delayed complications, including valgus and posterolateral rotatory elbow instability, longitudinal forearm instability, and osteoarthrosis.

- Fractures that extend into the radial neck are also treated with plate fixation (Fig. 12A and 12B). A variety of mini-condylar, T-shaped, L-shaped, and precontoured plates are available.
- Direct visualization and fluoroscopy are used to judge the reduction and concentricity of the radiocapitellar joint (Fig. 13) (see RH Fx Fluoro View videos 1 and 2).
- Fluoroscopy can also be use prior to radial head internal fixation to assess:
  - The status of the ulnar collateral ligament (i.e., valgus stress resulting in widening of the medial joint line) (Fig. 14)

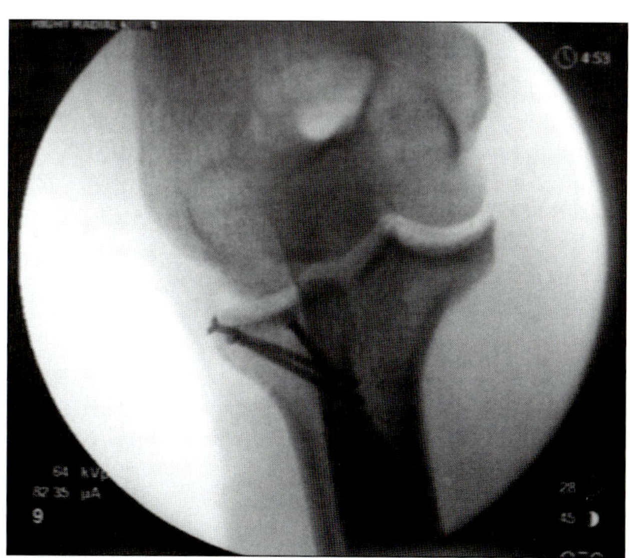

FIGURE 13

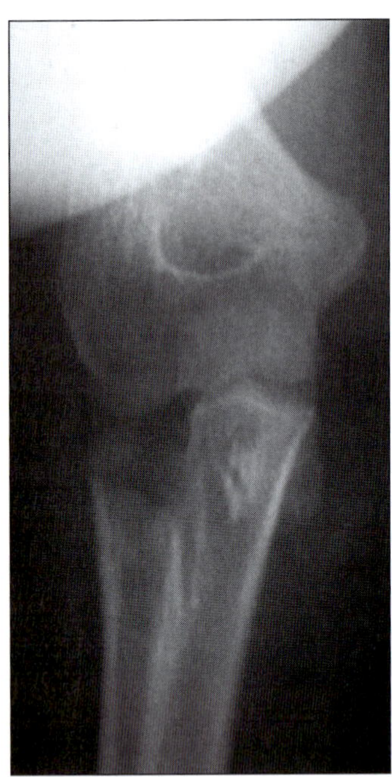

FIGURE 14

Pearls

- *When repairing the LUCL (transosseous tunnels), the suture passer is placed from anterior to posterior and a looped suture is passed from posterior to anterior. The looped suture is then used to pass the #2 nonabsorbable LUCL sutures from anterior to posterior.*
- *Following tensioning of, but prior to tying, the LUCL transosseous sutures, the elbow is examined under fluoroscopy to ensure that both the ulnohumeral and radiocapitellar joints are concentrically reduced. If residual posterolateral sagging of the radiocapitellar joint is noted, new bone tunnels can be placed slightly more superiorly to further tension the LUCL repair.*

Pitfalls

- *Anatomic repair of the LUCL complex is critical.*
- *Fixation of the ligamentous complex posterior to the isometric point can lead to subluxation of the ulnohumeral joint in extension.*

- The status of the interosseous membrane (IOM)
  - Longitudinal compression of ≥ 3 mm indicates disruption of the IOM
  - Longitudinal compression of greater than 6 mm indicates disruption of the IOM and triangular fibrocartilage
- The forearm and elbow are taken through a full range of motion to assess the fracture fixation stability and potential mechanical block to motion (see RH Fx Final Fixation video).
- The results are checked on AP (Fig. 15A) and lateral (Fig. 15B) radiographs.

Step 3

- If needed, the lateral collateral ligament complex is repaired to the lateral humeral epicondyle using heavy (#2) nonabsorbable sutures. Transosseous lateral epicondylar bone tunnels (Fig. 16) or commercially available suture anchors can be used.
  - Grasping sutures (two #2 nonabsorbable braided sutures) are placed into the lateral collateral ligament complex.
  - Two bone tunnels are placed, one superior and one inferior to the isometric point, in an anterior-to-posterior direction.
  - A suture passer is used to pass the #2 braided sutures from anterior to posterior.

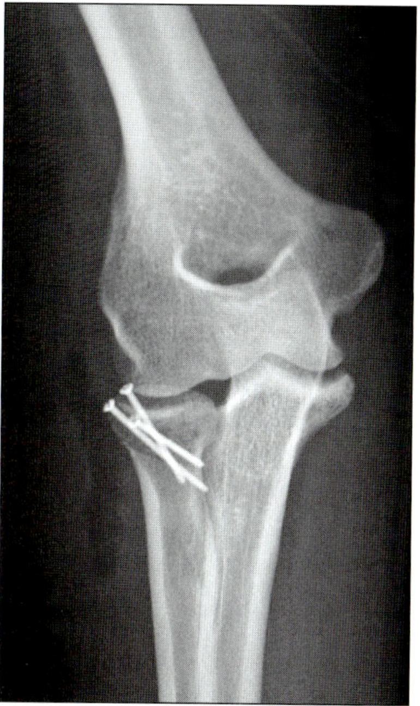

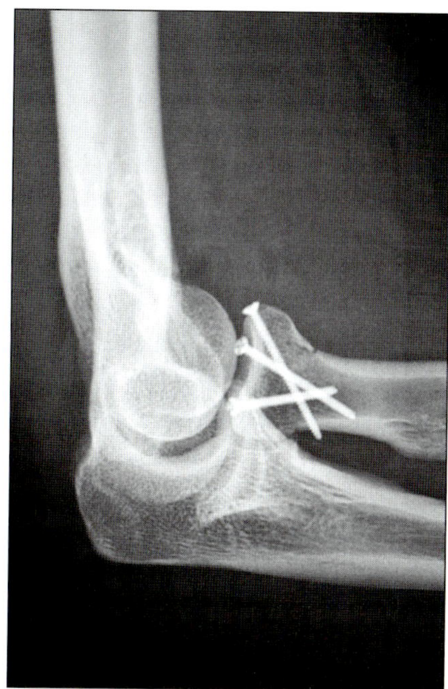

A B

FIGURE 15

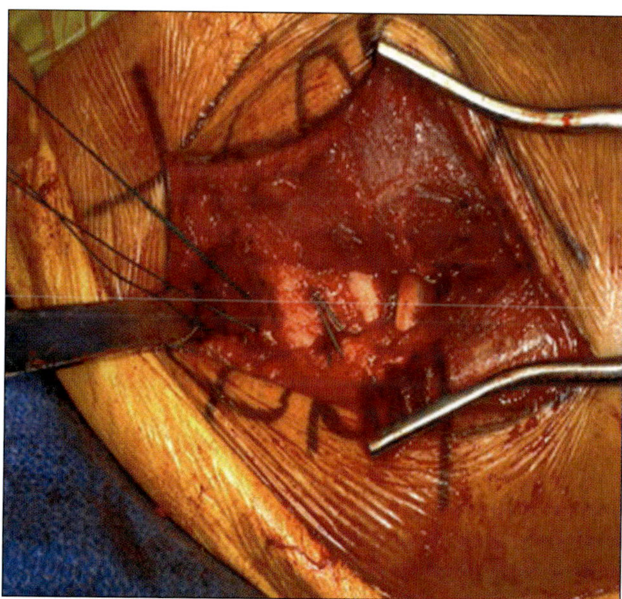

FIGURE 16

Instrumentation/ Implantation

- In cases of elbow fracture-dislocation, a hinged external fixator should be available in the event that elbow reduction cannot be maintained after bony and soft tissue repair.

- The sutures are tied on the posterior aspect of the lateral epicondyle.

■ Using fluoroscopy, the ulnohumeral joint is confirmed to be congruent throughout the range of motion. Forearm pronation and elbow flexion typically improves the stability of the radiocapitellar joint and ulnohumeral joint, respectively.

Controversies

- Repair of the medial (ulnar) collateral ligament is typically not necessary unless the elbow remains unstable after bony and lateral ligamentous repair.

- In cases of complex elbow fracture-dislocation, with residual ulnohumeral instability, particularly in extension, an anterior capsulodesis can be performed (Fig. 17).
  - Two #2 nonabsorbable braided grasping sutures are placed in the anterior capsule (Fig. 17, *black arrow*). Care is taken not to release the anterior capsular insertion off the anterior distal humerus.
  - Two transosseous holes are created from the subcutaneous border of the ulna (Fig. 17, *yellow arrow*) toward the coronoid process (*blue arrow*).
  - The holes in the coronoid process should be placed adjacent to the articular surface, helping to reinforce the anterior buttress effect of the coronoid process.

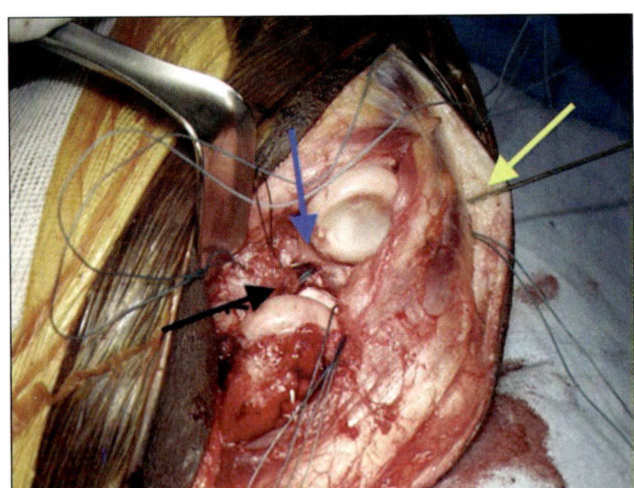

FIGURE 17

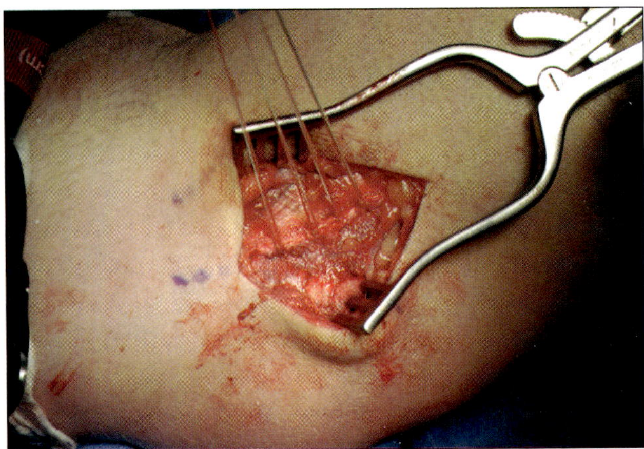

FIGURE 18

Pearls

- *The intraoperative assessment of elbow stability is critical for determining the postoperative therapy regimen, particularly in elbow fracture-dislocations.*
- *If there is residual posterolateral sagging of the radiocapitellar joint, postoperative rehabilitation is performed with the forearm in pronation.*

Pitfalls

- *Splinting the elbow for more than a few days will lead to elbow stiffness and a potential poor outcome.*

Controversies

- Indomethacin and/or irradiation can be used to reduce the incidence of heterotopic ossification in high-risk patients.

  - A suture passer is used to pass the grasping sutures in the anterior capsule from the coronoid process to the subcutaneous border of the ulna.
  - The sutures are tied over a bony bridge on the subcutaneous border of the ulna.
- The annular ligament (see RH Fx Annular Ligament Repair video) and overlying fascia (Fig. 18) (see RH Fx Fascial Repair video) and skin are closed in standard fashion.
- A sterile dressing is incorporated into a well-padded long-arm splint.

Postoperative Care and Expected Outcomes

- Patients are instructed in immediate digital and shoulder range of motion
- The long-arm splint applied at the end of surgery is removed 3–5 days postoperatively, a removable long-arm Thermoplast splint is applied (Fig. 19), and the patient is instructed in gentle passive and active-assisted elbow range of motion (Fig. 20A and 20B).
- Skin sutures are removed at 8–10 days postoperatively.
- Complications include loss of elbow motion, particularly terminal extension; heterotopic ossification; malreduction; loss of fixation/reduction; infection; and osteoarthrosis.

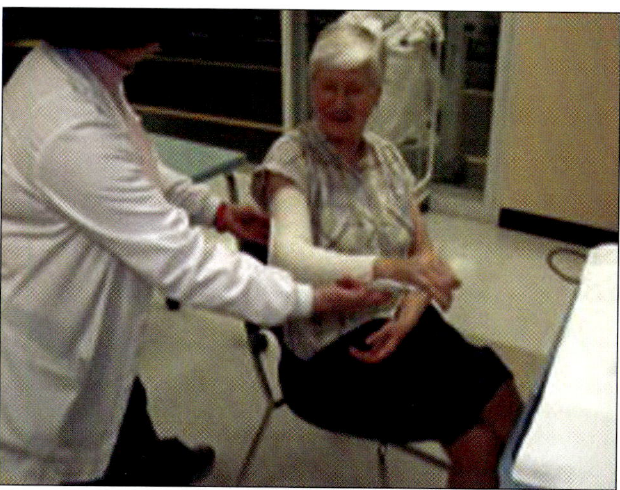

FIGURE 19

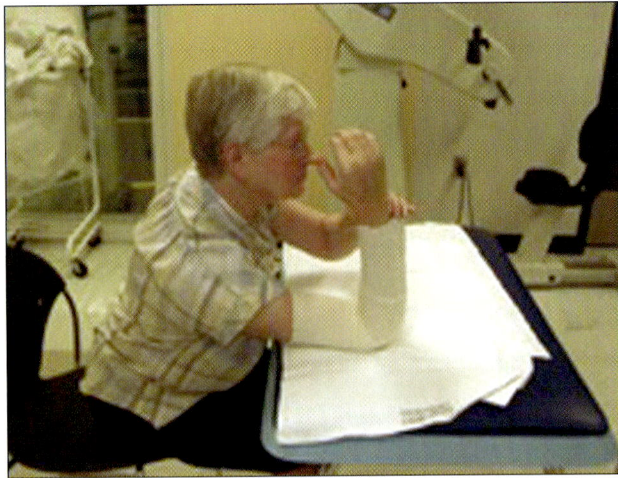
A

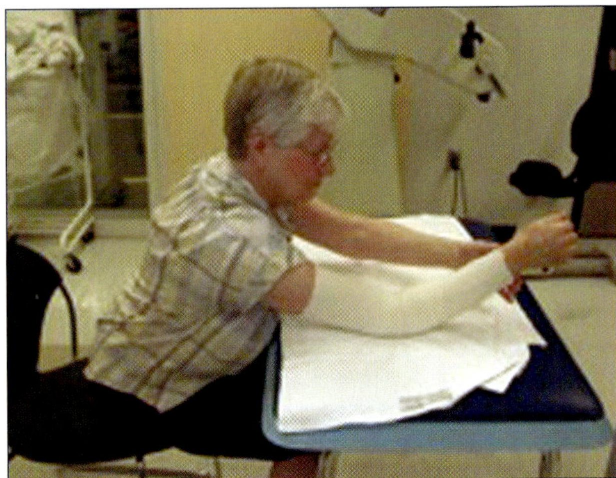
B

FIGURE 20

Evidence

Caputo AE, Mazzocca AD, Santoro VM. The nonarticulating portion of the radial head: anatomic and clinical correlations for internal fixation. J Hand Surg [Am]. 1998;23:1082-90.

The authors studied 24 cadaveric elbows to determine the nonarticular portion of the proximal radius for placement of fixation. They identified the safe zone as a 90° angle localized by palpation of the radial styloid and Lister's tubercle.

Ikeda M, Sugiyama K, Kang C, et al. Comminuted fractures of the radial head: comparison of resection and internal fixation. J Bone Joint Surg [Am]. 2005;87:76-84.

The authors performed a retrospective review of 28 patients who underwent either radial head excision or open reduction and internal fixation (ORIF) of comminuted radial head fractures. The patients who underwent ORIF demonstrated better strength, motion, and function than the patients who underwent excision. (Level IV evidence)

Lee DH, Weikert DW, Watson JT. Anterior elbow capsulodesis. Tech Shoulder Elbow Surg. 2006;7:72-6.

The authors described the technique of performing an anterior elbow capsulodesis for elbow instability.

Morrey BF, Tanaka S, An KN. Valgus stability of the elbow: a definition of primary and secondary constraints. Clin Orthop Relat Res. 1991;(265):187-95.

This classic biomechanical study demonstrated the importance of the radial head as a secondary stabilizer of the elbow.

Ring D, Quintero J, Jupiter JB. Open reduction and internal fixation of fractures of the radial head. J Bone Joint Surg [Am]. 2002;84:1811-5.

The authors retrospectively reviewed 56 patients who underwent ORIF of radial head fractures. Thirteen of 14 patients with Mason III fractures of more than three articular fragments had a poor result, and therefore the authors recommended excision or radial head replacement in such patients. (Level IV evidence)

Smith AM, Urbanosky LR, Castle JA, Rushing JT, Ruch DS. Radius pull test: Predictor of longitudinal forearm instability. J Bone Joint Surg 2002;84-:1970-1976.

This cadaveric biomechanical study showed that, following a radial head resection, ≥ 3 mm of proximal radial migration with longitudinal traction indicated disruption of the interosseous membrane, and ≥ 6 mm of proximal radial migration indicated gross longitudinal instability with disruption of all ligamentous structures of the forearm.

PROCEDURE 58

Open Treatment of Complex Traumatic Elbow Instability

George S. M. Dyer and David Ring

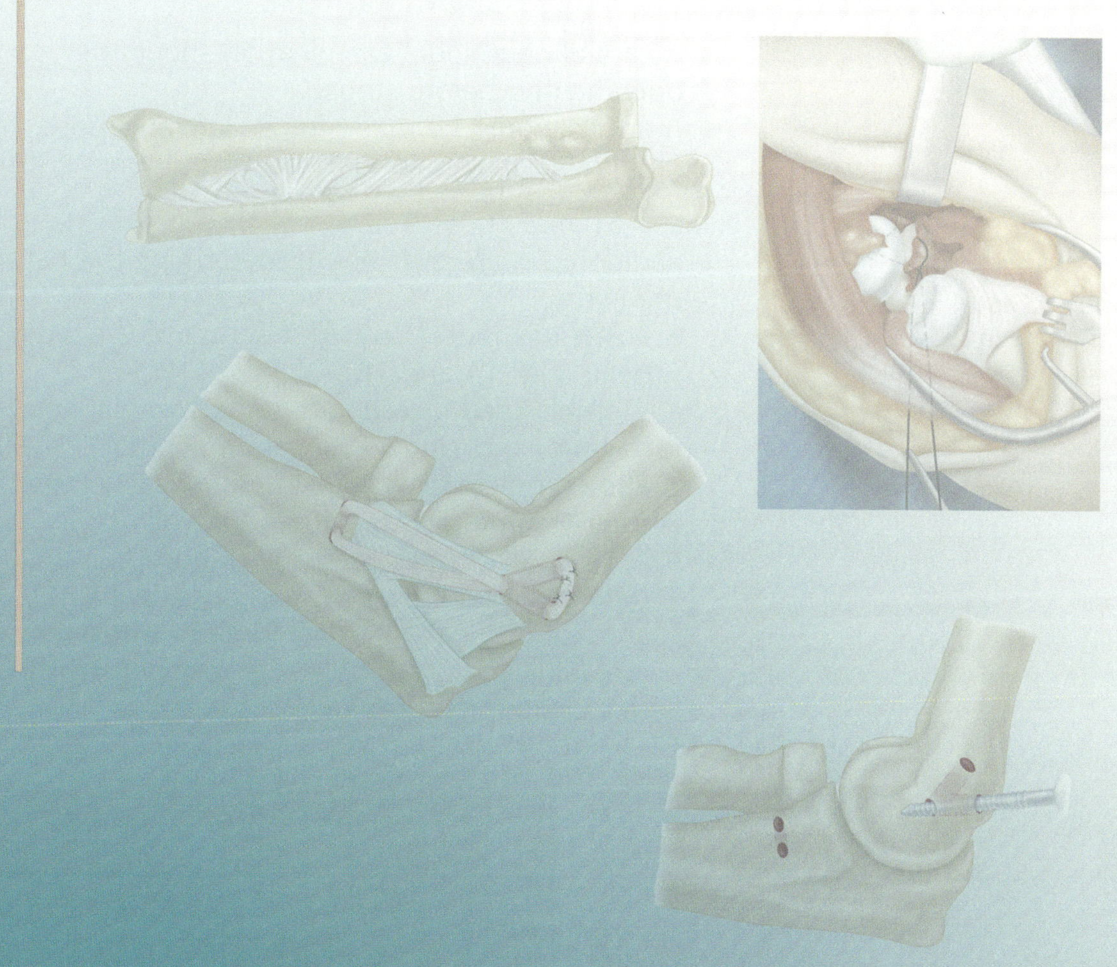

Figures 13–15 reprinted from Mathew PK, King GJW, Athwal GS. Terrible triad injuries of the elbow. In Schemitsch E (ed). Operative Techniques: Orthopaedic Trauma Surgery. Philadelphia: Elsevier, 2009:143, 151.

PITFALLS

- *Misclassification of a complex proximal ulna fracture as an "olecranon fracture"*
- *Failure to recognize or appreciate all of the important elements of the injury—proximal radius, proximal ulna, coronoid, distal humerus, and collateral ligaments*

Controversies

- Is there a role for nonoperative treatment of frequently troublesome injuries (e.g., "terrible triad" injuries and fractures of the anteromedial facet of the coronoid process)? When is it safe to consider?
- Repair versus replacement of the radial head.
- When do small coronoid fractures benefit from repair?
- When should the medial collateral ligament be repaired?
- The role of hinged external fixation.

Indications

- Any combination of fractures and ligament injuries that results in persistent subluxation or dislocation of the elbow after closed treatment (manipulative reduction)
- Injuries (such as a displaced radial head fracture) that might affect elbow function independent of stability issues

Examination/Imaging

Physical Examination

- A careful neurologic examination should be documented before surgery.
- A check should be made for ipsilateral injuries.
- The physician should look for wounds and abrasions.

Imaging Studies

- Radiographs are obtained to determine the nature of the injury.
  - Posterior dislocation with fracture of the radial head (Fig. 1A and 1B).
  - "Terrible triad": coronoid fracture, radial head fracture, and elbow dislocation (Fig. 2A). There is also complete capsuloligamentous failure and usually some muscle damage as well.
  - Anterior olecranon (trans-olecranon) fracture-dislocation (Fig. 3). In this injury, there is anterior dislocation of the forearm without radioulnar dislocation. Realignment of the ulna reduces the radiocapitellar joint.

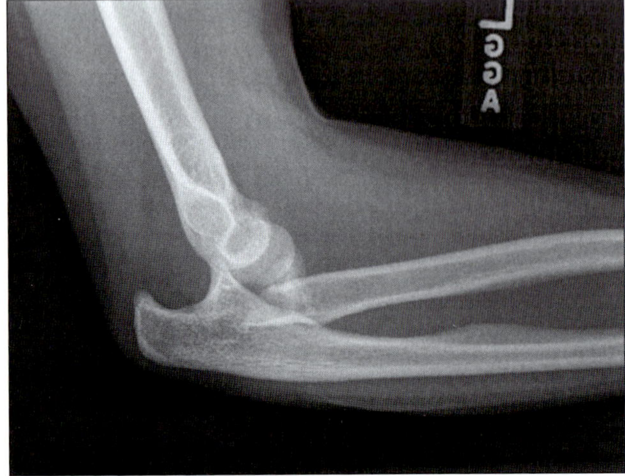

A

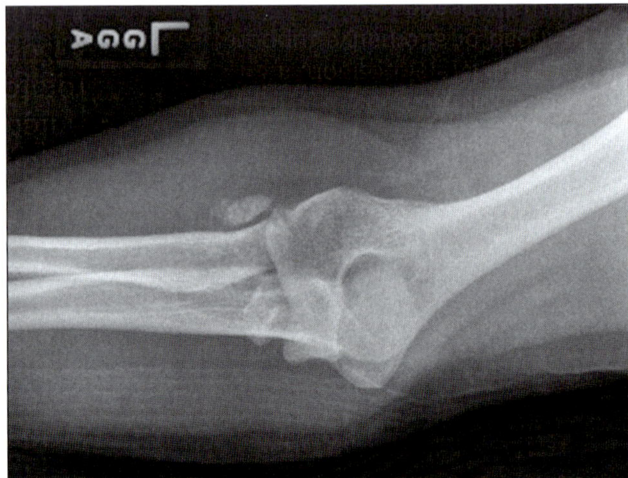

B

FIGURE 1

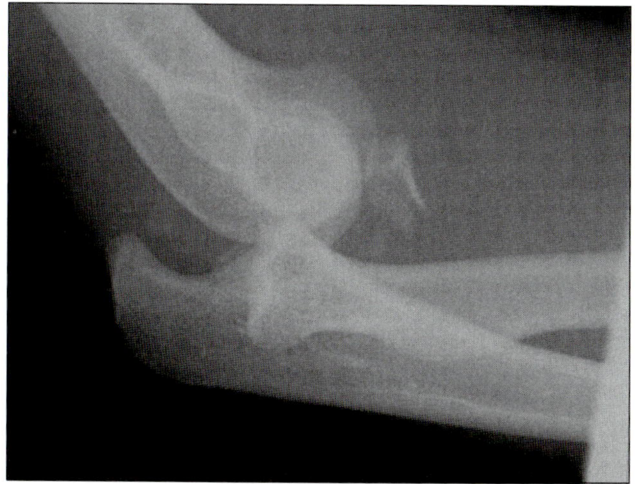

A

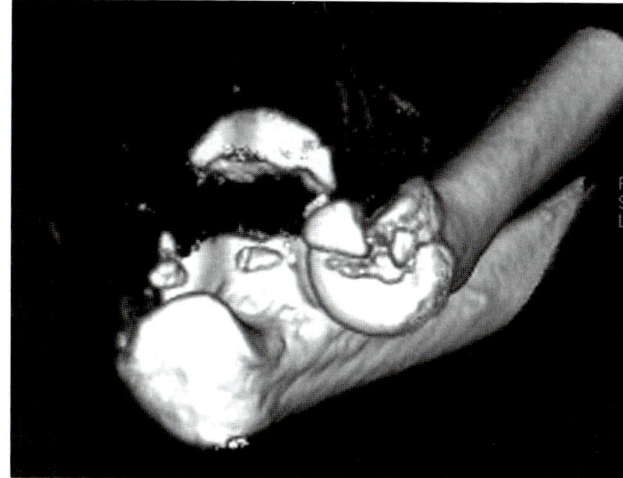

B

FIGURE 2

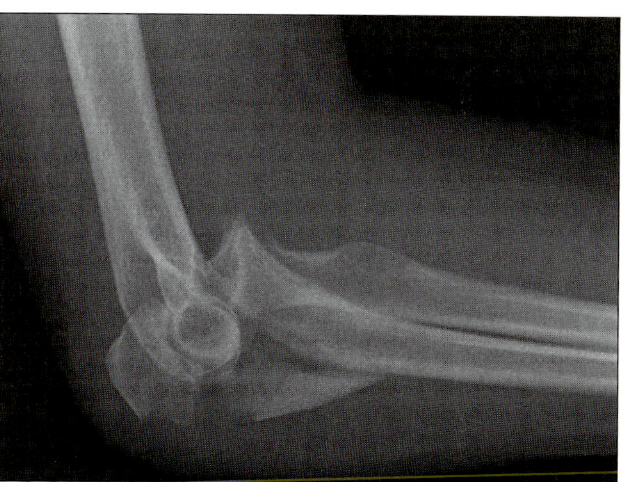

FIGURE 3

- Posterior olecranon fracture-dislocation (posterior Monteggia fracture) (Fig. 4). This injury is an apex posterior proximal ulna fracture with posterior dislocation of the radiocapitellar joint. The radioulnar relationships are relatively maintained in the metaphyseal- and articular-level fractures. This injury compromises both forearm and elbow function.
- Anteromedial facet fracture of the coronoid with avulsion of the lateral collateral ligament (LCL) origin (posteromedial varus rotational instability) (Fig. 5).
- Dislocation of the elbow with fracture of the capitellum/trochlea (Fig. 6).

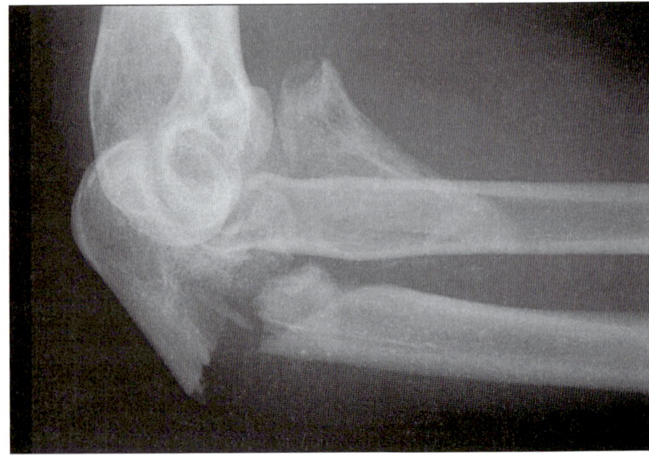

FIGURE 4

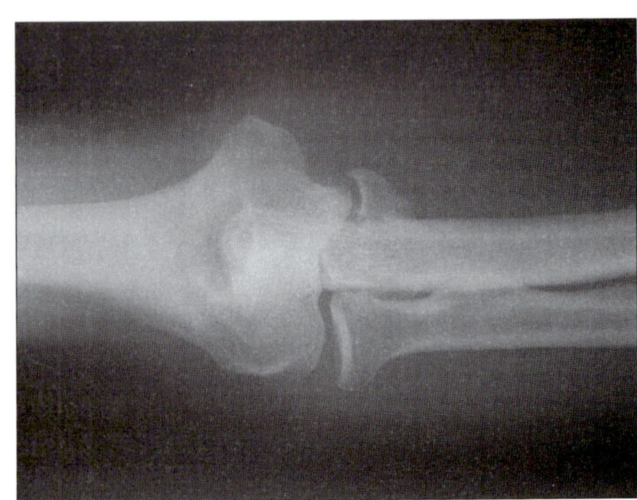

FIGURE 5

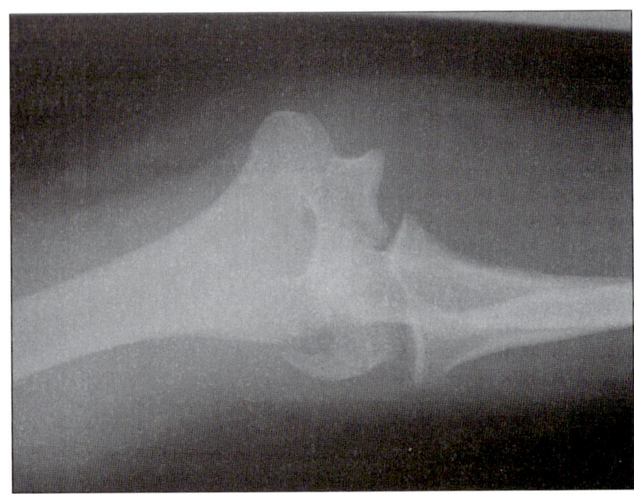

FIGURE 6

- A computed tomography scan, particularly a three-dimensional reconstruction if available, is very helpful in planning exposure and management of specific injury components (Fig. 2B). The unfractured bones can be removed digitally to improve fracture visualization.

Surgical Anatomy

- Repair of complex traumatic elbow injuries requires knowledge of the effects on the anatomy of the medial and lateral elbow.
- Medial elbow injuries (Fig. 7)
  - In the terrible triad injury, there is typically a small transverse fracture, an average of 39% of the total height of the coronoid (Ring et al., 1997). This always includes the capsular insertion.
  - Weakness of the medial collateral ligament (MCL) by itself does not cause recurrent dislocation (Ring and Jupiter, 2002).
- Lateral elbow injuries
  - The LCL is usually avulsed from the lateral epicondyle (about 50% of posterior olecranon fracture-dislocations).
  - In terrible triad injuries, the radial head is irreparably damaged about 60% of the time. Resecting it makes the coronoid much easier to see.
  - The common extensor origin is disrupted in about 60% of cases.

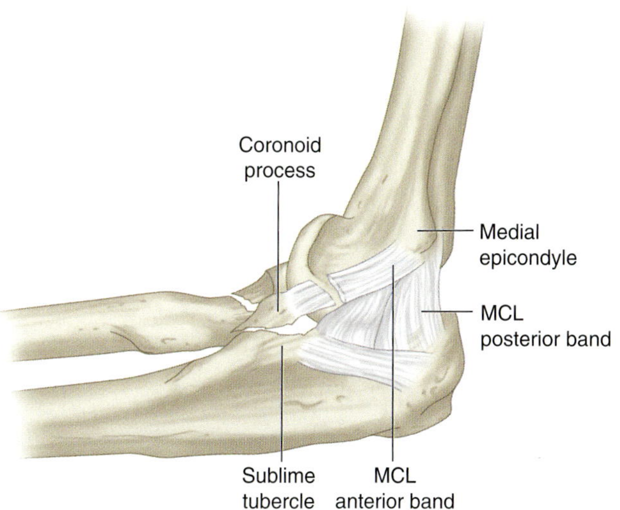

FIGURE 7

Anatomy to be Addressed

- Terrible triad injury
  - Rotatory elbow dislocation, including coronoid fracture or avulsion
  - LCL disruption
  - Radial head fracture
- Trans-olecranon fracture-dislocation
  - Fracture of olecranon
  - Anterior translation of main body of ulnar shaft
  - Anterior dislocation of radial head from capitellum
- Posterior Monteggia fractures
  - Radial head dislocation, with or without fracture
  - Proximal ulna fracture
  - Annular ligament disruption
  - Proximal radioulnar joint disruption
- Anteromedial coronoid facet fracture–posteromedial rotatory instability
  - Fracture of coronoid process of the ulna.
  - Other structures may be injured as well: LCL, olecranon, radial head, MCL.
  - Even when not evident, most anteromedial facet coronoid fractures are associated with LCL injury.

Pearls

- *If necessary, the arm can be supported over the patient's body for the posterior work and supported on a hand table for the anteromedial or anterolateral work.*
- *Use a sterile tourniquet.*

Pitfalls

- *Be certain the image intensifier has adequate access.*

Positioning

- Lateral or semilateral if exclusively posterior approach is anticipated (olecranon fracture-dislocation only)
- Supine with hand table for medial and lateral approach to anterior structures
- Terrible triad injury
  - Supine on hand table
  - Sterile tourniquet
- Trans-olecranon fracture-dislocation
  - Lateral or semilateral position with arm draped across bolster on body for posterior access (Fig. 8)

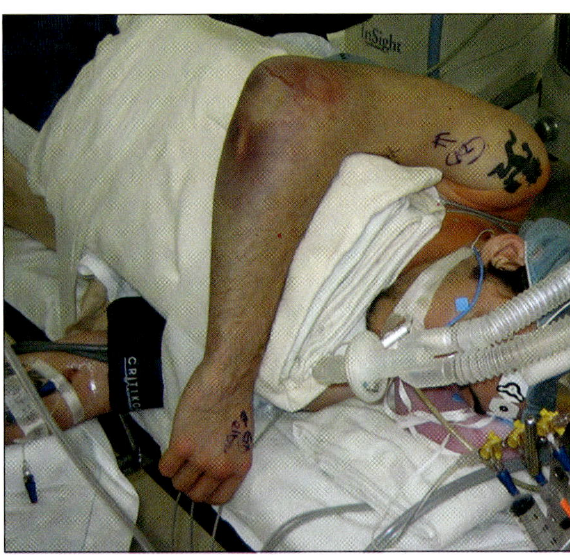

FIGURE 8

Equipment

- A few blankets or a beanbag can be used for support in a semilateral position.
- For a full lateral position, a beanbag or alternative support is usually needed.

- Posterior Monteggia fractures
  - Supine/semilateral with blankets to allow adduction for posterior access to elbow
- Anteromedial coronoid facet fracture–posteromedial rotatory instability
  - Supine on hand table
  - Sterile tourniquet

Portals/Exposures

Skin Incision

- A long posterior incision provides access to nearly the entire elbow via medial and lateral skin flaps, with the least risk to cutaneous nerves.
- Separate medial and lateral incisions may also be used and are preferred by some because they create a smaller subcutaneous pocket for the accumulation of hematoma or seroma.

Lateral Exposure

- Several lateral intervals are described for access to the radial head, the capitellum, the lateral collateral ligaments and the common extensor origin, as well as to the lateral aspect of the coronoid.
- Kocher interval (Fig. 9)
  - The Kocher interval between the anconeus and extensor carpi ulnaris is the most posterior interval.
  - It offers good protection of the posterior interosseous nerve, which is more anterior, but it places the LCL complex at greater risk.
  - The anconeus should not be elevated posteriorly, and the elbow capsule and annular ligament

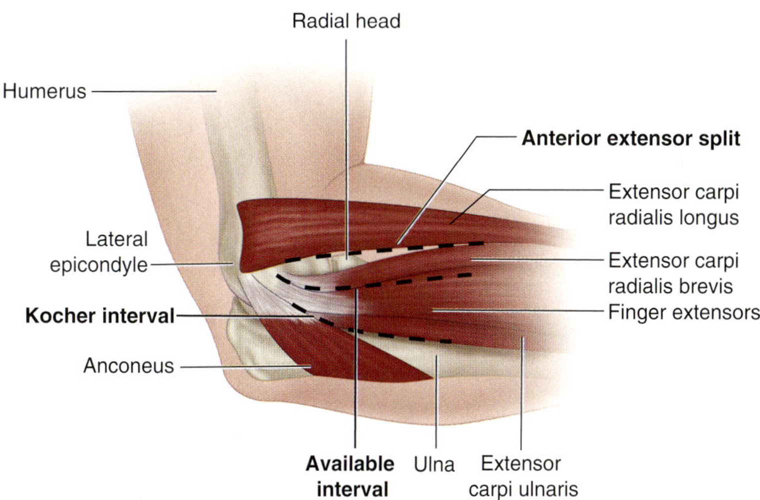

FIGURE 9

Pearls

- *Lateral exposure*
  - *An avulsion of the LCL or a fracture of the lateral epicondyle can greatly facilitate exposure.*
  - *A rent in the lateral soft tissues can indicate the best lateral muscle interval.*
  - *Preoperative planning will determine the best interval to use.*
  - *Several intervals can be used if the fracture proves more complex than anticipated.*
- *Medial exposure*
  - *Plan preoperatively which of these three exposures to use, depending on the fragment size, location, and fixation planned.*
  - *It is acceptable to use more than one interval if necessary, however.*

should be incised diagonally, in line with the posterior margin of the extensor carpi ulnaris.

- Anterior extensor split (more anterior approach) (see Fig. 9)
  - This approach is useful for injuries in which the radial head is fractured or displaced anteriorly, and for lateral access to the coronoid.
  - The posterior interosseous nerve is at greater risk, but the LCL complex is better protected.
  - A useful technique for choosing a good interval and protecting the LCL complex was described by Hotchkiss (1997).
    - Starting at the supracondylar ridge of the distal humerus, the origin of the extensor carpi radialis is incised and elevated, and the underlying elbow capsule is incised. It is then possible to see the capitellum and radial head.
    - The interval for more distal dissection should be just anterior to a line bisecting the radial head in the anteroposterior plane.
- "Available interval" approach (see Fig. 9)
  - The injury to ligaments, muscle, and tendon associated with fracture-dislocations of the elbow often presents the surgeon with a convenient window of disrupted structures.
  - The LCL almost always avulses from the lateral epicondyle.
  - A split in the common extensor origin that begins with the bare spot on the lateral epicondyle can be developed distally into a muscle-splitting interval.
  - A low lateral column fracture can serve as an osteotomy, reflecting the lateral ulnar collateral ligament and extensor origin back and allowing access.
  - In the setting of a posterior olecranon fracture-dislocation or posterior Monteggia fracture, the radial head often displaces posteriorly through capsule and muscle. Accentuation of the injury deformity usually brings the radial head up into the wound.
    - In some cases, the surgeon will extend the posterior muscle injury in order to mobilize the olecranon fracture proximally to expose and manipulate the coronoid fracture through the elbow articulation. Slight additional dissection between the radius and the ulna is acceptable given the usually extensive injury in this region,

but extensive new dissection in this area has been suggested to increase the risk of proximal radioulnar synostosis.

Medial Exposure

- A medial flap is developed using the universal posterior skin incision.
- Three intervals are described for access to the coronoid.
  - Small fragment, anterior to the sublime tubercle (Fig. 10) (described by Hotchkiss as the "medial over-the-top exposure")
    - The flexor-pronator mass is split longitudinally.
    - The proximal muscle bellies are retracted and the medial capsule incised longitudinally, in line with its fibers and anterior to the anterior band of the MCL.
    - This gives direct access to the apical portion of the coronoid.
  - Larger fragment, including the sublime tubercle (Fig. 11)

Pitfalls

- *Lateral exposure*
  - *Don't place retractors over the neck of the radius.*
  - *If implants are to be placed on the radial neck, pronate the forearm and consider identifying the posterior interosseous nerve if the implants are more than 4–5 cm down the neck.*
  - *To see the coronoid from the lateral side, remove the radial head fragments, release the origin of the extensor carpal radialis longus from the supracondylar ridge, and elevate the brachialis and brachioradialis from the anterior humerus.*
  - *Ulnar nerve palsy is common after dissection and retraction of the ulnar nerve.*
- *Medial exposure*
  - *In the FCU "natural split" approach, the FCU must be split much more distally than is typical when decompressing the ulnar nerve.*
  - *The first few posterior branches of the ulnar nerve to the FCU may be sacrificed if needed, but many large posterior branches will make it difficult to mobilize the nerve anteriorly.*
  - *Extensive mobilization in order to formally transpose the nerve may be associated with increased incidence of ulnar palsy.*

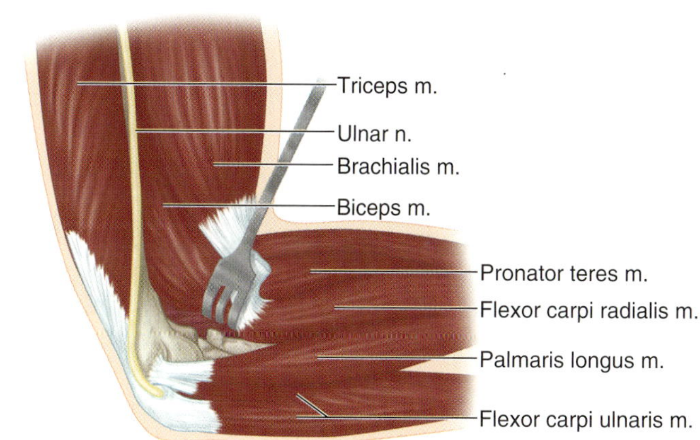

FIGURE 10

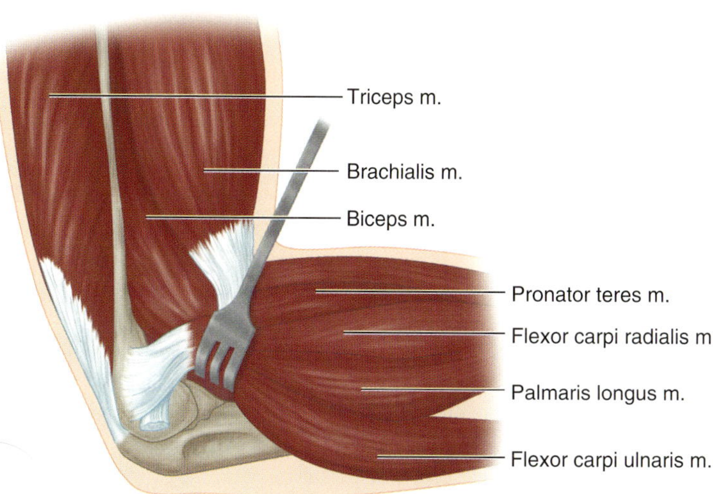

FIGURE 11

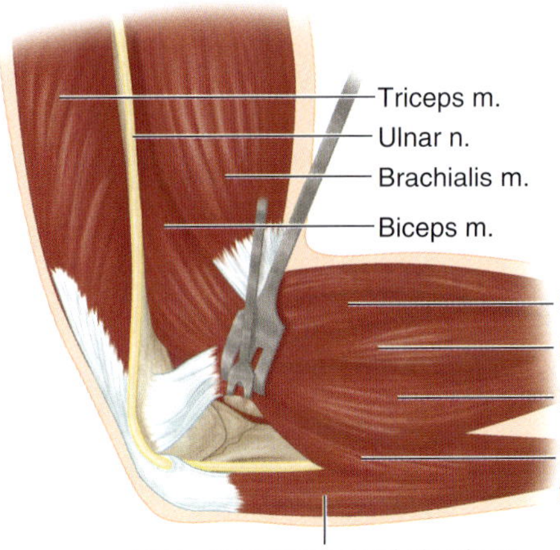

FIGURE 12

Instrumentation

- Z knee retractors are useful in the anterior elbow.

Controversies

- On the medial side: retract the ulnar nerve or leave it in situ and work with oscillating drills?
- When is it worthwhile to release muscle or ligament origins? As a rule, we will release a structure if it improves visualization for reducing or stably fixing fracture fragments. However, we would leave intact anything that can reasonably be worked around.

Pearls

- *Reduce the elbow during lateral exposure to ensure proper understanding of the anatomy.*

    - The "natural split" between the heads of the flexor carpi ulnaris (FCU) where the ulnar nerve lies is developed.
    - The two portions of this muscle are retracted apart from one another, taking care not to injure the crossing branches of the nerve.
    - This gives access to most of the medial aspect of the coronoid and is useful for medial buttress plating.
- Coronoid base fracture, including the whole coronoid (Fig. 12) (exposure credited to Taylor and Scham, 1967)
    - The entire flexor-pronator mass is elevated from posterior to anterior.
    - This reveals the medial coronoid, including the base.

Procedure: "Terrible Triad" Injury

Step 1: Lateral Exposure

- A posterior or direct lateral skin incision is made.
- There is usually extensive avulsion of the origins of the common extensor and LCL from the lateral epicondyle that facilitates exposure.
- In most patients, a very small rent in the fascia will direct the surgeon to the appropriate interval to develop in the common extensors. Alternatively, one can identify the supracondylar ridge and elevate the origin of the extensor carpi radialis longus, gaining access to the anterior distal humerus.
- Working distally, one will enter the joint and see the capitellum.

Pearls

- *The anatomic attachment point for the anterior capsule is on the anterior surface of the coronoid, but not at the very tip.*
- *Crossing the tunnels through the proximal ulna and coronoid base can make it easier to keep from skiving off the angled bone of the proximal ulna diaphyseal-metaphyseal junction and make it easier to stay within the bone.*
- *If possible, place the drill holes slightly off the very ridge of the ulna to avoid prominence of the suture knot.*

Pitfalls

- *The median nerve may be just anterior to the elbow joint capsule at the level of the stitch—a very superficial bite of the capsule is sufficient.*

Instrumentation/Implantation

- Z knee retractors or cobra retractors
- Trans-tibial tunnel guide for the ACL
- Suture retriever, or suture loop on a Keith needle, to pass the sutures for the coronoid

Pearls

- *The radial neck is easier to instrument and the radial head is easier to replace if the elbow is permitted to dislocate again for this step.*

Instrumentation/Implantation

- Implants for repairing or replacing the fractured radial head

- The muscle interval should split the common extensors 50:50 with respect to the center of rotation of the capitellum.

Step 2: Anterior Stability—Coronoid

- The transverse tip fractures of the coronoid that are typically associated with a terrible triad injury can be addressed through the lateral exposure.
- Exposure to the coronoid is improved by displacing or removing fragments of the fractured radial head and by releasing the origin of the extensor carpi radialis longus from the supracondylar ridge of the distal humerus.
- Once this exposure has been performed, it is safe to place retractors anterior to the distal humerus, but placement anterior to the radial head and neck should be avoided.
- We rely on suture repair for the vast majority of the small transverse coronoid fractures associated with terrible triad injuries. Sutures passed through drill holes in the proximal ulnar metaphysis and coronoid base are passed through the anterior capsular attachments to the coronoid.
- A drill guide, such as the guide used to drill the tibial tunnel in anterior cruciate ligament (ACL) reconstruction, can facilitate accurate placement of the tunnels for suture passage (Fig. 13).
- For relatively large coronoid fracture fragments, the sutures can be passed through drill holes in the coronoid fracture fragment (Fig. 14).
- The suture ends are retrieved dorsally and tied after all of the injuries have been addressed (Fig. 15).

Step 3: Repair or Replace Radial Head

- See Procedure 57 on radial head fracture.

Step 4: Reattach Origin of LCL to Lateral Epicondyle

- The LCL usually avulses from its attachment point on the lateral epicondyle (Fig. 16).
- The middle or isometric point of this bare area must be identified. It is usually at the anterior-inferior point of a nubbin on the epicondyle.
- Either a bone anchor or transosseous drill holes, tying suture posterior to the lateral ridge of the humerus, may be used for reattachment (Fig. 17).

Step 5: Reduction and Tensioning

- The ulnohumeral and radiocapitellar joints are reduced.
- The coronoid and LCL sutures are tensioned and tied.

Pearls

- *The LCL attachment point can be surprisingly anterior on the humerus.*

Instrumentation/ Implantation

- Suture anchors to repair the LCL

Pearls

- *Cycle the elbow (flexion and extension) with gentle tension on the sutures to get them securely tight.*
- *One of us (DR) likes to leave the tails long enough to pass under some FCU fascia to hide the knot in an attempt to make it less irritating.*

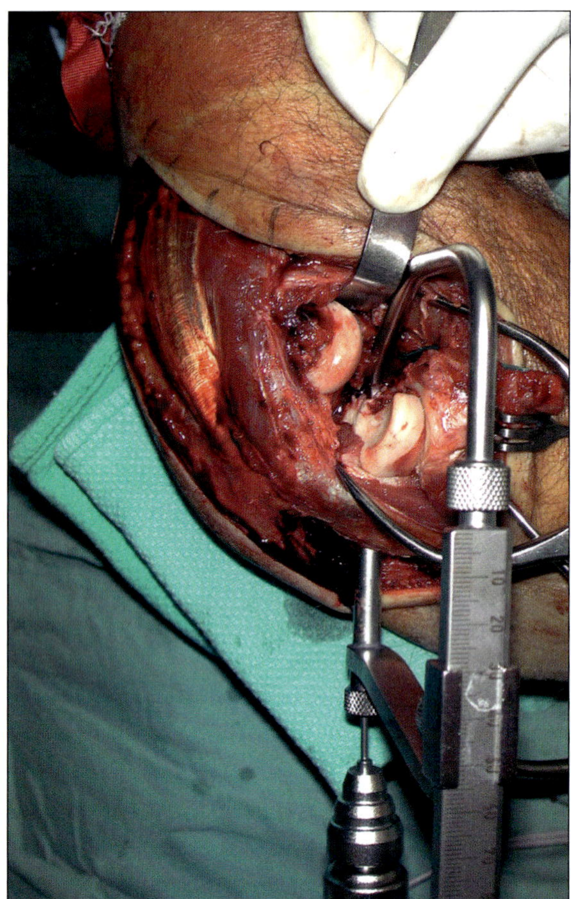

FIGURE 13

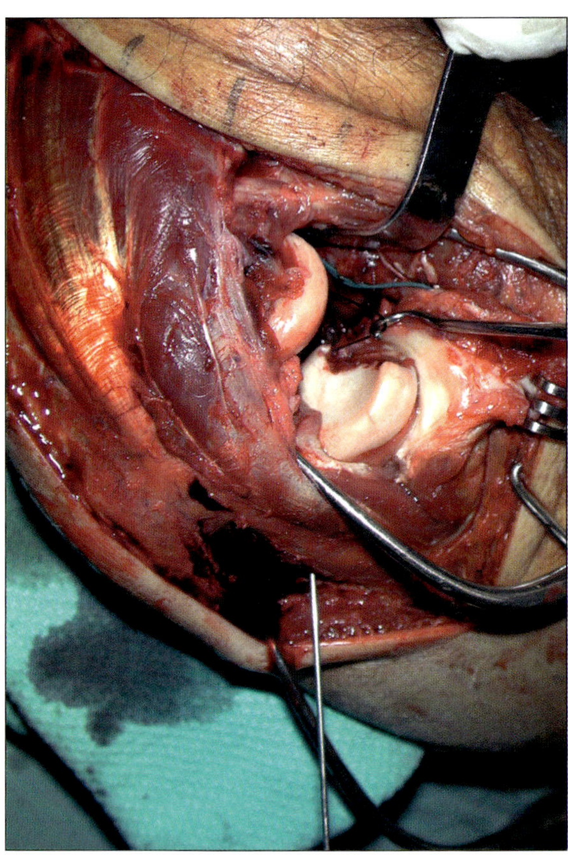

FIGURE 14

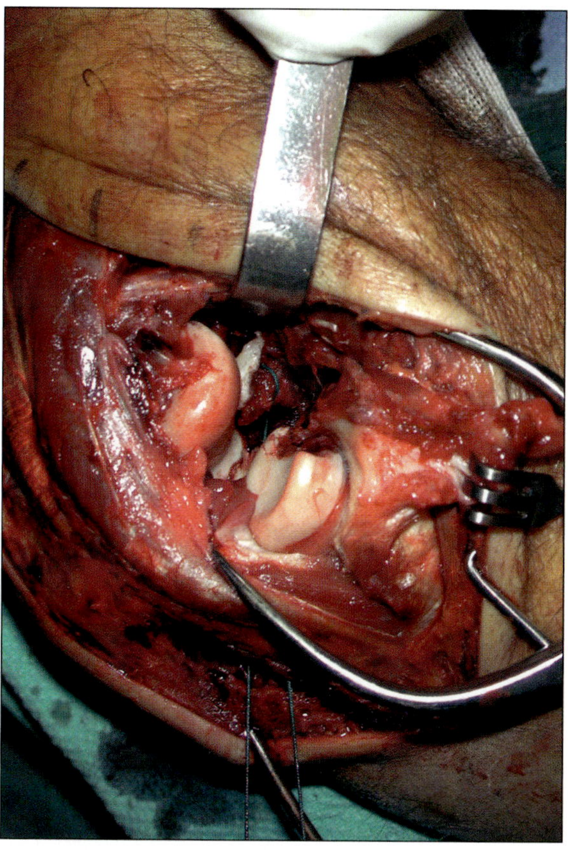

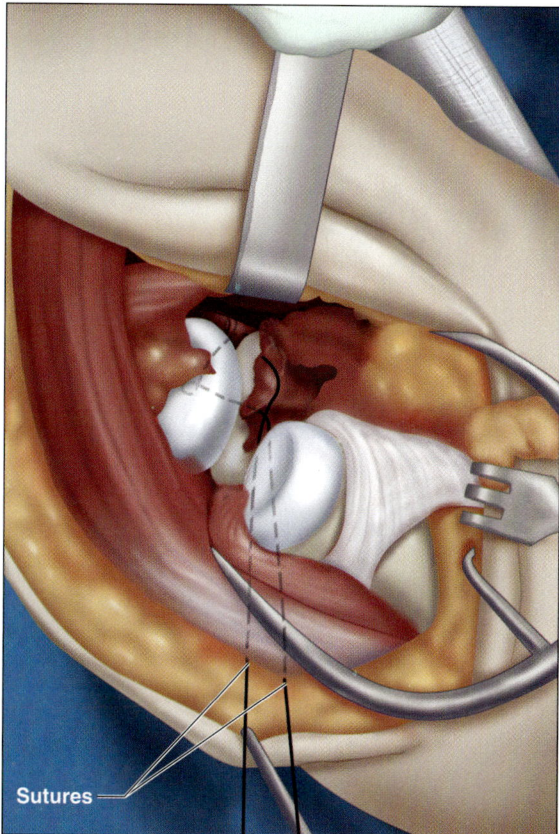

FIGURE 15

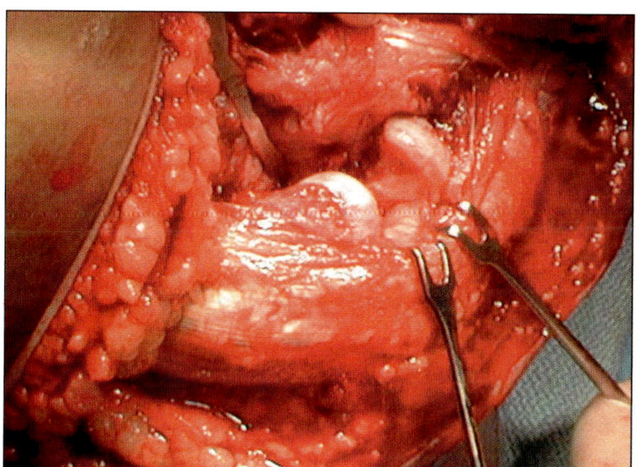

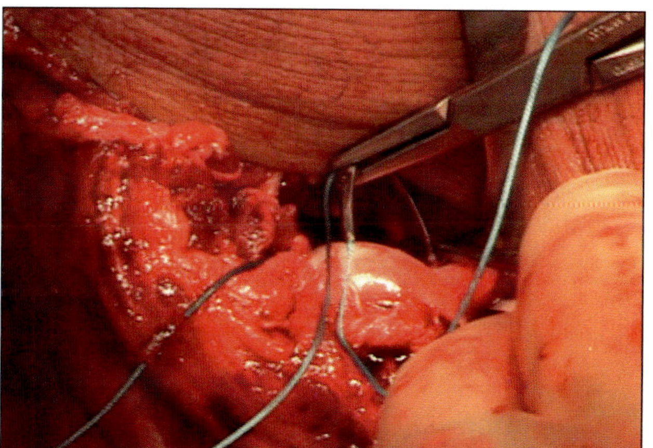

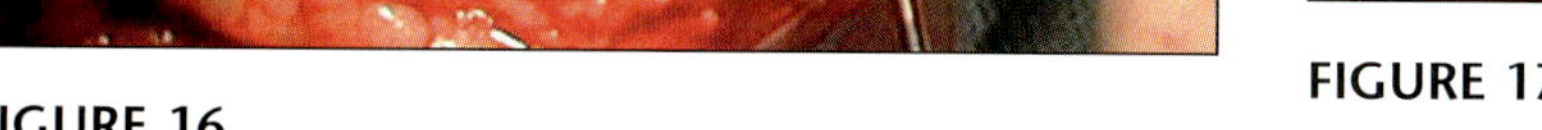

FIGURE 16

FIGURE 17

Controversies

- With careful reconstruction of the coronoid, the radial head, and the LCL, we have seldom found the need to separately repair the MCL. In cases in which the elbow remains unstable despite the reconstruction described in this procedure, one can consider repair of the MCL, hinged or static external fixation, or cross-pinning of the joint.
- Some surgeons prefer to formally isolate and/or transpose the ulnar nerve during or before working on the ulnar side of the elbow. One of us (GD) has found that, at least in some cases, extensive handling of the nerve was associated with an increased rate of ulnar palsy or injury.

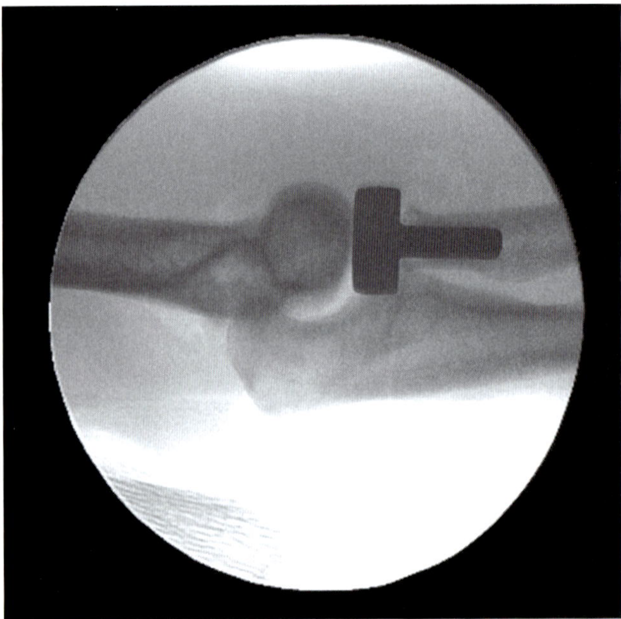

A

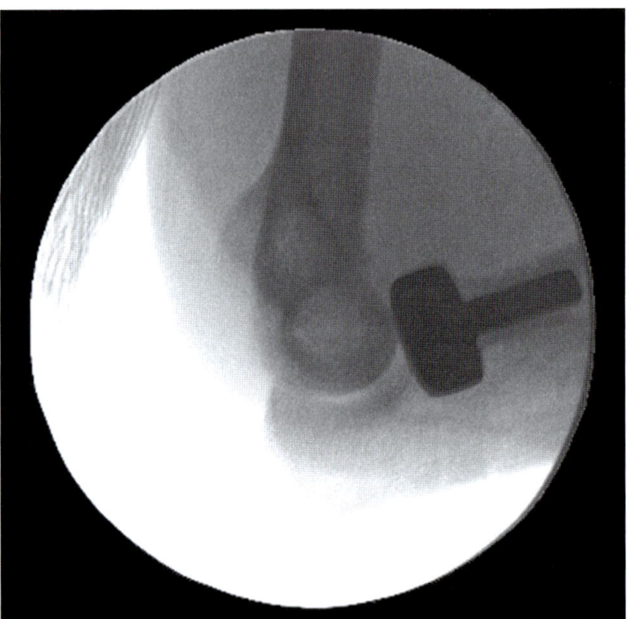

B

FIGURE 18

Step 6: Assess Stability

- Test final stability by placing the elbow in full gravity extension with the forearm in neutral and checking a lateral image. A small degree of 'sag' may be seen on the lateral image. It can be expected to resolve spontaneously in the first week or two (Fig. 18A and 18B). If a "clunk" or reduction from this position occurs or if there is subluxation or disocation on the image, additional treatments can be considered.

Pearls

- *Work through the olecranon fracture to inspect the radial head, evaluate and realign the coronoid process, evaluate the collateral ligaments, and clear out bone fragments or other debris from the ulnohumeral and radiocapitellar joints.*

Procedure: Trans-olecranon Fracture-Dislocation (Anterior Olecranon Fracture-Dislocation)

Step 1: Exposure

- A longitudinal posterior incision is used for exposure.
- Medial and lateral skin flaps are raised.

Step 2: Reduction

- Realignment of the proximal ulna fracture should reduce the radial head to its appropriate relationship with the capitellum.
  - Associated radial head fracture is rare with anterior olecranon fracture-dislocations.
  - Fracture fragments of the olecranon must be defined.
  - Reduction of the ulna is determined.

Pearls

- *There is often a roughly diamond-shaped fragment from the medial wall of the proximal ulna that serves as a guide for length and rotation of the proximal fragment to the proximal shaft. It is not necessary to key this in precisely, particularly if doing so would compromise its blood supply.*
- *Capsuloligamentous structures are usually preserved in anterior-type fracture-dislocations.*

Pitfalls

- *Take care not to narrow the trochlear notch.*
- *Comminution of the ulna will require a plate rather than any kind of tension band for fixation.*
- *When the olecranon process is fragmented, use a wire engaging the triceps insertion to ensure adequate fixation.*

Instrumentation/Implantation

- Specially designed olecranon plates, or plates that can be contoured to this purpose
- K-wires for provisional fixation
- Small screws

Pearls

- *The radial head fracture should be addressed before reduction and fixation of the ulna fracture as the displacement provided by the ulna fracture can facilitate exposure of the radial head.*
- *Once the radial head has been addressed, restoration of radiocapitellar alignment should help to realign the ulna.*

Pearls

- *If the radiocapitellar joint is unstable, the most likely reason is imperfect reduction of the ulna.*

Step 3: Fixation

- Once basic reduction and orientation are determined, a long Kirschner wire (K-wire) passed down the shaft is useful for provisional fixation. Alternatively, the olecranon fragment may be provisionally pinned to the trochlea, using the trochlea as a template for restoration of the proper contour and dimensions of the trochlear notch.
- The ulna is then fixed with a plate.
- Once the ulna is fixed with a plate and screws, the elbow should be congruent and stable.

Procedure: Dorsal Exposure, Reduction, and Plating of Posterior Monteggia Fractures (Posterior Olecranon Fracture-Dislocation)

Step 1: Exposure

- A posterior approach to the ulna is used (see above).

Step 2: Assess Radial Head and Neck

- If the radial head is uninjured (or has minimal injury), anatomic reduction of the ulna may be all that is required.
- The LCL sometimes requires repair, but the annular ligament generally does not require formal repair.
- With this fracture pattern, one can usually address the radial head through the posterior damage, although a separate exposure may be helpful on occasion.

Step 3: Reduce and Fix Ulna

- See Steps 2 and 3 for Procedure 2 above.

Step 4: Test Stability

- Test elbow and radioulnar stability through a complete range of forearm rotation as well as flexion-extension.

Procedure: Anteromedial Coronoid Facet Fracture–Posteromedial Rotatory Instability

Step 1: Exposure of Coronoid

- Medial exposure of the coronoid is employed.

Pearls

- *Suture fixation—in larger fragments it may be possible to drill through the fragment as well as the ulna. Carefully lining up these holes will allow the suture to act like a lag screw as it is tied down.*
- *Buttress plate fixation*
  - *The plate must be well fixed to the ulna distally for mechanical stability, but it can stand off the bone in some areas proximally as long as compression is achieved.*
  - *While placing screws, placing the screw just proximal to the fracture first, then rotating the plate slightly and placing a more distal screw in a compression mode, will often improve fixation.*

Pitfalls

- *For large medial fragments, use a plate even when the fragment seems large enough for screw-only fixation. This will help prevent catastrophic failure under medial shearing forces.*

Step 2: Fracture Fixation

- Small fragments may be secured with sutures only, capturing the attachment point in the anterior capsule with a grasping stitch and passing the sutures through tunnels in the ulna and tying them over the dorsal surface (see Procedure 1 above).
- Larger fragments may be amenable to medial buttress plating with either fragment-specific plates, T plates, or contoured small straight or recon plates.
  - Reduce and provisionally fix the fragment with a K-wire.
  - Select a plate and plan its position.
  - The proximal portion of the plate will often lie directly under the ulnar nerve—this is acceptable.

Instrumentation/Implantation

- Small plates to apply a medial buttress to the coronoid may be helpful.
- For small fractures best repaired with sutures, use the equipment described for Procedure 1 above.
- Suture anchors or other soft tissue fixation can be used for the LCL if needed.

Pitfalls

- *Supination is more commonly lost than pronation, and it is harder to live without. Patients can abduct the shoulder to achieve pronation if needed.*

Postoperative Care and Expected Outcomes

- Finger motion is initiated immediately. Patients should repeatedly squeeze a tight fist and open the hand with tension to squeeze out edema.
- When adequate fixation has been obtained or a hinged fixator applied to reduce stress on a more tenuous fixation, active-assisted elbow and forearm exercises are initiated as soon as the patient is comfortable. A brief rest is reasonable (maximum 7 days) for very uncomfortable patients.

- When the fixation is tenuous, it is reasonable to delay exercises for a month. Stiffness is more easily addressed than loss of fixation or articular injury.
- When the LCL has been repaired, shoulder abduction (varus stress) should be avoided for 1 month. Active exercises can be done with the elbow at the side or overhead (gravity assisted).

Evidence

Cohen MS, Hastings H 2nd. Rotatory instability of the elbow: the anatomy and role of the lateral stabilizers. J Bone Joint Surg [Am]. 1997;79:225-33.

Forty fresh cadavera were studied to define the ligamentous anatomy of the lateral aspect of the elbow specifically as it relates to rotatory instability. There is a broad conjoined insertion of the lateral collateral and annular ligaments onto the proximal aspect of the ulna. Serial sectioning studies revealed primary and secondary stabilizers of the lateral aspect of the elbow. In addition to the lateral collateral ligament and the annular ligament, the extensor muscle origins provide stability through fascial bands and intermuscular septa.

Doornberg JN, Ring D. Coronoid fracture patterns. J Hand Surg [Am]. 2006;31:45-52.

Large fractures of the coronoid process are associated with with anterior and posterior olecranon fracture-dislocations, small transverse fractures are associated with terrible-triad injuries, and anteromedial facet fractures are associated with varus posteromedial rotational instability pattern injuries. Terrible-triad injuries had small (<50%) coronoid fractures. (Level IV evidence)

Doornberg JN, van Duijn J, Ring D. Coronoid fracture height in terrible-triad injuries. J Hand Surg [Am]. 2006;31:794-7.

The total height of the coronoid process of the ulna averaged 19 mm. The average height of the coronoid fracture fragment was 7 mm. This corresponds to an average of 35% of the total height of the coronoid process. The transverse coronoid fractures associated with terrible-triad elbow injuries have a variable height that may not be easy to classify according to the system of Regan and Morrey. Classification of coronoid fractures according to fracture morphology and injury pattern may be preferable. (Level IV evidence)

Dowdy PA, Bain GI, King GJ, Patterson SD. The midline posterior elbow incision: an anatomical appraisal. J Bone Joint Surg [Br]. 1995;77:696-9.

Cutaneous nerves are at considerable risk of injury when medial or lateral incisions are used to approach the elbow, but the posterior approach carries less hazard. The routine use of the posterior incision may reduce the incidence of symptomatic paraesthesia and the formation of a painful neuroma after operation.

Hotchkiss RN. Displaced fractures of the radial head: internal fixation or excision? J Am Acad Orthop Surg. 1997;5:1-10.

Displaced fractures of the radial head in the young active patient should no longer be routinely treated with excision of the radial head. Better techniques of imaging, surgical exposure, and implant placement have improved the likelihood of preserving the head. Associated injuries may make preservation of the radial head important for both acute and long-term stability. In patients with suspected injury to the interosseous ligament of the forearm, saving the radial head may prevent pathologic proximal migration. Rigid internal fixation, permitting early mobilization, can be applied to the radial head and neck in a "safe zone" that does not impede motion. Radial-head excision should be performed in patients with grossly comminuted fractures and in those with low demand on their upper extremities.

McKee MD, Pugh DM, Wild LM, Schemitsch EH, King GJ. Standard surgical protocol to treat elbow dislocations with radial head and coronoid fractures: surgical technique. J Bone Joint Surg [Am]. 2005;87(Suppl 1, Pt 1):22-32.

A standard surgical protocol includes fixation or replacement of the radial head, fixation of the coronoid fracture if possible, repair of associated capsular and lateral ligamentous injuries, and in selected cases repair of the medial collateral ligament and/or adjuvant-hinged external fixation. Use of this protocol for elbow dislocations with associated radial head and coronoid fractures restores sufficient elbow stability to allow early motion postoperatively, enhancing the functional outcome. (Level IV evidence)

O'Driscoll SW. Elbow instability. Hand Clin. 1994;10:405-15.

Elbow instability is a spectrum from subluxation to dislocation, with corresponding clinical and pathologic features and therapeutic implications. A classification that unifies these aspects is presented. Posterolateral rotational displacement of the ulna (with the radius) on the humerus appears to be the common mechanism. Acute dislocations can be reduced in supination and tested for valgus stability in pronation. Treatment is determined by the stability following reduction. When there are fractures, the principle is to fix the bones so that the only limitation is the ligaments and then to repair them if the elbow is not stable enough to permit early motion. The three prerequisites for stability of the ulnohumeral articulation are an intact joint surface, anterior medial collateral ligament, and ulnar part of the lateral collateral ligament. Recurrent instability is usually due to insufficiency of the ulnar part of the lateral collateral ligament complex, the lateral ulnar collateral ligament (LUCL), with attenuation of the other secondary soft tissue constraints on the lateral side. Reconstruction of the lateral ulnar collateral ligament typically corrects the problem. Chronic dislocations are treated by similar techniques after releasing contractures and resurfacing the joint with biologic tissue if it is irreversibly damaged.

Ring D, Doornberg JN. Fracture of the anteromedial facet of the coronoid process: surgical technique. J Bone Joint Surg [Am]. 2007;89(Suppl 2, Pt 2):267-83.

Anteromedial fractures of the coronoid are associated with either subluxation or complete dislocation of the elbow in most patients. Secure fixation of the coronoid fracture usually restores good elbow function. (Level IV evidence)

Ring D, Jupiter JB. Fracture-dislocation of the elbow. Hand Clin. 2002;18:55-63.

Recognition of the pattern of an elbow fracture-dislocation allows immediate knowledge of the treatment principles, pitfalls, and prognosis of the injury. Specific techniques for each injury component increase the surgeon's ability to restore stability to the elbow. When complications are anticipated and avoided or addressed expediently, it is possible to restore elbow function in spite of the complexity of these injuries. (Level IV evidence)

Ring D, Jupiter JB, Sanders RW, Mast J, Simpson NS. Transolecranon fracture-dislocation of the elbow. J Orthop Trauma. 1997;11:545-50.

Anterior elbow dislocations occur most often as a fracture-dislocation in which the distal humerus is driven through the olecranon, thereby causing a complex, comminuted fracture of the proximal ulna. This injury is frequently confused with anterior Monteggia lesions by virtue of the readily apparent radiocapitellar dislocation. Stable restoration of the appropriate contour and dimensions of the trochlear notch of the ulna will lead to a good result in most cases. (Level IV evidence)

Sotereanos DG, Darlis NA, Wright TW, Goitz RJ, King GJ. Unstable fracture-dislocations of the elbow. Instr Course Lect. 2007;56:369-76.

Patterns of unstable fracture-dislocations include the "terrible triad" injury of the elbow (elbow dislocation, radial head fracture, and coronoid fracture), transolecranon fracture-dislocations, and the posterior Monteggia lesion. The proximal ulna must be anatomically reduced and internally fixed, the radial head must be repaired or replaced, and substantial coronoid fractures must be repaired or reconstructed. The lateral ulnar collateral ligament and extensor origin reattachment can be easily performed. If the elbow remains unstable, application of a hinged elbow external fixator or repair of the medial collateral ligament must be considered. The goal of reconstruction is early mobilization within a stable arc of motion. This treatment protocol has the potential to improve the suboptimal outcomes reported in the literature for such injuries.

Steinmann SP. Coronoid process fracture. J Am Acad Orthop Surg. 2008;16:519-29.

The coronoid process is one of the main constraints providing ulnohumeral joint stability. Surgical approaches to coronoid fractures depend on the condition of the radial head. When an associated radial head fracture is present, a lateral approach to the coronoid fracture is often performed. An isolated coronal fracture is typically approached from the medial side. Intraoperative stress testing may be helpful in assessing the need for surgery and choosing the surgical approach.

Tan V, Daluiski A, Simic P, Hotchkiss RN. Outcome of open release for post-traumatic elbow stiffness. J Trauma. 2006;61:673-8.

Open elbow release with excision of tethers and blocks is a valuable procedure for post-traumatic stiffness. Recurrence in postoperative period is common but is responsive to manipulation under anesthesia and repeat releases. (Level IV evidence)

PROCEDURE 59

Surgical Reconstruction of Longitudinal Radioulnar Dissociation (Essex-Lopresti Injury)

Julie E. Adams and A. Lee Osterman

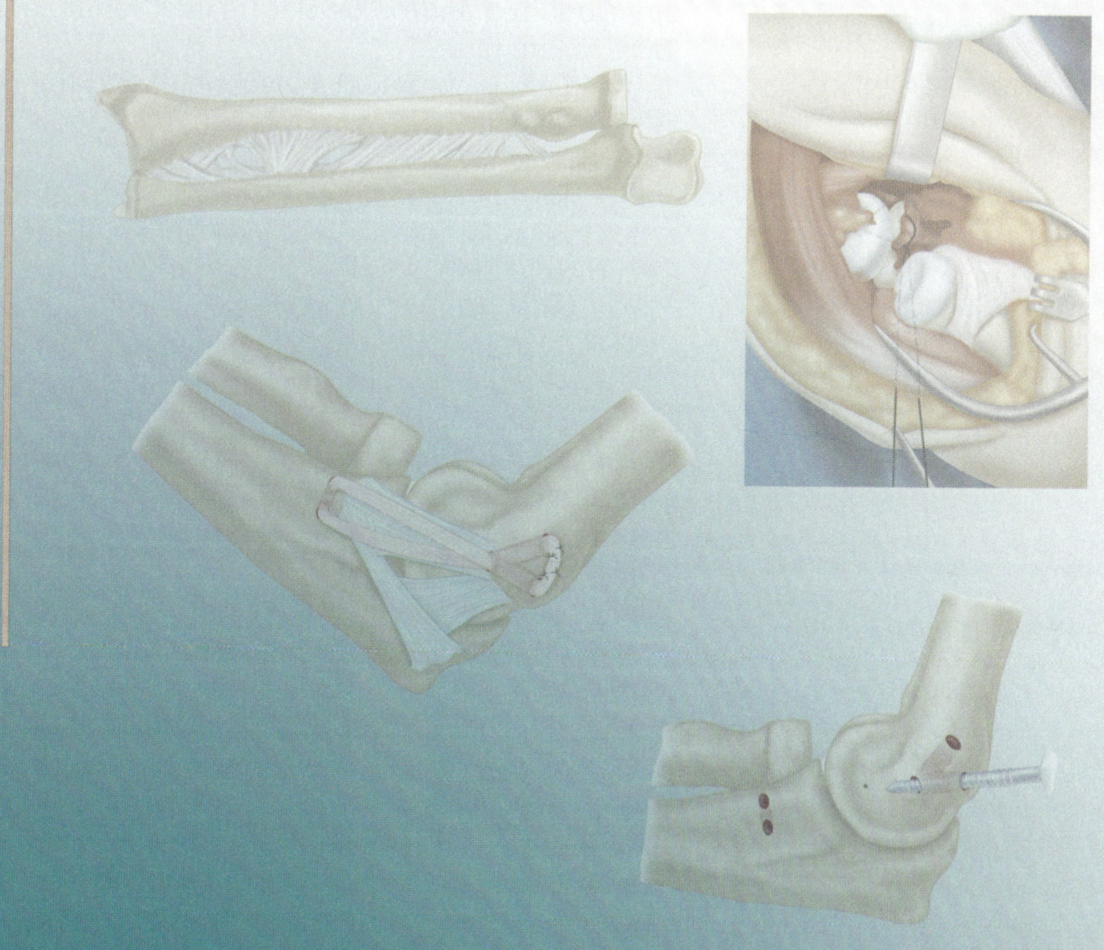

Figure 1 redrawn from Poitevin, LA: Anatomy and biomechanics of the interosseous membrane: its importance in the longitudinal stability of the forearm. Hand Clinics 17(1): 97-110. Feb 2001.
Figure 2 redrawn from Marcotte and Osterman Longitudinal radioulnar dissociation: identification and treatment of acute and chronic injuries. Hand Clin 23(2007)195-208. P 197, figure 2

Pitfalls

- *The Essex-Lopresti injury is a continuum from radial head fracture to longitudinal radioulnar dissociation. Therefore, it is critical to examine the forearm entirely to rule out potentially unrecognized associated injuries in addition to an isolated radial head fracture.*

Controversies

- When longitudinal radioulnar dissociation is diagnosed, if the injury is acute (<4 weeks old), the considerations include re-establishing the radiocapitellar articulation by radial head open reduction and internal fixation or radial head arthroplasty. **Excision should be avoided.** The DRUJ should be secured in supination or semi-supination for 4–8 weeks. This may be done with splint or cast immobilization if the DRUJ is stable, or transfixing the joint with Kirschner wires or 3.5-mm screws. Consideration may be given to acute repair or reconstruction of the interosseous ligament.

Indications

- Symptomatic chronic longitudinal radioulnar dissociation
- Acute longitudinal radioulnar dissociation, or the Essex-Lopresti injury, results from an axial compression force with injury to the radial head, interosseous membrane (IOM), and distal radioulnar joint (DRUJ). With recognition and appropriate treatment of the multiple components of this injury, good results are seen in up to 80% of cases; however, the great majority of cases go unrecognized and/or are not treated, resulting in an 80% failure rate.
- If the injury is chronic (>4 weeks old) and the patient is symptomatic, the wrist, forearm, and elbow should be addressed.
  - Consideration should be given to wrist arthroscopy for evaluation of the triangular fibrocartilage complex (TFCC) and evaluation for evidence of ulnar impaction. During the same setting, the TFCC can be débrided or repaired, and ulnar shortening osteotomy performed for ulnar impaction.
  - Forearm instability is addressed with reconstruction of the IOM.
  - In many cases of chronic but previously inappropriately treated Essex-Lopresti lesions, there will be symptomatic capitellar or radiocapitellar arthritis, which may be worsened if arthroplasty alone is performed; these patients may do better with radial head excision provided a stable forearm reconstruction is performed.

Examination/Imaging

- The history is taken, and physical examination includes attention to the wrist, forearm, and elbow.
  - The arc of flexion and extension of the elbow is assessed, as well as varus and valgus stability of elbow.
  - The wrist is examined with attention to TFCC click, extensor carpi ulnaris (ECU) subluxation, shuck test, LT ballottement, and Watson's manuever.
- The arc of pronation and supination and the stability of the DRUJ are then assessed. Under image intensification, axial loading is placed to assess impaction at the wrist and elbow. The axial load test

Treatment Options

- Because of the poor healing potential of the IOM, various methods of reconstructing or repairing the forearm have been suggested. Although in the acute setting, radial head reconstruction or replacement and stabilization of the DRUJ may be sufficient to allow for healing of the soft tissues, management in the chronic setting is more difficult.
- Treatment options for chronic longitudinal radioulnar dissociation include one or more of the following components: addressing the ulnar impaction with ulnar shortening and or transfixion of the DRUJ, radial head arthroplasty to prevent further proximal migration, and/or reconstruction of the IOM with a variety of allograft, autograft, or synthetic materials. Although initial results of reconstruction with an allograft radial head replacement were promising, further investigations demonstrated less satisfactory and less durable results. The ultimate salvage is creation of a radioulnar synostosis or single-bone forearm.

is performed under image intensification at the elbow and wrist; more than 5 mm of proximal migration is indicative of forearm instability.

- Appropriate imaging, including lateral and posteroanterior (PA) grip views of the wrist with contralateral comparison films, is obtained, and consideration is given to magnetic resonance imaging or ultrasound to evaluate the interosseous membrane.

Surgical Anatomy

- The IOM complex is composed of several components: a membranous portion, a proximal interosseous band, and a consistently present and functionally important strong central band (Fig. 1). The latter is the functionally significant structural support that preserves longitudinal stability of the forearm.
  - Figure 2 is a schematic demonstrating the origin and insertion of the central band of the IOM. The ulnar origin is at the junction of the distal and middle thirds of the ulna, an average of 7.7 cm distal to the radial head. The radial insertion is 60% of the radial length from the radial styloid, about 13.7 cm from the olecranon tip. The fibers are oriented approximately 21° distal and ulnar to the axis of the forearm.

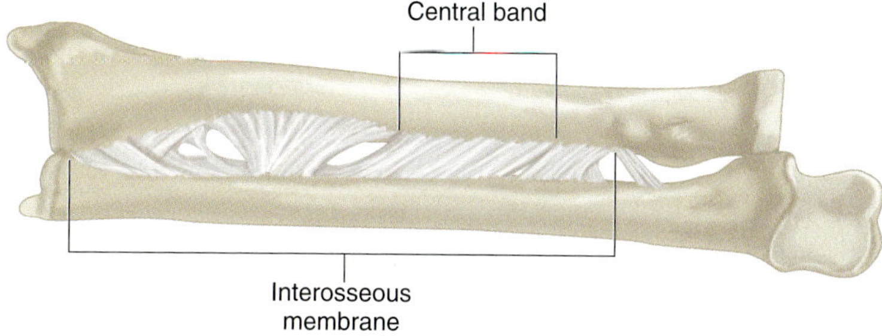

FIGURE 1

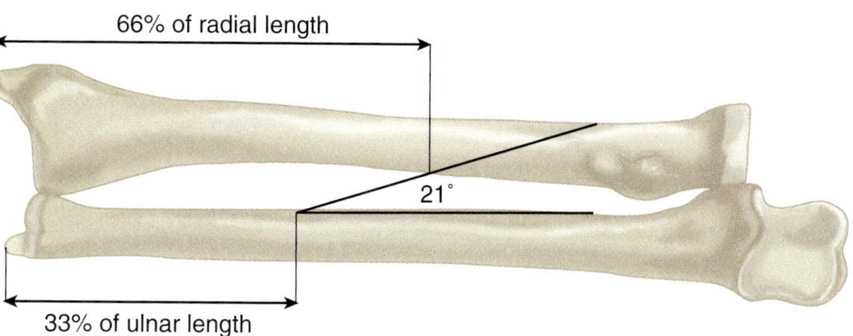

FIGURE 2

- The average width of the central band is 1.1 cm, and its thickness is approximately 1 mm (Chandler 2003; Hotchkiss et al., 1989; McGinley 2004; Marcotte and Osterman, 2007; Skaken et al., 1997).

- It has been suggested that the term *interosseous "membrane"* is a misnomer. This structure is a complex conglomerate of multiple parts; in particular, the important and functionally strong central band acts more like a ligament, and some have suggested it should be called the interosseous ligament and the interosseous membrane conglomerate should be termed the *interosseous ligament complex.* For clarity in this discussion, we will continue to refer to the *interosseous membrane.*
- Because the IOM is composed of organized collagen like other ligaments, it has little capacity to heal with structural integrity after injury, particularly in the setting of ongoing forearm instability (Marcotte and Osterman, 2007).

Equipment

- Wrist traction tower with four finger traps
- Radiolucent arm table
- Mini–C-arm

Controversies

- Some surgeons inflate the tourniquet at the start of wrist arthroscopy; however, the authors do not. In most cases, adequate visualization is possible, and synovitis is more apparent than when the tourniquet is inflated.

Positioning

- The patient is positioned supine with all bony prominences padded.
- A well-padded tourniquet is applied high upon the operative extremity
- If a bone–patellar tendon–bone autograft is to be used, the operative lower extremity is prepped from the thigh to the foot and draped in the usual fashion, and a sterile tourniquet is applied to the thigh.
- The prepped arm and hand are secured in a wrist traction tower with finger traps applied to each of the digits and suspended by 10–15 pounds of traction for wrist arthroscopy (Fig. 3).
- It is useful to have an armboard set up to support the arm and traction tower and for use after wrist arthroscopy for forearm reconstruction.

Portals/Exposures

- Diagnostic and therapeutic wrist arthroscopy proceeds with joint entry at the 3-4 portal. This portal is the one used for initial visualization and then later as a working portal.
  - A 6R portal is useful as a working and visualization portal.

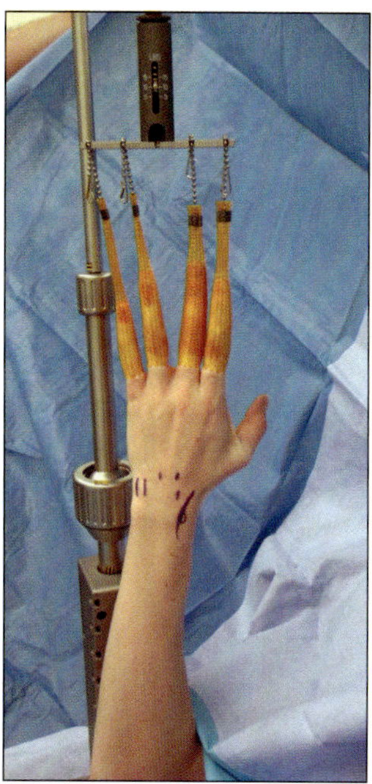

FIGURE 3

- The 6U portal is reserved for an outflow portal.
- Radial and ulnar midcarpal portals are used for midcarpal arthroscopy.

- A 10-cm incision over the ulnar border is used for ulnar shortening osteotomy.
- Incisions for forearm bone-ligament-bone reconstruction are included in the ulnar shortening osteotomy incision for the ulnar side (approximately 13.7 cm distal to the olecranon) and at approximately 7.7 cm distal to the radial head for the radial incision.
- The dorsal radial incision of approximately 5 cm is made between the brachioradialis and the extensor carpi radialis longus (ECRL) at the level of the pronator.
- The reconstruction parallels the normal fibers of the IOM central band and goes under the plane of the extensors.

Procedure

Step 1: Diagnostic and Therapeutic Arthroscopy

- Diagnostic wrist arthroscopy proceeds in the radiocarpal joint with assessment of the radial extrinsic ligaments, the scapholunate ligament, and the articular surfaces of the radius and carpus. Ulnarly, attention is turned to the TFCC and ulnar extrinsic ligaments, with assessment of the articular surfaces of the carpal bones and the lunotriquetral ligament.

- Introduction of air and fluid into the intended midcarpal portals with a syringe and 18-gauge needle is performed while visualizing the scapholunate and lunotriquetral ligaments to assess the competence of these interosseous ligaments.
- The midcarpal joint arthroscopy is approached next, and the integrity of the scapholunate and lunotriquetal interosseous ligaments is again assessed. The chondral surfaces are inspected, particularly at the capitohamate region, for evidence of ulnar impaction.
- In the radiocarpal joint, débridement of synovitis and either débridement or repair of the TFCC are performed.
- After diagnostic and therapeutic arthroscopy is completed, attention is turned to the ulnar shortening osteotomy.

Pitfalls

- *Care must be taken to identify and preserve the dorsal ulnar sensory nerve.*
- *Care must be taken to avoid injury to the ulnar neurovascular bundle.*

Step 2: Ulnar Shortening Osteotomy

- Ulnar shortening osteotomy is performed for treatment of ulnar impaction.
- The arm is exsanguinated and the tourniquet inflated to 250 mm Hg.
- A 10-cm incision is made over the distal ulnar border of the forearm through the interval between the flexor carpi ulnaris and the ECU (Fig. 4).
- Skin flaps are elevated, and bleeding is controlled with bipolar cautery.
- The bone is exposed subperiosteally, with care taken not to dissect the ECU from its sheath.

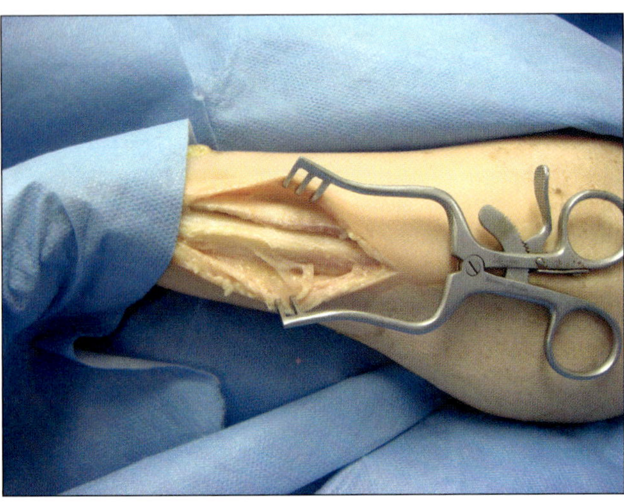

FIGURE 4

Controversies

- Either an allograft from the bone bank may be used or a bone–patellar tendon–bone autograft harvested. If an autograft is chosen, the operative leg is prepped from the thigh to the foot and draped in the usual fashion and a sterile tourniquet applied to the thigh. The tourniquet is inflated, and a midline incision is made to harvest a bone-ligament-bone central graft much as one would harvest for anterior cruciate ligament reconstruction. The wound is closed and, after the procedure is completed, a knee immobilizer is used postoperatively.

- The plate is chosen. A number of ulnar shortening plate systems are available; alternatively, a 6-hole 3.5-mm DCP plate is adequate.
- The osteotomy site is determined and marked.
  - It is preferable to make the osteotomy in an oblique fashion to increase the bone contact surface and promote healing.
  - It is helpful to longitudinally score the bone such that rotation is marked, facilitating restoration of normal alignment one the osteotomy is fixed and plated.
- Using the preoperative films (including those from the contralateral normal side) and preoperative plans, the amount of bone necessary to create 1–2 mm of ulnar negative variance is calculated.
- Either a commercial system allowing for a defined bone resection or the stacked blades technique can be used. The AO compression device is useful to compress the osteotomy site and to maintain alignment after the osteotomy is made.
- The osteotomy is made and the plate applied with compression across the osteotomy site.
- Image intensification is used to assess the appropriate amount of shortening to achieve slight ulnar variance and to check the alignment of the DRUJ.
- Bone wedges from the osteotomy site can be morselized and applied as bone graft.
- Assessment of pronation-supination and DRUJ stability is made, as well as assessing for TFCC click.

Step 3: IOM Reconstruction

- A Kelly clamp is passed from the distal ulna to proximal radius at approximately 21° of angulation to the shaft to replicate the fiber orientation of the central band (Fig. 5). Care must be taken to protect the posterior and anterior interosseous nerves.
- A proximal counter-incision of approximately 5 cm is made over the radius and then the Kelly clamp is passed beneath the radial wrist extensors to the interval between the brachioradialis (volar in Fig. 6) and the extensor carpi radialis longus (dorsal in Fig. 6), identifying and protecting the dorsal radial sensory nerve.
- With the nerves protected, the interval between the brachioradialis and the ECRL is exposed. Measurements are taken and a trough in the radius is made at the level of the pronator. The trough is designed such that the graft would fit into it.

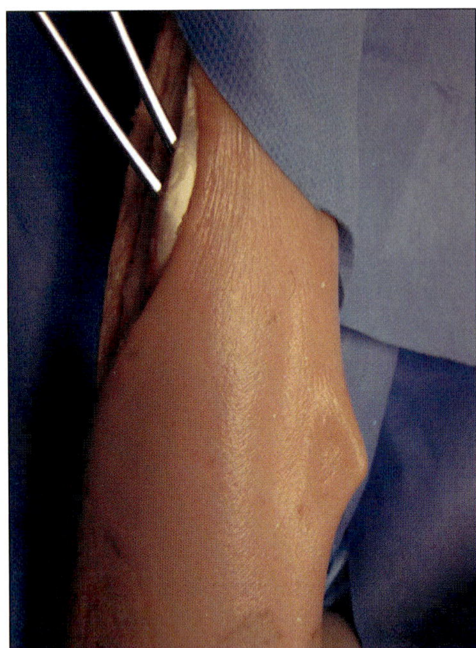

FIGURE 5

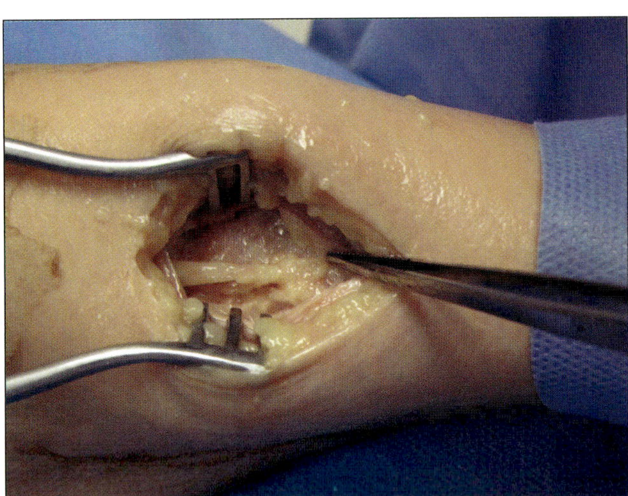

FIGURE 6

- A bone–patellar tendon–bone autograft is used in the reconstruction (Fig. 7).
  - The graft is secured to the ulna with an AO 3.5-mm screw and confirmed under image intensification.
  - The free end is then passed to the radial wound and the forearm is placed in semi-supination. The graft is tensioned maximally and the proximal radial graft is secured into its bony trough with an AO screw.
- Checking under image intensification, axial loading should indicate absence of axial instability of the radius.

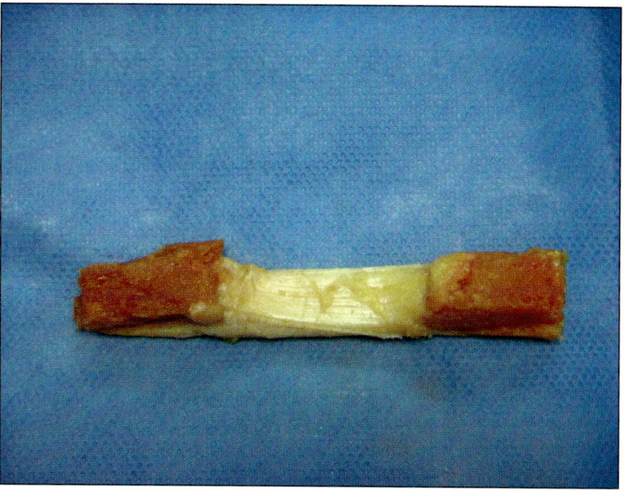

FIGURE 7

- The range of motion in the pronation and supination arc is assessed.
- The stability of the osteotomy, the DRUJ, and the screw length and stability of the IOM reconstruction are assessed.

STEP 4: CLOSURE

- The tourniquet is released and bleeding is controlled with bipolar cautery.
- The skin wounds are closed in layers, with a subcuticular closure of the radial and ulnar wounds with 4-0 Vicryl followed by a running Prolene suture. The arthroscopy portals are closed with 4-0 nylon sutures.
- Final radiographs are obtained, including PA, lateral, and oblique views of the forearm and of the wrist.
  - Figure 8A–C shows postoperative images demonstrating ulnar shortening osteotomy and reconstruction of the IOM with a bone–patellar tendon–bone allograft. This patient had undergone prior radial head arthroplasty which was unsuccessful in preventing radioulnar longitudinal instability and ulnar impaction.
- Sterile dressings are applied and a long-arm splint supporting the hand, wrist, and forearm is placed.

Postoperative Care and Expected Outcomes

- Patients are seen at 1 week postoperatively for removal of splint and sutures, and clinical examination. Routine radiographs are obtained of the forearm and wrist.

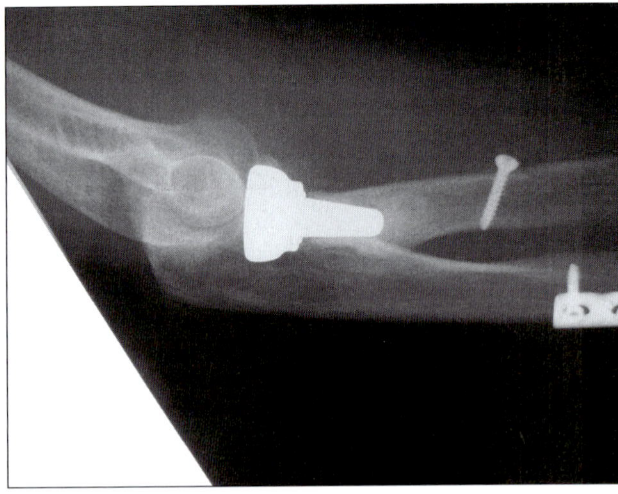
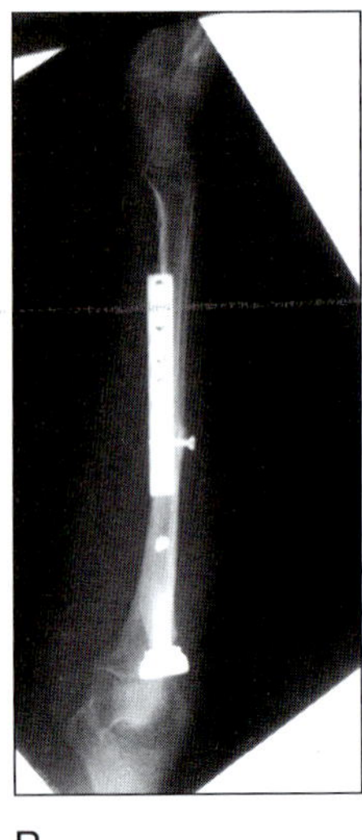
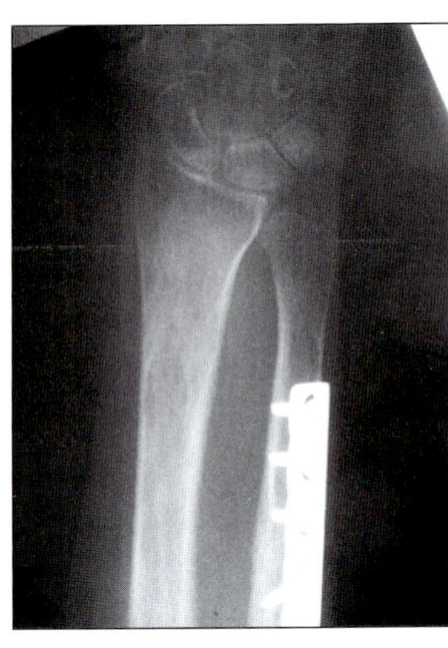

A B C

FIGURE 8

- The patient is either placed into a short-arm cast or then referred to physical/occupational therapy for application of a thermoplastic splint for immobilization purposes. Physiotherapy for digital mobilization and mobilization of the elbow in the flexion and extension arc is recommended. Supination and pronation are excluded.
- The patient is then seen at 4–5 weeks postoperatively for cast or splint removal, clinical examination, and radiographs. At this point, the patient is placed in a removable forearm splint and started on gentle therapy, including forearm rotation. Patients are sent to physical/occupational therapy to begin active range of motion, including forearm rotation. Eventually, weaning of the splint is allowed in order to improve forearm rotation.

Evidence

Because of the rarity of this injury complex, few evidence-based clinical trials exist; most reports document results in a series of patients or deal with biomechanical studies.

Essex-Lopresti P. Fractures of the radial head with distal radio-ulnar dislocation; report of two cases. J Bone Joint Surg [Br]. 1951;33:244-7.

This cases series by the author whose name is associated with this lesion described two patients with injury to the radial head, IOM, and DRUJ. Despite the many years that have passed since this was published, his recommendations hold true today for treatment of the acute Essex-Lopresti lesion: the radial head should be preserved by open reduction and internal fixation if possible; if this is not possible, radial head replacement is mandated. (Level IV evidence)

Chandler JW, Stabile KG, Pfaeffle HJ, Li ZM, et al. Anatomic parameters for planning of interosseous ligament reconstruction using computer-assisted techniques. J Hand Surg [Am]. 2003;28(1):111-16.

Hotchkiss RN, An KN, Sowa DT, Basta S, Weiland AJ. An anatomic and mechanical study of the interosseous membrane of the forearm: pathomechanics of proximal migration of the radius. J Hand Surg [Am]. 1989;14(2 Pt 1):256-61.

The authors investigated the relative contributions to longitudinal stiffness of the forearm after radial head excision in a cadaveric model. They found that the IOM was responsible for 71% of longitudinal stiffness of the forearm. In contrast, sectioning of the TFCC only resulted in a loss of 8% of the stiffness of the forearm; incising the TFCC and IOM proximal to the central band decreased stiffness by 11%. (Level III evidence)

Marcotte AL, Osterman AL. Longitudinal radioulnar dissociation: identification and treatment of acute and chronic injuries. Hand Clin. 2007;23:195-208.

This review article documented the senior author's approach to diagnosis and treatment for acute and chronic radioulnar longitudinal instability. In addition, a review of the senior author's experience with 16 chronic cases treated with patellar bone-ligament-bone graft reconstruction of the IOM was presented. Twenty-five percent of patients complained of knee aches with weather changes, but 94% stated that wrist discomfort had improved, and grip strength improved 31% from pre- to postoperative values. Elbow discomfort was improved, and ulnar variance was altered from preoperative +3 mm to postoperative −2 mm, which was preserved as an average of −1.5 mm at final follow-up. There was no recurrent instability. The authors recommended use of an allograft to avoid the high rate of knee discomfort. (Level IV evidence)

McGinley JC, Roach N, Gaughan JP, Kozin SH. Forearm interosseous membrane imaging and anatomy. Skeletal Radiol. 2004;33(10):561-8. Epub 2004 Aug 25.

Pfaeffle HJ, Stabile KJ, Li ZM, Tomaino MM. Reconstruction of the interosseous ligament restores normal forearm compressive load transfer in cadavers. J Hand Surg [Am]. 2005;30:319-25.

The authors investigated the effect of reconstruction of the IOM with a single or double flexor carpi radialis (FCR) graft when the radial head was intact. The native IOM central band insertions were marked and transosseous tunnels were used to attach the FCR graft with #2 suture, which was then tied to a 2.7-mm cortical screw post at the (distal) radial attachment. After pre-tensioning, the graft was then secured in a similar fashion to the (proximal) ulnar insertion. Reconstruction using a double but not single FCR graft resulted in normalization of forearm force transmission in this cadaveric model. (Level III evidence)

Poitevin LA. Anatomy and biomechanics of the interosseous membrane: its importance in the longitudinal stability of the forearm. Hand Clin. 2001;17:97-110.

The author found that reconstruction of the central band of the IOM was sufficient to restore longitudinal stability of the forearm in a case report of one patient. Transfer of the extensor indicis proprius (EIP) to the proximal radius in conjunction with primary repair of the IOM in the acute setting was proposed. The membrane was repaired with #1 PDS sutures, and the EIP was harvested just proximal to the metacarpal phalange and rerouted to the radius in a proximal oblique direction and attached under maximal tension to the radius through bony tunnels, replicating the central band's orientation. The author noted good results and stability at 2 months' follow-up, but thereafter the patient was lost to follow-up. (Level III evidence)

Ruch DS, Chang DS, Koman LA. Reconstruction of longitudinal stability of the forearm after disruption of interosseous ligament and radial head excision (Essex-Lopresti lesion). J South Orthop Assoc. 1999;8:47-52.

This paper described IOM reconstruction with a patellar bone-ligament-bone complex in a late case in which silicone arthroplasty of the radial head had failed. The Silastic radial head was removed and replaced with a metallic prosthesis, and the IOM was reconstructed with a bone–patellar tendon–bone autograft and secured with 3.5-mm cortical screws at either end. Distally, a TFCC tear was repaired and a screw was placed through the DRUJ for 3 months. Postoperatively, longitudinal stability was restored and range of motion was near full, lacking only 5° short of full extension and 20° short of full supination. (Level IV evidence)

Sellman DC, Seitz WH Jr, Postak PD, Greenwald AS. Reconstructive strategies for radioulnar dissociation: a biomechanical study. J Orthop Trauma. 1995;9:516-22.

This paper described a procedure for reconstruction of the central band of the IOM with a braided polyester cord placed at the anatomic location of the central band. Biomechanical testing in cadavers with simulated longitudinal compression demonstrated that stiffness was restored to 94% of the normal intact membrane. Radial head replacement alone with use of a silicone prosthesis was ineffective; however, the replacement with a metallic implant restored 89% of stiffness. Use of a metallic radial head in conjunction with membrane reconstruction restored stiffness to 145% of the normal value. (Level III evidence)

Skahen JR 3rd, Palmer AK, Werner FW, Fortino MD. Reconstruction of the interosseous membrane of the forearm in cadavers. J Hand Surg [Am]. 1997;22:986-94.

The authors described reconstruction of the IOM with an FCR graft in the setting of radial head excision in a cadaver model; this reduced proximal radial migration but did not completely restore forearm stability. (Level III evidence)

Trousdale RT, Amadio PC, Cooney WP, Morrey BF. Radio-ulnar dissociation. A review of twenty cases. J Bone Joint Surg [Am]. 1992;74:1486-97.

This series described treatment results in acutely recognized and unrecognized cases of radioulnar dissociation. Results of appropriate treatment when the injury is recognized early are good in 80% of cases; however, 80% of those patients who go unrecognized acutely fail treatment. (Level III evidence)

PROCEDURE 60

Ulnar Collateral Ligament Reconstruction Using the Modified Jobe Technique

Benton A. Emblom, James R. Andrews, and Leonard C. Macrina

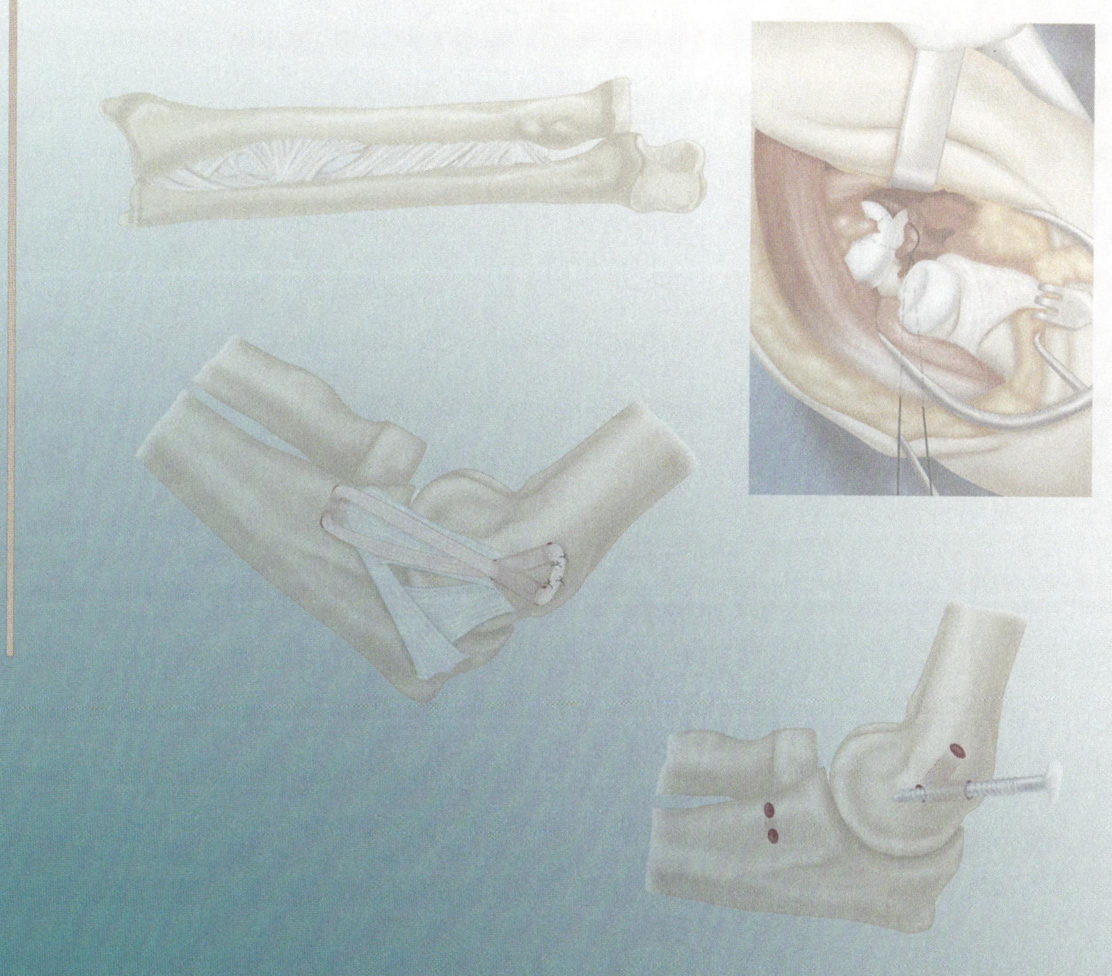

PITFALLS

- *Medial elbow pain at times other than overhead throwing or valgus stress.*
- *No desire to continue overhead athletics, particularly pitching, gymnastics, javelin throwing, wrestling, tennis, or sports that place increased repetitive stress on the medial side of the elbow.*
- *Failure to undergo a trial of active rest and focused rehabilitation. However, in some cases of complete disruption, acute reconstruction is indicated.*

Controversies

- UCL reconstruction in unproven athletes (i.e., high school level)
- Baseball players other than those at the pitching or catcher position

Indications

- Medial elbow instability due to injury to the anterior band of the ulnar collateral ligament (UCL) in high-level overhead athletes who desire to continue competition at their current or higher level of performance.

Examination/Imaging

- A standard elbow examination should be performed, including carrying angle assessment, range of motion in all planes, and motor and sensory evaluation. A UCL examination should include palpation (medial epicondyle, sublime tubercle, and midsubstance), moving valgus stress test (O'Driscoll et al., 2005), the milking maneuver, and the seated, supine, and prone valgus stress test.
- Signs of valgus extension overload should be noted, including reproducible posteromedial pain with valgus and forced passive extension, posteromedial impingement, and tenderness over the olecranon associated with olecranon stress fractures.
- An ulnar nerve examination should be conducted to rule out an associated neurapraxia or a subluxating ulnar nerve.
- Lateral compression testing should be done to evaluate for chondromalacia of the radiocapitellar joint or osteochondritis dissecans of the capitellum in younger patients.
- The presence of a palmaris longus tendon can be tested by opposing the thumb while actively flexing the wrist (Fig. 1).
- A thorough shoulder examination should also be performed in order to detect any associated or contributing pathology, particularly internal rotation contracture or glenohumeral internal rotation deficit.
- Conventional radiography
    - Anteroposterior, lateral, obliques, and axial views should be obtained.
    - Radiographs should be evaluated for ossification within the UCL (Fig. 2), avulsion fractures of the sublime tubercle (Fig. 3), posteromedial olecranon osteophytes (Fig. 4), and loose bodies.
- Stress radiography
    - Comparison valgus stress views can be used to measure side-to-side difference; a difference of greater than 2 mm is considered significant (Fig. 5).

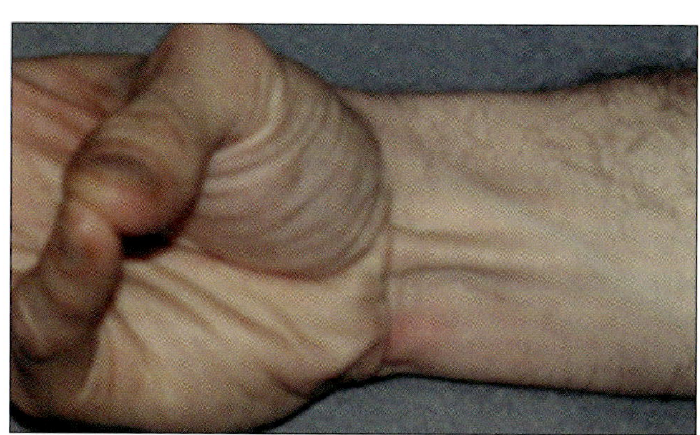

FIGURE 1

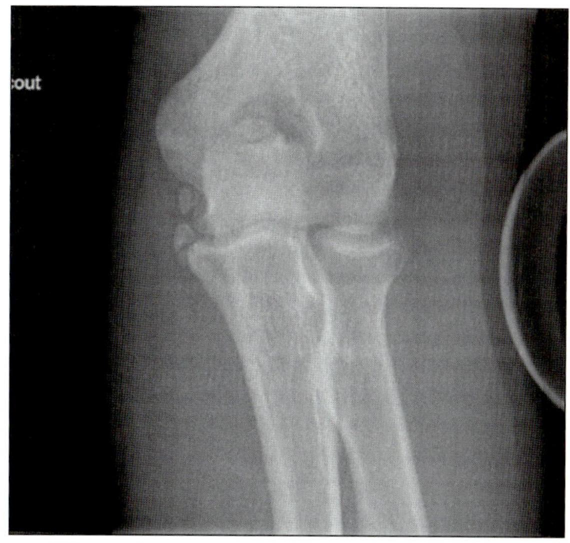

FIGURE 2

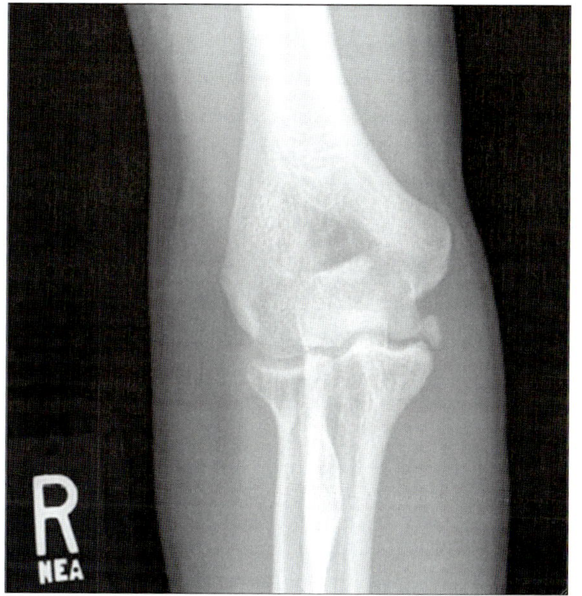

FIGURE 3

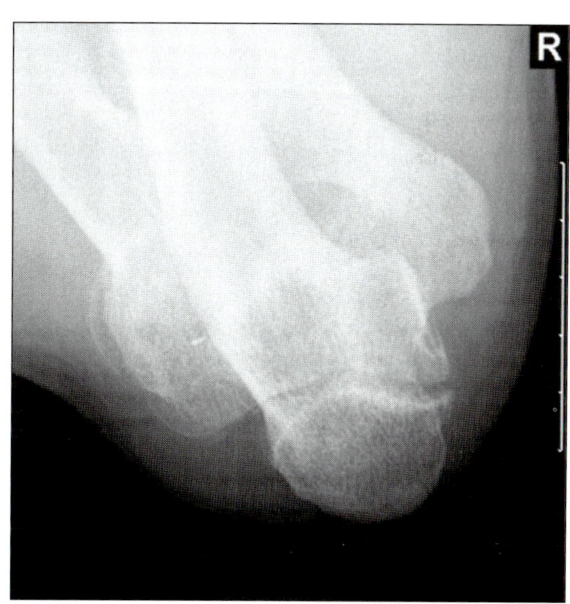

FIGURE 4

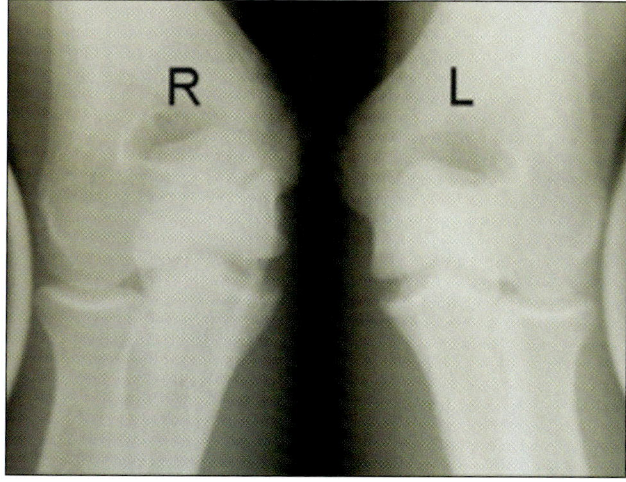

FIGURE 5

Treatment Options

- Nonoperative treatment will sometimes allow athletes with partial ruptures to return to play, but results are less predictable than those with reconstruction in athletes with complete ruptures (Rettig et al., 2001).
- Surgical reconstruction techniques
  - Modified Jobe (described here)
  - Docking technique (Rohrbough et al., 2002)
  - DANE TJ technique (Dines et al., 2007)
  - Interference screw

- Magnetic resonance imaging (MRI) arthrography
  - Intra-articular contrast (gadolinium or saline) has been advocated (Timmerman et al., 1994). However, noncontrast has been shown to be effective as well (Potter, 2000). We do utilize intra-articular contrast.
    - The contrast-enhanced coronal MRI in Figure 6A shows the "t-sign" associated with a distal UCL tear.
    - The contrast-enhanced coronal MRI in Figure 6B shows a proximal tear of the UCL.
  - The coronal sections are most appropriate for visualizing the UCL.
- Diagnostic elbow arthroscopy
  - Diagnostic arthroscopy can be utilized in conjunction with the arthroscopic valgus test (Field and Altchek, 1996) to visualize the laxity of the anterior band of the UCL. While visualized from the anterolateral portal, 1–2 mm of ulnohumeral opening is considered significant. We do not currently perform diagnostic arthroscopy on all elbows undergoing UCL reconstruction unless the diagnosis is in doubt.
  - In addition to diagnostic purposes, associated conditions such as posteromedial osteophytes or loose bodies can be addressed concurrently.

Surgical Anatomy

- The UCL's proximal attachment is a broad footprint over the inferior and medial surface of the medial epicondyle. The anterior band's distal attachment is the sublime tubercle of the ulna. The posterior band's distal attachment is the medial margin of the semilunar notch of the ulna (Fig. 7).
- The flexor-pronator mass includes the pronator teres, flexor carpi radialis, palmaris longus, flexor digitorum superficialis (FDS), and flexor carpi ulnaris (FCU) (Fig. 8).
  - The humeral head of the FCU originates from the medial epicondyle immediately superficial and superomedial to the UCL.
  - A portion of the FDS originates from the anterior band of the UCL. The most medial aspect of the origin on the anterior band is demarcated by a raphe. This raphe is the medial margin of the anterior band of the UCL (Fig. 9).

Pearls

- *Prep in the hand in order to prevent breaching sterility when harvesting the palmaris longus graft (see Fig. 10).*
- *Be sure to drape as high as possible in order to get adequate exposure for a complete ulnar nerve decompression and transposition.*
- *We utilize Ioban draping when performing ligament reconstruction and when we anticipate being in or around a joint.*

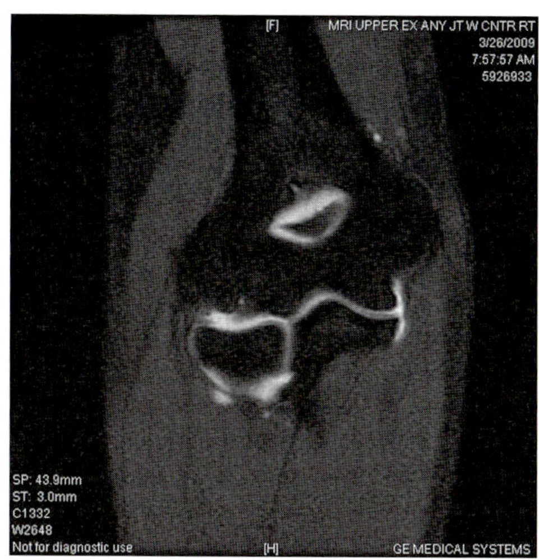

A

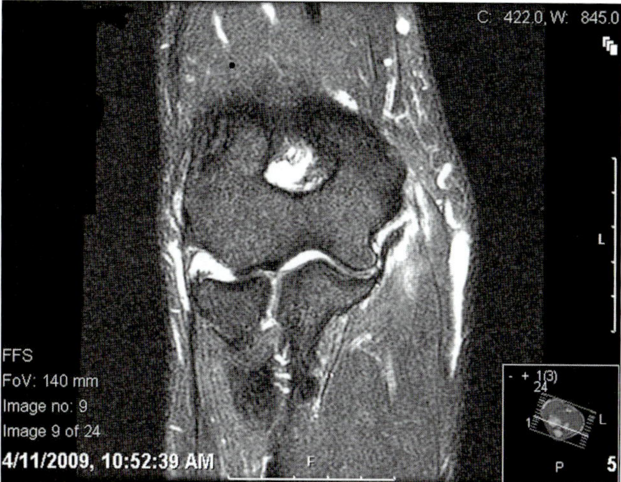

B

FIGURE 6

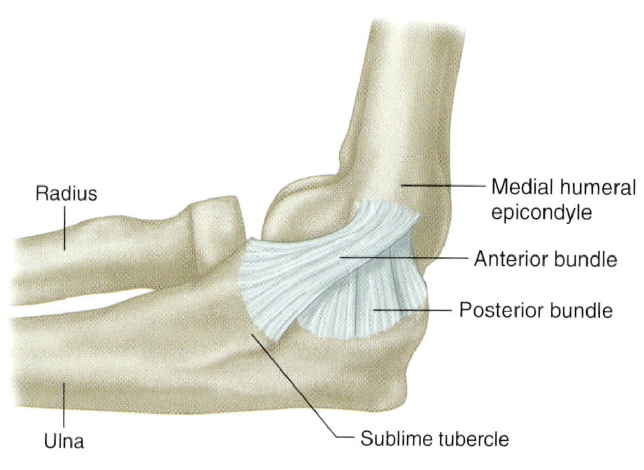

FIGURE 7

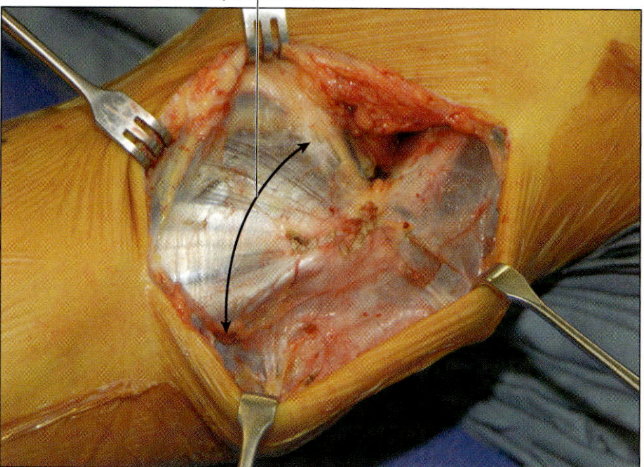

FIGURE 8

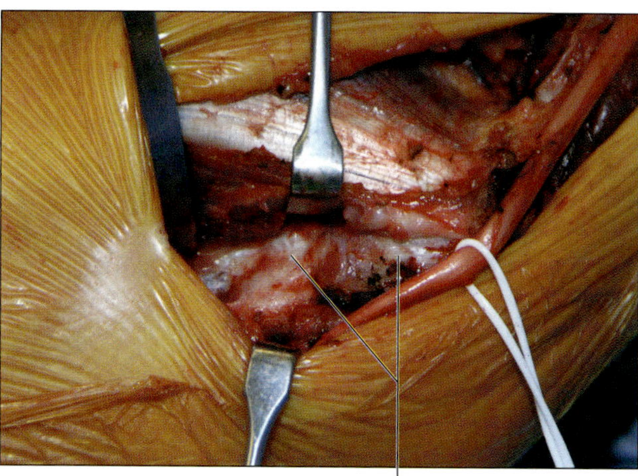

FIGURE 9

Pearls

- *The ulnar nerve must be adequately decompressed and released proximally and distally to prevent secondary compression.*
- *This dissection is done by first identifying the sublime tubercle attachment of the ligament and proceeding from distal to proximal up to the ligament's attachment on the medial epicondyle.*
- *The anterior band of the UCL flares anteriorly and medially as it attaches to the medial epicondyle. Angling the knife blade toward the ceiling when moving proximally (during elevation of the FDS from the capsule) helps prevent violating the anterior band.*

Pitfalls

- *Overzealous retraction (primarily distally) can injure the ulnar nerve.*
- *Be careful not to dissect the FDS and associated flexor-pronator mass too anteriorly off of the capsule and subsequently off of the medial epicondyle.*
- *Avoid dissection posterior to the medial epicondyle. This can lead to excessive bleeding, postoperative hematoma, and subsequent posteromedial calcification and extension block.*

Positioning

- The patient is positioned supine with an arm table utilized on the operative side (Fig. 10).
- A nonsterile arm tourniquet is placed high on the arm and set at 250 mm Hg.

Portals/Exposures

- A 6-cm longitudinal incision is made from the medial epicondyle to just below the sublime tubercle, and a 3- to 4-cm limb is made proximal to the medial epicondyle.
  - Care is taken to preserve the medial antebrachial cutaneous nerve.
- The ulnar nerve is identified and released in order to facilitate an anterior subcutaneous transposition. In our approach, the nerve is transposed to facilitate exposure of the UCL from distal to proximal underneath the flexor muscle mass.
  - A slip of medial intermuscular septum is taken down in order to eliminate contact compression on the transposed ulnar nerve and also to function as a stabilization sling for the transposition.
  - The small veins intimately associated with the ulnar nerve should be cauterized with an electrocautery device to prevent postoperative bleeding.
- The two heads of the FCU are split bluntly with a small elevator, and the ulnar attachment of the FCU is elevated off the sublime tubercle with a key elevator, exposing the distal attachment of the anterior band of the UCL.
- The FDS is sharply elevated off the capsule, up to the medial epicondyle (Fig. 11). Care is taken not to release any tendinous origin of the flexor-pronator mass.
- The anterior band is incised longitudinally approximately 2 mm anterolateral to the raphe from the sublime tubercle to the medial epicondyle (Fig. 12). The substance of the anterior band can be inspected as well as the underlying ulnohumeral joint.

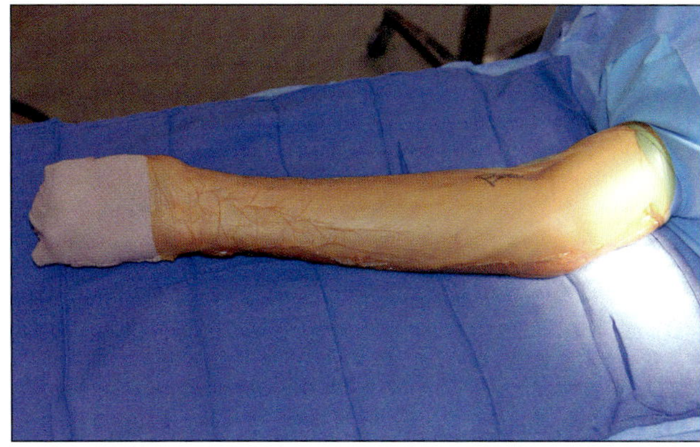

FIGURE 10

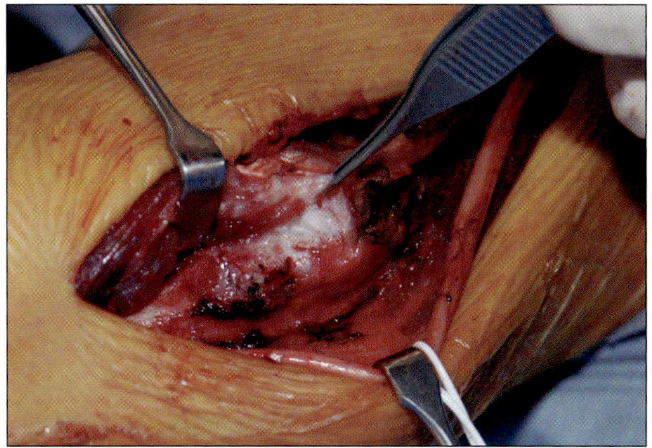

FIGURE 11

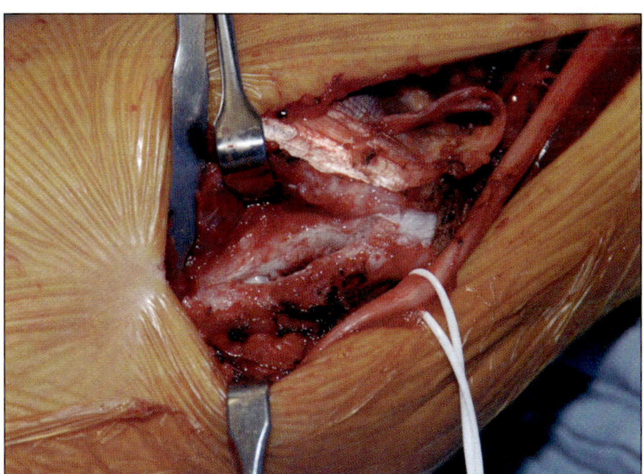

FIGURE 12

Procedure

Step 1

- Harvesting the graft is performed once the decision to reconstruct the UCL has been made.
- The ipsilateral palmaris longus tendon is identified preoperatively (see Fig. 1). If the patient does not have a palmaris longus (10–20%), we typically utilize the contralateral gracilis tendon.
- Two distal, transverse 1-cm incisions are made over the palmaris longus tendon, approximately 2 cm apart, one at the level of the middle wrist flexion crease and the other at the proximal wrist flexion crease. The tendon is carefully identified and elevated with the use of two small hemostats (Fig. 13).
- The most distal extent of the tendon is sharply incised and released. The tendon is then flipped out of the proximal of the two incisions. A #0 Ticron suture is then placed in a limited Krackow fashion in the distal end of the tendon.
- Tension is placed on the tendon and the myotendinous junction is palpated. This is typically at the junction of the proximal and middle one third of the forearm. A 1-cm transverse incision is then made at this level. The fascia is incised and the tendon identified.
- The tendon is then pulled out through the wound (Fig. 14) and amputated at the myotendinous junction. This end of the tendon is stripped of any residual muscle and prepared like the distal end.
- The fascia and skin are then closed.

Pearls

- *Placing the graft in a saline-soaked lap sponge prevents drying out during the procedure.*

Pitfalls

- *At least 13 cm of tendon is needed in order to adequately pass the graft.*
- *If the palmaris tendon is too short, the gracilis is then used.*

Controversies

- Some prefer utilizing a tendon harvester, limiting the incisions to two.

Step 2

- The ulnar tunnel is created.
  - The sublime tubercle is again identified on the proximal ulna.
  - A 3.6-mm drill bit is used to create two holes, approximately 5 mm off the joint line, immediately anterior and posterior to the sublime tubercle, and leaving a bone bridge of approximately 1.5 cm (Fig. 15).
  - Curved curettes (size 0 and 1) are then sequentially used to connect the holes and create a continuous curved tunnel.
- A manually curved Hewson suture passer is used to pass the graft through the ulnar tunnel.
- The distal two thirds of the incised UCL is reapproximated with a #0 Ticron suture (Fig. 16).

Pearls

- *Curved curettes allow straight drill paths to be converted into a curved tunnel.*
- *The native UCL is not reapproximated until after the drilling of the ulnar tunnel in order to facilitate visualization of the ulnohumeral joint.*

Pitfalls

- *Excessive retraction during preparation of the ulnar tunnel can damage the ulnar nerve.*
- *Utilizing a soft tissue protector also protects the ulnar nerve and any soft tissue in close proximity.*

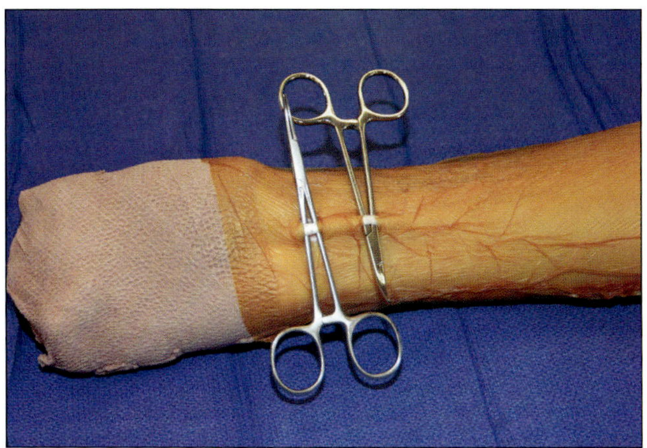
FIGURE 13

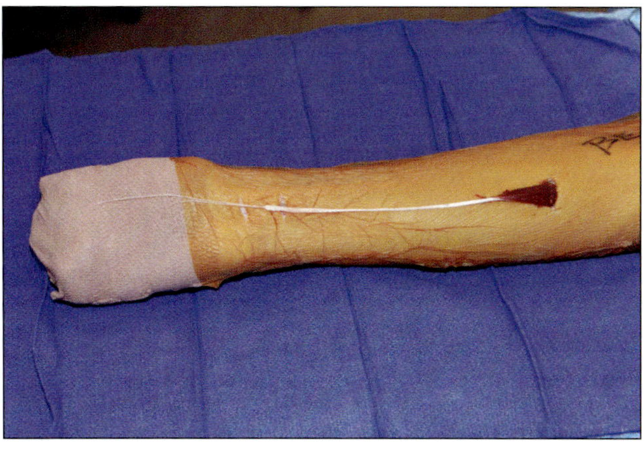
FIGURE 14

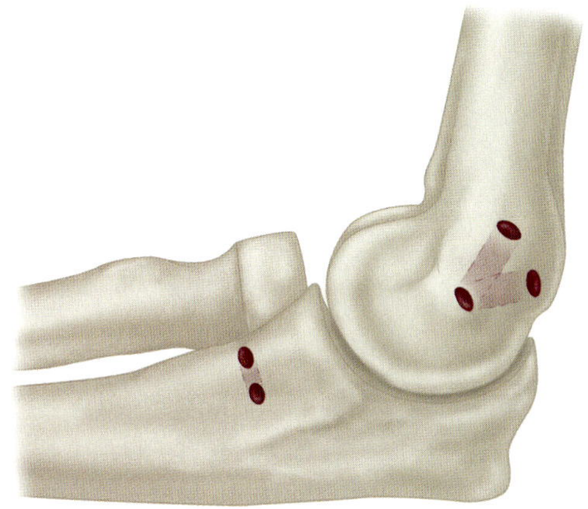
FIGURE 15

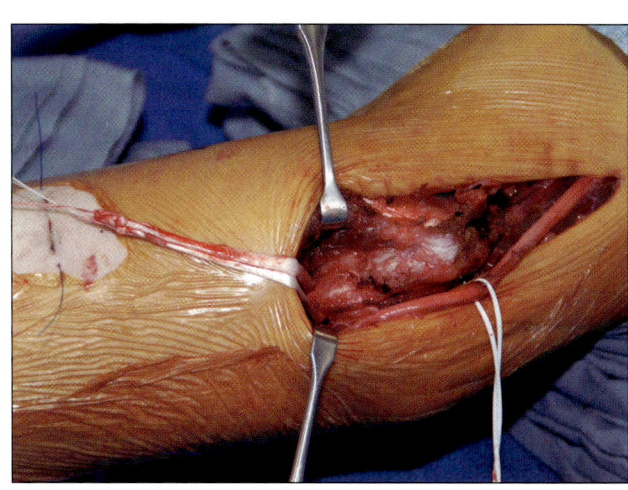
FIGURE 16

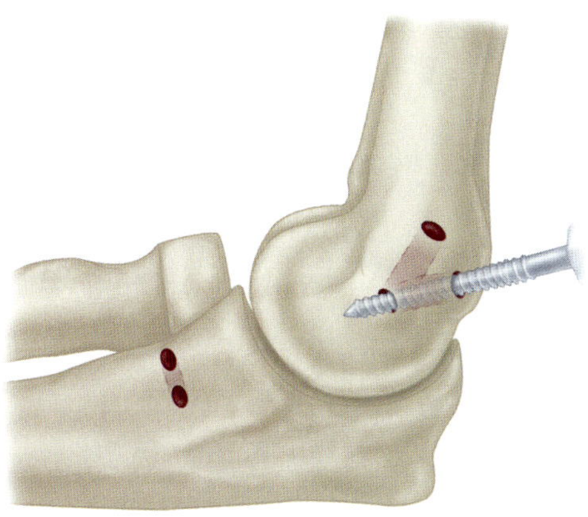
FIGURE 17

Step 3

- The humeral tunnels are created.
  - The center of the proximal UCL attachment is identified through the incised anterior band.
  - A 3.6-mm drill bit is directed retrograde from the proximal attachment, parallel to the humerus, up to the cortex at the junction of the medial epicondyle and the medial supracondylar ridge.
  - A size 0 straight curette is inserted into the tunnel.
  - The drill is then brought antegrade from the junction of the medial epicondyle and medial supracondylar ridge. It is advanced until it makes contact with the aforementioned curette.
  - The drill is then placed approximately 1.5 cm down the epicondyle distally and directed toward the original tunnel. This creates a Y-shaped tunnel in the humerus (Fig. 17; see also Fig. 15).
  - Straight curettes are then used sequentially to clear the path in the tunnels and to remove any residual debris.

Instrumentation/ Implantation

- When using a palmaris graft, a 3.6-mm drill bit is used, followed by size 0 and 1 curettes.
- When using a gracilis graft, a 4.0-mm drill bit is used, followed by size 1 and 2 curettes.
- The Hewson suture passer is curved to match the curve of a small towel clip.

Pearls

- *The most proximal aspect of the native UCL was not reapproximated in order to facilitate appropriate tunnel placement.*
- *The second arm of the humeral tunnel is placed slightly posteromedial on the epicondyle.*
- *If passing the graft is difficult, mineral oil can be used to facilitate easier passage.*

Pitfalls

- *If the initial arm of the humeral tunnel is drilled in one pass retrograde, the ulnar nerve can be inadvertently wrapped up in the drill bit.*
- *Be careful not to place the initial arm of the humeral tunnel too medially. This can limit the bone bridge between it and the second arm.*

Instrumentation/ Implantation

- When using a palmaris graft, a 3.6-mm drill bit is used, followed by size 0 and 1 curettes.
- When using a gracilis graft, a 4.0-mm drill bit is used, followed by size 1 and 2 curettes.

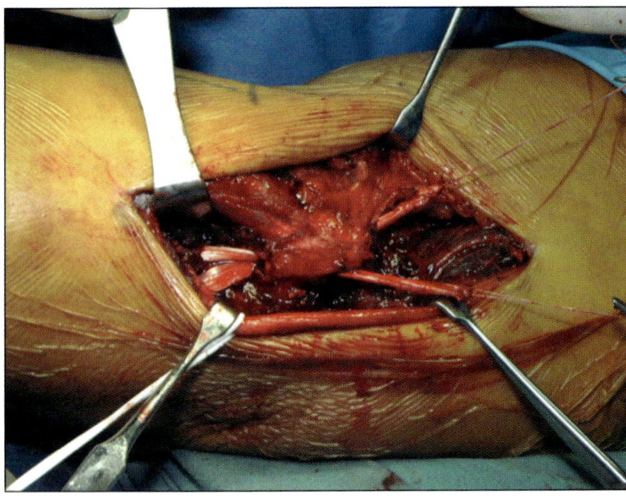

FIGURE 18

- Bulb irrigation is then utilized to clear any small bone chips from the tunnel and wound.
- A Hewson suture passer is used to pass the graft in a figure-of-8 fashion into the humerus (Fig. 18).

Step 4

- The graft is tensioned and secured.
  - The elbow is placed in 30° of flexion and a stack of towels is placed under the wrist to offset any resting valgus load.
  - Hemostats are clamped to each end of the graft (Fig. 19).
  - With tension applied to each end, a #0 Ticron suture is used to stitch the graft to itself in a simple side-to-side fashion over the back of the medial epicondyle (Fig. 20A and 20B). This is repeated five to six times. The excess is then cut sharply.
- The two arms of the graft traversing the ulnohumeral joint are also sewn to each other with a #0 Ticron suture (Fig. 21). This is repeated five to six times also.

Step 5

- The fasciotomy of the FCU is stabilized with a #0 Vicryl stitch.
- The cubital tunnel is closed down with two or three simple stitches of #0 Vicryl.
- The ulnar nerve is secured anteriorly and subcutaneously utilizing the medial intermuscular septum sling. Two stitches of 3-0 Ticron are used to secure the sling to the flexor-pronator fascia (Fig. 22).
- The wound is irrigated copiously and the tourniquet is released. All bleeding should be controlled.

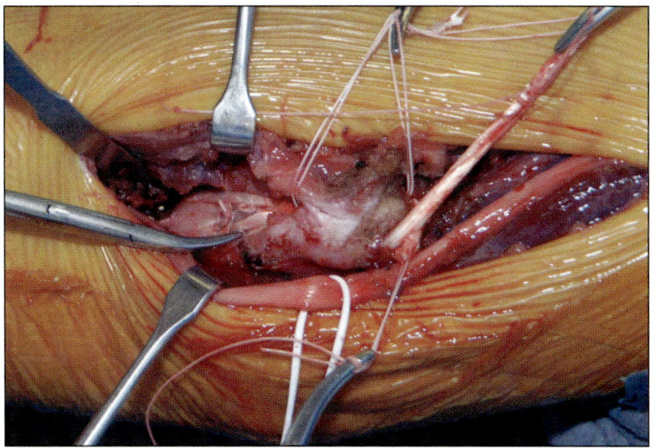

FIGURE 19

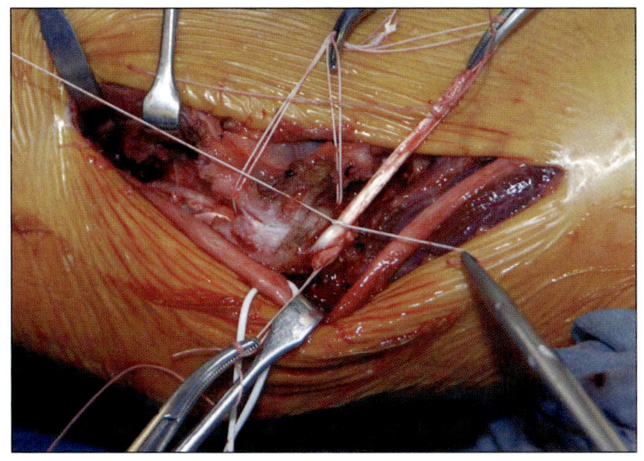

A

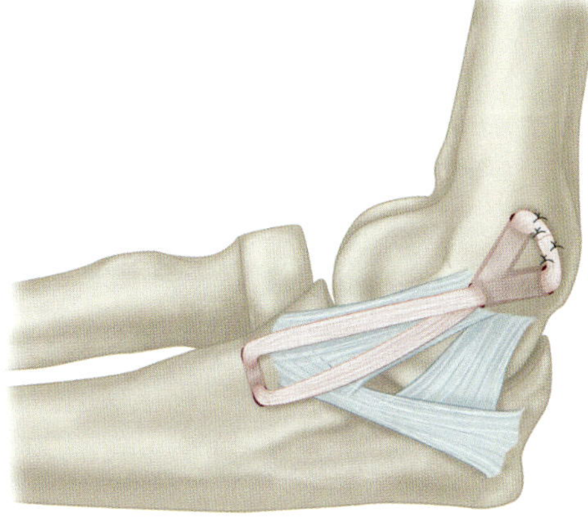

B

FIGURE 20

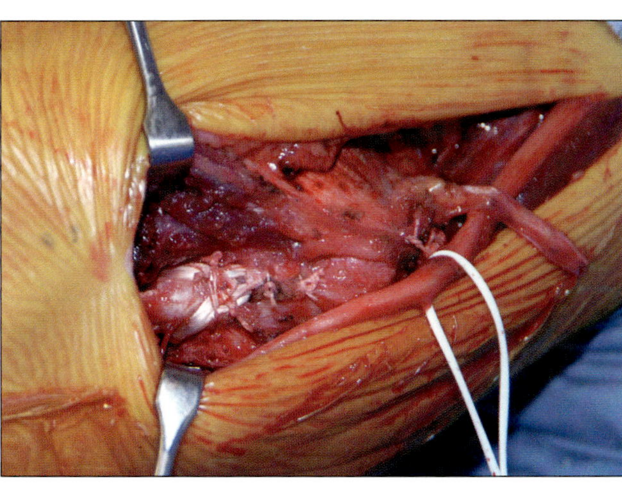

FIGURE 21

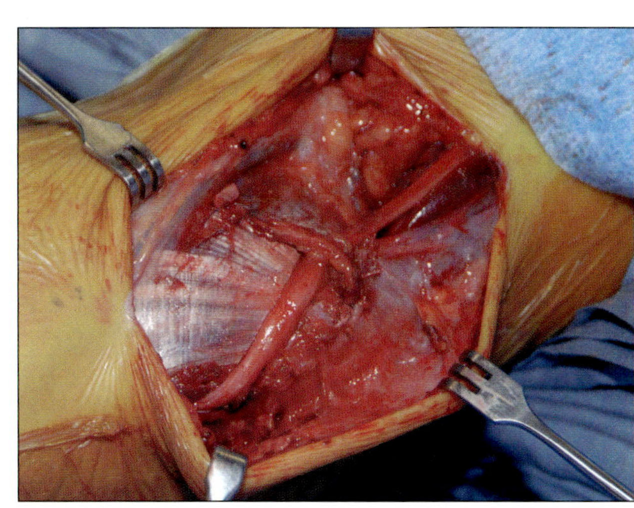

FIGURE 22

- A medium Hemovac drain is placed in the wound and the fascia, subcutaneous layer, and skin are closed in standard fashion.
- The arm is splinted in 75–90° of elbow flexion and neutral forearm rotation.

PITFALLS

- *Avoid valgus stress to the elbow during initial rotator cuff and weight-training exercises for the first 6 weeks.*
- *Obtain early passive extension to prevent flexion contracture and long-term range of motion restrictions.*
- *If a gracilis graft is used, allow 4–6 weeks before initiating hamstring stretching and strengthening to prevent irritation of the hamstring muscle belly.*

Postoperative Care and Expected Outcomes

- The postoperative splint is removed 5–7 days after surgery and a hinged elbow brace is applied, with active motion allowed from 30° to 100°. Hand and wrist strengthening are started once the splint is removed.
- The brace settings should be increased weekly to allow full motion by 5 weeks. Flexion is increased 10° per week and extension by 5° per week. In more stable cases with secure graft fixation, a more rapid increase in range of motion to normal in 2–3 weeks is recommended.
- Shoulder conditioning exercises begin at the third week.
- Elbow flexion and extension strengthening begins during the fifth week with the elbow at the side.
- Shoulder and elbow strengthening is progressed at the 6-week point with the initiation of the Thrower's 10 program. This is continually progressed throughout the rehabilitation process.
- Plyometric and sport-specific training follows strengthening during weeks 10–16. An interval hitting program can be started at 12 weeks.
- An interval throwing program begins around week 16 after successful completion of the previous phases of rehabilitation. A 6- to 8-week progressive long toss program precedes an interval mound program.
- Athletes should anticipate return to sport in 9–12 months after their reconstruction.
- A recent report by Cain et al. (2009) showed 84% return to previous or higher level of play after UCL reconstruction. This includes 1288 patients, 743 of whom had minimum 2-year follow-up.

Evidence

Azar FM, Andrews JR, Wilk KE, et al. Operative treatment of ulnar collateral ligament injuries of the elbow in athletes. Am J Sports Med. 2000;28:16-23.

This study was a retrospective review of 91 UCL reconstructions by the senior author. Follow-up averaged just under 3 years, and outcome was judged based on return to play. (Level IV evidence [case series])

Cain EL, Andrews JR, Wilk KE, et al. Ulnar collateral ligament reconstruction of the elbow in 1281 patients: results with minimum 2 year follow-up. Am J Sports Med. 2009, Submitted.

This study was a retrospective review of 1281 UCL reconstructions by the senior author. Minimum follow-up was 2 years, and outcome was judged based on return to play. (Level IV evidence [case series])

Conway JE, Jobe FW, Glousman RE, Pink M. Medial instability of the elbow in throwing athletes: treatment by repair or reconstruction of the ulnar collateral ligament. J Bone Joint Surg [Am]. 1992;74:67-83.

This study reported results of repair and reconstruction of the UCL in 68 patients with average follow-up of over 6 years. (Level IV evidence [case series])

Field LD, Altchek DW. Evaluation of the arthroscopic valgus instability test of the elbow. Am J Sports Med. 1996;24:177-81.

This laboratory study evaluated the optimal positioning of the elbow during arthroscopic evaluation and detailed the arthroscopic instability test of the elbow.

Dines JS, ElAttrache NS, Conway JE, et al. Clinical outcomes of the DANE TJ technique to treat ulnar collateral ligament insufficiency of the elbow. Am J Sports Med. 2007;35:2039-44.

This study was a prospective analysis of 22 patients with UCL insufficiency treated with the DANE TJ technique for UCL reconstruction. Average follow-up of 36 months and outcomes were classified using the modified Conway scale. The data compared favorably with other published techniques and supported the use of this technique for revision cases and those with sublime tubercle insufficiency.

O'Driscoll SW, Lawton RL, Smith AM. The "moving valgus stress test" for medial collateral ligament tears of the elbow. Am J Sports Med. 2005;33:231-9.

This study presented a correlation between the moving valgus stress test and surgical findings. (Level II evidence [cohort study])

Potter HG. Imaging of post-traumatic and soft tissue dysfunction of the elbow. Clin Orthop Relat Res. 2000;(370):9-18.

This paper presented a diagnostic imaging algorithm for the injured elbow. (Level V evidence [expert opinion])

Rettig AC, Sherrill C, Snead DS, Mendler JC, Mieling P. Non-operative treatment of ulnar collateral ligament injuries in throwing athletes. Am J Sports Med. 2001;29: 15-7.

This study reported on patients with UCL insufficiency treated nonoperatively. They were followed for a minimum of 3 months with conservative treatment. Determination of return to play was then evaluated. (Level IV evidence [case series])

Rohrbough JT, Altchek DW, Hyman J, et al. Medial collateral ligament reconstruction of the elbow using the docking technique. Am J Sports Med. 2002;30:541-8.

This study was a retrospective review of 36 patients undergoing UCL reconstruction with the docking technique. Average follow-up was 3.3 years and outcome was based on return to play. (Level IV evidence [case series])

Timmerman LA, Schwartz ML, Andrews JR. Preoperative evaluation of the ulnar collateral ligament by magnetic resonance imaging and computed tomography arthrography: evaluation in 25 baseball players with surgical confirmation. Am J Sports Med. 1994;22:26-31.

This study reported MRI and computed tomography accuracy in evaluating the UCL compared to surgical findings ("gold standard"). (Level II evidence)

PROCEDURE 61

Lateral Ulnar Collateral Ligament Reconstruction

Robert J. Schoderbek, Jr., Steven W. Meisterling, and James R. Andrews

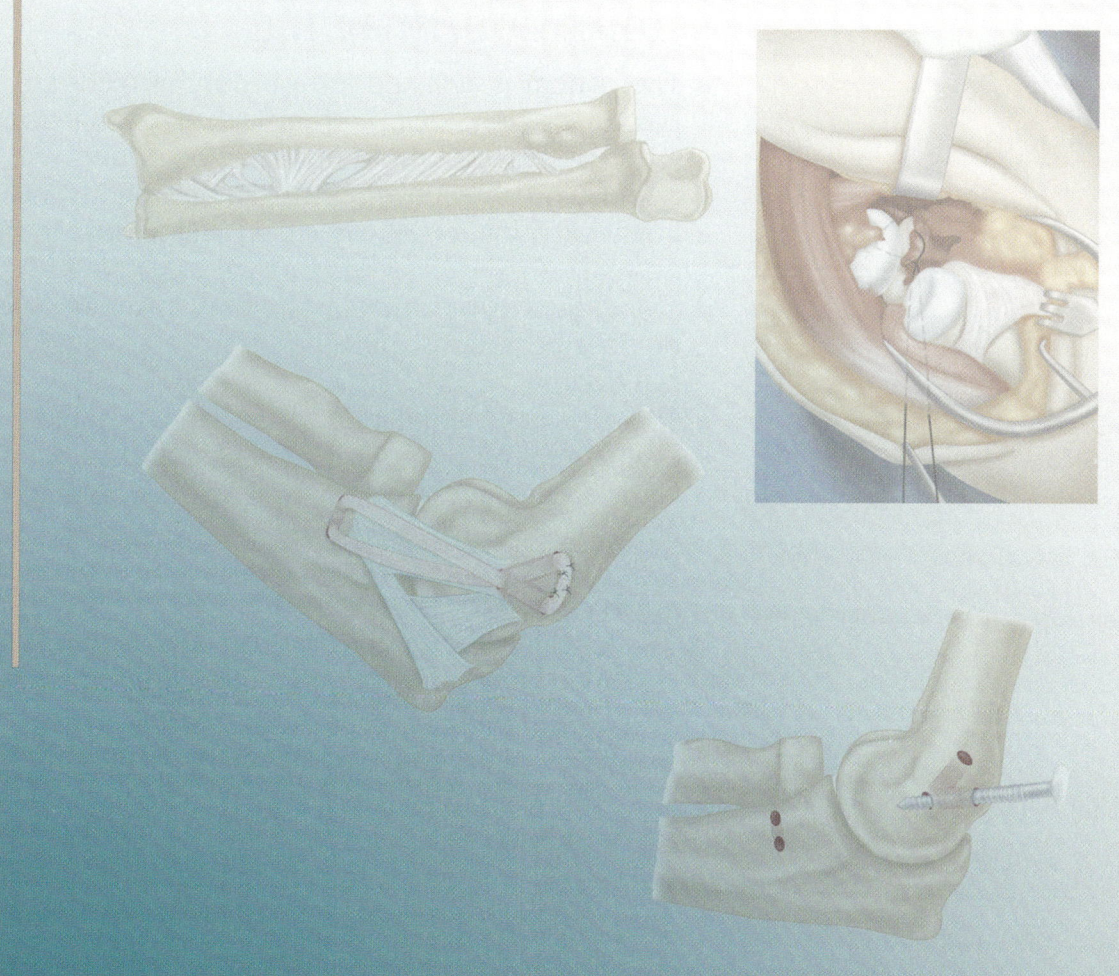

PITFALLS

- *Relative contraindications include children with open physes, generalized ligamentous laxity, concomitant arthritis of the elbow joint, voluntary recurrent dislocations, and ongoing infection.*

Indications

- Symptomatic recurrent posterolateral subluxation of the radioulnar joint in a patient with a history of a dislocation that was treated by closed reduction or reduced spontaneously, indicating an injury to the lateral ulnar collateral ligament (LUCL).
- Failure of the lateral collateral ligament complex to adequately heal in its anatomic position after a dislocation or recurrent subluxation of the elbow, resulting in posterolateral rotatory instability (PLRI).

Examination/Imaging

- The patient is assessed for a history of recurrent painful clicking, snapping, or locking of the elbow with the expression of apprehension about performing activities that precipitate the instability.
- Initial examination of the elbow will appear to be normal.
- The patient will complain of elbow instability when doing a push-up or pushing off from a seated position.
- The physical examination of the elbow should evaluate range of motion, strength, and stability with varus and valgus stress, as well as the presence or absence of PLRI.
  - Posterolateral rotatory instability test (Fig. 1A and 1B)
    - A "clunk" or shift will occur with testing.
    - Reproduction of the patient's symptoms along with apprehension is a positive result.

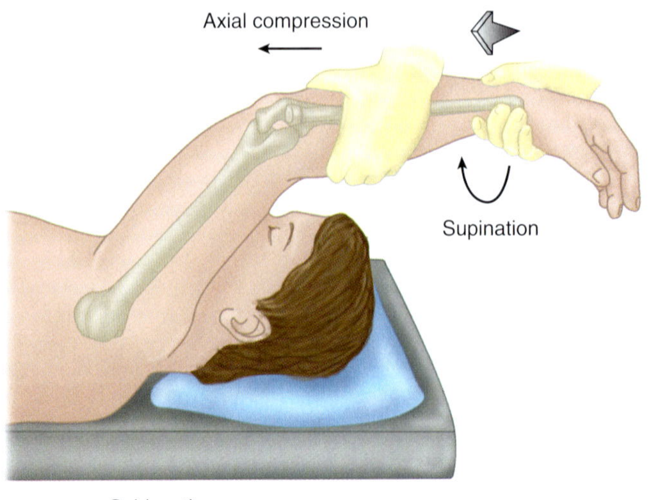

A

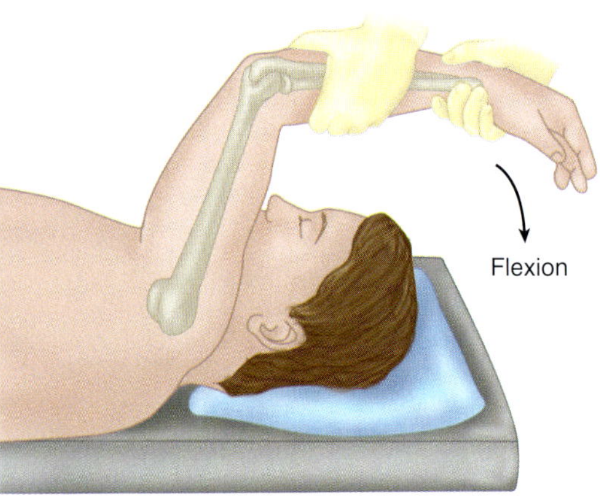

B

FIGURE 1

Treatment Options

- Acute initial subluxation or dislocation events are treated conservatively with a splint or brace, making sure to stabilize the forearm in a pronated position, which reduces the posterolateral subluxation and allows the lateral collateral ligament complex to heal. Progressive rehabilitation is performed.
- Primary surgical repair may provide appropriate restoration of the lateral collateral ligament complex and prevent chronic instability.
- Chronic injuries with associated recurrent instability usually do not respond well to conservative measures and quite often require reconstruction of the LUCL.
- Other techniques exist for operative treatment in addition to the modified O'Driscoll technique that is described here.

        - There may only be a positive test when the patient is under anesthesia.
    - Posterolateral drawer test
    - Prone push-up test
    - Armchair push-up test
- Plain radiographs
    - Anteroposterior, lateral, internal and external oblique, and axial views should be obtained to evaluate for
        - Subtle subluxation with ulnohumeral joint space widening
        - Impaction defect in the posterolateral capitellum from a radial head dislocation (Hills-Sach lesion of the elbow)
- Stress radiographs can demonstrate radial head subluxation and ulnohumeral joint widening.
- Fluoroscopic evaluation
    - Posterolateral rotatory instability test with local anesthetic infiltration into the joint or under conscious sedation
    - Stressed fluoroscopic radiographic evaluation
- Magnetic resonance imaging
    - Contrast imaging has been advocated.
    - Thin-cut pulse sequences should be obtained to evaluate for lateral collateral ligament complex injury.
- Elbow arthroscopy is used to evaluate the stability of the elbow.
    - If physical examination is not conclusive, arthroscopy is a useful adjunct to assess the level of instability. Arthroscopy also allows for identification and débridement of associated osteochondral injuries to the capitellum or radial head.
    - The arthroscopic PLRI test and stress testing are performed by viewing the lateral elbow in the lateral or posterior portal. Subluxation of the radial head or lateral joint widening with stress testing is indicative of instability.
    - The arthroscopic valgus stress test is also performed by viewing the medial elbow from the lateral portal and applying a valgus stress to the elbow. Opening of the medial joint line more than 1–2 mm is indicative of medial instability and indicates the need for reconstruction of both the LUCL and the ulnar collateral ligament.

Surgical Anatomy

- The lateral collateral ligament complex consist of four components (Fig. 2):
  - Lateral (radial) collateral ligament
    - Originates from the lateral epicondyle and fans out to merge with the annular ligament.
    - Functions as a varus restraint and stabilizes the annular ligament.
  - Lateral ulnar collateral ligament
    - Is a thickening of the capsule that originates from the isometric point of the lateral epicondyle and attaches distally to the tubercle of the supinator crest of the ulna.
    - Is the primary lateral stabilizer of the ulnohumeral joint and acts as a posterior buttress for the radial head to prevent subluxation associate with PLRI.
  - Accessory lateral collateral ligament
    - Blends proximally with the fibers of the annular ligament and is attached to the tubercle of the supinator crest.
    - Stabilizes the annular ligament during varus stress.
  - Annular ligament
    - Attaches to the anterior and posterior margins of the sigmoid notch, stabilizing the radial head.
- The mobile wad and extensor musculature attach to the lateral supracondylar ridge and the lateral epicondyle.
  - The mobile wad consists of the brachioradialis, extensor carpi radialis longus, and extensor carpi radialis brevis and attaches to the lateral supracondylar ridge and superior portion of the lateral epicondyle.
  - The extensor musculature consists of the extensor digitorum communis, extensor indicis, extensor digiti minimi, extensor carpi ulnaris (ECU), and anconeus muscles and attaches to the lateral epicondyle.
- The Kocher interval is an internervous plane that exists between the anconeus muscle and the ECU that allows exposure of the lateral collateral ligament complex with minimal muscle damage and avoidance of an osteotomy (Fig. 3).
  - The anconeus muscle lies posterior to the interval and is innervated by a branch of the radial nerve.
  - The ECU lies anterior to the interval and is innervated by the posterior interosseous nerve.

Pearls

- *Elbow arthroscopy is utilized to assist with the diagnosis of PLRI if clinical examination and examination under anesthesia are not conclusive.*
- *It is important to allow for free range of motion of the injured upper extremity to perform arthroscopic PLRI testing and stress testing. These tests cannot be performed appropriately if the extremity is stabilized in a positioning device.*
- *Regardless of the type of upper extremity hand table used, proper positioning and centering of the elbow on the table is essential for comfort and ease of the procedure.*

Pitfalls

- *Performing arthroscopy without the extremity stabilized in a positioning device can be cumbersome at times and requires a surgical assistant to perform the procedure.*
- *It is important to recognize that, with supine positioning, the shoulder is internally rotated, resulting in varus stress on the elbow. This varus stress must be corrected during the final stages of reconstruction.*

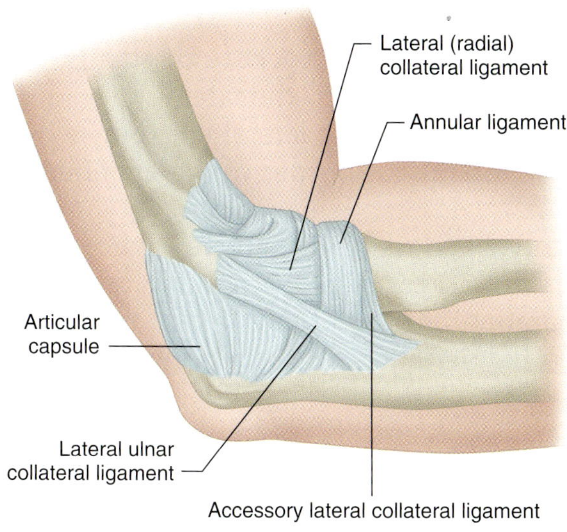

FIGURE 2

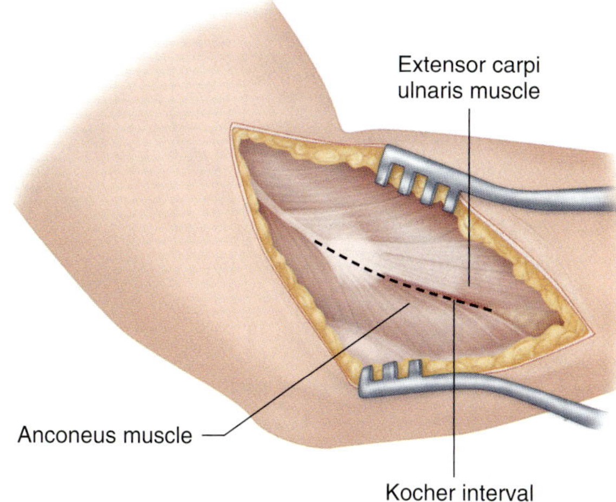

FIGURE 3

Positioning

- Examination under anesthesia is performed first for confirmation of a positive PLRI test.
- The patient is placed in the supine position with the affected extremity placed on the upper extremity hand table.
  - Secure the upper extremity hand table to the operating room table prior to the arthroscopic portion of the procedure.
- A sterile tourniquet is preferred.
- The important arm structures are labeled and the surgical incisions, including the arthroscopic portals, are marked (Fig. 4).
- Arthroscopy is performed if needed to assist with the diagnosis of PLRI, with the patient supine and the upper extremity held in place by a surgical assistant.
- After arthroscopy is completed, the arm is positioned on the upper extremity hand table for open ligament reconstruction.

Equipment

- There are many types of upper extremity hand tables on the market to assist with surgical treatment of upper extremity injuries. Be sure to utilize a table that provides the most comfort and stability for both elbow arthroscopy and open elbow reconstruction.

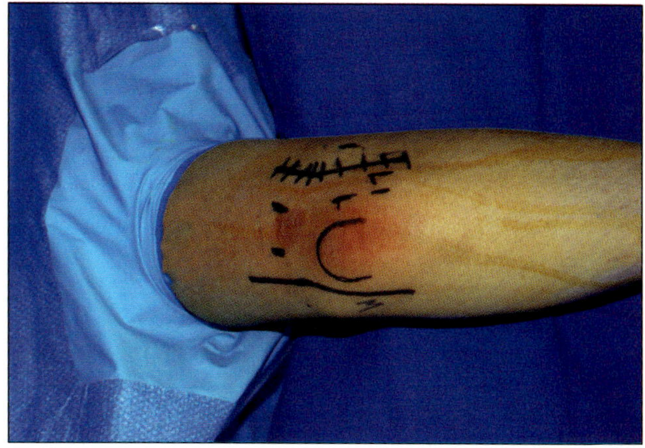

FIGURE 4

Pearls

- *It is very important to preserve the LUCL remnant and the anterior capsule while elevating the ECU and common extensor tendon anteriorly. By starting the dissection distally and using a Freer elevator rather than a knife during the dissection, injury to the lateral collateral ligament complex can be avoided.*
- *The PLRI test can be performed after exposure of the LUCL to assess stability and capsular deficiency.*

Pitfalls

- *Aggressive exposure of the lateral collateral ligament complex can result in damage to important anatomic structures and poor tissue quality for repair or reconstruction.*

Portals/Exposures

- An 8- to 10-cm posterolateral (Kocher) incision is made starting 3 cm proximal to the lateral epicondyle, extending over the lateral epicondyle and then along the anterior border of the anconeus distally (Fig. 5).
- The Kocher interval is developed between the anconeus and the ECU by identifying a thin fat strip or distinct separation between the different muscle planes that can be identified through the overlying fascia (Fig. 6).
- The proximal anconeus and the distal triceps are reflected from the lateral supracondylar ridge and lateral epicondyle to improve the exposure.
- The ECU is elevated off of the annular ligament and the common extensor tendon is elevated off the anterior aspect of the lateral epicondyle to expose the lateral collateral ligament complex.
- The LUCL is then inspected and assessed for tissue quality and stability to determine if a primary repair can be performed or ligamentous graft reconstruction is indicated (Fig. 7).

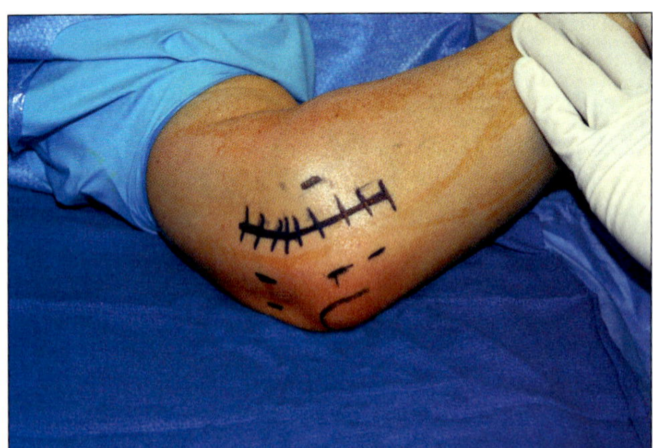

FIGURE 5

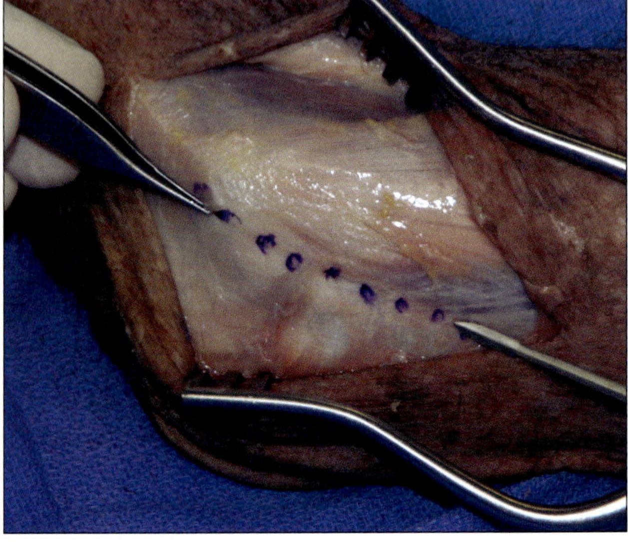

FIGURE 6

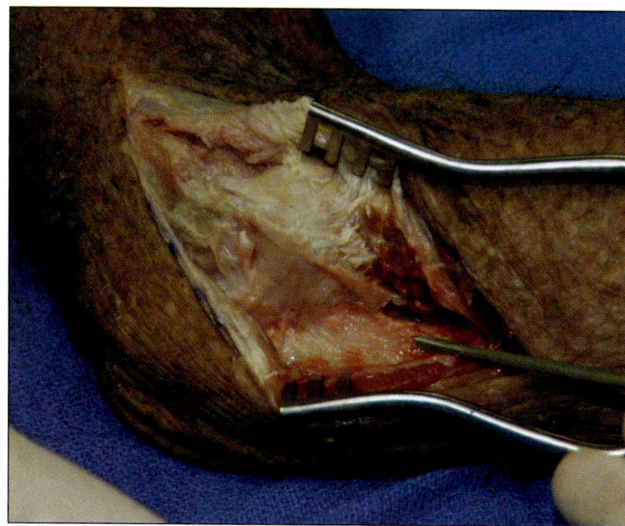

FIGURE 7

Procedure

Step 1

- Primary repair of the lateral collateral ligament complex should be performed if adequate-quality tissue is available for repair, especially if avulsed from the lateral epicondyle.
- Repair of the lateral collateral ligament complex can be achieved by performing the transosseous suture technique or suture anchor placement at the anatomic origin of the LUCL in the inferior posterior portion of the lateral epicondyle.
  - Nonabsorbable sutures are passed using a locked running stitch technique placed down the ligament remnant and back up the contralateral side and tied to itself to secure the injured ligament (Fig. 8).
- The forearm is splinted in pronation with the elbow flexed in 70–90° of flexion for 7–10 days, followed by gentle range of motion in a hinged elbow brace and progressive rehabilitation.

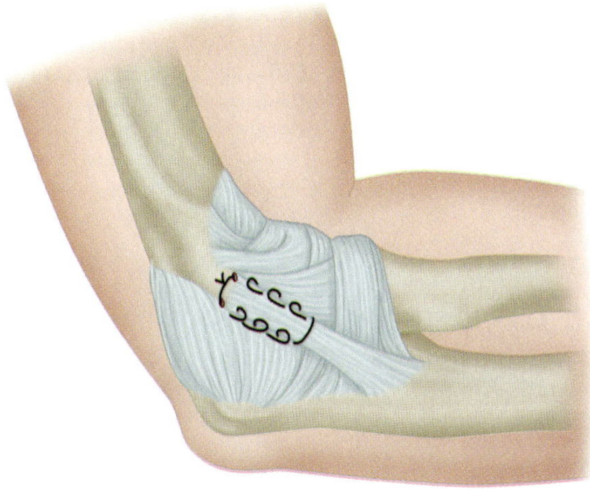

FIGURE 8

Pearls

- *The transosseous suture technique utilizes two drill holes placed in the midportion of the lateral epicondyle at the origin of the LUCL.*
- *Suture anchor placement for repair of the LUCL occurs at the midportion of the lateral epicondyle at the origin of the LUCL.*
- *Anterior and posterior capsular plication can also be performed to help provide some addition stabilization of the lateral collateral ligament complex.*
- *It is important to splint the elbow in a position of pronation and valgus stress because it reduces the lateral joint structures and prevents the stress of posterolateral subluxation.*

Pitfalls

- *Make sure that the transosseous drill holes are separated by at least 1 cm to avoid tunnel breakage.*

Instrumentation/ Implantation

- A 2.0-mm drill should be used to drill the transosseous holes.

Pearls

- *There are numerous graft sources, including the palmaris longus, gracilis hamstring, toe extensors, and perhaps an allograft.*
- *The required length of the graft is approximately 17–20 cm. It is imperative that the palmaris longus graft is excised as proximal and distal as possible to obtain the maximum length of graft (Fig. 12).*

Step 2

- Harvesting of the graft is done after exposure of the lateral collateral ligament complex and determination that reconstruction of the LUCL is necessary due to deficient tissue.
- Preoperative identification of an ipsilateral palmaris longus tendon is performed to ensure that it is present. If the tendon is not present, contralateral gracilis hamstring can be utilized.
- The palmaris longus tendon is harvested using the pull-through technique (Fig. 9).
  - Three 1-cm transverse incisions are made along the course of the palmaris longus tendon to assist with harvest. The initial incision is made 1 cm proximal to the proximal wrist crease, a second incision is made 3 cm proximal to the initial incision, and a third incision is made at the muscle-tendon junction approximately 12 cm proximal to the second incision.
  - The tendon is first identified in the two distal-most incisions and separated from the underlying soft tissue. Curved mosquito hemostats are used to deliver the tendon from the incisions. The wrist is flexed and the tendon is tenotomized as distal as possible. The tendon is then pulled out the second incision and a locking whipstitch is placed in the distal end using a 1-0 nonabsorbable suture to assist with graft passage (Fig. 10).
  - The tendon is then identified in the third incision and separated from the surrounding soft tissue. The tendon is then delivered through the proximal incision. The connecting muscle is then elevated off the tendon with a #15 blade, and the tendon is transected as proximal as possible (Fig. 11).

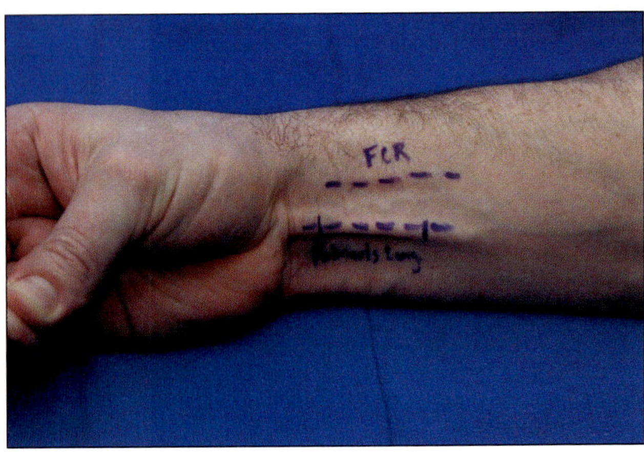

FIGURE 9

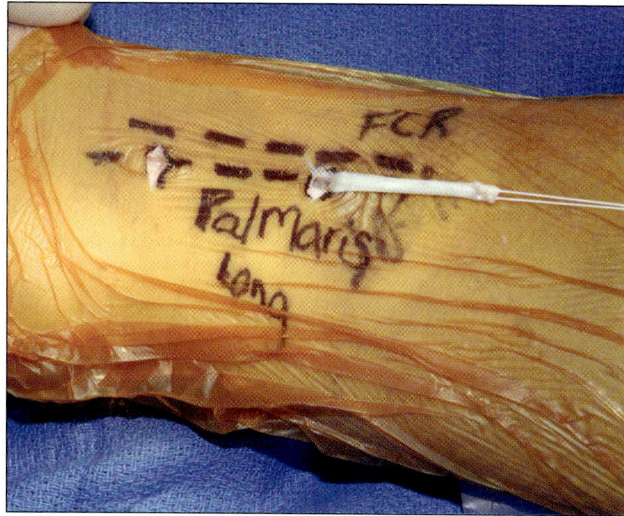

FIGURE 10

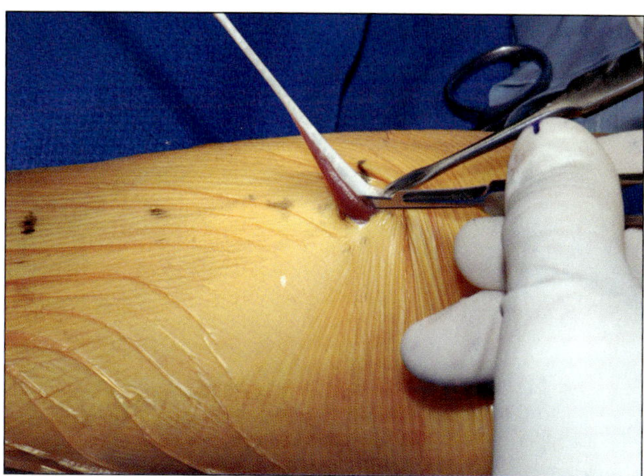

FIGURE 11

- The graft is prepared by stripping the residual muscle from the tendon and placing another locking stitch at the proximal end of the graft.
- The graft is then wrapped in a moist sponge and placed securely in the center of the instrument table until needed for the reconstruction.

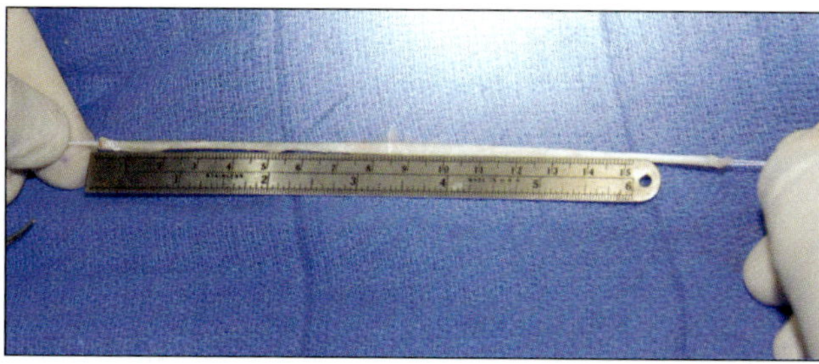

FIGURE 12

Controversies

- The palmaris longus tendon can also be harvested using a tendon-stripping technique described in Procedure 62.

Pearls

- *To lessen the likelihood of rupture of the osseous cortical tunnel roof, make sure that an adequate bone bridge of at least 1–1.5 cm is maintained when drilling both sets of tunnels. Do not be too aggressive with the curettes when trying to enlarge the tunnels for graft passage.*
- *Make sure that the convergent drill holes in the lateral epicondyle are separated by at least 1.5 cm to avoid tunnel failure.*
- *Meticulous identification of the isometric point in the lateral epicondyle is needed to provide stability with the reconstruction.*
- *When identifying the isometric point of the lateral epicondyle, make sure that the two suture strands are tight symmetrically, especially in extension, because PLRI primarily tends to occur in when the elbow is being brought from a flexed to an extended position.*
- *Err more anterior than posterior when identifying the distal isometric drill hole, and enlarge the drill hole in the anterior and proximal direction to ensure that the graft is tight in extension.*

Pitfalls

- *Aggressive enlargement of the tunnels and poor placement of the drill holes may result in tunnel fracture and therefore graft failure.*
- *Persistent instability can often be attributed to a posteriorly placed tunnel in the humerus, causing the graft to be lax in extension.*

Step 3

- The ulnar tunnels are created with a 3.6-mm drill.
  - The first drill hole is angled medially, posteriorly, and proximally and is made at the tubercle of the supinator crest of the ulna just distal to the lateral attachment of the capsule. A curved hemostat is then placed in this drill hole to identify the trajectory of the initial drilling.
  - The second drill hole is placed 1–1.5 cm posterior and proximal to the initial drill hole such that the connecting tunnel is perpendicular to the axis of the LUCL (Fig. 13). The drill bit is angled in a manner so that the drill comes into contact with the hemostat, indicating that the drill holes connect.
  - Two curved curettes are used to connect the drill holes and slightly enlarge the tunnel.
- A Hewson suture passer is then used to pass a free stitch and a looped stitch through the tunnel drilled in the tubercle of the supinator crest (Fig. 14).
- The free suture is connected with a hemostat to help identify the isometric attachment of the lateral collateral ligament complex on the lateral epicondyle (Fig. 15).
  - The hemostat is placed on the lateral epicondyle and the elbow is flexed and extended to identify the isometric point.
  - This point should correspond with the center of the capitellum on a lateral radiograph.
- The lateral epicondyle tunnels are created with a 3.6-mm drill.
  - The distal hole is placed at the isometric point, angling the drill medially and proximally toward the lateral supracondylar ridge. A straight curette is then placed in this drill hole to assist with connecting of the convergent drill holes.
  - Two convergent drill holes, one anterior and one posterior to the lateral supracondylar ridge, are then drilled 1.5 cm proximal to the distal isometric hole (Fig. 16). The drill is angled so that it comes in contact with the straight curette placed in the distal isometric hole, indicating that the drill holes are in continuity.
  - Straight and curved curettes are then used to make sure that the drill holes are in continuity and to enlarge the tunnels.
  - This drilling technique creates a Y-shaped convergent tunnel in the lateral epicondyle (Fig. 17).

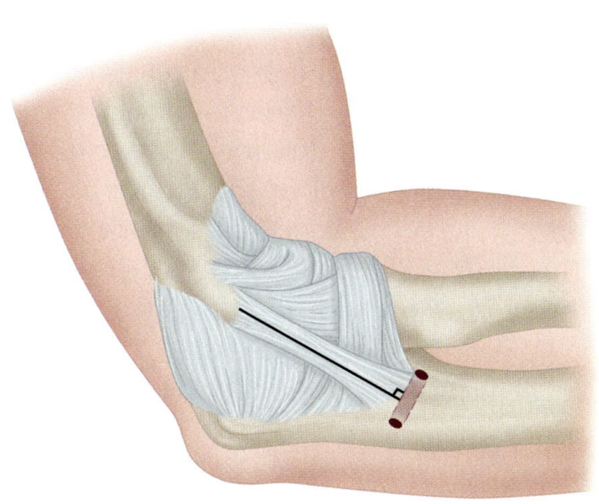

FIGURE 13

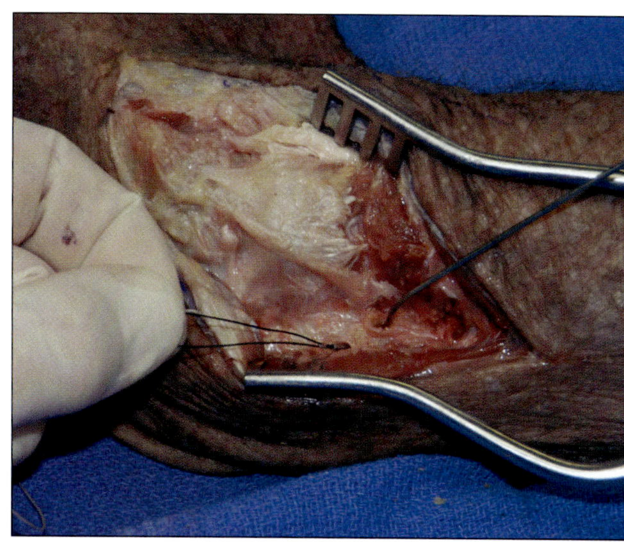

FIGURE 14

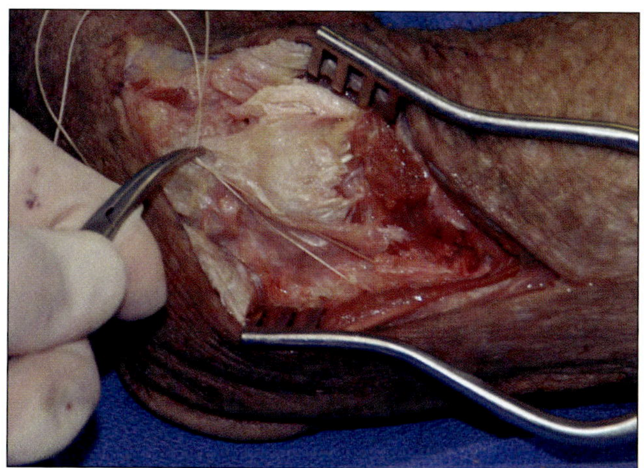

FIGURE 15

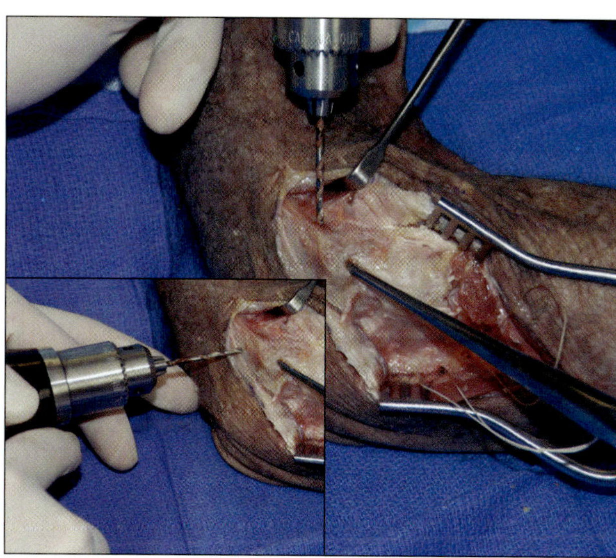

FIGURE 16

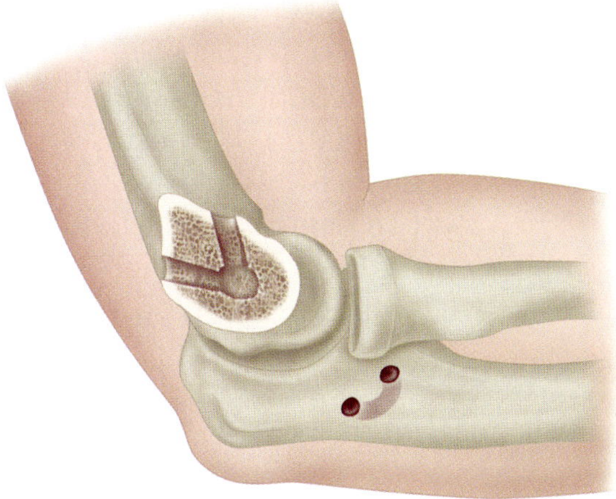

FIGURE 17

Instrumentation/ Implantation

- A 3.6-mm drill is used when reconstructing with the palmaris longus graft and a 4.0-mm drill is used when reconstructing with a gracilis hamstring graft.
- Curved curettes are helpful because they allow creation of a larger angle for the tunnel underneath the cortical bone with less levering required outside the bone.

Controversies

- Other procedures have been described for LUCL reconstruction. If one of these techniques is utilized, then the placement and number of tunnels may be altered.

Pearls

- *Sterile mineral oil can assist with graft passage if resistance is met during delivery of the graft through the tunnels drilled in the ulna and lateral epicondyle.*
- *It may be easier to deliver each limb of the graft separately through the convergent drill holes in the lateral epicondyle and supracondylar ridge to avoid damaging the graft.*

Pitfalls

- *Graft damage can occur during passage if the tunnels are not enlarged enough.*
- *Tunnel failure can occur during graft passage if the tunnels are enlarged too aggressively.*

Step 4

- Passing and securing of the graft follows tunnel placement.
- The graft is passed through the ulnar tunnel using the looped suture already present in the tunnel.
- A Hewson suture passer is then threaded through the hole drilled in the anterior aspect of the lateral supracondylar ridge and out the distal isometric hole. The sutures of the graft exiting the posterior limb of the tunnel drilled in the ulna are then delivered out the anterior hole drilled in the lateral supracondylar ridge using the positioned Hewson suture passer.
- A Hewson suture passer is then threaded through the hole drilled in the posterior aspect of the lateral supracondylar ridge and out the distal isometric hole. The sutures of the graft exiting the anterior limb of the tunnel drilled in the ulna are then delivered out the posterior hole drilled in the lateral supracondylar ridge using the positioned Hewson suture passer.
- The grafts are then delivered through the prospective tunnels, creating a figure-of-8 pattern of the graft (Fig. 18A and 18B).
- The graft is tensioned by crossing each limb over the supracondylar ridge with the arm positioned in maximum pronation and the elbow flexed to 30–40°. The graft is secured to itself with multiple 1-0 nonabsorbable sutures to secure its tension (Fig. 19).
- The graft is further tensioned by suturing the double-limb graft to itself, to the underlying capsule, and to the deficient LUCL starting at the isometric drill hole in the lateral epicondyle and ending where the graft limbs enter the ulnar tunnels (Fig. 20).

Step 5

- The wound is copiously irrigated and the tourniquet is deflated. Hemostasis is obtained prior to wound closure.
- The overlying soft tissues are then closed in layers in the standard fashion.
- An above-the-elbow splint is placed posteriorly with the forearm in pronation and the elbow flexed at 90°.

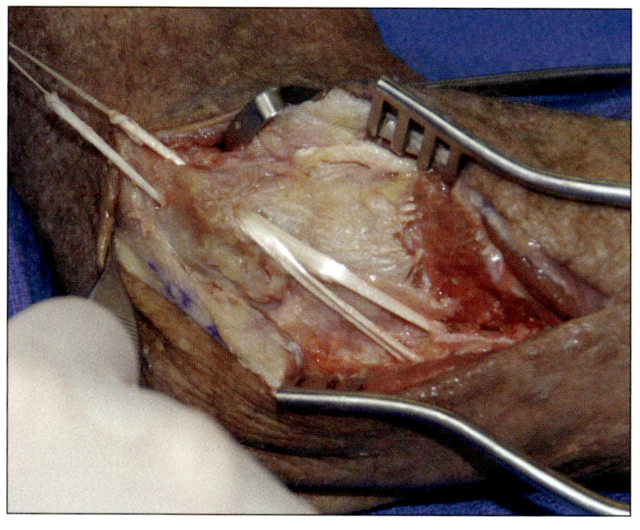
A

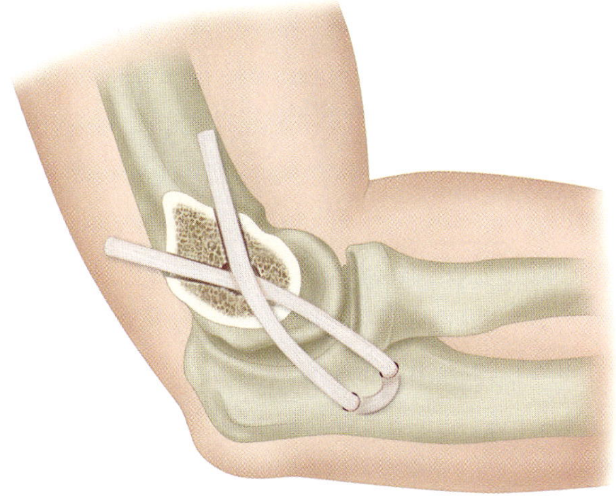
B

FIGURE 18

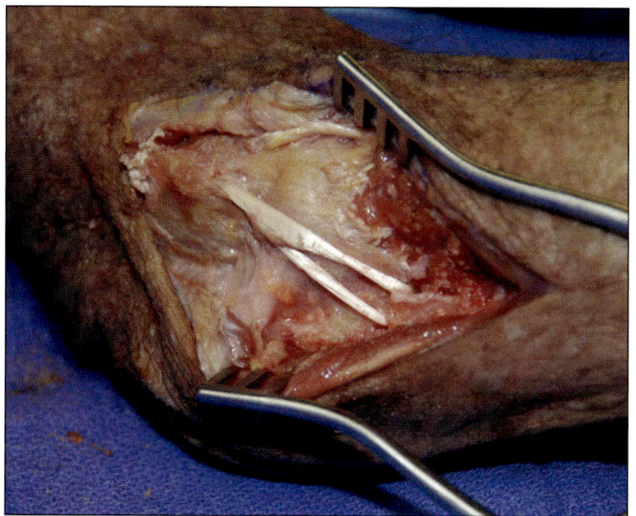
FIGURE 19

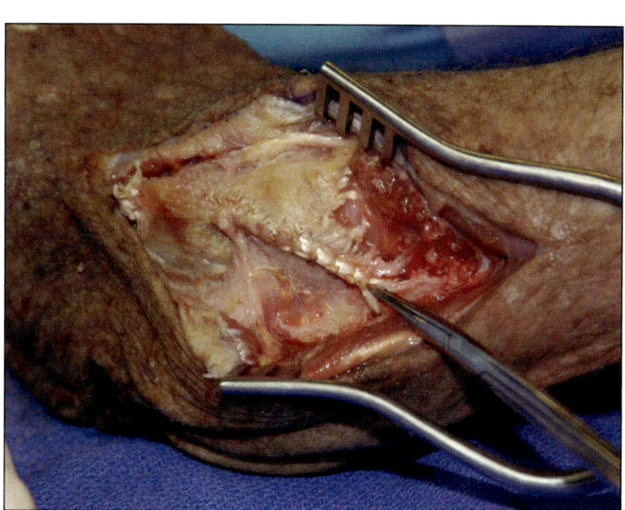
FIGURE 20

Instrumentation/ Implantation

- The Hewson suture passer is needed to assist with graft passage. It should be bent appropriately to maneuver through the desired drill holes.

Controversies

- Other procedures have been described for LUCL reconstruction. If one of these techniques is utilized, then the passage of the graft will be different than described here.

Postoperative Care and Expected Outcomes

- The postoperative splint is removed 1 week after surgery and a hinged elbow brace is applied with a 30° extension block for 6 weeks.
- Active elbow motion, rotator cuff muscle strengthening, and scapular stabilization exercises are initiated during second to third week.
- Biceps and triceps strengthening exercises are initiated during the fifth week with light resisted flexion and extension exercises.
- Full range of motion in the hinged elbow brace is initiated at 6 weeks.

PEARLS

- *Each patient's rehabilitation program should be curtailed to his or her functional activity and compliance and the strength of the repair.*

PITFALLS

- *Aggressive therapy can result in reconstruction failure.*

- If full motion is not restored by 8 weeks, then stretching exercises are initiated to the end of the active range of motion to increase the overall range of motion.
- Bracing is usually discontinued after 3 months.
- A strengthening program is then initiated at 3 months within the pain-free limits of function.
- Full recovery is expected after 6–9 months.

Evidence

Cohen MS, Hastings II H. Rotatory instability of the elbow: the anatomy and role of the lateral elbow stabilizers. J Bone Joint Surg [Am]. 1997;79:225-33.

Lee BP, Teo LH. Surgical reconstruction for posterolateral instability of the elbow. J Shoulder Elbow Surg. 2003;12:476-80.

Mehta JA, Bain IG. Posterolateral rotatory instability of the elbow. J Am Acad Orthop Surg. 2004;12:405-15.

Nester BJ, O'Driscoll SW, Morrey BF. Ligamentous reconstruction for posterolateral rotatory instability of the elbow. J Bone Joint Surg [Am]. 1992;74:1235-41.

O'Driscoll SW, Bell DF, Morrey BF. Posterolateral rotatory instability of the elbow. J Bone Joint Surg [Am]. 1991;73:440-6.

Rightmire E, Safran M. Surgical treatment of posterolateral instability of the elbow. In Cole BJ, Sekiya JK (eds). Surgical Technique of the Shoulder, Elbow, and Knee in Sports Medicine. Philadelphia: Saunders Elsevier, 2008:371-8.

Sanchez-Sotelo J, Morrey BF, O'Driscoll SW. Ligamentous repair and reconstruction for posterolateral rotatory instability of the elbow. J Bone Joint Surg [Br]. 2005;87:54-61.

Singleton SB, Conway JE. PLRI: posterolateral instability of the elbow. Clin Sports Med. 2004;23:629-42.

Smith 3rd JP, Savoie 3rd FH, Field LD. Posterolateral rotatory instability of the elbow. Clin Sports Med. 2001;20:47-58.

Yadao MA, Savoie 3rd FH, Field LD. Posterolateral rotatory instability of the elbow. Instr Course Lect. 2004;23:629-42.

SECTION II

ELBOW
Miscellaneous

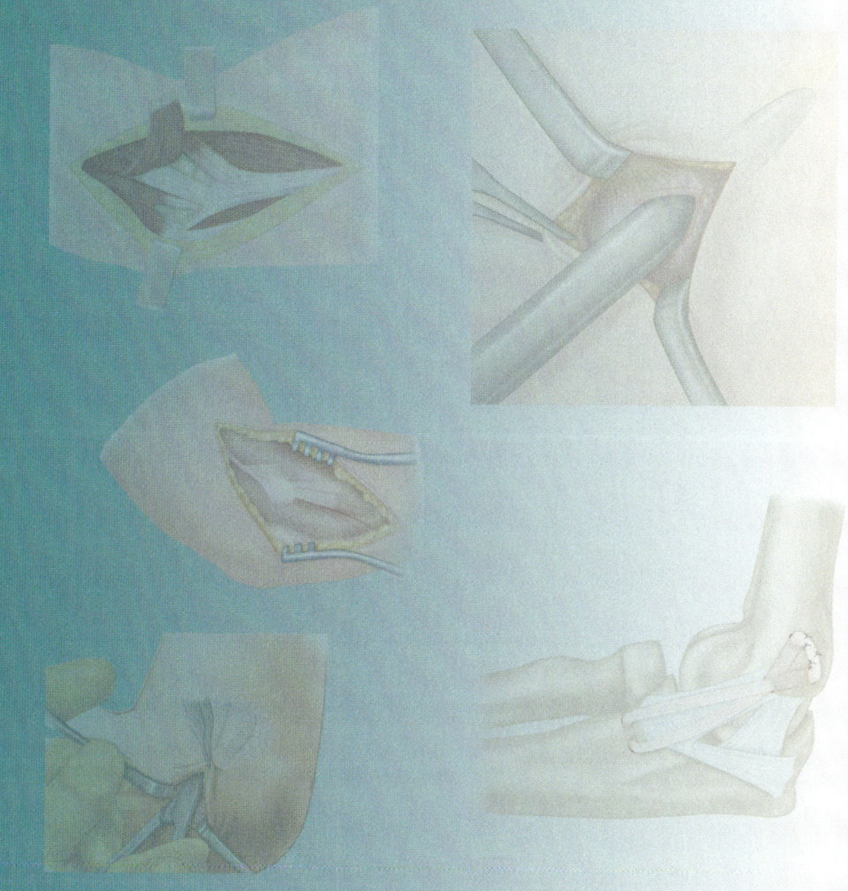

PROCEDURE 62

Soft Tissue Coverage I: Radial Forearm Flap

Wesley P. Thayer and R. Bruce Shack

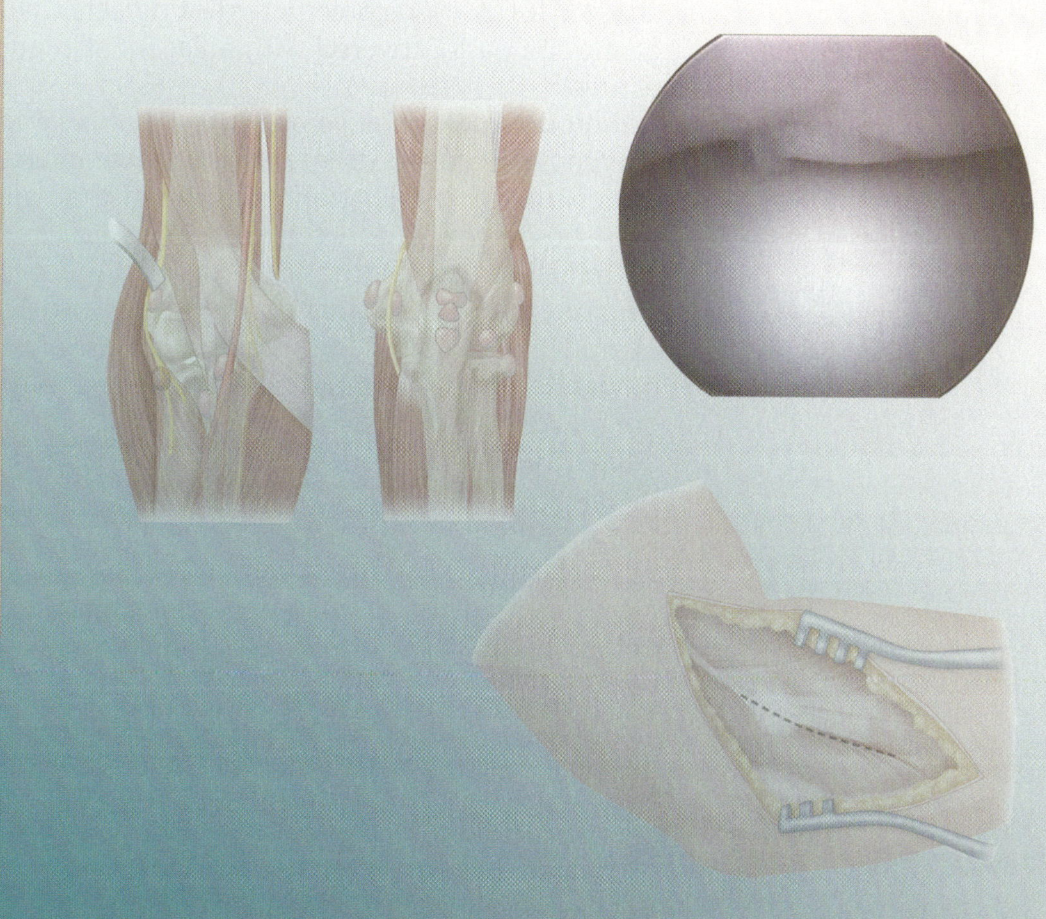

Elbow Coverage: Introduction

- Elbow injuries can be complex and involve bone, muscle, soft tissue, and nerves. The repair strategy should allow for all elements to be repaired in a timely fashion. The reconstruction should also permit early motion as elbow immobilization is poorly tolerated. The size of the wound, the presence of infection or contamination, and the complexity of the injury directly affect the technical aspects and timing of coverage. The procedures discussed in this chapter focus on reconstruction of defects that cannot be easily covered with adjacent skin and soft tissues.
- A thorough preoperative evaluation is crucial to maximize outcomes. The extent of bone injury, associated nerve injury, and the size of the wound must be determined. A complete physical examination focusing on the elbow, adjacent structures, and nerve function will help with operative planning. Radiographs and possibly magnetic resonance imaging are required, but operative inspection and washout help to formally define the soft tissue defect and initiate operative planning. Cultures can be taken to rule out infection and guide antibiotic therapy. Optimally, these wounds should be closed within 2–3 days of the injury. If gross contamination is present, serial débridements with intravenous antibiotics are required.
- The types of operations available for elbow coverage are briefly reviewed below.
  - Local flaps such a Z-plasty or rhomboid flaps are occasionally sufficient to cover elbow defects. Layered closure with wide mobilization can occasionally suffice. If these techniques are employed for posterior wounds, the surgeon must ensure that the closure tension is not excessive with the elbow flexed.
  - Axial flaps rely on named vascular inflow vessels that supply a skin paddle that can be mobilized and rotated into the defect. The best example of this is the radial forearm flap, and this is our favored flap for elbow coverage. It is described in detail in this part of the Soft Tissue Coverage Procedure. Other axial flaps include the posterior interosseous flap (Part III of the procedure), the

lateral arm flap (Part V of the procedure), and the ulnar artery flap.

- Of the pedicled muscle flaps, one stands out as an excellent choice for elbow coverage. The latissimus dorsi pedicle flap is commonly used for large to moderate elbow defects. It is second only to the radial forearm flap in our practice (see Part II of the Soft Tissue Coverage Procedure). The muscle bulk of this flap allows for elbow coverage when there is a very large wound. By using a muscle flap, the dead space is more easily filled, and the vascularity of this flap is exceptional. The flap can reach the olecranon with the insertion intact and can extend to cover defects up to 6 cm distal to the olecranon when the insertion is released. A skin graft is required for muscle coverage in most cases.
- Local muscle flaps are often an excellent choice for moderate to small defects. The brachioradialis is a large muscle that can cover lateral and anterior defects (see Part IV of the Soft Tissue Coverage Procedure). A skin graft may be needed as an adjunctive procedure. Other examples are the extensor carpi radialis longus, the flexor carpi ulnaris, and the anconeus. The key to successful use of these flaps is to ensure that the arc of rotation will be sufficient to cover the defect.
- Other pedicled flaps require staged procedures. They are rarely used for elbow reconstruction due to the prolonged period of immobilization. Examples include the thoracoepigastric flap, the groin flap, the external oblique flap, and a pedicled rectus flap. The requirement for up to 2 weeks of immobilization with complex pedicle care, with the need for flap division and inset at a second stage, limits the utility of these flaps. This is particularly true given the availability of free tissue transfer.
- Free tissue transfers should be considered when local tissues or flaps are not available. Although technically more complex, outcomes are excellent in trained hands. The options include free fascial flaps (such as the temporoparietal flap or the radial forearm fascial flap), fasciocutaneous flaps (such as the radial forearm, lateral arm flap, anterolateral thigh flap, and free groin flap), free muscle flaps (such as free rectus abdominus, latissimus dorsi, or gracilis flap), or even composite flaps. Donor site

morbidity and defect characteristics must be considered. Adjunctive angiography is helpful during operative planning. When joint space or hardware is exposed, muscle is an excellent choice with an overlying skin graft.

Pitfalls

- *The resulting scar can be both painful and aesthetically unappealing.*
- *Tendon exposure can occur at the donor site. This will prolong healing and often requires additional surgery.*

Controversies

- Use of the osteocutaneous modification of the radial forearm flap in elderly patients increases the incidence of postoperative distal radius fracture.

Treatment Options

- Local flap alternatives for elbow coverage include the latissimus dorsi flap, the posterior interosseous flap, the reverse lateral arm flap, the flexor carpi ulnaris flap, and the brachioradialis flap.
- Rarely, a wound vacuum-assisted closure device with or without Integra is indicated for elbow coverage.
- Free tissue transfer may be required if local tissues are damaged and if the latissimus flap is not available.

Indications

- The radial forearm flap is a workhorse flap for elbow coverage, providing up to 10 × 30 cm of soft tissue that can cover medial, lateral, or posterior defects. Most forearms will easily accommodate a 6 × 15-cm skin paddle. It can even be used to provide circumferential elbow coverage. The flap can be taken as skin only or as a composite graft including tendon and/or bone. This versatility makes this flap mainstay in elbow coverage.

Examination/Imaging

- The patient must have an acceptable ipsilateral ulnar artery providing adequate flow to the hand and all digits as determined by a preoperative Allen test. Particular attention should be paid to thumb and index finger perfusion via ulnar perfusion during the Allen test to verify patency of the deep palmar arch. Finger Doppler evaluation during the examination may be beneficial. This must be determined preoperatively as incomplete collateral flow prevents the use of this flap for reconstruction.
- In patients for whom there is concern, preoperative arteriography can be used to assess the vascularity of the upper extremity via magnetic resonance angiography, computed tomographic angiography, or standard arteriography. In either case, the Allen test must be used to verify patency of the palmar arch.

Surgical Anatomy

- Vascular anatomy
  - The dominant pedicle is the radial artery.
    - This is a branch of the brachial artery where it divides just distal to the elbow crease in the antecubital fossa. It travels deep to the brachioradialis in the proximal forearm and can be found between the flexor carpi radialis (FCR) and brachioradialis muscles (Fig. 1: BR, brachioradialis; FCU, flexor carpi ulnaris; FDS,

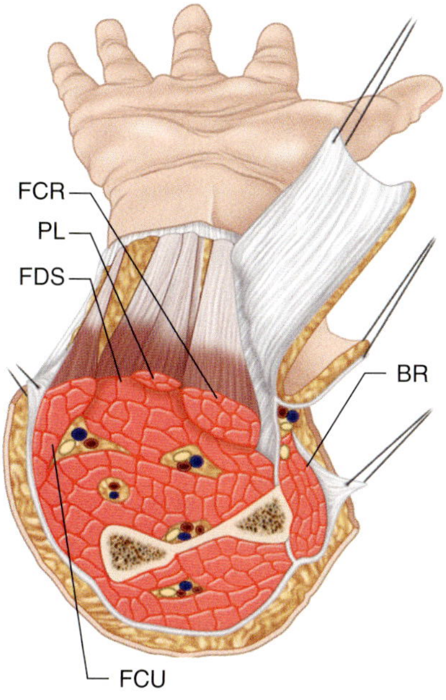

FIGURE 1

PEARLS

- *A hand surgery table is essential to safely harvest the flap.*
- *To inset the flap for a posterior defect, place the patient's hand over the abdomen.*

PITFALLS

- *Failure to prep the entire arm can result in contamination during flap inset.*
- *Particular attention should be paid to thumb and index finger perfusion via ulnar perfusion during the Allen test to verify patency of collateral flow to the digits and hand. This flap should not be used if the Allen test reveals inadequate collateral flow to the hand and/or digits.*

flexor digitorum superficialis; PL, palmaris longus).
    - The average length is 20 cm and the diameter range is 2–3 mm.
  - Venous outflow is dual from the deep and superficial system.
    - Deep—venae comitantes of the radial artery
    - Superficial—cephalic vein, which runs with the lateral antebrachial cutaneous nerve (both of these structures are often divided during flap elevation)
- Nerve supply is from the lateral and medial antebrachial cutaneous nerves.

Positioning

- The patient is supine with the arm abducted on a hand surgery table.
- The patient is prepped from the axilla to the fingertips and an extremity drape is used.
- A padded sterile tourniquet is placed high above the elbow.
- A site to harvest a split-thickness skin graft to cover the flap donor site (usually the lateral thigh) is prepared.

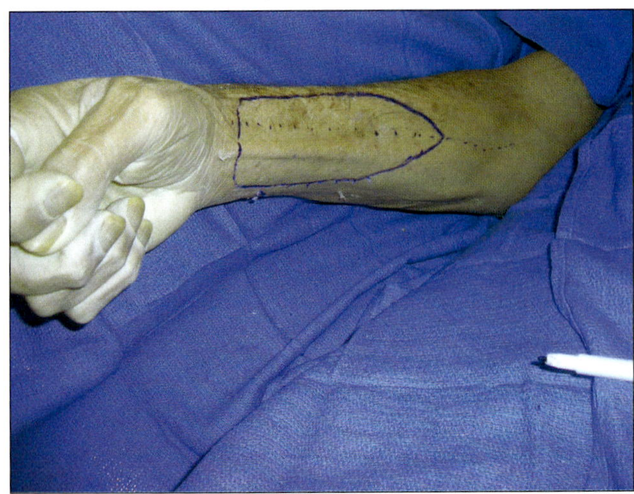

FIGURE 2

Pearls

- *The defect determines the paddle size. Using a paper template fashioned from surgical glove packaging can prevent raising an inadequate flap.*

Pitfalls

- *When the flap is raised on the ulnar aspect of the forearm, the ulnar artery can be accidentally raised with the fascia.*
- *In smokers, the ulnar portion of the flap is more likely to necrose.*
- *Harvesting a skin paddle too distal can increase the chance of tendon exposure.*
- *Harvesting a small flap dramatically increases the risk of division of the septocutaneous perforators.*

Controversies

- The donor site scar for this flap is substantial and difficult to hide unless wearing a long-sleeved shirt. Some surgeons view this as a distinct disadvantage.

Portals/Exposures

- Almost any size of flap can be marked between the wrist and antecubital fossa.
  - For elbow coverage, a distal flap centered over the radial artery that encompasses the distal two thirds of the volar forearm is best (Fig. 2).
- The distal marking should be placed 2 cm proximal to the wrist crease, and the proximal extent of the flap is determined by the defect size; however, a typical flap design is a 6 × 15-cm oval.

Procedure

Step 1: Flap Elevation

- The standard radial forearm flap is raised from distal to proximal. The first incision can be made on either the radial or ulnar aspect, but should be carried down to the level of muscle. The fascia should be included with the flap. Paratenon must be left behind. The safest place to get to the proper level is from the ulnar border of the skin paddle over the FCR muscle belly. A branch of the medial antebrachial cutaneous nerve will be found superficially here and can be divided. Dissection should proceed distally, keeping the fascia with the skin and taking care not to elevate the ulnar artery and nerve. By dissecting from ulnar to radial, the majority of the flap comes up with little resistance.
- The palmaris longus and FCR tendons are often incorporated into the fascia and must be dissected off, taking care not to injure the radial artery. The paratenon is preserved with the tendons. The

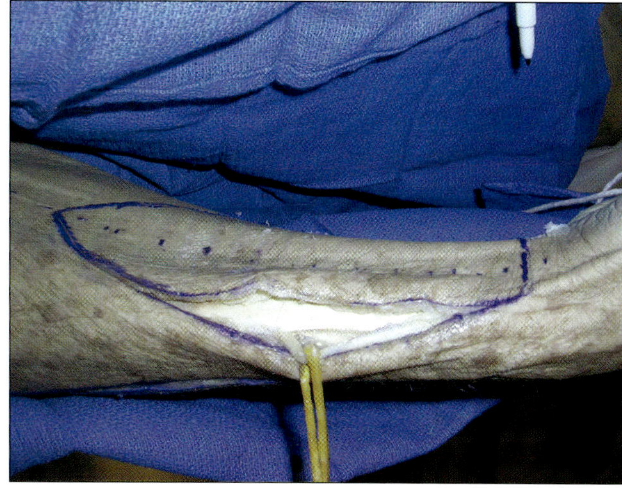

FIGURE 3

perforators lie within an intramuscular septum between the FCR and the brachioradialis.

- Once at this point, the radial incision is made and dissection proceeds down to the brachioradialis. Proximally at the skin level, the cephalic vein will be present and may be ligated and divided. The superficial sensory branch of the radial nerve is found distally on the radial aspect of the flap and should be preserved (Fig. 3).
- The distal incisions are connected and the distal radial artery and venae comitantes are identified (Fig. 4). This is a good time to clamp the vessels and let down the tourniquet to verify that the ulnar system can support the digits.
- Retraction is now essential for continued proximal dissection as the radial artery in the midforearm is

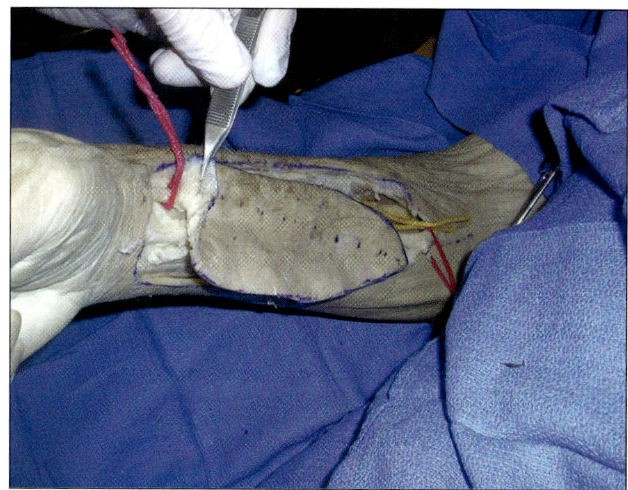

FIGURE 4

Pearls

- *Raise the flap from distal to proximal and take care not to put traction on the septocutaneous perforators.*
- *When making the ulnar and radial incisions for the skin paddle, go all the way down to and include the muscle fascia. This is essential to preserve the septocutaneous perforators.*
- *For the proximal dissection, the brachioradialis must be retracted radially to expose the radial artery underneath.*
- *Septocutaneous perforators can arise from the portion of the radial artery under the brachioradialis and feed the skin paddle distal to the muscle belly.*
- *Use loupe magnification.*
- *Use a tourniquet, but exsanguinate only with elevation to ensure that the veins are full to assist with identification.*

Pitfalls

- *Raising the flap from proximal to distal can result in separation ot the skin paddle from the radial artery.*
- *Before dividing the radial artery, let down the tourniquet and verify finger vascularity with the radial artery clamped.*

Controversies

- Exsanguination before placing the tourniquet can result in difficulty visualizing the venae comitantes.

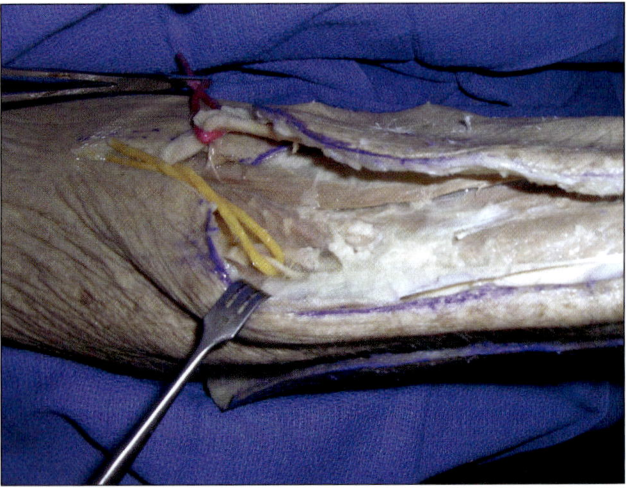

FIGURE 5

deep to the brachioradialis (Fig. 5). The brachioradialis tendon and muscle belly must be retracted radially to preserve the septum. The FCR can be retracted ulnarly. By keeping a cuff of subcutaneous tissue from this area with the flap, the more proximal perforators can more easily be preserved. The superficial branch of the radial nerve is also found under the brachioradialis at this level and should be identified and preserved (see Fig. 5). The lateral antebrachial cutaneous nerve is a superficial structure and is suitable for innervated flap transfer in free tissue cases.

- The dissection is now carried proximally to the bifurcation of the brachial artery. The veins in this area are complex but will coalesce into a more dominant vessel proximal to the antecubital fossa for free tissue transfer cases. The recurrent radial artery can also be identified in its typical position just distal to the origin of the radial artery from the brachial.
- If it has not already been done, the tourniquet is let down and ulnar flow to the digits is verified with a distal clamp on the radial artery. Once this is done, the radial artery is divided at the wrist level between ties. With the tourniquet down, hemostasis is obtained and preparation made for inset.

Step 2: Flap Inset

- The flap is rotated into place in a manner that minimizes kinking of the pedicle (Fig. 6). This may require incising tissue between the donor site and the defect.
- A two-layer closure using deep absorbable suture and either staples or nylon stitches is preferred.

Pearls

- *For a deep defect, design a larger flap; also, the tip or edge of the flap can be de-epithelialized and tucked into the void to fill the dead space.*

Pitfalls

- *Kinking or tunneling under a tight skin bridge can result in vascular pedicle insufficiency.*

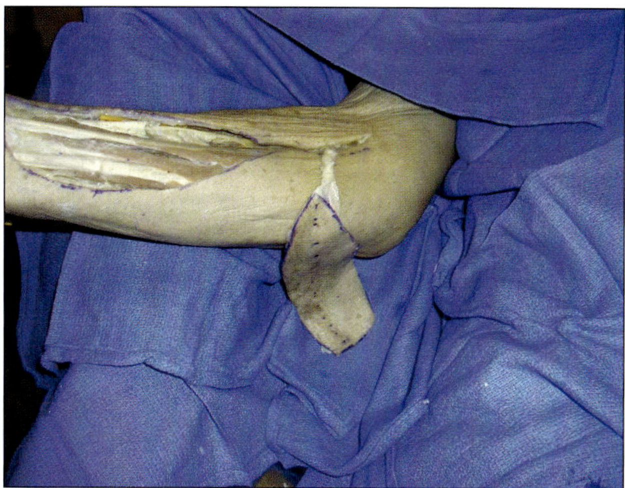

FIGURE 6

- The flap is typically inset over a closed suction drain. A soft dressing is typically applied directly over the flap that can easily be removed for flap inspection.
- Elbow splinting is optional but can impinge on the flap's blood supply. If casting is required because of underlying bone or ligament reconstruction, a large window should be created to visualize the flap postoperatively.

STEP 3: DONOR SITE CLOSURE

- The proximal donor site can be approximated if an elliptical flap design is utilized. Distally, the muscle bellies of the FCR and brachioradialis can be approximated to facilitate tendon coverage and reduce the incidence of tendon exposure.
- A split-thickness skin graft is almost always required unless tissue expanders are used preoperatively. Typically, the graft is either pie-crusted or meshed and a bolster is applied for 5 days. A safe position splint is also essential to prevent shearing of the skin graft from the underlying muscle and tendon.

PEARLS

- *Tendon exposure can often be overcome with conservative dressing changes and attention to wound care.*

PITFALLS

- *Poor postoperative positioning can result in flap compromise and failure.*
- *Tendon exposure may require reoperation for coverage, possibly even tendon excision.*

Postoperative Care and Expected Outcomes

- Postoperatively, the arm is elevated and the flap is routinely examined for hematoma formation, venous congestion, and later for infection or dehiscence. The drains are removed once output is appropriate, usually on day 1. The fingers are examined postoperatively for capillary refill and sensation. Adjustments may need to be made to the splint or dressing if it impinges on the forearm or the flap itself.

- On postoperative day 5, the bolster is taken down to inspect the skin graft. Any areas of graft loss are treated conservatively with nonadherent dressing changes. The splint should be reapplied for a total of 7 days to prevent shearing of the graft. Afterward, therapy is initiated as appropriate.
- Success rates for radial forearm flap coverage of elbow defects range from 90% to 100%. The most commonly reported complication is donor site breakdown with tendon exposure; however, hematoma, infection, and vascular insufficiency can occur requiring intervention. If the flap develops congestion that fails to respond to position changes, some stitches should be removed. If this fails to alleviate the problem, a re-exploration is warranted for pedicle kinking. The cephalic vein may need to be anastomosed to drain the flap and/or leech therapy can be considered. Arterial insufficiency is most likely due to septal perforator injury or spasm. If it does not resolve with warming and time, the flap may be lost.

Evidence

Bishop A. Soft tissue loss about the elbow: selecting optimal coverage. Hand Clin. 1994;10:531-542.

This review article delineated the techniques involved for elbow coverage and offered a useful algorithm for treatment decisions. (Grade C recommendation; Level V evidence)

Green DP, Hotchkiss RN, Pederson WC, Wolfe SW. Green's Operative Hand Surgery, ed 5. Philadelphia: Elsevier, 2005.

This text provides a thorough review of the topic of elbow coverage and provides technical descriptions of the surgeries. (Grade C recommendation; level V evidence studies referenced)

Mathes SJ, Nahai F. Reconstructive Surgery: Principles, Anatomy, and Technique. New York: Churchill Livingstone, 1997.

This text provides a thorough review of the topic of elbow coverage and provides technical descriptions of the surgeries. (Grade C recommendation; level V evidence studies referenced)

Timmons MJ. The vascular basis of the radial forearm flap. Plast Reconstr Surg. 1986;77:80.

This cadaveric study demonstrated the relevant anatomy of the radial forearm flap.

Tizian C, Sanner F, Berger A. The proximally pedicled arteria radialis forearm flap in the treatment of soft tissue defects of the dorsal elbow. Ann Plast Surg. 1991;26:40.

This case series included 14 patients in whom the flap was used for coverage of dorsal elbow defects. (Grade C recommendation; Level V evidence)

PROCEDURE 62

Soft Tissue Coverage II: Latissimus Dorsi Flap

Wesley P. Thayer and R. Bruce Shack

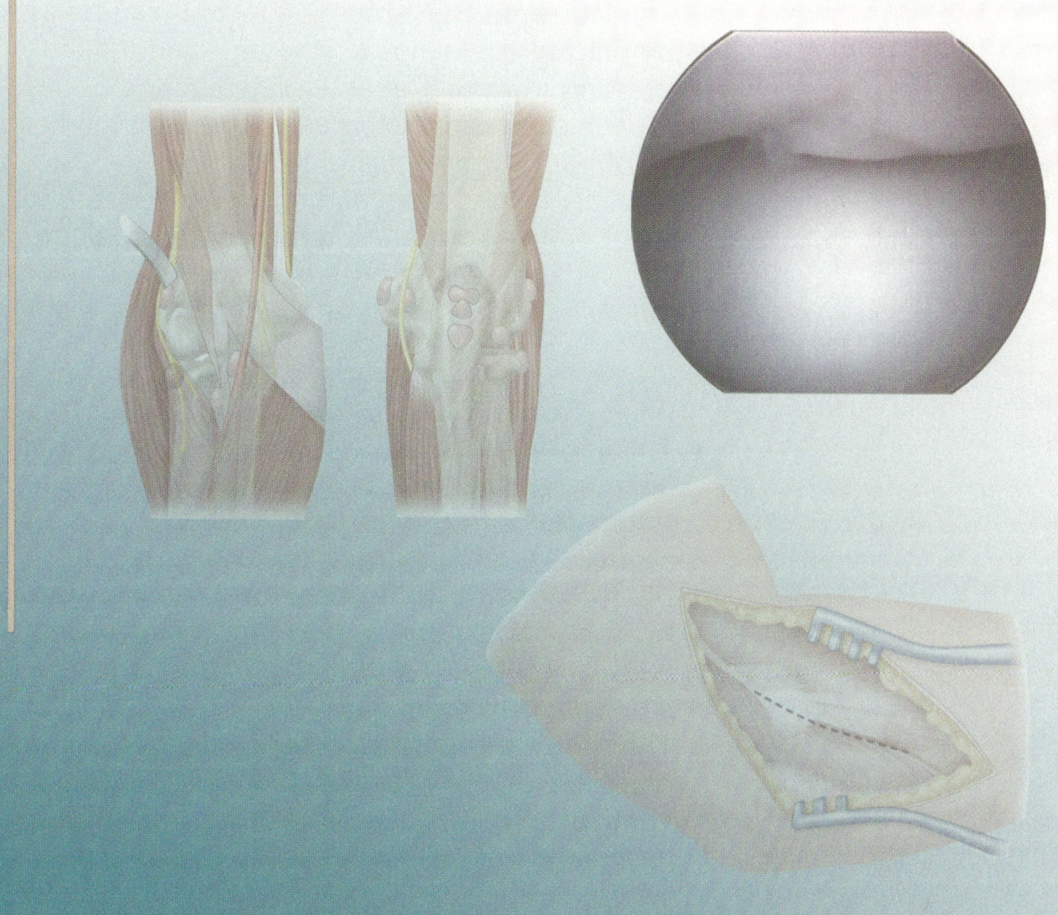

Pitfalls

- *The muscle can reach beyond the elbow, but the skin paddle rarely will. Closure almost always requires the use of a skin graft.*
- *This is not a good choice for circumferential defects.*

Controversies

- This flap should be avoided in patients with ipsilateral shoulder injuries.
- Also, avoid this flap in patients with contralateral upper extremity weakness or paraplegics in whom the loss of function will potentially be more functionally limiting.

Treatment Options

- Local flap alternatives for elbow coverage include the radial forearm flap, the posterior interosseous flap, the reverse lateral arm flap, the flexor carpi ulnaris flap, and the brachioradialis flap.
- Rarely, a wound vacuum-assisted closure device with or without Integra is indicated for elbow coverage.
- Free tissue transfer may be required if local tissues are damaged and if the latissimus flap is not available.

Indications

- The pedicled latissimus dorsi flap is best used for elbow coverage when there is a very large wound. By using a muscle flap, the dead space is more easily filled, and the vascularity of this flap is exceptional. The flap can easily reach the olecranon with the insertion intact and can extend to cover defects up to 6 cm distal to the olecranon when the insertion is released.

Examination/Imaging

- The latissimus dorsi muscle function can be assessed by placing the hands on the hips and forcefully pressing inward. The anterolateral edge of the muscle can be palpated and should be marked to assist with surgical planning.
- In patients who have had an axillary dissection, preoperative computed tomographic angiography can verify patency of the thoracodorsal vascular inflow.

Surgical Anatomy

- The latissimus dorsi muscle covers the lower and lateral aspects of the posterior trunk. The muscle originates from the posterior iliac crest, the lower six thoracic vertebrae, and the sacral vertebrae via a broad aponeurosis. It inserts into the intertubercular groove of the humerus and functions to adduct and internally rotate the shoulder. In an adult, the muscle size is approximately 25 × 35 cm.
- The dominant vascular pedicle to the latissimus dorsi muscle is the thoracodorsal artery and venae comitantes, which are branches of the subscapular artery and vein (Fig. 1A and 1B). Secondary segmental pedicles supply the muscle medially via both the posterior intercostal and the lumbar systems.
- The nerve supply to the latissimus dorsi muscle is via the thoracodorsal nerve, which travels through the posterior axilla; sensory innervation to the overlying skin is via intercostal branches (see Fig. 6 later).

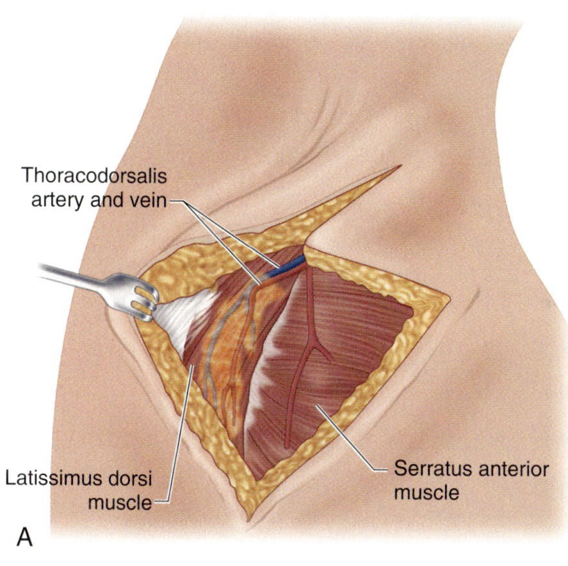

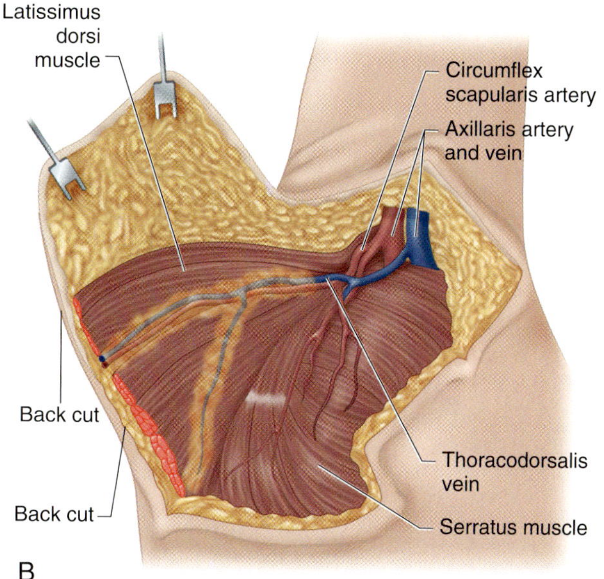

FIGURE 1

Pearls

- *By bringing in a sterile, padded Mayo stand once the flap has been elevated, the arm can be best positioned for flap inset without altering the patient's position and can allow for simultaneous inset and closure.*

Pitfalls

- *The absence of the surgeon during patient positioning often leads to an inappropriately prepped and positioned patient.*
- *An axillary roll is mandatory for lateral decubitus positioning to prevent nerve injury.*

Equipment

- Beanbag
- Axillary roll

Positioning

- For cases in which the latissimus dorsi is to be used for elbow coverage, the patient's entire arm, axilla, and back from the spine to the iliac crest should be included in the operative field. This is best accomplished by using a beanbag or a tailored bump under the patient to generate the full lateral decubitus position.

Portals/Exposures

- The anterolateral edge of the latissimus dorsi muscle can be palpated by placing the hands on the hips and forcefully pressing inward. It should be marked to assist with surgical planning. Next, mark the tip of the scapula to determine the superior margin of the flap (V-shaped mark in Fig. 2). The spinous processes of the spine denote the medial border, and inferiorly, the muscle margin is at the iliac crest.
- If no skin island is needed, a central oblique incision can be marked once the lateral margins of the muscle have been identified. The incision can be lengthened as needed to increase exposure.
- For cases in which a skin paddle is desired, the entire skin overlying the muscle can be taken; however, to allow for primary closure, a maximum width of 8–10 cm for the flap should be observed.
  - The typical paddle is 8 × 15 cm and is centered over the body of the muscle. The paddle can be

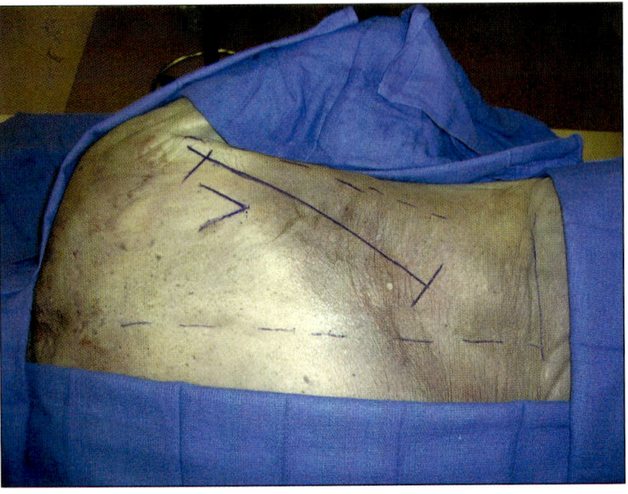

FIGURE 2

placed in either a superior, oblique, or vertical fashion as desired.

- Again, for elbow coverage, the use of a latissimus skin island pedicle is limited because the paddle should not include any skin closer than 8 cm to the iliac crest to ensure tissue viability. This limitation usually means that the skin island will not rotate enough to easily inset, unless local tissue at the elbow can be adequately rearranged.

PEARLS

- *Although muscle coverage of the elbow is excellent with the latissimus flap, skin islands can be bulky and are difficult to inset at the level of the elbow. Skin grafts are almost always needed with this flap. Unless radiation is planned, it is best to only rotate muscle and then cover the flap with a meshed split-thickness skin graft for elbow coverage cases.*

Procedure

Step 1: Flap Elevation

- A beveled incision is made around the circumference of the skin to maximize musculocutaneous perforating vessels if a skin paddle is to be rotated with the flap. Otherwise, one can simply cut down to the muscle itself. The medial skin is then elevated off the muscle toward the midline, stopping 1–2 cm from the spinous processes of the vertebrae, which can be palpated if they are prepped into the field. A similar inferior dissection is carried out toward the iliac crest. The lateral aspect of the latissimus muscle is the easiest to identify and, once noted, the elevation of the inferior portion of the flap can be initiated. Superiorly, the trapezius muscle's junction with the latissimus dorsi should be clearly identified near the tip of the scapula (Fig. 3; note that the skin has been cut away in this cadaveric dissection).
- Once the more superficial portion of the dissection is completed with identification of the above landmarks, the flap can be divided inferiorly from the

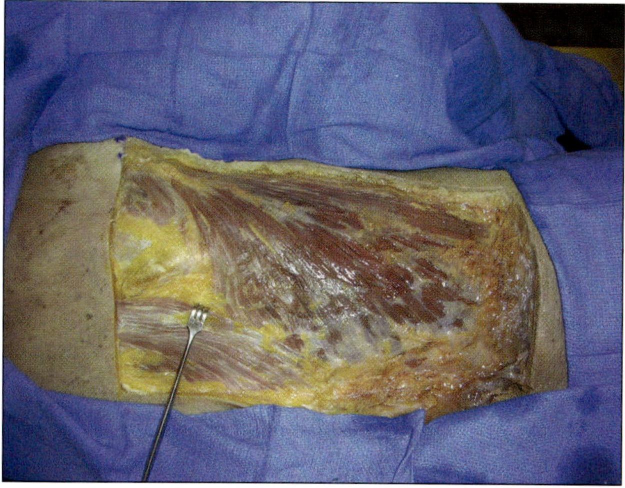

FIGURE 3

lumbosacral fascia and medially from the paraspinous fascia with cautery. Medially, veins will require ligation with clips or ties.

- Once free at its origin, the muscle can be flipped up and freed up on its deep surface primarily with blunt dissection techniques. The serratus can easily be erroneously elevated with the latissimus dorsi if care is not taken in this region; note the junction of the serratus anterior and the latissimus dorsi in Figure 4.
- The thoracodorsal vessels are found during this part of the dissection on the deep surface of the latissimus muscle once the dissection nears the serratus. It is essential to protect the vessels, which can be accomplished by preserving the fatty tissue plane that encases them. Small venous branches to

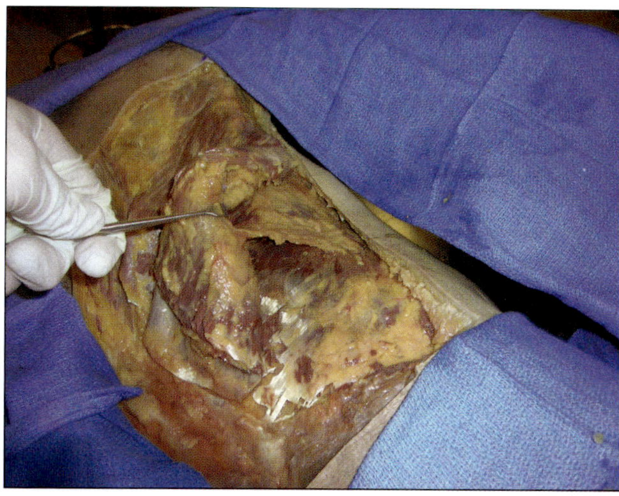

FIGURE 4

Pearls

- *By separating up to 90% of the muscle at the insertion, enough tissue is left to prevent traction injury to the pedicle, but will allow increased mobilization and will reduce the intensity of postoperative muscle contractions.*
- *The serratus branch to the latissimus dorsi should not be divided until the thoracodorsal system is identified and preserved because the flap can survive on reverse flow from the serratus. However, for elbow coverage, the arc of rotation will be decreased in this situation and this may limit the ability of the latissimus to cover distal defects.*
- *An assistant is critical to help with retraction during the proximal dissection. Extend the incision proximally as needed to gain adequate exposure of the proximal vessels.*

Pitfalls

- *Carefully separate the latissimus from underlying fascia over the scapula as the serratus can be inadvertently raised with the latissimus in this region.*

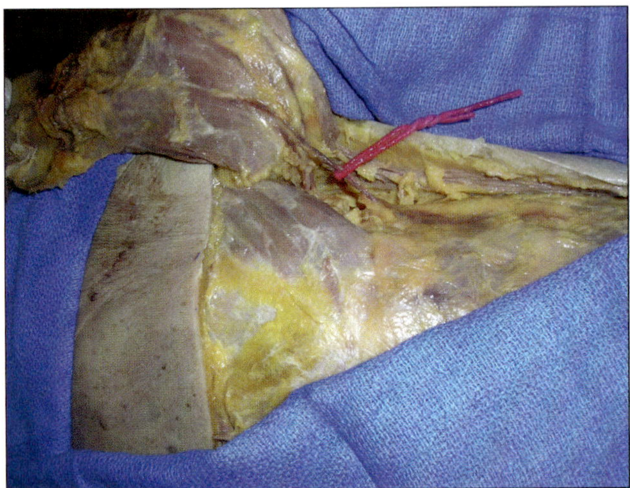

FIGURE 5

the deeper structures will require ligation. The branch to the serratus (Fig. 5) is preserved during the dissection as it can be used as an alternate source of inflow in some cases if the thoracodorsal pedicle is injured.

- The superior superficial dissection has to be carefully performed since the inflow can be transected when the deep vessels veer toward the axilla and the latissimus muscle courses toward its insertion on the humerus (Fig. 6; note the thoracodorsal nerve, artery, and vein separately looped).
- Once the inflow has been verified and mobilized, the vascular branches to the serratus can be divided (shown divided in Fig. 6). Also up to 90% of the muscle insertion can be divided to increase the arc of rotation. If all of the muscle is to be divided, this

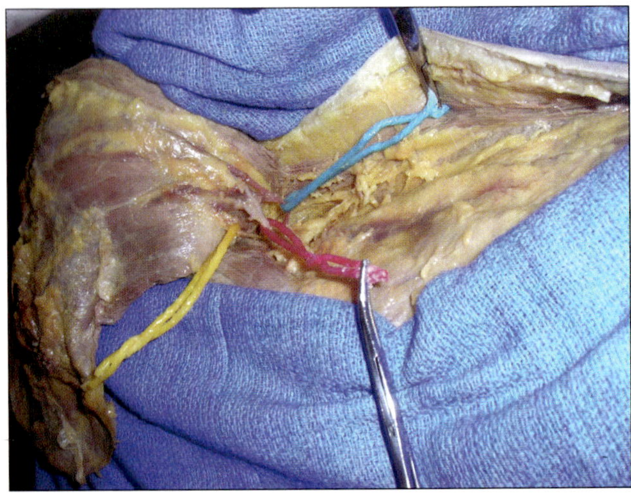

FIGURE 6

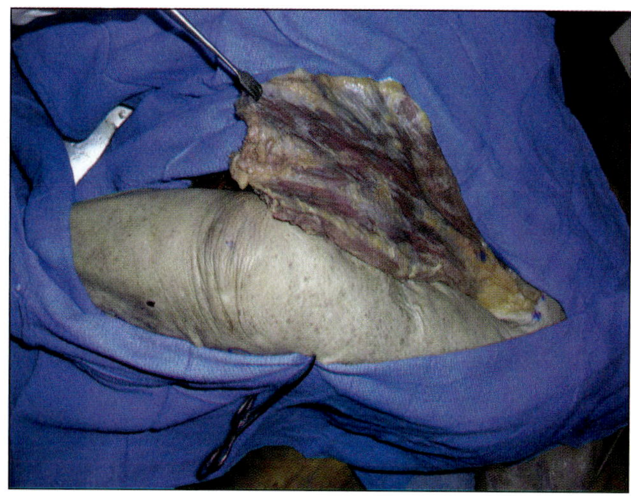

FIGURE 7

should be performed as late as possible in the surgery to prevent inadvertent vessel avulsion during inset or passage of the flap though a subcutaneous tunnel. Also, the muscle should be denervated to reduce aberrant muscle activation.

Step 2: Flap Inset

- The muscle can now be rotated to the defect with the insertion intact (Fig. 7).
- With the insertion divided, the muscle can cover defects up to 6 cm distal to the olecranon (Fig. 8). Caution must be used because the pedicle is easily avulsed once the insertion is released!
  - The flap should be inset over a drain, preferably with the muscle edge deep to viable elbow soft tissue. If the muscle is tunneled though the upper

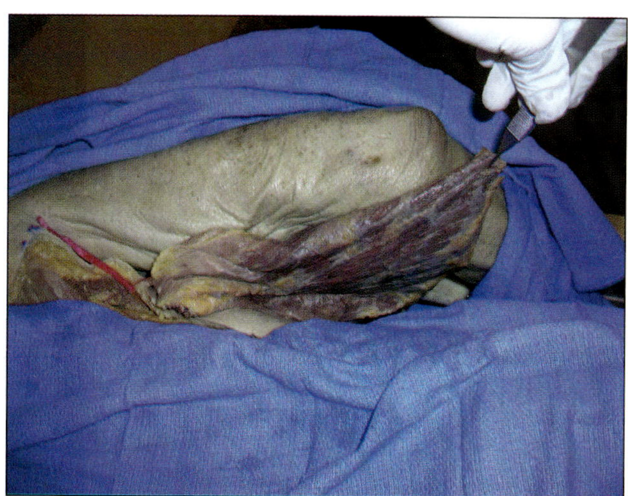

FIGURE 8

Pearls

- *Adequate tunnel creation is essential to prevent compression of the blood supply to the flap. A Z-plasty of the upper arm skin may be required to release the tunnel, and the resulting exposed muscle can be covered with a skin graft.*
- *Verify vascularity of the flap both by visual inspection of flap color and with Doppler analysis after inset.*
- *If left innervated, this flap can be used both to provide coverage of upper arm defects and as a functional muscle transfer.*
- *If the patient is in the lateral decubitus position with the arm on a sterile, padded Mayo stand, the inset and closure can be performed simultaneously.*

Pitfalls

- *If the insertion is divided, the blood supply can be easily disrupted due to excessive tension.*
- *Twisting of the pedicle can lead to venous or even arterial insufficiency.*

arm, it must not be rotated to prevent vascular ischemia.
- The arm may need to be opened to prevent venous insufficiency if the flap is congested. A Z-plasty incision in the upper arm can be used to transpose soft tissues proximally to prevent this flap constriction, and then the resulting defect distally can be covered with a meshed split-thickness skin graft.
- In almost all cases, a meshed split-thickness skin graft is placed over the muscle distally, with a bolster or a wound vacuum-assisted closure device and splint for 3–5 days.

- A splint can be applied to prevent the flap and skin graft from being sheared away form the elbow. This should not be placed directly over the flap, and the wrap over the split should not be tight.

Step 3: Donor Site Closure

- Direct closure of the donor site is recommended because the overlying skin will easily close, even when a large skin panel is taken. Also, skin grafts on the posterior chest wall leave a deforming scar.
- Drains are required due to the high seroma rate at the donor site.

Postoperative Care and Expected Outcomes

- Postoperatively, these patients must be admitted to the hospital for observation and pain control.
- Frequent flap evaluation for venous congestion (although rare) can result in flap salvage by re-exploration. Hematomas may also require exploration for evacuation.
- Other potential complications include seroma formation at the donor site, infection, and dissatisfaction with the donor site scar. Seromas at the donor site are the most common complication, with up to 20–79% incidence. They almost always require drainage. Quilting sutures may help reduce the risk of seroma formation, and suction drains should also be left in place until the output drops below 30 ml/day. Recalcitrant seromas may respond to sclerotherapy.
- Patients do experience mild weakness and a slight decrease in range of motion of the shoulder, but most tolerate these limitations well.

Pearls

- *Congestion of the flap in the early postoperative period warrants immediate re-exploration to release any potential kinks in the pedicle.*

Pitfalls

- *If the flap is inset over devitalized or infected bone, the resulting infection can limit the flap's ability cover the wound.*
- *Premature discontinuation of the drains or failure to place donor site drains can lead to seroma formation.*

Evidence

Bartlett SP, May JW, Yaremchuk MJ. The latissimus dorsi muscle: a fresh cadaver study of the primary neurovascular pedicle. Plast Reconstr Surg. 1981;67:631.

This cadaveric study demonstrated the relevant anatomy of the latissimus dorsi muscle.

Laitung JFG, Peck F. Shoulder function following the loss of the latissimus dorsi muscle. Br J Plast Surg. 1985;38:375.

This study reviewed the functional consequences of latisimus transfer. (Grade C recommendation; Level V evidence)

Jamara FNA, Akel S, Shamma AR. Repair of major defect of the upper extremity with a latissimus dorsi myocutaneous flap. Br J Plast Surg. 1981;34:121.

The authors presented a case report with anatomic description. (Grade C recommendation; Level V evidence)

Sadove RC, Vasconez HC, Arthur KR, Draud JW, Burgess RC. Immediate closure of traumatic upper arm and forearm injuries with the latissimus dorsi island myocutaneous pedicle flap. Plast Reconstr Surg. 1991;88:115.

The authors presented a case series of 11 patients with latissimus dorsi island myocutaneous pedicle flap application. (Grade C recommendation; Level V evidence)

PROCEDURE 62

Soft Tissue Coverage III: Posterior Interosseous Flap

Wesley P. Thayer and R. Bruce Shack

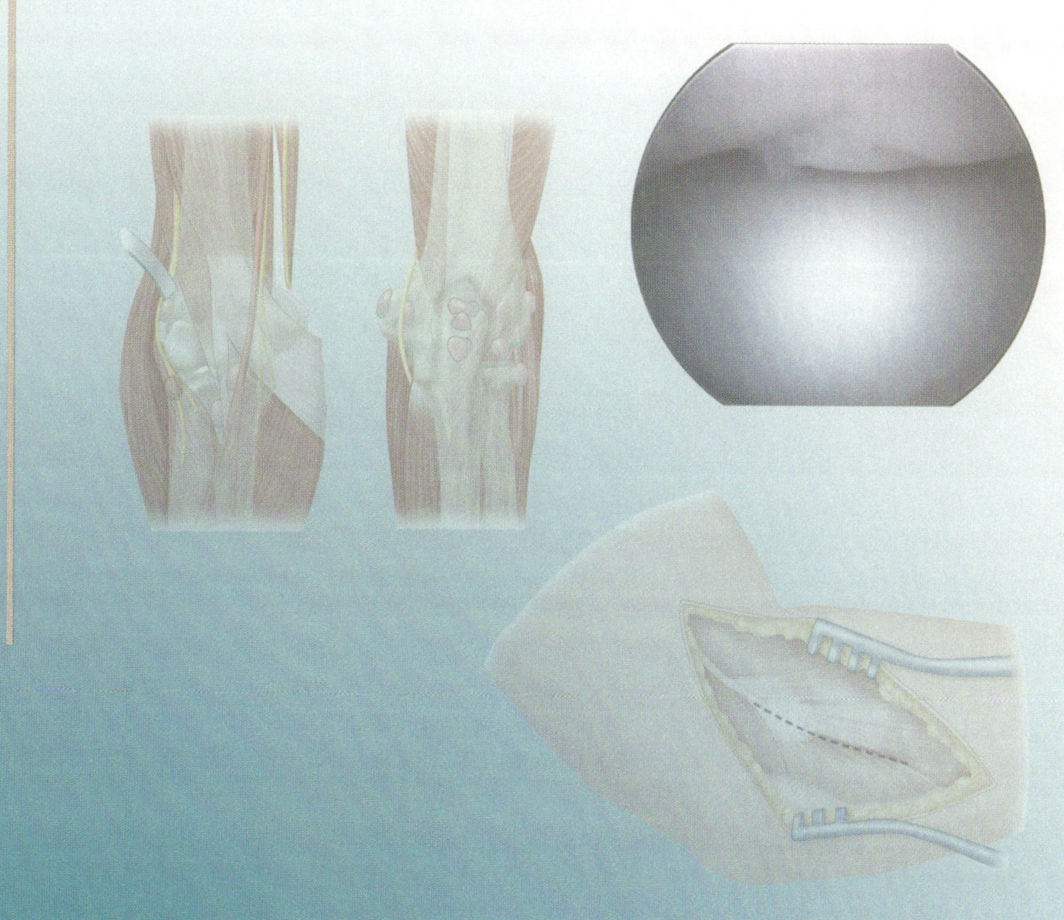

PITFALLS

- *Medial elbow defects may be difficult to cover.*

Controversies

- If the defect is larger than that which can be closed with a 5 × 6-cm paddle, primary donor site closure is difficult.

Treatment Options

- Local flap alternatives for elbow coverage include the radial forearm flap, the latissimus dorsi muscle flap, the reverse lateral arm flap, the flexor carpi ulnaris flap, and the brachioradialis flap.
- Rarely, a wound vacuum-assisted closure device with or without Integra is indicated for elbow coverage.
- Free tissue transfer may be required if local tissues are damaged and if the latissimus flap is not available.

Indications

- Although the radial forearm flap is the most versatile flap for elbow coverage, vascular insufficiency or associated trauma may preclude its use. With a skin paddle size of up to 8 × 18 cm, the standard posterior interosseous flap can adequately cover defects of the antecubital fossa and elbow.
- A vascularized segment of ulna can be taken with this flap in conjunction with a portion of the insertion of both the abductor pollicis longus and the extensor pollicis longus, both of which receive their blood supply from the posterior interosseous artery (PIA).

Examination/Imaging

- Preoperative evaluation of the dorsal forearm should verify that the donor site soft tissue has not been traumatized. Doppler evaluation is rarely helpful.

Surgical Anatomy

- This fasciocutaneous flap allows for a maximum skin paddle size of 8 × 18 cm. Typically a 5 × 6-cm paddle is designed to allow for primary donor site closure. This flap is located dorsally on the distal two thirds of the forearm between the radius and ulna.
- The PIA is a branch of the common interosseous artery that originates from the ulnar artery in the volar forearm. The PIA courses into the dorsal forearm proximal to the interosseous membrane and continues deep to the supinator (Fig. 1). The septocutaneous blood supply to the skin paddle typically runs between the extensor carpi ulnaris and the extensor digiti minimi.
- The majority of the sensory innervation to this paddle is provided by a branch of the dorsal antebrachial cutaneous nerve. The medial antebrachial cutaneous nerve also contributes.

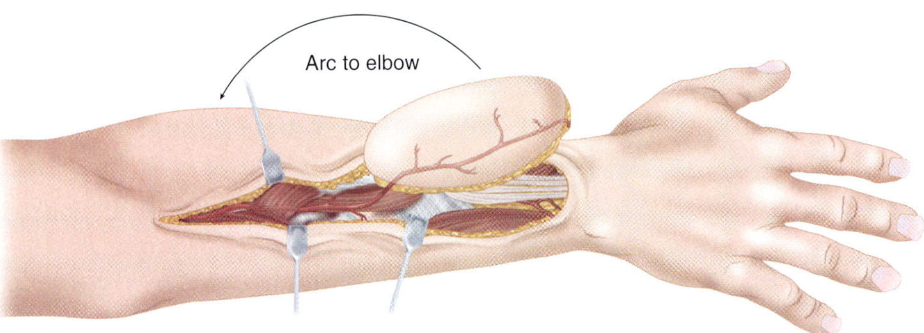

FIGURE 1

PEARLS

- *The surgeon should sit on the cranial side of the armboard.*

PITFALLS

- *Application of a nonsterile tourniquet can result in inadequate exposure of the elbow for inset.*

Equipment

- Armboard
- Sterile tourniquet

PEARLS

- *Using a template based on the actual wound size can minimize donor site size and possibly allow for donor site primary closure.*

PITFALLS

- *Coverage of medial or circumferential defects can be limited.*
- *When planning the arc of rotation, keep in mind that kinking of the pedicle can result in flap failure.*

Positioning

- The patient should be in a supine position with the arm abducted on an arm table.
- The arm is placed on a standard armboard and is prepped to the shoulder.
- A sterile tourniquet is required for this dissection.

Portals/Exposures

- The flap is located in the distal portion of the dorsal forearm. Up to an 8 × 18-cm skin paddle can be designed (Fig. 2).
- The flaps are centered on a line drawn from the ulnar styloid to the lateral epicondyle of the humerus. The proximal aspect of the skin paddle should not extend significantly proximal to the domain of the supinator muscle. This is roughly 6 cm distal to the lateral epicondyle. The distal aspect of the flap should be proximal to the distal radioulnar joint.
- For elbow defects, the design should allow for inset without a tunnel if possible and can include preservation of the proximal skin and dermis to allow for better vascular outflow.

Procedure

STEP 1: FLAP ELEVATION

- Once the skin paddle is marked, using tourniquet control, the distal portion of the incision is made down to and including the deep fascia.
- By identifying and retracting the extensor digiti minimi and extensor carpi ulnaris distally (both are marked with white loops and retracted in Fig. 3), the

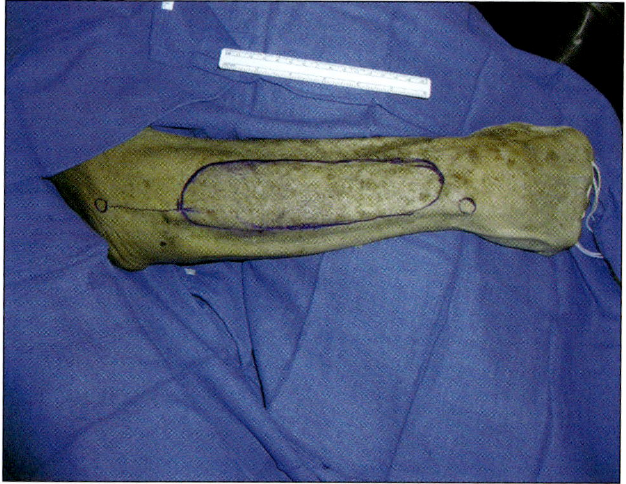

FIGURE 2

Pearls

- *Venous congestion can be avoided by leaving the cutaneous base of the flap intact.*
- *If venous congestion does develop, a microsurgical venous anastamosis may be required to salvage the flap.*
- *The pedicle can be extended by dissecting along the inferior edge of the supinator muscle, but the vessels can be easily injured.*

Pitfalls

- *Rarely, the pedicle for this flap is aberrantly located between the abductor pollicis longus, extensor pollicis longus, and extensor indicis proprius. Separation of the pedicle from the skin paddle can be avoided by identification of the vessels distally to ensure proper pedicle dissection.*
- *The motor branch to the extensor carpi ulnaris occasionally travels superficial to the PIA at the level of the inferior supinator, which can limit the arc of rotation.*
- *If paratenon is taken, the donor site skin graft will not take.*

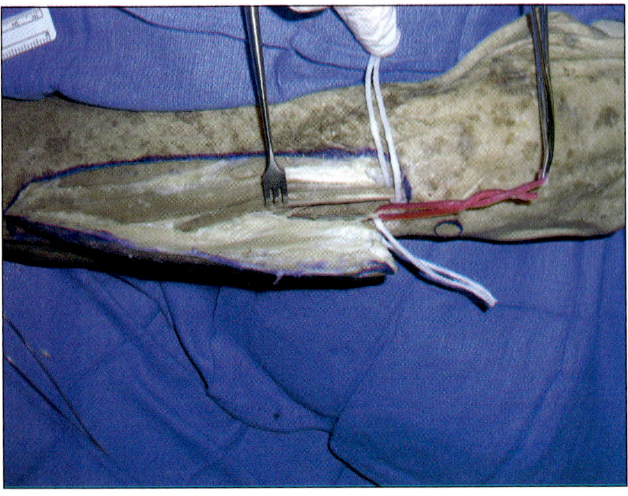

FIGURE 3

distal posterior interosseous vessel can be identified and divided along with its venae comitantes (see Fig. 3).

- The pedicle proximal to this can be elevated with the flap back to the level of the supinator muscle, where the pedicle enters the dorsal forearm through the interosseous membrane (Fig. 4). Note that the pedicle is very small and the septocutaneous perforators are fragile and can be accidentally separated. The posterior interosseous nerve (shown with the yellow loop in Fig. 4) must be preserved. The flap rotates around this point, which is typically 6 cm distal to the lateral epicondyle.
- Although the flap can be taken as an island flap, venous congestion can be avoided by leaving the cutaneous base of the flap intact.

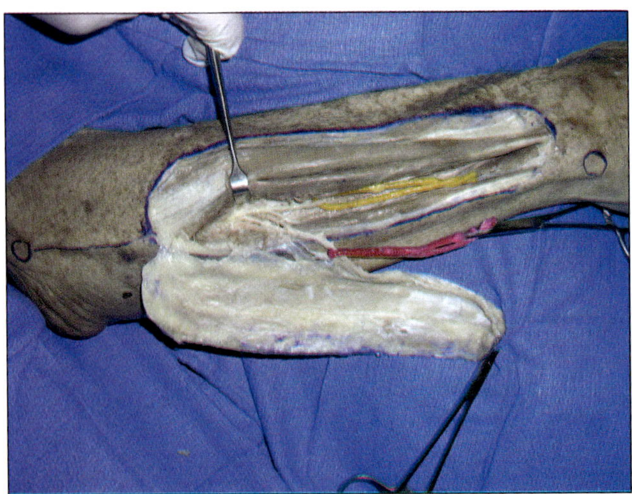

FIGURE 4

Pearls

- *Negative pressure dressings over the donor site skin graft for 3–5 days, with a splint to immobilize the fingers for 7–10 days, will prevent shearing and increase graft take.*
- *If possible, primarily close the distal flap harvest sites to prevent exposure of the ulna and the extensor tendons.*

Pitfalls

- *Excessive tension at the donor site can result in wound breakdown and subsequent exposure.*

Step 2: Flap Inset

- These flaps rarely require a tunnel for elbow defect closure, but if used the surgeon must ensure that the passageway is adequate.
- The flap can be rotated to cover most moderate-sized defects of the anterior (Fig. 5A), posterior (Fig. 5B), or lateral (Fig. 5C) elbow.
- The flap can be inset with a series of deep dermal interrupted, buried absorbable sutures. Over that, staples or sutures can be used to approximate the skin edges. A drain can be used deep to the flap.

Step 3: Donor Site Closure

- The donor site can be closed primarily if a smaller skin paddle has been harvested. If not, a skin graft can be applied.

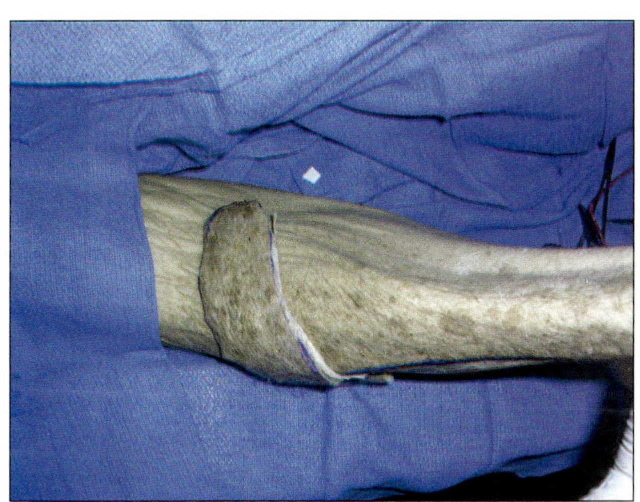

A

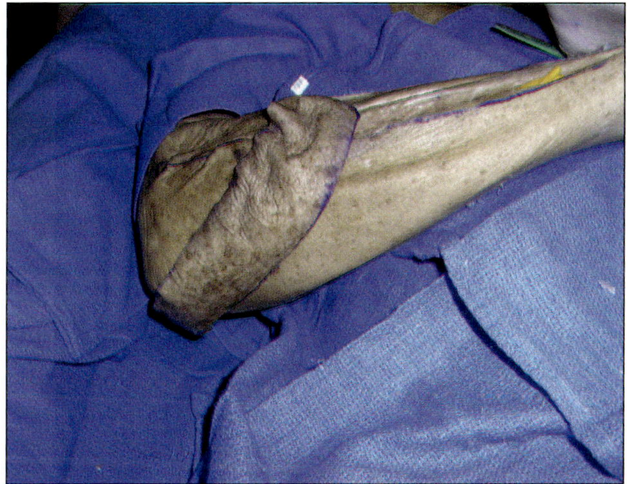

B

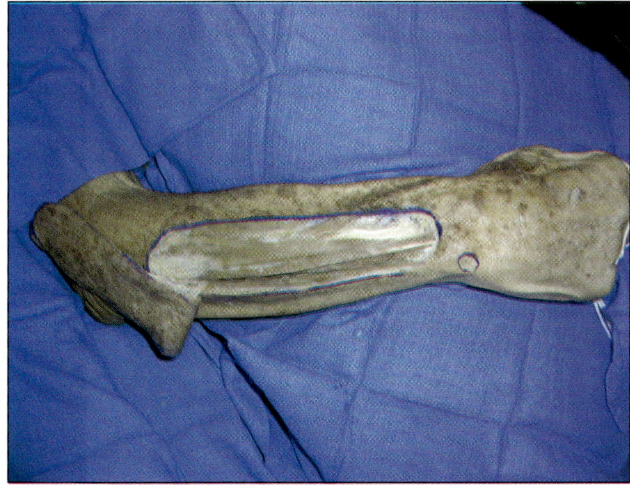

C

FIGURE 5

- Meshed split-thickness grafts have a high success rate, but exposure of extensor tendons or of the ulna can require secondary procedures.

PEARLS

- *If venous congestion develops, stitch removal might allow better outflow. If noted in the operating room, a microscopic venous anastomosis may augment outflow. Also, leech therapy may be used to salvage the flap.*

PITFALLS

- *A negative pressure dressing or a bolster will improve donor site skin graft adherence, but without a hand/wrist splint, shearing of the skin graft can still occur.*

Postoperative Care and Expected Outcomes

- The arm should be elevated to control edema, and the recipient site should be splinted to avoid direct pressure on the flap itself. Also, the hand and wrist should be put in a safe position splint not only for comfort and edema control, but to allow the donor site skin graft to adhere.
- The flap should be monitored for the development of venous congestion. If suture release does not relieve the congestion, leech therapy or a microscopic venous anastomosis may be required.
- Once the reconstruction permits, therapy should be initiated.
- The most troublesome complication aside from flap failure is donor site exposure that can require prolonged wound care, distal tissue rearrangement, or additional skin grafting. Integra may be required for persistent wounds.

Evidence

Costa H, Comba S, Martins A, Rodriques J, Reis J, Amarante J. Further experience with posterior interosseous flap. Br J Plast Surg. 1991;44:449.

Using a cadaver model, the blood supply to the posterior interosseous artery flap is described. A case series including 21 patients using this flap was also described. (Grade C recommendation; Level V evidence)

Costa H, Soutar DS. The distally based island posterior interoseous flap. Br J Plast Surg. 1988;41:221.

Using cadaver models, the authors precisely described the vascular anatomy of the posterior interosseous artery and its potential as a distally based fasciocutaneous flap. Three cases were described using the flap. (Grade C recommendation; Level V evidence)

PROCEDURE 62

Soft Tissue Coverage IV: Brachioradialis Muscle Flap

Wesley P. Thayer and R. Bruce Shack

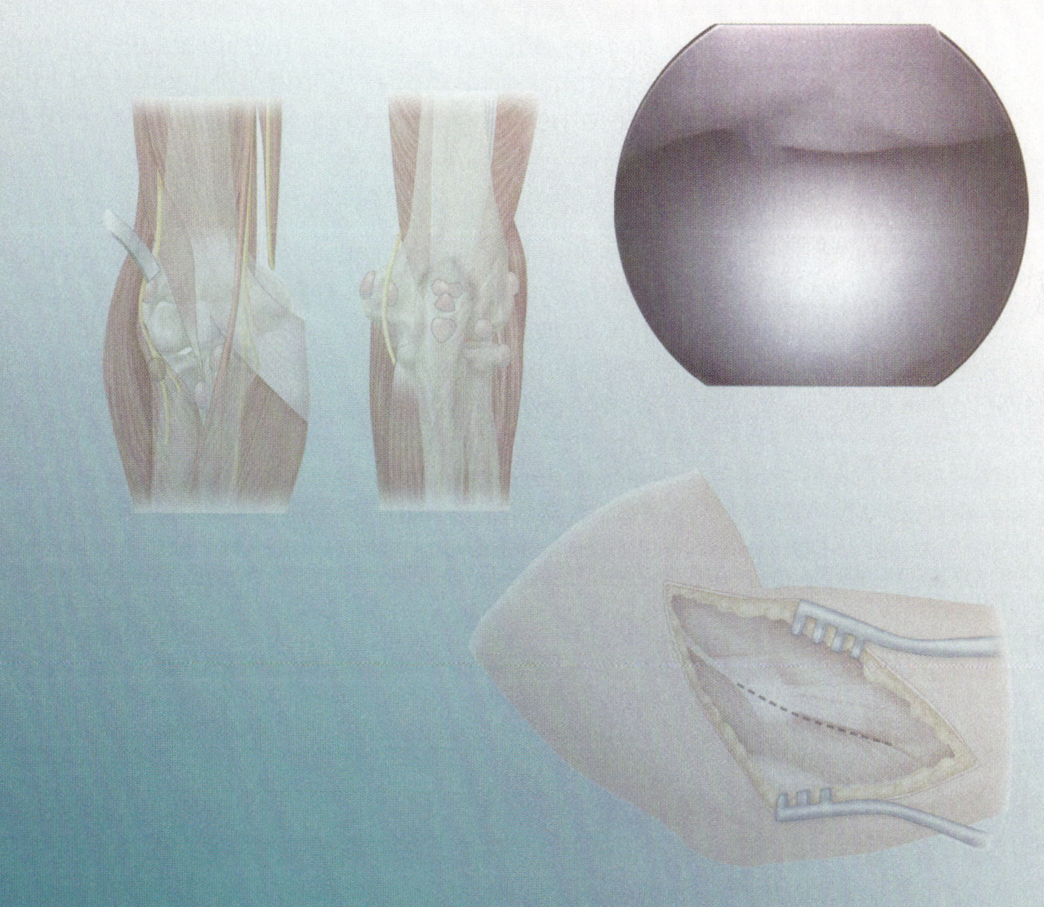

PITFALLS

- *This flap is a poor choice for medial, posterior, or large defects.*

Controversies

- Although a myocutaneous version of the flap can be rotated to close the defect, this typically results in a bulky tissue deformity.
- If concomitant injury to the other elbow flexors is present, this flap is a poor choice.

Treatment Options

- Local flap alternatives for elbow coverage include the radial forearm flap, the latissimus dorsi flap, the posterior interosseous flap, the reverse lateral arm flap, and the flexor carpi ulnaris flap.
- Rarely, a wound vacuum-assisted closure device with or without Integra is indicated for elbow coverage.
- Free tissue transfer may be required if local tissues or flaps are not available.

Indications

- Although the radial forearm flap is the most versatile flap for elbow coverage, its donor site scar is substantial. For cases where the defect is small and is located more in the anterolateral or posterolateral elbow, the brachioradialis muscle flap may be a more appropriate choice. Most surgeons choose to use this flap as a muscle flap only, with an overlying skin graft.

Examination/Imaging

- The radial aspect of the forearm must be examined to rule out injury to the brachioradialis. Doppler examination is not required. Concomitant injury to the other elbow flexors precludes the use of this flap.

Surgical Anatomy

- The brachioradialis muscle flap can be designed as either a purely muscle or a musculocutaneous flap. The primary function of this muscle is elbow flexion, and it also provides pronation or supination depending on the position of the forearm.
- The dominant pedicle for this flap is the radial recurrent artery and venae comitantes (Fig. 1A and 1B). Average length of this vessel is approximately 3 cm; it typically has a diameter of 1 mm. The radial recurrent artery is a branch of the radial artery in the proximal forearm and is located at the level of the insertion of the biceps to the radius. There is also a minor pedicle to this muscle via the radial collateral

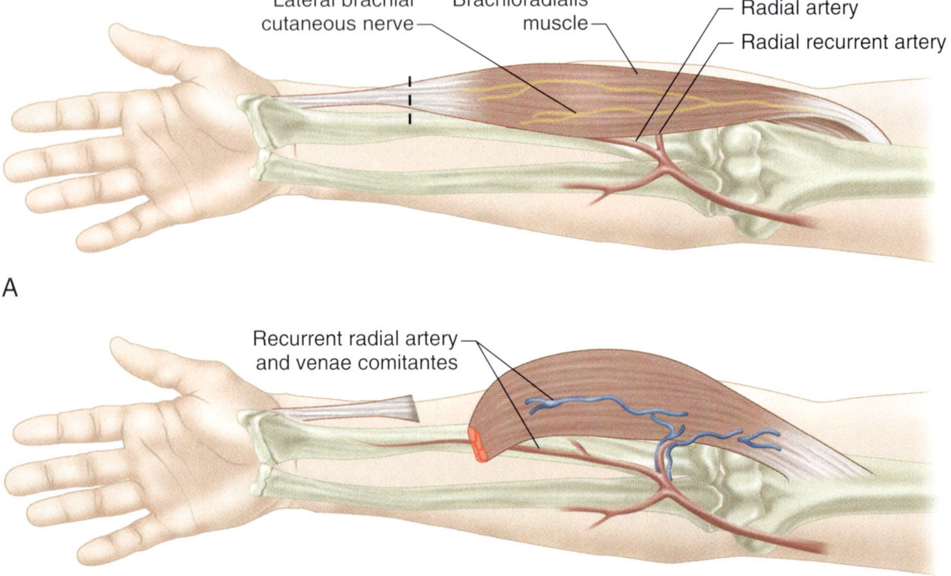

FIGURE 1

artery located between the brachioradialis and brachialis muscles. Finally, muscular branches of the radial artery and vein provide segmental flow to the middle and distal third of the muscle belly.

- The lateral muscular branches of the radial nerve supply motor innervation to the brachioradialis muscle. Sensation to the region overlying the brachioradialis muscle is from the lateral antebrachial cutaneous nerve.

Positioning

- The patient is placed in supine position.
- The arm is placed on a standard armboard and is prepped to the shoulder.
- A sterile tourniquet is required for this dissection.

Pearls

- *Do not forget to prep the donor site for an overlay skin graft.*

Pitfalls

- *Application of a nonsterile tourniquet can result in inadequate exposure of the elbow for inset.*

Equipment

- Armboard
- Sterile tourniquet

Portals/Exposures

- The brachioradialis muscle is located in the radial forearm and has a total length of approximately 15 cm. Its narrows in the distal third of the forearm, where it begins to insert on the radius.
- For a muscle flap, the incision starts just beyond the lateral epicondyles and extends to the distal forearm. If desired, a skin territory for this flap is located directly over the muscle. The muscle can be palpated in the lateral forearm with elbow flexion against resistance. The muscle transitions to tendon in the distal forearm.

Pearls

- *If possible, mark the incision preoperatively with active elbow flexion against resistance to identify the muscle belly.*

Pitfalls

- *Coverage of posterior, medial, or circumferential defects can be limited due to the thin nature of this muscle distally and due to the limited arc of rotation.*

Procedure

Step 1: Flap Elevation

- Once the incision is marked, using tourniquet control, an incision is made directly down to the muscle belly. If a skin paddle is desired, preserve a wide fascial base and approach the muscle from the sides, rather than risking separation of the skin paddle from the muscle. If possible, extend the skin incision into the defect.
- For the simple muscle flap, the incision starts proximally and extends distally. The dorsal and medial antebrachial cutaneous nerves on the superficial surface of the muscle belly must be identified and protected. Distally the tendon insertion is identified (Fig. 2; the white loop is the distal tendon, the yellow loop is the superficial sensory branch of the radial nerve). From the volar aspect,

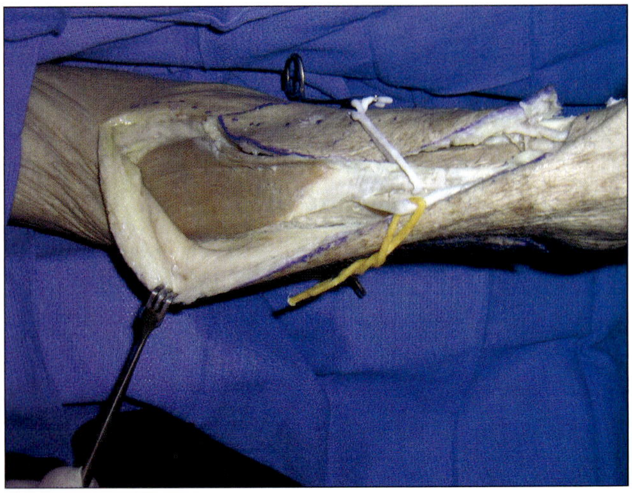

FIGURE 2

the insertion of the muscle can be sharply separated from the radius using a #15 blade.

- The insertion can now be retracted and the minor pedicles from the radial artery can be divided with bipolar cautery. Care must be taken to preserve the superficial sensory branch of the radial nerve, which lies deep to the brachioradialis (see Fig. 2). Blunt dissection should be used in the proximal third of the forearm with loupe magnification to identify the recurrent radial artery.
- The muscle is now ready to inset.

PEARLS

- *The blood flow to this flap enters distal to the muscle origin. As a result, there is no advantage to releasing the origin or dissecting proximal to the flap's dominant blood supply, the recurrent radial artery.*

PITFALLS

- *During dissection, the superficial branch of the radial nerve is at risk of injury. This is also true for the deep branch of the radial nerve in the proximal forearm.*

STEP 2: FLAP INSET

- If the muscle flap is used, it is rotated 90° and tacked down to cover the soft tissue defect with absorbable sutures.
    - The muscle is best suited for coverage of small lateral defects. In Figure 3, rotation to the lateral elbow is noted.

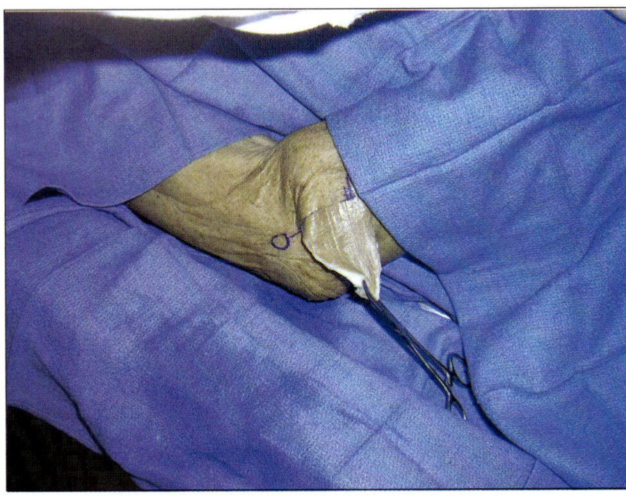

FIGURE 3

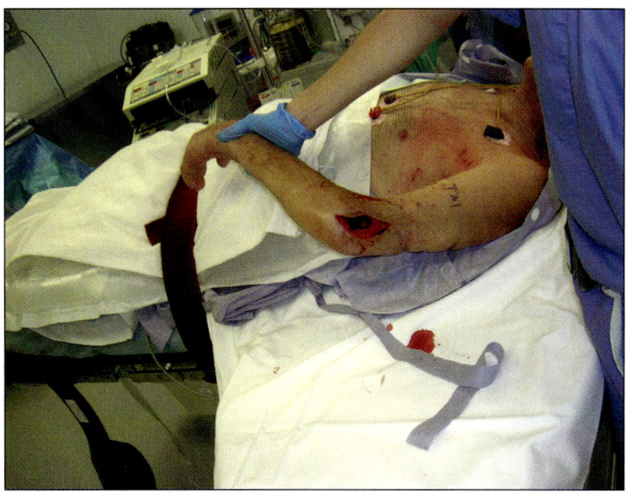

FIGURE 4

PITFALLS

- *Although a tunnel may be used to transpose the muscle to the soft tissue defect, this may result in flap compromise due to excessive tension or twisting.*

- We have successfully used this flap for coverage of a lateral elbow defect over an area of osteomyelitis (Fig. 4).
- Once elevated (Fig. 5A), the muscle can be rotated laterally (Fig. 5B) and inset over a drain (Fig. 5C).

- If a skin island has been designed, once the muscle has been inset, the skin edges can be approximated. This is best accomplished by extending the donor site incision to the point where it joins the soft tissue defect.

PEARLS

- *Using a negative-pressure dressing over the donor site skin graft for 3–5 days with a splint to immobilize the fingers for 7–10 days will prevent shearing and increase graft take.*
- *Primarily close the distal flap harvest site if no skin paddle was taken.*

PITFALLS

- *If the myocutaneous portion of the flap is used, a skin graft is often required to close the donor site.*

STEP 3: CLOSURE

- A meshed split-thickness skin graft can then be placed over the brachioradialis muscle. The result shown in Figure 6 is on postoperative day 7, at 2 days after takedown of the negative pressure dressing.

Postoperative Care and Expected Outcomes

- The arm should be elevated to control edema, and the recipient site should be splinted to avoid direct pressure on the flap itself.
- Although hematomas, infection, and vascular insufficiency can occur, the worst complication is failure to close the defect, requiring an additional procedure.
  - If the flap develops congestion that fails to respond to position changes, some stitches should be removed, or the skin tunnel should be released. If this fails to alleviate the problem, a

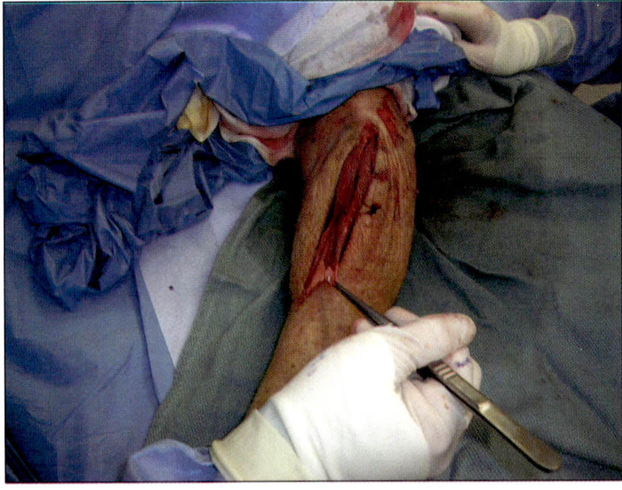
A

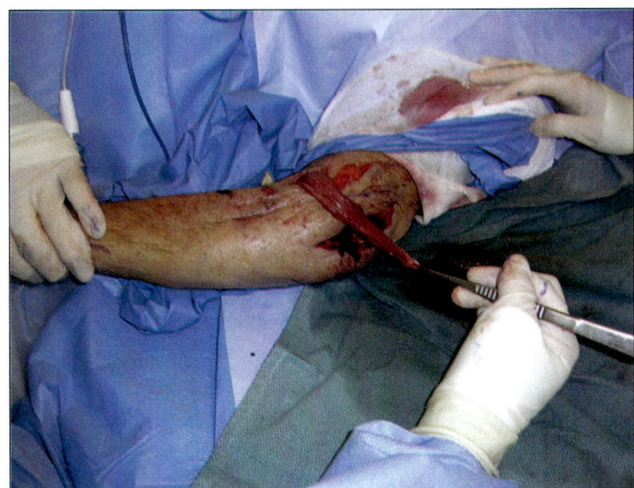
B

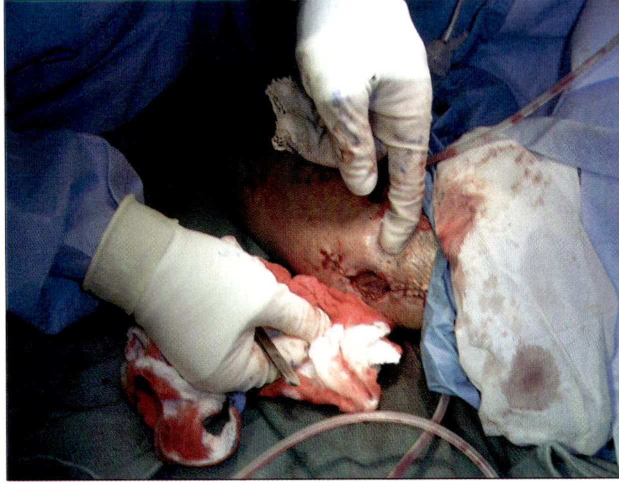
C

FIGURE 5

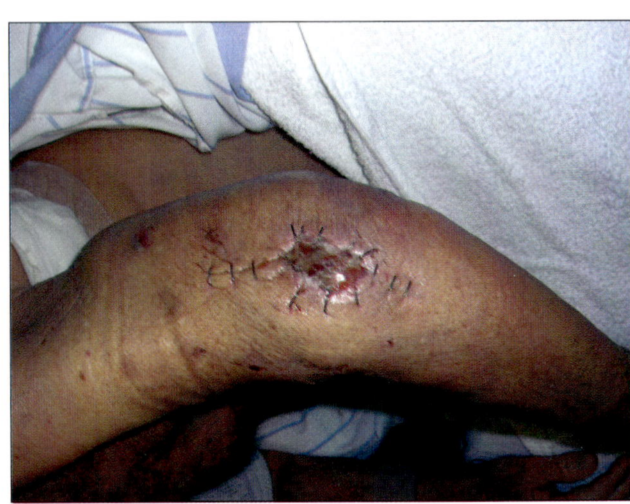

FIGURE 6

Pearls

- *At least 1 week of immobilization is required before initiating therapy if the skin graft is used.*

Pitfalls

- *A negative-pressure dressing or a bolster will improve donor site skin graft adherence, but without an elbow splint, shearing of the skin graft can still occur.*

re-exploration is warranted for pedicle kinking. If these interventions fail, a second coverage procedure may be required.
  - A negative-pressure dressing applied over the skin graft, which is itself covered with a Xeroform dressing, will increase the graft take and help control serous drainage. Occasionally, a small persistent defect can be resolved using the negative-pressure dressing without additional operative intervention.
- Once the reconstruction permits and the skin graft is adherent, therapy should be initiated.

Evidence

Hodgkinson DJ, Shepard GH. Muscle, musculocutaneous, and fasciocutaneous flaps in forearm reconstruction. Ann Plast Surg. 1983;10:400.

Four cases were presented, and the anatomy and clinical applications of the flaps were discussed. (Grade C recommendation; Level V evidence)

Lai MF, Krishna BV, Pelly AD. The brachioradialis myocutaneous flap. B J Plast Surg. 1981;34:431.

This cadaveric study demonstrated the relevant anatomy of the brachioradialis myocutaneous flap, with case reports. (Grade C recommendation; Level V evidence)

Lendrum J. Alternatives to amputation. Ann R Coll Surg Engl. 1980;62:95.

This case series described the author's use of muscle flaps to salvage limbs with chronic osteomyelitis. (Grade C recommendation; Level V evidence)

PROCEDURE 62

Soft Tissue Coverage V: Reverse Lateral Arm Flap

Wesley P. Thayer and R. Bruce Shack

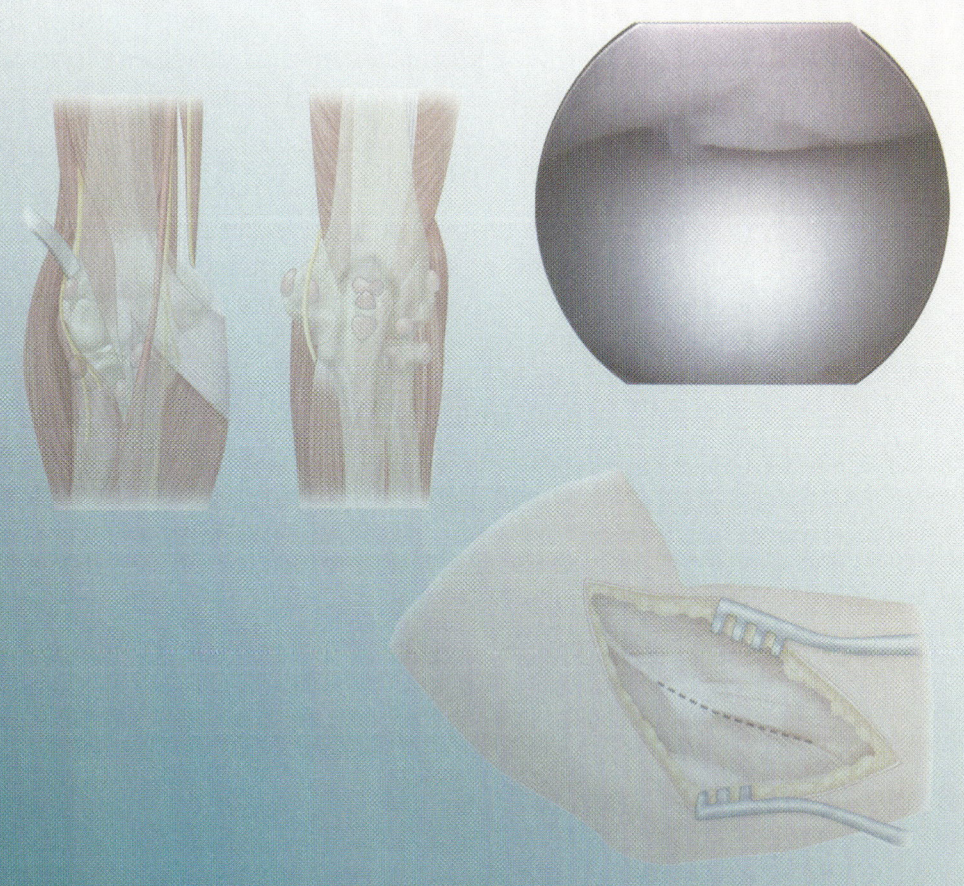

Pitfalls

- *This flap should not be used when significant trauma has occurred proximal to the lateral epicondyles as the recurrent radial artery will be in the zone of injury.*
- *This flap is a poor choice for medial defects due to an inadequate arc of rotation.*

Controversies

- Although a skin paddle as large as 8 × 15 cm can be designed, if the width of the flap is over 6 cm, the donor site cannot be primarily closed.
- Patients who have undergone prior elbow procedures may have had the radial recurrent artery sacrificed during their earlier procedures.

Treatment Options

- Local flap alternatives for elbow coverage include the radial forearm flap, the posterior interosseous flap, the latissimus dorsi flap, the flexor carpi ulnaris flap, and the brachioradialis flap.
- Rarely, a negative-pressure dressing with or without Integra is indicated for elbow coverage.
- Free tissue transfer may be required if local tissues are damaged and if the latissimus flap is not available.

Indications

- The reverse lateral arm flap may be used to cover defects of the antecubital fossa, distal lateral elbow, and posterior elbow. This fasciocutaneous flap is most frequently used in free tissue transfer cases, but can be used for elbow coverage when its blood supply is not in the zone of injury. It is best suited for cases in which the lateral epicondyle is not included in the zone of injury and when the defect is either mostly anterior or mostly posterior.
- There are number of advantages to using this flap, including the lack of an associated functional impairment at the donor site, no need to sacrifice a major blood vessel, and a better blood supply than local fasciocutaneous flaps.

Examination/Imaging

- The elbow must be examined to ensure that the zone of injury does not include the blood supply for this flap, the radial recurrent artery. This vessel anastomoses with the radial collateral artery just posterior to the lateral epicondyle.
- It is critical to perform a Doppler examination before the dissection is initiated to ensure that the radial collateral vessel can be identified in the intermuscular septum. Preoperative angiography can be performed if there is any question to ensure that the blood supply is intact.

Surgical Anatomy

- This fasciocutaneous flap allows for a maximum skin paddle size of 8 × 15 cm. This includes an area of skin in the distal two thirds of the lateral arm between the lateral epicondyles and the insertion of the deltoid. It is centered over the lateral intermuscular septum.
- The dominant pedicle to this flap is the radial collateral artery, which is a branch of the profunda brachii artery (Fig. 1). When designed as a standard flap, this pedicle has a length of 7 cm. However, for elbow coverage the reverse flap must be designed. In this case, the blood supply comes from a minor pedicle, the radial recurrent artery. The radial recurrent artery is a branch of the radial artery and arises in the cubital fossa. It courses laterally and then superiorly along the brachioradialis. Just

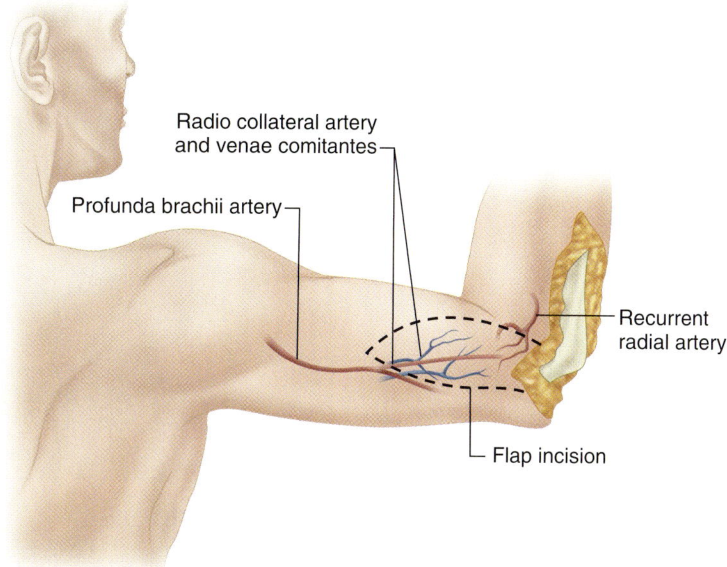

FIGURE 1

proximal to the lateral epicondyles the radial recurrent artery forms an anastomosis with the radial collateral artery.

- Musculocutaneous perforating arteries also provide minor pedicle blood supply to this region of skin directly from the triceps and brachialis muscles. These are divided during the dissection.

- The majority of the sensory innervation is from the posterior brachial cutaneous nerve. This is a branch of the radial nerve and, when used for free tissue transfer, this nerve can be used to generate a sensate flap. The posterior antebrachial cutaneous nerve is also a branch of the radial nerve and it courses with the posterior radial collateral artery. The nerve divides in the distal arm and generates branches that supply the lateral and posterior arm.

PEARLS

- *Although this flap can be harvested with the patient in the supine position using a standard arm table, continuous retraction from an assistant will be needed for the more posterior aspects of the dissection and during inset.*

PITFALLS

- *Application of a nonsterile tourniquet will result in inadequate exposure.*

Equipment

- Sterile tourniquet

Positioning

- The patient is placed in the supine position, and arm is positioned with the elbow flexed and the forearm laying over the abdomen.
- The entire arm and axilla are prepped into the field, and a sterile tourniquet is used.

PEARLS

- *The Doppler examination is critical to validate blood flow to the flap, particularly in patients who have had prior elbow surgery or have significant lateral elbow trauma.*

PITFALLS

- *Coverage of medial defects can be limited due to insufficient arc of rotation.*

Portals/Exposures

- The flap is located between the insertion of the deltoid and the lateral epicondyle of the humerus. Both of these can be palpated on examination. The

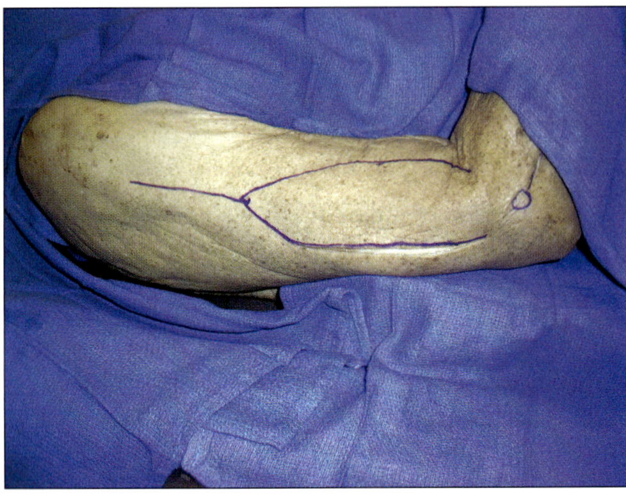

FIGURE 2

flap is centered over line between the mid-deltoid and the lateral epicondyle. The maximum width of the flap is 8 cm; however, it is more typically designed with a 6-cm width. The length of the flap can be up to 15 cm long for the standard flap; however, for the reverse flap is typically less than 12 cm.

- The radial collateral artery should be evaluated with Doppler ultrasound to validate flap design. This vessel is located in the lateral intermuscular septum and courses lateral to the posterior edge of the deltoid muscle under the lateral head of the triceps.
- If at all possible, a distal skin bridge or fascial bridge is designed with the flap to provide improved venous outflow (Fig. 2).

PEARLS

- *By using a sterile tourniquet, more accurate dissection of the vascular pedicle and radial nerve can be achieved.*

PITFALLS

- *The radial nerve is subject to injury during flap elevation. This is particularly true at the level of the deltoid insertion. The radial nerve passes deep to the posterior radial collateral artery in the spiral groove of the humerus. The nerve continues inferiorly beneath the brachialis and brachioradialis muscles. It must be identified and protected during the dissection. Retraction on the nerve must be gentle to prevent postoperative deficit.*
- *Prior injury or trauma may result in compromise of the retrograde flow that is required for perfusion of the reversed lateral arm flap. For this reason, a skin bridge of 3+ cm should be maintained to allow for improved outflow.*

Procedure

STEP 1: FLAP ELEVATION

- Once the skin paddle is marked, the initial incision is made proximal to the actual skin paddle. This vertical extension is located at the posterior edge of the deltoid muscle. This is used to identify and expose the proximal vasculature of the pedicle, the radial collateral artery and vein. Once these are identified, they can be more easily preserved during the more distal dissection.
- The dissection is then continued on the posterior arm. The incision is carried down to and through the deep fascia overlying the triceps muscle (Fig. 3). The fascia is divided directly beneath the posterior aspect of the skin paddle. The fascia is then sutured to the

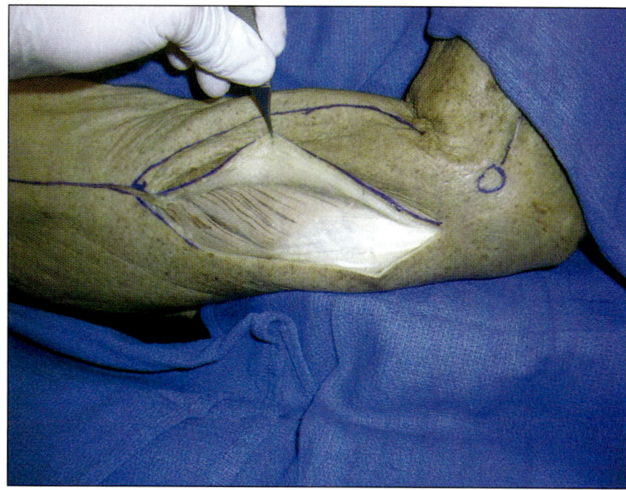

FIGURE 3

Controversies

- Microsurgical anastomosis may be required to improve venous outflow if it is insufficient. This is more commonly noted when the arc of rotation required approaches 180°, and can be avoided by designing a skin bridge with the flap.

deep dermal layer of the skin. The fascia is then elevated off the muscle belly of the triceps toward the intermuscular septum.

- At this point the posterior radial collateral artery, which had been located during the more proximal dissection, can be identified where it continues in the lateral intermuscular septum.
- The anterior dissection is made now through the skin and the fascia overlying the brachialis muscle. Again this fascia is tacked to the overlying skin, and the dissection is continued laterally toward the lateral intermuscular septum.
- The posterior radial collateral artery must now be mobilized away from the radial nerve. The radial nerve can be located just anterior to the radial collateral artery. Care must be taken to prevent injury to this nerve during the remainder of this flap dissection (Fig. 4).

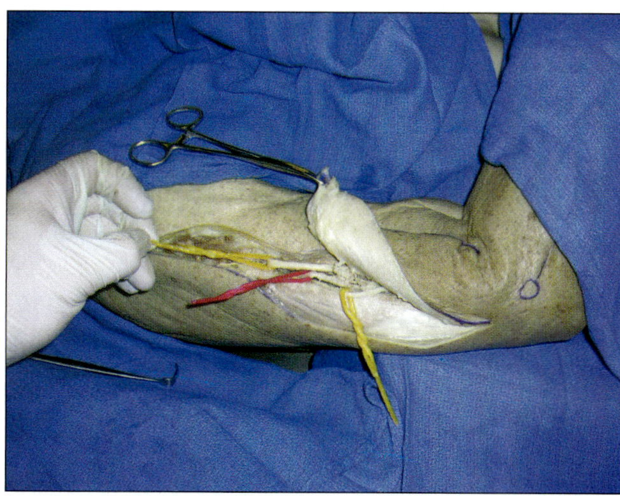

FIGURE 4

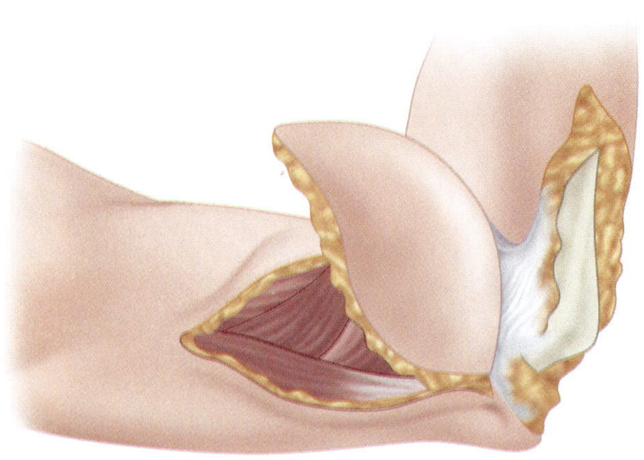

A

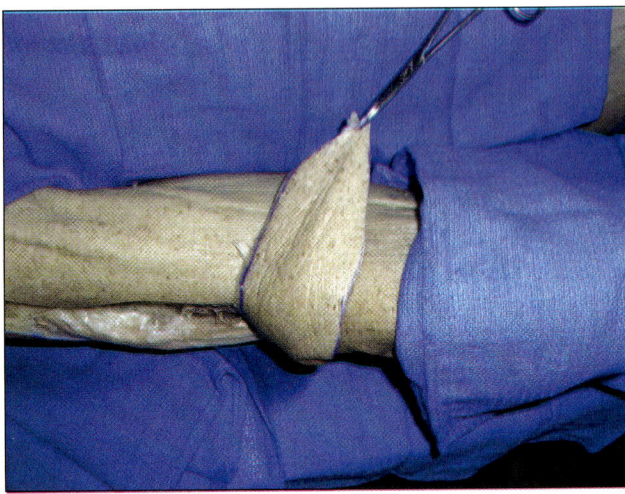

B

FIGURE 5

> **PEARLS**
>
> - *If during inset venous congestion is noted and cannot be overcome, the flap may need to be set back in its original position and inset delayed for 1–2 weeks. A negative-pressure dressing can be placed at the recipient site and regularly changed while the flap is allowed to mature.*

> **PITFALLS**
>
> - *If the donor site is over 6 cm in width, a skin graft may not be required for closure. If a skin graft is used, the elbow should be immobilized for at least 7 days to prevent shearing of the skin graft.*

- Any muscular branches to the skin paddle are divided. The intermuscular septum is kept with the skin paddle along with the radial collateral vessel. Once this vessel has been identified proximally, it is divided to facilitate the more distal dissection. Also, the intermuscular septum is divided sharply and elevated away from the humerus, taking care to preserve the vasculature in the intermuscular septum with the skin paddle.
- The dissection is continued more distally were the radial collateral artery joins the radial recurrent artery. If at all possible, a skin bridge of 3+ cm is kept over the lateral epicondyles to help preserve the distal blood supply to the flap.

STEP 2: FLAP INSET

- The anterior arc of rotation allows for coverage of antecubital defects (Fig. 5A and 5B).
- These flaps are typically inset over a drain.

STEP 3 CLOSURE

- The closure is usually two layers, with a deep absorbable stitch and then a more superficial either nylon or stapled closure (Fig. 6; skin graft is shown at donor site).

Postoperative Care and Expected Outcomes

- The arm should be elevated to control edema, and the recipient site should be splinted to avoid direct pressure on the flap itself.

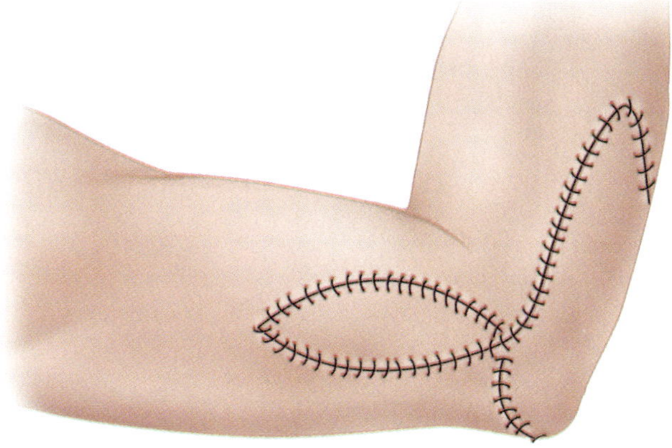

FIGURE 6

PEARLS

- *If no skin graft is applied, therapy can be in the early postoperative period.*

PITFALLS

- *The flap should be monitored for venous congestion. Stitches may need to be removed in order to allow flow, or the flap may even need to be delayed if inadequate outflow develops.*

- The drain is typically removed on postoperative day 1.
- The flap should be monitored for the development of venous congestion and stitches released if needed.
- Hematomas, infection, and vascular insufficiency can also occur. Occasionally, the tip of the flap will necrose, resulting in failure to close the defect. If this occurs, débridement followed by a negative-pressure dressing application may alleviate the need for a more complex procedure.
- Once the reconstruction permits, therapy should be initiated.

Evidence

Culbertson JH, Mutimer K. The reverse lateral upper arm flap for elbow coverage. Ann Plast Surg. 1987;18:62.

The authors reported a case series including the use of two radial recurrent fasciocutaneous flaps. (Grade C recommendation; Level V evidence)

Maruyama Y, Takeuchi S: The radial recurrent fasciocutaneous flap: reverse upper arm flap. Br J Plast Surg. 1986;39:458-61.

The authors reported a case series including the use of three radial recurrent fasciocutaneous flaps. (Grade C recommendation; Level V evidence)

PROCEDURE 63

Operative Treatment of Olecranon Bursitis

Donald H. Lee and John M. Erickson

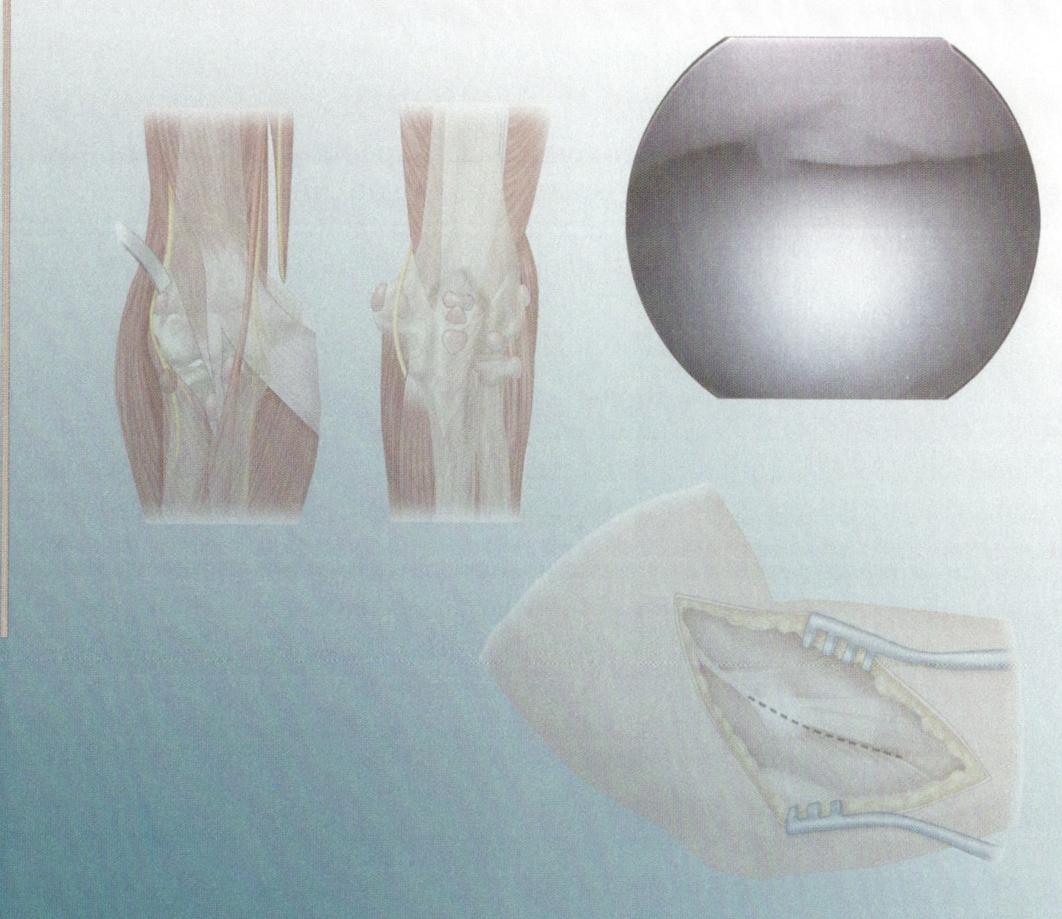

Pitfalls

- *Potential postoperative complications include wound healing problems, seroma or hematoma formation, recurrence of bursa, and chronic fistula.*

Controversies

- Rule out disruption of the triceps tendon insertion masquerading as olecranon bursitis.

Treatment Options

- Other treatment options for a chronic bursa include aspiration with or without steroid injection and use of an indwelling catheter and compression dressing.

Pearls

- *Use of an S-shaped incision may allow for mobilization of flaps proximally and distally to allow for wound closure if needed (see Fig. 5).*

Indications

- Chronic olecranon bursitis, refractory to nonoperative measures, interfering with daily or occupational activities
- Septic olecranon bursitis
- Olecranon bursitis related to chronic inflammatory conditions (e.g., rheumatoid arthritis, gout)

Examination/Imaging

- Anteroposterior (Fig. 1A) and lateral (Fig. 1B) radiographs of the elbow are taken to look for an olecranon osteophyte.

Surgical Anatomy

- There are several superficial and deep bursae around the elbow (Fig. 2A and 2B).
- The superficial subcutaneous olecranon bursa is the most clinically important (Fig. 3A and 3B).

Positioning

- Supine with arm table
- Alternatively, supine with arm across chest

Portals/Exposures

- A posterior approach is made using a curvilinear longitudinal incision (Fig. 4).
- Alternatively, an S-shaped incision is made, centered over the olecranon bursa (Fig. 5).

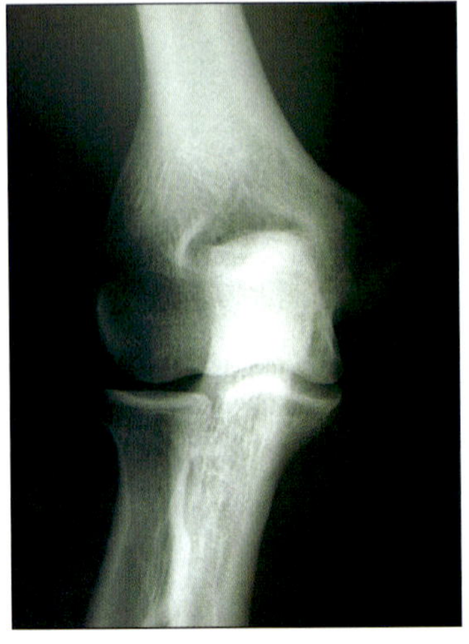

A

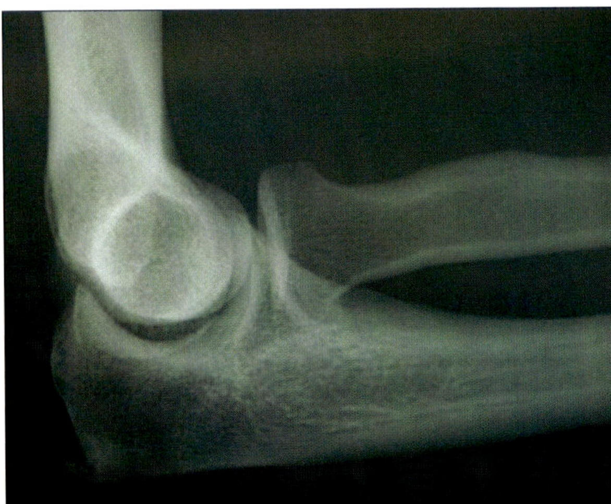

B

FIGURE 1

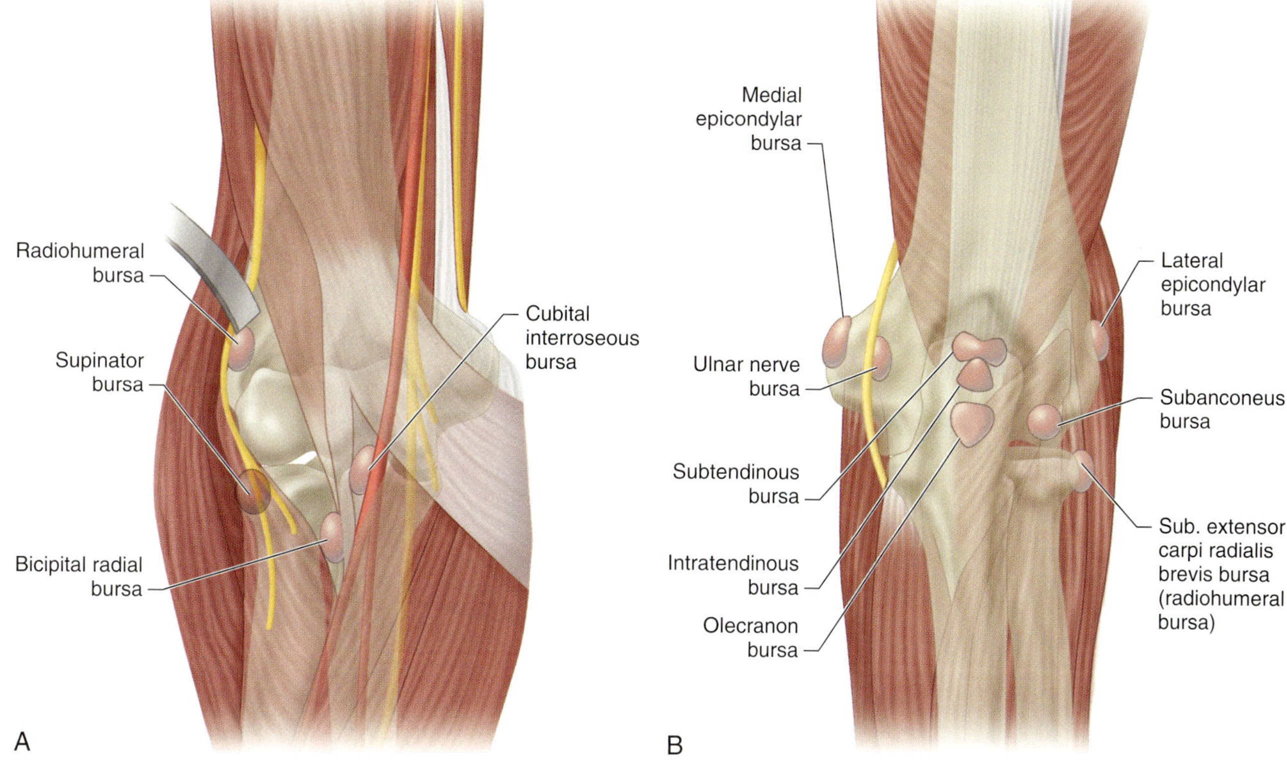

FIGURE 2

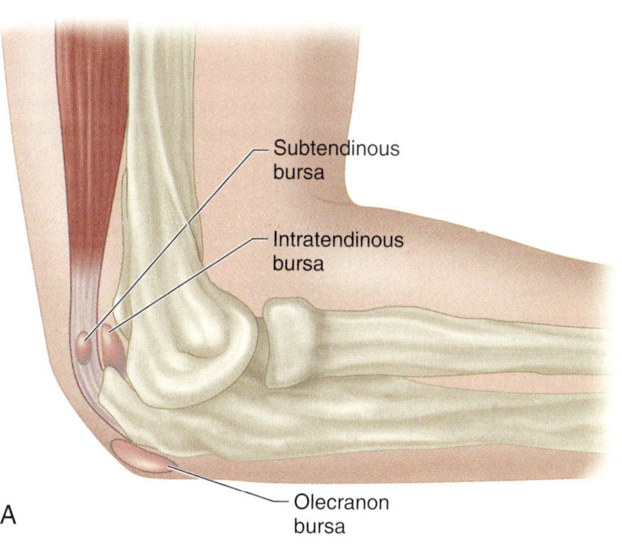

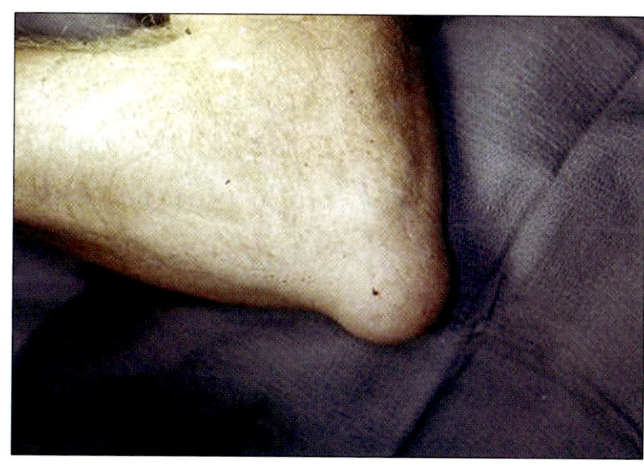

FIGURE 3

Procedure

Step 1: Bursal Drainage and Resection

- After Esmarch exsanguination, an arm tourniquet is elevated to 250 mm Hg.
- Methylene blue can be used to coat the inner layer of the olecranon bursa.

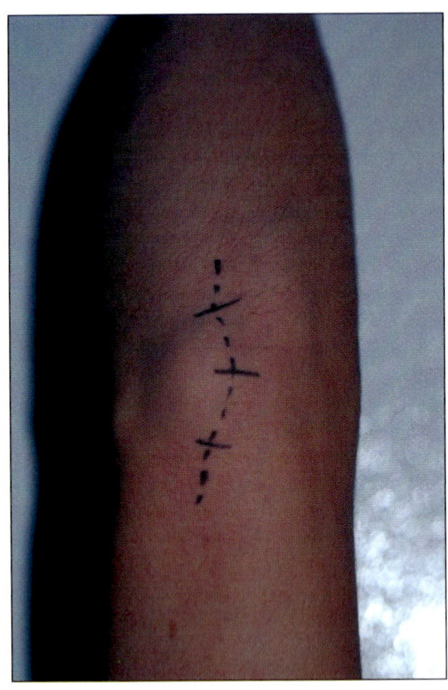

FIGURE 4

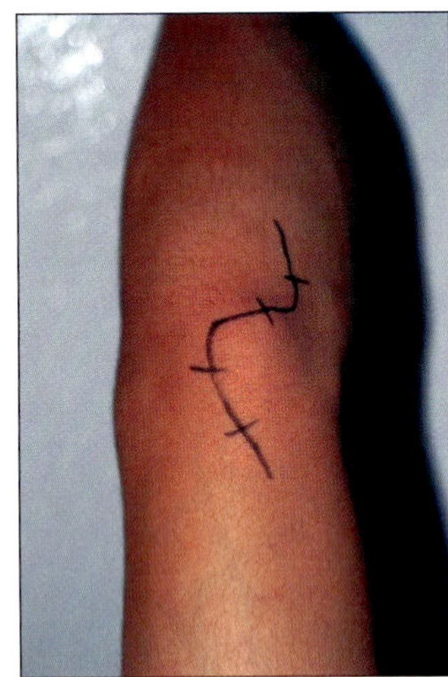

FIGURE 5

PEARLS

- *If wound healing is a potential problem, using an S-shaped incision allows for mobilization of proximal and distal flaps.*

PITFALLS

- *The majority of the methylene blue fluid is re-aspirated to prevent extravasation of a large amount of methylene blue outside of the bursa, coating the outer layer of the bursa.*
- *Alternatively, the methylene blue can be diluted with saline.*

- An empty 20- or 60-ml syringe with an 18-gauge hypodermic needle is used to aspirate the olecranon bursal fluid (Fig. 6).
- After the bursa is drained, the syringe is taken off the needle and the needle tip is left in place within the bursa.
- The clinician may choose to send the aspirate for culture, cytology, and/or crystals.
- Approximately 5 ml of methylene blue is injected through the same needle and as much of the methylene blue is re-aspirated (Fig. 7A and 7B).

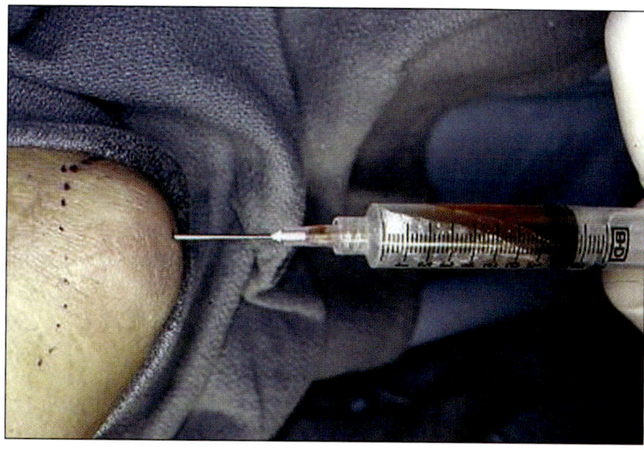

FIGURE 6

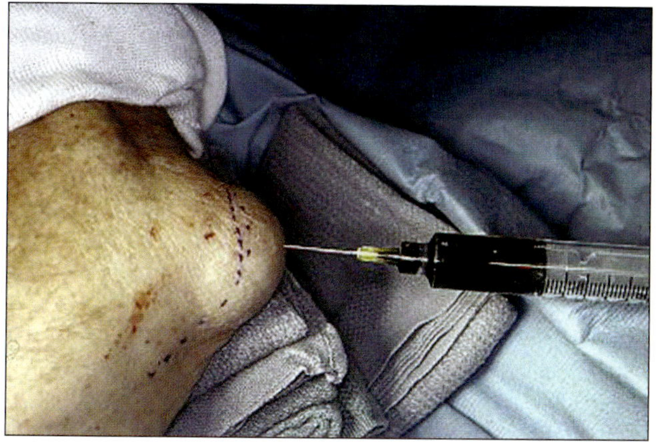

A

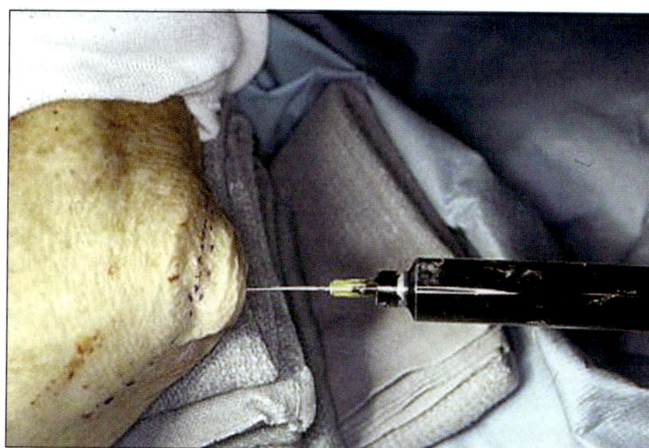

B

FIGURE 7

Instrumentation/ Implantation

- Arm tourniquet (sterile or nonsterile)
- 20- or 60-ml syringe with 18-gauge hypodermic needle
- Methylene blue

Controversies

- Arthroscopic bursectomy has been described.
- Septic bursitis may be treated with bursal fluid drainage and intravenous antibiotics.

  - The needle is carefully removed to prevent extravasation of the methylene blue.
  - The inner layer of the bursa is now coated, making dissection of the bursa easier.
- A posterior elbow incision is made using a curvilinear longitudinal incision around the tip of the olecranon process (see Fig. 4) or an S-shaped incision with the transverse portion of the incision centered over the olecranon bursa or tip of the olecranon process (Fig. 8).
  - The bursa is carefully dissected from the overlying subcutaneous tissue and underlying fascia and triceps tendon (Fig. 9).
  - The bursa can usually be resected intact (Fig. 10).
  - With cases of septic bursitis, the clinician may elect to leave the wound open with wound packing or add a wound vacuum-assisted closure device.

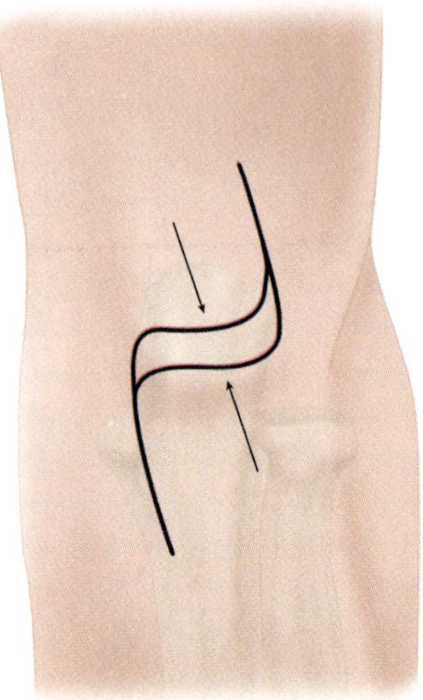

FIGURE 8

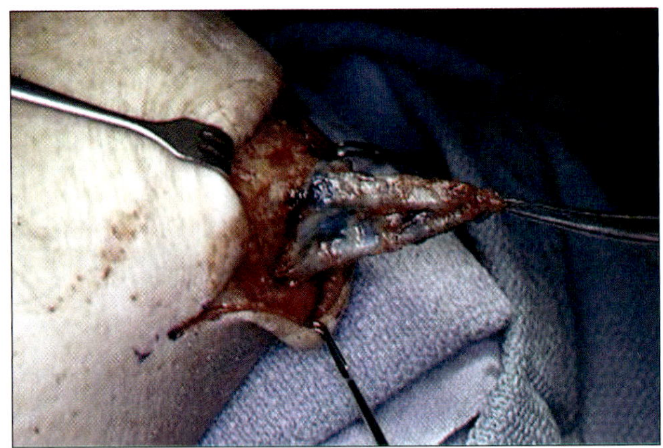

FIGURE 9

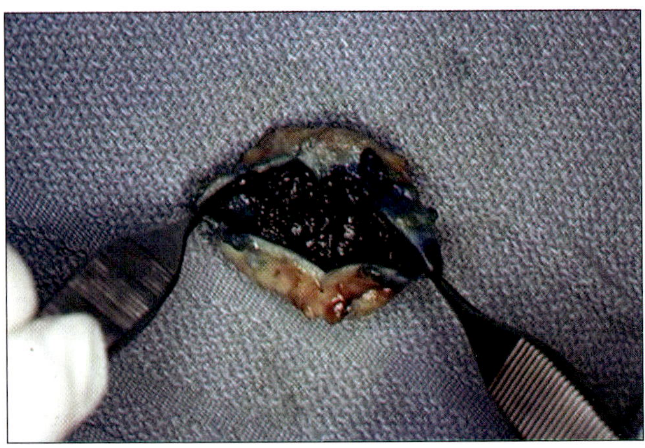

FIGURE 10

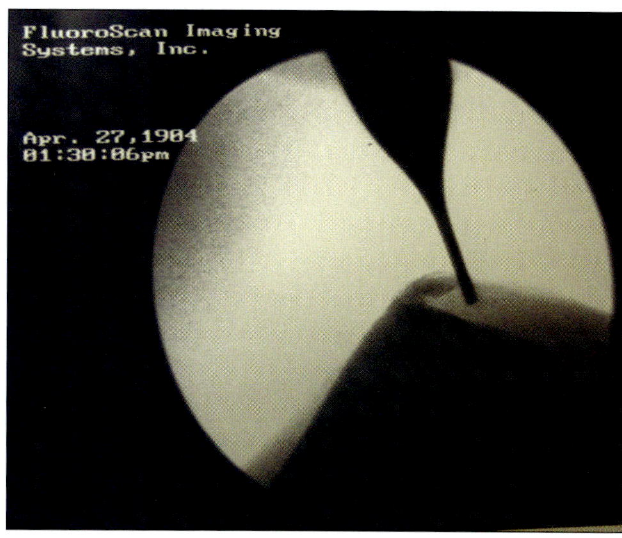

FIGURE 11

Controversies

- Removal of a portion of the olecranon process (without an olecranon osteophyte) has been described.

Pearls

- *If wound closure is difficult or a postoperative wound complication occurs:*
  - *A lateral random rotation flap and skin graft can be used.*
  - *A muscle flap (e.g., anconeus flap) has also been described.*

Step 2: Removal of Olecranon Osteophyte (if Present)

- The osteophyte is identified and overlying soft tissue is elevated. The triceps tendon insertion is split longitudinally over the osteophyte.
- Intraoperative fluoroscopy is helpful in localizing the osteophyte (Fig. 11) and confirming its complete removal.
- An osteotome (Fig. 12) or rongeur is used to resect the osteophyte.
- The longitudinal rent in the triceps tendon is repaired.

Step 3: Wound Closure

- The tourniquet is released.
- Careful hemostasis is required (Fig. 13).

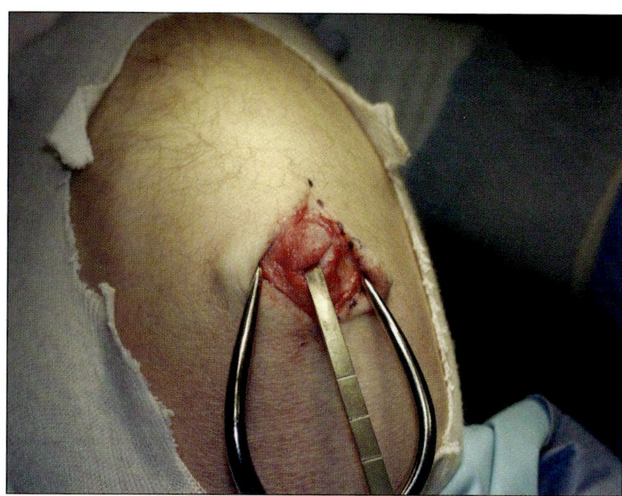

FIGURE 12

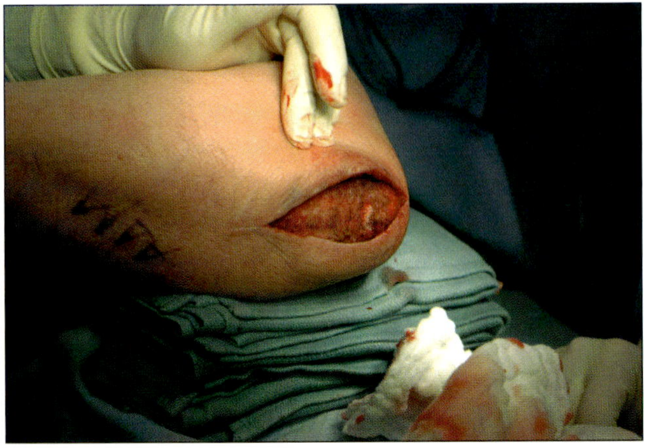

FIGURE 13

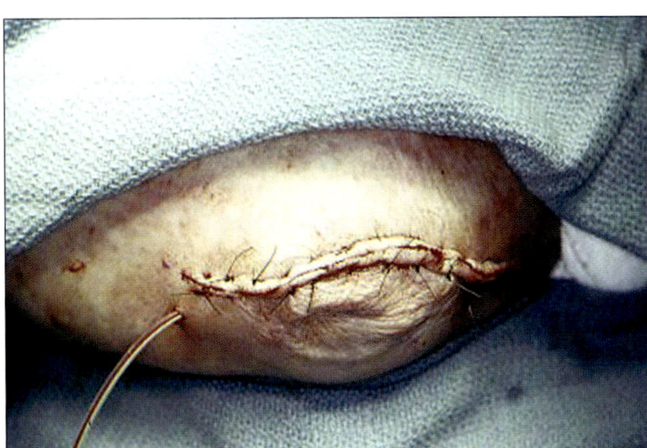

FIGURE 14

- The elevated skin flaps are sutured down to the underlying fascia to minimize open dead space.
- A flexible suction drain is recommended (Fig. 14).
- The skin closed in layers.

Postoperative Care and Expected Outcomes

- A long-arm splint is recommended.
- The suction drain is removed when drainage is minimal (may be done on an outpatient basis).
- Gentle range-of-motion exercises are started when the wound is stable.

> **PEARLS**
>
> - *In cases of a postoperative seroma or hematoma formation, a re-aspiration can be performed.*
> - *The arm is immobilized in a removable long-arm splint or cast.*

Evidence

Canoso JJ. Idiopathic or traumatic olecranon bursitis: clinical features and bursal fluid analysis. Arthritis Rheum. 1977;20:1213-6.

Bursal fluid analysis of aseptic olecranon bursitis was presented in a case series of 30 patients. (Level IV evidence)

Degreef I, De Smet L. Complications following resection of the olecranon bursa. Acta Orthop Belg. 2006;72:400-3.

The authors retrospectively reviewed 37 patients who underwent surgical treatment for olecranon bursitis, highlighting the high complication rate associated with olecranon bursectomy. They reported a 27% incidence of wound healing complications and 22% recurrence rate. (Level IV evidence)

Ho G Jr, Tice AD, Kaplan SR. Septic bursitis in the prepatellar and olecranon bursae: an analysis of 25 cases. Ann Intern Med. 1978;89:21-7.

In this study, 20 patients with septic olecranon bursitis were presented. The authors reported successful eradication of the infection with intravenous antibiotics and drainage of the bursae, emphasizing prompt recognition and treatment to reduce complications. (Level IV evidence)

Kerr DR, Carpenter CW. Arthroscopic resection of olecranon and prepatellar bursae. Arthroscopy. 1990;6:86-8.

Six patients with aseptic olecranon bursitis were treated with arthroscopic bursectomy and reviewed at an average of 6 months postoperatively. Unsatisfactory results were noted in two patients with an underlying inflammatory arthropathy. (Level IV evidence)

Knight JM, Thomas JC, Maurer RC. Treatment of septic olecranon and prepatellar bursitis with percutaneous placement of a suction-irrigation system: a report of 12 cases. Clin Orthop Relat Res. 1986;(206):90-3.

Ten cases of septic olecranon bursitis were satisfactorily treated with percutaneously placed suction and antibiotic irrigation systems. No complications or recurrences were reported by the authors. (Level IV evidence)

Quayle JB, Robinson MP. A useful procedure in the treatment of chronic olecranon bursitis. Injury. 1978;9:299-302.

The authors reviewed 11 patients who were treated with resection of an olecranon spur with preservation of the olecanon bursae. They reported no wound complications and a satisfactory outcome in all patients. (Level IV evidence)

Smith DL, McAfee JH, Lucas LM, Kumar KL, Romney DM. Treatment of nonseptic olecranon bursitis: a controlled, blinded prospective trial. Arch Intern Med. 1989;149:2527-30.

The authors conducted a prospective, randomized controlled trial of 42 patients evaluating the effectiveness of methylprednisolone acetate injection alone or in conjunction with nonsteroidal anti-inflammatory medications versus an oral placebo. They concluded that steroid injection alone was superior to both an oral placebo and steroid injection combined with anti-inflammatory medications. No complications were reported in any treatment group. (Level II evidence)

Stell IM. Management of acute bursitis: outcome study of a structured approach. J R Soc Med. 1999;92:516-21.

The authors presented a prospective cohort of 29 patients with septic and aseptic olecranon bursitis treated in an emergency department setting. Most patients were treated successfully with aspiration and oral antibiotics. Surgical intervention was required in one case. (Level III evidence)

Stewart NJ, Manzanares JB, Morrey BF. Surgical treatment of aseptic olecranon bursitis. J Shoulder Elbow Surg. 1997;6:49-53.

The authors retrospectively reviewed 21 cases of olecranon bursitis managed surgically over a 10-year period with average 5 years' follow-up. Surgical treatment of patients without rheumatoid arthritis provided complete and long-lasting relief in most cases. (Level IV evidence)

Weinstein PS, Canoso JJ, Wohlgethan JR. Long-term follow-up of corticosteroid injection for traumatic olecranon bursitis. Ann Rheum Dis. 1984;43:44-6.

In this study, 47 patients with aseptic olecranon bursitis were retrospectively reviewed at an average of 31 months' follow-up. Patients were nonrandomly treated with either aspiration alone or aspiration and injection of triamcinolone hexacetonide. The authors noted a high rate of long-term complications in patients receiving steroid injections, including subcutaneous atrophy (five patients), septic bursitis (three patients), and chronic pain (seven patients). (Level IV evidence)

PROCEDURE 64

Elbow Arthroscopic Débridement for Osteochondritis Dissecans

Michael J. O'Brien and Matthew L. Ramsey

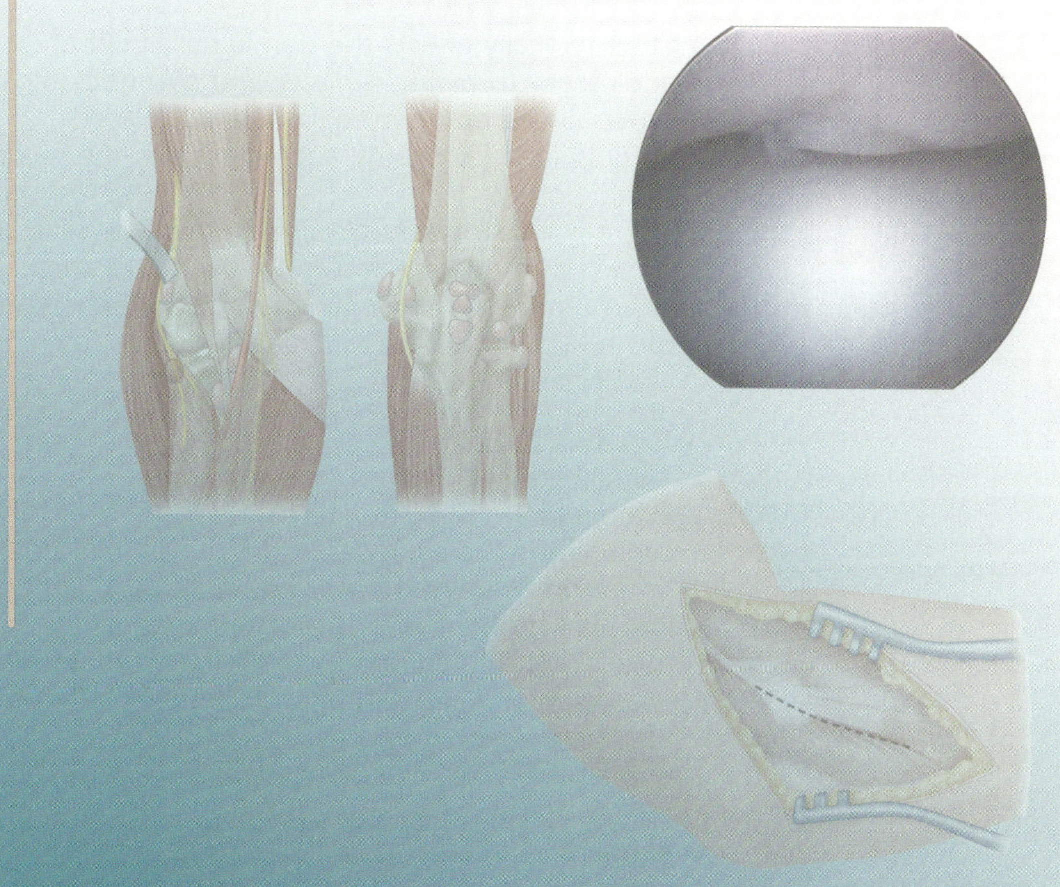

Figures 7 and 9 reprinted from Field LD, Pokabla C. Arthroscopic management of osteochondritis dissecans of the elbow. In Reider B, Terry MA, Provencher MT (eds). Operative Techniques: Sports Medicine Surgery. Philadelphia: Elsevier, 2009:341, 343, with permission.

PITFALLS

- *OCD is sometimes confused with Panner's disease, which is osteonecrosis of the ossific nucleus of the capitellum.*
- *Panner's disease affects a younger age group, typically children from 6 to 10 years of age.*
- *Treatment of Panner's disease consists of rest from vigorous activity, with complete resolution of symptoms and no long-term sequelae.*

Controversies

- Contraindications include severe medical comorbidities and active infection.
- In patients with open physes, nonsurgical management can be successful in the early stages of the disease.

Indications

- Failed nonsurgical management of osteochondritis dissecans (OCD) with persistent symptoms
- Evidence of unstable osteochondral fragment or loose bodies
- Mechanical symptoms of locking, popping, or catching
- Articular cartilage fracture
- Progressive joint contracture or fixed joint contracture with elbow pain

Examination/Imaging

- OCD typically affects the dominant elbow of adolescent throwing athletes and gymnasts. It is especially common in male baseball players.
- OCD is seen from early adolescence to the second decade of life.
- There is a history of pain and stiffness for several weeks, with possible history of overuse. Patients often report lateral elbow pain, loss of extension, and mechanical symptoms such as popping, catching, and locking.

Physical Examination

- A small effusion may be present.
- Examination reveals tenderness directly over the capitellum. The elbow should be examined in 20–90° of flexion to unlock the olecrannon fossa. Limited range of motion, with loss of terminal extension, is most common. Pain may be elicited with passive pronation and supination of the forearm. Crepitus may be present.
- The elbow is examined for signs of instability and medial collateral ligament insufficiency.
- Range of motion and carrying angle should be compared to that in the contralateral extremity.
- Paresthesias and nocturnal pain are uncommon.

Imaging Studies

- Plain radiographs
  - Anteroposterior (AP), lateral, and radiocapitellar views should be obtained.
  - Comparison radiographs of the contralateral elbow can help identify subtle differences.
  - A focal area of lucency is seen in the subchondral bone, localized to the anterior-distal aspect of the capitellum. A focal lesion surrounded by

Treatment Options

- Intact stable lesions are best managed nonoperatively.
  - A hinged elbow brace eliminates stress at the radiocapitellar joint.
  - Activity modification with rest from strenuous activities is instituted for 3–6 weeks, followed by return to activities in 3–6 months.
- Unstable or displaced fragments and presence of loose bodies requires operative treatment, either open or arthroscopically. Unstable fragments may be secured with internal fixation using headless screws.
- For large lesions, or following failed arthroscopic débridement with chondroplasty, osteochondral transplantation with either allograft or autograft remains an option. Fetal cartilage transplantation and autologous cartilage transplantation remain techniques of filling the defect with chondrocytes; however, there are no long-term data on the efficacy of these procedures.

subchondral sclerosis may be further demarcated by a characteristic semilunar rarefied zone called the crescent sign. The AP radiograph in Figure 1 demonstrates an OCD lesion and crescent sign.

- Loose body formation is common.
- Older lesions may demonstrate a sclerotic border.
- Irregularity and enlargement of the radial head may be noted.
- In Panner's disease, there is fissuring, fragmentation, or decreased size of the entire capitellum. The capitellum demonstrates a fragmented, ruffled border with lucencies and irregular ossification of the entire capitellum.

- Magnetic resonance imaging (MRI)
  - MRI is the preferred method for evaluating OCD lesions. It has high sensitivity and specificity.
  - Early changes of marrow edema in the capitellum are often evident before changes on plain radiographs. Late changes include subchondral collapse, flattening of the capitellum, fragmentation, and possible loose body formation. Unstable lesions demonstrate intervening fluid on T_2-weighted images.
  - MRI arthrography can provide information about the presence of loose bodies.
- Computed tomography (CT)
  - CT can help define bony anatomy and is helpful in cases of loose body formation.
  - Thin slices (1–3 mm) are needed.

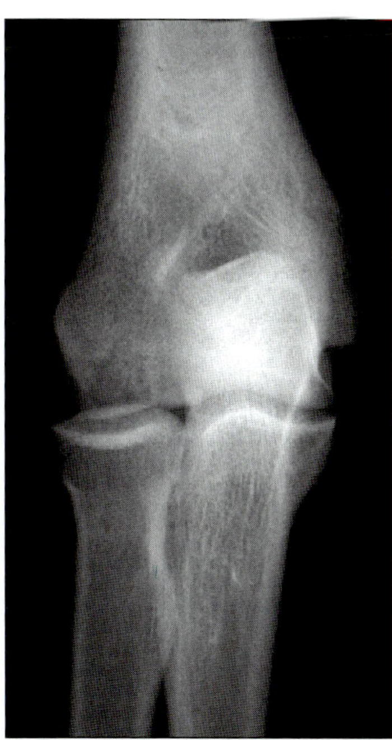

FIGURE 1

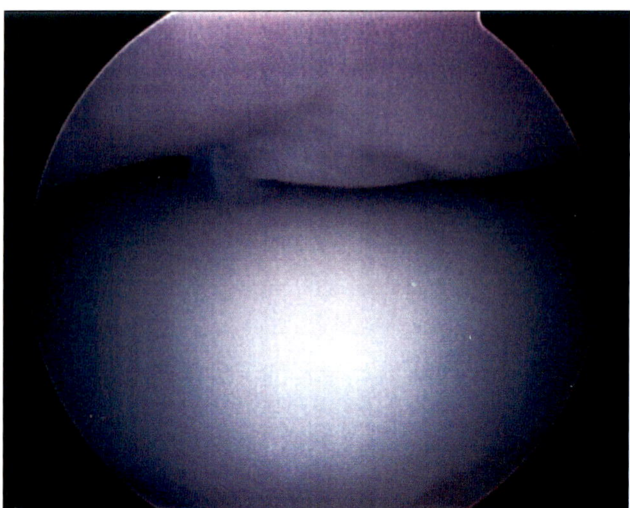

FIGURE 2

- Technetium-99m bone scans are highly sensitive for detecting bony changes. However, they have low specificity and not very useful in establishing the diagnosis.
- Arthroscopy of the elbow provides direct visualization of the OCD lesion, as well as the radial head and entire articular surface. It can be used to determine stability of the fragment, as seen in the arthroscopic view of an OCD from the "soft-spot" portal in Figure 2. It also offers the potential of therapeutic intervention.

Surgical Anatomy

- The ulnar nerve, median nerve, and medial antebrachial cutaneous (MABC) nerve are all at risk with placement of the anteromedial and proximal anteromedial portals. Injury to the ulnar nerve must be prevented by keeping the medial portal anterior to the medial intermuscular septum.
- The lateral antebrachial cutaneous (LABC) nerve, the posterior antebrachial cutaneous nerve, the posterior interosseous nerve (PIN), and the radial nerve are all at risk during placement of the anterolateral and proximal anterolateral portals.
- The radial nerve, median nerve, and brachial artery are at risk in the anterior compartment, especially during arthroscopic anterior capsular release.
- The lateral ulnar collateral ligament, part of the lateral collateral ligament complex, originates on the inferior lateral epicondyle of the humerus and inserts on the proximal ulna on the tubercle of the

supinator crest. This structure is at risk during open lateral approaches to the elbow.

Positioning

Supine-Suspended Position

- Originally described by Andrews and Carson in 1985, the patient is positioned supine with the shoulder in 90° of abduction, the elbow flexed 90°, and the forearm, wrist, and hand suspended over the body by a mechanical traction device.
- A nonsterile tourniquet is placed high on the arm.
- Pros:
  - Access for airway management is easy.
  - The elbow anatomy is presented in a familiar orientation, with the anterior compartment facing up and the posterior compartment facing down.
  - It allows for easy conversion to open procedures.
- Cons:
  - Access to the posterior compartment is difficult.
  - The elbow is relatively unstable in the traction device, which can increase the difficulty of surgery.

Prone Position

- Originally described by Poehling et al. (1989), the patient is positioned prone on chest rolls, and the arm is stabilized by a stationary armholder and allowed to hang off the table. The shoulder is abducted to 90°, and the elbow flexed to 90°.
- A nonsterile tourniquet is placed high on the arm. A compressive wrap is placed around the hand, wrist, and forearm to prevent excessive swelling of the soft tissues from fluid extravasation and the pull of gravity.
- Pros:
  - It eliminates the need for traction, and places the elbow in a stable position.
  - It allows significantly improved access to and visualization of the posterior aspect of the joint.
  - It allows for easy conversion to open procedures through a posterior approach.
- Cons:
  - Elbow anatomy is reversed, with the anterior compartment facing down and the posterior compartment facing up, making surgery less intuitive.
  - General anesthesia is required.
  - There is poor access to the airway for the anesthesiologist.

Pearls

- *Supine-Suspended Position: With the arm suspended over the chest, the anterior neurovascular structures drop away from the anterior capsule, making work on the anterior compartment easier and safer.*
- *Lateral Decubitus Position: The arm should be abducted away from the body, with the elbow positioned slightly higher than the shoulder. This prevents traction on the brachial plexus, and allows the arthroscopic instruments to clear the abdominal wall.*

Equipment

- Several commercially available arthroscopic armholders are available for prone and lateral decubitus positioning. They should be low profile and allow the extremity to be free or fixed within the holder based on surgeon preference.
- Several mechanical armholders are available, including the McConnell arm holder (McConnell Orthopaedic Manufacturing Company, Greenville, TX) and the Spider hydraulic arm holder (Spider Limb Positioner; Tenet Medical Engineering, Calgary, Alberta, Canada).

Lateral Decubitus Position

- Originally described by O'Driscoll and Morrey (1992), it attempts to maximize the advantages of both the supine and prone positions.
- The patient is positioned lateral with the unaffected side down, either on a beanbag or with chest and flank supports. An axillary roll must be placed to prevent a brachial plexus traction injury on the unaffected side. The shoulder is placed in 90° of flexion, and the elbow is placed in a stationary armholder at 90° of flexion (Fig. 3).
- A nonsterile tourniquet is placed high on the arm. A compressive wrap is placed around the hand, wrist, and forearm to prevent excessive swelling of the soft tissues from fluid extravasation and the pull of gravity.
- Pros:
  - It eliminates the need for traction, and places the elbow in a stable position.
  - It allows significantly improved access to and visualization of the posterior aspect of the joint.
  - It allows a full range of elbow flexion, extension, and rotation.
  - A regional anesthetic may be used, and pulmonary function is less compromised than the prone position.
- Cons:
  - There is potential for abutment of the arthroscopic instruments against the patient's abdomen.
  - Access to the anterior compartment may require repositioning.

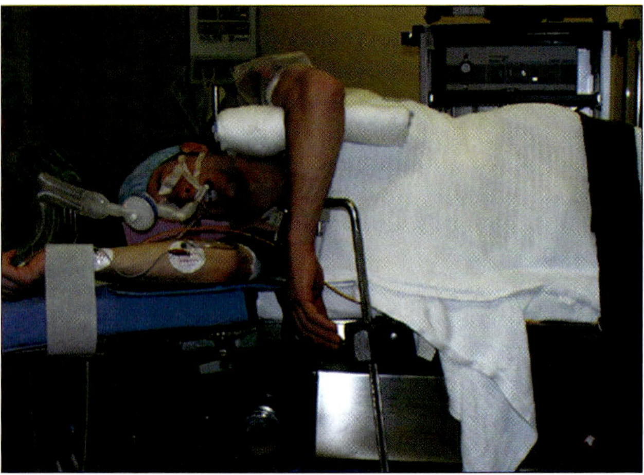

FIGURE 3

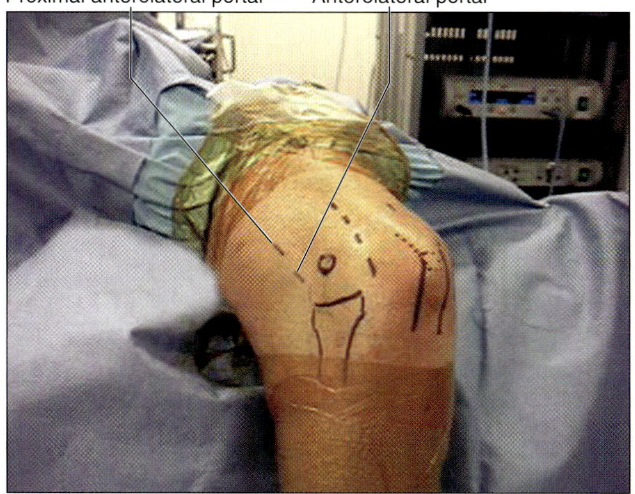

A

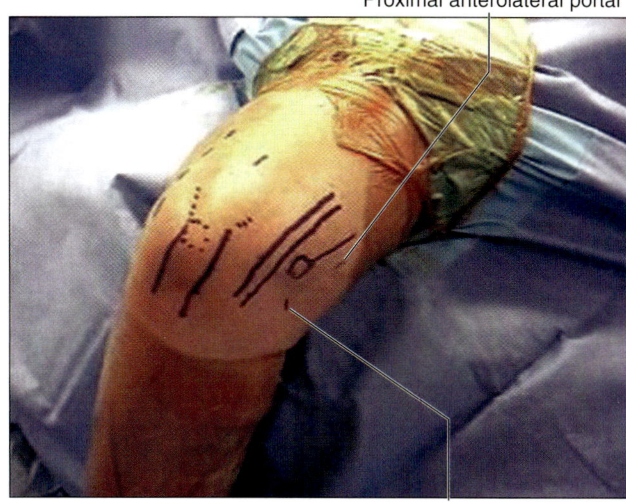

B

FIGURE 4

> **PEARLS**
>
> - *Typically, the proximal anteromedial portal is created first. A small skin incision is made, making sure to keep the scalpel blade superficial. The blunt trocar is used to flick the medial intermuscular septum, and advanced anterior to the intermuscular septum, thereby protecting the ulnar nerve. The blunt trocar is advanced along the anterior humerus, directed toward the center of the joint.*
> - *The other portals are then made under direct visualization, using a spinal needle to localize correct portal placement.*
> - *The distance from the radial nerve is increased by placing a portal more proximally toward the anterior cortex of the humerus.*
> - *No portal should be placed distal to the radiocapitellar joint.*
> - *The anterolateral portal may be preferred over the proximal anterolateral portal in elbows with osteochondral lesions, where access to the fragment may be limited with a more proximal portal placement.*

Portals/Exposures

Anterior Portals

- Four anterior portals have been described (Fig. 4A and 4B).
- Anterolateral portal
  - This portal is located at the anterior radiocapitellar joint, typically 1 cm distal and 1 cm anterior to the lateral epicondyle.
  - This is a common working portal for instrumentation, and is also useful for viewing the medial joint, including the distal humerus, trochlea, and medial radial head.
  - To limit potential radial nerve injury, the portal should enter the joint anterior to the radiocapitellar joint line.
- Proximal anterolateral portal
  - Created to provide a lateral entry point farther away from the radial nerve than the anterolateral portal, this portal is 2 cm proximal and 1 cm anterior to the lateral epicondyle.
  - It provides excellent visualization of the entire anterior joint, including the capitellum and anterior and lateral radial head. Flexion and extension of the elbow allow examination of the coronoid process, and elbow extension provides an excellent view of the medial and lateral trochlea.
  - This is an excellent working portal for most anterior joint procedures, and the preferred lateral portal of many surgeons.

Pitfalls

- *The LABC nerve, the anterior branch of the posterior antebrachial cutaneous nerve, and the radial nerve are all at risk during placement of the anterolateral and proximal anterolateral portals.*
- *The PIN travels immediately adjacent to the elbow capsule just anterior to the radial head and is therefore at risk during placement of the anterolateral portal.*
- *The ulnar, median, and MABC nerves are all at risk with placement of the anteromedial and proximal anteromedial portals.*
- *Prior ulnar nerve transposition, especially a submuscular or intramuscular transposition, is a relative contraindication to placement of an anteromedial or proximal anteromedial portal. In these instances, a limited open medial exposure is necessary to identify the ulnar nerve.*

- Anteromedial portal
  - This portal is placed just anterior to the ulnohumeral joint line, approximately 1–2 cm anterior to the medial epicondyle.
  - With the elbow distended and flexed to 90°, the portal is established with a blunt trocar directed toward the center of the joint.
  - It allows visualization of almost the entire anterior compartment, including the radiocapitellar and ulnohumeral joints and the coronoid fossa.
- Proximal anteromedial portal
  - This portal is established 2 cm proximal to the medial epicondyle and 1 cm anterior to the medial intermuscular septum.
  - With the elbow distended and flexed to 90°, the portal is established with a blunt trocar directed toward the center of the joint.
  - It allows visualization of almost the entire anterior joint.
  - It may be safer than the anteromedial portal, as the MABC and median nerves are farther away from the portal.

Posterior Portals

- Six major portals are commonly used. Posterior portals are generally safer than anterior portals because they are farther away from the neurovascular structures (Fig. 5).

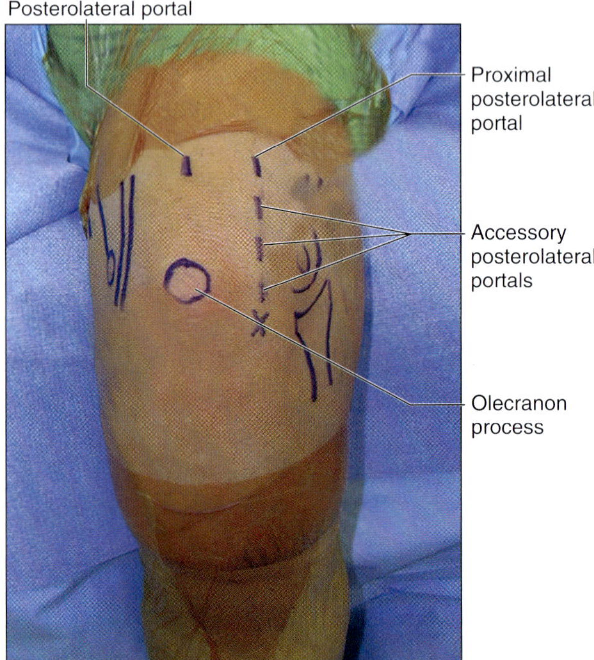

FIGURE 5

Instrumentation

- Portals may be established using an outside-in technique, utilizing an 18-gauge spinal needle to localize portal placement.
- When establishing portals, a guidewire or switching stick may be used to gain entry into the joint. A cannulated dilator can be inserted over the switching stick prior to insertion of a cannula into the portal.
- In full-grown patients, a 4.5-mm arthroscope is generally used. In smaller patients or pediatric patients, a 2.7-mm arthroscope may allow easier access to the joint but does limit the field of view.

- Proximal posterolateral portal
  - This portal is established 2–3 cm proximal to the olecranon tip and just lateral to the triceps.
  - The elbow is held at 45° of flexion to relax the triceps, and the trocar is advanced against the posterior humerus toward the olecranon fossa.
  - This is the primary posterior viewing portal, as it allows visualization of the entire posterior compartment.
- Posterolateral portal
  - This portal is established several millimeters lateral and proximal to the posterolateral corner of the olecranon.
  - It can be used to remove olecranon osteophytes and débride the olecranon fossa.
  - It may be used to visualize the posterior radiocapitellar joint.
- Posterior portal
  - Sometimes called the direct posterior portal, this portal is established by entering the joint through the triceps tendon 3 cm proximal to the tip of the olecranon, and advancing the blunt trocar toward the olecranon fossa.
  - It is routinely used as a working portal for osteophyte removal and débridement, loose body removal, and posterior synovectomy.
- Proximal posterior portal
  - This portal is established 2–3 cm proximal to the posterior portal.
  - It is useful for retracting the posteromedial capsule and the ulnar nerve.
- Midlateral portal
  - This is the "soft spot" portal, located at the center of the triangle formed by the radial head, olecranon, and lateral epicondyle (Fig. 6).
  - It is frequently used to insufflate the joint prior to portal placement.
  - It allows access to the posterior capitellum and radial head.
- Accessory midlateral portal
  - This portal is established 1–2 cm from the midlateral portal.
  - It may be useful for capitellar débridement.

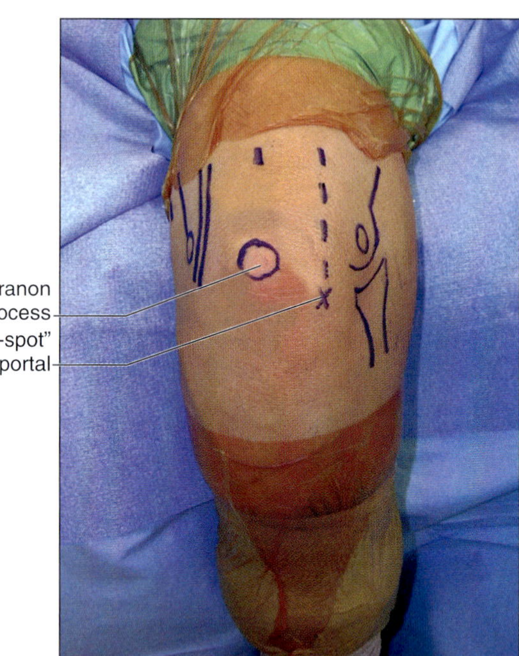

FIGURE 6

Pearls

- *When making the medial skin incision, keep the blade superficial to avoid damage to underlying neurovascular structures.*
- *Make sure to stay anterior to the medial intermuscular septum to avoid injury to the ulnar nerve.*
- *Approximately 75% of the radial head can be visualized with pronation and supination of the forearm.*

Pitfalls

- *During the preoperative examination, make sure to examine for a subluxating ulnar nerve.*
- *Once the medial portal is established, always maintain a cannula for safe instrumentation of the joint. Repeatedly re-establishing the medial portal, especially if the joint becomes swollen, risks injury to the ulnar nerve.*

Procedure

Step 1

- An 18-gauge needle is inserted into the elbow joint through the midlateral or "soft-spot" portal. The capsule is distended with 25–35 ml of normal saline or lactated Ringer's solution (Fig. 7).
- A proximal anteromedial portal is established.
  - The medial intermuscular septum is palpated, and a small skin incision is made 2 cm proximal to the

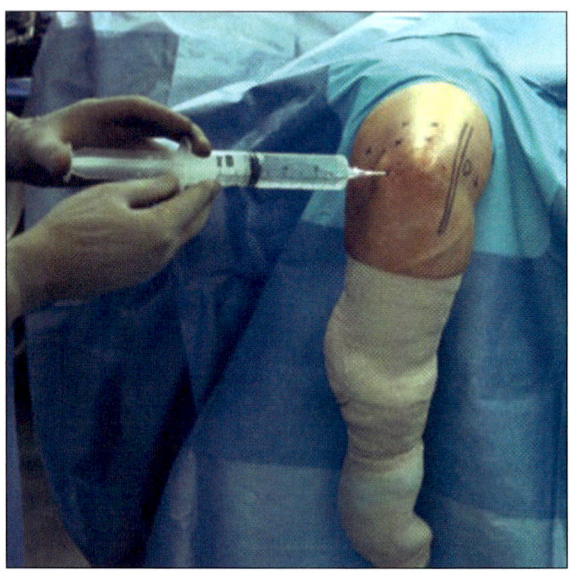

FIGURE 7

- medial epicondyle and 1 cm anterior to the intermuscular septum.
  - Using the blunt trocar, the intermuscular septum is gently flicked, and the trocar is advanced anterior to the intermuscular septum. The trocar is passed along the anterior aspect of the humerus, aiming for the center of the joint, and penetrates through the joint capsule.
  - The blunt trocar is removed and the arthroscope placed into the metal cannula.
- Through the proximal anteromedial portal, a diagnostic arthroscopy of the anterior compartment is performed. The anterior radiocapitellar joint, the radial head, the coronoid process, and the anterior trochlea are inspected for intra-articular pathology (see Video).

Pearls

- *To limit potential radial nerve injury, the anterolateral portal should enter the joint anterior to the radiocapitellar joint line.*

Instrumentation/ Implantation

- Generally a small (2.9-mm) shaver can be used for débridement of the OCD lesion. Use of the small shaver limits damage to surrounding healthy cartilage.

Step 2

- If pathology needs to be addressed in the anterior compartment, an anterolateral portal can be established.
- An 18-gauge spinal needle can be used to localize portal placement utilizing an outside-in technique. Alternatively, an inside-out technique can be used by pressing the arthroscope just anterior to the radiocapitellar joint line, and marking the light source from the scope on the exterior skin.
- Accessory portals can be created, using a spinal needle to localize the optimal position to address the pathology.
  - A diagnostic arthroscopy can also be performed to evaluate the articular cartilage and synovium and to look for loose bodies (Fig. 8).
  - Working instruments can be placed in the anterolateral portal to remove loose bodies and débride unstable fragments of articular cartilage. A small basket forceps and a small shaver can be used to smooth the base of the crater and the edge of the articular cartilage.
- If elected, drilling of the lesion or microfracture can be performed through the same anterolateral or midlateral portals.

Step 3

- Posterior portals can be created to inspect for loose bodies in the posterior compartment, as loose bodies are often found in the posterior aspect of the joint.
- A proximal posterolateral portal can be created for the arthroscope to visualize the posterior

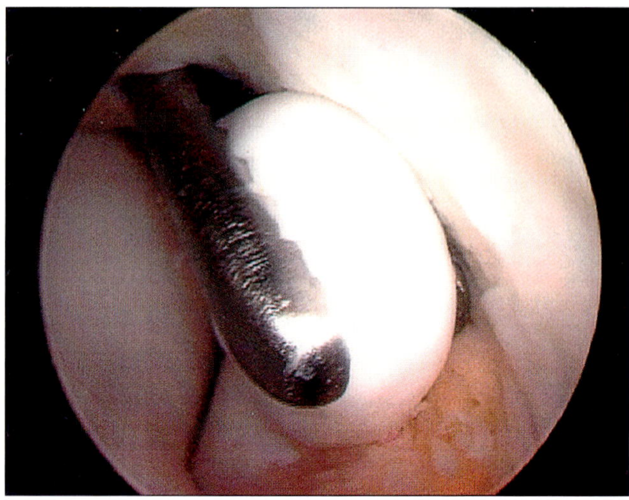

FIGURE 8

compartment. The blunt trocar is directed along the posterior aspect of the humerus, aiming toward the olecranon fossa.

- A direct posterior or posterolateral portal can then be established, and a small shaver introduced to remove the fat pad from the olecranon fossa. Perform a diagnostic arthroscopy of the posterior compartment. Any loose bodies that are identified can be removed (Fig. 9).

Pearls

- *Place the posterolateral portal off the lateral aspect of the triceps at the level of the olecranon tip when the elbow is flexed to 90°. This portal can be used to instrument the posterior compartment as well as the posterolateral gutter.*

Pitfalls

- *Do not place posterior portals medial to the midline in order to avoid injury to the ulnar nerve.*

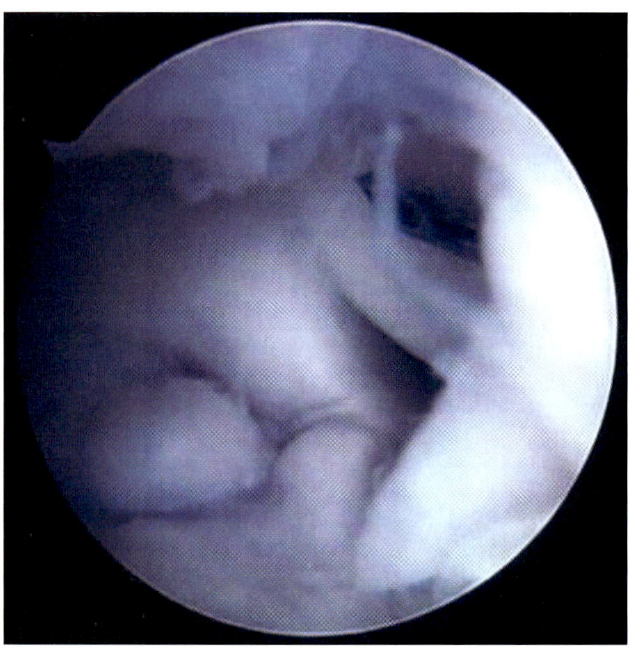

FIGURE 9

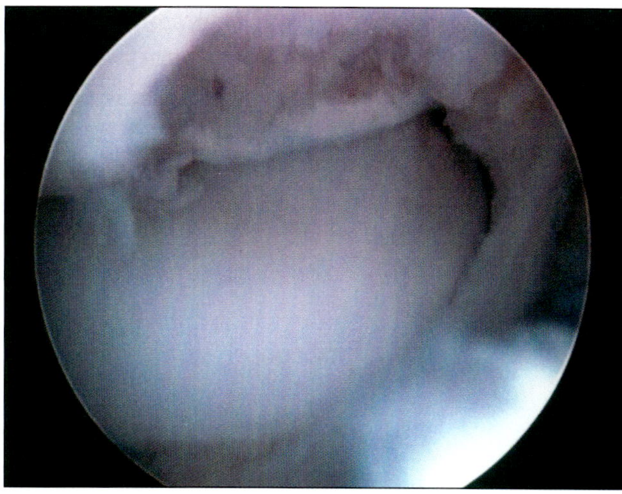

FIGURE 10

STEP 4

- The midlateral or "soft-spot" portal can be utilized to inspect the posterior surface of the capitellum and proximal radioulnar joint.
- This portal is well suited for visualization of the OCD lesion.
- An accessory midlateral portal in combination with a midlateral portal provides excellent access to most osteochondral lesions.

STEP 5

- Débridement of the OCD lesion requires removal of any loose fragments of bone and cartilage and débridement of the bed of the lesion to stable tissue (Fig. 10).
- The margins of the OCD lesion should be freshened to a sharp, well-circumscribed border. Ring currettes work particularly well.
- Chondral picks or small drill bits create channels into the subchondral bone. Bleeding should be confirmed by shutting off the fluid inflow and looking for pallasading bleeding.

PEARLS

- *Begin early range-of-motion exercises to prevent postoperative stiffness.*

PITFALLS

- *Progressive postoperative contracture may develop in select patients. The etiology of this uncommon condition is unknown.*

Postoperative Care and Expected Outcomes

- Range-of-motion exercises are initiated immediately after surgery. A full active and passive range-of-motion protocol can be used. Formal physical therapy is usually initiated 3–5 days after surgery.
- No postoperative bracing is required.
- Postoperative prophylaxis for heterotopic ossification is not necessary.

- Catching and locking, if present preoperatively, should be gone immediately.
- Results of surgery are typically very good, with decreased pain, improved range of motion, flexion contractures improving up to 14°, and 87–100% excellent results.

Evidence

Andrews JR, Carson WG. Arthroscopy of the elbow. Arthroscopy. 2009;195;2:97-107.

A preliminary study describing the technique of elbow arthroscopy in twelve patients. The authors described a variety of portals for performing elbow arthroscopy. The best results were obtained in patients with loose bodies while less satisfactory results were obtained in patients undergoing chondroplasty. The authors highlighted the need for meticulous technique in order to safely perform arthroscopy of the elbow.

Arai Y, Hara K, Fujiwara H, Minami G, Nakagawa S, Kubo T. A new arthroscopic-assisted drilling method through the radius in a distal-to-proximal direction for osteochondritis dissecans of the elbow. Arthroscopy. 2008;24:237.e1-4.

The authors described a new arthroscopic-assisted drilling method through the radius in a distal-to-proximal direction for OCD of the elbow. Only one drill hole is created in the radius by use of a single 1.8-mm Kirschner wire inserted from the shaft of the radius approximately 3 cm distal to the radiocapitellar joint, which allows drilling of the entire OCD lesion through flexion/extension of the elbow, and pronation/supination of the forearm. With this technique, the entire lesion can be vertically drilled under arthroscopic guidance.

Baumgarten TE, Andrews JR, Satterwhite YE. The arthroscopic classification and treatment of osteochondritis dissecans of the capitellum. Am J Sports Med. 1998;26:520-3.

A retrospective review of 16 patients (17 elbows) was performed, with mean follow-up of 48 months. All patients underwent abrasion chondroplasty of the lesion and removal of any loose bodies and osteophytes when present. Postoperatively, the average flexion contracture decreased by 14°, and the average extension contracture decreased by 6°. Seven of nine patients returned to their preoperative levels of activity.

Brownlow HC, O'Connor-Read LM, Perko M. Arthroscopic treatment of osteochondritis dissecans of the capitellum. Knee Surg Sports Traumatol Arthrosc. 2006;14:198-202.

The authors described the results of arthroscopic débridement and loose body removal for OCD of the capitellum in 29 symptomatic patients. At a mean follow-up of 77 months, the majority of patients had mild or no pain. All were capable of performing simple activities of daily living, and all but one had good or excellent outcomes and rated their satisfaction high.

Byrd JW, Elrod BF, Jones KS. Elbow arthroscopy for neglected osteochondritis dissecans of the capitellum. J South Orthop Assoc. 2001;10(1):12-6.

Ten patients (11 elbows) underwent elbow arthroscopy for neglected OCD of the capitellum. Symptoms were present for at least 2 years' duration. All patients returned to preoperative activities, though only 8 of 10 believed that surgery resulted in improvement. Elbow arthroscopy for neglected OCD can result in functional improvement. However, results are not as good as those reported with earlier intervention.

Byrd JW, Jones KS. Arthroscopic surgery for isolated capitellar osteochondritis dissecans in adolescent baseball players: minimum three-year follow-up. Am J Sports Med. 2002;30:474-8.

Arthroscopic surgery was performed on 10 baseball players (average age, 13.8 years) with OCD whose symptoms had been apparent for an average of 9 months before the operation. Follow-up averaged 3.9 years. All 10 patients had excellent results.

Chettouane I, Kohler R, Dohin B, Brunet-Guedj E, Lecoq C, Chrestian P. Osteochondral autograft for osteochondritis dissecans of the capitulum in adolescents: report of six cases and review of the literature. Rev Chir Orthop Reparatrice Appar Mot. 2008;94:449-55.

This paper presented the cases of six adolescent gymnasts with OCD of the capitellum who were treated with an en bloc osteochondral autograft. The graft was harvested from the ipsilateral knee from a non–weight-bearing zone of the lateral condyle. Graft integration was confirmed in all six patients on the 3-month plain radiographs, CT, or MRI. Four of the six gymnasts resumed their high-level sports activities at 1 year (at 6 months for one of them).

Mihara K, Tsutsui H, Nishinaka N, Yamaguchi K. Nonoperative treatment for osteochondritis dissecans of the capitellum. Am J Sports Med. 2009;37:298-304.

This retrospective case series examined 39 baseball players (mean age 12.8 years) with OCD of the capitellum who were treated conservatively. On final radiography, 25 of 30 early-stage lesions were assessed as healed, while only 1 of 9 advanced-stage lesions was assessed as healed. Healing of lesions occurred in 16 of 17 patients with an open growth plate, and in 11 of 22 patients with a closed growth plate. The spontaneous healing potential of OCD in early lesions, especially in patients with open capitellar growth plates, appeared high, and nonoperative treatment was appropriate. (Level IV evidence)

O'Driscoll SW, Morrey BF. Arthroscopy of the elbow: diagnostic and therapeutic benefits and hazards. J Bone Joint Surg [Am]. 1992;74:84-94.

In this article, results were reported on 71 arthroscopies performed in 70 elbows, with mean follow-up of 34 months. Fifty-one (73%) of the 70 patients benefited in some way. The procedure was successful in four elbows in which loose body removal had been performed for OCD.

Poehling GG, Whipple TL, Sisco L, Goldman B. Elbow arthroscopy: a new technique. Arthroscopy. 1989;5:222-4.

A modification to traditional elbow arthroscopy was described, by placing the patient in a prone position and using a proximal medial portal. Use of the prone position improved scope mobility, facilitated joint manipulation, and provided more complete intra-articular visualization.

Rahusen FT, Brinkman JM, Eygendaal D. Results of arthroscopic debridement for osteochondritis dissecans of the elbow. Br J Sports Med. 2006;40:966-9.

This prospective cohort study evaluated 15 patients (mean age 28 years) with OCD of the elbow treated with arthroscopic débridement. The function of the elbow, as reflected by the MAESS score, improved from poor to excellent, the mean level of pain at rest decreased from 3 to 1, and the level of pain after provocation decreased from 7 to 2. All patients were able to return to work 3 months after surgery, and 80% were able to resume their preinjury level of sport activity.

Ruch DS, Cory JW, Poehling GG. The arthroscopic management of osteochondritis dissecans of the adolescent elbow. Arthroscopy. 1998;14:797-803.

This article was a retrospective analysis of 12 patients (mean age 14.5 years) who underwent arthroscopic débridement alone followed by early range of motion. Follow-up at a mean of 3.2 years indicated that the average flexion contracture decreased by 13°. All patients had remodeling of the capitellum by plain radiographs; however, five patients had associated enlargement of the radial head.

Stubbs MJ, Field LD, Savoie FH 3rd. Osteochondritis dissecans of the elbow. Clin Sports Med. 2001;20:1-9.

The authors noted that conservative treatment regimens will provide complete resolution of symptoms in many patients with OCD; however, surgical management may be carried out when indicated. Unstable lesions can be treated primarily by excision of the fragment, accompanied by drilling or burring of the base of the lesion. Symptoms usually improve significantly, but approximately half of all patients will continue to experience chronic pain or limitation of elbow motion.

Takahara M, Mura N, Sasaki J, Harada M, Ogino T. Classification, treatment, and outcome of osteochondritis dissecans of the humeral capitellum. J Bone Joint Surg [Am]. 2007;89:1205-14.

The cases of 106 patients (mean age 15.3 years) with OCD of the capitellum were studied retrospectively. An OCD lesion with an open capitellar physis and a good range of elbow motion resulted in a good outcome. Continued elbow stress resulted in the worst outcome in terms of pain and radiographic findings. In patients with a closed capitellar physis, surgery provided significantly better results than elbow rest. Fragment fixation or reconstruction provided significantly better results than fragment removal alone. The results of removal alone were dependent on the size of the defect in the capitellum. (Level II evidence)

INDEX

Note: Page numbers followed by f refer to figures.

A

B

C

E

F

G

H

N

O

P

Q

R

S

T

U